P9-CBH-760

Foundations of Psychiatric Mental Health Nursing

Elizabeth M. Varcarolis, R.N., M.A.
Professor
Coordinator of Psychiatric Nursing
School of Nursing
Borough of Manhattan Community College
City University of New York
New York, New York

W.B. SAUNDERS COMPANY
Harcourt Brace Jovanovich, Inc.
Philadelphia London Toronto Montreal Sydney Tokyo

W. B. SAUNDERS COMPANY
Harcourt Brace Jovanovich, Inc.

The Curtis Center
Independence Square West
Philadelphia, PA 19106

Library of Congress Cataloging in Publication Data

Varcarolis, Elizabeth M.
Foundations of psychiatric-mental health nursing / Elizabeth M. Varcarolis.
p. cm.
ISBN 0-7216-1976-2
1. Psychiatric nursing. I. Title.
[DNLM: 1. Mental Disorders—nursing. 2. Psychiatric Nursing. WY 160 V289f]
RC440.V37 1990
610.73'68—dc20
DNLM/DLC 89-70091

Editor: Ilze S. Rader
Designer: Bill Donnelly
Production Manager: Carolyn Naylor
Manuscript Editor: Martha Tanner
Illustration Coordinator: Brett MacNaughton
Indexer: Kathy Garcia
Cover Designer: W. B. Saunders Staff

FOUNDATIONS OF PSYCHIATRIC NURSING ISBN 0-7216-1976-2

Printed in the United States of America

Last digit is print number: 9 8 7 6 5 4 3 2

With Love I Dedicate this Work to
Josiah *and* Ruth Merrill
Who Gave Me Life and Opportunity
and to
Paul S. Varcarolis
Who Gave Me Love and Taught Me How to Share It

Contributors

Helene S. Charron, R.N., M.S.N.
Professor of Nursing and Chairperson, Department of Nursing, Monroe Community College, Rochester, New York
Repetitive and Ineffective "Neurotic Defenses"

Brenda Lewis Cleary, R.N.C., Ph.D.
Associate Professor, Texas Tech University Health Sciences Center School of Nursing, Odessa, Texas; Faculty Practice at New Horizon Nursing Center, Odessa, Texas
Organic Mental Syndromes and Disorders

Michelle J. Conant, R.N., M.S.N.
Adjunct Faculty, Borough of Manhattan Community College and Lehman University, New York, New York, and Farleigh Dickinson University, Madison, New Jersey; Private Practice, Livingston, New Jersey
People Who Defend Against Anxiety Through Eating Disorders

Jeffrey S. Grunberg, M.A.
Assistant Professor in Clinical Psychology, Department of Psychiatry, Columbia University, College of Physicians and Surgeons, New York, New York; Vice President, Social Services Grand Central Partnership, New York, New York
The Mentally Ill Who Are Chronically Homeless

Mary Ursula Guthormsen, R.N., Ph.D.
Nursing Education Consultant, Board of Registered Nursing, Sacramento, California
Legal and Ethical Issues

Doris Hadley, R.N., M.N.
Infectious Control Coordinator, Veterans Administration Medical Center, San Francisco, California
A Nurse Speaks

Mary Jane Herron, Ph.D.
Adjunct Professor, Seton Hall University, South Orange, New Jersey; Private Practice, Woodcliff Lake, New Jersey
Adult Relationships and Sexuality

William G. Herron, Ph.D.
Professor, Department of Psychology, St. John's University, Jamaica, New York; Private Practice, Woodcliff Lake, New Jersey
Adult Relationships and Sexuality

Sally Kennedy Holzapfel, R.N.C., M.S.N., G.N.P.
Clinical Nurse Specialist in Gerontology, Veterans Administration Medical Center, Lyons, New Jersey
Evidence of Maladaptive Responses to Crisis: Elder Abuse; The Elderly

Suzanne Lego, R.N., Ph.D., C.S.
Associate Professor of Clinical Nursing, Graduate Program in Psychiatric Nursing, Columbia University School of Nursing, New York, New York; Private Practice, Demarest, New Jersey
Personality Disorders—Borderline

Kem B. Louie, R.N., C.S., Ph.D.
Assistant Professor, Lehman College–City University of New York, Division of Nursing, Bronx, New York; Joint faculty position, Assistant Professor, Albert

Einstein College of Medicine, Department of Psychiatry, Bronx, New York
Personality Disorders—Antisocial and Borderline

Mary McAndrew, R.N., M.S.
Hospital Administrator, Mount Carmel Guild Hospital, Newark, New Jersey
People Who Depend Upon Substances Other Than Alcohol

Jane Bryant Neese, M.S., R.N.
Formerly University of South Carolina Medical School, Hana Lou, South Carolina
The Hospitalized Person

John Payne, R.N., M.A.
Senior Management Consultant for Nursing and Long-Term Care, N.Y.C. Health and Hospitals Corporation, New York, New York
A Nurse Speaks

Hildegard E. Peplau
Professor Emerita, Rutgers, The State University of New Jersey, New Brunswick, New Jersey
Evolution of Nursing in Psychiatric Settings

Miriam Perez, B.S.
Bronx, New York
A Nurse Speaks

Margaret H. Pipchick, R.N., M.A., C.S.
Adjunct Faculty, Fairleigh Dickenson University School of Nursing, Rutherford, New Jersey; Private Practice, Cranford, New Jersey
Children and Adolescents

Sharon Shisler, R.N., C.S., M.A.
New York Hospital—Westchester Division, Westchester, New York
A Nurse Speaks

Kathleen Smith-DiJulio, R.N., M.A., C.S.
Psychosocial Clinical Nurse Specialist, Group Health Cooperative, Seattle, Washington
Evidence of Maladaptive Responses to Crisis: Child Abuse; Evidence of Maladaptive Responses to Crisis: Spouse Abuse; Evidence of Maladaptive Responses to Crisis: Rape; People Who Depend Upon Alcohol

Ardis R. Swanson, Ph.D., R.N.
Associate Professor, New York University, New York, New York
Psychophysiological Disorders

Juliet L. Tien-Hyatt, D.N.Sc., R.N., C.S.
Formerly Principal Investigator/Project Director, NIMH Ethnic Mental Health Nurse Specialist Program; formerly Professor at UCLA School of Nursing, University of California, Los Angeles, California; President, Institute of Holistic Health, Santa Monica, California
Mental Health Considerations Across Cultures

Julius Trubowitz, Ph.D.
Assistant Professor, Queens College, City University of New York, Queens, New York; Private Practice, New York, New York
Historical Overview—Classification—Trends; Personality Theories and Therapies

Lorenza M. Valvo, R.N., J.D.
Senior Hospital Negotiator, California Medical Assistance Commission, Sacramento, California
Legal and Ethical Issues

Sara Withgott, R.N., M.S.
Arizona State University, Tempe, Arizona
A Nurse Speaks

Preface

The purpose of this text is to provide beginning students with a concise yet comprehensive psychiatric–mental health nursing text. Since nursing students today are often nontraditional learners, a variety of features are included to provide visual as well as cognitive learning tools.

Nurses come into contact with people involved in the complex issues of society. Skill in dealing with psychosocial needs is basic to nursing practice, whether that practice is in a mental health setting, an emergency room, an acute care hospital, or the home and community. For that reason, social issues related to mental health needs and care are covered in depth in this book. Individual issues relating to *interpersonal violence* (child, spouse, and elder abuse and rape) are covered in several chapters. Comprehensive coverage of *substance use disorders* is included. Psychosocial needs of people with AIDS and their families are addressed. The process of *homelessness* is explored, along with information on the role of the nurse and other nursing considerations useful when working with the homeless population.

The book is composed of three parts: (1) Foundations in Theory, (2) Foundations in Practice: The Anxiety Continuum, and (3) Mental Health Issues: Special Populations. Every chapter includes an outline, key terms and concepts, stated objectives, self-study questions, and a summary highlighting the important concepts introduced in the chapter.

PART ONE *includes Chapters 1 through 9* and is made up of two units that focus on *theory*. Unit I (Chapters 1 through 4) is designed to provide *basic psychiatric concepts* that all mental health workers use in clinical practice. Unit II (Chapters 5 through 9) provides *basic concepts in psychiatric–mental health nursing*. It deals directly with nursing and nursing theory and presents concepts used in working with clients in a general hospital or a mental health setting. Chapters 8 and 9 introduce the framework for the clinical chapters. The material presented in the clinical chapters follows a schematic of an *anxiety continuum*, from mild to moderate, moderate to severe, and severe to panic. Chapter 8 discusses the concept of anxiety, while Chapter 9 provides a brief overview of the clinical syndromes and mental disorders discussed in this text.

PART TWO, *which is the heart of the book*, presents the *clinical chapters* (*Chapters 10 through 25*) in four units (*Units III through VI*). The information in these clinical chapters is organized according to the *Standards of Psychiatric and Mental Health Nursing Practice*, which are printed on the inside front cover of the book for easy reference. In addition, all clinical chapters include practical examples in the form of either *case studies* or *vignettes*. Each clinical chapter also provides at least one *nursing care plan*. The case studies, vignettes, and nursing care plans help to translate theory into practice and enhance student comprehension of the chapter topic by providing specific examples and concrete applications of the general, sometimes abstract information presented in the chapter. Special sections highlighting experiences of practicing nurses in various clinical settings (*A Nurse Speaks*) provide students with personal glimpses into the experience of nursing.

All clinical chapters follow the nursing process. It is presented both within the framework of the *Standards of Psychiatric and Mental Health Nursing* and within each case study. Assessment, diagnosis, planning, intervention, and evaluation are each clearly identified. *Nursing diagnoses are presented using only those approved by the North American Nursing Diagnosis Association* (NANDA).

The intervention component of the nursing process is discussed with reference to the relevant subcategories of Standard V: Intervention (e.g., V-A: Psychotherapeutic Interventions, V-B: Health Teaching, V-C: Activities of Daily Living, V-D: Somatic Therapies, V-E: Therapeutic Environment, V-F: Psychotherapy). Medications are discussed (when relevant) under V-D: Somatic Therapies.

The planning component of the nursing process is divided into *planning on the content level* (planning goals) and *planning on the process level* (nurses' reactions and feelings). Planning on the process level incorporates common reactions and countertransferential reactions of nurses and other health care professionals to specific client behaviors prominent in various disorders or situations. Guidelines for nursing action and alternative ways of responding are offered. In those chapters that discuss specific mental disorders, DSM III-R criteria are provided. Evaluation is covered both in text and care plans, so that beginning students learn to incorporate this important part of the nursing process into their thinking.

PART THREE (*Chapters 26 through 30*) *takes a closer look at mental health issues faced by special populations*. These chapters emphasize a balance of theory and practice. These special populations include hospitalized clients, children and adolescents, adults, elderly clients, and the homeless. In many clinical settings, nurses working with these populations have advanced education. Therefore, these chapters are designed to acquaint the beginning student with various issues (e.g., emotional needs and social problems) affecting each group, to outline relevant nursing considerations, and to provide a foundation for further learning.

Acknowledgments

It was Suzanne Lego who inadvertently got me started on this project, many years ago. Throughout the years she has given me advice, support, suggestions for authors, and more advice and support. I am deeply grateful.

I am lucky to have found such able, knowledgeable, and responsible authors, for they have surely given this book its authenticity and credibility along with its easy-to-read style. These chapters reflect a lot of work, and I offer these authors my sincerest thanks.

There are many individuals who have truly extended themselves on my behalf. Many of the clinical examples came from experienced clinicians in the field. Grace Patounis submitted clinical case studies for the crisis and anxiety chapters. Kathy Lala wrote the clinical case studies for the chapters on schizophrenia and mania.

The photographs were taken by my nephew, Jimmy Varcarolis, who tirelessly scouted for just the right photo. The idea for "A Nurse Speaks" came from Bill Burgower long before the personality of this book was formulated and it found a home at W. B. Saunders.

The typing and retyping reams of annotated manuscript through two and three drafts always "to be done yesterday" were cheerfully and faithfully executed by Pattie Romo, my traveling typist. I thank her and her husband, Chris, for their helpfulness and friendship.

It was the humor, wisdom, and creativity of Ilze Rader, my editor, who kept me at this task; I often had other plans. Her role as facilitator, "What would happen if . . . " "Have you thought about . . . " "What do you think of adding . . . " "Have you heard about . . . " kept me on my toes and added richness to the text. I also thank Marie Thomas, editorial assistant, for her good humor and quick response to numerous and sometimes repetitive requests, which kept things moving along. The book also owes much to the skills of Martha Tanner, who served as developmental editor and copy editor. She kept the many threads of the text in sharp focus.

Thanks also go to the teachers who have reviewed manuscript through several drafts and given me the benefit of their insights and experience: Charlene Bradham, RN, MNSc, CS, University of Arkansas, Little Rock, Arkansas; Helene S. Charron, RN, MS, Monroe Community College, Rochester, New York; Anita Deitrick, RN, BSN, Des Moines Area Community College, Ankeny, Iowa; Carol Grabow, RN, MSN, Indiana University, Kokomo, Indiana; Diane F. Greslick, RN, BSN, MSN, Southern Maine Medical Center, Portland, Maine; Barbara Light, RN, MS, John Tyler Community College, Chester, Virginia; Carol R. Marcus, RN, MS, State University of New York, Farmingdale, New York; Ann G. Ross, ARNP, MN, CS, Shoreline Community College, Seattle, Washington; Linda Smith, RN, MSN, Editorial Director, AD *Nurse*, Franksville, Wisconsin; Maureen Theroux, RN, MN, EdD, Manatee Community College, Bradenton, Florida; Mary Ware, RN, MEd, MSN, Mississippi University for Women, Columbus, Mississippi; Sara Withgott, RN, MS, Mesa Community College, Mesa, Arizona; Mary E. Wynn, RN, MSN, Pasadena City College, Pasadena, California. I have been fortunate to have had such excellent reviewers, whose creative ideas and comments, expertise, and perception provided excellent feedback and guidance.

The nurses for "A Nurse Speaks" contributed a human and warm touch. Their love and dedication to nursing are reflected in their anecdotal pieces. Such love and dedication are what nursing is all about; sometimes we forget.

I acknowledge my thanks to numerous friends and colleagues who offered frequent support and encouragement for this project. In particular, to both Aubrey Robinson, my chairperson, and Martha A. Small, a supportive colleague and partner with whom I work most closely, I offer thanks for their flexibility, concern, and support through the years. I owe a special debt of gratitude to Mattie Collins, a friend and colleague, whose enthusiasm from the very beginning of this project was always a lift. Dr. Collins has generously contributed verbatim excerpts from her text, *Communication in Health Care* (1983), which appear in Chapter 6.

And through it all, my husband, Paul, offered constant love, humor, and patience simultaneously with dinner and housework; I am truly blessed.

Brief Contents

Contents

Contents

PART ONE

FOUNDATIONS IN THEORY

BASIC PSYCHIATRIC CONCEPTS

UNIT I

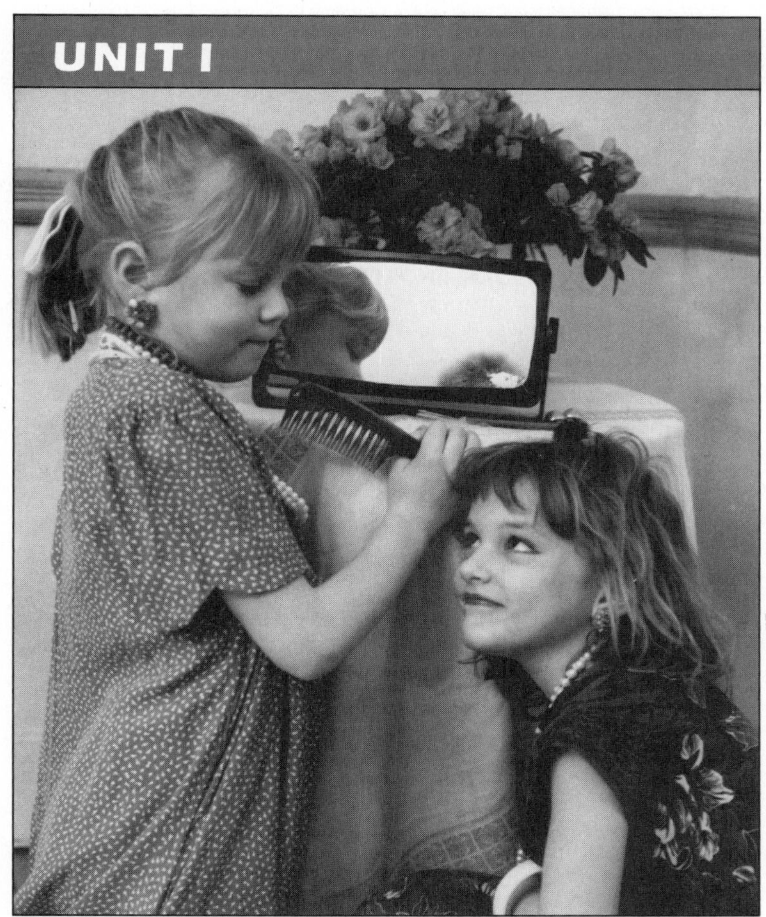

What you are to be you are now becoming.

A Nurse Speaks

by Juliet L. Tien-Hyatt

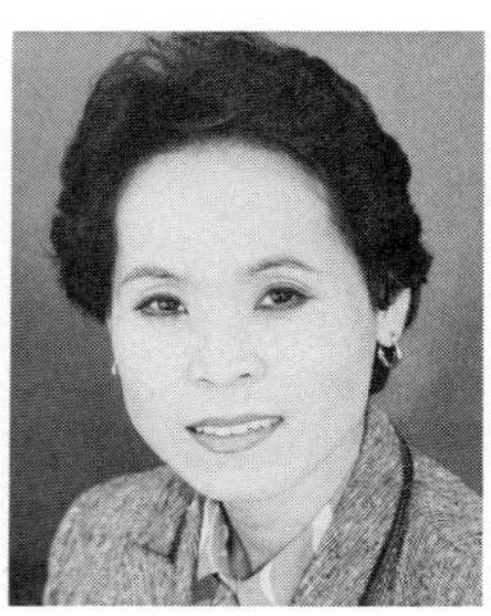

Writing the chapter *Mental Health Considerations Across Cultures* was a unique experience. It gave me an opportunity to review and integrate my personal, professional, and cultural experiences.

I grew up as a post-war farm girl; I fully understand poverty and the struggle for freedom from it. Educated as a nurse both in Taiwan and in the United States, I am in tune with the issue of health and illness across cultures. I am presently established as an educator, researcher, administrator, entrepreneur, and radio broadcaster; I am cognizant of the many dimensions of life.

My experiences as a human being in general, and as a first-generation immigrant in particular, have enabled me to explore the meaning of life in depth and to help myself and others grow and expand in a cultural context. Since 1966, when I first entered nursing school at the National Taiwan University, I have had unending curiosity and a desire for the knowledge of the interactions among mind, body, and spirit. I have spent thousands of hours studying various religions, human spirituality, and alternative health care practices such as acupressure, hypnotherapy, and nutritional therapy. Each new method I have learned has enhanced my nursing practice.

I feel fortunate to have received my graduate education in the United States. Even though I experienced a stress-induced life-threatening allergic reaction on the day that I received my master's degree and I was devastated when I initially failed the preliminary examinations for the doctorate program at the University of California, I have learned and grown tremendously from these adversities. After struggling and surviving through a series of difficult and overwhelming life events, I grew stronger and wiser.

My experience as the Principal Investigator/Project Director of the NIMH-funded Ethnic Mental Health Nurse Specialist Program and as Assistant Professor at the UCLA School of Nursing for six years taught me a lot. The politics, competition, and subtle yet ever-present racial discrimination were some of the elements that made me critically evaluate my personal goals and my career goals.

In 1987, I moved from teaching nursing to establishing the Institute of Holistic Health (IHH), a public-benefit, non-profit organization. Currently, IHH is staffed with physicians, nurses, psychologists, social workers, acupuncturists, chiropractors, and nutritionists. IHH combines the best of Eastern and Western health practices and offers a choice of services to the client. Although I am working 16 hours a day Monday through Saturday and 8 hours on Sunday, I feel I have found my true love. As president of IHH, I now can play a multifaceted role as clinician, administrator, researcher, educator, and radio broadcaster. I am the master of my personal and professional life! The joy, the excitement, and the expansion of my personal and private life are indescribable.

Being a nurse is an ever-challenging experience. As one philosopher said, "I am not afraid of tomorrow, for I have seen yesterday, and I love today."

CHAPTER 1

Historical Overview—Classification—Trends

Julius Trubowitz

OUTLINE

HISTORICAL OVERVIEW
Primitive Cultures
Greek and Roman Beliefs
Medieval Period
The Renaissance
The 17th and 18th Centuries
Mid-18th and Early 19th Centuries
The Emergence of Dynamic Psychiatry

MENTAL HEALTH, MENTAL ILLNESS, AND THE *DSM III-R*
Concepts of Mental Health and Mental Illness
DSM-III and *DSM III-R*

MAJOR TRENDS IN MENTAL HEALTH CARE

SUMMARY

KEY TERMS, CONCEPTS, AND PEOPLE

The key terms, concepts, and people listed here also appear in bold where they are defined or discussed in this chapter.

PSYCHIATRY
HIPPOCRATES
PLATO
ARISTOTLE
ASCLEPIADES
JOHANN WEYER
PHILLIPPE PINEL
BENJAMIN RUSH
PIERRE JANET
FRANZ ANTON MESMER
DIAGNOSTIC AND STATISTICAL MANUAL OF MENTAL DISORDERS (DSM III-R)

OBJECTIVES

After studying this chapter, the student will be able to:

1. Discuss the historical parallels between the concept of mental illness and psychiatric practice.
2. Name one contribution of each of the following figures:
   A. Hippocrates
   B. Plato
   C. Aristotle
   D. Asclepiades

E. Johann Weyer
F. Phillippe Pinel
G. Benjamin Rush
3. Assess his or her own mental health by examining five important signs of mental health.
4. Identify the strengths and weaknesses of the *DSM III-R* classification of mental disorders.
5. Identify strengths and weaknesses of four trends in the mental health care system seen in the 1980's.

Historical Overview

Psychiatry can trace its origins to the beginning of the history of humanity. Its earliest roots are found in primitive peoples' conception of illness and treatment. In the pre-scientific era of primitive humanity, the approach to illness and treatment was based on magic and superstition (as were all life's phenomena). It was only with the development of scientific medicine during the Greek era that psychiatry moved out of the realm of the supernatural and established a true scientific beginning. The Greeks perceived disease as a natural development, and mental illness was observed and studied as a disease phenomenon. It was the great scholars of Ancient Greece, Hippocrates, Plato, and Aristotle, who influenced the development of psychiatry through the modern era.

The value of clinical observation, the beginning of personality theory, the relationship between mental health and mental illness, and the first steps in the humane treatment of the mentally ill client were all contributions of Greek thinking.

In this chapter, the development of psychiatry will be examined, from the era of Ancient Greece, the Middle Ages, the Renaissance, and the seventeenth and eighteenth centuries to the emergence of the movement called dynamic psychiatry. The ideas of Mesmer, Charcot, and Janet and how they ultimately came together in the work of Sigmund Freud will be discussed.

Psychiatry is the science of curing or healing disorders of the psyche. It is the medical specialty that is derived from the study, diagnosis, treatment, and prevention of mental disorders (Hinsie and Campbell 1973). Follow the narrative by using Table 1–1 as a guide.

PRIMITIVE CULTURES

The field of psychiatry evolved from our first primitive attempts to understand and treat our own illnesses and abnormal behaviors. All physical or mental disorders had superstitious or supernatural explanations. Whether the client suffered from headaches and fever or displayed aberrant, bizarre thinking and behavior, primitive humanity attributed it all to the intervention of supernatural forces such as evil spirits, gods, witches, or magicians. Disease was understood to be the work of sorcerers or ghosts who stole the soul from the body, or it was thought to occur when evil spirits penetrated a person's body and took possession. When this happened, the individual suddenly lost his identity and became another person, taking the character, looks, and even the voice of the supposed intruder. Primitive humanity believed that illness resulted from violations of the group's laws and taboos.

Treatment methods and techniques of primitive medicine belong in the realm of the magical. The role of treating illness was vested in the medicine man, the shaman, or the healer. The ancient healer approached his client in a highly ritualized manner. The healing procedure was carefully prepared and well structured. Taking place in the presence of men, women, and children, it had the quality of a theatrical performance.

GREEK AND ROMAN BELIEFS

The true history of psychiatry, like that of scientific medicine, begins with the Greeks. The Greeks are generally credited with providing the first scientific view of mental disorders. It was the medical community of Greece that brought a scientific outlook to mental disease.

Hippocrates (460–377 B.C.) epitomized the movement away from the supernatural toward the natural explanation of mental illness. Called the Father of Medicine, Hippocrates, who devised an oath of ethical behavior that has guided physicians for centuries, advocated the separation of medicine from philosophy and theology. He vehemently attacked magical and religious explanations of illness. Although the gods were still revered and were thought to control the course of

Table 1-1 • HISTORICAL OVERVIEW—MENTAL HEALTH DEVELOPMENT

CONCEPTIONS OF ABNORMAL BEHAVIOR			CONTRIBUTIONS	
Culture	**Principal Theories of Causation**	**Characteristic Methods of Helping**	**Positive**	**Negative**
Primitive cultures	Possession by evil spirits, sorcerers, ghosts	Magic, exorcism		
Ancient Greece	Supernatural forces and divine intervention; beginning of naturalistic explanation of sickness	Clinical observation replaces superstition; still mainly primitive physical methods; start of humane treatment approaches	Beginning of concern with humanity of individual	Continuation of confinement; little recognition of psychological or social factors
Medieval period	Possession by devils and sorcerers	Harsh, primitive methods; banishment; first hospitals established	Establishment of first hospitals	Movement back to irrational explanation and harsh treatment of mentally ill
Renaissance	Sorcery, witchcraft, and naturalistic explanation of sickness	Harsh physical punishment; death; rebirth of humane attitude; clinical observation and description	Forerunner of modern clinical description	Ruthless persecution of the mentally ill
17th & 18th centuries	Irrationality and social deviance	Isolation and inhumane physical treatment		Isolation and harsh physical treatment
Mid-18th & early 19th centuries	Sickness; mental illness	Humane treatment; discovery of animal magnetism and hypnosis impetus for psychotherapy	Pinel—"breaking the chains," changes in mental hospitals, less barbaric treatment	
Late 19th & early 20th centuries	Intrapsychic, usually unconscious conflict	Emergence of psychotherapy; analysis and interpretation of free associations, dreams, and other behaviors	Recognition of importance of motivation and early childhood development	Overemphasis on past and unconscious factors as compared with interpersonal and social factors
Mid-20th century	Conflicts between individuals; family, community, and social forces	Marital, family, and community interventions designed to deal with problems of interaction between and among people	Recognition of importance of interaction among individual, family, and society	Interpersonal-social approach can ignore biological and other individual factors
1970-1980's	Biochemical abnormalities in combination with psychological factors	Chemical therapies	Discovery and application of scientific data on biochemical factors	Overemphasis on view that "it all comes down to chemistry"

From Altrocchi J. Abnormal Psychology. New York: Harcourt Brace Jovanovich, 1980, p. 30.

human events, the medical profession increasingly saw illness as stemming from natural causes.

Plato (427?-347 B.C.) believed that an individual's entire life merited study. According to Plato, one could write a psychological biography of a man from his earliest years, when "the soul is easily molded" (Plato's *Republic*), through his relationship with other members of his family and his educational process. There are striking parallels between Plato's three-part division of the human soul and Freud's theories. According to Plato, the soul is divided into three parts: it has a rational portion, a libidinal portion where our desires reside, and a "spirited" portion. This three-part division and the Freudian model of id, ego, and superego (to be discussed more fully later) are strikingly similar.

Aristotle, Plato's pupil (384-322 B.C.), made a significant contribution to the use of clinical observation. Although he is thought of as a great philosopher, Aristotle was a physician who observed a continuum in psychological reactions from normal to pathological behavior. Aristotle viewed psychological reactions as expressions of the total person rather than manifestations of a specific diseased part (Zilboorg and Henry 1941). This point has contemporary relevance in light of the current emphasis on holistic medicine.

Clinical observation was further developed and emphasized by **Asclepiades** (around 100 B.C.), whom some have called the Father of Psychiatry (Lewis 1942). As a pioneer in the application of humane treatment methods, Asclepiades opposed the use of mechanical restraints, an issue that was to loom large in later history of the treatment of the mentally ill. Asclepiades prescribed occupational therapy to increase attention span and memory and introduced music therapy for calming agitated clients (Major 1954).

MEDIEVAL PERIOD

Although there were attempts to preserve the Greek traditions of psychiatry, there were few positive developments during the Middle Ages, a period of about 1000 years from the fifth century to the fifteenth century. It was a period characterized by a breakdown of social conditions, with wars, plagues, and migrations. Life was unpredictable and precarious. Anxiety was rampant. Surgery was taken up by barbers and their assistants, obstetrics was handled by ignorant midwives, and psychiatry was practiced by exorcising priests and witch-hunting clerics. Clerics gradually assumed an increasingly important role in medical writing and practice, and pertinent clinical observation on mental illness began to dwindle. The mentally ill inspired great fear and were regarded as being possessed by the devil and by evil spirits. Harsh physical treatment and severe punishment were used to purge the mentally ill of their evil spirits. The severely mentally ill were often turned out of their houses and left to fend for themselves. In Central Europe, they were placed on boats, "ships of fools," to wander along the rivers of that region. The boat became a symbol of the wandering mind deprived of guidance.

However, in the fourth century, general hospitals were established, and a few possessed separate sections for the mentally ill. According to Lewis (1942), a hospital specifically for clients with mental disease opened in Jerusalem in the year 490 A.D.

THE RENAISSANCE

Three major conflicting trends regarding the care of the mentally ill developed during the Renaissance. They were (1) the increase of witch hunting, (2) the rebirth of humane attitudes toward the mentally ill, and (3) greater progress toward a scientific explanation of mental illness.

This period was one of profound contradictions. On one hand there was the ruthless persecution of the mentally ill as witches. Those who showed the slightest psychological deviation or peculiarity were suspected of being witches or sorcerers. Not only mental illness but almost any affliction of the body (impotence, sterility, deformity, infant mortality) and all of life's misfortunes (a poor harvest, death, or a broken marriage) were seen as the work of the devil.

A textbook, *The Witch Hammer*, was published in 1489 by two German theologians. Fanatical in their approach, the theologians had as their goal the extermination of witches. With political, religious, and scientific support and the authority of Pope Innocent VIII in 1484 (Zilboorg and Henry 1941), they set out on a witch hunt. Thousands of mentally ill people were put to death, along with those who were political and religious dissenters (who were then deemed witches) (Bromberg 1954).

In sharp contrast to this callous, cruel persecution, the Renaissance later brought a rebirth of a humane attitude toward the mentally ill. A deep sympathy for the unfortunate sick was nurtured.

Johann Weyer (1515–1588), a major figure identified with humane treatment of the mentally ill, is regarded as having made the greatest contribution to psychiatry during the Renaissance (Zilboorg and Henry 1941). Weyer, considered today to be the Father of Modern Psychiatry (Mora 1967), recognized that "witches" and those "possessed" were mentally ill and demanded that they be treated by doctors rather than by priests.

Another contribution to psychiatry during this time was made by Paracelsus (1493–1541). He has been credited with having made the first reference to unconscious motivation in mental illness (Zilboorg and Henry 1941). Carl Jung, the famous Swiss psychoanalyst, was one of those who considered Paracelsus a pioneer in the psychology of the unconscious.

THE 17TH AND 18TH CENTURIES

During the seventeenth and eighteenth centuries, two historic developments changed the way the mentally ill were perceived and treated. First, beginning in the seventeenth century, reason came to prevail in science, philosophy, and religion. Reason took the place of God. The attitude toward mental illness in seventeenth- and eighteenth-century Western Europe was one of shame, because mental illness did not fit the scheme of reason.

Second, as the mentally ill populations became less identified with the devil and witchcraft, they, along with the poor, were viewed as a social problem. The governments decided to resolve their social crisis by putting all these unfortunates in prison. In France these prisons were called "Hôpital Général"; in Germany "Zuchthaus"; in Great Britain "workhouse." Four years after its opening, the General Hospital in Paris housed 6000 people, including beggars, vagrants, prostitutes, criminals, cripples, old people, orphans, those suffering from venereal disease, homosexuals, "unbelievers," and the mentally ill. Although previously the mentally ill were only rarely kept in prison, this became the rule under governments of the mid-seventeenth century. Thus approval was given to the principle that the mentally ill should be kept in places of confinement by laymen, not by physicians.

In these institutions the mentally ill were chained, and doctors were practically never consulted. During this period, physical treatment methods designed to serve as shock therapy for the mentally ill were actively developed. One such treatment was "ducking." The client was plunged again and again into water as a shock measure. Another measure involved the use of the twirling stool in which a state of unconsciousness was produced through spinning. It was thought that the shock would result in mental reorganization leading to normalization.

MID-18TH AND EARLY 19TH CENTURIES

Phillippe Pinel (1745–1826) is credited with the beginning of humane treatment of the mentally ill. In 1793, Pinel was put in charge of the Bicetre asylum and, in 1795, the Salpetriere, both in Paris. He was a reformer and humanitarian. He opposed the traditional view of punishment for the mentally ill. He objected to bloodletting; he opposed indiscriminate prescription of drugs; he rejected beatings. Pinel described ducking as a "medical delirium, more serious than the delirium of patients" (Ackerknecht 1968). He directed restraints to be removed and chains to be broken.

Pinel was also a gifted therapist. He sought to make contact with, and understand the inner experiences of, his mentally ill clients. His concerned attitude and his emphasis on establishing a trusting relationship with his clients have led some historians to consider Pinel a pioneer in the use of psychotherapy for the severely mentally ill (Reik 1956).

Pinel made daily rounds, examining clients, observing their behavior, and taking notes on their conversations. Historians trace the development of psychiatric case reports and case histories to Pinel's observational methods (Zilboorg and Henry 1941).

Under Pinel's leadership, the hospital became the main tool in treating the mentally ill client. Psychotherapeutic measures were to be based strictly on the authority and expert knowledge of the physician. More humane treatment methods were introduced, appropriate segregation of types of mental clients was instituted, and occupational and recreational therapeutic programs were established in the hospital regimen.

Benjamin Rush, a similar leader, called the Father of American Psychiatry, wrote the first American textbook of psychiatry in 1812.

THE EMERGENCE OF DYNAMIC PSYCHIATRY

Psychiatry had made great strides since the era of primitive medicine. But still, the way the mind functioned remained largely an uncharted, undiscovered world.

Franz Anton Mesmer (1734–1815), a controversial Austrian physician, presented a theory of mental operations that, though flawed, led toward the understanding of the workings of the mind. He claimed that through his mysterious powers, called animal magnetism, he could cure a whole range of physical and mental disorders. He was able to provoke the appearance of symptoms in clients by his physical presence or by his gestures. The magnetizer, as Mesmer called it, had first to establish a rapport, a tuning in, with the client. Then the magnetizer, sitting in front of the client, looking directly into the client's eyes, would transmit his animal magnetism into the client's body, evoking what Mesmer called a crisis.

It was a disciple of Mesmer, Marquis de Puysegur (1751–1825), who made the discovery that provided the impetus for the development of the movement called Dynamic Psychiatry. Puysegur "magnetized" a young peasant named Victor Race, who fell into a strange sleep in which he seemed to be more awake and aware than in his normal waking state. Victor retained no memory of that state once it had passed.

Puysegur's discovery provided a new understanding of the unknown mind. Mental life began to be seen as a dynamic energy system of forces. The therapeutic implications of the psychological tie between the client and magnetizer (later hypnotist and then psychotherapist) came into the mainstream of psychiatry a century later in the work of Jean-Martin Charcot (1835–1893) and his contemporaries. Jean-Martin Charcot, a leading neurologist, conferred a scientific dignity on hypnosis when he read his famous paper on hypnosis at the Academie des Sciences in Paris in 1882.

It was **Pierre Janet** (1859–1947) who advanced the knowledge of the functioning of the mind and whose contributions brought a rich harvest of ideas to dynamic psychiatry. Mainly using hypnosis, Janet was the first to demonstrate that many symptoms of hysteria and other "neuroses" lay in what he called "subconscious fixed ideas" (Ellenberger 1970). In the development of dynamic psychiatry from Charcot and Janet, the path leads to Sigmund Freud.

Mental Health, Mental Illness, and the *DSM III-R*

CONCEPTS OF MENTAL HEALTH AND MENTAL ILLNESS

Mental health professionals are constantly faced with the problem of defining mental illness and mental health. Agreement on the definition of mental illness and mental health has been elusive throughout history. In the past, definitions of mental illness and mental health have used statistical measures. Mental illness was applied to behaviors, described as strange and different, that deviated from an established norm. However, such criteria are inadequate since they may suggest that mental health is based on conformity. By using such definitions, nonconformists and independent thinkers, such as Abraham Lincoln, Mahatma Gandhi, Socrates, and Martin Luther King, Jr., would be adjudged mentally ill.

One approach in defining mental illness and mental health is based on evaluating individual behavior in two dimensions:

1. On a continuum from *adaptive* to *maladaptive*.
2. On a continuum from *constructive* to *destructive*.

Along the **adaptive-maladaptive continuum,** behaviors are assessed to the degree that they contribute or are detrimental to the individual's psychological well-being. For example, does the behavior widen or restrict the range of possible responses to a problem of living? Does it raise or lower self-esteem? Does it create situations in which the individual or others are more likely to experience relief of tension or stress?

Maladaptive behavior allows a problem to continue and often generates new problems, interfering significantly—often over an extended period of time—with an individual's ability to function in such important areas of life as health, work, love, or interpersonal relationships. On the other hand, **adaptive behavior** solves problems in living and enhances an individual's life.

Table 1-2 identifies important aspects of mental health on a continuum. These aspects include degree of (1) happiness, (2) control over behavior, (3) appraisal of reality, (4) effectiveness in work, and (5) self-concept.

Regarding the second dimension, behavior along the **constructive-destructive continuum** often affects others as much as the individual. *Destructive behavior* not only results in failure to deal with a problem—and thus is maladaptive—but also undermines or destroys the psychological and often biological well-being of the individual and others. Such behavior—whether it occurs once or repeatedly—may seriously undermine health, significantly increase chances of (or actually bring about) death, or drastically affect psychological functioning in the individual or others. On the other hand, *constructive behavior* contributes to psychological growth and biological well-being. It improves the health and positively influences the psychological functioning of the individual and others.

To carry out their professional responsibilities, clinicians and researchers need accurate and clear-cut guidelines for identifying and categorizing mental illness. Such guidelines help clinicians plan and evaluate the success or failure of a treatment plan for their clients. Several elements are necessary to identify and clearly categorize types of mental illness. There must be agreement as to what specific behaviors—along the adaptive-maladaptive and constructive-destructive lines—constitute mental illness. A common language has to be agreed upon so that behaviors can be properly identified and organized into acceptable diagnostic categories.

The field of mental illness is plagued by a host of myths and misconceptions. One myth is that to be mentally ill is to be different and odd. Another misconception is that to be healthy one must be logical and rational. But many of those suffering from mental illness are not different and odd, and no "healthy" human being is fully logical and rational. There are people who show extremely abnormal behavior and are characterized as mentally ill who are far more like the rest of us than different from us. There is no obvious and consistent line between mental illness and mental health. In fact, all human behavior lies somewhere along a continuum of mental health and mental illness.

DSM-III AND *DSM III-R*

In 1952, the American Psychiatric Association set out to classify abnormal behavior and provide an official manual of mental disorders including descriptions of diagnostic categories. It is called the ***Diagnostic and Statistical Manual of Mental Disorders*** **(DSM)** and is now the most widely accepted system of classifying abnormal behavior in the United States today, consistent in most respects with the World Health Organization (WHO) and the International Classification of Diseases (ICD). The manual is the system used by trained professionals in most United States hospitals and other clinical settings.

There have been revisions to the original 1952 manual, DSM-II in 1968, DSM-III in 1980, and **DSM III-R** (revised)— in 1987. The changes that have been made include moving away from any particular theoretical

Table 1–2 • EXTREMES ON THE MENTAL HEALTH CONTINUUM

SIGNS OF MENTAL HEALTH	EXTREMES IN MENTAL ILLNESS
Happiness A. Finds life enjoyable. B. Can see in objects, people, and activities their possibilities for meeting one's needs.	**Major Depressive Episode** A. Loss of interest or pleasure in all or almost all usual activities and pastimes. B. Mood as described by person is depressed, sad, hopeless, discouraged, "down in the dumps."
Control Over Behavior A. Can recognize and act upon cues to existing limits. B. Can respond to the rules, routines, and customs of any group to which one belongs.	**Control Disorder, Undersocialized, Aggressive** A. A repetitive and persistent pattern of aggressive conduct in which the basic rights of others are violated.
Good Appraisal of Reality A. Accurate picture of what is happening around one. B. Good sense of the consequences, both good and bad, that will follow one's acts. C. Can see the difference between the "as if" and "for real" in situations.	**Schizophrenic Disorder** A. Bizarre delusions, such as delusions of being controlled. B. Auditory hallucinations. C. Delusions with persecutory or jealous content.
Effectiveness in Work A. Within limits set by abilities, can do well in tasks attempted. B. When meeting mild failure, persists until determines whether or not one can do the job.	**Adjustment Disorder with Work (or Academic) Inhibition** A. Inhibition in work or academic functioning where previously there was adequate performance.
A Good Self-Concept A. Sees self as approaching one's ideals, as capable of meeting demands. B. Reasonable degree of self-confidence helps in being resourceful under stress.	**Dependent Personality Disorder** A. Passively allows others to assume responsibility for major areas of life because of inability to function independently. B. Lacks self-confidence, e.g., sees self as helpless, stupid.

Data from Redl F, Wattenberg W. Mental Hygiene in Teaching. New York: Harcourt, Brace & World, 1959, pp. 198–201, and American Psychiatric Association. Diagnostic and Statistical Manual of Mental Disorders (DSM III-R), 3d ed., revised. Washington, DC: American Psychiatric Association, 1987.

framework for understanding mental disorders and establishing more specific criteria to identify disorders.

In the DSM-III (1980) and the DSM III-R (1987), for the first time, the criteria for classification of mental disorders are sufficiently detailed for clinical, teaching, and research purposes. For example, DSM III-R provides the following specific criteria for the diagnosis of generalized anxiety disorder:

Generalized Anxiety Disorder

A. Generalized, persistent anxiety is manifested by symptoms from *three of the following four categories*: (a) *motor tension*: shakiness, jitteriness, jumpiness, trembling, tension, muscle aches, fatigability, inability to relax, eyelid twitch, furrowed brow, strained face, fidgeting, restlessness, easy startle; (b) *autonomic hyperactivity*: sweating, heart pounding or racing, cold, clammy hands, dry mouth, dizziness, light-headedness, paresthesia (tingling in hands or feet), upset stomach, hot or cold spells, frequent urination, diarrhea, discomfort in the pit of the stomach, lump in the throat, flushing, pallor, high resting pulse and respiration rate; (c) *apprehensive expectation*: anxiety, worry, fear, rumination, anticipation of misfortune to self or others; (d) *vigilance and scanning*: hyperattentiveness resulting in distractibility, difficulty in concentration, insomnia, feeling "on edge," irritability, impatience.

B. The anxious mood has been continuous for at least one month.

C. Not due to another mental disorder, such as Depressive Disorder or Schizophrenia.

D. At least 18 years of age.

Furthermore, the DSM-III and DSM III-R introduced a new, multiaxial system of classification to allow for multiple complexities of people's lives. Each individual case is evaluated on five dimensions (Table 1–3).

The term *clinical syndrome* in Axis I refers to the collec-

Table 1–3 • DSM III-R MULTIAXIAL SYSTEM OF EVALUATION

AXIS I	Clinical syndromes
AXIS II	Personality disorders and developmental disorders (personality traits may also be noted)
AXIS III	Physical disorders and conditions
AXIS IV	Severity of psychosocial stressors
AXIS V	Highest level of adaptive functioning

Reprinted with permission from the *Diagnostic and Statistical Manual of Mental Disorders*, Third Edition, Revised. Copyright 1987 American Psychiatric Association.

tion of signs and symptoms that together constitute a particular disorder. Axis II refers to *long-term patterns of behavior and coping*. Axis III notes any *current physical disorder* or condition potentially relevant to understanding and helping the person. Axis IV refers to *stressful life events*, either acute events or enduring events, such as death of a loved one, divorce, or loss of a job. Severity is rated on a scale of 1 to 7 (from "none" to "catastrophic"). Axis V gives an indication of the *person's best level of psychological, social, and occupational functioning* during the preceding year, rated on a scale of 1 to 7 (from "superior" to "grossly impaired").

According to the latest report from the American Psychiatric Association's Task Force on Nomenclature and Statistics, Axes I, II, and III constitute the official DSM III-R diagnosis; Axes IV and V provide additional information that may be useful in decisions about the therapeutic intervention and in the prediction of likely outcome.

Evaluation and revising are ongoing processes, and a task force is presently at work on DSM IV, to be published in the 1990's. However, caution needs to be exercised in diagnosing or labeling whether a medical diagnosis or a nursing diagnosis is being formulated.

The premise that every society has its own view of health and illness and its own classification of diseases has long been observed by anthropologists, historians, and students of cross-cultural society (Klerman 1986). However, the DSM-III and DSM III-R have been criticized for their lack of emphasis on the individual within his or her cultural context (Rothblum et al. 1986). Although the authors of DSM-III state that abnormality is continuous with wellness, the medical perspective reflected in DSM III-R can lead to a search for pathological characteristics in those who might otherwise be considered healthy individuals (Rothblum et al. 1986).

The process of psychiatric labeling can have harmful effects on an individual and his or her family, especially if the diagnosis was made on insufficient evidence and proves faulty. A cross-national study of the diagnosis of mental disorders demonstrates, for example, a dramatic difference between British and American psychiatrists. The study revealed that London psychiatrists tend to "diagnose" people more frequently as manic or having character disorders, whereas New York psychiatrists use the diagnosis schizophrenia much more readily (Rothblum et al. 1986). Psychiatric classifications presently are based mostly on clinical observations, to some degree on theoretical viewpoints, and least of all on empirical studies (Boxer 1987).

An example of cultural and social bias influencing psychiatric diagnosis is the fact that homosexuality was labeled a psychiatric disease in DSM-I and DSM-II. *All* research consistently failed to demonstrate that people with a homosexual orientation were any more maladjusted than heterosexuals. Despite the research data, change occurred in the medical community only when Gay Rights activists advocated an end to discrimination against lesbians and gay men. No longer is homosexuality classified as a mental disorder.

Bias in a social system extends to many minority groups. Some examples include blacks, elderly, children, women, and those with homosexual orientation. These biases are often reflected in our power structures and the political system of the time.

Presently, a new category thought by many to reflect social bias is *self-defeating personality disorder*, found in the appendix to the DSM III-R (1987). Most people who would come under this category are women. The American Psychological Association has declared this new diagnosis potentially dangerous to women and without scientific basis (Boxer 1987).

A syndrome often takes different superficial forms in different cultures. Also, people from minority or migrant populations may have good reason to be distrustful, and it should not be assumed too quickly that these clients are suffering from paranoia or paranoid schizophrenia (Westermeyer 1986).

Awareness of the cultural bias and dangers inherent in labeling has enormous implications for nursing practice, especially in the field of mental health, since nurses often take their cues from the medical structure. Doctors diagnose "diseases." Nurses diagnose "a perceived difficulty or need" (ANA 1980). The more objectively we as nurses observe, assess, and diagnose the individuals under our care, the more effectively we shall administer our skills.

Major Trends in Mental Health Care

It has been the goal of mental health advocates and concerned citizens to raise the level of the human condition. The major thrust of their efforts in recent times has been directed toward community mental health programs designed to help those in need to cope better with problems and achieve a better quality of life.

These goals were manifested in the Community Mental Health Centers (CMHC's) Act of 1965, which laid the basis for the delivery of services in the areas of mental health and mental illness. By the 1980's this government-funded program had resulted in the establishment of 760 CMHC's, each encompassing geographic areas of approximately 100,000 persons, providing approximately 3.1 million patient contacts yearly (Klerman 1981). The centers receive about 25% of state mental health dollars and are involved in 75% of all psychiatric contacts (Andrulis and Mazade 1983).

Within the community-based mental health programs of today, a number of trends have been identified. **First, the so-called paraprofessional has moved into what is called the "new" professional status and has taken over more and more aspects of the care and treatment of the mentally ill.** There has been a huge increase in the number of nontraditionally trained (and sometimes untrained) personnel in the human services fields (Riessman 1980). At the same time, Ph.D. level psychologists and psychiatrists are having less and less to do with the care and treatment of the severely mentally ill and constitute a decreasing percentage of community mental health workers (Berlin et al. 1981). Some observers have pointed to the paucity of psychiatric involvement as a crisis in patient care (Fink and Weinstein 1979; Langsley 1980; Winslow 1982).

Second, greater consideration is being given to combining the delivery of health and mental health services in one setting. Including mental health services within health centers, which already have a long tradition of serving needy populations, is seen as more effective and more consistent with a holistic approach to health.

Third, the field of prevention of mental illness, including both policy and activities, remains undeveloped and neglected. Although there have also been isolated attempts, such as the establishment of preventive components in the New York and Michigan State Departments of Mental Health, prevention programs remain at a low priority level.

Fourth, a major community development in the mental health field in the 1980's was the rise of self-help groups throughout the United States. In 1981, it was reported that there were 500,000 self-help programs in the United States with a membership of 23,000,000 people (Katz 1981), and they continue to proliferate today. These programs are made up of persons experiencing similar circumstances or misfortune either directly or indirectly concerned with mental health, such as Alcoholics Anonymous, Mothers Against Drunk Drivers (MADD), Parents Without Partners, and Gamblers Anonymous. The self-help groups function as a source of information as well as psychological support. The self-help group initiators and members perceive that existing social institutions or agencies fail to meet their needs. Unlike clinicians, who focus on the individualistic, introspective basis of problems, self-help groups focus on the social origins of problems.

A controversial social and mental health issue of the 1980's has been the process of deinstitutionalization, in which vast numbers of mental patients have been discharged from mental hospitals. Discharge from the institution, in many cases, has resulted in increased exposure to a hostile environment, lack of health care, and deterioration of living conditions (Gruenberg and Archer 1979; Rose 1979; Lamb 1981; Miller 1981). Returning mental patients to the community has highlighted the importance of the social support systems, family involvement, and the need to provide suitable living conditions to maintain the chronically ill in the community. A critical question to be resolved in mental health care today is whether the deinstitutionalized are better off in terms of life and health status.

Finally, mental health care in the 1990's is confronted with the issue of the neglect of populations that have been traditionally underserved and unserved, such as women, children, the aged, and those in rural populations. It has been calculated that 10% of the population at any one time is in need of mental health services and that only about one-third of this group comes to the attention of any sort of mental health treatment facility (Iscoe and Harris 1984). The fate (good or bad) of the rest of this population is as yet undetermined. Women are still underserved, particularly when their problems run counter to societal stereotypes, such as the female alcoholic. Two out of three seriously disturbed children in the United States are not receiving the mental health services they need. Generally, there are few mental health services in rural areas. By the year 2000, one out of every six Americans will be over the age of 65, presenting greater demands for mental health services. Indeed, the current challenge to the mental health community and society is to meet the needs of the vast numbers of underserved and unserved populations by the end of the twentieth century.

Summary

The history of psychiatry dates back to primitive man. Great progress in the understanding of mental illness and the treatment of the mentally ill was made in Ancient Greece.

Subsequently, the development of psychiatry has been influenced by many factors. Religious fanaticism resulted in many mentally ill persons' being condemned as witches. Later, the mentally ill were viewed as social problems to be kept in places of confinement. Changes in the treatment of the mentally ill and a more humane attitude were advanced by Phillippe Pinel in the late eighteenth and early nineteenth centuries. Psychiatry moved into the modern era with the emergence of dynamic psychiatry through the works of Mesmer, Puysegur, Charcot, and Janet, culminating in Freud's contributions.

Defining mental illness or recognizing mental health may change with the culture, the time in history, the political system and power, and the person or group doing the defining. There is no question that mental health and mental illness do exist on a continuum. One continuum is called adaptive-maladaptive; another is termed constructive-destructive. General indications of a mentally healthy person can be assessed by the degree of (1) happiness, (2) control over behavior, (3) appraisal of reality, (4) effectiveness in work, and (5) self-concept (see Table 1–2).

The DSM-III and DSM III-R provide specific behavioral criteria for each diagnostic category of mental disorder and include axes to incorporate other data relevant in best diagnosing and planning appropriate care. However, caution in adopting labels is advised, and some problems in applying information from the DSM III-R were identified, such as the diagnostician's potential or actual bias toward specific minority groups and the need to incorporate cultural norms when making a diagnosis. Awareness of these biases and caution in adopting and promoting labeling have enormous implications for nurses.

To be sure, there are great deficiencies in numbers and types of services available to people needing mental health care. Political and monetary reasons explain some of the deficits. Some trends seen during the 1980's were trying to fill this need (increased paraprofessionals, self-help groups, and the inclusion of mental health centers within existing health care centers). The eighties experienced the reverberation of deinstitutionalization, which increased the numbers of people needing extensive mental health care in areas already overextended. The fact that a great majority of our population (women, children, the aged, refugees, those living in rural areas, and those of African descent) are still grossly underserved is of great concern to those working in the field of mental health. Deficiencies in addressing the mental health needs of these populations persist into the 1990's.

References

Ackerknecht EH. A Short History of Psychiatry, 2nd rev. ed., S. Wolff, Trans. New York: Hafner Publishing Company, 1968. (Original work published 1959.)

American Nurses' Association. Nursing: A social policy statement. Kansas City, MO: American Nurses' Association, 1980.

American Psychiatric Association. Diagnostic and Statistical Manual of Mental Disorders (DSM III-R), 3d ed., revised. Washington, DC: American Psychiatric Association, 1987.

Andrulis DP, Mazade NA. American mental health policy: Changing directions in the 80s. Hospital Community Psychiatry, 34:601, 1983.

Berlin RM, Kales JD, Humphrey FJ II, Kales A. The patient care crisis in community mental health centers: A need for more psychiatric involvement. American Journal of Psychiatry, 138:450, 1981.

Boxer S. The parable of the check turners and the check-smiters. Discover, 8(6):80, 1987.

Bromberg W. Man Above Humanity. Philadelphia: J.B. Lippincott Company, 1954.

Cornford FM. The Republic of Plato. Oxford, MA: Oxford University Press, 1970.

Davison GC, Neale JM. Abnormal Psychology: An Experimental Clinical Approach. New York: John Wiley & Sons, 1982.

Ellenberger HF. The Discovery of the Unconscious: The History and Evolution of Dynamic Psychiatry. New York: Basic Books, 1970.

Fink P, Weinstein S. Whatever happened to psychiatry? The deprofessionalization of community mental health centers. American Journal of Psychiatry, 136:406, 1979.

Gruenberg EM, Archer J. Abandonment of responsibility for the seriously mentally ill. Milbank Memorial Fund Quarterly. Health and Society, 57:485, 1979.

Hinsie LE, Campbell RJ. Psychiatric Dictionary, 4th ed. New York: Oxford University Press, 1973.

Iscoe I, Harris LC. Social and community interventions. Annual Review of Psychology, 35:333, 1984.

Katz AH. Self-help and mutual aid: An emerging social movement. Annual Review of Psychology, 7:129, 1981.

Klerman G. Report of the administrator: Alcohol and drug abuse and mental health administration, 1980. DHHS Publications, 81-1165, 1981.

Klerman GL. Historical perspectives on contemporary schools of psychotherapy. *In* Millon T, Klerman GL (eds). Contemporary Directions in Psychopathology Towards the DSM IV. New York: The Guilford Press, 1986.

Lamb HR. What did we really expect from deinstitutionalization? Hospital Community Psychiatry, 32:105, 1981.

Langsley DG. The community mental health center. Does it treat patients? Hospital Community Psychiatry, 31:815, 1980.

Lewis NDC. A Short History of Psychiatric Achievement. London: Chapman & Hall, 1942.

Major RH. A History of Medicine. Springfield, IL: Charles C Thomas, 1954.

Miller GE. Barriers to serving the chronically mentally ill. Psychiatric Quarterly, 54:118, 1981.

Mora G. From demonology to the Narrenturm. *In* Gladstone I (ed). Historical Derivations of Modern Psychiatry. New York: McGraw-Hill, 1967, pp. 41–73.

Reik LE. The historical foundations of psychotherapy in schizophrenias. American Journal of Psychology, 10:241, 1956.

Riessman F. The role of paraprofessional in the mental health crisis. Paraprofessional Journal, 1:1, 1980.

Rose SM. Deciphering and deinstitutionalization: Complexities in policy and program analysis. Milbank Memorial Fund Quarterly. Health and Society, 57:429, 1979.

Rothblum ED, Solomon LJ, Albee GW. A sociological perspective of the DSM III. *In* Millon T, Klerman GL (eds). Contemporary Directions in Psychopathology Towards the DSM IV. New York: The Guilford Press, 1986.

Schneck JM. A History of Psychiatry. Springfield, IL: Charles C Thomas, 1960.

Westermeyer J. Cross cultural diagnosis. The Harvard Medical School Mental Health Letter, 2(12):4, 1986.

Winslow WW. Changing trends in CMHCs: Keys to survival in the eighties. Hospital Community Psychiatry, 3:273, 1982.

Zilboorg G, Henry GW. A History of Medical Psychology. New York: W.W. Norton, 1941.

Self-Study Exercises

Match the major contribution to mental health development with the correct time or person.

1. ________ Called the Father of Medicine. Encouraged the thinking that mental illness had a natural explanation and was not caused by evil spirits.
2. ________ Called the Father of Psychiatry. Placed emphasis on clinical observation. First to prescribe music and occupational therapy.
3. ________ Although a barbaric time dominated by superstition, wars, and plagues, this period saw the establishment of the first hospitals.
4. ________ Time when mentally ill were isolated and banished to prisons and workhouses and treated atrociously.
5. ________ A reformer and humanitarian. A gifted therapist. First to keep case records. Treated the mentally ill with respect and compassion.
6. ________ Introduced hypnosis to psychiatry as a useful tool.
7. ________ A humanitarian called the Father of American Psychiatry.
8. ________ Known for humane treatment of the mentally ill. Called the Father of Modern Psychiatry.

A. Asclepiades
B. Phillippe Pinel
C. Hippocrates
D. Benjamin Rush
E. Medieval period
F. Pierre Janet
G. Johann Weyer
H. 17th and 18th centuries
I. Harry Stack Sullivan

True or false. Correct the false statements.

9. ________ Happiness, control of behavior, sound reality testing, ability to work effectively, and good self-concept are measures of mental health.
10. ________ Behaviors that allow problems to continue and that interfere with an individual's health and ability to function in work, love, or interpersonal relationships are deemed maladaptive behaviors.
11. ________ Destructive behaviors undermine or destroy the psychological or physical well-being of a person or others around him or her.
12. ________ The DSM-III and DSM III-R do provide specific diagnostic criteria as guides for diagnosis of mental disorders.
13. ________ The DSM III-R is free of cultural, social, and political bias and always provides accurate labels.

CHAPTER 2

Personality Theories and Therapies

Julius Trubowitz

OUTLINE

KEY TERMS AND CONCEPTS

The key terms and concepts listed here also appear in bold where they are defined or discussed in this chapter.

CONSCIOUS
PRECONSCIOUS
UNCONSCIOUS
ID
EGO
SUPEREGO
DEFENSE MECHANISMS
PSYCHOSEXUAL STAGES OF DEVELOPMENT
Oral Stage
Anal Stage
Phallic Stage
Latency Stage
Genital Stage
PLEASURE PRINCIPLE
PRIMARY PROCESS
REALITY PRINCIPLE
SECONDARY PROCESS
SUBLIMATION
SELECTIVE INATTENTION
DISSOCIATION
ASSIMILATION

ACCOMMODATION
SOMATIC THERAPY
PSYCHOTROPIC DRUGS
ANTIPSYCHOTIC DRUGS
Neuroleptics — Major Tranquilizers
ANTIANXIETY DRUGS
Anxiolytics — Minor Tranquilizers
ANTIDEPRESSANT DRUGS
ANTIMANIC DRUGS
INDIVIDUAL THERAPY
Classical Psychoanalysis
Psychoanalytic Psychotherapy
Short-term Dynamic Psychotherapy
Transactional Analysis (TA)
Behavior Modification
Gestalt Therapy
FREE ASSOCIATION
TRANSFERENCE FEELING
GROUP THERAPIES
Analytic Group
Psychodrama
Family Therapy
OTHER APPROACHES
Sex Therapy
Hypnotherapy
Crisis Therapy
Milieu Therapy

OBJECTIVES

After studying this chapter, the student will be able to:

1. Identify Freud's basic assumptions of personality development and discuss his development of personality as it relates to
   A. Levels of awareness.
   B. Agencies of the mind (id, ego, superego).
   C. Defenses against anxiety.
2. Compare and contrast the developmental stages of Freud, Erikson, and Piaget.
3. Relate Sullivan's security operations to a personal experience.
4. Examine the basic assumptions of cognitive theory.
5. Compare and contrast the four major groups of psychotropic drugs used today.
6. Describe the treatment style of each of the six individual subtypes of therapy discussed in this text.
7. Discuss three group modalities in terms of their advantages, indication, and method of effecting change.
8. Identify specific indications for sex therapy, hypnotherapy, crisis intervention, and milieu therapy.

Major Theories of Personality

All people go through a series of stages in their development from infancy through old age. Each stage has its own character and offers its own unique opportunities for growth. The meaning of particular events and relationships is deeply influenced by the stage in the life cycle in which they occur. Although each of us is unique, we all go through the same basic stages of growth. Each has its own special contribution to the individual as a whole. Hebrew, Chinese, and Greek documents dating back over 2000 years attest to our interest in and observation of the "stages of man." Each document has identified similar stages in the human life cycle (Levison and Gooden 1985).

Different theorists view the life cycle through their own disciplines and individual theories of personality development. Nurses draw on relevant theories of personality and human development as a basis for assessment, nursing diagnosis, planning, intervention, and evaluation.

The contributions of Freud, Erikson, Sullivan, Piaget, and the cognitive theorists form important theoretical foundations used in all medical and nursing practices, not just in the specialties of psychiatry or psychiatric nursing.

FREUD

Sigmund Freud (1856–1939), an Austrian psychiatrist and the founder of psychoanalysis, developed a complex theoretical formulation of the nature of the human personality. The following major components of his theory will be discussed: (1) levels of awareness, (2) agencies of the mind (id, ego, and superego), (3) concept of anxiety and defense mechanisms, and (4) psychosexual stages of development.

Levels of Awareness—Topography of the Mind

Essentially, Freud's levels of awareness are divided into three parts: (1) conscious, (2) preconscious, and (3) unconscious.

CONSCIOUS. Conscious level of awareness includes all experiences that are within a person's awareness. For example, all intellectual, emotional, and interpersonal aspects of a person's behavior that a *person is aware of and is able to control* are within conscious awareness. All information that is easily remembered and immediately available to an individual is in the conscious mind. The conscious mind is logical and, according to Freud, regulated by the reality principle.

PRECONSCIOUS. Preconscious includes experiences, thoughts, feelings, or desires that might not be in immediate awareness but can be recalled to consciousness. The preconscious (sometimes called subconscious) can help screen out extraneous information and can enhance concentration. The preconscious can censor certain wishes and thinking and helps repress unpleasant thoughts or feelings.

UNCONSCIOUS. Although Freud cannot be credited with discovering the unconscious, it was Freud who developed the concept of the unconscious in clear, rich, and original terms. Freud described the mind as an iceberg to convey the relationship between the conscious and the unconscious. The surface of water represents the boundary between conscious and unconscious, with nine-tenths of the mind submerged under water (Fig. 2–1).

The **unconscious** refers to all memories, feelings, thoughts, or wishes that are not available to the conscious mind. Often these repressed memories, thoughts, feelings, or wishes could, if made prematurely conscious, trigger enormous anxiety. However, unconscious material often does become manifest in dreams, slips of the tongue or jokes, or through the use of hypnosis, therapy, or certain drugs (e.g., sodium pentothal, hallucinogens).

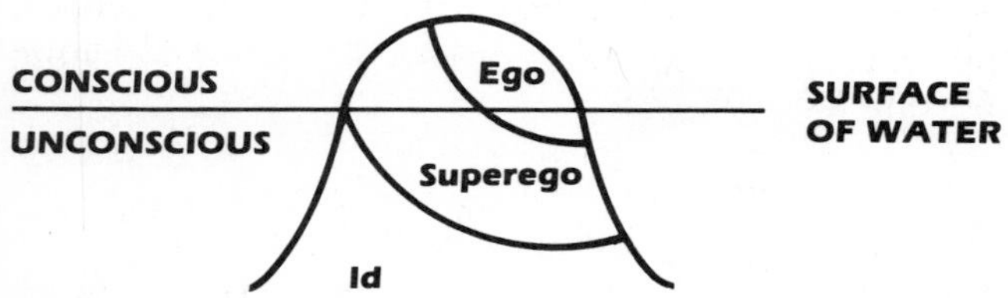

Figure 2–1. *The mind as an iceberg.*

The unconscious exists comfortably with extreme contradictions and ambivalence (love and hate toward the same object), intense emotions, and strong sexual urges. The unconscious is not logical, has no conception of time, and is governed by what Freud calls the pleasure principle.

Conscious, preconscious, and unconscious are not mental processes or systems. They are adjectives that describe the quality of psychological activity.

Agencies of the Mind—Freud's Structure of Personality

Freud sought to describe what he called the "anatomy of the mental personality." He isolated three categories of experience—the id, the ego, and the superego—which represent a method of looking at the way an individual functions. They are not separate entities or sections of the mind. Very roughly, they may be identified as biologically driven energy (id), ways of coping with reality (ego), and finally, conscience (superego). The way the three interact, the conflicts they produce, and their blendings provide a comprehensive picture of the behavior of the individual.

THE ID. The **id** is the "core of our being." It is the source of all drives; the reservoir of instincts. The id is the oldest and the first original function of the personality, and it is the basis out of which the ego and the superego develop. The id includes all of our genetic inheritance, our reflexes, and our capacities to respond, including our instincts, basic drives, needs, and wishes that motivate us. It is the reservoir of psychic energy and furnishes all of the power for the operation of the other two systems. It is with us at birth.

The id operates according to the **pleasure principle** and uses primary processes. The pleasure principle refers to seeking immediate tension reduction. The id cannot tolerate increases in libido, or tension, which are experienced as uncomfortable states. Therefore, the id seeks to discharge the tension and return to a more comfortable constant level of energy. In endeavoring to avoid painful tension and obtain pleasure, the id acts immediately in an impulsive, irrational way. It pays no attention to the consequences of its actions and, therefore, often behaves in ways harmful to self and others.

Freud makes a distinction between primary process thinking and secondary process thinking. **Primary process** is a psychological activity in which the id attempts to reduce tension by hallucinating or forming an image of the object that will satisfy its needs and remove the tension. For example, the primary process provides the hungry individual with a mental picture of food. Picturing a hamburger momentarily reduces hunger pangs. This hallucinatory experience in which the desired object is present in the form of a memory image is called wish-fulfillment. This activity is present in the mental functioning of newborns, in nocturnal dreams, and in the hallucinations of psychotics. Picturing a bottle or the breast partially pacifies the hungry infant, but it does not satisfy his need. The primary process by itself is not capable of reducing tension. The hungry infant cannot eat mental images of food. A new or secondary psychological process must develop if the individual is to survive. When this occurs, the structure of the second system of the personality, the ego, begins to take form.

THE EGO. The **ego** emerges because the needs, wishes, and demands of the id require appropriate exchanges with the outside world of reality. The hungry person has to be able to seek, find, and eat food for himself in order to meet his needs and survive. The ego emerges out of the id and acts as an intermediary between the id and the external world. The ego is said to begin its development during the fourth or fifth month of life. The ego distinguishes between things in the mind and things in the external world, whereas the id knows only the subjective reality of the mind. *Reality testing is one function of the ego.*

The ego follows the reality principle and operates by means of the **secondary process,** that is, realistic thinking. The aim of the reality principle is to satisfy the id's impulses in the external world with an object that is suitable. The **reality principle** determines whether an experience is true or false and whether it has external existence or not. While the id employs fantasies and wishes of the primary process to satisfy a need, the ego uses the realistic thinking characteristic of the secondary process. Using the secondary process, the ego devises a plan and then tests the plan, usually by some kind of action, to see whether it will work. *Problem solving, then, is another function of the ego.* For example, the hungry person figures out where he may find food and then proceeds to look for it in that place.

The ego has been called the executive of the personality. The ego becomes the mediator between the organism and the outer world. Through the use of mental functions of judgment and intelligence, the ego selects the parts of the environment to which it will respond, and decides what instincts will be satisfied, and in what fashion. Carrying out its executive function is not an easy task for the ego. The ego has to try to integrate the often conflicting demands of its "three harsh masters" —external reality, the id, and the superego.

THE SUPEREGO. The third and last system of personality to be developed is the **superego.** It is the internal representative of the values, ideals, and moral standards of society. It comes from the interactions with one's parents during the extended period of childhood dependency. From a system of rewards and punishments originally imposed on the child from without, the child internalizes the moral standards of parents and society. The superego is the moral arm of personality; it strives for perfection rather than pleasure; it represents the ideal rather than the real.

The superego consists of two subsystems: the conscience and the ego-ideal. What parents view as improper and what they punish the child for doing become incorporated into the child's conscience. The conscience refers to the capacity for self-evaluation and criticism. When moral codes are violated, the conscience punishes the person by instilling guilt. A maladaptive example of this behavior is seen in the extreme condition of depression, in which people berate themselves cruelly for minor actions and trivial shortcomings.

What parents approve of and what they reward the child for doing become incorporated as the ego-ideal. The mechanism by which this incorporation takes place is called introjection. Living up to one's ego-ideal results in the person's feeling proud and increases self-esteem.

The development of the superego is a necessary part of socialization, since the young children's egos are too weak to control their impulses. Parental "Thou shalt nots" are needed for a period of time. But a harsh superego can be uncompromising and may lead to blocking necessary and reasonable satisfactions. Furthermore, a rigid superego can create feelings of inferiority, expressed as "I'm a bad person," when the individual fails to meet parental dictates. The superego is said to have its development during Freud's phallic stage (3–5 years).

The three systems of the personality, the id, the ego, and the superego, are names for the psychological processes that follow different operating principles. In a mature and well-adjusted personality, they work together as a team under the administrative leadership of the ego. However, development does not always proceed smoothly. Too powerful an id or superego may gain control, and imbalance and maladjustment may be the result. Let's take a look at a hypothetical situation and consider the roles of the id, ego, and superego. In the case of a young man or woman out on a date with an attractive member of the opposite sex with whom he or she might wish to have a sexual relationship, the id would declare, "I want, I want!" while the superego might assert, "Thou shalt not!" The ego would be faced with the problem of meeting the id's demands within the limitation and standards of society. A solution might involve the young person's waiting until he or she becomes better acquainted with the other individual or some other social norm is met.

The Defense Mechanism

Freud believed that anxiety was an inevitable part of living. The environment, physical and social, presents dangers and insecurities; threats and satisfactions. It can produce pain and increases in tension, as well as pleasure and reductions in tension. Everyone must cope with anxiety. The ego develops defenses, or **defense mechanisms,** to ward off anxiety by preventing conscious awareness of threatening feelings. Without defense mechanisms, anxiety might overwhelm and paralyze us and interfere with daily living.

Defense mechanisms share two common features: (1) they operate on an unconscious level (except suppression) so that we are not aware of their operation, and (2) they deny, falsify, or distort reality to make it less threatening. We cannot survive without defense mechanisms. However, should they become too extreme in distorting reality, then interference in healthy adjustment and personal growth may occur. A fuller discussion of defense mechanisms is found in Chapter 8. Table 2–1 includes an overview of some common defense mechanisms and a brief description of their characteristics, with examples from daily living.

Psychosexual Stages of Development

Freud believed that human development proceeds through a series of stages, from infancy to adulthood. Each stage is characterized by the inborn tendency of all individuals to reduce tension and seek pleasure. Each stage of development during the first five years is defined and named for those parts of the body (erogenous zones) that produce the main source of gratification during that stage. Each stage is associated with a particular conflict that must be resolved before the child can move successfully to the next stage. Freud felt that the experiences during the early stages determine an individual's adjustment patterns and the personality traits that person has as an adult. In fact, Freud felt the personality was rather well formed by the time the child entered school and that subsequent growth consisted of elaborating this basic structure.

The three early stages, collectively called the pregenital stage, are the **oral, anal,** and **phallic** stages. The child then goes into a prolonged **latency** period, the quiet years in which the dynamics become more or less stabilized. With the arrival of adolescence, there is a burst of libidinal forces, primitive impulses from the id,

Table 2–1 • COMMON DEFENSE MECHANISMS

DEFENSE MECHANISM	CHARACTERISTICS	EXAMPLE
Repression	Blocking a wish or desire from conscious expression	Forgetting the name of someone for whom you have intense negative feelings
Projection	Attributing an unconscious impulse, attitude, or behavior to someone else (blaming or scapegoating behavior)	A man who is attracted to his friend's wife on an unconscious level accuses his wife of flirting with his friend
Reaction formation	An intense feeling regarding an object, person, or feeling is beyond awareness and acted out consciously in an opposite manner	Treating someone whom you unconsciously intensely dislike in an overly friendly manner
Regression	Returning to an earlier form of expressing an impulse	Resuming bed-wetting after having long since stopped (after the birth of a child, a baby brother)
Rationalization	Unconsciously falsifying an experience by giving a "rational" explanation	A student who did not study for an exam blamed his failure on the teacher's poor lecture material and the unfairness of the exam
Identification	Modeling behavior after someone else	A six-year-old girl dresses up in her mother's dress and high heeled shoes
Displacement	Discharging intense feelings for one person onto another object or person who is less threatening, thereby satisfying an impulse with a substitute object	A child who has been scolded by her mother hits her doll with a hairbrush
Sublimation	Rechanneling an impulse into a more socially desirable outlet	Satisfying sexual curiosity by conducting sophisticated research into sexual behaviors

which upsets the stabilization of the latency period and gradually comes under control as the adolescent moves into adulthood. The final developmental stage of adolescence and adulthood is the **genital** stage. Table 2–2 summarizes Freud's psychosexual stages of development and can be used to follow the narrative.

ORAL STAGE (0–1 year). The first stage is the **oral stage,** which lasts from birth to age one year. The baby is "all mouth," getting most of his or her gratification from sucking. The erogenous zones are the lips and mouth, through which the infant receives nourishment, has the closest contact with the mother (in breast feeding), and discovers information about the world.

During this stage, which Freud called "primary narcissism," the infant is concerned only with his or her own gratification. The infant is all id, operating on the pleasure principle and striving for immediate gratification of needs. The ego begins to emerge during this time (fourth or fifth month of life), as the infant begins to see himself as separate from the mothering one. This is the beginning of the development of a "sense of self." When the infant experiences gratification of basic needs, a sense of trust and security begins.

ANAL STAGE (1–3 years). Freud's second psychosexual stage is the **anal stage,** which is experienced in the second year of life. Generally, toilet training occurs during this period. According to Freud, the child gains pleasure both from the elimination of the feces and from their retention. Toilet training involves converting an involuntary activity, the elimination of bodily wastes, into a voluntary one. Until this time, the infant presumably has experienced few demands from others,

Table 2–2 • FREUD'S PSYCHOSEXUAL STAGES OF DEVELOPMENT

STAGE (AGE)	SOURCE OF SATISFACTION	PRIMARY CONFLICT	TASKS	DESIRED OUTCOME	OTHER POSSIBLE PERSONALITY TRAITS
Oral (0–1 year)	Mouth (sucking, biting, chewing)	Weaning	Mastery of gratification of oral needs; **beginning of ego development (4–5 months)**	Trust in the environment develops with the realization that needs can be met	Fixation at the oral stage is associated with passivity, gullibility and dependence, the use of sarcasm, and the development of orally focused habits (e.g., smoking, nailbiting)
Anal (1–3 years)	Anal region (expulsion and retention of feces)	Toilet training	Beginning to gain a sense of control over instinctual drives; learns to delay immediate gratification to gain a future goal	Control over impulses	Fixation associated with anal retentiveness (stinginess, rigid thought patterns, obsessive-compulsive disorder) or anal expulsive character (messiness, destructiveness, cruelty)
Phallic (3–6 years)	Genitals (masturbation)	Oedipus and Electra complexes	Sexual identity with parent of same sex; **beginning of superego development**	Identification with parent of same sex	Unresolved outcomes may result in difficulties with sexual identity and difficulties with authority figures
Latency (6–12 years)	—	—	Growth of ego functions (social, intellectual, mechanical) and the ability to care about and relate to others outside the home (peers of the same sex)	The development of skills needed to cope with the environment	Fixations can result in difficulty in identifying with others and in developing social skills, resulting in a sense of inadequacy and inferiority
Genital (13–20 years)	Genitals (sexual intercourse)	—	Developing satisfying sexual and emotional relationships with members of the opposite sex; emancipation from parents—planning life goals and gaining a strong sense of personal identity	The ability to be creative and find pleasure in "love and work"	Inability to negotiate this stage could result in difficulties in becoming emotionally and financially independent, lack of strong personal identity and future goals, and inability to form satisfying intimate relationships

Data from Gleitman H. Psychology. New York: W.W. Norton, 1981.

but now there appear to be direct attempts by the parents to interfere with the pleasure obtained from the excretory functions. Thus the conflict of this stage is between those demands from society in the persons of the parents and the sensations of pleasure associated with the anus.

Parents' reactions during this stage may have far-reaching effects upon the formation of specific traits and values. According to Freud, if the mother is very strict and repressive in her methods, the child may hold back his feces in defiance and become constipated. If this mode of reaction generalizes to other forms of behavior, the child will develop a retentive character, that is, he will become stubborn and stingy, unwilling to give. Or, under the pressure of coercive measures in toilet training, the child may vent his rage by expelling his feces at the most inappropriate times. This can become the original model for all kinds of expulsive traits — cruelty, malicious destructiveness, temper tantrums, and messy disorderliness. On the other hand, if the mother is warm and sensitive in her urging and extravagantly praises the child in toilet activity, the child will acquire the notion that the whole activity of producing feces is extremely important. This idea may be the basis for creativity and productivity. The child learns to delay immediate gratification (expelling feces) to obtain a future goal (parental approval).

PHALLIC STAGE (3–6 years). The **phallic stage** of development occurs between the ages of three and six years. The child experiences both pleasurable and conflicting feelings associated with the genital organs. At this time, children devote much energy to examining their genitalia, masturbating, and expressing interest in sexual matters. Children are curious about everything, including anatomical differences between the sexes and the origin of babies. They create unconscious fantasies about the sexual act itself and the birth process. Their ideas are frequently inaccurate and unrealistic, such as believing that a pregnant woman has eaten her baby and that a baby is expelled through the mouth or anus.

The pleasures of masturbation and the fantasy life of children set the stage for the Oedipus complex, which Freud considered to be one of his greatest contributions to the study of personality development. Freud's concept of the Oedipus complex was suggested by the Greek tragedy of Sophocles in which King Oedipus unwittingly murdered his father and married his mother. To Freud, the Greek myth symbolized the unconscious psychological conflict that each child faces: the child's unconscious sexual attraction to, and wish to possess, the parent of the opposite sex, and the hostility and desire to remove the parent of the same sex, as well as subsequent guilt for these wishes. The conflict is resolved when the child identifies with the parent of the same sex.

According to Freud, the emergence of the superego is both the solution to, and the result of, these intense forbidden impulses. Since these intense erotic and murderous impulses have no prospect of succeeding, the child channels this emotional energy through the defense mechanisms of identification and introjection. As a result, the child not only identifies with the parent of the same sex but also incorporates into his or her own belief system the values and social standards of his or her parents and those of his or her culture and subculture.

LATENCY PERIOD (6–12 years). After the phallic stage, the child enters elementary school and begins what Freud termed the **latency stage.** This period, encompassing approximately six years between the phallic and genital stages, is marked by a tapering off of conscious biological and sexual urges. The sexual impulses, which are unacceptable in their direct expression, are channeled and elevated into more culturally accepted levels of activity, such as sports, intellectual interests, and peer relations. Freud was relatively silent about the latency period. He did not consider it a genuine psychosexual stage, but rather a period of transition and comparative sexual quiescence.

Today, Freud's view of latency has been questioned by most critics. They feel that it is more accurate to observe that during this period children learn to hide their sexuality from disapproving adults.

GENITAL STAGE (13–20 years). Freud's final stage is termed the **genital stage** and emerges at adolescence with the onset of puberty, when the genital organs mature. The impulses of the pregenital period are narcissistic in character, that is, the individual gains gratification from his or her own body. The child values other people because they satisfy his or her narcissistic pleasures. During adolescence some of this self-love or narcissism becomes redirected toward gratification involving genuine interaction with other people. Sexual attraction, socialization, group activities, vocational planning, and preparation for marrying and raising a family begin to manifest themselves. By the end of adolescence, the person becomes transformed from what was originally a pleasure-seeking individual to a more reality-oriented, socialized adult.

A mature individual is one who has reached conventional genital sexuality; one who satisfies his or her needs in socially approved ways; one who is able, in Freud's words, "to love and to work."

Although Freud differentiated five stages of personality growth, he did not assume that there were any sharp breaks or abrupt transitions in proceeding from one stage into another. The final organization of personality represents contributions from all stages.

ERIKSON'S PSYCHOSOCIAL STAGES OF DEVELOPMENT

Erik Erikson, an American psychoanalyst and a close follower of Freud, broadened Freud's theory of human development. First, Erikson stressed the role of the ego, or the rational part of the personality, whereas Freud concentrated largely on the nonrational, instinctual parts of the personality (the id). Second, Erikson viewed the growing individual within the larger social setting of the family and its cultural heritage rather than in the more restricted triangle of mother-child-father. Third, Erikson's stages span the full life cycle, in contrast to Freudian theory, which views basic personality as established by age five years. Fourth, Erikson differed from Freud in that he studied healthy personalities to arrive at his theory, rather than analyzing neurotic clients, as Freud had done.

In summary, Erikson remolded Freud's psychosexual stages of development into psychosocial stages, emphasizing the growth of individuals as they establish new ways of understanding and relating to themselves and to their changing social world throughout the whole life cycle.

Erikson's recognition that humans continue to develop throughout their life span resulted in a developmental scheme of eight stages, extending from infancy to old age. Erikson states that at each stage individuals are faced with a particular crisis or conflict, which can have a positive or a negative outcome.

The stages listed in Table 2–3 are the major stages in the life cycle as described by Erikson. They clearly build on Freud's psychosexual stages, but they emphasize the social determinants of personality development.

Table 2–3 • ERIKSON'S EIGHT STAGES OF MAN

APPROXIMATE AGE	DEVELOPMENTAL TASK	PSYCHOSOCIAL CRISIS	SUCCESSFUL RESOLUTION OF CRISIS	UNSUCCESSFUL RESOLUTION OF CRISIS
0–1½ years	Attachment to mother, which lays foundations for later trust in others	Trust versus mistrust	Sound basis for relating to other people; trust in people; faith and hope about the environment and the future	General difficulties relating to people effectively; suspicion; trust-fear conflict; fear of the future
1½–3 years	Gaining some basic control of self and environment (e.g., toilet training, exploration)	Autonomy versus shame and doubt	Sense of self-control and adequacy; willpower	Independence-fear conflict; severe feelings of self-doubt
3–6 years	Becoming purposeful and directive	Initiative versus guilt	Ability to initiate one's own activities; sense of purpose	Aggression-fear conflict; sense of inadequacy or guilt
6 years–puberty	Developing social, physical, and school skills	Industry versus inferiority	Competence; ability to learn and work	Sense of inferiority; difficulty learning and working
Adolescence	Making transition from childhood to adulthood; developing a sense of identity	Identity versus role confusion	Sense of personal identity; fidelity	Confusion about who one is; identity submerged in relationships or group memberships
Early adulthood	Establishing intimate bonds of love and friendship	Intimacy versus isolation	Ability to love deeply and commit oneself	Emotional isolation; egocentricity
Middle age	Fulfilling life goals that involve family, career, and society; developing concerns that embrace future generations	Generativity versus self-absorption	Ability to give and care for others	Self-absorption; inability to grow as a person
Later years	Looking back over one's life and accepting its meaning	Integrity versus despair	Sense of integrity and fulfillment; willingness to face death; wisdom	Dissatisfaction with life; denial of or despair over prospect of death

Adapted from Erikson EH. Childhood and Society. New York: W.W. Norton, 1963, and Altrocchi J. Abnormal Psychology. New York: Harcourt Brace Jovanovich, 1980, p. 196.

The conflicts are not simply caused by frustration of instinctual drives early in one's life; they take into account the roles that society and the individual play throughout life in the formation of the personality. Furthermore, Erikson's view of the individual is an optimistic one in that he demonstrates that each phase of growth has its strengths as well as its weaknesses and that failures at one stage of development can be rectified by successes at later stages.

SULLIVAN'S INTERPERSONAL THEORY

Harry Stack Sullivan (1892–1949), American-born theorist in dynamic psychiatry, early in his career used the Freudian framework. Later he developed a new concept of personality. Sullivan stopped trying to deal with what he considered unseen and private mental processes within the individual (Freud's intrapsychic processes) and began to focus on interpersonal processes that could be observed in a social framework. The basis of his theory was the contention that personality can be observed and studied only when a person is actually behaving in relation to one or more other individuals. Thus, Sullivan defines personality as "the group of characteristic ways in which an individual relates to others" (Sullivan 1953). According to Sullivan, personality consists of behavior that an observer can see, hear, and feel.

Sullivan believes that individuals are motivated by two sets of purposes or goals: (1) the pursuit of satisfactions and (2) the pursuit of security. Satisfactions refer to biological needs, including sleep and rest, sexual fulfillment, food and drink, and physical closeness to other human beings. Security was used by Sullivan to refer to a state of well-being, of belonging, of being accepted. Sullivan used the term "dynamism" to describe those characteristic patterns of interpersonal behavior that the individual develops in the pursuit of those two goals—satisfaction and security.

Anxiety and the Self or Self-System

Anxiety is a key concept in Sullivan's interpersonal psychiatry. It refers to any painful feeling or emotion. It comes from tension that arises from social insecurity or blocks to satisfaction (organic needs). According to Sullivan there are a number of characteristics of anxiety. First, it is interpersonal in origin. For example, a mother's anxious feelings can be transmitted to a child. Second, anxiety can be described, and behaviors stemming from anxiety can be observed. The anxious person can tell how he or she feels, and behavior resulting from anxiety can be observed and studied. Third, individuals strive to reduce anxiety. For example, the child learns that he can avoid anxiety that comes from punishment and the threat to his security by conforming to his parent's wishes.

Sullivan used the term "security operations" to describe those measures that the individual employs to reduce anxiety and enhance security. Collectively, all of the security operations an individual uses to defend himself against anxiety and ensure self-esteem make up the "self-system."

There are many parallels between Sullivan's notion of security operations and Freud's concept of defense mechanism. Both are processes of which we are unaware, and both are ways in which we reduce anxiety. Although at times the concepts overlap, the major difference between security operations and defense mechanisms is Sullivan's emphasis on what is observable. For example, Freud's defense mechanism of repression is an *intrapsychic* activity, whereas Sullivan's security operations are *interpersonal* relationship activities that can be observed. Some examples of the observable manifestations of security operations are sublimation, selective inattention, and dissociation.

SUBLIMATION. When a child's behavior brings disapproval, he experiences anxiety and threats to his self-esteem. He learns to reduce the anxiety by behaving in a more acceptable manner. For example, the child learns to express anger verbally instead of biting, hitting, or kicking the person with whom he is angry. This expression of unacceptable drives into more acceptable behaviors is called **sublimation.**

SELECTIVE INATTENTION. Sullivan states that **selective inattention** refers to an individual who "doesn't happen to notice an almost infinite series of more-or-less meaningful details of one's living" that might cause anxiety (1953). For example, a husband may not notice his wife's seductive behavior toward other men because it threatens his own self-esteem.

DISSOCIATION. Some things are so threatening to the security of the self that they cannot be faced by the individual. For example, the abused child, needy, helpless, and dependent upon the abusing parent, blocks out or dissociates the experience of hate or anger toward his or her parent(s). Such feelings are excluded from conscious awareness before they are able to trigger overwhelming and intolerable anxiety. Thus **dissociation** is similar to the defense Freud referred to as repression.

Sullivan's interpersonal theory has had a great impact on the direction of nursing practice. Hildegard Peplau, influenced by the work of Sullivan and learning theory, developed the first systematic theoretical framework in psychiatric nursing. In her book *Interpersonal Relationships in Nursing*, Peplau laid the foundation for the professional practice of psychiatric nursing and has continued to enrich psychiatric nursing theory and the advancement of nursing practice. The discussions of the one-to-one nurse-client relationship and the clinical interview (Chapter 6) illustrate how Peplau's theoretical framework has become a cornerstone for the practice of psychiatric nursing and consequently all nursing practice.

PIAGET

Piaget (1896–1980), after earning a doctorate in zoology in his home town in Switzerland, went on to explore the field of psychology. Piaget believed that just as other living organisms *adapt* to their environment biologically, so, too, do human beings adapt to their environment psychologically. He considered cognitive acts as ways in which the mind organizes and adapts to its environment. Piaget uses the word *schema* to refer to the child's cognitive structure or framework of thought. Schemata are categories that people form in their minds to organize and understand the world. At the beginning, the young child has only a few schemata with which to understand the world. Gradually these are increased. Adults use a wide variety of schemata to comprehend the world.

Two complementary processes of adaptation help in the development of schemata: assimilation and accommodation. **Assimilation** refers to the ability to incorporate new ideas, objects, and experiences into the framework of one's thoughts. Through assimilation the growing child will perceive and give meaning to new information according to what he or she already knows and understands. Assimilation is conservative in that its main function is to make the unfamiliar familiar, to reduce the new to the old. In contrast, **accommodation** refers to the ability to change one's schema in order to introduce new ideas, objects, or experiences. Whereas the process of assimilation molds the object or event to fit the child's existing frame of reference, accommodation changes the mental structure in order that new experiences may be added. These two processes are constantly working together to produce changes in the growing child's understanding of the world.

The acquisition of knowledge is an active process that depends upon interaction between the child and his or her environment. Children do not passively receive stimulation from the environment. They learn about the world through active encounters with it. The development of the child's thinking relies on changes made in the mental structure of the child as he or she interacts with the environment. The true measure of a child's intellectual growth depends on his or her ability to change old ways of thinking to solve new problems.

Piaget's Stages of Cognitive Development

The development of children's thinking progresses through a sequence of four major stages, each of which is very different from the others. They are (1) sensorimotor period (0 to 2 years), (2) preoperational period (2 to 7 years), (3) period of concrete operations (7 to 11 years), and (4) period of formal operations (age 11 years through adulthood) (Table 2–4).

The sequence of these four stages and of the substages they comprise never varies; no stage is ever skipped, since each one further develops the preceding stage and lays the groundwork for the next. The stages are somewhat related to chronological age. As with all development, however, each individual reaches each stage according to his or her own timetable. For this reason—and also because there is considerable overlapping between the stages of retention, and some characteristics from preceding stages occur in those that follow—all age norms must be considered approximate.

COGNITIVE THEORISTS

A more recent approach to understanding personality development and mental illness, called cognitive psychology, has shifted attention away from the individual's biology and the dynamic mind. It focuses on the individual's thought processes. The aim of cognitive theorists is to understand the individual through an examination of his or her cognition (thought processes) and cognitive development. In growing up, individuals learn certain thoughts about themselves and their world. These learned thoughts become the basis for emotions and behavior. This approach assumes that it is the individual's faulty thought processes that are at the basis of his or her mental disorder. For example, Albert Ellis (1957) states that an individual may learn that "it is a dire necessity . . . to be approved or loved by almost everyone for almost everything he does," or that "it is terrible, horrible, and catastrophic when things are not the way one would like them to be." With these thoughts, an individual may feel excessively anxious and dependent. He may look to others for approval

Table 2–4 • PIAGET'S STAGES OF COGNITIVE DEVELOPMENT

PERIOD	CHARACTERISTICS OF THE PERIOD	MAJOR CHANGE OF THE PERIOD
Sensorimotor (0–2 years)	—	
Stage 1 (0–1 month)	Reflex activity only; no differentiation	Development proceeds from reflex activity to representation and sensorimotor solutions to problems
Stage 2 (1–4 months)	Hand-mouth coordination; differentiation via sucking reflex	
Stage 3 (4–8 months)	Hand-eye coordination; repeats unusual events	
Stage 4 (8–12 months)	Coordination of two schemata; object permanence attained	
Stage 5 (12–18 months)	New means through experimentation—follows sequential displacements	
Stage 6 (18–24 months)	Internal representation; new means through mental combinations	
Preoperational (2–7 years)	Problems solved through representation; language development (2–4 years); thought and language both egocentric; cannot solve conservation problems	Development proceeds from sensorimotor representation to prelogical thought and solutions to problems
Concrete Operational (7–11 years)	Reversibility attained; can solve conservation problems—logical operations developed and applied to concrete problems; cannot solve complex verbal problems	Development proceeds from prelogical thought to logical solutions to concrete problems
Formal Operational (11 years–adulthood)	Logically solves all types of problems—thinks scientifically; solves complex verbal problems; cognitive structures mature	Development proceeds from logical solutions to concrete problems to logical solutions to all classes of problems

and feel unworthy when he does not get it. In addition, such thoughts may lead to frustration and an inability to deal with thwarting and unexpected events.

Aaron Beck, one of the major proponents of the cognitive approach, maintains that it is the individual's fallacious thinking, due to faulty learning during development, that is at the root of mental disorders. Beck (1976) states that individuals with faulty thoughts use the following thinking processes: (1) they are likely to distort reality, (2) they have unreasonable attitudes, (3) they make incorrect inferences on the basis of inadequate and incorrect information, (4) they have trouble distinguishing between imagination and reality, (5) they use incorrect premises and assumptions in making judgments and decisions.

Cognitive theorists affirm that this new approach to mental disorders changes our perspectives on ourselves and our problems. Instead of viewing ourselves as helpless in the face of our biological reactions or swayed by unconscious drives and impulses, we can regard ourselves as products of faulty learning and self-defeating ideas who are thus capable of unlearning and correcting faulty thinking. Changing self-defeating ideas can open the way to more adaptive and self-rewarding behaviors.

Major Somatic Treatments and Psychotherapeutic Approaches

Like all diseases, diseases of the mind (mental disorders) necessitate a variety of treatment approaches. The following section provides an overview of some of the more prevalent treatments. Within individual chapters covering specific mental disorders, these approaches are discussed in more detail, involving the relevance for nursing practice and outlining the nurse's responsibilities. Predominant therapies to be covered are outlined in Table 2–5.

Two broad approaches to the treatment of mental disorders are practiced today: *somatic therapy* and *psychotherapy*.

Somatic therapy involves various manipulations of the body. It constitutes medicine's classic attack on mental disease through the use of medications and electroconvulsive therapy (ECT). The second approach continues the tradition of Freud and his followers, who initially developed psychotherapy to help people with their inner conflict and "neurotic" behaviors.

Table 2–5 • PREDOMINANT THERAPIES

PREDOMINANT SOMATIC THERAPY	INDIVIDUAL PSYCHOTHERAPY	GROUP PSYCHOTHERAPY	OTHER THERAPIES
Psychopharmacological therapy, electroconvulsive therapy (ECT)	Classical psychoanalysis, psychoanalytically oriented psychotherapy, brief psychotherapy, transactional analysis (TA), behavior therapy, gestalt therapy	Analytic group therapy, psychodrama, family therapy	Sex therapy, hypnotherapy, crisis therapy, milieu therapy

Psychotherapy can be defined as "a process by which one or more mental health professionals help, through psychological methods, one or more other people who have significant psychological difficulties in living" (Altrocchi 1980).

SOMATIC THERAPY

Two major areas of treatment involving the body are discussed: (1) psychopharmacological therapy and (2) electroconvulsive therapy (ECT).

Psychopharmacological Therapy

Since 1955, psychopharmacology has become an important scientific discipline in its own right and, through the development of new chemical agents, a major treatment method for a variety of mental disorders. The use of psychopharmaceuticals has radically improved the treatment of the mentally ill both within and outside the hospital. With their use, it has become possible for some families to hold together and for some individuals to hold jobs and/or make use of psychotherapy.

Drugs that have an effect on psychic function, behavior, or experience are called **psychotropic drugs.** Most of the prescribed medication for people with some form of mental disorder come under the category of psychotropic drugs.

Since the advent of psychotropic drugs in psychiatry, nurses must accept the responsibility of evaluating therapeutic effects, observing for and teaching clients about potential harmful effects, and administering these drugs. An overview of the four categories of psychotropic drugs—antipsychotic, antianxiety, antidepressant, and antimanic (lithium carbonate)—is provided in this chapter. These drugs are discussed in detail in the clinical chapters addressing the disorders for which they are indicated. Psychotropic drugs are discussed under *Standard* V-D: *Somatic Therapies* in each of the clinical chapters.

ANTIPSYCHOTIC DRUGS. This group of drugs, often called **neuroleptics** or **major tranquilizers,** have the ability to:

1. Decrease psychotic, paranoid, and disorganized thinking.
2. Alter bizarre behavior.
3. Decrease dangerous levels of hyperactivity.
4. Increase activity level of severely withdrawn individuals.

These drugs are believed to be effective because of their action in reducing the effect of the neurotransmitter dopamine by blocking the dopamine receptors. This has the effect of reducing distorted perceptions and misinterpretations of reality. These drugs are useful in acute psychotic episodes (e.g., schizophrenia, manic phase of manic depression, agitated psychotic depressions, and organic brain syndromes). Examples of these drugs include the phenothiazines (e.g., Thorazine), the thioxanthenes, and the butyrophenones. The antipsychotic (neuroleptic) drugs and specific side effects, nursing implications, and responsibilities are discussed at length in Chapter 20.

Antiparkinsonian drugs are often given to prevent or minimize the extrapyramidal side effects (EPS) of neuroleptic therapy. They are assumed to work by their anticholinergic effects. Antiparkinsonian drugs are not helpful in the prevention or treatment of tardive dyskinesia. Popular examples include benztropine mesylate (Cogentin), biperiden (Akineton), and trihexyphenidyl (Artane).

ANTIANXIETY DRUGS. These drugs are also referred to as **anxiolytics** or **minor tranquilizers.** Essentially these drugs are used for

1. Management of anxiety disorders.
2. Short-term relief of anxiety.
3. Reduction of anxiety associated with depression.

The most widely used antianxiety or anxiolytic drugs used today are the benzodiazepines. These drugs are central nervous system (CNS) depressants. The calming effect appears to be related to their affect on the limbic system and reticular formation. Common drugs in this group include chlordiazepoxide hydrochloride (Librium), diazepam (Valium), lorazepam (Ativan), and oxazepam (Serax). Many of these drugs are used as muscle relaxants or anticonvulsants, and in acute alcohol withdrawal. Tolerance to these drugs develops, and withdrawal should be gradual. (See Chapter 16 for a fuller discussion.)

ANTIDEPRESSANT DRUGS. Essentially, these drugs are used for the treatment of depression. Some desired effects of the drugs include

1. Heightened mood.
2. Increased concentration.
3. Increased socialization.
4. Increased energy levels.

There are two major categories of antidepressants: (1) the tricyclics (TCA's) and (2) the monoamine oxidase inhibitors (MAOI's). In special instances, the tricyclic antidepressants are used in the treatment of phobias and childhood neuroses. Popular tricyclics include amitriptyline hydrochloride (Elavil), imipramine hydrochloride (Tofranil), and doxepin hydrochloride (Sinequan). Of the MAOI's, isocarboxazid (Marplan), phenelzine sulfate (Nardil), and tranylcypromine sulfate (Parnate) are used. Other antidepressant drugs that do not resemble either MAOI's or TCA's have recently come on the market. Trazodone hydrochloride, triazolobenzodiazepine, alprazolam (Alprazolam), and fluoxetine hydrochloride (Prozac) are currently proving successful. The side effects, actions, and nursing responsibilities regarding antidepressant drugs are covered in Chapter 18.

ANTIMANIC DRUGS. Lithium carbonate is the drug of choice for treating individuals with acute manic behavior and for preventing the recurrence of manic-depressive episodes. Essentially, lithium helps normalize some of the following behaviors in a client with a manic depressive disorder:

1. An elevated, unstable mood.
2. Grandiosity and aggressiveness.
3. Psychomotor agitation.
4. Extreme talkativeness (logorrhea).
5. Extreme irritability.

It is thought that lithium acts by altering the sodium transport in the nerve and muscle cells, causing a shift toward intraneural metabolism of catecholamines. The contraindications for the drug, along with the actions and side effects, are covered at length in Chapter 19.

More recently, increasing attention has been given to the use of anticonvulsant medications to promote mood stabilization in people with a bipolar (manic-depressive) disorder. Carbamazepine (Tegretol), valproic acid (Depakene), and clonazepam (Klonopin) are examples of anticonvulsants proven successful in the treatment of manic excitement.

Electroconvulsive Therapy

Electroconvulsive therapy (ECT) is one of the most effective treatments for treating severe depressions, especially for people who are acutely suicidal, are unwilling to eat, do not respond to the TCA's or MAOI's (antidepressants), and are unable to tolerate medication.

Since the introduction of ECT in 1938, its popularity has waxed and waned, but today ECT is becoming more widely and successfully used in many parts of the country. Essentially, while the client is under the effects of anesthesia and muscle relaxants, an electrical stimulus is passed through the temporal lobes, causing seizure activity in the brain. The client is usually hospitalized during the course of the treatment. Short-term memory loss is experienced. Nursing responsibilities and implications in relation to ECT are discussed in Chapter 18.

Insulin shock/coma therapy, once popular in the 1930's, has been supplemented by psychotropic drugs and ECT. Psychosurgery is another procedure used before the advent of psychotropic drugs. Psychosurgery has been dramatized to the lay public in *One Flew Over The Cuckoo's Nest*. Prefrontal lobotomies are rarely used today. There are potential complications and negative side effects, and they are thought by many to be unethical and unacceptable. Their use is indicated for chronic clients with intractable assaultiveness when all other approaches have failed.

PSYCHOTHERAPY

There are many different schools of psychotherapy. According to one author, there were 36 different systems in 1959 (Harper 1974). This number has substantially increased since then. Different systems of psychotherapy vary in goals and techniques. The following discussion separates major psychotherapies practiced today into three categories: (1) individual psychotherapy, (2) group psychotherapy, and (3) other therapeutic approaches. Refer to Table 2–5 for an overview of the therapies to be discussed.

Individual Psychotherapy

Six subtypes of psychotherapy conducted with individual clients are discussed subsequently: classical psychoanalysis, psychoanalytically oriented psychotherapy, short-term dynamic psychotherapy, transactional analysis (or TA), behavior therapy, and gestalt therapy.

CLASSICAL PSYCHOANALYSIS. The term psychoanalysis describes the school and the system of therapy based on Freud's theory of personality and developed from Freud's treatment methods with neurotic clients in Vienna at the beginning of the twentieth century.

A number of techniques are employed by the analyst to uncover unconscious feelings and thoughts that interfere with the client's living a fuller life. One such technique is called **free association.** When a client free associates, he or she is encouraged to say anything that comes to mind, without censoring thoughts or feelings. Another method of uncovering unconscious material is through dream analysis. During sleep, one's defenses are weakened, and unconscious material often becomes conscious, although in symbolic forms.

During treatment the client traditionally lies on a couch, in a relaxed posture, which helps bring unconscious processes to the surface. The client faces away from the analyst and is encouraged to project his or her fantasies onto the unseen, relatively neutral analyst. Through development of transference, the client experiences the therapist as if he or she were a significant person in the client's life and transfers feelings for that person or persons onto the analyst. The client reexperiences childhood conflicts that are inappropriate to his or her adult life. The analyst facilitates awareness of these **transference feelings** and fantasies. The process of repeated interpretation to the person of his or her unconscious processes has the effect of bringing about change and is called "working through."

PSYCHOANALYTIC PSYCHOTHERAPY. The psychoanalytic model of psychotherapy uses many of the tools of psychoanalysis, such as free association, dream analysis, and transference, but the therapist is much more involved and interacts with the client more freely. Lego (1984) states the nurse/therapist works with the client to uncover unconscious material that appears in the form of symptoms or unsatisfactory life patterns. This is done through an intimate professional relationship between the nurse/therapist and the client over a period of time. The process proceeds through stages—the introductory, working, and termination stages. These stages are described with examples in Chapter 6.

SHORT-TERM DYNAMIC PSYCHOTHERAPY. Short-term dynamic psychotherapy (STDP) is usually indicated when a person has a specific symptom or interpersonal problem he or she wants to work on. The therapist participates actively and influences the direction of the content more than in either of the models discussed previously.

Although many of the tools employed in traditional psychotherapy are used, such as uncovering unconscious process through transference and dream interpretations, other methods such as free association are discouraged. Sessions are held weekly, and the total number of sessions to be held (anywhere from 12 to 30) is determined at the outset of therapy. This type of intervention is successful for highly motivated individuals who have insight and who indicate a positive relationship with the therapist from the beginning.

TRANSACTIONAL ANALYSIS. Transactional analysis (TA) is a theory and a therapeutic approach developed by Eric Berne in the late 1950's. As a personality theory, transactional analysis incorporates concepts from orthodox Freudian psychoanalysis and ego psychology. Berne states that each person has three ego states or personality parts:

1. The child—immature, need-gratifying aspects.
2. The parent—moralistic, rigid, standard-setting aspect.
3. The adult—mature, reality-based aspect.

Berne says problems come about when there is an incongruency between the ego states when people relate to one another. One example is on responding like a child or a parent cor istently with one's peers or friends. As a therapeutic approach, transactional analysis can be used among groups and families, as well as in individual therapy. The client is taught to be able to identify his or her ego states, evaluate which ego states (child, adult, or parent) are operating in a given situation, and identify the pattern of his or her communication with others. Maladaptive patterns, which Berne calls games, interfere with relationships and effective functioning.

The continuation of maladaptive communication patterns is often rewarded positively or negatively with "strokes," and the client is taught how to identify these reinforcers and initiate alternate methods of getting the needed reinforcement. In effect, the therapist works with the client using here-and-now experiences to work through four stages:

1. Structural analysis.
2. Transactional analysis.
3. Games analysis.
4. Script analysis.

BEHAVIOR MODIFICATION. Behavior therapies have evolved from the work of Pavlov, Watson, and, later, Thorndike and Skinner. Skinner believed that man is motivated not only by freedom of choice but also by positive and negative reinforcements. Behaviorists restrict their attention to directly observable stimuli, the response, and the effects of reinforcement of a particular response.

One such method of affecting behavior is to reward desired behaviors. This is called positive reinforcement. Positive reinforcement is thought to be one of the most direct ways to increase desired behaviors. Therefore, whenever the desired behavior is performed, a positive reward is given, which in turn elicits the desired behavior. Skinner called this process operant conditioning. Operant conditioning methods have proved effective with improving verbal performance of mute, autistic, and mentally defective children, stutterers, and enuretic children. In hospital settings, clearly specified goals are reinforced with "token economies." Clients are rewarded with a token when desired behaviors are performed, and they can exchange these tokens for food, small luxuries, or privileges. Long-term hospital clients have increased levels of self-care, levels of social behaviors, and attendance in group activities when token economies are well planned and thoughtfully executed by hospital staff (Kolb and Brodie 1982).

Systematic desensitization is another form of behavior modification. For example, a client who has a fear, or phobia, of a particular situation or object will be introduced gradually to low doses of the phobic object or situation in a relaxed state over a period of time until the anxiety or fear of the object or situation has ceased. This is a common treatment for a variety of phobias (e.g., school phobia, fear of flying, fear of closed spaces). Refer to Chapter 16 for application of systematic desensitization.

Aversive "conditioning," or negative reinforcement, is another technique used to change behavior. One example of the use of aversion therapy has been employed with people who have drinking problems. Each time the person takes a drink, he or she is given an electric shock or an emetic. Over time, it is hoped that the taking of a drink will be associated with an unpleasant experience, which will eventually override the desire for a drink. Antabuse (disulfiram) works on the same principle (see Chapter 23).

Aaron Beck uses a behavioral approach for depressed persons, believing that depression is a learned response that can be changed through relearning.

GESTALT THERAPY. The evolution of gestalt therapy is closely related to the work of Fritz Perles (1893–1970). Although Perles was trained in the psychoanalytic tradition, he turned away from many of the basic proponents of psychoanalytic training. For example, gestalt therapy emphasizes the creative and expressive aspects of people, rather than the negative and distorted features. Another example is that the emphasis of living is on the "here and now," not the "then and there." Intellectual understanding of dysfunctional behavior is considered useless, because the gestaltists state that only present behavior can be changed, not history.

Gestalt therapy is noted for a variety of techniques that are geared toward uncovering repressed feelings and needs. For example, clients might be asked to carry out a dialogue between different parts of their personality. Another technique is to have a person behave the opposite to the way he or she feels, presuming that a person can then come in contact with a submerged part of the self. When dealing with dreams, a gestalt therapist might ask the client to play the part of various persons or objects in the dream in order to get in touch with a variety of repressed feelings.

Perles settled at Esalen, a center for humanistic therapy at Big Sur, California, where his ideas and techniques of therapy have grown and been applied to group modalities (Davison and Neale 1982).

Group Psychotherapy

Therapeutic work in groups provides an individual with opportunities not often possible in individual therapy. For example, distortions in interpersonal relationships revealed by peers may arouse less resistance than those revealed by an authority figure (therapist). The group provides validation from a variety of sources for erroneous thinking or distortions. A person may share with peers, perhaps for the first time, disturbing thoughts or feelings, thereby decreasing feelings of isolation. A group also provides the opportunity for participants to try out new ways of relating in a "safe environment." Group therapy is more economical, since the therapist can work with more than one person at a time. Three major group approaches are presented in this chapter: analytic group therapy, psychodrama, and family therapy.

ANALYTIC GROUP THERAPY. Problems of individuals in groups seem to parallel interpersonal problems and distortions in thinking that individuals first experienced in their family of origin. The psychoanalytically oriented group therapists use the phenomena of transference, resistance, interpretation, and working through as critical tools in group therapy. The goal is for people to work out unconscious conflicts within the group setting, in which the group members take an active role. Although called a leader, the therapist acts more as a facilitator of the group process.

Psychoanalytically oriented group therapy provides an atmosphere in which clients (usually seven or eight) gain reassurance in the knowledge that they are not alone or that their feelings, thoughts, and problems are not unique. The variety of group members enables an individual to form multiple transferences, which highlight unresolved emotional conflicts from childhood. The group provides a forum for recognizing and changing outmoded behaviors and adopting alternate and more satisfying styles of relating. Over time, group members are able to identify change and growth in themselves and others, reinforcing group cohesiveness and commitment toward growth.

PSYCHODRAMA. J. L. Moreno (1946) thought that emotional difficulties and maladaptive patterns could be seen and treated more readily in situations that involve action rather than just conversation. Using a play-like format, group members use dramatic techniques such as role playing, role reversal, and soliloquies to portray intrapsychic and interpersonal conflicts and to play out pent-up feelings. Other members of the group serve as actors in each person's psychodrama. Role-switching within each psychodrama attempts to increase empathy and heighten the emotional reality of the scene. The therapist (called director) then works with group members to fantasize and play out more satisfying and constructive ways of dealing with their problems. Psychodrama is used effectively in prison settings.

FAMILY THERAPY. Family therapy is based on the premise that the transactions within the family system determine the stability and later social adaptations of its members (Kolb and Brodie 1982). It is within the family structure that people learn to trust, love, communicate, and function positively. If the family structure is faulty, then each member suffers. Dysfunctional patterns of one individual—say, a child—are thought to be a result of a dysfunctional family. Therefore, the dysfunctional member is said to be the "identified patient," or the one who acts out the pain in the family.

A family therapist might ask the family members about extended members of their family and about problems, such as personality traits and relationships. The therapist can then construct a chart visualizing generational relationships. This chart is called a genogram (see Chapter 27). Dysfunctional relationship problems are often handed down from one generation to another, and an understanding of complex relationships can help the therapist and the family better identify the process of faulty communication and erroneous beliefs. There are a variety of approaches therapists use in order to improve faulty communication, help families change dysfunctional behaviors, and develop support and satisfaction within the family unit.

Goldenberg and Goldenberg (1980) have identified several situations in which family therapy is preferred over individual therapy:

- When individual therapy has been ineffective.
- When improvement by one family member in individual therapy causes distress in other family members.
- For intergenerational conflicts.
- When the primary problem is related to marital conflict or sibling rivalry.
- For various family-related crises (e.g., divorce, death).

Family therapy is contraindicated, however, in the following situations:

- When key family members are unavailable or unwilling to cooperate.
- When one family member is so grossly disturbed that his or her behaviors make family therapy impossible.
- When one family member's maladaptive behaviors—though affecting the family—are unrelated to family structure or process.

Many of the disorders discussed in this text suggest family therapy as one of a variety of appropriate treatment approaches.

Other Therapeutic Approaches

Four major treatment approaches that meet special needs or unique situations are discussed here: sex therapy, hypnotherapy, crisis therapy, and milieu therapy.

SEX THERAPY. Sex therapy is essentially limited to the relief of a person's or a couple's sexual symptoms and is geared toward improvement of sexual functioning. Sex therapy employs a combination of prescribed sexual experiences and psychotherapy sessions. Sex therapy is considered completed when a couple's sexual difficulty is relieved.

Sex therapy aims to remove immediate obstacles to sexual functioning without seeking change in either the overall personality structure of the individuals or the fundamental nature of the marital relationship. It deals specifically with the present sexual aspects of the relationship that directly interfere with sexual functioning. Its goal is to improve a partner's or a couple's ability to communicate sexual feelings and sensations, wishes and fears to each other.

Treatment includes psychotherapy sessions and prescribed experiences, to be conducted by the couple when they are alone together. The psychotherapeutic sessions and prescribed experiences both help to reveal and resolve the sexual blocks, thereby allowing a more satisfying sexual relationship. At times hidden marital difficulties are revealed, and referrals for an appropriate therapeutic modality (e.g., individual, family, or couples) are made.

The Masters and Johnson (1966, 1970) treatment program has served as a model for sex therapy treatment formats. Generally, only couples are accepted for treatment. Masters and Johnson advocate a treatment program of a limited period, usually two weeks, conducted by co-therapists of both genders. During the treatment period, the couple resides away from their home, near the treatment center. Masters and Johnson feel that effective sex therapy requires clients to be free of the usual pressures of home and business, necessitating a change of environment. Other programs do not require change of residence, utilize a single therapist of either gender, and do not place a time limit on length of treatment (see Chapter 28).

HYPNOTHERAPY. Hypnosis has been successfully used by therapists to relieve specific target symptoms in their clients. Some therapeutic uses of hypnosis are (Kennedy 1984)

- Pain relief — may be used for some types of surgical anesthesia.
- Anxiety and stress reduction.
- Removal of undesirable habits (smoking, overeating, phobias).
- In conjunction with some therapies in unusual circumstances (age regression, multiple personality).
- Change in physiological mechanisms (blood pressure, heart rate).

Hypnosis should be used only by trained individuals and often in conjunction with reconstructive forms of psychotherapy. Some disadvantages of hypnosis follow:

- Not all people can be hypnotized.
- Suggestions may lose their effect over time.
- A client may become dependent on hypnosis instead of developing his or her own problem-solving skills.
- There is some concern that some individuals may substitute a more harmful symptom if the underlying conflicts are not properly addressed.

CRISIS THERAPY. Crisis therapy is covered in depth in Chapter 10. Essentially, crisis therapy is indicated for "normal" people whose usual coping patterns are not adequate when faced with a change they perceive as overwhelming. Crises can include maturational crisis (mid-life, adolescence), situational crisis (death, loss of a job), or an adventitious crisis (flood, tornado). Crisis therapy is short term (usually 4 to 6 weeks), and the goal is to return people to their pre-crisis level of functioning. Some people during crisis learn more mature adaptive patterns of functioning, whereas others (usually those lacking support from others) may come out at a lower level of functioning.

MILIEU THERAPY. Milieu therapy was developed by Bruno Bettelheim (1967, 1974) in his work with autistic children. At the Sonia Shankman Orthogenic School at the University of Chicago, Bettelheim created a comfortable, secure environment (or milieu) where psychotic children were helped to form a new world. Staff members were trained to provide 24-hour support and understanding for each child on an individual basis. It was Bettelheim's goal ". . . to create for (each child) a world that is totally different from the one he abandoned in despair, and moreover a world he can enter right now" (Bettelheim 1967).

There are certain basic characteristics of milieu therapy whether the setting involves psychotic children, clients in a psychiatric hospital, drug abusers in a residential treatment center, or psychiatric clients in a day hospital. **Milieu therapy** consists of the establishment of an environment that is adapted to the individual client's needs but that also provides greater comfort and freedom of expression than he or she has experienced in the past. The environment is staffed by persons who are trained to provide support and understanding and give individual attention. All members of the environment contribute to the planning and functioning of the setting. The power hierarchy is diminished, as all members are viewed as significant and valuable members of the community. Clients assume more responsibility, differential status is blurred, and communication is more open.

Despite the wide variations in the approaches to milieu therapy, milieu therapies are based on three common assumptions (Gutheil 1985):

1. That clients and staff have meaningful impact on each other and are therefore interactive models.
2. That mental operations (e.g., defense mechanisms and regressions) are experienced by both clients and staff, although with differences in degree and frequency.
3. That the process of milieu therapy is dynamic and ongoing and that vigilance and attention are needed to preserve the therapeutic effect against negative influences.

An overview of the major theoretical schools of thought, some major theorists, research emphases, and therapeutic approaches are depicted in Table 2–6.

Summary

Sigmund Freud advanced the first theory of personality development, which in part still influences the thinking of mental health workers today. He articulated levels of awareness (unconscious, preconscious, conscious) and demonstrated the influence of one's unconscious on behavior in everyday life as evidenced through the use of defense mechanisms. Freud identified three psycho-

Table 2–6 • SUMMARY OF SCHOOLS, THEORISTS, AND THERAPIES

SCHOOL	SOME U.S. THEORISTS	THEORETICAL INFLUENCES	RESEARCH EMPHASIS	THERAPEUTIC APPROACHES
Biological	—	—	Genetic studies; CNS research	Pharmacotherapy
Psychoanalytic	Erikson, Mahler, Kernberg	Freudian concepts and modifications, e.g., ego psychology	Personality disorders	Intensive insight psychotherapy and psychoanalysis
Interpersonal	Fromm-Reichmann, Ariete, Peplau	Sullivan	Adult relations, e.g., marriage, work, and community	Broadened psychotherapeutic frameworks, e.g., families and groups; psychotherapy expanded for use with schizophrenia, depression, and other disorders
Social	Lindemann, Caplan, Meyer	Derived from sociology, anthropology, and other social sciences	Epidemiological studies and large-scale social analysis	Community mental health centers, e.g., crisis therapies
Behavioral-cognitive	Wolpe, Ellis, Beck	Based on Pavlovian and Skinnerian theories	Behavioral analysis of symptoms; learning theory	Behavioral therapies and learning theories, e.g., positive reinforcement, operant conditioning, systematic desensitization, aversion "conditioning"

Adapted from Klerman G. Historical perspectives on contemporary schools of psychopathology. *In* Millon T, Klerman G (eds). Contemporary Directions in Psychopathology Towards the DSM IV. New York: The Guilford Press, 1986, p. 8.

logic processes of personality (id, ego, and superego) and described how they operate and develop. Freud proposed one of the first modern developmental theories of personality based on five psychosexual stages of human growth from infancy to adulthood.

Erik Erikson viewed the growth of the individual in terms of the social setting (family, community, and culture). Erikson expanded on Freud's developmental stages to include middle age through old age. Erikson called his stages psychosocial and emphasized the social aspect of personality development.

Harry Stack Sullivan proposed the interpersonal theory of personality development, which focuses on interpersonal processes that can be observed in a social framework. Anxiety is a key concept in Sullivan's theory, and he described certain "security operations" people use to decrease anxiety, such as sublimation, selective inattention, and dissociation. Hildegard Peplau was influenced by Sullivan's interpersonal theory. Peplau's theoretical framework in psychiatric nursing has become the foundation of all psychiatric nursing practice.

Piaget added to the understanding of personality development by identifying four cognitive stages in an individual's development. These are (1) sensorimotor, (2) preoperational, (3) period of concrete operations, and (4) period of formal operations. All stages follow this sequence and each stage lays the groundwork for the next stage.

Cognitive theorists focus on an individual's thoughts, with the premise that thoughts become the basis for emotions and behaviors. Cognitive therapy is based on the assumption that if one changes patterns of thinking, changes in behavior will follow. Much of cognitive theory is based on the work of Pavlov and B. F. Skinner.

Four major pharmacological approaches for treating mental disorders are (1) antipsychotics (neuroleptics), (2) antianxiety agents (anxiolytics), (3) antidepressants, and (4) antimanic drugs (for manic episodes in manic-depressive disorders). These are all discussed in detail in subsequent chapters in the book.

Electroconvulsive therapy (ECT) is extremely effective, especially in major depressive disorders and in acutely suicidal clients, clients who are not eating, and those for whom medication is not effective.

An overview of some individual, group, and other psychotherapies has been provided. Many of the psychotherapies will also be explained in more detail within those chapters that deal with specific mental disorders. The therapies introduced under *individual* are (1) classical psychoanalysis, (2) psychoanalytically oriented psychotherapy, (3) short-term dynamic psychotherapy, (4) transactional analysis (TA), (5) behavior therapy, and (6) gestalt therapy.

Group therapies covered were (1) analytic, (2) psychodrama, and (3) family therapy. For each, the method of approach, the role of the participants, and the role of the therapist were mentioned.

Other therapies useful in certain situations are (1) sex therapy, (2) hypnotherapy, (3) crisis therapy, and (4) milieu therapy. Conditions, indications, and contraindications for some were mentioned.

References

Aguilera DC. Crisis intervention. *In* Herink R (ed). The Psychotherapy Handbook: The A to Z Guide to More Than 250 Different Therapies in Use Today. New York: New American Library, 1980.

Altrocchi J. Abnormal Psychology. New York: Harcourt Brace Jovanovich, 1980.

Beck AJ. Cognitive Therapy and the Emotional Disorders. New York: The New American Library, 1976.

Bettelheim B. The Empty Fortress. New York: Free Press, 1967.

Bettelheim B. A Home for the Heart. New York: Knopf, 1974.

Chapman AN. Harry Stack Sullivan: His Life and Work. New York: Putnam, 1976.

Davison GC, Neale JM. Abnormal Psychology: An Experimental Clinical Approach. New York: John Wiley & Sons, 1982.

Ellis A. How to Live With a Neurotic. New York: Crown, 1957.

Engler B. Personality Theories: An Introduction. Boston: Houghton Mifflin, 1979.

Erikson EH. Studies in the interpretation of play—Part I: Clinical observations of play disruption in young children. Genetic Psychology Monograph, 22:557, 1940.

Erikson EH. Ego development and historical change. *In* Greenacre P, et al. (eds). The Psychoanalytic Study of the Child, Vol II. New York: International Universities Press, 1946, pp. 359–396.

Erikson EH. Sex differences in the play configurations of pre-adolescents. American Journal of Orthopsychiatry, 21(4):667, 1951.

Erikson EH. Childhood and Society, 2nd ed. New York: W.W. Norton, 1963.

Gleitman H. Psychology. New York: W.W. Norton, 1981.

Goldenberg I, Goldenberg H. Family Therapy: An Overview. Monterey, CA: Brooks/Cole, 1980.

Groddeck G. The Book of the Id (English trans). New York: Funk & Wagnalls, 1950. (Original work published in 1923.)

Gutheil TG. The therapeutic milieu: Changing themes and theories. Hospital and Community Psychiatry, 36(12):1279, 1985.

Harper RA. Psychoanalysis and Psychotherapy—36 Systems. New York: Jason Aronson, 1974.

Kennedy MS. Hypnosis. *In* Lego S (ed). The American Handbook of Psychiatric Nursing. Philadelphia: J.B. Lippincott Company, 1984.

Kolb LC, Brodie HK. Modern Clinical Psychiatry, 10th ed. Philadelphia: W.B. Saunders Company, 1982.

Lego S. Individual therapy. *In* Lego S (ed). The American Handbook of Psychiatric Nursing. Philadelphia: J.B. Lippincott Company, 1984.

Levison DJ, Gooden WE. Theoretical trends in psychiatry. *In* Kaplan HI, Saddock BJ (eds). Comprehensive Textbook of Psychiatry, 4th ed. Baltimore: Williams & Wilkins, 1985.

Masters WH, Johnson VE. Human Sexual Response. Boston: Little, Brown, 1966.

Masters WH, Johnson VE. Human Sexual Inadequacy. Boston: Little, Brown, 1970.

Moreno JL. Psychodrama. New York: Beacon, 1946.

Piaget J. The Construction of Reality in the Child. New York: Basic Books, 1954.

Piaget J. The Psychology of Intelligence. Paterson NJ: Littlefield Adama, 1963.

Piaget J. Six Psychological Studies. New York: Random House, 1967.

Strachey J (ed and trans). The Standard Edition of the Complete Psychological Works of Sigmund Freud. London: The Hogarth Press, 1961. (Original work published 1923.)

Sullivan HS. The Interpersonal Theory of Psychiatry. New York: W.W. Norton, 1953.

Wadsworth BJ. Piaget's Theory of Cognitive Development: An Introduction for Students of Psychology and Education. New York: David McKay, 1971.

Self-Study Exercises

Choose the answer that most accurately completes the statement.

1. The psychoanalytic theory of Freud placed major emphasis on

   A. sex instincts
   B. unconscious motivation
   C. fixation in psychosexual stages
   D. all of the above

2. Freud called the structure of personality that represents our basic drives, needs, and wishes

   A. the id
   B. the ego
   C. the superego
   D. the unconscious

3. According to Freud, the ego

   A. is totally conscious
   B. obeys the pleasure principle
   C. follows the reality principle
   D. is in control of the personality

4. The order in which Freud's three personality components appear as a result of the division of psychic energy is

   A. ego, id, superego
   B. superego, ego, id
   C. id, ego, superego
   D. ego, superego, id

5. Defense mechanisms

   A. ward off anxiety
   B. occur on an unconscious level
   C. deny or distort reality
   D. all of the above

6. According to Freud, anxiety

   A. is an inevitable aspect of the human condition
   B. is a cultural and social product
   C. has its source in the birth trauma
   D. invariably leads to severe neurosis

7. A child identifies with the parent of the same sex and starts to take on the values and standards of his or her parents (superego) during the

   A. oral stage
   B. anal stage
   C. phallic (Oedipal) stage
   D. genital stage

Match the stage of psychosocial development (Erikson) with the correct age group.

8. __________ Initiative versus guilt.
9. __________ Identity versus role confusion.
10. __________ Generativity versus stagnation.
11. __________ Integrity versus despair.
12. __________ Autonomy versus shame.
13. __________ Intimacy versus isolation.
14. __________ Trust versus mistrust.
15. __________ Industry versus inferiority.

A. Birth to 12–18 months
B. Second year to third
C. Third to fifth years
D. Sixth year to puberty
E. Adolescence
F. Early adulthood
G. Middle adulthood
H. Old age

Choose the answer that most accurately completes the statement.

16. The stage that is NOT one of the four major stages of cognitive development according to Piaget is

   A. sensorimotor (0–2 years)
   B. preoperational period (2–7 years)

C. period of concrete operations (7 – 11 years)
D. period of adolescence (11 – 21 years)

17. According to Piaget's theory, children progress from one stage to another

A. in an orderly and invariant sequence
B. on the basis of chronological age
C. and occasionally may skip a stage
D. only when their behavior is consistent with the final stage

18. Sullivan believed that anxiety

A. usually leads to ineffective relationships
B. results from failure to satisfy physiological needs
C. is interpersonal in origin
D. enhances an individual's self-esteem

19. The security operation in which one fails to observe some factor in interpersonal relations that might cause anxiety is termed

A. sublimation
B. selective inattention
C. "as if"
D. suppression

20. Cognitive theories of personality emphasize

A. unconscious modes of perception and awareness
B. motivational factors in personality development
C. behavioral responses to the environment
D. processes of knowing and understanding the world

Match the following:

21. __________ Are useful for short-term relief of anxiety, management of anxiety disorders, and alcohol withdrawal.

22. __________ Help normalize behaviors (e.g., grandiosity, psychomotor agitation, elevated unstable mood) in people in a manic state of a manic-depressive illness.

23. __________ Used primarily for treating depressive disorders.

24. __________ Can decrease bizarre behaviors and disorganized thinking and increase activity in severely withdrawn clients.

A. Antimanic drugs (lithium)
B. Antipsychotics (neuroleptics or major tranquilizers)
C. Antianxiety drugs (anxiolytics or minor tranquilizers)
D. TCA's and MAOI's

Complete the statements by filling in the appropriate missing information.

25. Receiving a reward for a desired behavior is a form of ________________ therapy.
26. Techniques used to get people in touch with different aspects of themselves

with emphasis on the "here and now" rather than the "then and there" is part of ________________ therapy.

27. Lying on a couch, free associating to a neutral analyst upon whom transference feelings are directed, is part of ________________.
28. Identification of specific personality parts (child, parent, adult) and the types of interactions (games) and recognizing maladaptive parental influences (scripts) are integral to ________________.
29. Therapy is limited in time, and although certain tools (e.g., transference, dream interpretation) are used, the therapist often influences the direction of the content. This is called ________________.
30. The therapist interacts actively with the client within the context of an intimate professional relationship to change symptoms or uncover unsatisfactory life patterns. This is called ________________.

Write a short answer to the questions that follow:

31. Indicate the advantage of each of the following:

    A. Group therapy: ________________

    B. Family therapy: ________________

    C. Psychodrama: ________________

32. For each of the following therapeutic modalities, identify a circumstance that would indicate its use:

    A. Sex therapy: ________________
    B. Hypnotherapy: ________________
    C. Crisis therapy: ________________
    D. Milieu therapy: ________________

CHAPTER 3

Legal and Ethical Issues

Lorenza M. Valvo
Mary Ursula Guthormsen

OUTLINE

ETHICAL CONCEPTS
Mental Illness and the Social Norm

MENTAL HEALTH LAWS
Admissions to the Hospital
Release From the Hospital
Civil Rights and Other Patient Rights

GENERAL PRINCIPLES OF TORT LAW
Intentional Torts
Negligence

THE DUTY OF CARE: DETERMINING A STANDARD OF CARE FOR PSYCHIATRIC NURSING PRACTICE

THE DUTY TO INTERVENE

DOCUMENTATION OF CARE/ RECORDKEEPING

MAINTAINING PATIENT CONFIDENTIALITY
Ethical Considerations: ANA Code for Nurses
Legal Considerations
Exceptions to the Rule: Duty to Warn Third Parties
Exceptions to the Rule: Child Abuse/ Elder Abuse Reporting Statutes

PATIENTS' RIGHTS
Due Process Rights in Civil Commitment
Right to Treatment
Informed Consent
The Right to Refuse Treatment

SUMMARY

KEY TERMS AND CONCEPTS

The key terms and concepts listed here also appear in bold where they are defined or discussed in this chapter.

TORTS

INTENTIONAL TORT

BATTERY

ASSAULT

FALSE IMPRISONMENT

NEGLIGENCE

RIGHT TO PRIVACY/ CONFIDENTIALITY

TARASOFF HOLDING: DUTY TO WARN THIRD PARTIES

CHILD ABUSE/ELDER ABUSE REPORTING STATUTES

LEAST RESTRICTIVE ALTERNATIVE DOCTRINE

RIGHT TO TREATMENT STATUTE

INFORMED CONSENT

RIGHT TO REFUSE TREATMENT

ETHICS/BIOETHICS

VOLUNTARY HOSPITAL ADMISSION

INVOLUNTARY HOSPITAL ADMISSION

CONDITIONAL RELEASE

DISCHARGE

OBJECTIVES

After studying this chapter, the student will be able to:

1. Define the following terms:
   A. Ethics/bioethics
   B. Torts
   C. Battery
   D. Assault
   E. False imprisonment
   F. Negligence
2. Summarize the relationships between social norms, ethics, and mental deviation.
3. Contrast (a) voluntary admission with two types of involuntary admission and (b) conditional release with discharge.
4. Discuss and give examples of what is meant by a client's civil rights, especially as they pertain to restraint and seclusion.
5. Discuss the Standards of Care for Psychiatric Nursing Practice.
6. Describe the balance between patient's rights and legal concepts relevant in nursing and psychiatric nursing:
   A. Right to intervene
   B. Documentation/charting
   C. Confidentiality
   D. Right to treatment
   E. Right to refuse treatment
   F. Informed consent

Through licensure, the state confers upon the registered nurse the privilege to practice the profession of nursing in that state. Implicit in this right to practice nursing is the responsibility to practice safely and competently and in a manner consistent with state laws and regulations. Each state has a licensing agency, a state board of nursing, which is charged with the implementation of the nursing practice act in that state. The state law sets forth the legal parameters of the practice of nursing, minimum qualifications for practicing nursing, and actionable offenses for disciplinary purposes.

The underlying premise of this chapter is that the patient's rights and the nurse's responsibilities are necessarily intertwined. Knowledge of the nursing practice act is merely a starting point, for there are numerous statutes, regulations, and court decisions that may affect the way a nurse practices. This is particularly true in the area of psychiatric nursing practice because every state has enacted mental health laws regarding the care and treatment of the mentally ill.

The purpose of this chapter is to introduce the student to current legal and ethical issues that the student may encounter in the practice of psychiatric nursing. Because the law is dynamic and evolving, it does not often lend itself to clear yes or no answers. Accordingly, where the law is not clearly stated by statute, regulation, or court decision, the nurse is often in an ethical dilemma, that is, a situation that requires a choice between morally conflicting alternatives.

The fundamental concept in any legal or ethical issue confronting the nurse in a psychiatric setting is striking the balance between the individual patient's rights and the rights of society at large. This chapter is designed to assist the student in identifying competing ethical or legal interests involved in various nursing interventions and considering their impact in decision making.

Although the New York and California statutes and cases cited in the chapter might not be from the reader's particular state, New York and California statutes are representative of modern mental hygiene law in the United States. Different state cases are cited to demonstrate different principles of law. **The reader is encouraged to be aware of the mental health statutes in his or her own state.**

Ethical Concepts

Ethics, the discipline concerned with the moral good, and specifically, **bioethics,** which studies the relationship of the moral good and moral customs and beliefs, helps to provide knowledge and understanding with guidelines for action. **Bioethics** in psychiatric nursing is the application of principles within the scope of the psychiatric nursing practice setting.

Four principles of bioethics are (1) beneficence, (2) autonomy, (3) justice, and (4) fidelity. Beneficence is the doing of good for charity; autonomy is the respect for others' rights to make decisions; justice is to give one just due; and fidelity is the strictest observance of personal and professional beliefs or ethics.

Beneficence is the doing of good, for example, the decision to donate a body organ in the event of a fatal accident. Respecting others' rights to make treatment decisions that are not in conformity with the recommendation of the staff is an example of *autonomy*. Assuring that equal staff attention is given to the depressed, disgruntled, disagreeable patient is an example of *justice*. And an example of *fidelity* is demonstrated by the nurse's commitment to clinical expertise through participating in continuing education.

Ethics is not new. It has been within the society of humankind at least since the time of Socrates, the moral philosopher. The Hippocratic oath, known to every physician, gives testimony to the longevity of humankind's acknowledgment of ethics. The Hippocratic oath continues to be symbolic of the physician's commitment to the good of humankind.

Centuries later nursing ethics emerged with the initial emphasis on obedience, honor, and selflessness. The religious roots of nursing are reflected in the Florence Nightingale pledge, which addresses purity, confidentiality, loyalty to the physician, and devotion to the patient. Today's Code for Nurses encompasses not only the rights of a person as an individual member of a family in society but also the nurses' responsibilities and continued competence in their practice.

Everyone has an inner set of standards, the result of the influences of family and teachers, as well as life's experiences. The development of a value system is a dynamic process, and exposure to different values gives opportunity for reordering and incorporating new values. Self-exploration to identify one's belief system through reading, questioning, and discussing ethical issues, that is, clarifying one's own value system, is an essential element in the process of becoming a professional. Knowledge of one's value system helps formulate a sturdy foundation for professional development. Without this knowledge, one becomes vulnerable and possibly confused when confronted in work settings that present a different set of values.

When one's behavior is consistent with one's professional beliefs and behavior, harmony exists. On the other hand, conflict arises when a situation develops that jars one's personal value system. Not always do professional persons find themselves in harmony with the prevailing institutional value system. For example, the nurse may experience conflict in a setting where there is an abundant use of tranquilizers for treatment of the elderly or depressed patient. Whenever one's value system is compromised, increased stress results.

Ethics, though lacking the clarity and power of law, does serve as a field guide for decision making. As each generation advances in both knowledge and technology, society inherits increased options. Choices exist today that were nonexistent just ten years ago. Such dynamic progress promotes more questions than answers. In such a society, the most limited, and thus the most dangerous, way of proceeding is to assume with moral certitude that there is only one "right" or "correct" thing to do. The nurse's role as a patient advocate is a prime example of the need to be able to view a situation from another vantage point, that is, through the eyes of the patient. Clearly, this is not always a simple exercise; rather, it is one that demands empathy and understanding of all the critical elements of the situation.

MENTAL ILLNESS AND THE SOCIAL NORM

Social norms are known to every society, and most of the members of the society conform to these norms. There are those who do not conform. What happens to those who do not conform? Must all people conform?

Thomas Szasz, a psychiatrist, questioned the basic concepts of mental illness (Szasz 1961, 1970, cited in Fenner 1980). He suggested that committing people to institutions for treatment was a mechanism used by society to come to terms with those who do not conform to society's mores. Thus, the issue was society's "dealing with" rather than "caring for" the deviants.

Does society need the nonconformist, the artist, the scientist, and the inventor? Does the majority have the right to impose its will on the individual?

What about the freedom of the individual to do what he or she wants to do when he or she wants to do it? When is the right of the individual curtailed for the benefit of society? Take, for example, the street lady who for years has been unobtrusively pilfering trash containers every evening. The behavior, though not desirable, is acceptable. Eventually she takes to rummaging after midnight, and as the noise level escalates, the community responds by notifying the authorities of the violations of the peace. What once was tolerable behavior becomes unacceptable. Davis and Aroskar (1978), when discussing mental illness, state that deviance is not the quality of the act the person commits but is a consequence of the application by others of rules or sanctions to the offender.

Therapy is always directed at restoring some functions and suppressing others. According to Haring (1975), almost every therapeutic act contains some element of manipulating or restructuring some biologic or psychologic functions. The objective of psychotherapy is to modify undesirable behavior and to increase the person's repertoire of more socially acceptable behavior. The formulation of desirable or acceptable behaviors of the individual is decided upon by the norming group.

Methods of changing human behavior include behavior modification techniques as well as psychotropic drugs. All brain activity has a chemical component that affects behavior. We now have available a wide range of medications to alter behavior, including psychotherapeutic drugs, tranquilizers, energizers, and hypnotics. Other methods of modifying behavior include behavior modification techniques, psychosurgery, and electric shock therapy—all tremendously powerful means to treat the brain, the essence of the human being.

The brain is more than millions of neurons interfacing with one another. The brain is the center of the thought process of the individual and has the capability for expression of thoughts and ideas. Freedom of expression is a fundamental value of our society, a right embodied in our Constitution. Many psychiatric treatment modalities alter the individual's thought processes, challenging our fundamental societal values.

A very real risk in a highly specialized society is reducing the dignity of the whole person. Therefore, great weight must be given by the health professionals to judicious use of these treatments after a full disclosure to, and informed consent by, the patient. The legal issues presented by forcible use of antipsychotic drugs is explored later in the chapter.

In summary, essential to understanding ethical questions and issues is a knowledge of one's personal value system, the professional code of ethics, and societal values. In the area of mental health and psychiatric nursing, in addition, it is further necessary to understand the mental health laws.

Mental Health Laws

A fundamental component of psychiatric nursing care is understanding the legal framework for the delivery and provision of mental health services in the particular state in which the nurse practices.

Laws have been enacted in each state regarding the care and treatment of the mentally ill. Many of these laws have undergone major revision in the past 25 years to reflect a shift in emphasis from state institutional care of the mentally ill to community-based care, heralded by the enactment of the Community Mental Health Center Act in 1963 under President Kennedy. Along with this shift in emphasis has come the more widespread use of psychotropic drugs in the treatment of mental illness—enabling many people to integrate more readily into the larger community—and an increasing awareness of providing the mentally ill with humane care that respected their civil rights.

An example of this shifting emphasis in patient care is found in Section 5001 of the *California Welfare and Institutions Code*, in which the legislature declares its intent

- To end the inappropriate, indefinite, and involuntary commitment of mentally disordered persons, developmentally disabled persons, and persons impaired by chronic alcoholism, and to eliminate legal disabilities;
- To provide prompt evaluation and treatment of persons with serious mental disorders or impaired by chronic alcoholism;
- To guarantee and protect public safety;
- To safeguard individual rights through judicial review;
- To provide individualized treatment, supervision, and placement services by a conservatorship program for gravely disabled persons;
- To encourage the full use of all existing agencies, professional personnel, and public funds to accomplish these objectives and to prevent duplication of services and unnecessary expenditures;
- To protect mentally disordered persons and prevent mentally disabled persons from commiting criminal acts.

This statement of intent illustrates the breadth of issues covered in the California statutes and the competing interests between protection of the individual patient's rights and protection of the public safety. State laws are extensive, with a range in topics including types of admissions; appointment of conservators and guardians; treatment of minors; informed consent for electroconvulsive therapy, psychosurgery, and medication administration; civil rights; and disordered sex offenders.

The following section of this chapter provides an overview of the types of hospital admissions and discharges. This section will compare selected provisions of the New York Mental Hygiene Law and the California Mental Health Act in order to provide the student with a basis for understanding some common features of the states' statutory scheme. **All students are encouraged to become familiar with the important provisions of the laws in their own state regarding admissions, discharges, patient rights, and informed consent,** since a state-by-state review of the law is beyond the scope of this chapter.

ADMISSIONS TO THE HOSPITAL

Admissions to mental institutions are governed by statutes that vary from state to state. Generally, admissions are voluntary or involuntary, and this categorization affects a patient's rights to release, notice, and treatment.

VOLUNTARY HOSPITALIZATION. Generally, **voluntary admission** is sought by the patient or the patient's guardian through a written application to the facility. Voluntary patients have the right to demand and obtain release. However, few states require voluntary patients to be notified of the rights associated with their status. Additionally, many states require that a patient submit a written release notice to the facility administrator and further require a waiting period prior to release. This requirement provides time for the facility staff to re-evaluate the patient's condition for possible conversion to involuntary status according to criteria established by the state law.

A minority of state statutes provide for a less restricted form of voluntary admission, informal admission. Informal admission permits a patient to make a verbal application for admission similar to that for hospital admission for medical treatment.

INVOLUNTARY HOSPITALIZATION. Involuntary admission presupposes the patient's lack of consent. Though criteria vary from state to state, there are two common threads found in state law justifying involuntary commitment. Involuntary admission is necessary when a person is a danger to himself or others as a result of a mental disorder or when a person is in need of psychiatric treatment or care. Three different procedures are commonly available: judicial determination, administrative/agency determination, and certification by a specified number of physicians that a person's mental health justifies detention and treatment.

Involuntary hospitalization can be further categorized by the nature and the purpose of the involuntary admission. The majority of the states provide for emergency involuntary hospitalization for a specified period of time (3 to 10 days on the average) to prevent dangerous behavior likely to cause harm to self or others. Police officers, physicians, and mental health professionals may be designated by statute to authorize detention of a mentally ill person who is a danger to himself or others.

Observational or Temporary Involuntary Hospitalization. Observational or temporary involuntary hospitalization is of longer duration than emergency hospitalization. The primary purpose of the hospitalization is observation, diagnosis, and treatment of persons who suffer from mental illness or pose a danger to themselves or others. The length of time is specified by statute and varies markedly from state to state. Application for this type of admission can be made by a guardian, family member, physician, or other public health officer. Some states permit any citizen to make an application for aid for another. States vary as to their procedural requirements for this type of involuntary admission. Medical certification by two or more physicians that a person is mentally ill and in need of treatment or a judicial or administrative review and order are often required for involuntary admission.

Indeterminate or Extended Involuntary Hospitalization. Indeterminate or extended involuntary hospitalization has as its primary purpose extended care and treatment of the mentally ill. Like observational involuntary patients, extended treatment involuntary patients are committed solely through judicial or administrative action or medical certification. States that do not require a judicial hearing prior to commitment often provide the patient with an opportunity for a judicial review after commitment procedures. This type of involuntary hospitalization generally lasts from 60 to 180 days or may be for an indeterminate length of time.

RELEASE FROM THE HOSPITAL

Release from hospitalization depends on the patient's admission status. Informal or voluntary patients, as previously discussed, have the right to demand and receive release. Some states, however, do provide for conditional release of voluntary patients, which enables the treating physician or administrator to order continued treatment on an outpatient basis if the clinical needs of the client warrant further care.

CONDITIONAL RELEASE. Conditional release usually requires outpatient treatment for a specified period of time to determine the client's compliance with medication protocols, ability to meet his or her basic needs, and ability to reintegrate into the community. Generally, a voluntary patient conditionally released cannot be reinstitutionalized without consent unless the institution complies with the procedures for involuntary hospitalization. An involuntary patient conditionally released, however, may be reinstitutionalized at any time without re-commencement of formal admission procedures.

DISCHARGE. Discharge, or unconditional release, is a termination of patient-institution relationship. This release may be court-ordered or administratively ordered by the institution's officials. Generally, the administrative officer of an institution has the discretion to discharge, but the patient, as a rule, cannot initiate an administrative discharge. In a majority of states, a patient can institute a court proceeding to seek a judicial discharge.

Tables 3–1 and 3–2 compare the admission, release, and right to notice and hearing provisions within the New York Mental Hygiene Law and the California Mental Health Act, respectively.

CIVIL RIGHTS AND OTHER PATIENT RIGHTS

New York specifically prohibits any person from depriving a recipient of mental health services of his or her civil rights, including the right to vote, right to civil service ranking, rights related to granting, forfeit, or denial of license, privilege, permit, or other benefit of law. New York further requires that each patient receive an annual medical, dental, and psychiatric examination and evaluation. Proper orders for specific therapies and treatments are required and must be documented in the patient's chart. The section also requires consent for surgery, shock treatment, or the use of experimental drugs or procedures.

Another section of the law states that patients have the right to communicate fully and privately with those outside of the facility. Patients have a right to have visitors, have reasonable access to phones and mail, and receive unopened correspondence.

Similar California laws state that persons with mental illness have the same rights guaranteed under the federal and state constitutions as any other citizen. The statute lists a right to treatment provided by the least restrictive means, the right to prompt medical care and treatment, the right to be free from hazardous procedures, and the right to dignity, privacy, and humane care.

The law also provides a right to be free from harm, which includes freedom from unnecessary or excessive physical restraint, isolation, medication, abuse, or neglect. Use of medications for staff convenience, as a punishment, or as a substitute for treatment programs is explicitly prohibited. The statute also includes the right to religious freedom and practice, the right to social interaction, and the right to exercise and recreational opportunities.

Additionally, another statute specifies rights of voluntary and involuntary mental health patients. These include the right to wear personal clothing, to keep and use personal possessions, to have access to storage space, to see visitors every day, to have reasonable access to telephones, to make and receive confidential calls, to receive and mail unopened correspondence, and to have access to letter-writing materials and stamps. This statute also gives the patient the specific right to refuse convulsive treatment, insulin coma treatment, and psychosurgery.

RESTRAINT AND SECLUSION. Behavioral restraints and seclusion are authorized as an intervention (1) to control behavior that is physically harmful to the patient or a third party, (2) when the disruptive behavior presents a danger to the facility, and (3) when alternative or less restrictive measures are insufficient in protecting the patients or others from harm.

As previously indicated, the California law prohibits the use of unnecessary physical restraint or isolation. Use of seclusion and restraints is permitted only on the written order of a physician, which must be reviewed and renewed every 24 hours and which must also specify the type of restraint to be used. PRN orders are prohibited.

In an emergency, the charge nurse may place a patient in seclusion or restraint and obtain a written or verbal order as soon as possible thereafter. The patient must be removed from restraints when safer and quieter behavior is observed. While in restraints, the patient must be protected from all sources of harm. Behavior leading to restraint or seclusion, the time the patient is placed in and released from restraint, and observations of the patient in restraint must be documented at regular and frequent intervals (for example, every 15 to 30 minutes).

New York's statutory provisions are very similar to California's regulatory requirements. In New York the patient may be restrained only on the written order of an M.D., following a psychiatric examination. Restraints may be used to prevent the patient from harming self or others and only if less restrictive techniques have been determined to be clinically inappropriate or insufficient to avoid an injury. The statute also expressly prohibits the use of restraints as a punishment.

While restrained, the patient must be assessed every 30 minutes (or more frequently upon a physician's order) for physical needs, safety, and comfort. The patient must be released from restraint every two hours, and the duration of the restraint is set at a maximum of four hours unless the patient is placed in restraint at

Table 3–1 • NEW YORK MENTAL HYGIENE LAW: SELECTED PROVISIONS COMPARED*

	INFORMAL ADMISSION	VOLUNTARY ADMISSION	INVOLUNTARY ADMISSION	EMERGENCY ADMISSION
Admission Criteria	Person in need of care and treatment	Person in need of care and treatment	Statement of facts alleging mental illness Person in need of care and treatment Less restrictive alternatives must be considered by M.D.'s	Mental illness likely to result in serious harm to self Person in need of immediate observation, care, and treatment
Admission Procedure	No written application by patient required	Written application of patient	Certification by two M.D.'s and application Application executed 10 days prior to admission by specified persons Peace officer may take patient into custody and transport upon request of certifying M.D.	Exam by M.D. Second exam by M.D. confirming findings within 48 hours.
Duration of Confinement	—	—	Court-ordered confinement not to exceed 6 months from date of order Director application for court order within 60 days of admission on medical certification or within 30 days from court's denial of patient application for release	15 days
Notice of Rights	Given to patient on admission Every 120 days patient notified of rights and status; consent obtained for continued treatment On conversion of status Rights include the notice of availability of mental hygiene legal services	Given to patient on admission Every 120 days patient notified of rights and status; consent obtained for continued treatment On conversion of status Rights include notice of availability of mental hygiene legal services	Given to patient on admission Notice of status to mental hygiene legal services Within 5 days, notice of admission to nearest relative and/or 3 other persons	Notice of status to patient, 3 others, and mental hygiene legal services
Right to Hearing	—	If court order sought to determine suitability or willingness of patient to be a voluntary patient	Any time prior to 60 days after admission on written request by patient, relative, friend, legal services to director Upon notice of application by director to seek continued retention For review of court authorization to retain involuntary patient, within 30 days by patient or family for determination by jury trial	Hearing within 5 days on written request

Table 3–1 • NEW YORK MENTAL HYGIENE LAW: SELECTED PROVISIONS COMPARED* *Continued*

	INFORMAL ADMISSION	VOLUNTARY ADMISSION	INVOLUNTARY ADMISSION	EMERGENCY ADMISSION
Release	Free to leave at any time	Written notice to director, prompt release. EXCEPTION: Reasonable grounds for involuntary treatment, may hold for 72 hours • Court order to retain for 72 hours • Hearing held within 3 days of order if demanded • May be held 60 days on court order	—	Release within 15 days if not in need of involuntary treatment If in need of further treatment, must be admitted upon application by medical certification and given attendant notice and hearing rights
	Administrative discharge	Court-ordered release Administrative discharge	Court-ordered release Administrative discharge	Court-ordered release
Conditional Release	—	Conditional release for patients who require outpatient care but no longer need inpatient care Conditional release for remainder of any authorized retention period and only 12 months after placement on conditional release status without review and patient consent Must be discharged if unwilling to continue on status Voluntary patient conditional release may be withdrawn and patient ordered to inpatient treatment only with patient consent; if no consent, must be pursuant to involuntary admission requirements Notice every 120 days of status and right to legal mental health staff	Conditional release for patients who require outpatient care but no longer need inpatient care. Conditional release can be terminated and patient ordered to facility to finish authorized retention period Written notice to mental hygiene service, and right to hearing within 30 days in accordance with provisions of involuntary commitment if requested	—

* New York Mental Hygiene Law, §7.07, 9.13, 9.15, 9.19, 9.25, 9.27, 9.31, 9.33, 9.35, 9.39, 29.15 (McKinney 1986).

Table 3–2 • CALIFORNIA MENTAL HEALTH ACT: SELECTED PROVISIONS COMPARED*

	VOLUNTARY ADMISSION	INVOLUNTARY ADMISSION	EMERGENCY ADMISSION
Admission Criteria	—	Certification for 14-day intensive treatment: Danger to self, others, or gravely disabled as a result of mental disorder Needs continued treatment after 72-hour hold Post-certification treatment, confinement for treatment after 14 days: If as result of mental disorder made attempt or serious threat of harm to self or another or inflicted serious harm on self or another during 14-day treatment	Danger to self, others, or gravely disabled as a result of mental disorder
Admission Procedure	Direct personal application to any private or public agency or practitioner for mental health services Or by referral from private or public agency or practitioner	Certification by facility administrator and evaluating psychiatrist or psychologist for 14-day intensive treatment Petition by facility administrator to court for post-certification treatment	Written application by health professional, peace officer, or attending staff of facts stating that there is probable cause to believe that the person, as result of mental disorder, is danger to self or others or gravely disabled Evaluation as soon as possible after admission
Duration of Confinement	—	14-day intensive treatment: Total 17 days involuntary treatment including intervening voluntary treatment Post-certification treatment: Not to exceed additional 180 days	72 hours
Notice of Rights	At time of admission Given copy of handbook In language patient can understand	At time of admission Given copy of handbook In language patient can understand Notice of status must also inform of right to counsel and right to habeas corpus hearing at time of certification for 14-day intensive treatment	At time of admission Given copy of handbook In language patient can understand
Right to Hearing	—	All persons certified for 14-day intensive treatment entitled to probable cause hearing within 7 days of detention Right to a jury trial within 4 days of administrator's filing of petition for post-certification treatment Right to hearing within 15 days of revocation of outpatient status Right to habeas corpus hearing	—
Release	May leave at any time after giving notice to any staff Must complete hospital departure procedures	Unconditional release prior to expiration of 180 days at discretion of M.D. Release from post-certification treatment after 180 days unless new petition for certification filed	At conclusion of 72 hours or before if no longer in need of treatment Referral for voluntary treatment if needed Certified for intensive treatment if needed

Table 3-2 • CALIFORNIA MENTAL HEALTH ACT: SELECTED PROVISIONS COMPARED* *Continued*

	VOLUNTARY ADMISSION	INVOLUNTARY ADMISSION	EMERGENCY ADMISSION
Conditional Release		Release prior to, or at conclusion of, 14-day treatment if no longer in need of involuntary treatment; may be converted to voluntary status with consent Court-ordered termination of involuntary status if no probable cause for further detention; may be converted to voluntary status with consent Conditional release to outpatient status from post-certification treatment prior to conclusion of 180 days Outpatient status may be revoked	

* California Welfare & Institutions Code, § 5150, 5152, 5200, 5250, 5256.5, 5257, 5260, 5275, 5300, 5302, 5304, 5306, 5325 (West 1985).

9:00 p.m., in which case the restraint may continue until 9:00 a.m. Documentation is required. New York permits only a camisole or full or partial restraining sheet or less restrictive restraints. As in California, in an emergency, a senior staff member may place a patient in restraint and notify the physician as soon as possible thereafter.

General Principles of Tort Law

While the statutes governing the delivery of mental health services clearly affect the rights of mental patients and the responsibilities of caregivers, the law, which has evolved through court decisions, plays an equally important role in defining rights and responsibilities generally.

Torts are civil wrongs for which money damages are collected by the injured party (the plaintiff) from the wrongdoer, the defendant. The injury can be to persons, property, or reputations. Because tort law has general applicability to nursing practice, this section may represent a review of material previously covered elsewhere in the student's nursing curriculum.

In a psychiatric setting, nurses are more likely to encounter provocative, threatening, or violent behavior. Such behavior might require the use of restraints or seclusion until a patient demonstrates quieter and safer behavior. Accordingly, the nurse in the psychiatric setting should understand the intentional torts of battery, assault, and false imprisonment.

INTENTIONAL TORTS

An **intentional tort** requires a voluntary act and an intent to bring about a physical consequence. In the most basic terms, a voluntary act is a voluntary movement of the body. The requirement for intent is met when the defendant acts purposefully to achieve a result or is substantially certain that the result will occur. If the party consents to an act, there can be no intentional tort. Likewise, self-defense and defense of others are privileges that can be used to defend successfully against a court action for intentional torts.

BATTERY. A **battery** is a harmful or offensive touching of another's person. Based on this definition, do the following examples constitute an actionable battery?

- Prince Charming kisses Sleeping Beauty on the cheek.
- Ms. P, an epileptic patient, has a grand mal seizure and strikes Nurse A.

Prince Charming acts purposefully in kissing Sleeping Beauty on the cheek. While his kiss may not be harmful, it is probably offensive in that a kiss, without consent, would probably offend the reasonable person's sense of dignity. In the second example, Ms. P, during a grand mal seizure, did not commit a voluntary act in striking Nurse A and did not act purposefully to strike Nurse A. Therefore, there is no battery.

ASSAULT. An **assault** is an act resulting in the plaintiff's apprehension of an immediate harmful or offensive touching (battery). In an assault there is no actual contact. The defendant's act must amount to a threat to use force, though threatening words alone are not enough. The defendant also must have the opportunity and ability to carry out the threatened act immediately. Based on the definition of assault, are the following examples actionable assaults?

- Prince Charming kisses Sleeping Beauty.
- An 80-pound, elderly female patient raises her fist to strike the 200-pound male orderly while he transfers her from her bed to a bed scale.

There is no actionable assault in the first example. Sleeping Beauty is asleep and therefore has no knowledge or apprehension of an immediate battery. The second example is an actionable assault. While the orderly may have no fear of being hurt, he does have an awareness of the elderly patient's present ability and opportunity to strike him.

FALSE IMPRISONMENT. False imprisonment is an act with the intent to confine a person to a specific area. Based on this definition, do the following examples constitute an action for false imprisonment?

- Mr. D is confused and combative. Nurse B restrains him without a physician's order.
- Mrs. J wants to leave the hospital against medical advice. Nurse C prohibits her leaving by calling the security guard.

In the first example, the nurse has a defense to the false imprisonment action, although the nurse acted with the intent to confine Mr. D. The nurse acted to prevent Mr. D's harm to himself or to another and will prevail in the lawsuit. However, appropriate nursing action would require that the nurse obtain an order to restrain Mr. D as soon as possible.

The second example is an actionable false imprisonment. Generally, institutions have no right to detain patients against their will. However, a psychiatric patient's admission and release status is affected by statutory criteria as previously discussed.

PUNITIVE DAMAGES. Punitive damages may be recoverable by an injured party in an intentional tort action. Because these damages are designed to punish and make an example, punitive damages awards can be very large. Often the plaintiff's actual damages are insignificant, and nominal damages may be awarded in the sum of $1. However, intentional acts are not covered by malpractice insurance, making intentional torts a less attractive theory of liability for injured patients to pursue against health professionals and hospitals. The following case, *Plumadore v. State of New York* (1980), is illustrative of the use of intentional tort theory in the psychiatric setting.

Mrs. Plumadore was admitted to the Saranac Lake General Hospital for a gall bladder condition. Her medical workup revealed emotional problems stemming from marital difficulties resulting in suicide attempts several years prior to her admission. After a series of consultations and tests, she was advised by the attending surgeon that she was scheduled for gall bladder surgery later that day. Following the surgeon's visit, a consulting psychiatrist who had examined her directed her to dress and pack her belongings, since he had arranged to have her admitted to a state hospital at Ogdensburg.

Subsequently, two uniformed state troopers handcuffed her and strapped her into the back seat of a patrol car. She was also accompanied by a female hospital employee and transported to the state hospital. Upon arrival, the admitting psychiatrist recognized that the referring psychiatrist lacked the requisite authority to order her involuntary commitment. He therefore requested her signature on a voluntary admission form, which she refused to do. Despite Mrs. Plumadore's protests regarding her admission to the state hospital, the psychiatrist assigned her to a ward without a physical or psychiatric examination and without the opportunity to contact her family or her medical doctor. The record of her admission to the state hospital reflected "informal," which is a patient-initiated voluntary admission in New York.

The court awarded $40,000 to Mrs. Plumadore for false imprisonment, negligence, and malpractice.

NEGLIGENCE

Knowledge of the basic elements of negligence and thus of professional negligence is an important foundation for understanding the legal effect of one's conduct. A nurse's involvement in a law suit for professional negligence is by no means commonplace. The far greater impact professional negligence can have on a nurse is a curtailment of the privilege to practice nursing through licensure suspension or revocation by the state board of nursing. State law definitions of incompetence and professional negligence vary but share a common thread in the tort of negligence.

Negligence is an act or an omission to act that breaches the duty of due care and results in or is responsible for a person's injuries. Five elements in the definition required to prove a negligence action are (1) duty, (2) breach of duty, (3) cause in fact, (4) proximate cause, and (5) damages.

Duty is measured by a standard of care. Generally, the duty owed is to act as a reasonable person would in the same or similar circumstances. The reasonable person is a legal fiction representing a community ideal of reasonable behavior against which conduct is measured. For example, the duty owed in driving a car is to drive as a reasonable person would drive. Those persons possessing superior knowledge and skills, such as members of a profession like nursing, will be held to a higher standard of care in the practice of that profession.

Breach of duty is the conduct that exposes another to an unreasonable risk of harm. If a person is driving 65 miles per hour in a blizzard, he or she is falling short of the duty to drive as a reasonable person would. *Cause in fact* is the actual cause of injury: "But for" defendant's act, plaintiff would not be injured. *Proximate cause* is the legal cause. This complex legal concept can be simply understood as a policy consideration for who should bear the loss for unexpected injuries or for expected injuries that are caused in an unexpected way. The question of foreseeability of harm is critical to the outcome of the case because it will determine whether a person is liable for the harm. *Damages* include actual damages, such as lost earnings, medical expenses, and property damage, as well as pain and suffering. Table 3–3 explains the elements of negligence.

All nurses are liable for their own acts of negligence, but those acts can be imputed to the hospital or employer under the doctrine of *respondent superior*. Under this theory, the employer will be held liable for negligent acts of its employees performed within the scope of their employment. As a practical matter, this theory is most frequently used because the hospital has the assets to satisfy a judgment in the plaintiff's favor.

NEGLIGENCE PER SE. *Negligence per se* is failure to perform an act or duty or otherwise meet minimum standards, and it constitutes a breach of duty. In such an action, the violation of a statute creates a presumption of liability. The other elements of cause in fact, proximate cause, and damages must be proven.

States may have several health-related statutes that specify minimum standards of conduct. An example of such a law is the New York statute previously discussed, which sets forth the frequency of nursing assessments required on restrained psychiatric patients.

The Duty of Care: Determining a Standard of Care for Psychiatric Nursing Practice

Professional standards of practice determined by professional associations differ from the minimum qualifi-

Table 3–3 • UNDERSTANDING THE ELEMENTS OF NEGLIGENCE

Medication Order:	Doxepin hydrochloride i tablet po qd	Tylenol x gr po q4h prn for headache
Nursing Intervention:	Nurse gives Colace i tablet po	Nurse gives aspirin x gr po; patient chart stamped "Allergic ASPIRIN"
ELEMENTS	**ANALYSIS**	**ANALYSIS**
Duty	Nurse has a duty to the patient to administer • Right medication • By right route • At the right time • In the right dosage	Nurse has a duty to the patient to administer • Right medication • By right route • At the right time • In the right dosage
Breach of duty	Nurse gives the wrong medication to the patient and falls short of the duty owed.	Nurse gives the wrong medication to the patient and falls short of the duty owed.
Cause in fact	The act causes the outcome. But for the administration of a stool softener, the patient would not have a soft BM.	The act causes the outcome. But for the administration of the wrong medication, the aspirin, the patient would not suffer an allergic reaction.
Proximate cause	It is foreseeable that injury could result from the wrong medication administration.	It is foreseeable that injury could result from the wrong medication administration.
Damages	Patient has a BM, the intended result.	Patient suffers anaphylactic shock and dies.
CONCLUSION	Nurse is negligent for failing to meet the standard of care, but nurse is not liable because patient suffered no harm. Thus, the damage element is missing. There is a causal connection between the medication error and the patient's BM, but the intended result was achieved.	Nurse is negligent and liable for the patient's death.

cations set forth by state licensure for entry into the profession of nursing. The American Nurses' Association has developed general professional practice standards and rationale and assessment factors identifying the nursing actions necessary to meet the standards. Additionally, the American Nurses' Association has established standards for psychiatric nursing practice and credentialing of clinical psychiatric nurse specialists.

Standards for psychiatric nursing practice differ markedly from minimum state requirements because the primary purposes for setting the qualifications are different. The state's qualifications for practice provide consumer protection in assuring the public that all practicing nurses have successfully completed an approved nursing program and passed the national licensing exam. The professional association's primary focus is to elevate the practice of its members by setting standards of excellence. The ANA Standards of Psychiatric and Mental Health Nursing are provided inside the front cover of this book.

Nurses are held to a standard of care exercised by other nurses possessing the same degree of skill or knowledge in the same or similar circumstances. The standard of care, as was previously discussed, is the standard against which a person's conduct is measured in a negligence action. This is a higher standard of care than the "reasonable person" test generally used in negligence actions because nurses possess expert knowledge in their field.

A closely related concept of law requires that persons representing themselves as possessing special skills will be measured by that standard. This is known as "holding one's self out."

A standard of care can be established at trial or at a disciplinary hearing before the state board of nursing through a combination of methods. A discussion of these methods is useful in assessing the factors that constitute competent practice generally. The most common method for establishing a standard of care is through the use of an expert witness. The expert witnesses testify as to their opinions and conclusions based on a hypothetical fact pattern that is presented by counsel and that resembles the fact pattern of the actual case. This testimony differs from that of other witnesses, who are able to testify as to facts only, their opinions and conclusions being inadmissible.

In a professional negligence case or a disciplinary action, the expert witness testifying should be a member of the profession about which he or she is testifying. An expert is qualified as an expert by reason of education, clinical practice, and research.

Professional standards of practice for nursing promulgated by the ANA and other specialty nursing organizations are being advocated as a means of establishing a standard of care (Eccard 1977). This method, coupled with the use of a nurse expert, most accurately reflects nursing's view of appropriate intervention based on the use of the nursing process.

Hospital policies and procedures set up institutional criteria for care, and these criteria, such as the frequency of rounds on seclusion patients, may be introduced to prove a standard that the nurse met or failed to meet. The shortcoming of this method is that the hospital policy in and of itself may be substandard. For example, the state licensing laws for institutions might set a minimum requirement for staffing or frequency of rounds on certain patients, and the hospital policy might fall below that minimum. Substandard institutional policies do not absolve the individual nurse of responsibility to practice based upon professional standards of nursing care.

Custom can be used similarly to hospital policy and procedures as evidence of a standard of care. For example, in the absence of a written policy on use of restraints, testimony might be offered regarding the customary use of restraints in emergency situations where the combative, violent, or confused patient poses a threat of harm to self or others. In *Chalmers-Frances v. Nelson* (1936), a California case, custom was used to establish that the administration of anesthesia under the supervision of a physician was within the scope of nursing practice. The state statute at that time did not define the parameters of nursing practice.

Custom, however, is not conclusive and may suffer from the same defect as the use of hospital policy or procedures. Expert testimony was introduced as to the standard of care and custom to forego glaucoma testing in patients under 40 years of age because it was so rare. In *Helling v. Carey* (1974), a Washington state case, two ophthalmologists were sued for negligence in failing to diagnose a 32-year-old patient's glaucoma after nine years of treatment and repeated difficulty with the fit of her contact lenses. The Washington court ruled that the standard itself, to forego testing, was negligent because the test was simple, painless, and inexpensive.

QUESTIONS FOR DISCUSSION

The distinction between minimum entry practice standards and professional practice standards is important in a discussion of a standard of care for psychiatric nurses. Consider the legal and ethical issues posed by the following situation:

Nurse A has worked in a psychiatric setting for five years since being licensed by the state. She arrives at work on her unit and is informed that the nursing office has requested a nurse from the psychiatric unit to assist the ICU staff in caring for an agitated car accident victim with a history of schizophrenia. Nurse A works with Nurse B in caring for the patient. While the patient is sleeping, Nurse B leaves the unit for a coffee break. Nurse A, unfamiliar with the telemetry equipment, fails to recognize an arrhythmia, and the patient has a cardiopulmonary arrest. The patient is successfully resuscitated after six minutes and suffers permanent brain damage.

- *Can* Nurse A *legally practice, that is, does her license permit her to practice in an* ICU?
- *Does the ability to legally practice in an area differ from the ability to competently practice in that area?*
- Did Nurse A *have any legal or ethical grounds to refuse the assignment to the* ICU?
- *What are the risks in accepting an assignment to a specialty practice area in which you are professionally unprepared to practice?*
- *What are the risks in refusing an assignment to a specialty practice area in which you are professionally unprepared to practice?*
- *Would there have been any way for* Nurse A *to minimize the risk of an action for insubordination by the employer had she refused the assignment?*
- *What action could* Nurse A *have taken to protect the patient and herself when* Nurse B *left the unit for a coffee break?*
- *If* Nurse A *is negligent, is the hospital liable for any harm to the patient caused by* Nurse A?

A 40-year-old man, admitted to the emergency room for a severe nosebleed, had both nares packed. Because of a history of alcoholism and probability of ensuing delirium tremens, the patient was transferred to the psychiatric unit. He was admitted to a private room, placed in four-point restraint, and checked by an R.N. every hour per physician order. While unattended, the patient suffocated by apparently inhaling the nasal packing, which had become dislodged from the nares. On the next one-hour check, the nurse found the patient without pulse or respirations.

A state statute requires that a restrained patient on a psychiatric unit be assessed by a nurse every hour for safety, comfort, and physical needs.

- *If not otherwise specified, do statutory requirements set forth minimum or maximum standards?*
- *Does the nurse's compliance with the state statute relieve her of liability in the patient's death?*
- *Does the nurse's compliance with the* M.D. *order relieve her of liability in the patient's death?*
- *Was the order for the type of restraint appropriate for this patient?*
- *What factors did you consider in making your determination?*
- *Was the frequency of rounds for assessment of patient needs appropriate in this situation?*
- *Did the nurse's conduct meet the standard of care for psychiatric nurses? Why or why not?*
- *What nursing action should the nurse have taken to protect the patient from harm?*

The Duty to Intervene

As previously discussed, the nurse-patient relationship creates a legal obligation to provide the care that a reasonable nurse would provide in the same or similar circumstances. The duty of due care is owed to the patient—and not to the hospital or physician—by virtue of this nurse-patient relationship. The landmark 1965 case, *Darling v. Charleston Community Memorial Hospital*, illustrates this duty.

A young athlete was injured playing football and treated for a fractured leg in an emergency room by the physician on call. He was admitted to the hospital after having his leg casted. Shortly thereafter he experienced pain in his toes, and the toes became swollen and dark in color. The next evening the physician notched the cast around the toes. The following afternoon the physician cut the cast three inches from the toes. Three days following admission, the cast was cut on both sides with a Stryker saw. The nurses noted blood and seepage from the cast, as well as a foul odor. Finally, two weeks after admission, the young man was transferred to another hospital where he underwent surgery for below-the-knee amputation of the injured leg.

The court ruled that the nurses had a duty to recognize the signs and symptoms of impaired circulation and the duty to inform the physician. However, the court further declared that if the physician failed to act, the nurse had a duty to advise the hospital administration so that appropriate action might be taken to protect the patient.

The duty to intervene on the patient's behalf poses many legal and ethical dilemmas for the nurse in the workplace. Institutions that have a chain-of-command policy or other reporting mechanisms offer some assurance that the proper authorities in the administration are notified. Most patient care issues regarding physician orders or treatments usually can be settled fairly early in the process, with the nurse discussing her or his concerns with the physician. If further intervention by the nurse is required to protect the patient, the next step in the chain of command can be initiated. Generally, the nurse then notifies her immediate nursing supervisor, and the supervisor discusses the problem with the physician and then the chief of staff of a particular service until a resolution is reached. If there is not time to resolve the issue through the normal process because of the life-threatening nature of the situation, the nurse must act to protect the patient's life.

The issues become more complex when a professional colleague's conduct is criminally unlawful, involving the diversion of drugs from the hospital or sexual misconduct with patients. Increasing media attention and recognition of substance abuse as an occupational hazard for health professionals has led to substance abuse programs in many states. These programs provide appropriate treatment of impaired professionals in order to protect the public from harm and rehabilitate the professional. Programs were first initiated as an alternative to disciplinary action by medical licensing boards for drug-impaired physicians. Florida and California were the first states to extend such programs to nurses.

The problem of reporting impaired colleagues becomes a very difficult one, particularly when no direct patient harm has occurred. Concern for professional reputations, damaged careers, and personal privacy rather than public protection has generated a code of silence regarding substance abuse among health professionals. New York, Florida, and Massachusetts are examples of the very few states that require reporting of impaired or incompetent colleagues to the professional licensing boards. Without this legal mandate, the question of reporting and to whom becomes an ethical one.

QUESTIONS FOR DISCUSSION

Assume that there are no mandatory reporting laws for impaired or incompetent colleagues in the following clinical situations:

Jane Smith, 45 years old, was admitted to the surgical unit for a biopsy of the thyroid gland. Her admitting physician has recommended a psychiatric consultation because Mrs. Smith has had a history of pronounced mood swings for the past three months following the break-up of her marriage of 20 years. The nurse introduces the patient to the psychiatrist and is called away because of a new admission. Within the hour, the nurse is summoned to Mrs. Smith's room and finds the patient alone, agitated, and crying. The nurse encourages Mrs. Smith to share her concerns, and the patient then states that the doctor touched her "private areas" while talking with her and exposed himself to her. She states she pushed him away as he advanced toward her. She states she feels violated and humiliated. What action, if any, should the nurse take?

- *Should the nurse chart the incident?*
- *Should the nurse inform the admitting physician?*
- *Should the nurse inform the nursing supervisor?*
- *Should the nurse talk with the consulting psychiatrist about the patient's allegation?*
- *Should the nurse inform the chief of staff of psychiatry of the patient's reported incident?*
- *Should the nurse report the incident to the chairperson of the peer review committee of the hospital?*
- *If the nurse initiates the reporting mechanism in her facility, must she take any further action?*
- *Should the nurse report the psychiatrist to the medical board?*
- *Should the nurse notify the police?*

Two nurses, Joe and Beth, have worked for two years on the psychiatric unit. During the past six months Beth has confided to Joe that she has been going through a particularly difficult marital situation. Joe has noticed that for six months Beth has become increasingly irritable and at times difficult to work with. Joe notices that minor tranquilizers are missing frequently from the unit dose cart on the evening shift. Joe complains to the pharmacy and is informed that the drugs were stocked as ordered. A couple of the patients state that they have not been receiving their usual drugs. Joe finds that Beth has recorded that the drugs have been given as ordered. Joe also notices that the patients appear more agitated. Joe suspects that Beth is diverting drugs. What action, if any, should Joe take?

- *Should Joe confront Beth with his suspicion?*
- *Should Joe make his concern known to the nursing supervisor directly by identifying Beth or state his concern in general terms?*
- *Should Joe report his suspicions to the board of nursing?*
- *Does the fact that the harm to the patients is limited to increased agitation affect your responses?*

Documentation of Care/ Recordkeeping

PURPOSE

The purpose of the medical record is to provide accurate and complete information regarding the care and treatment of patients and a means for health care personnel responsible for that care to communicate with each other. A record's usefulness is determined by how accurately and completely it portrays the patient's status at the time it was written when read at a later date.

Accrediting agencies, such as the Joint Commission of Hospital Associations (JCHA) and state regulatory agencies, require health care facilities to maintain records on patients' care and treatment. Noncompliance with recordkeeping responsibilities may result in fines or loss of accreditation or both.

USE OF MEDICAL RECORDS

The medical record has many uses other than providing information on the course of the patient's care and treatment to health care professionals. Retrospective chart review can provide valuable information to the facility for determining the quality of care provided and improving that care. Accordingly, the chart may be reviewed to evaluate care for quality assurance or peer review. Utilization review analysts make use of the chart to determine appropriate utilization of hospital and staff resources consistent with reimbursement schedules.

Retrospective chart review can be performed for educational research and investigative purposes. Additionally, a facility may conduct reviews for risk management purposes to determine areas of potential liability for the facility and to evaluate methods used to reduce the facility's exposure to liability. These are just a few of many examples of the internal uses of the medical record.

THE MEDICAL RECORD AS EVIDENCE

From a legal perspective, the chart is a recording of data and opinion made in the normal course of the patient's hospital care. It is deemed to be good evidence because it is presumed to be true, honest, and untainted by memory lapses. Accordingly, the medical record finds its way into a variety of legal cases for a variety of reasons. Some examples of its use include personal injury cases, such as auto accidents, to determine the extent of the patient's damages and pain and suffering; child abuse or elder abuse cases to determine the nature and extent of injuries; disability cases to determine the nature and extent of physical or mental disability; workers' compensation to determine the nature and extent of injury and rehabilitative potential.

Medical records may also be used in police investigations, civil conservatorship proceedings, competency hearings, and commitment procedures. In those states that mandate a mental health legal services or patients' rights advocacy program, audits may be performed to determine the facility's compliance with state laws or violation of patients' rights. And finally, medical records may be used in professional and hospital negligence cases.

During the discovery phase of litigation, the medical record is a pivotal source of information for attorneys in determining whether a cause of action exists in a professional negligence or hospital negligence case. Evidence of the nursing care rendered will be reflected in what the nurse charted at the time. Incomplete or poor notes will raise suspicion about the quality of care delivered.

NURSING CONSIDERATIONS: GUIDELINES FOR CHARTING

Accurate, descriptive, and legible nursing notes serve the best interests of the patient, nurse, and institution. In providing complete information regarding the care and treatment of patients, communication among health professionals through the medical record is enhanced. Internal, institutional audits of the record can improve the quality of care rendered. Following the guidelines in Box 3–1 will improve your charting.

QUESTIONS FOR DISCUSSION

A 23-year-old woman in an agitated state was admitted to a psychiatric unit and placed in a seclusion room without furniture, per physician order. Four days after admission a bed frame inexplicably arrived in the room. On the ninth day of hospitalization, her psychosis became more acute, and the staff intensified their care. The following day the patient reported to the staff that she heard voices telling her to hurt herself. The patient was sedated and locked in her room. Four hours later the room was unlocked and the patient was found unconscious with her head wedged between the bed frame and side rails. She suffered severe neurological damage. The following day the director of nurses ordered the staff to remove the original charting, rewrite their notes, and replace the falsified notes in the chart.

- *Which acts or omissions by the staff breach the staff's duty to provide the patient with a safe environment?*
- *What nursing action should the staff have taken after sedating the patient to protect her from harm?*
- *Discuss the legal and ethical ramifications of the staff's falsification of the patient's record on the director of nurse's order.*

Box 3-1. DO'S AND DON'TS OF CHARTING

Do

- Be familiar with the nursing documentation policy in your facility and conform your charting to this standard. The policy will generally state the method of charting (e.g., SOAP, systems review, chronological block), the frequency, pertinent assessments, interventions, and outcomes.
- Chart legibly in ink.
- Chart facts fully, descriptively, and accurately.
- Chart what you see, hear, feel, and smell.
- Chart a total patient assessment on each shift and on admission, discharge, and transfer.
- Chart pertinent observations: psychosocial, physical symptoms pertinent to the medical diagnosis, behaviors pertinent to the nursing diagnosis.
- Chart fully the facts surrounding unusual occurrences and incidents, but do **not** notate in the chart that an incident report was filed. This form is generally a privileged communication between the hospital and hospital attorney. Charting it may destroy the privileged nature of the communication.
- Chart ALL nursing interventions, treatments, and outcomes, including teaching efforts and patient response, and safety and patient protection interventions.
- Chart patient's expressed subjective feelings.
- Chart each time you notify a physician, the reason for notification, what was communicated, the accurate time, instructions or orders, and the follow-up activity.
- Chart M.D. visits and treatments.
- Chart discharge medications and instructions given for use.

Do Not

- Chart before an event occurs.
- Chart generalizations, suppositions, or "pat phrases."
- Obliterate, erase, alter, or destroy a record. If an error is made, draw one line through the error, write "error," and initial.
- Leave blank spaces for chronological notes. If you must chart out of sequence, chart "late entry." Identify the time and date of entry and the time and date of occurrence.

The clinical situation above is taken from the facts in a Connecticut case. In *Pisel v. Stamford Hospital* (1980), the falsification of the record was not disclosed until after a lawsuit had been filed. The Connecticut Supreme Court in upholding a $3.6 million award for the patient decided that the jury was entitled to consider the falsified record as evidence that the hospital was conscious of its negligence.

Maintaining Patient Confidentiality

ETHICAL CONSIDERATIONS: ANA CODE FOR NURSES

The ANA Code for Nurses states: "The nurse safeguards the client's right to privacy by judiciously protecting information of a confidential nature" (1985). The applicable interpretive statement provides further explanation for maintaining patient confidentiality and recognizes the distinction between legal and ethical obligations. The interpretive statement follows:

> The right of privacy is an inalienable right of all persons, and the nurse has a clear obligation to safeguard any confidential information about the client acquired from any source. The nurse-client relationship is built on trust. This relationship could be destroyed and the client's welfare and reputation jeopardized by injudicious disclosing of information provided in confidence. Since the concept of confidentiality has legal as well as ethical implications, an inappropriate breach of confidentiality may also expose the nurse to liability.

As previously stated, a profession's code of ethics is the basic moral tenant upon which the profession is based. Though often consistent with codified, statutory requirements, constitutional principles of law, or judicial decisions, a code of ethics is separate and distinct from legal requirements and may often differ markedly from legal obligations imposed on the profession by states.

LEGAL CONSIDERATIONS

The fundamental principle underlying the ANA code on **confidentiality** is a person's constitutional **right to privacy.** Generally, the nurse's legal duty to maintain confidentiality is to act to protect the patient's right to privacy. Therefore, disclosures of information obtained from the patient or in the medical record beyond those necessary to carry out a patient's treatment plan are impermissible without the patient's consent.

For example, the nurse's release of information to the patient's employer regarding the patient's condition without the patient's consent is a breach of confidentiality subjecting the nurse to liability for the tort of invasion of privacy. On the other hand, discussion of a patient's history with other staff members to ascertain a consistent treatment approach is not a breach of confidentiality.

Many states have enacted privileged communication statutes that prohibit specified health professionals from disclosing patient information unless the patient has either consented to the disclosure or waived the privilege. Those state statutes differ markedly.

Generally, to create the privilege, a patient–health professional relationship must exist, and the information must relate to the care and treatment of the patient. The health professional often may assert the privilege on the patient's behalf. However, the patient is the holder of the privilege, and health professionals cannot raise the privilege for their own defense or benefit. The privilege usually applies in quasi-judicial or judicial proceedings. California Evidence Code, Section 1014, is an example of such a statute.

> Section 1014, **Psychotherapists-patient privilege; application to individual entities,** . . . the patient, whether or not the party, has a privilege to refuse to disclose, and to prevent another from disclosing, a confidential communication between patient and psychotherapist if the privilege is claimed by:
> (a) The holder of the privilege;
> (b) A person who is authorized to claim the privilege by the holder of the privilege; or
> (c) The person who is the psychotherapist at the time of the confidential communication, but such person may not claim the privilege if there is no holder of the privilege in existence or he is otherwise instructed by a person authorized to permit disclosure . . . .

EXCEPTIONS TO THE RULE: DUTY TO WARN THIRD PARTIES

The California Supreme Court in its 1976 landmark decision *Tarasoff v. The Regents of University of California* ruled that a psychotherapist had the **duty to warn** his or her client's potential victim of potential harm. This decision created much controversy and confusion in the psychiatric and medical community over breach of patient confidentiality and its impact on the therapeutic relationship in psychiatric care and the psychotherapist's ability to predict patient dangerousness. This trend continues as other jurisdictions have adopted or modified the California rule, despite the psychiatric community's objections, viewing the public safety issue paramount to the privacy issue in narrowly defined circumstances.

In the *Tarasoff* case, the patient, Mr. Poddar, told Dr. Moore, a psychologist at the University of California, that he intended to kill Ms. Tarasoff, a former girlfriend. Dr. Moore notified campus police, who detained Mr. Poddar but released him after a short time since he appeared rational. Dr. Moore's recommendation to the police that Mr. Poddar be confined was overruled by Dr. Moore's superior, who then directed the staff to take no further action. Mr. Poddar killed Ms. Tarasoff, and her parents sued the police, therapists, and the University of California for their failure to confine Poddar under the state's commitment law and their failure to warn Ms. Tarasoff of the danger.

While acknowledging that generally there is no duty to aid third persons at common law unless special relationships exist, the court found the patient-therapist relationship between Dr. Moore and Mr. Poddar sufficient to create a duty to aid Ms. Tarasoff. The duty to protect the intended victim from danger arises when the therapist determines—or, pursuant to professional standards, should have determined—that the patient presents a serious danger to another. Any action reasonably necessary under the circumstances, including notification of the potential victim, the victim's family, and the police, discharges the therapist's duty to the potential victim.

Arguing that predictions of future violence are inaccurate at best and speculative at worst, the psychiatric community raised concerns over the use of a professional standard to determine when a therapist should have known of the client's future violence toward another, as required by *Tarasoff*. The courts and other legal commentators have recognized the difficulty in the therapist's forecast of violence but have also noted that the therapist's prediction of violence is used in civil commitment procedures in California to determine whether a client or patient poses a threat to others.

The psychologist's diagnostic function, a professional service rendered within the legal scope of practice, was central to the California Supreme Court's ruling in *Hedlum v. Superior Court of Orange County* (1983). The court stated that the duty to warn was composed of two elements: (1) the duty to diagnose and predict the client's danger of violence and (2) the duty to take appropriate action to protect the identified victim. The court stated that " . . . a negligent failure to diagnose dangerousness in a Tarasoff action is as much a basis for liability as is a negligent failure to warn a known victim once such a diagnosis has been made."

A limited duty to investigate the patient's history was enunciated in *Jablonski v. United States* (1983), a federal court case decided following California law. Though not binding on California courts, it will be influential in the consideration of similar factual situations by California and other jurisdictions. In *Jablonski v. United States* (1983), Ms. Kimble's mother notified police that Mr. Jablonski had attempted to rape her. Ms. Kimble was, at the time, Mr. Jablonski's girlfriend. Mr. Jablonski agreed to undergo psychiatric treatment, and the police subsequently notified the chief psychiatrist that Mr. Jablonski had a prior criminal record, was threatening others, and recommended that he be treated on an inpatient basis. The chief psychiatrist indicated he would transmit the information to the treating psychiatrist, which he failed to do. Mr. Jablonski underwent outpatient care when he refused to voluntarily commit himself, and the treating physician, while noting his potential for violence, did not believe the patient met the civil commitment criteria.

During his initial interview with Mr. Jablonski, the treating psychiatrist learned of Mr. Jablonski's criminal record for raping his ex-wife, the recent rape attempt against his girlfriend's mother, and that he had undergone psychiatric treatment elsewhere. No attempt was made to locate the records that indicated that Mr. Jablonski had "homicidal ideations" toward his ex-wife and had tried to kill her. Prior to Mr. Jablonski's second appointment, the victim, Ms. Kimble, moved out of Mr. Jablonski's apartment, though she continued to see him and drove him to his second appointment. Again Mr. Jablonski refused voluntary inpatient treatment, made no specific threats toward the victim, and was scheduled for another outpatient appointment. Two days later he killed Ms. Kimble.

The court found that failure to obtain the patient's records and failure to record and communicate the telephone contact by the police were negligent acts. Although there was no specific threat toward Ms. Kimble, Mr. Jablonski's previous history indicated his violence would likely be directed toward her.

In California there is no affirmative duty to warn third persons of potential violence when the victim is not a "known, identifiable victim." In another California case, *Thomas v. County of Alameda* (1980), a juvenile with dangerous and violent propensities toward young children was released from custody of the county to custody of his mother for a home visit. While home, he killed a neighborhood child, and the deceased child's parents sued the county for wrongful death, alleging that the county had a duty to warn the police, the juvenile's mother, and other local parents. The court held that there was no duty to warn, since the victim was a "member of a large amorphous public group of potential targets and not a known, identifiable victim." This is distinguishable from *Jablonski*, where sufficient information existed to identify the victim.

Other states that have considered the therapist's duty to warn potential victims include Minnesota, Georgia, Iowa, and federal district courts in Nebraska and California.

Nursing Considerations

As this trend to impose a therapist's duty to warn third persons of potential harm continues to gain wider acceptance in other jurisdictions, it is important for students and nurses to understand the implications for nursing practice. While none of these cases to date has dealt with nurses, it is fair to assume that in those jurisdictions that have adopted the *Tarasoff* doctrine, the duty to warn third persons will be applied to clinical psychiatric nurse specialists in private practice who engage in individual therapy.

It is unlikely that a duty to warn potential victims would be extended to staff psychiatric nurses working in the institutional setting, since the nurse does not have primary case management responsibilities. However, the failure of a staff psychiatric nurse who is a member of a team of psychiatrists, psychologists, psychiatric social workers, and other psychiatric nurses to report patient threats of harm against specified victims or classes of victims to the team or the patient's managing psychotherapist for assessment and evaluation is likely to be considered substandard nursing care.

So, too, the failure to communicate and record relevant information from police, relatives, or the patient's old records might also be deemed negligent. Breach of patient-nurse confidentiality should not pose ethical or legal dilemmas for the nurses in these situations, since a team approach to delivery of psychiatric care presumes communication of pertinent information to other staff members to develop a treatment plan in the patient's best interest.

EXCEPTIONS TO THE RULE: CHILD ABUSE/ELDER ABUSE REPORTING STATUTES

Because of the states' interest in protecting children, all 50 states, and the District of Columbia, have enacted **child abuse reporting statutes.** While these statutes differ from state to state, they generally include a definition of child abuse, a list of persons required or encouraged to report, and the governmental agency designated to receive and investigate the reports. Most statutes include civil and criminal immunity clauses for those professionals required to report, as well as criminal or civil penalties for failure to report. Many states specifically require nurses to report cases of suspected abuse.

The New York State Social Services Law, Section 411, provides in part:

> The following persons and officials are required to report or cause a report to be made in accordance with this title when they have reasonable cause to *suspect* that a child coming before them in their professional or official capacity is an abused or maltreated child, or when they have reasonable cause to *suspect* that a child is an abused or maltreated child where the parent, guardian, custodian or other person legally responsible for such child, comes before them in their professional or official capacity and states from personal knowledge, facts, conditions or circumstances which, if correct, wound render the child an abused or maltreated child; any physician, surgeon, . . . nurse . . . .

There is a conflict between federal and state law with respect to child abuse reporting when the health professional discovers child abuse or neglect during the suspected abuser's alcohol or drug abuse treatment. Federal laws and regulations governing confidentiality of patient records, which apply to almost all drug abuse and alcohol treatment providers, prohibit any disclosure without court order. In this case, federal law supersedes state reporting laws, though compliance with the state law may be maintained if a court order is obtained pursuant to the regulations, or if a report can be made without identifying the abuser as a patient in an alcohol drug treatment program, or if the report is made anonymously.

As reported incidents of abuse to other persons in society surface, states may require health professionals to report other kinds of abuse. California recently enacted an **elder abuse reporting law,** which requires registered nurses and others to report cases of abuse of the elderly. The elderly are defined as adults 65 years of age and older. The law also applies to dependent adults—that is, adults between 18 and 64 years of age whose physical or mental limitations restrict their ability to carry out normal activities or protect themselves—when the R.N. has actual knowledge that the person has been the victim of physical abuse. Additionally, the R.N. may report knowledge of, or "reasonable suspicion" of, mental abuse or suffering. Both dependent adults and elders are protected by the law from purposeful physical or fiduciary neglect or abandonment.

Mandatory reports must be made by telephone as soon as possible and in writing within 36 hours to the state department of social services, the nursing home ombudsman, the county welfare department, or the social services department. The California statute provides immunity from civil or criminal action for making the report. Failure to report is a misdemeanor, punishable by a $1000 fine, six months in county jail, or both.

Since state law requirements vary, **students are encouraged to become conversant with their own state requirements.**

Questions for Discussion

In a private psychiatric unit in California, a 15-year-old male is admitted voluntarily at the request of his parents because of violent, explosive behavior which seems to stem from his father's recent remarriage following his parents' divorce. A few days following admission, while in group therapy, he has an explosive reaction to a discussion concerning weekend passes for Mother's Day. He screams about being abandoned and nobody caring about him. Several weeks later on the day before discharge, he elicits from the nurse a promise to keep confidential his plan to kill his mother.

Consider the ANA code of ethics on patient confidentiality, principles of psychiatric nursing, and the duty to warn cases in answering the following questions:

- *Did the nurse use appropriate nursing judgment in promising confidentiality?*
- *Discuss the bioethical principles of beneficence, justice, autonomy, and fidelity as they relate to the situation described.*
- *Does the nurse have a legal duty to warn the patient's mother of her son's threat?*
- *Is the duty owed to the patient's father and stepmother?*
- *Would a change in the admission status from voluntary to involuntary protect the patient's mother without violating the patient's confidentiality?*
- *Would your response be different by virtue of the state where the incident occurred? Why or why not?*
- *What nursing action, if any, should the nurse take upon the disclosure by the patient?*

How would your responses to the concepts in the previous questions differ in relation to the changes in the following clinical situation:

A 25-year-old female is attending a New York federally funded outpatient rehabilitative center for alcoholism after successful completion of the inpatient program. The patient's husband comments to the nurse that he believes his wife is showing improvement because she no longer beats his 3-year-old son. A few weeks later the son is admitted to the hospital with a fractured arm and several bruises and contusions over his body.

- *What nursing intervention, if any, should the nurse have taken upon disclosure of the patient's alleged child abuse?*
- *Does the nurse have a legal duty to report child abuse?*
- *Does the patient's participation in a federally funded rehabilitation program have any effect on the nurse's duty to report suspected child abuse?*

Patients' Rights

Nowhere is the conflict between the patient's expressed interests and the nurse's judgment of the patient's best interest more apparent than in the psychiatric setting. The nurse's role of patient advocate can be difficult to exercise in the psychiatric setting, given this inherent conflict. Questioning one's ability to be an effective advocate and separating one's clinical judgment of the patient's situation from the patient's expressed desires are essential.

Some facilities may employ a designated institution-based patient advocate to mediate such conflicts. As Davis and Aroskar (1978) point out, the effectiveness of an institution-based patient advocate depends upon access to hospital records, ability to call on qualified consultants, active participation in patient care conferences and quality of care committees, and direct access to the hospital administrator. This is an attempt to equalize the power of the individual within the institution.

Some states, recognizing mental patients' inability to assert their own rights effectively in the psychiatric setting, have developed ombudsmen programs for mental patients. State law in California mandates an independent patient advocate, and New York provides for mental health legal services. Both programs assure that patients' constitutional rights are protected and that their expressed interests are represented.

The single most important thing a nurse can do to protect patients' rights is to be familiar with state law provisions regarding the care and treatment of mental patients and any rights specified by the state. If state law mandates legal services for mental patients or a patients' rights advocate program, patient concerns regarding confinement, treatment, change in status, release, medication, and any other treatment modality can be referred to the appropriate offices.

Additionally, nurses should be familiar with their own hospital's policies regarding admission, change in status, release, medications, informed consent, and use of restraints. The next section will discuss patients' rights in depth.

DUE PROCESS RIGHTS IN CIVIL COMMITMENT

The courts have recognized that involuntary civil commitment to a mental hospital is a "massive curtailment of liberty" (*Humphrey v. Cady* 1972, p. 509) requiring due process protections in the civil commitment procedure. This right derives from the Fifth Amendment of the United States Constitution, which states that "no person shall . . . be deprived of life, liberty or property without due process of law." The Fourteenth Amendment explicitly prohibits states from depriving citizens of life, liberty, and property without due process of law. State civil commitment statutes, if challenged in the courts on constitutional grounds, will have to afford minimal due process protections to pass the court's scrutiny.

A state's power in enacting civil commitment procedure is based either on the *parens patriae* power or on state policy power. *Parens patriae* is the power of the state to act for the care, treatment, or protection of an individual or class of individuals who are unable to act on their own behalf in their own best interests.

For example, in an 1845 Massachusetts case, *In re Oakes*, the court found justification for depriving a person of liberty for his own safety and that of others when such restraint might be beneficial to him. Mr. Oakes, an elderly widower, was confined when he became engaged to a woman of questionable character and involved in speculative financial ventures following the death of his wife. This case is an example of early judicial application of the *parens patriae* doctrine to civil commitment of the mentally ill.

In contrast, the states' police power is a plenary power to make laws and regulations to protect the public health, safety, and welfare. Civil commitment statutes, which are enacted to protect societal interests rather than individual interests of the mentally ill, have their basis in the police power.

The privilege of the writ of habeas corpus and the least restrictive alternative doctrine are two other important concepts applicable to civil commitment cases. A writ of habeas corpus is the procedural mechanism, guaranteed by Article I, Section 9, of the United States Constitution, used to challenge an unlawful detention by the government. The **least restrictive alternative**

doctrine requires a less drastic means for achieving the same purpose.

RIGHT TO TREATMENT

With the enactment of the Hospitalization of Mentally Ill Act in 1964, the federal statutory **right to psychiatric treatment** in public hospitals was created. The statute requires that "a person hospitalized in a public hospital for a mental illness shall, during his hospitalization, be entitled to medical and psychiatric care and treatment."

While state courts and lower federal courts have opined that there may be a federal constitutional right to treatment, the United States Supreme Court has never firmly grounded the right to treatment in a constitutional principle. The evolution of these cases in the courts provides an interesting history of the development and shortcomings of our mental health delivery system.

The initial cases presenting the psychiatric patient's right to treatment arose in the criminal justice system. In *Rouse v. Cameron* (1966), the petitioner filed a writ of habeas corpus alleging that he was unlawfully detained and without psychiatric treatment after four years in a maximum security pavilion of St. Elizabeth Hospital. Mr. Rouse had pleaded not guilty by reason of insanity to a misdemeanor charge of having a dangerous weapon in his possession, which carried a one-year maximum sentence.

Pursuant to the District of Columbia's law, such a plea attached no criminal responsibility to the act but rather subjected the defendant to involuntary commitment in a psychiatric institution. The court ruled that without treatment the petitioner would be deprived of liberty in violation of the District of Columbia law and remanded the case to a lower court to determine whether the petitioner had received adequate treatment. The court, though reaching its conclusion based on state law and citing a federal statutory right, indicated that there might also be a constitutional basis for a right to treatment.

The next significant right to treatment case served as a sorry indictment of mental health state hospitals in Alabama. A class action suit was initiated by guardians of patients institutionalized in Alabama state hospitals, who sought an injunction against the institutions following the layoff of 99 employees. The central issue in *Wyatt v. Stickney* (1971) was the absence of adequate treatment for involuntarily committed patients. Five thousand patients were cared for by a professional staff of 17 M.D.'s, 21 registered nurses, 12 psychologists, 13 social workers, and a nonprofessional staff of 12 activity workers and 850 psychiatric aides.

The court found that the state hospitals lacked individualized patient treatment plans, adequate qualified professional staff to administer treatment, and a humane physical and psychological environment. In fashioning a remedy, the court issued several standards, including minimum staffing requirements, treatment in the least restrictive setting required by the individual, and development of a human rights committee in each institution. The court stated "when patients are so committed for treatment purposes, they unquestionably have a right to receive such individualized treatment as will give each of them a realistic opportunity to be cured or improve his or her mental condition" (*Wyatt v. Stickney* 1971, p. 784).

The court ruled that the state's failure to meet the standard set forth would deny the patients adequate treatment and necessitate their release. The court summarized by stating " . . . to deprive any citizen of his or her liberty upon the altruistic theory that confinement is for humane, therapeutic reasons and then fail to provide adequate treatment, violates the very fundamentals of due process" (*Wyatt v. Stickney* 1971, p. 785).

The Alabama governor and the mental health board appealed the lower court's order to implement standards, but the Federal Circuit Court affirmed the lower court's ruling on the standards issue (*Wyatt v. Aderholt* 1974).

The United States Supreme Court first considered the right to treatment issue in *O'Connor v. Donaldson* (1975).

In 1957, Mr. Donaldson was involuntarily committed to a Florida state hospital for care, treatment, and maintenance on his father's initiation. For 14 years prior to his commitment, he was gainfully employed. Despite posing no danger to himself or others, Mr. Donaldson's requests for ground privileges, occupational training, and an opportunity to discuss his case with the superintendent, Dr. O'Connor, or others were denied. During his 15 years of confinement he was not provided with any treatment.

Mr. Donaldson frequently requested his release, which the superintendent was authorized to grant even though Mr. Donaldson was lawfully confined, since even if he continued to be mentally ill, he posed no danger to himself or others. Between 1964 and 1968, Mr. Donaldson's friend requested on four separate occasions that he be released into his custody. These requests, and requests by a halfway house on Mr. Donaldson's behalf, were all denied by Dr. O'Connor, who believed that Mr. Donaldson should be released into his parents' custody. Dr. O'Connor further believed that

Mr. Donaldson's parents were too old and infirm to care for him adequately.

The lower court found Mr. Donaldson's care was merely custodial, since he received no treatment. He was not dangerous, community alternatives were available for him, and the doctor's refusal to release him was "malicious." On appeal, the Federal Court of Appeals ruled that there was a constitutional right to treatment and awarded Mr. Donaldson $38,000 in damages.

The United States Supreme Court, in declining to affirm the lower court's finding of damages and a broad constitutional right to treatment, narrowly defined the issue for consideration: whether a finding of mental illness alone can justify the state's indefinite custodial confinement of a mentally ill person against his will. The United States Supreme Court held " . . . [a] state cannot constitutionally confine a nondangerous individual who is capable of surviving safely in freedom by himself or with the help of willing and responsible family members or friends" (*O'Connor v. Donaldson* 1975, p. 576).

In 1982, the United States Supreme Court again considered an aspect of the right to treatment issue in *Youngberg v. Romeo*. The plaintiff, Romeo, a profoundly retarded 33-year-old with the development of an 18-month-old, was involuntarily committed to Pennhurst State Hospital. He alleged that he suffered physical harm perpetrated by himself and others and that he was unduly restrained while institutionalized.

The issue before the Supreme Court was whether involuntarily committed mentally retarded patients have a constitutionally protected interest in safety, freedom from undue restraint, and minimally adequate training. The court decided that the state has an obligation to provide safe conditions and reasonable amounts of physical freedom and minimally adequate or reasonable training. However, the court further noted that the substantive liberty interests established in the case were not absolute, and the patient's interest in liberty must be balanced against the state's reasons for restraint.

Though not specifically dealing with the rights of psychiatric patients, *Youngberg v. Romeo* has had an impact on cases regarding the psychiatric patient's right to refuse treatment.

INFORMED CONSENT

The principle of **informed consent** is based on a person's right to self-determination as enunciated in the landmark case *Canterbury v. Spence* (1972, p. 780):

> The root premise is the concept, fundamental in American jurisprudence, that every human being of adult years and sound mind has a right to determine what shall be done with his own body . . . true consent to what happens to one's self is the informed exercise of a choice, and that entails an opportunity to evaluate knowledgeably the options available and the risks attendant on each.

For consent to be effective legally, it must be informed. Generally, the informed consent of the patient or client must be obtained by the physician or other health professional to perform the treatment or procedure, and must include the nature of the patient's problem or condition, the nature and purpose of a proposed treatment, the risks and benefits of that treatment, alternative treatment options, probability that the proposed treatment will be successful, and risks of not consenting to the treatment.

New York is among those states that have enacted statutes delineating the requirements for informed consent. California, on the other hand, is among those states in which the courts have enunciated the parameters of informed consent. Both California and New York, as previously noted, have special statutory requirements for informed consent for institutionalized psychiatric patients.

The nurse has no legal duty to provide a patient with disclosure consistent with the legal requirements for informed consent, since nursing procedures generally are noninvasive and are commonly understood. The fact that the nurse does not have the legal duty to inform the patient of the risks associated with a particular procedure does not excuse the nurse from explaining the procedure to the patient and obtaining the patient's expressed consent.

THE RIGHT TO REFUSE TREATMENT

A corollary to the right to consent to treatment is the right to withhold consent. Retraction of consent previously given must be honored whether it is a verbal or written retraction. However, the mental patient's **right to refuse treatment** with psychotropic drugs has been debated in the courts, turning in part on the issue of mental patients' competency to give consent or withhold consent to treatment and their status under the civil commitment statutes. These cases, initiated by state hospital patients, consider principles of constitutional law, balancing competing state interests and societal interests against the patient's interest in autonomy and self-determination in the face of the often permanent and disfiguring side effects of psychotropic drugs. The analyses in these cases included medical, legal, and ethical considerations, such as pragmatic treatment problems, the doctrine of informed consent, and the bioethical principle of autonomy.

The United States Supreme Court, in two separate cases, *Mills v. Rogers* (1982) and *Rennie v. Klein* (1982), declined to rule on the issue of the involuntarily committed mental patient's right to refuse treatment with antipsychotic drugs. Even without the enunciations of a federal constitutional right by the United States Supreme Court, these cases have had a significant, if not uniform, impact on the evolution of mental patients' rights.

In *Rogers v. Okin* (1979), Rubie Rogers and six other mental patients involuntarily hospitalized at the Massachusetts State Hospital brought a class action suit in the Federal District Court of the District of Massachusetts against various officials and staff, alleging that their constitutional rights were violated by forcible medication with antipsychotic drugs. The district court ruled that patients involuntarily committed are not incompetent and have constitutionally protected liberty and privacy interests in making treatment decisions for themselves. Without consent by the patient or the patient's guardian, this right could not be overridden except in an emergency. Forcible administration of medication is justified when the "need to prevent violence outweighs the possibility of harm to the medicated individual" and reasonable alternatives to medication have been ruled out (*Rogers v. Okin* 1979, p. 1365).

The court of appeals (*Rogers v. Okin* 1980) affirmed the lower court's ruling that mental patients have the constitutionally protected right to make treatment decisions and refuse treatment. However, they differed with respect to the circumstances under which the state's police power interests in preventing violence and maintaining order in the institution and *parens patriae* interest in alleviating the suffering of the mentally ill and providing effective treatment override the patient's liberty interests.

The court of appeals ruled that the police power provides the hospital staff with substantial discretion in an emergency and the *parens patriae* doctrine justifies forcible administration of psychotropic medication to competent patients only when necessary to prevent further deterioration of a patient's mental health. The court of appeals reversed the lower court's conclusion that a guardian may make psychotropic drug treatment decisions for incompetent patients in nonemergency situations and instead decided that the patient's rights must be protected by a judicial determination of incompetency and application of the "substituted judgment rule," which would justify treatment with antipsychotic medication only if the patient, if competent, would have voluntarily accepted treatment.

Shortly after the United States Supreme Court accepted the case of *Mills v. Rogers* to determine whether involuntarily committed mental patients have a constitutionally protected liberty interest in refusing forcible medication, the Supreme Judicial Court of Massachusetts decided, based on state law, that noninstitutionalized mentally ill patients have the right to refuse antipsychotic drugs. After noting that procedural and substantive issues were entwined with issues of state law, and consistent with the policy to avoid unnecessary decisions of constitutional law, the United States Supreme Court sent the case back to the court of appeals to determine the effect of the Massachusetts case on its previous decision. The court of appeals then certified nine questions to the Massachusetts Supreme Judicial Court, focusing on the right of the involuntarily committed patient to refuse treatment and on standards and procedures that must be followed by institutions treating those patients.

Currently, Massachusetts prohibits nonconsensual, nonemergency forcible psychotropic drug treatment of involuntarily committed mental patients. The Supreme Judicial Court in *Rogers v. Commissioner of the Department of Mental Health* (1983) ruled the following:

1. Involuntarily committed mental patients are competent and have the right to make treatment decisions until adjudicated incompetent by a judge.
2. If such patients are adjudicated incompetent, a judge using the "substituted judgment" standard shall decide whether the patient would have consented to the administration of antipsychotic drugs.
3. Forcible administration of psychotropic drugs is only justified without patient consent or court approval when necessary to prevent "immediate, substantial and irreversible deterioration of a serious mental illness."

In upholding the institutionalized mental patient's right to bodily integrity, the Massachusetts court rejected physicians' assertions that they should have unqualified discretion in making treatment decisions. It further noted that informed consent and the right to privacy, which are the basis of the substituted judgment rule, outweigh institutional interests in forcible medication of patients to facilitate hospital administration, to reduce staff turnover, or to increase the number of patients treated and decrease the patient length of stay. Additionally, the court rejected the argument that physicians are the appropriate party to make substituted judgment because the court deemed forcible administration of antipsychotic drugs to be an extraordinary treatment.

The precedent for the *Rogers* decision was set in the case *In the Matter of the Guardianship of Richard Roe*, III (1981), which held that noninstitutionalized mental patients who are adjudicated incompetent have a right to refuse treatment with antipsychotic drugs by use of a substituted judgment rule. In this case, Richard Roe, a 21-year-old with a history of chronic schizophrenia since adolescence, had been hospitalized for observation. During that time the court appointed his father temporary guardian and decided, relying on the United States District Court's 1979 opinion in *Rogers v. Okin*, that as guardian, his father had the right to consent to the forcible administration of drugs. However, this authorization would not be effective until a permanent guardianship hearing was held. In the interim, Richard Roe was discharged to his family.

At the permanent guardianship hearing, the judge upheld his previous ruling, and the decision was appealed by the party responsible for representing Richard's interests in the matter. The Supreme Judicial Court of Massachusetts allowed the plaintiffs in *Rogers v. Okin* (1979) to become parties in the case because of the potential impact its decision might have on the outcome of their federal case. All parties agreed that any decision to forcibly medicate should be based on a substituted judgment rule. The court then ruled that the case was premature, since Richard's father sought continuing authority to medicate and was not planning to authorize immediate administration and substituted judgment can be made accurately only when an immediate proposed treatment is sought. Even though this decision was enough to dispose of the case, the court enunciated general standards for courts to use in applying substituted judgment.

The factors underlying the court's decision that guardians do not have inherent authority to consent to antipsychotic drug treatment for their wards are

- intrusiveness of the treatment,
- potential for side effects,
- absence of an emergency,
- nature and extent of prior judicial involvement,
- likelihood of conflicting interests.

In discussing intrusiveness of the treatment and the possibility of adverse side effects, the court stated that there are "few . . . medical procedures which are more intrusive than forcible injection of antipsychotic medication" since it affects the patient's thought processes and personality. It further noted that the very significant side effects "are frequently devastating and often irreversible" (*In Guardianship of Roe* 1981, p. 52).

After concluding that prior court approval was necessary in a substituted judgment, the court identified six relevant factors in applying this standard:

1. The person's expressed preferences regarding treatment when competent.
2. The person's religious belief.
3. The effect of treatment, or lack of it, on the person's family.
4. The probability of an adverse side effect.
5. The risks involved in the refusal of the treatment.
6. The prognosis with treatment.

In those instances in which forcible medication is sought to prevent violence to third persons, prevent suicide, or preserve security, the court noted that the medication is being used as a "chemical restraint" and justification for medication changes to public protection rather than individual treatment. Accordingly, the infringement on a person's liberty is at least equal to involuntary commitment. In this circumstance, the noninstitutionalized incompetent mental patient has the right, through substituted judgment, to determine whether to be involuntarily committed or to be medicated.

In New Jersey, involuntarily committed psychiatric patients also brought a suit in federal court alleging violation of their constitutional rights through forcible administration of antipsychotic drugs. The district court in *Rennie v. Klein* (1979) recognized a qualified constitutional right based on four factors: physical danger posed by a patient to other patients and staff; patient's mental capacity to decide a course of treatment; availability of a less restrictive treatment; and risk of permanent side effects.

Additionally, the court extended the right to refuse medication to voluntarily committed patients. On appeal, the right was reaffirmed but limited by the state's ability to forcibly medicate when the patient is a danger to himself or others, with the caveat that in nonemergency situations the patient must first be provided with procedural due process (*Rennie v. Klein* 1981). The United States Supreme Court declined again to decide whether mental patients have a right to refuse treatment with psychotropic drugs, but this time it set aside the judgment of the Third Circuit Court of Appeals with instructions to reconsider the case in light of the United States Supreme Court ruling in *Youngberg v. Romeo* (*Rennie v. Klein* 1982).

In applying the "accepted professional judgment standard" of the *Youngberg* ruling, the Third Circuit Court of Appeals narrowed its previous ruling. The court ruled that involuntarily committed patients have the right to refuse administration of antipsychotic drugs, and the decision to administer such drugs against the patient's will must be based on an accepted professional judgment and consistent with procedures delineated in the New Jersey regulations which satisfy due process requirements (*Rennie v. Klein*, 1983).

In the court's analysis, the patient's right to refuse medications is weighed against whether the patient presents a danger to himself or others. This evaluation is a product of a medical professional judgment. The decision of the medical staff would be presumed valid unless shown to be a "substantial departure from accepted practice." The factor to be considered is whether, and to what extent, the patient will suffer harmful side effects.

The contrast between the First and Third Circuit Court of Appeals' analyses is substantial. Whereas the court in *Rogers* recognizes the individual's autonomy and right to self-determination, even giving great weight to the incompetent patient's previously expressed preference through substituted judgment, the *Rennie* court substitutes the physician's professional judgment for that of the patient's expressed preference. Tables 3–4 and 3–5 summarize the Massachusetts and New Jersey right to refuse treatment cases.

Cases involving the right to refuse psychotropic drug treatment are still evolving. The California Supreme Court recently accepted a case concerning the right of involuntarily committed mental patients to refuse psychotropic drugs in a nonemergency situation.

Without clear direction from the United States Supreme Court, there will be different case outcomes in different jurisdictions. However, at this writing, the United States Supreme Court has accepted a Washington state case concerning a prisoner's right to refuse treatment with psychotropic drugs (*Harper v. State of Washington* 1988). The United States Supreme Court decision in this upcoming case may have far-reaching implications on state and federal right to refuse treatment cases.

The relationship between the right to refuse psychotropic drug treatment cases and the right to terminate life support/right to die cases presents compelling ethical, legal, and philosophical questions. The Massachusetts courts, using a substituted judgment rule, and the New York courts, based on common-law grounds, have honored incompetent medical patients' previously expressed desires to terminate life support made while they were competent. Other states, such as California, have enacted statutes that permit a person to designate a health care representative to consent to treatment should he or she become incompetent, with instructions delineating the patient's health care treatment desires.

These court cases and statutes are based on the individual's right to self-determination. The fundamental issue is whether there is a difference between medical and mental illness that justifies a distinction between the rights afforded to persons in making treatment decisions. The right to refuse medication cases have

Table 3–4 • RIGHT TO REFUSE TREATMENT: EVOLUTION OF MASSACHUSETTS CASE LAW TO PRESENT LAW

CASE	COURT	DECISION
Rogers v. Okin, 478 F. Supp. 1342 (D. Mass. 1979)	Federal District Court	Involuntary mental patients are competent and have the right to make treatment decisions Forcible medication administration is justified in an emergency if needed to prevent violence and if other alternatives have been ruled out Guardian may make treatment decisions for an incompetent patient
Rogers v. Okin, 634 F. 2d 650 (1st Cir. 1980)	Federal Court of Appeals	Affirmed involuntary mental patients are competent and have the right to make treatment decisions Staff has substantial discretion in an emergency Forcible medication also justified to prevent patient's deterioration Patient rights must be protected by judicial determination of incompetency
Mills v. Rogers, 457 U.S. 291 (1982)	United States Supreme Court	Set aside judgment of court of appeals with instructions to consider the effect of an intervening state court case
Rogers v. Commissioner of the Department of Mental Health, 458 N.E. 2d 308 (1983)	Massachusetts Supreme Judicial Court answering questions certified by the Federal Court of Appeals	Involuntary patients are competent and have the right to make treatment decisions unless judicially determined incompetent

Table 3–5 • RIGHT TO REFUSE TREATMENT: EVOLUTION OF NEW JERSEY CASE LAW TO PRESENT LAW

CASE	COURT	DECISION
Rennie v. Klein, 476 F. Supp. 1294 (D.N.J. 1979)	Federal District Court	Involuntary mental patients have a qualified constitutional right to refuse treatment with antipsychotic drugs Voluntary patients have an absolute right to refuse treatment with antipsychotic drugs under New Jersey law
Rennie v. Klein, 653 F. 2d 836 (3rd Cir. 1981)	Federal Court of Appeals	Involuntary mental patients have a constitutional right to refuse antipsychotic drug treatment The state may override a patient's right when the patient poses a danger to self or others Due process protections required prior to forcible medication of patients in nonemergency situations
Rennie v. Klein, 454 U.S. 1078 (1982)	United States Supreme Court	Set aside judgment of court of appeals with instructions to consider the case in light of the U.S.S.C. decision in *Youngberg v. Romeo*
Rennie v. Klein, 720 F. 2d 266 (3rd Cir. 1983)	Federal Court of Appeals	Involuntary mental patients have the right to refuse treatment with antipsychotic medication Decisions to forcibly medicate must be based on "accepted professional judgment" and must comply with due process requirements of the New Jersey regulations

pointed out the complex and difficult tasks of translating social policy concerns into a clearly articulated legal standard.

Summary

The states' power to enact laws for public health and safety and for the care of those unable to care for themselves often pits the rights of society against the rights of the individual. The complexities of these relationships can manifest as legal and ethical dilemmas in the psychiatric setting. More frequently, the nurse will encounter problems requiring ethical choices. The nurse's privilege to practice nursing carries with it the responsibility to practice safely, competently, and consistently with state laws. Knowledge of the law, the ANA Code for Nurses, and the Standards for Psychiatric Nursing Practice will enhance the nurse's ability to provide safe, effective psychiatric nursing care and will serve as a framework for decision making when the nurse is presented with complex problems involving competing interests.

References

American Nurses' Association. Standards of Psychiatric and Mental Health Nursing Practice. Kansas City, MO, 1982.

American Nurses' Association. Code for Nurses. Kansas City, MO, 1985.

Bellah v. Greenson, 81 C.A. 3d 614 (1978).

Brennan J, Ethics and Morals. New York: Harper and Row, 1973.

Canterbury v. Spence, 464 F. 2d 722 (D.C. Cir. 1972), quoting Schloendorf v. Society of N.Y. Hosp., 211 N.Y. 125 105 N.E. 2d 92, 93 (1914).

Chalmers-Frances v. Nelson, 6 C 2d 402 (1936).

Darling v. Charleston Community Memorial Hospital, 211 N.E. 2d 253 (Ill. 1965).

Davis A, Aroskar M. Ethical Dilemmas and Nursing Practice. New York: Appleton-Century-Crofts, 1978.

Eccard W. A revolution in white: New approaches to treating nurses as professionals. Vanderbilt Law Review, 30:839, 1977.

Fenner KM. Ethics and Law in Nursing. New York: Van Nostrand Reinhold, 1980.

Haring B. Ethics of Manipulation. New York: The Seabury Press, 1975.

Hawaii v. Standard Oil Company, 405 U.S. 251 (1972), quoting 3 W. Blackstone, Commentaries #47.

Hedlum v. Superior Court of Orange County, 34 C. 3d. 695 (1983).

Helling v. Carey, 83 Wash. 2d 514 (1974).

Humphrey v. Cady, 405 U.S. 504 (1972).

In Guardianship of Roe, 421 N.E. 2d 40 (Mass. 1981).

In re Detention of Harris, 654 P. 2d 109 (Wash. 1982).

In re Oakes, 8 Law Rep. 122 (Mass. 1845).

Jablonski v. U.S., 712 F. 2d 391 (9th Cir. 1983).

Lake v. Cameron, 364 F. 2d 657 (D.C. Cir. 1966).

Mavroudis v. Superior Court of San Mateo, 102 C.A. 3d 594 (1980).

Mills v. Rogers, 457 U.S. 291 (1982).

O'Connor v. Donaldson, 422 U.S. 563 (1975).

Pisel v. Stamford Hospital, 430 A. 2d 1 (Conn. 1980).
Plumadore v. State of New York, 427 N.Y. S. 2d 90 (1980).
Project Release v. Prevost, 722 F. 2d 960 (2nd Cir. 1983).
Rennie v. Klein, 476 F. Supp. 1294 (D.N.J. 1979).
Rennie v. Klein, 653 F. 2d 836 (3rd Cir. 1981).
Rennie v. Klein, 454 U.S. 1078 (1982).
Rennie v. Klein, 720 F. 2d 266 (3rd Cir. 1983).
Rogers v. Commissioner of the Department of Mental Health, 458 N.E. 2d 308 (Mass. 1983).
Rogers v. Okin, 478 F. Supp. 1342 (D. Mass. 1979).
Rogers v. Okin, 634 F. 2d 650 (1st Cir. 1980).
Rouse v. Cameron, 373 F. 2d 451 (D.C. Cir. 1966).
Tarasoff v. Regents of University of California, 17 C. 3d 425 (1976).
Thomas v. County of Alameda, 27 C. 3d 741 (1980).
Vitek v. Jones, 445 U.S. 480 (1980).
Wyatt v. Aderholt, 503 F. 2d 1305 (5th Cir. 1974).
Wyatt v. Stickney, 325 F. Supp. 781 (M.D. Ala. 1971).
Youngberg v. Romeo, 457 U.S. 307 (1982).

Bibliography

California Department of Mental Health. Patients' Rights Advocacy Manual. 1985.
Cole R. Patients' rights to refuse antipsychotic drugs. Law, Medicine & Health Care, 9(4):19, 1981.
Davis A. Ethical issues in nursing practice. Western Journal of Nursing Research, p. 135q, July 1980.
Davis A. Ethical issues in nursing research. Western Journal of Nursing Research, p. 760, Fall 1980.
Davis A. Ethical issues in nursing research. Western Journal of Nursing Research, p. 97, Winter 1983.
Development in the law: Civil commitment of the mentally ill. Harvard Law Review, 87:1193, 1974.
Fama AJ. Reporting incompetent physicians: A comparison of requirements in three states. Law, Medicine & Health Care, 11:111, 1983.
Furrow BR. Will psychotherapy be transformed in the 1980's? Law, Medicine & Health Care, 11:96, 1983.
Furrow BR. Public psychiatry and the right to refuse treatment: Toward an effective damage remedy. Harvard Civil Rights Civil Liberties Law Review, 19(1):20, 1984.
Gottlieb NR. Vitek v. Jones: Transfer of prisoners to mental institutions. American Journal of Law and Medicine, 8:175, 1982.
Greenlaw J. Documentation of patient care: An often underestimated responsibility. Law, Medicine & Health Care, 10:172, 1982.
Health Law Center. Nursing and the Law, 2nd ed. Rockville, MD: Aspen Publication, 1975.
Keeton WP, Dobbs DB, Keeton RE, Owen DG. Prosser and Keeton on Torts, 5th ed. St. Paul, MN: West Publishing Company, 1984.
Kjervik DK. The psychiatric nurse's duty to warn potential victims of homicidal psychotherapy outpatients. Law, Medicine & Health Care, 9(6):11, 1981.
Kravitz M. Informed consent: Must ethical responsibility conflict with professional conduct? Nursing Management, Nov. 1985.
Litman J. Note, a common law remedy for forcible medication for the institutionalized mentally ill. Columbia Law Review, 82:1720, 1982.
Monius E. Introduction to bioethics. Center Nurse, The Washington Hospital Center, 2(1):4, 1986.
Naisbitt J. Megatrends. New York: Warner Books Edition, 1982.
Rockford SH. More on the right to refuse treatment: Brother Fox and the mentally ill in New York. Law, Medicine & Health Care, 11(1):19, 1983.
Rosoff AJ. Informed Consent, A Guide for Health Care Providers. Rockville, MD: Aspen Publication, 1981.
Roth MD, Levin LJ. Dilemma of Tarasoff: Must physicians protect the public or their patients? Law, Medicine & Health Care, 11:104, 1983.
Selected recent court decision, involuntary treatment with antipsychotic drugs—Mills v. Rogers. American Journal of Law & Medicine, 8:216, 1982.
Selected recent court decision, mental patients—involuntary treatment—Rogers v. Commissioner of Department of Mental Health. American Journal of Law & Medicine, 9:522, 1984.
Southwick AF. The Law of Hospital and Health Care Administration. Health Administration Press, 1978.
Taub J. Psychiatric malpractice in the 1980's: A look at some areas of concerns. Law, Medicine & Health Care, 11:97, 1983.
Winslade W. Choosing Life or Death, A Guide for Patients, Families and Professionals. New York: Macmillan Publishing Company, 1986.

Self-Study Exercises

Match the word with the correct definition.

1. ________ Civil wrongs for which money damages are collected by the injured party.
2. ________ Harmful or offensive touching of another's person.
3. ________ The act or an omission to act that breaches the duty of care and is the actual or proximate cause of a person's injuries.
4. ________ Based on the principle of a person's right to self-determination.
5. ________ Verbal or written retraction of consent previously given must be honored.

A. Negligence
B. Assault
C. Battery
D. Torts
E. Bioethics
F. Right to refuse treatment
G. Informed consent

True or False

6. _________ Voluntary patients have the right to demand and obtain release.
7. _________ In many states, common criteria for involuntary admission to mental health facilities include need for psychiatric treatment and danger to self or others.

For discussion

8. Discuss what is meant by *client's civil rights*, and give examples.
9. Discuss some of the legal responsibilities of the nurse in the care and discharge of a client in seclusion/restraints, as identified in this chapter.
10. Name at least four standards of care for psychiatric nursing practice.

CHAPTER 4

Mental Health Considerations Across Cultures

Juliet L. Tien-Hyatt

OUTLINE

CULTURAL EXPLANATIONS OF MENTAL ILLNESS

NURSES' ATTITUDES TOWARD THE CULTURALLY DIFFERENT

THEORETICAL FRAMEWORK

GUIDELINES FOR CULTURAL ASSESSMENT

MENTAL HEALTH PROBLEMS ACROSS CULTURES

Schizophrenia

Depression

Alcoholism

Domestic Violence

INTERVENTIONS FOR MULTICULTURAL POPULATIONS

SUMMARY

KEY TERMS AND CONCEPTS

The key terms and concepts listed here also appear in bold where they are defined or discussed in this chapter.

CULTURE

RACE

ETHNICITY

NATION

FOLK GROUP

FOLK MEDICINE

OBJECTIVES

After studying this chapter, the student will be able to:

1. Define the following terms: culture, race, ethnicity, nation, folk group, and folk medicine.
2. Discuss four common cultural explanations of mental illness.
3. Identify differences and similarities in concepts of mental health and mental illness across cultures.
4. Recognize the effects of nurses' attitudes toward the culturally different.
5. Summarize four guidelines in making a cultural assessment.
6. Identify major differences across cultures for each of the following:
   A. Schizophrenia
   B. Depression
   C. Alcoholism
   D. Domestic violence
7. Compare and contrast at least six holistic approaches effective with multicultural clients.

With the increasing diversity of racial and ethnic groups in the United States, mental health professionals are facing great complexity in diagnosis and treatment of culturally different clients.

To achieve therapeutic effects, mental health professionals need to be cognizant of the fact that the cultural experience of the client does not remain static; in fact, it changes constantly and often imperceptibly. The race/ethnicity, nationality, socioeconomic status, religion, and cultural experiences of the client and therapist also interplay in a very complex manner in the course of mental health treatment.

A behavior that is socially acceptable in one culture may be perceived as dysfunctional in another. Mental health professionals need to be familiar with the distinct nature of mental health practices in the cultural groups with whom they are dealing. Acceptance of, and respect for, the differences in cultural beliefs and mental health practices are key factors contributing to a successful therapeutic outcome. While counseling the culturally different client, we should be aware of our own cultural beliefs, attitudes, and professional competence, as they are also important factors influencing the therapeutic outcome (Tien and Johnson, 1985). As the culture changes, life also changes; the intent of this chapter, therefore, is to induce critical thinking and further exploration, rather than to impart definitive information.

Some working definitions of the key concepts of this chapter may be helpful to mental health professionals who work closely with a culturally diverse population.

Culture, as defined by Kluckhohn (1968), is the total life way of a people, the social legacy the individual acquires from his or her group, or the environment that is the creation of humankind. Linton (1945) suggests that cultures change and grow, discarding certain elements and acquiring new ones in the course of their histories. In other words, *culture is a phenomenon through which norms and values are socially transmitted from generation to generation.* In the process of this transmission, changes occur constantly and often imperceptibly.

According to the *Webster's New Collegiate Dictionary* (1976, 950), **race** is a kind of people unified by community of interests, habits, or characteristics; or a division of humankind possessing traits that are transmissible by descent and sufficient to characterize the division as a distinct human type.

Typically, skin color, such as black, yellow, white, or red, is used as a major indicator of race.

Ethnicity is defined as affiliation due to a shared linguistic, racial, or cultural background (Werner 1979). Apparently there are overlaps between the definitions of race and ethnicity. The existing literature suggests that a race may encompass several ethnic groups. For example, Chinese and Japanese Americans are considered as a yellow race; Afro-Americans and some South Americans are classified as a black race; Irish and Italian Americans are regarded as a white race; and Native Americans are viewed as a red race.

A **nation** is a community of people composed of one or more ethnic groups and possessing a more or less defined territory and government (Webster 1976, 765). One ethnic group can spread out in several nations (e.g., mainland China and Taiwan, and East and West Germany), and one nation can be composed of several ethnic groups, (e.g., the United States and the United Kingdom).

Folk group is defined as the great proportion of the

members of a people that determines the group character and tends to preserve its characteristic form of civilization and its customs, arts and crafts, legends, traditions, and beliefs from generation to generation (Webster 1970, 446). A folk group does not necessarily have a common nationality, race, or ethnicity, but its members do share common beliefs. For instance, Chinese, Japanese, and Korean people can be regarded as a folk group because they share common Asian cultural beliefs; or Americans from the South can be seen as a folk group that represents a unique cultural orientation.

Folk medicine refers to syndromes from which members of a particular group claim to suffer and for which their culture provides the etiology, diagnosis, preventive measures, and regimens of healing (Rubel 1978). Folk medicine is usually passed from generation to generation, is not necessarily based on scientific medicine, and is not usually recognized by the American Medical Association.

These working definitions of the key concepts will provide a foundation for a better understanding of the discussion that follows.

Cultural Explanations of Mental Illness

Culture influences behavior. Each of us lives within an invisible sheath called culture. This sheath has many layers that have been formed by various factors, including race, ethnicity, national origin, geography, climate, neighborhood, and religion. These layers make imprints on each of us, sometimes lightly, often indelibly (Tseng and McDermott 1981).

Happy and mentally healthy individuals usually add new layers of culture. They do not totally discard previous values and behaviors. If old ways are discarded, it is because they are no longer useful or appropriate. Today we live in a world of travel, migration, and increasing interracial marriage. The individual's culture is constantly affected by other cultural groups. Therefore, the merging, conflicts, and acceptance or rejection of cultural values may increasingly influence the stresses in individual experiences and the way stress is handled (Tseng and McDermott 1981).

In counseling, although the ultimate focus is usually on the individual client and his or her family, it is also pertinent to consider culture in general. If we studied only one cultural group, we would have little idea whether a behavior was culturally shaped. The differences and similarities stand out more clearly when we compare and contrast behaviors across cultures.

What a culture perceives as the cause of mental illness dictates how healing is sought. The following explanations reflect some general concepts of mental illness (Tseng and McDermott 1981).

SOCIOPSYCHOLOGICAL EXPLANATIONS. Mental disorder may be perceived as a psychological reaction to the stress of the internal or external environment. For example, divorced women may attribute their "nervous condition" to single parenthood, inadequate income, and the struggle for career success. Many Americans believe that bottling up frustration and unexpressed emotions contributes to psychological tension.

PHYSICAL-MEDICAL EXPLANATIONS. Other reasons for mental illness are considered physical or physiological. For instance, many contemporary health professionals believe that senile plaques in the brain cause Alzheimer's disease, or senile dementia (Busse and Pfeiffer 1973), that excessive alcohol intake results in delirium tremens, and that chemical imbalance may cause depression or manic-depressive reactions (Solomon and Patch 1971).

SUPERNATURAL EXPLANATIONS. Many ethnic/racial groups believe that mental disorders are caused by supernatural powers. Mental illnesses can occur as the result of spirit intrusion or possession, soul loss, divine wrath, black magic, or violations of taboos (Tseng and McDermott 1981).

The spirits are said to be intelligent beings who reach perfection through many reincarnations. These spirits can be good or evil and can be in human or animal form (Ralph 1977). In the case of soul loss, the soul may wander or be stolen by spirits during sleep, fright, or injury. Divine wrath is the punishment by gods and is due to moral transgression. Black magic, or voodoo, is usually done by a sorcerer or witch who is hired by the enemy of the client. Violation of taboo is the breaking of a taboo or cultural rule such as incest, stealing, or eating forbidden foods. The punishment for this violation can cause illness (Tseng and McDermott 1981).

NATURAL EXPLANATIONS. These beliefs are concerned with natural phenomena and cosmic forces. Many cultures believe that human beings should maintain harmony with both the internal and the external environment. Within the human body, there are hot and cold or yin and yang elements. Imbalance of these elements may cause both physical and mental disorders (Currier 1978; Tien-Hyatt 1987). The improper location or construction of a dwelling or a graveyard of the ancestors is thought to be the cause of physical or mental illness, unhappiness, and misfortune. Many Chinese consult with *fung-shui* specialists (geomancers) to ensure that there is a smooth flow of wind and water in their dwellings (Potter 1970).

CAUSAL EXPLANATIONS. Many Asians believe in

causal relationship and reincarnation. Good deeds bring about positive results, whereas misdeeds lead to ill effects. This causal relationship can continue from generation to generation and from one life to another. This causal relationship is also called karma. Health or illness, fortune or misfortune is the result of karma. Karma can perpetuate unless the individual makes efforts to change the life course (Tien-Hyatt 1987).

The concepts of mental illness previously described are not mutually exclusive. They may overlap or coexist. These beliefs are also shared by all ethnic/racial groups to a greater or lesser degree.

Nurses' Attitudes Toward the Culturally Different

In dealing with culturally diverse people, nurses need to recognize the attitudes and the psychodynamics of prejudice. Prejudice is derived from the Latin *praejudicium*, which means prejudgment or a premature judgment. Thus, the term prejudice implies an attitude based on insufficient knowledge. According to Marmor (1977), prejudice can be acquired by passive adoption of environmental attitudes, usually from the parents or in-group. This is fundamentally part of the acculturation process of a child growing up in a prejudiced setting. Certain personality patterns are "prejudice-prone." Such personality patterns are particularly apt to develop within the context of families in which parents have been rigid, dominating, and authoritarian and have related to their children on the basis of power and fear rather than trust and love. Children growing up in such families tend to experience some of their impulses, particularly sexual, aggressive, or rebellious ones, as dangerous and therefore tend to repress a great deal of hostility and guilt with regard to these impulses. When given an appropriate scapegoat, individuals with such repressed emotions tend to project them onto the scapegoat. This leaves the prejudiced individual feeling "cleaner," "better," and "purer" than the scapegoat. Prejudiced individuals suffer from deep feelings of inadequacy, which are usually compensated for by false feelings of superiority and by virtue of their scapegoating of other groups.

The effects of prejudice are destructive both to the prejudiced person and to the victim of prejudice. In the prejudiced person prejudice causes false feelings of superiority, which often interfere with genuine accomplishment and self-fulfillment. The effects on the victim of prejudice are more obvious: impaired self-image, exhibition of the defensive attitudes of denial, withdrawal, passivity, self-deprecation, dissimulation, and identification with the aggressor (Marmor 1977).

I have observed that many nursing colleagues, including faculty, students, and therapists, exhibit prejudice against the culturally different (Tien 1982; Abdu-Saad et al. 1982). Although all people possess certain degrees of prejudice, we nurses need to critically examine our own attitudes toward the culturally different. If our attitudes tend to be negative, we need to recognize this and avoid prejudice in the counseling process. If we have difficulty remaining objective, we should cease engaging in cross-cultural counseling, and we ourselves should perhaps seek counseling or supervision. Only when we can show respect for all who deserve respect, regardless of ethnicity or race, can we achieve maximum therapeutic effects.

Theoretical Framework

The use of a theoretical framework is based largely on the nurse's philosophical beliefs, academic training, and professional experience. Whether the theories are labeled as nursing theories or not, the fact is that a large part of the body of theory used by nurses is borrowed from theories developed by other disciplines. Therefore, it is important to understand fully the origins of the theories or concepts to be used for nursing assessment, intervention, or research (Tien-Hyatt 1986).

All theories derived from other disciplines, especially psychology, anthropology, and sociology, ought to be applicable to a greater or lesser degree to nursing assessment, intervention, or research involving culturally different clients. However, in cross-cultural counseling, application of certain theories is essential to achieve better therapeutic effects. For instance, Husserl's (1962, 1970) phenomenology and Glasser and Strauss's (1967) grounded theory have been increasingly used to gather data based on the respondent's subjective experience and the impact of this experience on health care practices (Lynch-Sauer 1985; Stern 1985; Stern & Pyles 1985; Tien-Hyatt 1986). Myths or stereotypes can be clarified by using a consumer-centered approach based on these theories.

For instance, Acosta (1980) found that some Mexican and Black American clients terminated therapy prematurely because their symptoms were relieved and their life situations were improved. To the clients, the therapy was a success, and they simply did not see the need to continue it; to the therapists, the therapy was a failure because the client attended therapy for less than four sessions. Ironically, many studies and publications perpetuate the myth that minority clients tend to terminate therapy prematurely owing to, the researchers assume, negative reasons. Some studies are seriously misconceived because of the researcher's questionable definition of premature termination of the therapy.

It is not uncommon for culturally different clients, regardless of ethnicity and socioeconomic status, to come for two to three sessions of holistic therapy for the improvement of their life situation. When old problems recur or a new stressor occurs, they then come back for a few "booster" sessions. They perceive short-term therapy as very helpful and as what they need.

In nursing intervention, Carl Rogers's client-centered approach is quite helpful. The basic theory of client-centered therapy can be stated simply in the form of an "if-then" hypothesis. If certain conditions are present in the attitudes of the person designated "therapist" in a relationship, namely congruence, positive regard, and empathic understanding, then growthful change will take place in the person designated "client" (Meador and Rogers 1979). Client-centered therapy calls upon the whole range of the ongoing inner dynamics of the therapist and the client. The interaction of two persons arising out of an awareness of their individual inner responses provides the dynamics of the therapeutic relationship. Many concepts have been identified in this approach.

Client-centered theory stresses how the qualities of the therapist, namely, *empathy*, *positive regard*, and *genuineness*, can affect the client's self-actualization and growing process. Clients will develop awareness of their life situation and generate positive change if they are allowed to define their own goals. This is especially important when the therapist and client come from different sociocultural backgrounds.

Guidelines for Cultural Assessment

According to Leininger (1978), cultural assessment in nursing refers to a systematic appraisal or examination of individuals, groups, and communities as to their cultural beliefs, values, and practices to determine explicit needs and nursing interventions within the cultural context of the people being evaluated.

Several nursing assessment guides are available for a systematic cultural assessment. Davies and Yoshida (1981), Orque (1983), Bloch (1983), and Tripp-Reimer and her associates (1984) basically agree that in the process of cultural assessment, nurses should collect data in the following areas: cultural, sociological, psychological, and biological/physiological. A cultural assessment does not require information on every element of the culture. Nurses need to identify the major values, beliefs, and behaviors that influence and relate to a particular clinical setting or health problem.

In the case of mental health nursing assessment, nurses need to direct their special attention to the areas of ethnicity/race, folk beliefs, acculturation, and motivation.

ETHNICITY/RACE. Ethnic origin, or racial background, seems to have great influence on how a client views the mental health or mental illness process. Many ethnic/racial minorities who appear at community mental health centers or the offices of private practitioners tend to seek symptom relief. It is common that they terminate therapy after two or three sessions, thinking that they can function on their own. They may return to therapy when a new, difficult life situation occurs. They are simply not accustomed to a prolonged period of psychotherapy to work on personality change.

FOLK BELIEFS. This seems to be one of the most influential elements affecting the results of assessment and intervention. The client's deep-rooted beliefs in the etiology and prognosis of a mental illness cannot be changed by contemporary mental health theorists. Interestingly, the overwhelming majority of clients seen in my office hold beliefs in karma, reincarnation, or causal relationships to a greater or lesser degree, regardless of race or ethnicity, socioeconomic status, or religion. Some believe that their mental disturbance is the result of a curse, black magic, or bad deeds. The following questions may be helpful in assessing the client's folk beliefs:

1. What do you think is the cause of your problem?
2. What does your family think is the cause of your problem?
3. How severe does this problem seem to you?
4. What do you think will be most helpful in remedying your problem?
5. What do you expect to accomplish in the therapy sessions?

In many cases, the clients will not disclose their folk beliefs until they feel comfortable with the therapist. Therefore, the therapist may need to repeat the questions in several different situations in order to obtain sufficient information.

ACCULTURATION. Although research findings on the correlation between the acculturation level and the therapeutic outcome are not readily available, the acculturation level of the client seems to play an important role in the client's receptiveness to contemporary mental health practice. The 20-item *Tien-Hyatt Acculturation Scale* (Fig. 4–1) (Tien-Hyatt 1985) may be helpful in assessing the client's acculturation level and its correlation with the diagnosis, etiology, and prognosis of mental illness. As can be seen in Figure 4–1, the acculturation scale basically assesses the birthplace of the client and the client's parents, generation, place raised, language used, ethnic identity of the client and the client's parents, food preference, entertainment preferences, and ethnic pride.

MOTIVATION. Among all the factors, motivation seems to be of utmost importance. It is easier to stay negative and miserable than to make positive and constructive changes. Many clients hold onto their secondary gains and are resistant to change. To change their illness process is to give up control, and many are not ready to do so. Motivation is a cultural-free factor, and this factor seems to play an important role in the outcome of mental illness or mental health process.

After gathering data, nurses need to determine to what degree the client's behavior or mental health practice is culturally universal or culturally specific. This requires much knowledge and experience. If nurses had difficulty making this assessment, they should seek consultation from experts.

Mental Health Problems Across Cultures

The correlation between mental illness and ethnicity is very complex. This complexity has only begun to become evident through research during the past 30 to 40 years (Bullough and Bullough 1982). In a series of publications, Dohrenwend and Dohrenwend (1974, 1975) have analyzed the relationship between mental illness and social class, race, and life stress. Based on the available evidence, their conclusions are that major debilitating psychoses probably are not related to culture or ethnicity in any consistent fashion. Socioeconomic status may be linked with mental illness, but it is not clear whether this is a cause or a consequence. Carefully controlled research is still needed in this area. The following discussion on prevalent mental health problems across cultures considers the relationship between mental illness and culturally related factors.

SCHIZOPHRENIA

Schizophrenia remains very much a mystery in contemporary health systems. Comparing the prevalence of schizophrenia across cultures is indeed a great challenge. At this time, research findings on prevalence of schizophrenia across cultures during the same time period are not readily available. The available data indicate that the methodology of diagnosis plays an important role ultimately in the determination of schizophrenia's prevalence.

For example, in the United States, ethnic/racial minority groups tend to have a higher proportion of schizophrenic diagnoses than do nonminority groups. One study (Simon et al. 1973) examined 192 black and white clients who had been diagnosed with schizophrenia. These clients were re-interviewed by project psychiatrists using a structured mental status examination. The results indicate that the rates of schizophrenic diagnosis for blacks were significantly lower in the later diagnostic interviews.

Many researchers have found that the major difference in schizophrenic symptomatology across cultures is the outward expression of the illness. For instance, Katz and his associates (1969, 1973) have studied hospitalized schizophrenics of various ethnic groups in Hawaii. The report indicates that there are marked contrasts between the Hawaiian-Japanese and the Hawaiian-Caucasian patients. The greatest divergence is in the expression of emotional states: hostility, anxiety, depression, and apathy. The Hawaiian-Caucasian psychotic individual was more "emotional," whereas the Hawaiian-Japanese psychotic individual was more "schizoid, withdrawn, and retarded." Tseng and McDermott (1981) also assert that the main impact of culture is seen in the way emotions and behaviors are expressed and manifested. Although the patient's behavior varies by ethnic group, there is little change in the basic characteristics — in either cognitive or perceptual aspects of their psychoses. Certain "core" symptoms seem common to schizophrenics in most cultures. These include disturbances of perception, thinking, and affect. Cultural factors, however, operate in the content and expression of delusions and hallucinations.

The preceding discussions reflect that schizophrenia is not culture-caused. Rather, it is a disease process that is affected by a combination of various genetic and environmental factors.

For some clients, karma may be used to provide a logical explanation of how a schizophrenic person is genetically mixed up from one life to another, and how the environmental factors in this life can further influence the existing causal relationship. The explanation of karma can release a family from feelings of guilt and enable them to help their schizophrenic member in a more effective fashion.

DEPRESSION

The term depression is used loosely for a wide range of conditions. It may be used to denote normal, everyday

Figure 4-1 • TIEN-HYATT ACCULTURATION SCALE

PLEASE NOTE: 1. For Native American group, outside US—on reservation; in US—off reservation.
2. Ethnic—Chinese, Korean, Japanese, Philipino, Black, Mexican, Cuban, or Native.

1. Where were you born?
   A.______Outside U.S. (if native born on reservation)
   B.______Inside U.S. (if native born off reservation)

2. Where was your father born?
   A.______Outside U.S. (if native born on reservation)
   B.______Inside U.S. (if native born off reservation)

3. Where was your mother born?
   A.______Outside U.S. (if native born on reservation)
   B.______Inside U.S. (if native born off reservation)

4. Are you:
   A.______First generation (you were born outside U.S. or on reservation)?
   B.______Second generation (you were born in U.S. or off reservation and one or both parents were born outside U.S. or on reservation)?
   C.______Third generation (you and your parents were born in U.S. and one or more grandparents were born outside U.S. or on reservation)?
   D.______Fourth generation (you, your parents, and grandparents were born in U.S. and one or more great-grandparents were born outside U.S. or on reservation)?
   E.______Other (you, your parents, grandparents, great-grandparents, and beyond were born in U.S. or off reservation)?

5. Where were you before you were 18 years old?
   A.______Outside U.S. (on reservation) only.
   B.______Mostly outside U.S. (on reservation), partly inside U.S. (off reservation).
   C.______Equally outside U.S. (on reservation) and inside U.S. (off reservation).
   D.______Mostly inside U.S. (off reservation), partly outside U.S. (on reservation).
   E.______Inside U.S. (off reservation only).

6. What language(s) do you speak at home?
   A.______Mother tongue only (e.g., tribal language, dialect).
   B.______Mostly mother tongue, some English.
   C.______Equally mother tongue and English.
   D.______Mostly English, some mother tongue.
   E.______English only.

7. What language(s) do you speak at work?
   A.______Mother tongue only (e.g., tribal language, dialect).
   B.______Mostly mother tongue, some English.
   C.______Equally mother tongue and English.
   D.______Mostly English, some mother tongue.
   E.______English only.

8. What language(s) do you read?
   A.______Mother tongue only (e.g., tribal language, dialect).
   B.______Mostly mother tongue, some English.
   C.______Equally mother tongue and English.
   D.______Mostly English, some mother tongue.
   E.______English only.

9. What language(s) do you write?
   A.______Mother tongue only (e.g., tribal language, dialect).
   B.______Mostly mother tongue, some English.
   C.______Equally mother tongue and English.
   D.______Mostly English, some mother tongue.
   E.______English only.

10. In what language(s) do you think?
    A.______Mother tongue only (tribal language, dialect).
    B.______Mostly mother tongue, some English.
    C.______Equally mother tongue and English.
    D.______Mostly English, some mother tongue.
    E.______English only.

11. How do you identify yourself?
    A.______Ethnic (e.g., Chinese, Korean, Japanese, Philipino, Black, Mexican, Indian).
    B.______Ethnic-American.
    C.______American-Ethnic.
    D.______American.

12. How does (did) your father identify himself?
    A.______Ethnic (e.g., Chinese, Korean, Japanese, Philipino, Black, Mexican, Indian).
    B.______Ethnic-American.
    C.______American-Ethnic.
    D.______American.

13. How does (did) your mother identify herself?
    A.______Ethnic (e.g., Chinese, Korean, Japanese, Philipino, Black, Mexican, Indian).
    B.______Ethnic-American.
    C.______American-Ethnic.
    D.______American.

14. What is the ethnic origin of the people with whom you work now.
    A.______Almost exclusively my own ethnic/racial group.
    B.______Mostly my own ethnic/racial group.
    C.______Equally my own ethnic/racial group and Anglos or other ethnic/racial groups.
    D.______Mostly Anglos or other ethnic/racial groups.
    E.______Almost exclusively Anglos or other ethnic/racial groups.

15. What is the ethnic origin of the people with whom you socialize outside your work?
    A.______Almost exclusively my own ethnic/racial group.
    B.______Mostly my own ethnic/racial group.
    C.______Equally my own ethnic/racial group and Anglos or other ethnic/racial groups.
    D.______Mostly Anglos or other ethnic/racial groups.
    E.______Almost exclusively Anglos or other ethnic/racial groups.

16. What is your food preference?
    A.______Exclusively ethnic food (e.g., Chinese, Korean, Japanese, Philipino, Black, Mexican, Indian).
    B.______Mostly ethnic, partly American food.
    C.______Equally ethnic and American food.
    D.______Mostly American, partly ethnic food.
    E.______Exclusively American food.

17. What is your T.V./movie viewing preference?
    A.______In ethnic language only.
    B.______Mostly in ethnic language.
    C.______Equally in ethnic and English language.
    D.______Mostly in English.
    E.______English only.

Figure continued on following page

Figure 4–1 • TIEN-HYATT ACCULTURATION SCALE *(Continued)*

18. What is your music preference?
    A.______In ethnic language only.
    B.______Mostly in ethnic language.
    C.______Equally in ethnic and English language.
    D.______Mostly in English.
    E.______English only.

19. How much pride do you have in your ethnic/racial background?
    A.______Very proud.
    B.______Somewhat proud.
    C.______Neutral.
    D.______Somewhat ashamed.
    E.______Very ashamed.

20. How do you see yourself?
    A.______Very ethnic (e.g., Chinese, Korean, Japanese, Philipino, Black, Mexican, Cuban, Native).
    B.______Somewhat ethnic.
    C.______Equally ethnic and Americanized.
    D.______Somewhat Americanized.
    E.______Very Americanized.

Figure 4–1. *Tien-Hyatt Acculturation Scale.*

mood variations, mild but pathological depressive disorders, or severe psychotic depression. All have very different etiological natures and varying clinical implications.

Pfeiffer (1968) and Sartorius (1974, 1975) claim that the "core" symptoms of depression, such as mood change, disruption of physiological functions (e.g., sleep and appetite), and hypochondriacal symptoms, are similar across the cultures studied. The differences rest on the frequency of and intensity in expressions of feelings of guilt and suicidal tendencies.

Murphy and his associates (1967) propose that the higher incidence of guilt feelings in Western cultures is due to the influence of the Christian religion. However, after investigating the relationship of guilt, religion, and depression in Christian and Moslem patients in Cairo, El-Islam (1969) reports that the presence or absence of guilt feelings is associated with the level of education and degree of depression and is not significantly related to one's religion.

Manifestation of suicidal tendencies can be different among cultures. From clinical observations of depressive illness in Afghanistan, Waziri (1973) has found that depressed patients expressed death wishes instead of suicidal intentions or thoughts. In Afghanistan, most religions view suicide as a sin.

Many Asians believe in Buddhism, which dictates that suicide is an act that eliminates the resources that the individual could have possibly offered to parents, family, and society. Therefore, suicide may result in more misery in their following lives (reincarnation) or in hell. To avoid the burden of that sin, the depressed individuals may have death wishes so they can reincarnate into a better life.

How a community views death and dying and how it ritualizes its mourning may also affect the way in which depression is expressed. The grief-stricken White Americans may express their depressive moods in the symptoms of exhaustion, insomnia, anger, frustration, feelings of hopelessness and inadequacy, and lack of motivation. They often seek psychotherapists to work through "unfinished business" and to obtain clarification, reassurance, and comfort.

Many ethnic/racial minority groups express depression by manifesting more somatic symptoms. The following vignette by Kleinman and Mechanic (1981) reflects how a Chinese person may somatize and treat depression:

> One client was a 41-year-old man with headaches, pains in joints, insomnia, "too many dreams," loss of appetite, weakness, and the belief that there was something wrong with his brain that caused his scalp to sweat excessively. It seemed that this client had a depressive syndrome associated with a fixed idea, which could have been a somatic delusion. In treating him, the doctor diagnosed a skin disease of the scalp that was making the man depressed. He prescribed herbal medicine that he claimed would improve the scalp problem and the "brain function." That in turn, would cure the depression. In the entire interchange, doctor and client discussed illness and treatment solely in somatic terms.

In addition to taking care of the natural cause, some Asians also turn to supernatural resources, such as chanting and religious rituals, to exorcise the ghost or to reduce the bad karma. Some Black Americans interpret depressive symptoms as loss of energy or soul resulting from "fix," "hex," or "spell" cast by demons, evil spirits, or their enemies. Therefore, after experiencing ineffectiveness of Western treatment methods, they might turn to folk healers (root doctors) for herbs or magic rituals. These are said to dissolve spells and to eliminate physical and psychological symptoms. In many instances, the clients may receive treatment from Western-trained physicians and folk healers simultaneously to experience "double protection" (Scott 1978).

Many Hispanic Americans believe in supernatural and natural causes for depression. They may interpret the symptoms as the result of *susto* (fright) or *mal de ojo* (evil eye) or disharmony with nature. Therefore, they might seek curanderos for a cure. Curanderismo is eclectic and holistic; it is a mixture of the beliefs derived from Aztec, Spanish, spiritualistic, homeopathic, and modern "scientific" medicine (Maduro 1983).

Native Americans often manifest depression in the behaviors of drinking, drug abuse, aggression, and suicide. Usually the client will go to the medicine man (shaman) before he consults a Western physician. The medicine man is considered a doctor, counselor, priest, and historian. He uses incantations, charms, prayers, and religious rituals to treat psychosomatic symptoms and restore the wholeness of the sick person (Kunitz 1983).

ALCOHOLISM

The World Health Organization (WHO) Expert Committee on Mental Health has framed a general definition: "Alcoholics are those excessive drinkers whose dependence upon alcohol has attained such a degree that it shows a noticeable mental disturbance or an interference with their bodily and mental health, their interpersonal relations, and their smooth social and economic functioning; or who show prodromal signs of such development. They therefore require treatment." However, this definition is subject to cultural interpretations. What one society may perceive as interference in social functioning or a mental disturbance, another society may not. In many ways, the culture shapes the drinking consumption and recognition of drinking as a problem. The rates of alcoholism in different cultural areas may vary enormously. Even the rate within a culture is not necessarily fixed; the prevalence of alcoholism may double or triple within a decade with social changes (Tseng and McDermott 1981).

The United States includes thousands of subcultures and subgroups; consequently, the literature on alcoholism has been broad and general. Cahalan and Cisin (1976) present the most detailed overview of drinking behavior and problems in the United States. They define relatively heavy drinkers as those who drink nearly every day, with five or more drinks on each occasion at least once in a while, or those who drink about once a week, usually with five or more drinks each time. Among drinkers, they listed those most likely to drink heavily as men aged 45 to 49; people of lower social status; operatives and service workers; men who have completed high school but not college; single, divorced, or separated men and women; residents of the Middle Atlantic, New England, and Pacific regions; residents of the larger cities; Americans whose fathers were born in Ireland, Latin America, the Caribbean, or the United Kingdom; Protestants of no specific denomination; Catholics; and people without religions.

Accessibility seems to account heavily for the drinking problem in the United States. I have observed that in a community hospital located in Napa Valley, California, admission rates for alcohol detoxification rise on the day when welfare checks are received. Inexpensive alcoholic beverages and general encouragement of social drinking play a role in the formation of drinking behaviors.

Economic pressure and deculturation and acculturation stress also contribute to the drinking problems in American multicultural society. A classic study by Horton (1943) reveals that in all primitive societies, the primary function of drinking is to reduce anxiety. This is probably also true in contemporary societies.

Among all the ethnic/racial groups in the United States, Native Americans seem to have received more attention in the area of drinking problems. The introduction of alcohol and its problems occurred several hundred years ago when early settlers traded whiskey for Indian goods. According to FBI crime reports, the alcohol-related arrest rate for Native Americans is ten times higher than that for the white population (Lewis 1982), and Native Americans display more severe withdrawal symptoms than other groups (Brod 1975).

There have been a great many changes in the past two hundred years or so. Western civilization has almost replaced the natural world as the environment for Native Americans. In the process of this transition, the tradition has been weakened, the kinship has been disturbed, and the moral prestige of the elderly has eroded (Thomas 1981). In a study using participant observation, Topper (1981) obtained stories as told by drinkers. The subjects in the study revealed that drinking is not a central aspect of life to most Navajos. In fact, it is a form of "bad life" (*doo ya' at'eehgo iina'da*). Drinking is one of the many types of behavior that are considered to be antithetical to the way of life that was "given" to the Navajo people at the time of their creation (Topper 1978). Drinkers recognize that drinking is an escape from the psychological pain caused by some unpleasant person, condition, or experience (Topper 1981). Levy (1958) describes this as a "narcotizing" function.

Drinking problems in the Hispanic communities are considered "pervasive, widespread, and epidemic" (Alcocer 1982; Caetano 1983). For example, in New York City, cirrhosis of the liver was found to be the third leading cause of death among adult Puerto Ricans, preceded only by homicide and drug-related causes (Alers 1978). The pressures of unemployment, poverty, crowding, and discrimination have contributed to an increase in marital separations, divorces, and drinking problems (Pelto et al. 1982).

Black Americans also seem to have higher rates of alcohol abuse than their White American counterparts. Alcohol dependence is considered a major health and social problem among Black Americans. Drinking problems also precipitate more intense economic, social, physical, mental, and legal problems for this minority group. This vicious circle is often perceived as a result of oppression in a white-dominated society.

Asian Americans seem to have the lowest rates of alcohol dependence among all the ethnic/racial groups in the United States. Drinking is part of the culture in many Asian societies. Toasts and drinking games are common at banquets, especially those for new year celebrations, festivals, and special social occasions for Chinese, Japanese, and Korean people. Hanna (1978) has found that both Chinese people and Japanese people metabolize alcohol at a much higher rate than do Europeans. It is speculated that the low rate of alcoholism among Asian Americans has physiological rather than cultural influences. Some recent studies, however, show that there has been a sharp increase in alcoholism among Asian Americans since World War II. Yamamuro (1973) reveals that before the war, the Japanese annual per capita consumption of absolute alcohol was 2.4 liters, and in 1969 it increased to 4.3 liters. Kitano (1987) also reports that 25.8 percent of Korean Americans drink heavily as compared with 15.3 percent of their White American counterparts. As for other ethnic/racial groups, alcoholism is considered one of the major factors causing marital disruption for Korean Americans.

Among White Americans, Irish Americans seem to have received more attention than other subgroups in the area of alcohol abuse. Although the overall rate of mental illness among Irish Americans has fallen during the past 25 years, the Irish, both in Ireland and in the United States, continue to have a very high incidence of alcoholism (Clare 1974; DHEW 1971; Stivers 1976; Walsh and Walsh 1973). Alcoholism is tolerated as a "good man's weakness." Ireland's damp climate, which has forced people to be confined indoors, might be enough to make anyone seek to repress physical sensations with alcohol. In any event, alcohol has been their universal disqualifier and solution: it dulls the pain, keeps out the cold, cures the fever, eases the grief, enlivens the celebration, allows them all a manner of expression, and even cures a hangover. Because the Irish often claim not to be responsible for what is done under its influence, alcohol makes anything — but particularly aggression — permissible. Considerable alcohol use is tolerated, especially by men, without being seen as a difficulty. Alcohol dependence has thus become a serious problem for the Irish and the cause of much family disruption (McGoldrick 1982).

DOMESTIC VIOLENCE

Domestic violence is an alarming epidemic in the United States. One out of two families has experienced violence at least once in its lifetime. Domestic violence occurs in all ethnic/racial, age, and socioeconomic groups. Studies by Finkelhor and his associates (1983) reveal that at least six million men, women, and children are physically attacked each year by a family member and one out of four murder victims in the United States is killed by a member of his or her own family.

Each subgroup within the family system has the inherent potential for conflict, physical abuse, or emotional neglect. Domestic violence occurs in family subgroups such as spouse, sibling, child, and the elderly. The most common form of domestic violence is the battered woman syndrome. According to Getty (1981), the incidence rate of wife battering in the United States is between 40 and 50% of all families. This is certainly an underestimate of the true total, since domestic violence is one of the most underreported crimes in the nation owing to personal shame and fear of further injury. The following case anecdotes may shed some light on this phenomenon:

Case 1

A Chinese woman was married to a Jewish man. They were both Harvard graduates. The husband was a physician, and the wife had a Ph.D. in public health. They both worked in a renowned university as researchers. One year after the marriage, they had a baby girl. The conflict began when they argued whether their daughter should be raised according to Jewish or Chinese customs. Before the wife knew it, the husband had wrestled her down to the floor and had beaten her up with the doors locked. His parents watched the scene and enjoyed seeing that their son was "in charge." She reported this to the police, but the case was dismissed because there was no apparent injury. Due to embarrassment and fear, she did not seek any further help until she talked to a friend who was a therapist. She then pursued a divorce. Her husband hired a very powerful male attorney who intimidated her female attorney. Her attorney advised her to drop the charges, forget about child support, and move out of the area. She did, for the sake of peace of mind and a new life without battering and shame.

Case 2

A Philipino physician was married to a Philipino man. The husband had been unemployed for quite some time and had turned to alcohol for escape. He beat up his wife first when he was drunk and later when he was sober as well. After many years of struggle, the wife filed for divorce and found a new boyfriend. Shortly before her marriage to the new man, the jealous ex-husband killed her and himself with a gun in the parking lot near her office.

Case 3

A bright white woman was married to a white man for 16 years; the couple had three children. They were happy when they first married. By the time their third child was born, the husband had become an alcoholic and a drug abuser. Although he held a job, their financial situation was bleak. The wife decided to improve their family's situation by enrolling in a registered nursing program. She graduated with honors. However, her husband was threatened by her success, and he started to abuse her physically. She filed for divorce, and that only heightened her husband's instability. He beat her so badly that she was hospitalized. At that time, she filed a police report, and the husband was jailed for five days. She had her husband released because she feared that he would lose his job. Continuing to use the legal system, she filed a restraining order that forbade her husband to call or visit her at home or at work. However, on December 31, 1986, when she met him outside of work, both their lives ended; this orphaned three young girls.

The preceding vignettes reflect that domestic violence occurs regardless of ethnic/racial groups, inter- or intraracial marriages, or socioeconomic status. Domestic violence also has a strong correlation with alcohol and drug abuse.

An interview with the Director of the Program on Domestic Violence at the Los Angeles Indian Center revealed that 20% of the battered women they house in their shelter are Native Americans. Most of them are married to other Native Americans, but others are married to Mexican, Black, or White Americans. The low percentage of Native Americans treated is thought to be the result of stigma and reluctance to ask for help, not the lack of abuse in this particular population.

Most Hispanic American traditional cultures do not have strong taboos against a man having extramarital affairs and drinking excessively. These activities are seen as ways for men to demonstrate their masculinity and are considered acceptable behavior. The combined beliefs of machismo and the man as the head of the household mean that the husband has a right to discipline family members in any way that he sees fit. This may, at times, include using violence.

Many Asian Americans share a similar belief that wife and children are the husband's property; therefore, he has the right to hit them. Choy (1987) reports that many American-born Asians are still quite traditional. The traditional culture that permits a man to feel a sense of ownership over his wife and family might allow that same man, who has failed to learn how to control his anger, to express himself through physical violence. The Asian practice of "saving face" is a powerful incentive for a battered woman to remain in a life-threatening situation. The wife may initially seek help for her husband because his excessive drinking or gambling is tearing the family apart. The wife and family are usually mistakenly convinced that once the husband stops drinking and gambling, the violence will stop.

As in other ethnic/racial groups, no statistics are readily available for the occurrence of domestic violence in Black American families. One source reveals that one fourth of all black homicides in 1972 took place among family members, either killings between the spouses or killings between parent and child (Owens 1980). Historically, black males have had feelings of low self-esteem and powerlessness. This may make them prone to violent behavior. Yet domestic violence occurs no more nor less frequently in the black culture than in other cultures.

Interventions for Multicultural Populations

The concepts of mental illness that the individual employs determine the kind of mental health practice that he or she will adopt or accept. If the individual believes that mental disorder is caused by sociopsychological factors, counseling from a mental health professional would likely be sought. If the individual believes in physical-medical causes, medical treatment, such as ECT (electroconvulsive therapy) or psychotropic drugs, is more likely to be sought from psychiatrists or other medical professionals.

Despite the advancement of modern medicine, many Americans—especially the first-generation immigrants—believe in supernatural and natural causes and in causal relationships. They might, therefore, seek out folk healers in their communities for the treatment of mental illness. In most instances, the conventional medicine is tried first, and if it fails, the client or family may then seek nonconventional treatment such as exorcism, religious rituals, restoring the lost soul, dissolving the spell, or regaining harmony with nature by reorganizing their living arrangements. Sometimes the conventional treatment and folk remedies are sought simultaneously. These practices are shared by many ethnic/racial groups, including Asian (Tien-Hyatt 1987), Black (Spector 1985), Hispanic (Martinez 1978), and Native Americans (Attneave 1982).

Dealing with mental health problems of multicultural populations is a very complex and challenging task. A holistic approach with multicultural clients can include (1) psychological counseling, (2) hypnotherapy, (3) acupressure, (4) nutritional counseling, (5) exercise, (6) pharmacology, and/or (7) spiritual healing.

PSYCHOLOGICAL COUNSELING. Western schools of psychological counseling theories and techniques are helpful in dealing with mental health problems on the conscious level or the unconscious level or both. The psychoanalytic approach can be used to explore the causes of the mental health problem and help the client gain insights into the problem. Also, gestalt therapy, rational emotive therapy (RET), and behavioral therapy techniques can be used to guide the client to restructure his or her outlook on life and reconstruct coping mechanisms. Refer to Chapter 2 for further discussion of these therapies.

The following approaches can be highly effective in short-term therapies. They are particularly useful in counseling the ethnic/racial minorities, since minority members are apt to favor short-term treatment.

HYPNOTHERAPY. All hypnosis processes are self-hypnosis. Self-hypnosis techniques can be extremely effective in working through "unfinished business" and in developing positive attitudes and increasing internal locus of control. Historically, self-hypnosis has been used to treat various psychological and physical problems such as hysteria, depression, epilepsy, arthritis, and skin disease (Anderson-Evangelista 1980). Hypnosis can also be used as an adjunct in managing pain, both psychological and physical.

ACUPRESSURE. Acupressure is the application of pressure by fingers and hands on acupoints. The acupoints used for acupressure are basically the same as those for acupuncture (Warren 1976). The purpose of acupressure is to facilitate the energy flow and release endorphins. Endorphins are natural substances that function like opium. Endorphins can relieve pain and promote a general feeling of well-being. The use of acupressure is particularly welcomed by clients with psychophysiologic symptoms. For example, to the therapist, symptoms of pain may be psychogenic; however, to the client the pain is real and cannot be explained away. Acupressure can relieve pain and consequently provide the client with more energy for working on underlying conflicts and alternative solutions.

Many practitioners adopt the self-care model and teach clients to apply acupressure on themselves between office visits. This approach often helps relieve such symptoms as headaches, insomnia, anxiety, and gastrointestinal disturbance.

NUTRITIONAL COUNSELING. The type of nutritional counseling provided by some practitioners is using natural foods and vitamins to assist in the treatment of various psychosomatic symptoms. For example, if the client suffers from arthritic pain, a combination of carrot juice and celery juice and vitamin C and calcium would be suggested. If the client suffers from nervous stomach, a combination of papaya juice and pineapple juice would be recommended. Certain herbs are also used. For example, topical use of aloe vera may be suggested for a skin rash, or *dong quai* (a Chinese herb) may be recommended for premenstrual syndrome.

EXERCISE. As long as the client is not severely disabled or confined to a bed, exercise is also incorporated in the holistic treatment program. The client is encouraged to do any type of exercise that he or she can manage. Often the client will begin walking five to ten minutes a day and gradually increase to 30 minutes or more. Like acupressure, exercise facilitates the release of endorphins, which can reduce pain and promote a general feeling of well-being. Also, exercise increases blood circulation and oxygen supply to the brain, which can reduce fatigue. Most of all, exercise promotes fitness, which is highly valued by contemporary society. Many clients overeat because of depression, which in turn results in their becoming overweight. The weight problem may then compound the depression. Exercise helps break this vicious cycle.

PHARMACOLOGY. Many clients take prescribed medication. However, the dosage (especially with psychotropic drugs) should be closely monitored. For example, some Asian clients can develop adverse reactions or side effects easily, even with smaller dosages of psychotropic drugs than those normally prescribed (Tien 1984). Nurses should observe and document the behavioral changes induced by psychotropic drugs and suggest adjustment of the dosage to the prescribing physician if necessary. Sometimes after clients are exposed to holistic treatment, a prescribed dosage may be reduced or discontinued as dependence on chemical substances tends to diminish.

SPIRITUAL HEALING. Whether clients have any religious beliefs or not, they are encouraged to pray. They may create their own prayers if they wish. They are also instructed to pray for others as well, not just for themselves. Praying for the individuals with whom they have trouble is particularly encouraged. The therapist might suggest that while praying, the client should imagine a bright, warm, white energy or aura surrounding his or her entire body. The use of this guided imagery and prayer helps many clients reduce feelings of depression, anger, resentment, and negativity.

Some clients believe that their living quarters have been haunted by unsettled spirits. Consequently, they are encouraged to call on their religious leader to cleanse the house with holy water or to pray for these "felt" spirits.

CASE EXAMPLES. A variety of holistic approaches can be employed to help clients get well within the shortest time possible. A holistic approach is used within a cultural context. The following case examples may help to illustrate the use of culturally sensitive holistic approaches:

Case 1

A 56-year-old white woman had a well-paying job in a big financial company. She suffered from multiple injuries as a result of an automobile accident and falls in the office and at home. Despite frequent visits to her orthopedic and chiropractic doctors, her pain and depression persisted. After listening to a radio program discussing holistic medicine, she decided to try the holistic approach. In the first session, she revealed that she had consulted with a psychic and was told that her family and her husband's side of the family had been cursed. The psychic advised that helping her dissolve the spell would cost five thousand dollars. She refused to pay that amount of money and continued to search for better alternatives. Psychological counseling such as rational emotive therapy was employed to help reprogram her cognitive thinking. She was reminded to count her blessings and to redirect her energy to get well. Acupressure and hypnotherapy were also used to reduce her pain.

In the second session, she reported that her pain was reduced but that she was still depressed and had no energy. She believed that the curse was still working against her. She was taught more about acupressure treatment to reduce her pain further and to enhance energy flow. The content of her hypnosis tape was revised to induce deeper relaxation and more positive thinking. Vitamins, natural foods, herbs, and exercise (slow walking) were also recommended. Furthermore, it was explained to her that the curse would work only when she had a weak psychological and physical system. It was stressed that she was the one who could break that vicious cycle. It was also suggested that she might burn some white candles and pray for her enemies to dissolve the spell.

In the third session, she indicated that she had followed all regimens. She had also bought some white candles the day before. Interestingly, before she had had a chance to burn the candles, she felt much better. She "saw" that the aura of her house and her body was much brighter. After that, she decided to stop therapy for a while to see whether she could function on her own. Her decision was respected.

Case 2

A 40-year-old Japanese male musician had suffered from severe social phobia for 15 years. He reported that 15 years ago, when he was deeply involved in meditation, he got "meditation illness." From then on, he saw or felt shadows whenever he socialized with people, especially in a public area. He had seen a few psychiatrists and hypnotists, without satisfactory results. Despite his heavy use of Valium, the symptoms of horror, nervousness, shakes, and freezing worsened over the years. The only time he felt "normal" was when he taught piano lessons or performed in a concert.

The combination of gestalt therapy, rational emotive therapy, and behavioral therapy was used to reprogram his cognitive thinking and to recondition his behavior. Psychoanalytic theory was also used to help him understand the influence of his childhood experience on his phobic behavior. He recalled that his father was very stern and critical. He was always the second best in his father's eyes—no matter how hard he tried. Consequently, in his therapy sessions, he was instructed to "secretly" see his social partners as his piano students. That made him feel superior, confident, and respected in a social setting. Hypnotherapy was used to reduce his irrational fear, nervousness, and anxiety and to brighten the aura of his system.

The approach of graded exposure was employed. He was instructed to increase his exposure to social interactions gradually and to keep a diary. He was also encouraged to pray and meditate again. After 12 sessions, he showed marked improvements. He was able to go out with friends with minimal or no tranquilizers. He was also able to meditate and "tough it out" when the shadows appeared. After 16 sessions, the shadows totally disappeared, he no longer needed tranquilizers, and he was able to enjoy his life again.

Case 3

A 39-year-old black woman suffered from increasing conflicts with her boyfriend and her three daughters from her previous two marriages. Shortly after her father passed away, she moved in with her boyfriend, who was white. She felt that her boyfriend's mother distanced her because of her ethnicity. She also felt that the difficulty in adjusting to her new living situation prevented her from working through the grief over her father's death. At the time she entered treatment, she suffered from depression, allergies, and varicose veins.

Rational emotive therapy and gestalt therapy was

used to persuade her that she was an attractive woman and that she should not allow her "blackness" to get in the way. Hypnotherapy was used to reinforce positive thinking and attitudes. Vitamins C and E, herbs, and exercise were recommended to reduce the symptoms of varicose veins and allergies. Acupressure techniques were also taught to her to improve the blood circulation and energy flow. As to the grief over her father's death, she was instructed to pray for her father and imagine that her father was surrounded by bright, warm, white energy. Every time she performed this mental exercise, she was to see her father smiling calmly and peacefully.

After practicing this holistic approach diligently for two weeks, she dreamed that her father called her on the phone and told her that he was fine. A week later she had another dream. She dreamed that she was rushing to her father's funeral. By the time she got there, the coffin was closed. She frantically requested that the coffin be opened. The pastor opened it, and she saw her father lying there with a relaxed and peaceful smile. And, all of a sudden, he stood up! She cried out loud, "Dad, I thought you were dead!" The father replied, "I was just asleep." She woke up feeling relieved.

After seven sessions, she reported having better relationships with her boyfriend and daughters. Her physical symptoms were also subsiding.

Case 4

A 36-year-old Hispanic woman had conflicts with her colleagues and suffered from prolonged grief over her mother's death. She had been molested by her uncle during her preschool years. She attempted to tell her mother about the molestation in a very subtle way, but her mother did not get the message. Because of the fear of being grabbed by her uncle in the bathroom (which was next to her uncle's bedroom), she developed a bed-wetting problem. Her mother did not seek help for her bed-wetting problem. She interpreted her mother's behavior as not loving her. The molestation continued until her uncle was killed in an automobile accident. She was happy about the punishment her uncle received. Her bed-wetting problem diminished; however, her anger at her mother remained. Consequently, she had given her mother a "hard time" since childhood until her mother's death three years previously. After her mother suffered from a long-term illness and passed away, she began to be overwhelmed by guilt. She also manifested "victim's behavior" at work. She allowed her coworkers to take advantage of her and then became angry. Despite her advanced clerical skills, she had not stayed in the same job for more than two years. She was also 75 pounds overweight.

Rational emotive therapy, gestalt therapy, and hypnotherapy were used to help her accept her past and to redirect her energy to start a new life course. She was also instructed to send positive, bright, warm energy to her mother through guided imagery. After six sessions, she was able to "dialogue" with her deceased mother to achieve some mutual understanding, forgiveness, and love. She also quit her job, in which she felt that the presence of too many negative coworkers had made her perpetuate her "victim's behavior." After she found a new job, she wished to try to function on her own and terminated the therapy. Two months later she returned to therapy and decided to work on her weight. Through the combination of hypnotherapy, nutritional counseling, acupressure, and exercise, she lost 15 pounds in five weeks.

At the time of writing this report, she was still in therapy and losing more weight.

The preceding vignettes reflect that clients from different racial/ethnic backgrounds may have varying degrees of beliefs in medical, natural, or supernatural causes of illness, both physical and mental. After they feel comfortable with the therapist and disclose their beliefs, they are usually open to holistic treatment within a cultural context.

Summary

Understanding this chapter may be like sorting out a puzzle with many missing pieces. The lack of systematic research on mental health issues across cultures makes it extremely difficult to compare and contrast the differences and similarities among major cultural groups in the United States. It is hoped that the following "working" conclusions will stimulate critical thinking and induce more scientific research:

1. Culture is a phenomenon through which norms and values are socially transmitted from generation to generation. In the process of this transmission, changes occur constantly and often imperceptibly. Therefore, nurses should avoid stereotyping client behaviors. The rule of thumb is to check with and learn from the client and his or her family. Do not assume anything. Overgeneralization can be as dangerous as ignorance, if not more so.
2. The demographic trends among major racial/ethnic groups in the United States are changing rapidly. Although some racial/ethnic groups settle in certain geographical pockets, most of the major cities are populated by a blend of multicultural groups. The rapid population increases in various racial/ethnic

groups representing a diversity of sociocultural backgrounds has heightened demands for culturally specific mental health care.

3. The socioeconomic trends of major racial/ethnic groups in California reflect that Black, Native, and Hispanic Americans have higher percentages of low income families and unemployment. However, in terms of higher income families, all racial/ethnic minority groups, including Asian, Black, Hispanic, and Native Americans, have almost equal percentages. Therefore, stereotypes of "model minority" should be avoided.
4. The correlation between mental illness and ethnicity is very complex. The scanty research reflects that major debilitating mental illness probably is not related to culture or ethnicity in any consistent fashion. Studies of prevalent mental health problems (including schizophrenia, depression, alcoholism, and domestic violence) among Asian, Black, White, Hispanic, and Native Americans reveal that the manifestation of general symptoms may differ to a greater or lesser degree, but the "core" symptoms seem similar across cultures.
5. A client usually believes and employs more than one explanation for mental illness. The degree of beliefs in various explanations (including sociopsychological, physical-medical, supernatural, natural, and causal) is influenced by the client's acculturation level and personal exposure. Nurses should not impose their own beliefs or nonbeliefs on clients. Using the phenomenological and client-centered approaches, nurses should encourage clients to describe their personal beliefs.
6. In dealing with culturally diverse clients, nurses need to recognize their attitudes and the psychodynamics of prejudice. The effects of prejudice are destructive both to the prejudiced and to the victim of prejudice. Although all people possess certain degrees of prejudice, nurses need to examine critically their attitudes toward the culturally different and avoid prejudice in the counseling process. If nurses have difficulty in remaining objective, they should not engage in cross-cultural counseling, and they should perhaps seek counseling or supervision.
7. In mental health assessment, nurses should collect data in cultural, sociological, psychological, and biological/physiological areas. Special attention should be given to ethnicity/race, socioeconomic status, folk beliefs, acculturation, and motivation. The nurse should consider both general cultural traits and personal idiosyncrasies while assessing etiology, treatment, and prognosis.
8. In almost all cases, psychological and physical problems are interrelated, and the client often manifests both sets of symptoms concurrently. Therefore, a holistic approach dealing with both psychological and physical problems seems to be highly effective. When combining psychological counseling, hypnotherapy, acupressure, nutritional counseling, exercise, pharmacology, and spiritual healing, the client is treated as a whole person within the confines of his or her own culture. The fusion of the best of Western, Eastern, and folk medicine seems to be welcomed by all clients, regardless of ethnicity.

References

Abdu-Saad H, Kayser-Jones J, Tien JL. Asian nursing students in the United States. Journal of Nursing Education, 21:11, 1982.

Acosta FX. Self-described reasons for premature termination of psychotherapy by Mexican-American, Black-American and Anglo-American patients. Psychological Reports, 47:435, 1980.

Alcocer AM. Alcohol use and abuse among the Hispanic American population. Special Population Issues, Alcohol and Health, Monographs, 4:361, 1982.

Alers JO. Puerto Rican health: Findings from New York. Hispanic Research Center, Monograph Series no. 1. New York: Fordham University, 1978.

Anderson-Evangelista A. Hypnosis: A Journey into the Mind. New York: Arco Publishing, 1980.

Attneave C. American Indians and Alaska Native families: Emigrants in their own homeland. *In* McGoldrick M, Pearce JK, Giordano J (eds). Ethnicity & Family Therapy. New York: The Guilford Press, 1982, pp. 55–83.

Benjamin R, Benjamin M. Socio-cultural correlates of black drinking. Journal of Studies on Alcohol, 9:241, 1981.

Bloch B. Bloch's assessment guide for ethni/culture variations. *In* Orque MS, Bloch B (eds). Ethnic Nursing Care: A Multi-Cultural Approach. St. Louis, MO: C.V. Mosby Company, 1983, pp. 49–75.

Brod TM. Alcoholism as a mental health problem of Native Americans, a review of the literature. Archives of General Psychiatry, 32:1385, 1975.

Bullough VL, Bullough B. Mental health and mental illness. *In* Bullough VL, Bullough B. Health Care for Other Americans. New York: Appleton-Century-Crofts, 1982, pp. 157–177.

Busse EW, Pfeiffer E (eds). Mental Illness in Later Life. Washington DC: American Psychiatric Association, 1973.

Caetano R. Drinking patterns and alcoholic problems among Hispanics in the US: A review. Drug and Alcohol Dependence, 12:37, 1983.

Cahalan D, Cisin IH. Drinking behavior and drinking problems in the United States. *In* Kissin B, Begleiter H (eds). Social Aspects of Alcoholism. The Biology of Alcoholism, 4, New York: Plenum Press, 1976.

Choy M. Battered: Rise of domestic violence in the Asian American community. Asian Week, 12–13, December 5, 1986.

Clare A. Mental illness in the Irish emigrant. Journal of the Irish Medical Association, 67:225, 1974.

Collins JL, Rickman LE, Mathura CB. Frequency of schizophrenia and depression in a black inpatient population. Journal of the National Medical Association, 9:851, 1980.

Cooper JE, Kendall RE, Gurland BJ, Sartorius N, Farkas T. Cross-national study of diagnosis of the mental disorders: Some results from the first comparative investigation. American Journal of Psychiatry [Suppl.], 125:21, 1969.

Currier RL. The hot-cold syndrome and symbolic balance in Mexican and Spanish-American folk medicine. *In* Martinez RA (ed). Hispanic Culture and Health Care, St. Louis, MO: C.V. Mosby Company, 1978, pp. 138–151.

Davies M, Yoshida M. A model for cultural assessment. The Canadian Nurse, 226:22, 1981.

Department of Health, Education and Welfare. First Special Report to US Congress on Alcohol and Health. Washington DC: Health Services and Mental Health Authority, 1971.

Dohrenwend BS, Dohrenwend BP. Stressful Life Events: Their Nature and Effects. New York: Wiley and Sons, 1974.

Dohrenwend BS, Dohrenwend BP. Sociocultural and social-psychological factors in the genesis of mental disorders. Journal of Health and Social Behavior, 16:365, 1975.

El-Islam MF. Depression and guilt: A study at an Arab psychiatric clinic. Social Psychiatry, 4:56, 1969.

Feldstein S, Costello L. The Ordeal of Assimilation. New York: Anchor Press/Doubleday, 1974.

Finkelhor D, Gelles R, Hotaling G, Straus M. The Dark Side of Families. Beverly Hills: Sage, 1983.

Frederick C. Suicide, homicide and alcoholism among American Indians. National Institute of Mental Health, Pub. 58763-12. Washington DC: U.S. Government Printing Office, 1973.

Getty C, Humphreys W. Understanding the Family. New York: Appleton-Century-Crofts, 1981.

Glasser BG, Strauss AL. The Discovery of Grounded Theory: Strategies for Qualitative Research. New York: Aldine, 1967.

Goldberg EM, Morrison SL. Schizophrenia and social class. British Journal of Psychiatry, 109:785, 1963.

Hanna JM. Metabolic responses of Chinese, Japanese and Europeans to alcohol. Alcoholism: Clinical and Experimental Research, 2:89, 1978.

Hollingshead AB, Redlich FC. Social stratification and psychiatric disorders. American Sociological Review. 1:163, 1953.

Hollingshead AB, Redlich FC. Schizophrenia and social structure. American Journal of Psychiatry, 110:605, 1954.

Hollingshead AB, Redlich FC. Social Class and Mental Illness. New York: John Wiley & Sons, 1958.

Horton D. The functions of alcohol in primitive societies: A cross-cultural study. Quarterly Journal of Studies on Alcohol, 4:199, 1943.

Husserl E. Ideas: General Introduction to Pure Phenomenology. New York: Collies, 1962.

Husserl E. The Crisis of European Sciences and Transcendental Phenomenology. Evanston, Ill: Northwestern University Press, 1970.

Iu CR, Ethnic and economic correlates of marital satisfaction and attitudes towards divorce of Chinese American women. Doctoral Dissertation, Department of Social Welfare, University of California, Los Angeles, 1982.

Katz MM, Gudeman H, Sanborn K. Characterizing differences in psychopathology among ethnic groups: A preliminary report on Hawaiian-Japanese and Mainland-American schizophrenics. *In* Caudill W, Lin TY (eds). Mental Health Research in Asia and the Pacific. Honolulu, HI: East-West Center Press, 1969.

Katz MM, Sanborn KO. Multiethnic studies of psychopathology and normality in Hawaii. *In* Brown BS, Torrey EF (eds). International Collaboration in Mental Health. Bethesda, MD: National Institute of Mental Health, 1973.

Kitano H. Personal conversation. Professor at the University of California, Los Angeles, Department of Social Welfare, 1987.

Klaf FS, Hamilton JG. Schizophrenia—A hundred years ago and today. Journal of Mental Science, 107:819, 1961.

Kleinman A, Mechanic D. Mental illness and psychological aspects of medical problems in China. *In* Kleinman A, Lin T. (eds). Normal and Abnormal Behavior in Chinese Culture, p. 337, Boston: D. Reidel Publishing Company, 1981.

Kluckhohn C. Mirror for Man. Greenwich, CT: Fawcett Publishing, 1968.

Kunitz SJ. Disease Change and the Role of Medicine. The Navajo Experience. Berkeley, CA: University of California Press, 1983.

Lee K. Mother-in-law as the cause of family problems. Korean Street Journal, July 3, 1981.

Leininger M. Culturological assessment domains for nursing practices. *In* Leininger M (ed). Transcultural Nursing: Concepts, Theories and Practices. New York: John Wiley & Sons, 1978.

Levy JE, Kunitz SJ. Economic and political factors inhibiting the use of basic research findings in Indian alcoholism programs. *In* Heath DB, Waddell JO, Topper MD (eds). Journal of Studies on Alcohol [Suppl.], Washington DC: Smithsonian Institution, 1981, pp. 60–71.

Levy R. The psychodynamic functions of alcohol. Quarterly Journal of Alcohol, 19:649, 1958.

Lewis R. Alcoholism and the Native American—A review of the literature. Alcohol and Health Monograph 4—Special Population Issues, Washington DC: DHHS Publication no. ADM 82–1190, 1982.

Linton R. The Cultural Background of Personality. New York: Appleton-Century-Crofts, 1945.

Lynch-Sauer J. Using a phenomenological research method to study nursing phenomena. *In* Leininger M (ed). Qualitative Research Methods in Nursing. Orlando, FL: Grune & Stratton, 1985, pp. 93–109.

Maduro R. Curanderismo and Latino views of disease and curing. The Western Journal of Medicine, 139:868, 1983.

Marmor RW. The psychodynamics of prejudice. *In* Padilla ER, Padilla AM (eds). Transcultural Psychiatry: A Hispanic Perspective. Los Angeles: Spanish Speaking Mental Health Research Center, 1977, pp. 5–12.

Martinez RA. Hispanic Culture and Health Care: Fact, Fiction, Folklore. St. Louis, MO: C.V. Mosby Company, 1978.

McGoldrick M. Irish families. *In* McGoldrick M, Pearce JK, Giordano J (eds). Ethnicity & Family Therapy. New York: The Guilford Press, 1982, pp. 310–339.

Meador B, Rogers C. Person-centered therapy. *In* Corsini RJ (ed). Current Psychotherapies. Itasca, Ill: F.E. Peacock Publishers, 1979, pp. 131–184.

Murphy HBM, Wittkower ED, Chance NA. Cross-cultural inquiry into symptomology of depression: A preliminary report. International Journal of Psychiatry, 3:6, 1967.

Orque M. Orque's ethnic/cultural system: A framework for ethnic nursing care. *In* Orque MS, Bloch B (eds). Ethnic Nursing Care: A Multi-Cultural Approach. St. Louis, MO: C.V. Mosby Company, 1983, pp. 5–48.

Owens CE. Mental Health and Black Offenders. Lexington, MA: Lexington Books, 1980.

Pelto P, Roman M, Nelson L. Family structures in an urban Puerto Rican community. Urban Anthropology, 11:39, 1982.

Pfeiffer WM. The symptomology of depression viewed transculturally. Transcultural Psychiatric Research Review 5:121, 1968.

Potter J. Wind, water, bones and souls: The religious world of the Cantonese peasant. Journal of Oriental Studies, 8:139, 1970.

Ralph JA. Voodoo, spiritualism and psychiatry. (Monograph). Transcultural Psychiatry: A Hispanic Perspective, 4:97, 1977.

Rubel AJ. The epidemiology of a folk illness: Susto in Hispanic America. *In* Martinez RA (ed). Hispanic Culture and Health Care. St. Louis, MO: C.V. Mosby Company, 1978, pp. 75–91.

Sartorius N. Depressive illness as a world wide problem. *In* Kielholz P (ed). Depression in Everyday Practice. St. Moritz, (Huber, Berne/Stuttgart/Vienna): International Symposium, 1974.

Sartorius N. Epidemiology of depression. WHO Chronicle, 29:423, 1975.

Scott CS. Health and healing practices among five ethnic groups in Miami, Florida. *In* Bauwens EE (ed). The Anthropology of Health. St. Louis, MO: C.V. Mosby Company, 1978.

Simon RJ, Fleiss JL, Gurland BJ. Depression and schizophrenia in hospitalized black and white mental patients. Archives of General Psychiatry, 28:509, 1973.

Solomon P, Patch VD. Handbook of Psychiatry. Los Altos, CA: Lange Medical Publications, 1971.

Spector RE. Health and illness in the Black American community. *In* Spector RE. Cultural Diversity in Health and Illness, 2nd ed. Norwalk, CT: Appleton-Century-Crofts, 1985, pp. 141–159.

Stern PN. Using grounded theory method in nursing research. *In* Leininger M (ed). Qualitative Research Methods in Nursing. Orlando, FL: Grune & Stratton, 1985, pp. 149–161.

Stern PN, Pyles SH. Grounded theory: Its uses in the study of women's culturally based decisions about health care. *In* Stern PN (ed). Women, Health and Culture. New York: Hemisphere, 1985.

Stivers R. The hair of the dog: Irish drinking and American stereotypes. University Park, PA: Penn State University Press, 1976.

Thomas RK. The history of North American Indian alcohol use as a community based phenomenon. *In* Heath DB, Waddell JO, Topper MD (eds). Journal of Studies on Alcohol [Suppl. 9], Washington DC: Smithsonian Institution, 1981, pp. 29–39.

Tien JL. Surviving graduate nursing programs in the United States—A personal account of an Asian-American student. Journal of Nursing Education, 21:42, 1982.

Tien JL. Do Asians need less medication? Journal of Psychosocial Nursing and Mental Health Services, 22:19, 1984.

Tien JL, Johnson HL. Black mental health clients' preference for therapists. A new look at an old issue. International Journal of Social Psychiatry, 31:258, 1985.

Tien-Hyatt JL. Minority mental health clients' preference for therapists: A new look at an old issue. Research proposal submitted to the National Institute of Mental Health, 1985.

Tien-Hyatt JL. Methodological issues in cross-cultural nursing research. Paper presented at the conference International Nursing: The Cross-Cultural Context. Edmonton, Alberta, Canada, May 6, 1986.

Tien-Hyatt JL. Cultural issues in Asian health care. Nursing and Health Care, 8:268, 1987.

Topper MD. Not Navajo lie; mental "illness," psychotherapy and clinical anthropology among the Navajo. *In* Steinberg JL (ed). Cultural Factors in the Rehabilitation Process. Los Angeles: University of California, Department of Counsellor Education, 1978.

Topper MD. The drinker's story: An important but often forgotten source of data. *In* Heath DB, Waddell JO, Topper MD (eds). Journal of Studies of Alcohol [Suppl. 9]. Washington DC: Smithsonian Institution, 1981, pp. 73–86.

Tripp-Reimer T, Brink P, Saunders JM. Cultural assessment: Content and process. Nursing Outlook, 32:78, 1984.

Tseng W, McDermott JF, Jr. Culture, mind and therapy, New York: Brunner/Mazel, 1981.

Walsh B, Walsh B. Validity of indices of alcoholism: A comment from Irish experience. British Journal of Preventive and Social Medicine, 27:18, 1973.

Warren FZ. Freedom From Pain Through Acupressure. New York: Frederick Fell Publishers, 1976.

Waziri R. Symptomatology of depressive illness in Afghanistan. American Journal of Psychiatry. 130:213, 1973.

Webster's New Collegiate Dictionary. Springfield, MA: G & C Merriam Company, 1976.

Werner EE. Cross-cultural Child Development: A View from the Planet Earth. Monterey, CA: Brooks/Cole Publishing Company, 1979.

World Health Organization. Second report of the Alcoholism Subcommittee of the World Health Expert Committee on Mental Health. WHO Technical Report Series no. 48, 1952.

Yamamuro B. Alcoholism in Tokyo. Quarterly Journal of Alcohol, 34:950, 1973.

Annotated Bibliography

GENERAL

Branch M, Paxton P. Providing Safe Nursing Care for Ethnic People of Color. New York: Appleton-Century-Crofts, 1976.

This book describes how positive aspects of cultural health traditions have been ignored when discussing ethnic people of color. Ideas generally not held by American medicine, such as the holistic health view that is basic to Latino, black, Asian, and Indian cultures, are viewed as inferior. Ethnic people do not receive safe, effective nursing care when cultural differences are omitted from nursing care plans and medical programs. Ethnicity should be included in nursing ranks and in curricula of nursing schools. The three nursing education models—cultural diversity, humanistic attitudes, and patient advocate—are outlined for nursing curriculum use. Progress must be made in communication skills and adaptive nursing interventions.

ASIAN AMERICAN

Tien JL. Do Asians Need Less Medication? Journal of Psychosocial Nursing and Mental Health Services, 22:19, 1984.

Based on the author's observations, Asians can easily develop adverse reactions or side effects, even with smaller dosages of psychotropic drugs than normally prescribed. Therefore, the following suggestions were made: (1) to prevent further misuse and abuse, psychopharmacology should be included in the curriculum for psychiatric professionals, especially psychiatric interns, with clinical exposure to victims suffering from irreversible side effects; (2) alternative treatment modalities, such as exorcism, herbal medicine, acupressure, and so forth, should be considered by modern psychiatric professionals for patients and families who have the desire to use them and believe that they will be effective; and (3) scientific studies should be conducted to compare psychotropic drug responses between Asian and other groups and to determine the effectiveness of alternative treatment modalities.

BLACK AMERICAN

Hines P, Boyd-Franklin N. Black American families. *In* McGoldrick M, Pearce JK, Giordano J (eds). Ethnicity & Family Therapy. New York: The Guilford Press, 1982, pp. 55–83.

In this chapter the authors refer to previously written texts and articles that have described the Black experience as a family within white society and the long-term effects of slavery and racist oppression. They also elaborate the family pattern of kinship bonds and role flexibility, the need for extended kinship networks, and the importance of religion, work, and education. All have been survival techniques. The approach to family treatment is encouraged, and further suggestions are made to enhance family therapy. Increased sensitivity and less racist cultural awareness are stressed.

HISPANIC AMERICAN

Alvarez R. Delivery of Services for Latino Community Mental Health. California: University of California, Los Angeles, 1975.

This monograph states that the Spanish-speaking group of individuals is seriously underrepresented in mental health service facilities. Folk medicine and faith healers may be used as adjuncts to psychiatric treatment. Three models for improving services to the Spanish-speaking population are described: (1) professional adaptation model, (2) family adaptation model, and (3) barrio service center model. It is suggested that research support and efforts should be increased to improve mental health services to the Spanish-speaking population.

NATIVE AMERICAN

Vogel VJ. American Indian Medicine. Oklahoma: University of Oklahoma Press, Publishing Division, 1970.

This is a fascinating account of Indian medicinal practices in white civilization. Discussed are Indian theories of disease, such as soul loss and sorcery, and methods of combating disease. A list of Indian drugs that have won acceptance in the Pharmacopoeia of the United States *is also included. Drugs such as insulin and penicillin were used in rudimentary form by the aborigines, and coca leaves were used as anesthetics by Peruvian Indians hundreds of years before anesthesia was introduced in 1884. Methods of treating injuries, from fractures to snakebites, and even surgeries are presented. Also included is a discussion of the influence of Indian folklore upon domestic medicine.*

Self-Study Exercises

After reading the chapter, write a short paragraph in answer to each of the following questions:

1. What are the definitions of culture, race, ethnicity, nation, folk group, and folk medicine?

2. What are some of the concepts of mental health and mental illness across cultures?

3. How might a nurse's attitudes influence the therapeutic outcome when the nurse counsels the culturally different client?

4. What theoretical approaches may be useful in mental health nursing assessment with the culturally different client?

5. Which mental health problems are prevalent across cultures?

6. How can a holistic approach be used to treat a client within a cultural context?

BASIC CONCEPTS IN PSYCHIATRIC NURSING

UNIT II

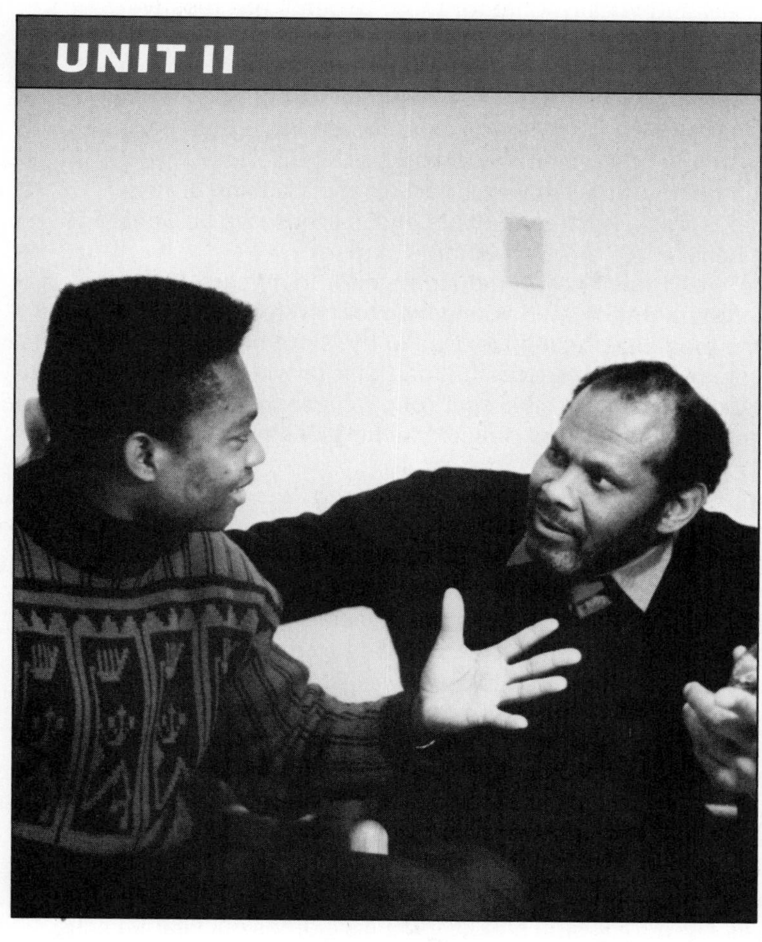

Individual growth can't take precedence over relationships; it can't because it ceases to be growth in the attempt.

HUGH PRATHER

A Nurse Speaks

by John A. Payne

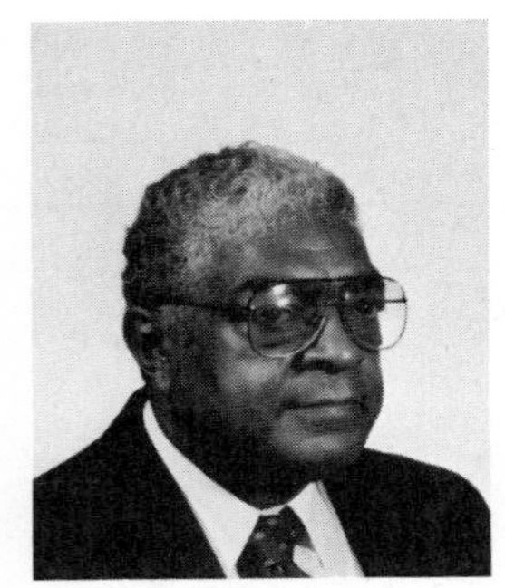

Forty years ago psychiatry was practiced in an environment vastly different from the one in which it is practiced today. Most patients were treated in large state hospitals, which were like small towns with their own store, restaurant, churches, farms, power plant, carpentry shop, and buildings housing thousands of patients and staff. There were buildings for admission, treatment, infirmaries, chronic quiet units, and chronic disturbed units.

As nursing students, we were taught to care for patients who were receiving sedation, insulin shock, electric shock, malaria therapy, continuous hydrotherapy, wet packs, supraorbital lobotomies, physical restraints, and seclusion. All of these treatments were designed to make the patients more amenable to psychotherapy or to calm them or for the safety of themselves or others. The disturbed wards were usually noisy and very active places in which patients acted out their psychoses both physically and vocally. Care for these patients was mostly custodial and involved keeping them clean, fed, safe, and calm.

I distinctly remember one patient who was almost continuously kept in seclusion because of bizarre and aggressive behavior. He would not keep his clothes on, could not safely use eating utensils, and roared like a lion. Because of his behavior, he was frequently referred to as the *Lion Man*.

Keeping him clean and fed was a major project for the staff and always required several people. It was a frustrating experience because we all wanted to help him and see him behave in a more acceptable manner.

During the Korean War, I was away in the air force for four years. For three years I was a part of a system that treated young men for psychiatric problems by using many of the same modalities that were used in the state hospitals. The treatment there was somewhat more successful than that provided in the state hospitals because most of the men's visible signs of psychoses were of recent origin, having been caused by the stress of basic training or the stress of being in battle.

In my fourth year, psychotropic drugs were introduced. We began to use them very cautiously on our patients, with very limited success. As the doctors became more familiar with the drugs and increased the dosages, the results showed much improved behavior with most patients. Gradually no patients were being put into packs, and the hydrotherapy room was seldom used.

After being discharged from the air force, I returned to the hospital in which I had trained. As I went to the different buildings, I was surprised to see that here too there had been a decrease in the use of the old treatment modalities. Patients for the most part appeared much calmer; no patients were in seclusion all of the time, not even the *Lion Man*.

One day while walking on the grounds with one of the charge attendants, he asked me if I knew who a patient sitting on a bench talking with another patient was. I said, "No. Who is he?" "That is the guy we used to call the *Lion Man*." What a change! He told me how they had given him Thorazine and how within one week he was out of seclusion and keeping his clothes on. Gradually he began to socialize with staff and other patients. Within one month he was playing checkers, and within one year he was granted ground privileges. Truly the psychotropic drugs revolutionized the treatment of psychiatric patients.

Some psychotherapeutic modalities that had been used in smaller settings began to be used in the state hospitals. Group therapy, milieu therapy, and remotivation therapy became the vogue, and with this the role of nursing became a more therapeutic one.

During President Kennedy's tenure in office, the Community Mental Health Bill was passed. This provided funds for moving the teatment of patients from the large state hospitals to the local hospital. Two things were significant about this legislation. First, all levels and modalities of treatment had to be provided to all residents within a specific "catchment area." And, second, all disciplines (including nursing) had to be represented on the treatment team.

States passed Patient's Rights Bills that released thousands of patients who had spent many years in state hospitals into the community. A part of the movement that was never adequate was the provision of group homes and follow-up supervision. This has led to our present situation of many actively psychotic ex-patients wandering our streets as homeless citizens. A change is going to come, and nursing is going to be an important part of that change. For now we have nurses in ever-increasing numbers who are becoming psychotherapists and psychiatric nurse practitioners. They will be leaders in providing care themselves and through mental health and/or psychiatric technicians—for nursing is still the only discipline that is proficient in providing 24-hour care to people in need.

CHAPTER 5

Evolution of Nursing in Psychiatric Settings

Hildegard E. Peplau

OUTLINE

KEY TERMS, CONCEPTS, AND PEOPLE

The key terms, concepts, and people listed here also appear in bold where they are defined or discussed in this chapter.

FLORENCE NIGHTINGALE
DOROTHEA DIX
LINDA RICHARDS
HARRIET BAILEY

HILDEGARD E. PEPLAU
NURSING: A SOCIAL POLICY STATEMENT
PHENOMENA RELATIVE TO PSYCHIATRIC NURSING
STANDARDS OF PSYCHIATRIC AND MENTAL HEALTH NURSING PRACTICE
NURSING PRACTICE ACTS
GENERAL STANDARDS
CODES OF ETHICS

OBJECTIVES

After studying this chapter, the student will be able to:

1. Place contemporary nursing within a perspective of the historical development of psychiatric nursing.
2. Recognize the role psychiatric nursing has played in the development of nursing as a whole.
3. Appreciate the gradual evolution of the workrole of nurses in psychiatric settings, in the light of changing societal circumstances.
4. Recognize major components in the work of other health care providers working in various psychiatric settings.
5. Know available contemporary guidelines for use in providing psychiatric nursing care.

History derives from many sources and serves important purposes. New opportunities and challenges arise with each era. Events, in those particular times, create new contexts in which choices are made, actively or by default. The narrative of history is rooted in such events. History consists not only in facts, dates, and circumstances of events, but also in trends, themes, and patterns that characterize those situations. All of these involve the participation of persons. One purpose of history is to pinpoint the continuities in the forward movement of people—of nurses—in society.

The history of psychiatric nursing is about the struggles, choices, and progress that nurses made over many years in developing this component of the field of nursing. It is the story of the continuities—the beginnings, forward steps that were taken, a report of how psychiatric nurses in the United States got to their present position in nursing and society. The whole history of psychiatric nursing has not yet been told. It is a long story—much longer than what is presented in this chapter, which primarily contains highlights in the development of psychiatric nursing in the United States.

There are always lessons to be learned from history. One such lesson is that there were very courageous nurses, working in psychiatric hospitals, who were willing to take a stand on unpopular issues of their day. At the turn of the twentieth century, and earlier, psychiatric nursing was an unpopular field of work. It shared the general stigma attached to mental illness and to the institutions that cared for psychiatric patients.

Another lesson to be learned is that after World War II, when a change in attitude toward the mentally ill occurred, the nursing profession was able to rise to this challenge. It was able to pursue opportunities promised in the provisions of the National Mental Health Act of 1946. Nursing's readiness occurred not so much by design but rather as a consequence of the persistence of a few psychiatric nursing leaders. In earlier years, from the beginning of organized nursing, they had spoken out, persuaded, and therefore helped to shape the general direction taken by the nursing profession. Their perspective, eventually adopted by the profession, was to include psychiatric nursing as an important component of the whole of nursing.

It is useful to learn lessons such as these, seeing how they emerged from the context of earlier times and with the evolution of psychiatric nursing. It is not the lessons per se that have contemporary relevance but rather the fact that struggle, persistence, and choice shaped nursing's future. All nurses, wittingly and unwittingly, are in the same way agents of change and are therefore participants in shaping nursing for today and in the future. Fresh opportunities arise, political winds—inside and outside the profession—shift and blow in new directions, social forces impinge in new ways, all allowing or forcing choices that nurses make, individually and collectively. Such choices shape and reshape nursing.

Nursing leaders and all other nurses are in one way or another participants in the drama of making nursing's history. It is out of this ongoing history-making process that the present place, role, and function of psychiatric nursing have emerged. Nurses who know the history of psychiatric nursing gain a sense of cohesion, of continuity, between their nursing forebears and their own present-day work. Psychiatric nursing today can be more clearly understood when viewed from this historical perspective. The future of psychiatric nursing, which lies ahead, can be more clearly determined when its past is appreciated; that future lies in the hands of the present generation of nurses—especially those who care deeply about the needs of the mentally ill.

Brief History of Psychiatric Nursing

EARLY DEVELOPMENT: PRE-WORLD WAR II

Pennsylvania Hospital in Philadelphia was the first hospital to be built in the United States. Of the first two patients admitted, one was a mentally ill person. Thus, from the beginning of hospital health care, psychiatric care was a component of the whole. While this pattern did not continue uninterrupted, over the years psychiatric units in general hospitals eventually, in the 1950's, became the norm. In the interim period psychiatric services were split off as separate institutions were built for the mentally ill.

The nursing profession as such was not yet established in 1752 when Pennsylvania Hospital was opened. In the mid-eighteenth century and earlier, "nursing" was an expected function of all women. In earlier centuries, even as the medical profession was beginning to develop, it was women who "nursed" their sick family members in their homes. Later on, mostly as "good works," a religious duty, women began to provide nursing care as a voluntary activity to sick people in the community, convents, asylums, and institutions as these were built. During the Industrial Revolution, beginning in the eighteenth century, nursing began to be an occupation—apprenticeship training and employment for wages being two of its characteristics. Although nursing has been called a "profession," it is only in the twentieth century that criteria by which occupations are objectively judged to be a profession are being met by nursing.

In 1751, the year before Pennsylvania Hospital opened, ". . . a suitable Matron" to "take care of the House and of the sick" was appointed (Packard 1957). These two concepts, "Matron" and "House," have a very long history. During the Feudal period in Europe, when land was the major resource base, and well into the Victorian Era, when capital became the major economic resource, the great Houses of Europe were not generally called homes (Painter and Painter 1985). The term "House" referred to an institution for production of virtually everything needed for the survival of all occupants of an entire estate. The landowner was the "Master," a specified position held by the male owner of exceedingly large tracts of land. The Master had virtually complete authority over his wife, servants, children, and slaves. In his absence his wife, called "Mistress," was in charge; in her absence, a mature woman called "Matron" was in charge. This hierarchical arrangement later became the model for organization of the nuclear family, industries, asylums, and hospitals as these evolved in the eighteenth and nineteenth centuries. As in the Manor Houses, patients in early institutions had to perform some domestic work "for the good of the whole."

The title "Matron" was in use at Pennsylvania Hospital from 1752 to 1760. The first one, Elizabeth Gardner, held this position as long as the facility remained small. In 1756, a specific building to house more "sick poor" was built and called a hospital. In 1757 a man was appointed and given the title of "Steward," having the function of, but a status above, a Matron in Manor Houses (Packard 1957). When **Florence Nightingale** proposed her model for schools to educate nurses in 1860, she envisioned preparing nurses at two levels—Matrons and ordinary nurses.

From its inception, Pennsylvania Hospital admitted all sick persons who were in need. Their care was provided by attendants, who were called "nurses." Their work is the earliest root of psychiatric nursing in this country. In 1793, the staff, called "the hospital family," lived in "the picture house" until 1898 when a "nurses' home" was built. The term "nurses' residence" was used much later in public mental hospitals.

Public Mental Hospitals

The first public mental hospital in "British North America" opened in Williamsburg, Virginia, in 1773* (Zwilling 1985). At first, it was a small institution, having "24 cells,

*In 1885 this hospital burned down; in 1986 it was reconstructed as a part of Colonial Williamsburg, and it has exhibits on the mental health care that was provided in that facility from 1773 to 1885.

an apartment for a live-in keeper, and a meeting room for the overseeing court of directors." At about the same time, a church and a courthouse were erected within the city; the "Public Hospital," however, was located "like the gaol . . . on the edge of town for those poor souls that must live on the fringe of society" (Pappas 1985).

By 1885 there were more than 50 public mental hospitals in the United States. Virtually all of them were built on large tracts of land on the edge of or beyond a city, were hierarchically organized—much like the Manor Houses—and operated "for the good of the whole." Some of these institutions were almost totally self-contained communities. Some had their own police units, post offices, fire departments, and laundry. Some had railroad sidings to bring in coal and supplies. There were rooms, apartments, or houses for staff, distributed according to status and often rent-free. (By the 1950's such on-grounds living quarters for hospital staff began not to be provided.) Typically, at first, the Medical Superintendent had a very large apartment and the Director of Nursing a smaller one, usually within the administration or central building. Some hospitals had extensive farms or dairies that produced much of the food the compound required. Patients, supervised by employees, provided most, if not all, of the labor required for maintenance outside and within the hospital buildings: to raise, harvest, store, and serve the food and to keep the buildings and grounds in repair, clean, and often quite attractive. In keeping with a prevailing value that "idle hands do the devil's work," it was believed that keeping the patients busy was good for them. In an insightful paper published in 1961, Rouslin has described how patients as "chronic helpers" fit well into the continuing maintenance and economic effectiveness of the hospital but with perpetuation of their illness (Rouslin 1982).

There were, of course, some patients who could not, would not, or did not work. Many of these patients eventually were housed in "back" wards. The tendency was to move patients (or threaten to) periodically, from up-front units, such as admissions and other somewhat "better" wards (cleaner, open doors, larger staff, etc.), through a progression of units to the ones farthest back, where the long-term chronic patients were "warehoused." Medical Superintendents, masters over the entire compound, presided over these self-sufficient enclosures—almost "closed systems." The few physicians on staff prescribed medications, such as paraldehyde; treatments and/or hydrotherapy; seclusion or restraints; and often rules of conduct for staff. Attendants were, in effect, white collar workers who managed units, supervised domestic work by patients, and observed and reported patient behavior to R.N.'s and M.D.'s. Before the 1960's, untrained attendants greatly outnumbered R.N.'s, often were married to them, and bossed them in the name of male protection of women in dangerous situations. The ratio of staff to patients, sometimes 1 : 400, and the lack of nursing publications to provide adequate direction were among factors that eventuated in custodial care.

At psychiatric conventions into the 1960's, many mental hospital superintendents attended meetings planned for nurses. Apparently, they felt more comfortable in these situations than in meetings where their psychiatric colleagues were beginning to discuss treatments other than custody and "work therapy." Their concerns had more to do with crops, animal husbandry, farm equipment, and the problems of general management of an estate. With the nurses they could assert their authority, as a matter of custom, on whether what the nurses were saying was "right" or "wrong," for back at the House they had control over the nursing schools in Public Mental Hospitals, which finally closed in the late 1950's.

The Beginning of Psychiatric Nursing in the United States

The first school of nursing in the United States opened in 1872. A decade later, in 1882, the first school of nursing in a mental hospital opened at McLean Hospital, Belmont, Massachusetts. This marked the beginning of psychiatric nursing in this country. In 1886, the McLean Asylum Training School for Nurses graduated its first class of 15 women and admitted a first class of male nursing students (Mericle 1983). This provided the first opportunity for American men to become trained nurses (Mericle 1983). Thereafter, particularly in psychiatric settings, male nurses (and attendants) were most valued when control of aggression of patients or protection of nurses or physicians seemed necessary. In 1986, a century later, "the number of men enrolled in all types of nursing programs has increased steadily since 1978. In 1984, men accounted for 6.2 percent or 13,652 of total enrollment in R.N. programs. Overall, about 3 percent of nurses are male" (Rosenfeld 1986). Moreover, in recent decades, as nurturing behavior by men has become more acceptable, men in nursing are finding that the scope of their nursing work has broadened considerably.

Social Forces Leading to Mental Illness

The opening of the McLean School was a propitious event for both society and the nursing profession. In the

130 years between the opening of hospitals in Philadelphia and Williamsburg and the opening of the McLean School, a great many social forces were creating new challenges for the leaders of the country. As Pennsylvania Hospital opened its doors, the Industrial Revolution, already well under way in Europe, was beginning to change life in America. Philadelphia was already a thriving commercial city. Just after the turn of the nineteenth century, between 1813 and 1913, six million Slavs, particularly from German territories such as Poland, came to the United States. Many were recruited for work in the coal mines, steel mills, and iron foundries — industries that were springing up rapidly, particularly along the eastern part of the country. Capitalism, the concept of economic liberty, and other values, such as freedom and individualism — principles guiding development in America — were frightening and suspect to some immigrants. Those who had recently arrived from very small European villages — some still governed by remnants of Feudalism — were particularly vulnerable. Modern science, born during the Renaissance (14th to 17th centuries), was also being transplanted to America. Particularly in the nineteenth century in the eastern part of the country, but also with the moving frontier (immigrants edging westward), there existed great ferment, rapid population increases, and strains of the "melting pot" and upward mobility. Many people experienced stress, tension, anxiety, and conflict. It is therefore not surprising that many immigrants and others became mentally ill. Many mental hospitals, Pennsylvania (1752), Williamsburg (1773), McLean (1811), and others, attempted to meet this challenge. But, because of the rapidly increasing numbers of mentally ill patients, many of them were housed in jails.

Modern science had not yet progressed to the point of providing viable theories, explanatory of mental illness, that could guide corrective treatment. There were many speculations about causation: sin and the devil's influence, imbalance among the four humors — blood, phlegm, choler, and black bile (from Galen c. 130–200) — laziness and willfulness, focal infections, and others. None of these "theories" led to viable treatments.

"Moral Management" of Mentally Ill Patients

In the late seventeenth century, a physician named Edward Tyson (1651–1708) was appointed in charge of Bethlehem Hospital, built in England in the thirteenth century and often called "Bedlam." His first action was to bring in female "nurses" to care for patients; by this and other means he humanized care (Boorstin 1983). In the United States, at Pennsylvania Hospital, Benjamin Rush, a physician, also pioneered in humane care. At Williamsburg and elsewhere, a program of care called "moral treatment" was developing, often in reaction against the harsh, cruel, punitive, and coercive behavior of untrained attendants toward mentally ill patients.

Moral treatment, or "moral management," included the use of kindness, teaching self-control to patients by persuasion, work programs, and leisure time activities of various kinds — all provided in a climate of optimism and a benign environment. "The moral management movement attained full bloom in Williamsburg during the 1840's" (Painter and Painter 1985). Some psychiatric facilities (particularly small private ones) for care of patients from the enlarging middle class were called "retreats." This was in accord with the general ideal that "to get away from it all" in an attractive, humane, nondemanding environment would be curative. Nevertheless, the increasing numbers of mentally ill — many of them incarcerated in jails — became a public concern, particularly in the first half of the nineteenth century. Hospitals began to add beds and buildings. "Waning optimism, concern for costs, and an overriding fear of social deviancy" greatly damaged the humanitarian efforts (Chappell 1985).

Dorothea Dix's Crusade

In 1841, **Dorothea Dix** — who on July 10, 1861, was appointed Superintendent of Women "Nurses" in the Civil War — began a crusade to get the mentally ill out of jails. She traveled across the nation persuading legislatures to build hospitals for the mentally ill. And they did! Large and ever-larger public mental hospitals, most of them on palatial tracts of land, were built, often well removed from cities. Dix's cause was driven by humanitarian concerns, which she felt deeply. However, what Dix did not recognize nor take into account was the fragility of moral treatment, which was little understood and was effective only when carefully selected staff were in ample numbers. Moral treatment was soon crushed by an on-rushing, vast, bureaucratic, mental hospital system nationwide, which was well in place by the dawn of the twentieth century. Dix's concern, however, was not in understanding mental illness nor in the nature of treatment. No doubt she assumed that physicians in public mental hospitals had these concerns under control. At the time of Dix's crusade, medical education was often a hodgepodge, as shown by the Flexner report (1909). There were no nursing schools until 1872. There was no scientific understanding of mental illness. Dix's concern and her commendable crusade were aimed at getting patients out of jails, out of chains, away from association with criminals, and into hospitals.

Public hospitals were built away from cities, and as it turned out, away from families of patients. (This, of course, occurred a century before the view that "mental illness is a system effect" replaced the idea of mental illness as an intrapersonal disturbance.) Certainly, political decisions about locations turned on many factors: visibility of the mentally ill in cities at a time when able-bodied men, required for developing industries, were the nation's norm; fear of the behavior of social deviants particularly among upwardly mobile middle-class people; prevailing ideas that fresh air, rest, quiet, and work promoted health (one thing was surely proved—these factors are not curative of mental illness); and, no doubt, economic considerations—land was surely less expensive outside the cities than in them.

Training Schools

In 1841, **Linda Richards**—later America's "first trained nurse" and a champion of psychiatric nursing—was born in Potsdam, New York. In 1873, she graduated from the Training School, opened in 1872, at the New England Hospital for Women and Children. Ms. Richards then went to Bellevue Hospital in New York City as night superintendent. She was the first American trained woman to hold a hospital position. In 1878 she returned to Boston, where she collaborated with Dr. Edward Cowles in organizing the training of nurses at Boston City Hospital (Peplau 1982). In 1882, Cowles, by then superintendent at McLean Hospital, and Ms. Richards started the first formally organized training school for nurses in a hospital for the mentally ill. This event launched psychiatric nursing.

Before the turn of the twentieth century, McLean had its students in an "affiliation" experience in general nursing with Massachusetts General Hospital. This event signaled, from the outset, that the direction of American nursing was toward becoming one unified whole practice field. This is in contrast, for example, to the British experience, where the separate training of mental health nurses began in 1891 and continues to the present time. "Nightingale herself showed no desire to include asylums within the scope of nursing reform. The links with general nursing did not occur until later" (Carpenter 1980).

Although there had already been graduates of nurse training schools in America for almost a quarter-century, in 1895 two British nurses were employed at Pennsylvania Hospital. One, Lucy Walker, was superintendent of nurses; the other was her assistant. The reason for this reliance on England for nurses is unclear, but it may not be a total mystery. American women, active in the Civil War (1861 to 1865), were showing public interest in improving their status. Public high schools—some for girls—began to develop (1860 to 1880). Y.W.C.A.'s were opening (Boston, 1866). The National Women's Suffrage Association was organized (1869). A Nursing Society was organized by Friends (Quakers) in Philadelphia (1839). "Trained Nurses" were organizing nationally (NLN, 1893; ANA, 1897). Beginning in 1871, training schools for nurses were opening in hospitals all along the Eastern seaboard (549 schools by 1900) (Oderkirk 1985). The learned men at Pennsylvania Hospital were surely aware of these developments among "uppity women."

One historian suggests that the School of Nursing at Pennsylvania Hospital became one of America's most outstanding schools after Lucy Walker became superintendent (1895 to 1907). Ms. Walker brought "a heritage of British nursing methods—the emphasis on rigid discipline, hierarchical authority, efficient organization, and autonomy of nursing services" (Tomes 1984). Ms. Walker was born in 1860 and received her training at St. Bartholomew's in London, a school of the Nightingale model. She was a stern disciplinarian both of herself and of others. Like many career women of her day, she was frequently ill, had one "nervous breakdown," and resigned for health reasons. She would be considered something of a martinet by today's expectations of nurse executives. She expected unquestioning obedience and loyalty to her methods, and she forced resignations or fired nurses for even slight disobedience. She generated much resentment by unfavorable comparisons of American nurses with British ones. Gradually she developed a nursing staff composed of nurses who had graduated during her tenure at Pennsylvania; a "little world of our own," they called it. She set rules for students regarding "arising, eating, resting, studying and retiring," and about daily exercises, seniority among classes of students, room inspections, dress, school grades, and virtually every detail of work and personal life of students. She was especially a guardian of the moral character of students. The student population consisted mainly of Protestant (62%) young women (mostly ages 21 to 24) of less than high school education, but there were some (17%) who had had some private education. When Ms. Walker asked the Board of Managers to enlarge the nurses' home, she commented on what ". . . a severe ordeal" it was "for women of refinement to share their rooms" with such a mixed group of students. There were also some American nurse superintendents who patterned operation of their training schools along similar lines.

Developments Toward an Organized Profession

The last two decades of the nineteenth century saw considerable activity within nursing. "Training schools" were being established at a rapid rate. There were at least 35 in mental hospitals before the turn of the century; in 1936, 67 such schools were accredited by the American Psychiatric Association. The American Society of Superintendents of Training Schools (ASSTS—now the National League for Nursing) was formed in 1893. The Nurses' Associated Alumni of the United States and Canada (now the American Nurses' Association) was established in 1897. A course in Hospital Economics for Nurses was offered in 1889, by Teachers College, Columbia University—the entry point into universities for nursing education (Roberts 1954). In 1899 the International Council of Nurses was organized (Bridges 1967). All of these remarkable developments toward an organized profession occurred less than three decades after the establishment in 1872 of the first training school for nurses.

Reports of meetings of these organizations document the views held by nurses on pressing problems of the profession and they served as vehicles for wide dissemination of those views. At the first ASSTS meeting, an appeal was made to raise the standards of nursing in insane hospitals. Linda Richards, first President of ASSTS, called for standards and uniformity of training of *all* nurses. The issue then was the relation between general and psychiatric training schools. Snively commented that "schools attached to special hospitals" would ultimately benefit the entire profession. There were objections to having schools in mental hospitals, but these objections were mostly due to concern for having "all around" rather than specialty training for nurses in basic schools.

Kraepelin's System of Classification

Other events were occurring in the late 1800's that had a bearing on psychiatric nursing. Kraepelin's system of classification of mental diseases, introduced in 1896 by Adolph Meyer, was adopted for use in mental hospitals. Classification is a first step in making a field scientific. Kraepelin identified symptoms related to known categories of mental disease; as was then occurring in medicine, a search for causes of these symptoms was to follow, leading to definitive treatment. That search continues. Descriptive Psychiatry has prevailed, although there are now many developing theories of causation of mental illness. One beginning point occurred in 1895, when Breuer and Freud published "*Studies in Hysteria*." In 1909 Freud gave a lecture in the United States, at Clark University, which stimulated new thought about causation of mental illness among American psychiatrists and psychologists.

Exploring Integration of Psychiatric Nursing Training into Basic Nursing Programs

In 1909, the ASSTS appointed a "Sectional Committee of the Committee on Education." Members included Sara Parsons, Amy Hilliard, Linda Richards, and Elizabeth May—all nurse leaders who championed the cause of the mentally ill and promoted the development of psychiatric nursing. The committee recommended "affiliations" of general hospital students in psychiatric hospitals for three to nine months in their third year of training. There was not universal agreement on this recommendation; in fact, it took several decades before all basic nursing students had theory and clinical practice in psychiatric nursing included in their generic nursing education. The committee also proposed use of a list of books on "nursing the insane," all of which were written by non-nurses, for there were as yet no psychiatric nursing textbooks written by nurse authors.

The crucial question of whether to include affiliations in psychiatric nursing in all basic curricula was discussed at length many times during the first half of the twentieth century. The question was crucial, since inclusion of this component of nursing meant that nursing would then become one whole comprehensive field of nursing practice. General hospitals that conducted training schools did not, as a rule, accept psychiatric patients. Sending students away for several months of training in a psychiatric hospital suggested at least some erosion of the basic school's authority over them and possibly of the student's loyalty to the basic school. Parents were apprehensive, too, for they tended to share the prevailing social fear of mental patients. Training schools were generally viewed as safe, protective places that kept close watch on the "young girls" who entered them. Nevertheless, during the period between 1909 and 1943, when many schools opened, there were an increasing number of efforts toward favorable resolution of the question (Oderkirk 1985). Neuropsychiatric casualties (69,394) among those who served in World War I (1914 to 1918) helped to force the issue toward resolution.

Each of the three curriculum guides (1917, 1927, 1937) published by NLNE (now NLN) suggested, in succession, a greater emphasis on psychiatric nursing. In 1920, the first textbook on psychiatric nursing, *Nursing*

Mental Diseases, written by **Harriet Bailey,** a nurse, was published. "Postgraduate courses" offered by mental hospitals began to be provided—14 in 13 states by 1929—suggesting that R.N.'s had a need left unfilled by their basic nursing program. The Grading Committee reported that 88% of nursing students had less than two months' experience in psychiatric nursing services—73% had not yet spent one day with a psychiatric patient (Nursing Schools Today, 1934). Meanwhile, by 1930, more than half of the beds of all hospitals were for mentally ill patients. Moreover, these were the years of the Great Depression (1929 to 1935), when unemployment of nurses was excessive. Nurses were needed in public mental hospitals; however, in that era, training schools prepared for "private duty nursing." In big-city general hospitals, staff nursing was provided by student nurses, not by R.N.'s. "Free labor," Mrs. Robb called it (Robb 1897).

Evolution of the Nurse's Role

The history of nursing is full of attempts to define the workrole of nurses. In the earlier eras, the emphasis was mostly on the character of the student nurse. Patience, tact, and honesty were prime virtues. The morality of nurses was a major concern. Obedience and loyalty to the hospital were expected. Richards has described how students worked from 5:30 A.M. to 9 P.M., when they left to sleep in rooms adjacent to the wards in which they worked. The students had no evenings out, no study time, no recreation, were overworked, poorly fed, and had no supervision. Twice each year they went to church (Richards 1949). The "born nurse" was a person of impeccable moral character. The injunction toward moral character was buttressed by long lists of "duties of the nurse," do's and don'ts, things nurses should, ought, or must do or not do. Some "shoulds" were even called "principles." Staff nurses were called "general duty nurses."

In the 1930's the profession conducted a major study of the activities of nurses (Johns and Pfefferkorn 1934). This led to the publication of long lists of activities of nurses in various positions, such as general duty nurse, head nurse, supervisor, and instructor. These activities then began to appear in job descriptions and in activity-oriented definitions of nursing (Henderson 1961).

A decade or so later, the ANA embarked on a massive study of functions, which similarly provided long lists of functions connected with various nursing positions in employment situations. A publication resulted from this effort (Hughes 1958).

In the 1950's and 1960's, the sociological concept of *role* entered the picture. Discussion and publications began to describe the workrole and sub-roles of nurses. As can be seen from the foregoing accounts, the movement in describing the work of nurses has been from concrete "duties" toward more abstract ideas such as role.

In 1972, exactly one century after the training schools for nurses began in 1872, New York State adopted a revised Nursing Practice Act that is having far-reaching impact on nursing. In 1980, the ANA publication ***Nursing: A Social Policy Statement*** proposed a definition of nursing in terms of a trend—already evident in licensing laws in many states—that originated with the New York Practice Act. In the ANA publication, nursing is defined as "the diagnosis and treatment of human responses to actual and potential health problems" (ANA 1980). This definition represents a paradigm shift—a reformulation of the question "what do nurses do?" to "what *phenomena* do nurses fix, correct, ameliorate, relieve, or prevent by addressing nursing practices to them?" (Fig. 5–1).

The workrole of nurses in mental hospitals has evolved somewhat along the lines similar to those just described. Attendants in psychiatric institutions before and during the nineteenth century were called "cell keepers" and later "custodial attendants." Tucker, a nurse, decried the use of chains, iron chairs, handcuffs, straps, crib beds, and other primitive devices to restrain patients. Nurses were taught to use isolation, rest, diet, persuasion, and suggestion, with appeals to the intellect and will power of the patient. One nurse said: "We have to study, if we study blindly." That was the problem—limited knowledge, if any, about the phenomena observed by nurses, which, through nursing practices, they were expected to help correct in a way favorable for patients. In the absence of definitive nursing knowledge, nurses carried out medical prescriptions, assisted in medical treatments, provided recreational and diversional activities, often served as companions to patients, and promoted "habit training"—all within a framework of optimism, leniency, and patience.

LATER DEVELOPMENT: POST-WORLD WAR II

Wars produce profound social changes. World War II had far-reaching impact on nursing and particularly on psychiatric nursing. During the war there were enormous shortages of physicians, stateside and in both theaters of war. Consequently, registered nurses had out of necessity to take on far greater authority and responsibility than ever before. Never again, thereafter, would nurses be satisfied with their previous "handmaiden" status. The thrust toward professionalization of the occupation of nursing moved steadily and more

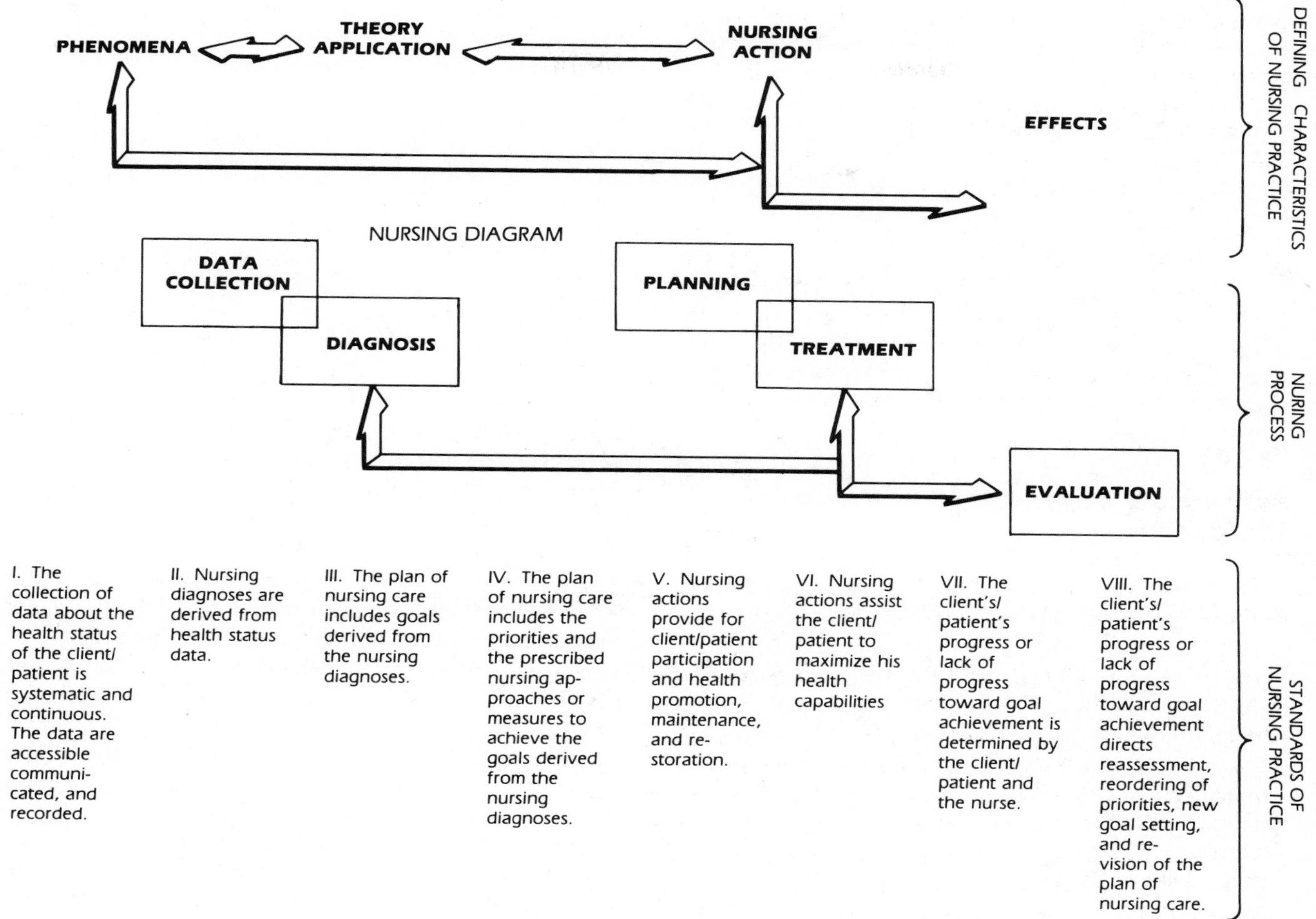

Figure 5–1. *Defining characteristics of nursing practice: relationship to the nursing process and the standards of nursing practice.* (From American Nurses' Association. *Nursing: A Social Policy Statement.* Kansas City, MO: American Nurses' Association, 1980.)

swiftly after World War II. Psychiatric nursing developed rapidly and provided considerable leadership in the profession as a whole during the four decades between the end of World War II and the publication of this book.

There had been many psychiatric casualties during World War I. Public opinion, not universally sympathetic, attributed these "breakdowns" to problems ranging from weak will power to cowardice. During and after World War II, public opinion turned on a new idea, namely "that everyone has his breaking point." During the war there were many efforts to treat "combat fatigue" and other psychiatric casualties, often just behind the lines of battle. Nurses participated in such medical treatments as narcosynthesis, subcoma insulin therapy, and Pentothal interviews.

After the war, the high rate of psychiatric casualties aroused public generosity and gave rise to unprecedented federal legislation intended to improve the nation's mental health (40th Anniversary 1986):

3 July 1946	National Mental Health Act signed by President Harry S. Truman
1 April 1949	National Institute of Mental Health established
28 July 1955	Mental Health Study Act signed by President Dwight D. Eisenhower
2 August 1956	Health Amendments Act signed by President Dwight D. Eisenhower
31 October 1963	Mental Retardation Facilities and Community Mental Health Centers Construction Act signed by President John F. Kennedy
8 November 1966	Narcotic Addiction Rehabilitation Act signed by President Lyndon B. Johnson
31 December 1970	Comprehensive Alcohol Abuse and Alcoholism Prevention, Treatment, and Rehabilitation Act signed by President Richard M. Nixon
21 March 1972	Drug Abuse Office and Treatment Act
And others . . .	

In the half-century before World War II, the development of psychiatric nursing was greatly influenced by prevailing norms: descriptive psychiatry, hospital financing and control of training schools, largely physician control of content of teaching, a somewhat tenuous relationship between psychiatric nursing and nursing as a whole field, and a paucity of well-educated psychiatric nurse leaders. In 1943, with funds allocated under the Bolton Act, three university-sponsored courses in psychiatric nursing were started. By 1956, there were 28 university programs — 20 on the master's level, two in schools of public health, and six at the undergraduate level (which soon were phased out). There are currently over 100 graduate programs in psychiatric nursing at the master's and doctoral levels.

Advanced Psychiatric Nursing Education

Between 1946 and in the 1970's, funds available under the National Mental Health Act provided support for academic-based programs in "advanced psychiatric nursing" and for the preparation of teachers and supervisors, with stipends for students. The GI Bill, which provided support for education of World War II veterans, also enabled many R.N.'s who had served their country to enter academic study. Furthermore, many states provided scholarships, particularly for nurses employed in public mental hospitals. In other words, in the late 1940's there was generous support for the development of psychiatric nursing and for the education of nurses. However, there were many constraints. There were exceedingly few psychiatric nurses who had the proper credentials to qualify as academic faculty.

These leaders and their students were among the early contributors to the literature in psychiatric nursing (Smoyak and Rouslin 1982):

Madge Bauman	Cecile Lediger
Barbara Bernard	Eleanor Lewis
Kathleen Black	Garland Lewis
Nora Cline	Marguerite Manfreda
Annie Laurie Crawford	Ruth Matheney*
Laura Fitzsimmons*	Ann K. McGibbon*
Lavonne Fry	Dorothy Mereness
Lee Fuller	Agnes B. Middleton
Esther A. Garrison	Tirzah Morgan*
Winifred Gibson	Theresa G. Muller*
Ruth Gilbert*	Hildegard E. Peplau
Rose Godbout	Mary Redmond*
Mildred Gottdank	Alice Robinson
Dorothy Gregg	Mary M. Schmitt
Anne Hargreaves	Katherine Steele*
Marion E. Kalkman	Dorris Stewart
Frances Theilbar*	Jeanette White*
Mary Topalis	
Ruth von Bergen	

*Deceased

There were enormous challenges of defining "advanced psychiatric nursing" and in determining new directions to be taken in teaching graduate students. There were very few psychiatric nursing textbooks, and none that addressed advanced practice until the Burd-Marshall book was published in 1963 (Osborne 1984; Burd and Marshall 1963).

Integration of Psychiatric Nursing Training into Basic Nursing Programs

Affiliations in psychiatric nursing had been progressing. By 1944 a basic experience was offered by 54% of the schools, but the prevailing idea was that the purpose of the exposure was to enrich general nursing practice. It was on June 21, 1952, that the NLN — acting on a petition from a group of psychiatric nurses — established an Interdivisional Council on Psychiatric and Mental Health Nursing. On January 21, 1953, the NLN adopted a recommendation that basic programs in nursing should prepare students for beginning positions in the care of all patients — including psychiatric patients. Thus, seven decades after the McLean school started a training school, psychiatric nursing was finally and fully accepted as a part of the whole of nursing. It was in the 1950's that schools of nursing in mental hospitals began closing at a fairly rapid rate. They had served a worthy purpose.

In this same period, the attendants in psychiatric hospitals began to be threatened by the encroachment of developments in psychiatric nursing. Training programs to develop the attendant's occupation in competition for nurse positions were being set up. There were two major workshops, which included physicians, psychiatric nurses, social scientists, and attendants, to discuss this matter — the first in 1951 in Peoria, and the second in 1952 in Manteno, Illinois. In 1953 the NLN declared that psychiatric attendants and aides were nursing personnel who were to be supervised by R.N.'s.

In order to promote interprogram consultation, develop some cohesion, and reduce isolation, meetings of Directors of Graduate Programs in Psychiatric Nursing were held: 1948 — at NLN, New York City; 1950 — University of Minnesota; 1951 — University of Cincinnati; 1952 — Philadelphia; 1956 — Williamsburg, Virginia; and others. Although many issues and concerns were debated in these meetings, the major question was whether or not psychiatric nurses should be prepared to provide psychotherapy for patients. In 1955, Rutgers University obtained a National Institute of Mental Health (NIMH) grant in support of preparation of only "clinical specialists in advanced psychiatric nursing"; all other programs at that time included teaching or supervision in addition to advanced nursing practice in their one academic year programs. The Rutgers program required two academic years of study plus one month and prepared nurses for individual, group, and family psychotherapy. Many academic programs eventually followed this pattern.

In 1952, the NIMH made grants of funds available to virtually all schools of nursing to enable them to employ a psychiatric nurse faculty member as "integrator." The purpose was to assist all clinical faculty to include basic sociopsychiatric concepts in their teaching. The aim was to sensitize all nurses to the psychosocial stresses inherent in all illness experiences of patients, not to reduce, replace, nor obviate the basic clinical educative experience students had with psychiatric patients. This latter effect occurred, however, in some schools in which faculty seemingly did not recognize the continuing need for more nurses as staff nurses and clinical specialists in psychiatric facilities.

Further Developments in Psychiatric Nursing

In the mid-1950's various psychotropic drugs became available for medicating psychiatric patients, particularly for the relief of anxiety. Simultaneously, Smith, Kline, and French (SKF) laboratories supported production of a film in 1958 entitled *Psychiatric Nursing: The Nurse-Patient Relationship*. This film, which received several awards, encouraged nurses to talk with patients, inasmuch as the new medications made patients more accessible for therapeutic communication. SKF distributed this film to virtually all schools of nursing and psychiatric hospitals at no cost to them. Before the 1950's, nurses generally were not encouraged to talk with patients — they were to keep busy "doing something."

In less than two decades after the Mental Health Act funds became available, developments in psychiatric nursing began to proceed more rapidly. In 1963, two journals addressed to the specific interests of psychiatric nurses began publication: *Perspectives in Psychiatric Care* and the *Journal of Psychiatric Nursing* (since renamed *Journal of Psychosocial Nursing and Mental Health Services*). In 1967, the ANA Division on Psychiatric and Mental Health Nursing published the *Statement on Psychiatric and Mental Health Nursing Practice*, which was revised in 1976. This statement provides a definition of psychiatric nursing, its roles, and its scope. The ANA Division also issued ***Standards of Psychiatric and Mental Health Nursing Practice*** in 1982, which are used widely by responsible nurses (see *front endsheet*). Currently, the ANA has a task force working on the "phenomena project," defining the nursing diagnoses of interest to psychiatric nursing. Table 5–1 summarizes many of the historic contributions to psychiatric nursing.

Overview of Nursing in Today's Psychiatric Settings

NATURE OF THE WORKROLE OF NURSES WITH PSYCHIATRIC PATIENTS

Nurses consider themselves to be enhancers of healing and health, primarily through the use of noninvasive, humanistically oriented nursing practices. In the care of the mentally ill, the main work requires nurses to understand, theoretically, those internal processes that have become dysfunctional. Nursing practices are addressed to these manifestations, when observed in their many patterns and variations, so as to establish a pull or to set these processes in a functional direction. These efforts by nurses help patients develop their capacities into intellectual and interpersonal competencies, such as focusing attention, describing experiences, and naming feelings. These nursing interventions are provided in all nurse-patient interactions: in informal contacts in the milieu and in structured relationships using various therapeutic and psychotherapeutic modalities.

Psychiatric patients additionally receive services from other health care providers — physicians, psychologists, social workers, occupational and recreational therapists, and others. It is generally nurses who plan a patient's daily schedule in accordance with the total treatment plan and the patient's interests. Thus, nurses schedule and often coordinate the services of others so that patients make the best use of them. Nurses accept responsibility for carrying out the prescriptions of physicians for medications and treatments patients are to receive while also maintaining accountability to check and verify the need for and accuracy of such prescriptions. Nurses are active members of interdisciplinary groups, which plan, record, review, and evaluate patient care, and provide peer review evaluations of each other's work.

Psychiatric inpatients are residents in a facility. Their activities of daily living, around-the-clock, are the re-

Text continued on page 102

Table 5–1 • SUMMARY OF HISTORIC CONTRIBUTIONS TO PSYCHIATRIC AND MENTAL HEALTH NURSING

PSYCHIATRIC NURSING LEADER	CONTRIBUTION
Pre-1860	
—	Nursing care for the young, ill, and helpless historically has existed as long as the human race. Care was given by family members, relatives, servants, neighbors, members of religious orders or humanitarian societies, or by convalescing patients or prisoners.
1860	
Florence Nightingale	Established Nightingale School at St. Thomas Hospital in London after Crimean War and worked with untrained women caring for soldiers. *Founder of modern-day nursing.*
1860–1880	
	Emphasized maintaining healthful environment, personal hygiene, cleanliness, and healthful living habits, such as adequate nutrition, exercise, and sleep so that nature could heal. Emphasized kindness toward patients along with custodial care.
Linda Richards	*First graduate nurse and first psychiatric nurse in the United States.* After study under Miss Nightingale, organized nursing services and educational programs in Boston City Hospital and in several state mental hospitals in Illinois.
Dorothea Lynde Dix	*Worked to reform psychiatric care in mental hospitals* and to correct overcrowding and the insufficient number of physicians and attendants.
1882	
—	First school to prepare nurses to care for acutely and chronically mentally ill opened at McLean Hospital, Waverly, Massachusetts, through collaboration of Linda Richards and Dr. Edward Cowles.
1890–1930	
—	Nurses recognized by some administrative psychiatrists in state and private hospitals for their preparation. Nurses relieved of menial housekeeping chores to engage in physical, custodial care of patients. Role primarily to assist physician or carry out procedures for physical care. Few psychological nursing skills. Psychologically concerned with maintaining kind, tolerant attitude and humane treatment.
1920	
Harriet Bailey	*First nurse educator to write a psychiatric nursing text,* Nursing Mental Diseases, 1920. She wrote of the importance of a nurse knowing mental illness and of teaching mental health nursing, and she worked for student experiences in psychiatry. She argued for more holistic care of patients.
1937	
—	The incorporation of psychiatric nursing was recommended by the National League for Nursing for inclusion in basic nursing curriculum.

Table 5-1 • SUMMARY OF HISTORIC CONTRIBUTIONS TO PSYCHIATRIC AND MENTAL HEALTH NURSING *Continued*

PSYCHIATRIC NURSING LEADER	CONTRIBUTION
1946	
—	National Mental Health Act passed, authorizing establishment of National Institute of Mental Health, with funds and programs to train professional psychiatric personnel, conduct psychiatric research, and aid in development of mental health programs at the state level. Provided impetus for psychiatric nursing as a specialty.
1950–1960	
—	Nurse's role included physical care and medications and maintenance of therapeutic milieu. Less emphasis on physical restraints.
Ruth Matheney Mary Topalis	Emphasized importance of milieu therapy and the nurse using this intervention.
1952	
Hildegard E. Peplau	*Formulated first systematic theoretical framework in psychiatric nursing; presented in* Interpersonal Relations in Nursing, 1952. Emphasized that nursing is an interpersonal process and that psychological techniques and theoretical concepts are essential to nursing practice. Emphasized steps in nurse-patient relationship: 1. Nurse helps patient examine situational factors through observation of behavior. 2. Nurse helps patient describe and analyze behavior. 3. Nurse formulates with patient connections between feelings and behavior. 4. Nurse encourages patient to improve interpersonal competence through testing new behavior. 5. Nurse validates with patient when new behavior is integrated into personality structure. Psychoanalytic, interpersonal, and communication theories utilized by nurses.
1953	
—	*The Therapeutic Community*, by Maxwell Jones in Great Britain, laid basis for movement in United States toward therapeutic milieu and nurse's role in this therapy.
1956	
—	National Conference on Graduate Education in Psychiatric Nursing introduced concept of psychiatric clinical nurse specialist. Theoreticians begin to differentiate functions based on master's level of preparation in nursing.
1957	
June Mellow	*Introduced second theoretical approach to psychiatric nursing, called* Nursing Therapy, utilizing psychoanalytic theory in one-to-one approach with schizophrenic patient. *Emphasized providing corrective emotional experience rather than investigating pathological processes or interpersonal developmental processes in order to facilitate integration of overwhelmed ego.*

Table continued on following page

Table 5-1 • SUMMARY OF HISTORIC CONTRIBUTIONS TO PSYCHIATRIC AND MENTAL HEALTH NURSING *Continued*

PSYCHIATRIC NURSING LEADER	CONTRIBUTION
1958	
—	American Nurses' Association established Conference Group on Psychiatric Nursing.
1959	
—	Accredited schools of nursing had to have own psychiatric nursing curriculum and instructor, per National League for Nursing. Could no longer buy services of hospitals to supply education.
1960–1970	
Hildegard E. Peplau Gertrude Ujhely Joyce Travelbee Shirley Burd Loretta Bermosk Joyce Hays Catherine Norris Gertrude Stokes Anne Hargreaves Dorothy Gregg Sheila Rouslin	Nursing leaders emphasized importance of self-awareness and use of self, nurse-patient relationships therapy, therapeutic communication, and psychosocial aspects of general nursing. Peplau formulated the manifestations of anxiety and steps in anxiety intervention, now used by all health care professions. All of these nursing leaders developed various psychological concepts into operational definitions for use in nursing.
1960	
Ida Orlando	*Initiated term* nursing process *and began to delineate its components.* Presented general theoretical framework for all nurse-patient relationships, with focus on client ascertaining meaning of behavior and explaining help needed. Wrote the classic book, *The Dynamic Nurse-Patient Relationship,* 1961.
—	Comprehensive Community Mental Health Act passed, 1960; provided impetus for nurses moving from hospital to community setting.
1961	
Anne Burgess Donna Aguilera	Engaged in crisis work and short-term therapy as well as in long-term therapy. *Applied crisis theory to psychiatric nursing.*
Hildegard E. Peplau	Promoted *primary role of nurse as psychotherapist or counselor* rather than as mother surrogate, socializer, or manager.
1967	
—	American Nurses' Association presented Position Paper on Psychiatric Nursing, endorsing role of clinical specialist as therapist in individual, group, family, and milieu therapies.
—	American Nurses' Association, Division in Psychiatric and Mental Health Nursing Practice published first *Statement on Psychiatric Nursing Practice.*
M. Meldman	Nurse psychotherapist moved into private practice.

Table 5–1 • SUMMARY OF HISTORIC CONTRIBUTIONS TO PSYCHIATRIC AND MENTAL HEALTH NURSING *Continued*

PSYCHIATRIC NURSING LEADER	CONTRIBUTION
1970–1980	
Sheila Rouslin	*Certification of clinical specialists in psychiatric nursing begun* by Division of Psychiatric Mental Health Nursing, New Jersey State Nurses' Association, *because of her leadership.* Later, certification developed by American Nurses' Association.
Shirley Smoyak	*Client defined as individual, group, family, or community;* nurse as family therapist. Expanding role of psychiatric nurse.
Gwen Marram Irene Burnside	*Group and family psychotherapy by graduate-prepared nurses* emphasized by nursing leaders.
Carolyn Clark	*Systems framework was used increasingly* by psychiatric nurses.
—	Change agent, health maintenance, and research roles emphasized in latter half of decade.
Bonnie Bullough	*Legal and ethical aspects of psychiatric care emphasized.*
Madeleine Leininger	*Care of whole person reemphasized. Introduced implications of cultural diversity for mental health services and psychiatric treatment.*
—	Practice as autonomous member of team and in independent or private practice increased in latter half of decade.
Hector Gonzales Doris Mosley Paulette D'Angi	Work with citizens, consumer groups, and consumer organizations increased toward end of decade.
1976	
—	American Nurses' Association Division on Psychiatric and Mental Health Nursing Practice published revised *Statement on Psychiatric and Mental Health Nursing Practice.*
1978	
—	President's Commission Report of 1978 concluded that effects of deinstitutionalization and discharge of patients to community facilities have not worked as expected because of lack of financial, social, medical, and nursing resources and lack of coordination of services.
1980's	
Anne Burgess	*Formulated theory of victimology,* based on extensive studies of adult and child victims of rape and abuse, child victims of neglect, and family violence of incest and battering. *Described rape trauma syndrome, silent rape trauma, and compounded reactions to rape.*
Lee Ann Hoff	*Expanded crisis theory to be used in nursing practice. Contributed to theory of suicidology.* Described battering syndrome after research on battered women and battered elderly.
1982	
—	American Nurses' Association Executive Committee and Standards Committee, Division on Psychiatric and Mental Health Nursing Practice, published *Standards of Psychiatric and Mental Health Nursing Practice.*

Table continued on following page

Table 5-1 • SUMMARY OF HISTORIC CONTRIBUTIONS TO PSYCHIATRIC AND MENTAL HEALTH NURSING *Continued*

PSYCHIATRIC NURSING LEADER	CONTRIBUTION
1986	
Suzanne Lego	Received the ANA Award for Clinical Excellence in Nursing Practice for her substantial contributions to the practice of psychiatric nursing.
1987	
Maxine E. Loomis Anita W. O'Toole Marie Scott Brown Patricia Pothier Patricia West Holly S. Wilson	Began the development of a classification system for Psychiatric and Mental Health Nursing, first published in Archives of Psychiatric Nursing, 1(1):16–24, 1987.

Adapted from Murray R. The nursing process and emotional care. *In* Murray R, Huelskoetter M (eds). Psychiatric Mental Health Nursing—Giving Emotional Care, 2nd ed. Norwalk, CT: Appleton & Lange, 1987, pp. 93–97.

sponsibility of nurses. All of the amenities and necessities of social living within an institution, having highly specialized educative and therapeutic aims, are also the concern of nurses. Nurses consult family members about supplies patients need and about plans for their release from the hospital. Nurses have a responsibility to patients that the living environment will be clean and safe; on these matters they consult with patients, the housekeeping, maintenance, security, and fire departments when necessary. Among other things, health is related to nutrition; thus, nurses observe patients' dietary habits—at meals and in-between—and take steps to educate patients about good nutrition. Many psychiatric patients tend to be isolated; nurses assist and support them in establishing friendships with other patients.

Specially prepared psychiatric nurses (usually M.S.N.'s) take a nursing history and make periodic assessments of patient patterns of difficulty and progress toward their resolution. In addition, psychiatric nurses

- provide situational counseling (e.g., arbitrating disputes among patients),
- conduct short-term scheduled counseling sessions,
- provide individual, group, or family psychotherapy in a series of scheduled sessions,
- engage in biofeedback training and behavior modification,
- participate in "token economics,"
- use hypnosis, psychodrama, and other modalities.

Health teaching is a function of nurses—both experiential teaching (using an experience described by or acted out by a patient) and didactic teaching, such as holding classes on sex education, anxiety, and stress management.

The interactions of patients with each other and with the staff members are of special interest to nurses. It is in this milieu that patients frequently seek partners in order to integrate relationships with them that are illness-maintaining and, therefore, comfortable and anxiety-relieving (Benfer and Schroeder 1985). Studying such pattern interactions and intervening are complex features of the work of psychiatric nurses. Managing structured aspects of the milieu, such as location of patients, rules of living, and ward governmental meetings, is part of the work of nurses.

All staff are involved in careful recording of observations, for these records are of particular importance in studying a patient's progress. They also have legal implications.

All of the foregoing components of the work of nurses in psychiatric settings can be sorted into roles or modalities, as a convenience in viewing the work in an organized way (Table 5-2) (Lego 1984). The division of work among nursing personnel, according to education, can similarly be shown.

RELATION BETWEEN WORKROLE AND EDUCATION

Education determines the kind and scope of practice that a particular nurse is capable of performing competently. This is not to say that work experience lacks

Table 5–2 • WORK OF NURSES IN PSYCHIATRIC SETTINGS

ROLES & MODALITIES	EXAMPLES	NURSING PERSONNEL*
"Mother surrogate"	Bathing, dressing, feeding, toileting, warning, disciplining, sleep routines, etc.	
Technical	Assisting with medications and medical treatment; giving enemas, catheterizing, performing other nursing procedures (TPR, BP, etc.)	
Socialization agent	Activities of daily living, ward games, grooming advice, promoting friendships, etc.	
Health Teaching		
Experiential	Eating habits, individual problems	
Didactic (classes)	Stress management, anxiety, sex education, sessions for families of patients	
Taking a nursing history	On admission	
Preparing, revising nursing care plan, evaluation		
Assignment of nursing personnel to patients; evaluation		
Discharge planning & follow-up		
Coordination	Rounds, preparing patient schedules, scheduling patient appointments, health team meetings	
Milieu	Study and record milieu interactions among patients, at ward government meetings, and during visitor-patient interactions	
Relaxation therapy		
Recording		
Behavior modification	Token economics, individual schedules	
Counseling	Situational Patient-patient disputes Incidents of violence, etc. Short-term therapy Scheduled interview sessions (up to 6)	
Individual psychotherapy	Scheduled sessions (more than 6)	
Group psychotherapy	Scheduled sessions	
Family psychotherapy	Scheduled sessions of a patient with family members	
Biofeedback		
Hypnosis		
Psychodrama		
Liaison/consultation		
Other		

*Psychiatric nursing faculty should advise students of those nursing performances for which their nursing education has fully prepared them.

value. However, educational credentials are what assure the public that a nurse has successfully completed systematic, supervised study at a particular level that distinguishes a range of nursing competence. Nurses who exceed the level of their education based upon diligent study and analysis of their work experience ought to seek higher-level academic credentials.

THEORY. *The central feature of nursing education programs is theory — concepts and processes that explain the phenomena that nurses observe in varied manifestations during clinical practice.* It is the theory that a nurse has — is able to recall and use — during a particular nurse-patient interaction that defines whether the nurse's response to the patient will set up a corrective pull in a direction favorable for the patient. *Concepts that explain anxiety, conflict, hallucinations, delusions, dissociation, self-system disturbances, language-thought disorders, and problems relating to attention or perception are of particular relevance for psychiatric nurses.* It is not enough for a nurse to know about these phenomena; the nurse must grasp the functioning of a phenomenon as a mechanism or process — what it is, how it works, purposes and functions it has served and still provides for the patient, and its many variations in patterning of presentation in behavior. Such in-depth knowledge is acquired in course work, through reading and study, and most particularly through clinical experience. For students in psychiatric nursing, that clinical experience consists primarily in nurse-patient relationship studies, interview sessions with psychiatric patients that occur regularly over a substantial period of time, followed by supervisory review of the details of interaction data with a qualified psychiatric nurse faculty member. In such lengthy review sessions, theory application by the student, for purposes of explanation of phenomena and determination of constructive responses to the patient, is examined, developed, and verified. Obviously, the length and depth of the studies and the numbers of different patients studied in this manner will differ substantially by associate, baccalaureate, and master's students who, during an educative program, are studying nursing practice in psychiatric settings. At each succeeding level of education in nursing, the scope and complexity of psychiatric phenomena that are studied increase (or should increase), as does the number of explanatory concepts that the nurse masters. The nurse's competence in using these concepts is tested, as is the nurse's ability to use constructively increasingly complicated modalities and techniques of psychiatric nursing practice. It is these significant differences in education that determine the level of competence in psychiatric nursing of a particular nurse.

PRACTICAL TECHNIQUES. Nursing education also includes practical techniques, already more or less fully accepted for their usefulness. Practical techniques, such as bathing, feeding, planning games and other diversional or recreational activities within a service unit, and assisting patients to establish friendships with other patients, require limited, if any, theory. They rest on age-old social practices, common sense, or long traditions in nursing. Technical procedures, such as giving medications, assisting in medical treatments, or carrying out nursing procedures, are theory-based but have been tested over many years. Principles that guide their use include efficiency, accuracy, economy of resources, and safety for patients. Most of these practical techniques and procedures used in psychiatric nursing are few in number and are the same as those used in general nursing. Special adaptation may have to be made in light of the psychiatric condition of the patient, such as feelings of suspicion and ideas of persecution.

Violence is an increasing problem in psychiatric settings. Patients are admitted to public mental hospitals when they are dangerous to themselves and others. Methods of anticipating violent outbursts—recognizing cues, early intervention—require that nurses who work in psychiatric settings also know ways to protect themselves from injury and how to restrain patients when necessary.

PROMOTING SELF-CARE. The emphasis in psychiatric nursing is on promoting self-care rather than taking care of or doing things for patients that they are able to do or learn to do. Virtually all patients are ambulatory and physically able to meet basic self-care needs. Failure to do so suggests psychological problems, such as low self-esteem, rebellion against authority, felt and learned helplessness, and long-standing dependency claims. These aspects of self-care difficulties do require theoretical understanding of the particular patient's dilemmas in order to design nursing approaches to the presenting problems. There are no research-tested nursing interventions that, for example, can be used with a patient who refuses or does not bathe regularly that will simultaneously help to resolve, in time, both the physical and psychological problems. One theory holds that if the behavior is changed first, inroads are made on underlying problems. Psychiatric patients who do not attend to their basic needs do require psychiatric nursing that helps meet those needs while minimizing dependency claims. The patient's objections to bathing can be talked about during the bathing scene and in other formal and informal nurse-patient contacts.

TALKING WITH PATIENTS. The following general principle is useful when applied in clinical work: **Anything that goes on may be talked about; events that are discussed are more likely to be understood; understanding is a basis for changing one's behavior.** Conversely, anything that goes on that is not talked about but is merely acted out is most likely subject to highly private, autistic interpretation by a patient, which may well contribute to psychopathology and its maintenance.

Another general principle follows: **Language influences thought; thought influences actions; feelings are emotional responses that arise in relation to thoughts and actions taken within events in which a person is a participant.**

On the basis of the two foregoing principles, it can be argued that talking with patients is the most important component of the work of psychiatric nurses. Such talk, however, is not of the same quality as in social conversations that a nurse might have outside of the clinical setting. Different purposes are served. The focus is one-way—on the life of the patient. The aims include helping patients to recall, describe, and clarify past experience and to put it in a new and more constructive perspective. The nurse listens, asks questions, seeks details, and so forth. Nurses who use the patient's time to talk about themselves or their own experiences put the patient in the position of audience, watcher, listener. Discussions with patients are guided not by such social aims as the nurse being liked, gaining a friend, or being complimented but by theoretical understanding

Table 5–3 • SETS OF BASIC SKILLS REQUIRED FOR PSYCHIATRIC NURSING: A PARTIAL LIST

INTELLECTUAL AND INTERPERSONAL SKILLS
Observation: Detached spectator; participant; empathic; sensing hunches.
Interviewing: Situational counseling; short-term therapeutic counseling; Listening, hearing details and communicated messages; Disciplined attention, to sustain a focus, to pursue a trend; Assessment of patient data for patient's ability to focus, to describe, to pursue relevant details, etc.; Selecting relevant verbal inputs—to promote description, continuity of thought in patient, etc.; Controlling nurse verbalizations—quantity, quality, confidentiality, purpose of therapy, timing of inputs, etc.
Self-reflection: Auditing and editing one's own behavior during nurse-patient relationships.
Recording: Narrative; systematic; audio- and videotaping of nurse-patient data; for purposes of review, analysis, study.
Data analysis: Decoding; abstracting themes, trends, patterns; seeing relationships, connections; processing patient data as nurse hears it.
Formulation: Summarizing succinctly, accurately; generalizing—inferences, working hypotheses, nursing diagnoses; revising.
Theory application: As observed framework; to explain observed phenomena; to choose interventions.
Planning: Short- and long-term goals; for discharge continuity and follow-up.
Validation: Verifying inferences with another nurse; consensual validation of inferences of patients.
Foreseeing: Upcoming problems of patients; possibilities and opportunities for change; foreseeable short- and long-term possible effects of current nursing actions.
Evaluation: Short- and long-term effects of nursing actions on problems of patients.
Arbitrating: Disputes of patients so neither patient loses.
Anticipatory intervention: For prepanic, previolent, presuicidal behavior.

From Peplau HE. List of intellectual and interpersonal basic skills. Nursing Times, 83:1, 1987.

of how talking by patients develops their intellectual and interpersonal competencies and increases their self-understanding. Table 5–3 summarizes pertinent basic skills required for the practice of psychiatric nursing.

THEORIES RELEVANT FOR PSYCHIATRIC NURSING

Psychiatric nurses are generating theories for psychiatric nursing through scholarship and research. Smoyak and Rouslin (1982) described these efforts:

> From 1952 onward, psychiatric nursing textbooks took a decided turn toward educated scrutiny of clinical work. With the publication of Peplau's book, *Interpersonal Relations in Nursing*, no subsequent psychiatric nursing text could ignore the influence of some notion of 'nurse-patient relationship,' the 'therapeutic interview' or the 'participant observer' role of the psychiatric nurse. The nurse was now to be seen as an active, knowledgeable, knowledge-seeking therapeutic agent in work with patients. In one way or another, the impact of Peplau's introduction of an interpersonal concept of psychiatric nursing was reflected in books in the 1950's and 1960's such as the following: Kalkman's *Introduction to Psychiatric Nursing*, Mereness and Karnosh's *Psychiatry for Nurses*, Burton's *Personal, Impersonal and Interpersonal Relations*, Schwartz and Schokley's *The Nurse and the Mental Patient*, Muller's *The Nature and Direction of Psychiatric Nursing*, Hofling and Leininger's *Basic Psychiatric Concepts in Nursing*, Orlando's *The Dynamic Nurse-Patient Relationship*, Armstrong and Rouslin's *Group Psychotherapy in Nursing Practice*. Burd and Marshall's *Some Clinical Approaches in Psychiatric Nursing*, Hays and Larsen's *Interacting with Patients*, Bermosk and Mordan's *Interviewing in Nursing*, Manaser and Werner's *Instruments for the Study of the Nurse-Patient Relationship*, and Ujhely's *Determinants of the Nurse-Patient Relationship*.*

At a conference entitled "The State of the Art of Psychiatric Nursing," sponsored by the NIMH and Rutgers University, a critical assessment of psychiatric nursing developments from 1946 to 1974 was made and published (Huey 1975). Since then, there has been a proliferation of journal articles and textbooks on psychiatric nursing. However, much research still needs to be conducted, particularly in defining the phenomena that fall within the purview of psychiatric nursing. These phenomena are currently being identified by an ANA Task Force. Meanwhile, there are psychiatric nursing and psychosocial nursing diagnoses in current publications of taxonomies of nursing (Gebbie and Lavin 1972). The **phenomena** to which the practices of psychiatric nurses are addressed for intended corrective effects also include processes such as attention, perception, memory,

*Reprinted by permission of Slack Incorporated, Thorofare, NJ.

language-thought, the self-system and hallucinations, delusions, ideas of reference, suspiciousness, incorporated identities, loneliness, depression, and others. *It is for these phenomena that nurses need theories—concepts and processes*—that define the mechanisms: what they are, how they arise and function, distortions and how they occur, purposes served in maintaining dysfunctional patterns, and so forth.

Nurses generate psychiatric nursing theories in two ways. The first is scholarly study, reformulation, and empirical testing in clinical work of any theory published by any established science—physical, social, or applied sciences (other professions). Nurses have access to all published scientific literature. Concepts drawn from sources become "nursing theory" when applied to nursing phenomena. The second way nursing theory is developed is from the results of nursing research. Nurses have a very large practical responsibility, the more so in psychiatric nursing, where their around-the-clock interactions with patients ought to be directed by theoretical understanding of psychopathology so that the nursing actions will tend toward correction of the patient's difficulties rather than toward the participation in illness maintenance.

Nurses work with other health care providers within psychiatric services. Although psychiatric nurses use nursing theories in their work, they do need to know and appreciate the theoretical orientations of their psychiatric colleagues. It is a fair question for any nurse working in a psychiatric facility to say, "I am interested and would appreciate it if you would share with me a brief overview of the theoretical orientation you use in your work with patients." By the same token, nurses ought to be able to state their own theoretical orientation simply and clearly.

There are many theoretical frameworks currently in use in psychiatric settings. Some professionals may use one exclusively, having an orientation to Freud, Jung, Adler, Horney, Sullivan, or one of many other psychiatric theorists' work. Some, if not most, psychiatrists or other professionals are eclectic in orientation. The following paragraphs provide brief descriptions of prevailing theoretical frameworks.

DESCRIPTIVE THEORIES. Descriptive theories of psychiatry primarily provide names for diagnostic categories of mental diseases and identify or describe the accompanying symptoms. Historically, most psychiatric nursing textbooks have followed this framework.

INTRAPERSONAL THEORIES. Intrapersonal theories present concepts to explain phenomena that purportedly go on within an individual. "Spectator observation" is used to notice the behavior of the individual being studied, without reference to others or to context. Many of Freud's intrapsychic concepts—id, ego, libido, repression—are intrapersonal constructs.

INTERPERSONAL THEORIES. Interpersonal theories include concepts that define "what goes on between two or more people, all but one of whom may be completely illusory" (Sullivan 1947). Thus hallucinations would be studied as an interaction between a patient and an autistically invented illusory figure, the interaction being a pattern-integration serving a purpose for the patient. The nurse-patient interaction would also be studied, by "participant observation," in order to notice relations, for instance, between nurse inputs and patient responses, and vice versa.

SYSTEMS THEORIES. Systems theories explain interactions among parts of a whole—a family, members of an inpatient milieu, an organization. Pattern interactions, strategies used to maintain them, formal and informal rules of organization, and the privileges of the system and how they are gained would be among the phenomena to be studied.

SOCIAL SCIENCE THEORIES. Social science theories—psychology, social psychology, sociology, anthropology, and others—derive from studies of some aspect of individual or collective human behavior, each discipline generally having areas and methods that are of special interest.

Psychiatrists seem to be moving away from the foregoing theoretical frameworks toward biological, physiological, biochemical, and genetic explanations of psychiatric phenomena. This trend is sometimes referred to as the "biomedicalization" of psychiatry, sometimes as their becoming "real doctors." A great deal of research is currently under way to identify brain dysfunction and biochemical, pathophysiological, and genetic "causes" of mental illness. In the history of medicine, this is not an entirely new thrust; such efforts have been made by physicians since the seventeenth and eighteenth centuries, if not before that (Scull 1981). It is quite probable that in the next several decades there will be new "medical treatments" of psychiatric patients, well beyond the present pharmaceutical management and including new forms of brain surgery (Valenstein 1986). In that event, no doubt, some nurses will go along with that trend, providing the nursing required following the application of technological medical practice. Hopefully, other psychiatric nurses will continue the development of their already well-established psychotherapeutic nursing practices.

OTHER MEMBERS OF THE MENTAL HEALTH TEAM

There are about 250 different health care occupations. Not all of them are represented in psychiatric institutions but are available in general hospitals having inpatient psychiatric units. The following are very brief descriptions of the *major* unique functions of coworkers and colleagues who do work alongside nurses in psychiatric settings.

PSYCHIATRISTS. Psychiatrists provide psychiatric diagnoses of patients for the official records, prescribe medications and medical treatments such as electroshock—which they administer—and some also provide psychotherapy.

PSYCHOLOGISTS. Psychologists administer psychological and other tests and therefore contribute to psychiatric diagnoses; some direct behavior modification and biofeedback programs; most engage in psychotherapy.

SOCIAL WORKERS. Social workers usually take an intake history, confer with families about admission, economic status, welfare problems, and discharge. Some also provide psychotherapy.

OCCUPATIONAL THERAPISTS. Occupational therapists generally provide for various activities, based upon the study of the needs of the patients, for diversion, to increase attention span, release emotions, develop hand-eye coordination, and so forth. Some may also provide vocational or work training or activities to help patients develop a hobby.

RECREATIONAL THERAPISTS. Recreational therapists provide socializing group activities, physical exercise programs, diversion, and so forth.

DANCE THERAPISTS. Dance therapists use bodily movement as a medium of expression of self and feelings and to release inhibitions in patients.

ART THERAPISTS. Art therapists employ art materials both to encourage externalization of difficulties symbolically, through art forms, and to release and use creative capacities of the patients.

CLERGY. The clergy provide religious solace, instruction, continuation of patients' religious interests, counseling about religious conflicts, last rites, and so forth. Some also provide psychotherapy.

SETTINGS IN WHICH NURSES PRACTICE WITH PSYCHIATRIC PATIENTS

The number and kinds of settings in which health care of psychiatric patients is provided have been increasing since the 1970's. Only the major settings are briefly described here.

PUBLIC MENTAL HOSPITALS. The patient population of public mental hospitals established by state government has changed. "Deinstitutionalization," which began in the 1970's, has reduced the patient population considerably by returning patients to their families, by transferring them to nursing homes, and by shifting some to the status of "homeless street people" (Dato and Rafferty 1985). Although there are still some older "chronic" patients, now there seem to be an increasing number of young persons admitted to mental hospitals, many of whom act out violence. In the past several decades, these institutions have been employing an increasing number of master's prepared clinical specialists in psychiatric nursing. Associate degree nurses, therefore, have opportunities in these hospitals to work under well-prepared clinical nurses.

PSYCHIATRIC UNITS. Psychiatric units in general hospitals are the norm. Such units are often specialized for children, adolescents, adults, alcohol or drug abuse, and so forth. The advantage for the patient is access to all of the assessment technology usually associated with a modern hospital. Some units are psychotherapeutically oriented; some are more biomedical in treatment approaches. Units associated with university teaching hospitals tend to be well staffed and generally engaged in research.

COMMUNITY MENTAL HEALTH CENTERS. Community mental health centers began to develop rapidly in 1963 as a "bold, new approach in attacking the societal problem of mental illness." Some centers have inpatient units as well as many outpatient services. Psychiatric nurses, especially clinical specialists, are employed for inpatient care and to provide psychotherapy.

OTHER FACILITIES. Psychiatric nurses are employed in many other psychiatric facilities: specialized centers for the treatment of alcohol and drug abuse; shelters for abused women or children; psychiatric clinics most often attached to general hospitals; crisis intervention hotlines and walk-in clinics; day and night care centers; sheltered workshops for discharged patients or persons who are mentally retarded; Veterans Administration hospitals; the military; prisons; and many others.

PRIVATE PRACTICE. Since the mid-1960's, psychiatric nurses have engaged in private practice, particularly clinical specialists who hold a graduate degree and are eligible for or hold ANA Certification in their specialty. Some psychiatric nurses practice independently, in solo or group practice with other nurses; others are in joint practice with other mental health professionals. Their practices include individual, group, or family psychotherapy, and other specialized services.

CONTEMPORARY GUIDELINES FOR PRACTICE

Nursing is a service to the public. Therefore, nurses do not have the option to practice solely in accordance with their personal wishes; the public interest must be safeguarded. Such safeguards are provided through the application of mandatory and voluntary guidelines for nursing practice.

NURSING PRACTICE ACTS. Nursing practice acts, contained in state laws, provide mandatory guidelines. In order to practice nursing and to use one of the various titles, such as LPN or RN, graduates of schools of nursing must take and pass a licensing examination and maintain a current license issued by a Board of Nursing.* The practice acts generally describe the parameters of practice allowed in a particular state. Additionally, the board establishes rules, regulations, and policies that govern the practice of nursing. The board is empowered to administer the acts, that is, to police, warn, discipline, or press legal charges for violations of the nursing act. All nurses should, upon employment in any state, obtain a license to practice in that state, and obtain and study a copy of the licensing law and of any rules and regulations then in force.

STANDARDS. Standards also govern the practice of nursing. Institutions in which nurses work generally have policies or standards that apply to personnel and their practices. On employment, every nurse should at once obtain a copy of such standards from the Director of Nursing, for study and use. Such standards describe and determine practices in local situations. Additionally, the State Nurses' Association usually has standards that apply to conduct and performances in that state, such standards representing a consensus of members in such voluntary organizations.

The purpose of standards is to ensure quality of nursing care to the public. Increasingly, the public is aggressively pursuing its right to quality health care by taking cases of alleged negligence to the courts. In a recent publication, which discusses one such case, the reported court judgment relied upon "national trends in nursing standards of care" rather than the "locality rule." This judgment signifies that nurses would be well advised to be fully acquainted with the national standards of care† (Fiesta 1986).

General standards of nursing care are presented in the paradigm from the ANA *Social Policy Statement* (see Fig. 5–1). Additionally, nurses who work with psychiatric patients use the ANA's *Standards of Psychiatric and Mental Health Nursing Practice* (see inside front cover). Nurses should also consult the ANA's *Statement on Psychiatric and Mental Health Nursing Practice.*

*The Board of Nursing (or similar title) is an arm of state government; many nurses fail to recognize that such boards are not the same as nor connected with the Board of Directors of the State Nurses' Association, a voluntary organization of nurses.

†The American Nurses' Association (2420 Pershing Road, Kansas City, MO, 64108, c/o Marketing) will send free to any nurse who requests it, their current *Catalog of Publications* which contains titles of all current national standards established by the ANA.

CODES OF ETHICS. Codes of ethics also serve as guides to nursing practice. There are many ethical issues that arise in psychiatric nursing practice: the patient's right to treatment, the right to be in the least restrictive environment, the right to refuse treatment (see Chapter 3). In making nursing judgments in practice and in collaborating in treatment prescribed or given by other professionals, nurse performances, choices, and decisions are made within the framework of the nursing profession's code of ethics. These codes are published

Box 5–1. ANA CODE FOR NURSES

1. The nurse provides services with respect for human dignity and the uniqueness of the client unrestricted by considerations of social or economic status, personal attributes, or the nature of health problems.
2. The nurse safeguards the client's right to privacy by judiciously protecting information of a confidential nature.
3. The nurse acts to safeguard the client and the public when health care and safety are affected by the incompetent, unethical, or illegal practice of any person.
4. The nurse assumes responsibility and accountability for individual nursing judgments and actions.
5. The nurse maintains competence in nursing.
6. The nurse exercises informed judgment and uses individual competence and qualifications as criteria in seeking consultations, accepting responsibilities, and delegating nursing activities to others.
7. The nurse participates in activities that contribute to the ongoing development of the profession's body of knowledge.
8. The nurse participates in the profession's efforts to implement and improve standards of nursing.
9. The nurse participates in the profession's efforts to establish and maintain conditions of employment conducive to high-quality nursing care.
10. The nurse participates in the profession's effort to protect the public from misinformation and misrepresentation and to maintain the integrity of nursing.
11. The nurse collaborates with members of the health profession and other citizens in promoting community and national efforts to meet the health needs of the public.

From American Nurses' Association. Code for Nurses With Interpretive Statements. Kansas City, MO: American Nurses' Association, 1985, p. 1.

by the American Nurses' Association and represent a consensus of the nurses in membership with the American Nurses' Association and the International Council of Nurses (Box 5–1).

Summary

The history of psychiatric nursing in the United States is just over one century old. In that short time a basic workrole has evolved, specialization has developed, and considerable influence has been exercised on nursing as a whole. The field has expanded in scope of practice, in numbers and kinds of practitioners, and in the variety of services and facilities in which psychiatric nursing is practiced. The continuing development of psychiatric nursing, however, depends upon present generation nurses becoming interested and competent in this component of nursing practice and in the preparation of many more psychiatric nurse clinical specialists and researchers.

References

Albee GA et al. The mental health disciplines. Hospital and Community Psychiatry, 27(7):492–495, 1976.

American Nurses' Association. Nursing: A Social Policy Statement. Kansas City, MO: American Nurses' Association, 1980.

Bailey H. Nursing Mental Disease. New York: Macmillan Publishing Company, 1920.

Benfer BA, Schroeder PJ. Nursing in the therapeutic milieu. Bulletin of the Menninger Clinic, 49(5):451, 1985.

Boorstin DJ. The Discoverers. New York: Random House, 1983.

Bridges DC. A History of the International Council of Nurses, 1899–1964: The First 65 Years. Geneva: International Council of Nurses. Philadelphia: J.B. Lippincott Company, 1967.

Burd SF, Marshall MA. Some Clinical Approaches to Psychiatric Nursing. New York: Macmillan Publishing Company, 1963.

Carpenter M. Asylum nursing before 1914: A chapter in the history of labor. *In* Davis C (ed). Rewriting Nursing History. London: Croom Helm, 1980.

Chappell EA, McDonald TC. Containing madness. Colonial Williamsburg, Spring, 1985.

Dato C, Rafferty M. The homeless mentally ill. International Nursing Review, 32(6):170, 1985.

Fiesta J. Look beyond your state for your standards of care. Nursing '86, 16(8):41, 1986.

40th Anniversary of the national mental health act. Organizing committee for the 40th anniversary commemoration, 1986.

Gebbie K, Lavin MA (eds). Classification of Nursing Diagnosis: Summary of the Second National Conference. St. Louis: Clearinghouse, 1972.

Henderson V. Basic Principles of Nursing Care. Geneva: International Council of Nurses, 1961.

Huey FL (ed). Psychiatric Nursing 1946 to 1974: A Report on the State of the Art. New York: American Journal of Nursing Company, 1975.

Hughes EC. Twenty Thousand Nurses Tell Their Story. Philadelphia: J.B. Lippincott Company, 1958.

Johns E, Pfefferkorn B. An Activity Analysis of Nursing. New York: Committee on the Grading of Nursing Schools, 1934.

Lego S (ed). The American Handbook of Psychiatric Nursing. Philadelphia: J.B. Lippincott Company, 1984.

Mericle B. The male as psychiatric nurse. Journal of Psychosocial Nursing, 21(11):30, 1983.

Nursing schools today and tomorrow: Final report of the committee on the grading of nursing schools. New York, 1934.

Oderkirk WW. Setting the records straight: A recount of late nineteenth-century training schools. Journal of Nursing History, 1(1):30, 1985.

Osborne OH. Intellectual traditions in psychiatric-mental health nursing: A review of selected textbooks. Journal of Psychosocial Nursing, 22(11):27, 1984.

Packard FR. Some Account of the Pennsylvania Hospital of Philadelphia from 1751–1956. Philadelphia: Pennsylvania Hospital, 1957.

Painter D, Painter TK. Building innovative nursing departments in turbulent times. Nursing Economics, 3:73, 1985.

Pappas NA. The public hospital: Its place in Williamsburg. Colonial Williamsburg, Summer, 1985.

Peplau HE. Historical development of psychiatric nursing: A preliminary statement of some facts and trends. *In* Smoyak SA, Rouslin S (eds). A Collection of Classics in Psychiatric Nursing Literature. Thorofare, NJ: Charles B. Slack, 1982.

Proceedings of the fifth annual convention of the National League of Nursing Education. New York: NLN, 1899.

Richards AJ. Reminiscences of Linda Richards: America's First Trained Nurse. Philadelphia: J.B. Lippincott Company, 1949.

Robb IH. Nursing in the smaller hospitals and in those devoted to the care of specialized forms of disease. Proceedings, page 59, 1897.

Roberts MM. American nursing: history and interpretation. New York: Macmillan Publishing Company, 1954.

Rosenfeld P. Nursing education: statistics you can use. Nursing and Health Care, 7(6):329, 1986.

Rouslin S. Coping with chronic helpfulness. *In* Smoyak S, Rouslin S (eds). A Collection of Classics in Nursing Literature. Thorofare, NJ: Charles B. Slack, 1982.

Scull A, (ed). Madhouses, Mad-doctors, and Madmen: The Social History of Psychiatry in the Victorian Era. Philadelphia: The University of Pennsylvania Press, 1981.

Smoyak S, Rouslin S. Introduction. *In* Smoyak S, Rouslin S (eds). A Collection of Classics in Psychiatric Nursing Literature. Thorofare, NJ: Charles B. Slack, 1982.

Snively MA. A uniform curriculum for training schools. Proceedings, page 24, 1895.

Sullivan HS. Conceptions of Modern Psychiatry. Washington DC: William Alanson White Institute, 1947.

Tomes N. Little world of our own: The Pennsylvania Hospital training school for nurses 1895–1907. *In* Leavitt JW (ed). Women and Health in America. Wisconsin: University of Wisconsin Press, 1984.

Valenstein ES. Great and Desperate Cures: The Rise and Decline of Psychosurgery and Other Radical Treatments for Mental Illness. New York: Basic Books, 1986.

Zwilling SS. Inside the public hospital. Colonial Williamsburg, Spring, 1985.

Self-Study Exercises

Write a short answer to the questions that follow:

1. What were the *themes* of attitude changes toward the mentally ill after World War I and World War II?
2. *Name* and give the *date* of the first hospital built in the United States; what *trend* initiated there was fully developed almost two centuries later?
3. What *three phases* in the process of nursing's development preceded its emergence as a profession?
4. Historically, *what* provided the *model* for the hierarchical arrangement of the organization of public mental hospitals; cite *three components* of the model.
5. Specify three or four *features* of nineteenth century public mental hospitals as "almost closed systems."
6. Cite three dimensions of "moral management" or "moral treatment."
7. In *what year* did Dorothea Dix begin her crusade to get mentally ill persons out of jails? What was society's response?
8. State three to four reasons why public mental hospitals were usually built on the edge or outside of cities.
9. What was Linda Richards's connection with psychiatric nursing?
10. What was the major method for getting psychiatric nursing included into all basic nursing curricula? *When* was it first proposed? *When* was it finally accomplished?
11. Who was the nurse author of the first textbook for psychiatric nurses? In contemporary terms, what is problematic about the book's title?
12. Identify six different emphases in the developing workrole of nurse that also applied in psychiatric nursing.
13. *Which* act provided funds to open *how many* university programs in psychiatric nursing in *what* year?
14. Cite four challenges faced by psychiatric nurse faculty in developing university programs in "advanced psychiatric nursing."
15. In what year did the NLN recommend that all schools of nursing prepare all nursing students for beginning positions in psychiatric facilities? How many decades intervened between that decision and the opening of the first school of nursing in an asylum?
16. What was one major issue concerning "advanced practice" decided by Graduate Program Directors? What was the resolution of that issue?
17. What was the purpose of the "integration grants"? Who got them? During what approximate time period?
18. In what year did psychiatric nursing get its own journals? How many? Name their current titles.
19. Compare the components of the workrole of nurses in psychiatric services *before* and *after* the 1950's.
20. *Formulate* and *state* the role of theory in the practice of psychiatric nursing.

21. Name as many components of the total workrole of nurses in psychiatric settings as you can. Indicate those for which your education has prepared you for competent functioning.
22. Cite two principles useful in practice with psychiatric patients. State why you accept them as important.
23. Name two ways in which nursing theory can be generated.
24. Name four to five theoretical frameworks that are used by providers of psychiatric services.
25. What do *you* think will be *your* position as a practicing nurse with regard to the relation between psychiatric nursing practice and the biomedicalization of psychiatry.
26. Identify six to eight other mental health care providers, and name one major unique function each performs in psychiatric settings.
27. If you had a family member or a friend who was seeking psychotherapy, would you refer that family member or friend to a qualified psychiatric nurse clinical specialist for psychotherapy? Justify your position.
28. What is the difference between a mandatory standard or guideline and a voluntary standard or guideline?
29. What is the significant difference between a "Board of Nursing" and a "Board of Directors" of a State Nurses' Association?
30. What standards do you plan to use in the practice of nursing in a psychiatric setting?

CHAPTER 6

Communication, the Nurse–Client Relationship, and Clinical Interview

Elizabeth M. Varcarolis with contributions by Mattie Collins

OUTLINE

KEY TERMS AND CONCEPTS

The key terms and concepts listed here also appear in bold where they are defined or discussed in this chapter.

COMMUNICATION MODEL (BERLO)
Referent
Sender
Message
Medium/Channel
Receiver
Feedback

Portions of this chapter first appeared in *Communication in Health Care: The Human Connection in the Life Cycle*, 2nd ed.; C.V. Mosby, 1983. We thank Dr. Mattie Collins for generously sharing her insights and ideas.

VERBAL COMMUNICATION
NONVERBAL COMMUNICATION/ BEHAVIORS
THERAPEUTIC TECHNIQUES
NONTHERAPEUTIC TECHNIQUES
PARAPHRASING
RESTATING
REFLECTING
USE OF SILENCE
ACTIVE LISTENING
SOCIAL RELATIONSHIP
INTIMATE RELATIONSHIP
THERAPEUTIC RELATIONSHIP
THERAPEUTIC ENCOUNTER
ORIENTATION PHASE OF NURSE-CLIENT RELATIONSHIP
CONTRACT
CONFIDENTIALITY
TRANSFERENCE
COUNTERTRANSFERENCE
WORKING PHASE OF NURSE-CLIENT RELATIONSHIP
TERMINATION PHASE OF NURSE-CLIENT RELATIONSHIP
PROCESS RECORDINGS

OBJECTIVES

After studying this chapter, the student will be able to:

1. Define the five components in Berlo's communication model.
2. Identify three personal factors that can impede accurate communication.
3. Identify two environmental factors that can impede accurate communication.
4. Discuss the differences between verbal and nonverbal communications and identify five (5) areas of nonverbal communication.
5. Identify four techniques that enhance communication and discuss what makes them effective.
6. Identify four techniques that hinder communication and discuss what makes them ineffective.
7. Contrast and compare the purpose, focus, communication styles, and goals for (a) a social relationship, (b) an intimate relationship, and (c) a therapeutic relationship.
8. Define and discuss the role of empathy and positive regard on the part of the nurse in a nurse-client relationship.
9. Identify two attitudes and four actions that may reflect the nurse's positive regard toward a client.
10. Summarize the three stages of the nurse-client relationship.
11. Discuss the purpose of clinical supervision.
12. Name four areas of concern the nurse should address during the first interview.
13. Identify four client behaviors a nurse can anticipate, and discuss possible nursing interventions for each behavior.

Effective communication is the foundation for a therapeutic nurse-client relationship. Communication is the medium through which the nursing process is realized. In this chapter, a review of the basics of communication is presented, followed by a discussion of the nurse-client relationship, and an introduction to a special form of communication — the clinical interview.

Communication

Simply put, communication is the process of sending a message to one or more persons. One way of thinking about the process of communication is a **communica-**

tion model, which identifies the parts of an interaction. Berlo's (1960) model has five parts: referent (stimulus), sender, message, channel (medium), and receiver.

The **referent** is that stimulus which begins communication. For example, a referent can be a need for information, comfort, or advice. A referent or stimulus in a nurse might be the perception in a client of discomfort or confusion. A referent or stimulus in a client could be the experience of anxiety, despair, or pain.

It is the **sender** who initiates interpersonal contact. The **message** is the information sent or expressed to another. The clearest messages are those that are well organized and expressed in a manner familiar to the receiver. The message can be sent through a variety of **mediums** or **channels.** A message can be sent through an auditory channel (hearing), a visual channel (seeing), or a tactile channel (touch). For example, a person may send a very clear message through silence, body language, or a hug, as well as the stated word.

The **receiver** is the person(s) who receives and interprets the message. Often the message from the sender may act as a stimulus or referent to the receiver. The receiver may then respond to the sender by giving **feedback** to the sender. The nature of the feedback often indicates whether the meaning of the message sent by the sender has been correctly interpreted by the receiver. When the receiver gives feedback to the sender, communication becomes reciprocal. Communication is most effective when the message sent is the same as the message received.

Figure 6–1 shows this simple model of communication. However, communication is a *complex* process involving a variety of personal and environmental factors that can distort both the sending and the receiving of messages.

Personal factors that can impede accurate transmission or interpreting of messages include emotional factors (anger, anxiety), physical factors (pain, illness), intellectual factors (knowledge levels, language use), and social factors (difference in culture, ethnic groups, and language).

Environmental factors include physical factors (background noise, lack of privacy, uncomfortable accommodations) and social factors (presence of others, expectations of others, and so forth) (Parkinson 1986).

Effective communication in helping relationships depends on knowing what you are trying to convey (the purpose of the message), communicating what you really mean to the client, and comprehending the meaning of what the client is intentionally or unintentionally conveying (Collins 1983). The success of such an interdependent activity can be evaluated by the de-

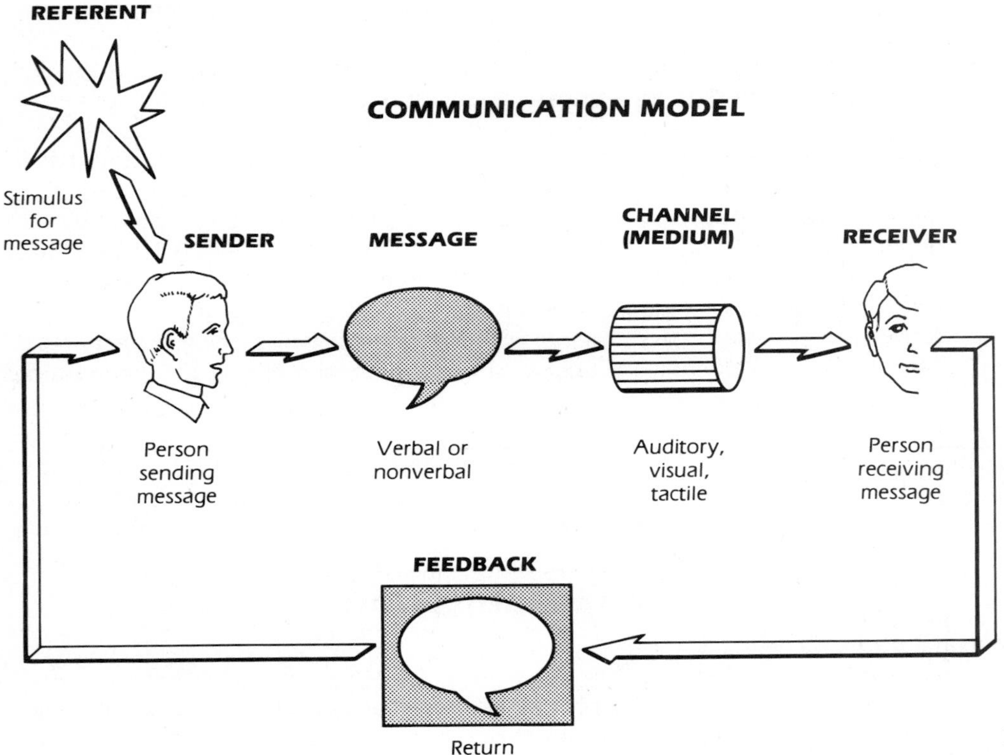

Figure 6–1. *The reciprocal process of communication.*

gree to which each person understands what was communicated and can show the other person that the message was understood.

Communication consists of verbal and nonverbal elements. It is said that communication is roughly 10 percent words and 90 percent nonverbal (Shea 1988). Therefore, learning to be an effective communicator means using both verbal and nonverbal cues.

VERBAL COMMUNICATION

Verbal communication consists of all words a person speaks. We live in a society of symbols, and our supreme social symbol is words. Talking is our most common activity, our public link with one another, the primary instrument of instruction, a need, an art, and one of the most personal aspects of our private life. When we speak, we communicate definitions of ourselves and our unique world (Gass 1979). Even if the nurse and the client have the same background, the mental image they have of a word may not be exactly the same. Although believing they are talking about the same thing, the nurse and the client may in reality be talking about two quite different things. The word *trip* shows the manner in which differences in mental images can produce misunderstanding. If you say to a client, "I heard you had some trip," the client will define *trip* according to the images that he or she has formed of the word from speaking, reading, writing, and listening. Depending on the client's past experience, the nurse's statement could convey interest or insult. Did the nurse think that the client stumbled and fell? Traveled to another city? Experimented with a drug? Tending to reflect the rapid, widespread changes in society, words often change meanings and are, therefore, best interpreted in accordance with the company they keep (Collins 1983).

Conversation between persons of different cultures can be confusing if one statement simultaneously conveys different messages. One of the messages is transmitted *explicitly*, or with the precise meaning of the sentence, whereas the other message is communicated by *implication*, or the meaning that the speaker wishes to convey at the moment. In our culture the question, "Why don't you drop in sometime?" is not a request for a visit. If it were a true invitation, a specific date and hour would be set. However, someone from a different background may take the hostess at her word and create an embarrassing situation for all concerned. That we can say one thing and at the same time mean another may be baffling to someone unfamiliar with the way we use words. Many remarks are no more than social phrases: "Nice day, isn't it?" or "Hi, how are you?" These remarks are made in passing, and the speaker neither expects to discuss the weather seriously nor really wants to know how you are. More information must be communicated either verbally or nonverbally to make the statement personally relevant (Collins 1983).

NONVERBAL COMMUNICATION

Nonverbal behaviors are the behaviors displayed by an individual rather than the actual content of speech (Shea 1988). Tone of voice and the manner in which a client paces his or her speech are examples of **nonverbal communication.** Other common examples of nonverbal cues come from facial expressions, body posture, amount of eye contact, hand gestures, sighs, fidgeting, yawning, and so forth.

INTERACTION OF VERBAL AND NONVERBAL COMMUNICATION. Communication thus involves two radically different but interdependent kinds of symbols: the deliberate impressions that one *gives* and the less deliberately controlled impressions that one *creates*. The first involves the *spoken word*, which is the best friend of our public self. Verbal assertions can be skillfully used to distort, conceal, deny, and generally disguise true feelings. The second, *nonverbal behaviors*, covers a wide range of human activities, from body movements to responses to the messages of others. How one listens and uses silence and the sense of touch may also convey important information about the private self that is not available from conversation alone (Collins 1983).

Table 6–1 gives examples of some types of nonverbal behavior. Some nonverbal communication seems to be inborn and is similar across cultures, for example, facial expressions. Others, such as how close people stand to each other to speak, depend on cultural conventions. Some nonverbal communication is formalized and has very specific meanings, e.g., the military salute or the Japanese bow.

Therefore, an interaction consists of both verbal and nonverbal messages. Often people have more conscious awareness of their verbal messages and are less aware of their nonverbal behavior. The verbal message is sometimes referred to as the **content** of the message, and the nonverbal behavior is called the **process** of the message. *When the content (verbal message) is congruent with (agrees with) the process (nonverbal behavior), the communication is more clearly understood and is considered healthy*. For example, if a student says that it is important that she earn high grades and proceeds to buy the text, read her notes, and study systematically, the content message is consistent with the process, or the nonverbal behaviors.

If, however, the verbal message is not reinforced or in fact is

Table 6–1 • AREAS OF NONVERBAL BEHAVIOR

POSSIBLE BEHAVIORS	EXAMPLE
Body Behaviors	
Posture, body movements, gestures, gait (e.g., pacing, coordination)	Client slumped in chair, face in hands, occasionally tapping right foot
Facial Expressions	
Frowns, smiles, grimaces, raised eyebrows, pursed lips, licking lips, tongue movements	Client grimaces when speaking to nurse; when alone, client smiles and giggles to self
Voice-Related Behaviors	
Tone, pitch, level, intensity, inflection, stuttering, pauses, silences, and fluency	Client talked in a loud sing-song voice
Observable Autonomic Physiologic Responses	
Increase in respirations, diaphoresis, pupil dilation, blushing, paleness	When the client mentioned discharge, he became pale, his respirations increased, and his face became diaphoretic
General Appearance	
Grooming, dress, hygiene	Client dressed in wrinkled shirt, and pants were stained; socks were dirty and he wore no shoes
Physical Characteristics	
Height, weight, physique, complexion	Client appeared grossly overweight, and muscle tone appeared flabby

contradicted by nonverbal behavior, then the message is confusing and not clear. If the student who stated that it was important to earn high grades did not purchase the text, did not clarify questions from her notes, and did not study, she would be sending out two different messages. This is known as a *double or mixed message.*

Nurses can make use of these two levels of communication to compare the client's dialogue with the client's nonverbal communication. What persons do either may express and reinforce or contradict and belie what they say. Thus we say that "actions speak louder than words," since actions often tell the true meaning of a person's intent, whether conscious or unconscious. The meaning of nonverbal cues depends on the context of the situation, the client, and the total pattern of both nonverbal and verbal behavior. The cues need to be considered together to form an accurate interpretation. The greater the cultural distance between the nurse and the client, the greater the probability of being incorrect (Collins 1983, 74).

The nurse learns by directed observation to become aware of a client's verbal and nonverbal communication. The nurse also learns that the content, or what the person says, is not always congruent with the person's nonverbal behaviors.

TECHNIQUES THAT ENHANCE OR HINDER COMMUNICATION

The goal of the nurse in the mental health setting is to help the client

1. identify and explore problems relating to others,
2. discover healthy ways of meeting emotional needs, and
3. experience a satisfying interpersonal relationship (Hays and Larson 1963).

Once specific needs and problems have been identified, the nurse can work with the client on increasing problem-solving skills, learning new coping behaviors, and experiencing more appropriate and satisfying ways of their relating to others.

In order to do this, the nurse needs to have a sound knowledge of communication skills. Therefore, nurses need to become more aware of their own interpersonal techniques. The nurse is then better able to eliminate nontherapeutic techniques and to apply additional responses that maximize nurse-client interactions. Appropriate techniques are neither therapeutic nor nontherapeutic in and of themelves. They can, when used in the context of respect and genuine interest, greatly facilitate open communication.

Peplau's book *Interpersonal Relations in Nursing* (1952) and groundbreaking article *Interpersonal Techniques: The Crux of Psychiatric Nursing* (1962) are the classic writings that defined our understanding of the relationship between nurse and patient.

Hays and Larson (1963) discussed and compiled from various sources and theorists examples of **therapeutic and nontherapeutic techniques,** which are basic to communication skills used by mental health personnel today. These communication techniques are used throughout the nurse-client relationship.

Techniques that may discourage open communication are often used in social relationships but may impede communications during a therapeutic relationship.

Table 6–2 identifies therapeutic techniques that may enhance communications. Read the description of the technique and the examples given. You may recognize some techniques that you already use. Throughout this

Table 6–2 • TECHNIQUES THAT ENHANCE COMMUNICATION

DISCUSSION	EXAMPLE
Using Silence	
Gives person time to collect thoughts or to think through a point.	Encouraging a person to talk by waiting for the answers.
Accepting	
Statements such as "I'm with you," "I follow what you say," "Uh hmm" indicate that the person has been understood. The statement does *not* necessarily indicate agreement but is nonjudgmental. However, the nurse does *not* imply she understands when she does *not* understand.	"Yes." "Uh hmm." "I follow what you say."
Giving Recognition	
Indicates awareness of change and personal efforts. Does not imply good or bad or right or wrong.	"Good morning Mr. James." "You've combed your hair today." "I notice that you shaved this morning."
Offering Self	
When a person is unable to communicate, the nurse can offer presence, interest, and a desire to understand. It is *not* offered to get the person to talk or behave in a specific way.	"I would like to spend time with you." "I'll stay here and sit with you for a while."
Offering General Leads	
Allows the other person to take direction in the discussion. Indicates that the nurse is interested in what comes next.	"Go on." "And then?" "Tell me about it."
Giving Broad Openings	
Clarifies that the lead is to be taken by the client. However, the nurse discourages pleasantries and small talk.	"Where would you like to begin?" "What are you thinking about?" "What would you like to discuss?"
Placing the Events in Time or Sequence	
Puts events and actions in better perspective. Notes cause and effect relationships and identifies patterns of interpersonal difficulties.	"What happened before?" "When did this happen?"

Table continued on following page

Table 6-2 • TECHNIQUES THAT ENHANCE COMMUNICATION *Continued*

DISCUSSION	EXAMPLE
Making Observations	
Nurse calls attention to person's behavior, e.g., trembling, biting nails, restless mannerisms. Encourages person to notice the behavior in order to describe thoughts and feelings for mutual understanding. Helpful with mute and withdrawn persons.	"You appear tense." "I notice you're biting your lips." "You appear nervous whenever Mr. X enters the room."
Encouraging Description of Perception	
Increases nurse's understanding of client's perceptions. Talking about feelings and difficulties can lessen the need to act them out inappropriately.	"What do the voices seem to be saying?" "What is happening now?" "Tell me when you feel anxious."
Encouraging Comparison	
Comparing experiences or interpersonal relationships brings out recurring themes. Helps person clarify similarities and differences.	"Has this ever happened before?" "Is this the way you felt when . . . ?" "Was this something like . . . ?"
Restating	
Repeating the main idea expressed. Gives the client an idea of what has been communicated. If misunderstood, client can clarify the message.	P: I can't sleep. I stay awake all night. N: You have difficulty sleeping?
Reflecting	
Directing questions, feelings, and ideas back to client. Encourages clients to accept their own ideas and feelings. Acknowledges the right to have opinions and make decisions and encourages clients to think of themselves as capable people.	P: Do you think I should? N: Do you think you should? P: My brother spends all my money and then has the nerve to ask for more. N: This causes you to feel angry?
Focusing	
Concentrating on a single point. Especially useful when client jumps from topic to topic. If a person is experiencing a severe or panic level of anxiety, the nurse *should not* persist until the anxiety lessens.	"This point seems worth looking at more closely."
Exploring	
Examining certain ideas, experiences, or relationships more fully. If the client chooses not to elaborate, the nurse does *not* probe or pry. In such a case, the nurse respects the client's wishes.	"Tell me more about that." "Would you describe it more fully?"
Giving Information	
Making available facts the person needs. Supplies knowledge from which decisions can be made or conclusions can be drawn. For example, the client needs to know the role of the nurse, the purpose of the nurse-client relationship, and the time, place, and duration of the meetings.	"My purpose in being here is . . ." "This medication is for . . ."
Seeking Clarification	
Clarifying unclear or vague communications can help clients clarify their own thoughts as well as maximize mutual understanding between the nurse and the client.	"I am not sure I follow you." "What would you say is the main point of what you just said?"

Table 6–2 • TECHNIQUES THAT ENHANCE COMMUNICATION *Continued*

DISCUSSION	EXAMPLE
Presenting Reality	
When a client misinterprets what is going on, the nurse indicates what is real. The nurse does not argue or try to convince the client. The nurse just describes personal perceptions or facts in the situation.	"I don't see anyone else in the room." "That sound was a car backfiring." "Your mother is not here; I am a nurse."
Voicing Doubt	
When distortions arise, the nurse can undermine the client's beliefs by not reinforcing the perceptions.	"Isn't that unusual?" "Really?" "That's hard to believe."
Seeking Consensual Validation	
Clarifies that both the nurse and client share mutual understanding of communications. Helps clients become clearer about what they are thinking.	"Tell me whether my understanding agrees with yours." "Are you using this word to convey . . . ?"
Verbalizing the Implied	
The nurse puts into concrete terms what the client implies, making the client's communication more explicit.	P: I can't talk to you or anyone else. It's a waste of time. N: Do you feel no one understands?
Encouraging Evaluation	
The nurse aids the client in considering people and events within his or her own set of values.	"How do you feel about . . . ?" "Does this contribute to your comfort?"
Attempting to Translate Into Feelings	
The nurse responds to the feelings expressed, not just the content. Often termed "desymbolizing" or "decoding."	P: I am dead. N: Are you saying that you feel lifeless? Does life seem meaningless to you?
Suggesting Collaboration	
Emphasis is placed on working *with* the client, not doing things for the client. Encourages the view that there is possibility of change through collaboration.	"Perhaps you and I can discover what produces your anxiety."
Summarizing	
Brings together important points of discussion to enhance understanding. It also allows for the opportunity to clarify communications so both go away with the same ideas in mind.	"Have I got this straight?" "You said that . . ." "During the past hour you and I have discussed . . ."
Encouraging Formulation of a Plan of Action	
Allows clients to identify alternative actions for interpersonal situations they find disturbing, e.g., when anger or anxiety are provoked.	"What could you do to let anger out harmlessly?" "Next time this comes up, what might you do to handle it?"

From Hays JS, Larson KH. Interacting With Patients. New York: Macmillan Publishing Company, 1963.

book in case studies and text, examples of verbal communication will be given. You can identify various therapeutic techniques as you read and learn to recognize and apply them in your practice.

Table 6–3 identifies techniques that may hinder communications and make understanding between two people difficult.

Students new to a mental health setting can become aware of their own communication patterns, identify their responses, and increase their ability to alter responses to maximize open communication. Some important therapeutic techniques will be discussed further, essentially (1) clarifying techniques, (2) the use of silence, and (3) active listening.

Table 6–3 • TECHNIQUES THAT HINDER COMMUNICATION

DISCUSSION	EXAMPLE
Reassuring	
Underrates a person's feelings and belittles a person's concerns. May cause clients to stop sharing feelings if they think they will be ridiculed or not taken seriously.	"I wouldn't worry about . . ." "Everything will be all right." "You're doing fine."
Giving Approval	
Saying that what the client is now doing is "good" implies that not doing it is "bad." When praise is given, potential learning may be closed because the client now seeks to gain the nurse's approval rather than to focus on the steps of learning.	"That's good." "I'm glad you . . ."
Rejection	
A client may feel rejected by the nurse when unable to express personal thoughts and feelings. Thus, the client avoids sharing thoughts or feelings to avoid the risk of further rejection.	"Let's not discuss . . ." "I don't want to hear about . . ."
Disapproving	
Implies the nurse has the right to judge the client's thoughts or actions. It further implies the client is expected to please the nurse. If the client's behavior is extreme or hurtful, the nurse shouldn't label the behavior.	"That's bad . . ." "I'd rather you wouldn't . . ." "You are upset now. We can't allow you to do this."
Agreeing	
When the nurse agrees with clients, they are denied an opportunity to change their point of view.	"That's right." "I agree."
Disagreeing	
Disagreeing often makes a person defensive. Defending one's ideas often tends to strengthen them. If a client has delusional thinking, defending such thinking prevents the exploration of feelings or refocusing energies into more productive activities or interactions.	"I don't believe that." "I disagree with that."
Advising	
Conveys that the nurse knows best and that clients cannot think for themselves. Fosters dependency and denies clients the right to think through their own problems.	"I think you should . . ." "Why don't you . . ."
Probing	
Clients may feel used and valued only for the information they can give. Most people resent persistent personal questions.	"Tell me about your dislike for your wife."

Table 6-3 • TECHNIQUES THAT HINDER COMMUNICATION *Continued*

DISCUSSION	EXAMPLE
Challenging	
Demanding proof from people tends to expand and strengthen their beliefs, especially if their beliefs serve an unmet need. Clients become more defensive and block attempts to discuss unmet needs.	"If you're dead, how come your heart is beating?"
Testing	
By testing, the nurse is saying, "Admit that you need help." Instead of asking questions such as "Can you remember?" the nurse could say "Tell me what took place."	"What day is this?" "Do you know what kind of hospital this is?"
Defending	
Protecting someone or something from verbal attack implies that the client has no right to express his or her impressions, opinions, or feelings. Defending could also imply to the client that the nurse is taking the others' side against the client.	"I am sure he only meant to help you." "No one here would lie to you."
Requesting an Explanation	
Asking people to provide reasons for thoughts or feelings can be intimidating. Actually, if people knew why they were losing weight or were anxious, they could probably deal with the situation. It is better to ask people to describe *what* is occurring rather than why it is occurring.	"Why do you feel this way?" "Why did you do that?"
Indicating an External Source	
Suggesting that a person's thoughts, feelings, or behaviors are caused by an outside force can have two detrimental outcomes. It encourages the use of projection (the devil made me do it), or it negates the client's responsibility for his or her own thoughts or actions. Better to ask, "What events led up to that conclusion?" than "What made you think that?"	"What would make you say that?" "Who told you that you were God?"
Belittling Feelings Expressed	
This is evident when the nurse is unable to empathize or understand another point of view. When a nurse tells a client to "buck up" or "cheer up," the client's feelings or experience is being belittled. This can cause a person to feel "small" or "insignificant." It is more useful to say, "You must feel upset," or "Would you like to talk about it?"	P: I wish I was dead. N: Everyone gets down once in a while. N: I know what you mean. N: I get that way sometimes.
Making Stereotypical Comments	
Cliches and trivial expressions lack value in the nurse-client relationship. Empty conversation by the nurse encourages empty responses by the client.	"It's for your own good." "Keep your chin up." "I'm fine, how are you?"
Giving Literal Responses	
Responding to a person's figurative statements as though they were statements of fact indicates the nurse's inability to understand the client's experience. This type of response prevents the nurse's working with the client to describe feelings.	P: I'm an Easter egg. N: What a shame. You don't look like an Easter egg. P: They are looking into my head with a TV. N: Try not to watch TV. What channel?

Table continued on following page

Table 6–3 • TECHNIQUES THAT HINDER COMMUNICATION *Continued*

DISCUSSION	EXAMPLE
Using Denial	
When the nurse uses denial, avenues of discussion are blocked, and clients are blocked from identifying and exploring their difficulties.	P: I am nothing. N: Of course you're something. Everybody is somebody.
Interpreting	
While a psychiatrist may interpret directly, the nurse is not prepared to deal with a client's unconscious perceptions.	"What you really mean is . . ." "Unconsciously you're saying . . ."
Introducing an Unrelated Topic	
This happens when the nurse changes the topic when a threatening or anxiety-provoking topic is brought up. It is important for the nurse to become aware of what precipitates these occurrences.	P: I'd like to die. N: Did you have visitors this weekend?

From Hays JS, Larson KH. Interacting with patients. New York: Macmillan Publishing Company, 1963.

Clarifying Techniques

Understanding depends on clear communication, which is aided by verifying with a client your interpretation of the client's messages. Requesting feedback on the accuracy of our listening and observations is essential to critical thinking. The use of clarifying techniques assists both participants in identifying major differences in their frame of reference, giving them the opportunity to correct misperceptions before they cause any serious misunderstandings. The client who is asked to elaborate on or clarify vague or ambiguous messages needs to know that the purpose is to promote mutual understanding (Collins 1983, 88).

PARAPHASING. For clarity, one might restate in newer and fewer words the basic content of a client's message. Using simple, precise, and culturally relevant terms, one may confirm without delay the interpretation of the client's previous message before the interview proceeds. Prefacing statements with a phrase such as, "I am not sure I understand . . . ?" or "In other words, you seem to be saying . . . " the nurse helps the client form a clearer perception of what may be a bewildering mass of details. After paraphrasing, the nurse must validate the accuracy of the restatement and its helpfulness to the discussion. The client may confirm or deny the perceptions through nonverbal cues or by directly responding to a question such as, "Was I correct in saying that . . . ?" As a result, the client is made aware of the face that the interviewer is actively involved in the search for understanding (Collins 1983, 88).

RESTATING. Using **restating,** the nurse mirrors the client's overt and covert messages. Thus, this technique may be used to echo content as well as feeling. In a manner different from paraphrasing, restating the content of the client's communication involves repetition of the same key words that the client has just spoken. As a corollary, should a client remark, "My life has been full of pain," additional information may be gained by restating, "Your life has been full of pain . . . " The purpose is to more thoroughly explore subjects that may be significant. However, too frequent and indiscriminate use of restating might be interpreted by clients as disinterest or inattention. To inappropriately parrot or mimic what another has said may be perceived as poking fun at the person, making this nondirective approach a definite drawback to communication (Collins 1983, 88).

REFLECTING. Another key to understanding is **reflecting** the feelings that messages convey. The interviewer describes briefly to the client the apparent meaning of the emotional tones of his or her verbal and nonverbal behavior. By way of example, to reflect to a client his feelings about his life, a good beginning might be, "You sound like you have had many disappointments" (Collins 1983, 88). Sharing **observations** with a client shows acceptance; the nurse helps bring the client's feelings into his awareness and encourages his ownership of them, for example, "You look sad." Preceiving that the nurse's concern may parallel his own, a client may more spontaneously share his feelings (Collins 1984, 89).

Use of Silence

In our society and in nursing there is an emphasis on action and "doing." In communication, we tend to expect a high level of verbal activity. Many students and practicing nurses find that when the flow of words stop, they become uncomfortable. Using silence well, however, is a good communication technique.

Instead of being the absence of communication, silence is a specific channel for transmitting and receiving messages. This awareness along may help the practitioner accept the use of silence as a significant means of influencing and being influenced by others.

In the initial interview, the client may be reluctant to speak because of the newness of the situation, the strangeness of the nurse, self-consciousness, embarrassment, or shyness. Talking is highly individualized; some find the telephone a nuisance, yet others believe they cannot live without it. One must recognize and respect individual differences in styles and tempos of responding. How else can we learn of another's nature and our own but by courtesy, care, and time? The quiet person, the person with a language barrier or speech impediment, the elderly, and persons who lack confidence in their ability to express themselves may be communicating through their silences a need for support and encouragement in acts of self-expression.

Although there is no universal rule concerning how much is too much silence, silence has been said to be "worthwhile" only as long as it is "serving some function and is not frightening to the patient" (Schulman 1974). Knowing when to speak during the interview is largely dependent on one's perception about what is being conveyed through the silence. Sometimes the topic under discussion has been exhausted; if the client does not begin anew, brief supportive comments or an open-ended question may stimulate conversation in another direction. Icy silence may be an expression of anger and hostility. Being ignored or "given the silent treatment" is recognized as an insult and a particularly hurtful form of communication.

Silence may also indicate emotional blocking. A client who feels pressured to talk about a subject that is too painful or delicate may react by changing the subject or looking away with stony silence as a form of defiance or resistance. One can intervene in a surefooted manner against resistance only when the relationship has built a reservoir of trust and intimacy so that it can withstand the strain. Timing is essential; the more positive experiences the participants have had together over time, the greater the likelihood of painful disclosures by the client. If the relationship has not reached the stage of mutual trust, more may be gained if the client's unreadiness is respected and the conversation is not pursued along the lines that evoked the initial reaction. Rather, silence can communicate strength and support in regaining composure and continuing the conversation at a more comfortable level. *Thus, silence can show respect for the client's right to choose the nature, circumstances, and the degree of openness in communication* (Collins 1983, 80).

Successful interviewing may be largely dependent on the nurse's "will to abstain"—refrain from talking more than is necessary. Solitude may provide meaningful moments of reflection for both participants. It gives them each an opportunity to contemplate thoughtfully what has been said and felt, to weigh alternatives, to formulate new ideas, and to gain a new perspective of the matter under discussion. If the nurse waits to speak and allows a client to break the silence first, the client may share thoughts and feelings that might otherwise have been withheld. Nurses who feel compelled to fill every void with words may often do so because of their own anxiety, self-consciousness, and embarrassment. When this occurs, the nurse's needs for comfort tend to take priority over the needs of clients (Collins 1983, 81).

On the other hand, prolonged and frequent silences by the nurse may hinder an interview that requires verbal articulation. Although the untalkative nurse may be comfortable with silence, this mode of communication may make the client feel used and like a fountain of information to be drained dry. Moreover, without feedback, a client has no way of knowing whether what he or she said was understood. Verbal patterns of students have been demonstrated to correlate with communication competence (Johnson 1964). The *appropriate* use of verbal techniques of interviewing helped the students focus more directly on the client's needs and elicit more emotional responses. The nurse who values silence highly may need to reassess the impact of nonverbal communication on the interviewing process. Without such a reassessment, there may be minimal use of the creative potential of mutuality, or working with the client toward goals (Collins 1983, 81).

Active Listening

Active listening is listening attentively and responding relevantly. This kind of listening can be of considerable help to persons working through a problem. Listening creates an interpersonal situation of maximal involvement that may allow clients to experience themselves more fully and freely. In the search for understanding, the nurse observes a client's total network of communication: body messages, tactile messages, silent messages, and the messages that may be plainly or symbolically verbalized. In turn, caring and concern for a client may be communicated by acknowledging understanding or misunderstanding of messages (Collins 1983, 81).

Listening helps strengthen a client's ability to solve personal problems. In the depths of one's fantasy world, one does not have to make any sense, but to reach an objective, whether relief from tension or gaining information, one usually has to place one's thoughts in some semblance of order to be able to identify the problem area more readily to others. Giving the client undivided attention, the nurse communicates that the client is not alone but with someone who will be thinking along with the client to understand and help. This kind of intervention enhances self-esteem and encourages the client to direct energy toward reaching the discussion objectives. Serving as a "sounding board," the nurse listens as the client tests thoughts by voicing them aloud. This form of interpersonal interaction often enables the client to clarify thinking, link ideas, and tentatively decide what should be done and how best to do it (Collins 1983, 82).

The Therapeutic Nurse-Client Relationship

TYPES OF RELATIONSHIPS

The term nurse-client relationship is often loosely defined within a hospital setting, but a therapeutic relationship incorporating principles of mental health nursing is more clearly defined and different from other relationships. There is an awareness that such a relationship develops over time and goes through specific stages. It is also acknowledged that specific phenomena occur during the process of the relationship.

A relationship is an interpersonal process between two or more people. Throughout life, we meet people in a variety of settings and share a variety of experiences. With some individuals, we develop relationships on either a short- or a long-term basis. The kinds of relationships we enter into vary with different people. Generally, they may be defined as (1) social, (2) intimate, or (3) therapeutic in nature.

Social Relationships

For our purposes, **social relationships** are primarily initiated for the purpose of friendship, socialization, enjoyment, or accomplishing a task. Mutual needs are met during social interaction, such as participants sharing ideas, feelings, and experiences. Communication skills include giving advice and, sometimes, meeting basic dependency needs, such as loaning money and helping with jobs. Often the content remains superficial. During social interactions, roles may shift. Within a social relationship, there is little emphasis on the evaluation of the interaction.

Intimate Relationships

An **intimate relationship** occurs between two individuals who have an emotional commitment to each other. Those in an intimate relationship usually react naturally to each other. Often the relationship is a partnership whereby each member cares about the other's needs for growth and satisfaction. Within the relationship, mutual needs are met, and intimate desires and fantasies are shared. Short- and long-range goals are usually mutually satisfying for both partners. Content shared between them may be personal and intimate. People may want an intimate relationship for many reasons, such as procreation, sexual or emotional satisfaction, economic security, social belonging, and reducing loneliness. Although transference and countertransference phenomena occur, they are usually not recognized or dealt with within the relationship. Depending on the style, level of maturity, or awareness of both parties, evaluation of the interactions may or may not be ongoing.

Therapeutic Relationships

A **therapeutic relationship** differs from either a social or an intimate relationship in that the nurse maximizes his or her communication skills, understanding of human behaviors, and personal strengths in order to enhance personal growth in the client. The focus of the relationship is on the client's ideas, experiences, and feelings (Smitherman 1982). Inherent in a therapeutic relationship is the nurse's focus on significant personal issues introduced by the client during the clinical interview. The nurse and the client identify areas that need exploration and periodically evaluate the degree of change in the client. The roles do not change, and the relationship is consistently focused on the client's problems. Communication skills and knowledge of the stages and phenomena occurring in a therapeutic relationship are crucial tools in the formation and maintenance of that relationship. Within the context of a therapeutic relationship, the needs of the client are identified, alternate problem-solving approaches are taken, and new coping skills may be developed.

King (1971) describes a therapeutic relationship as a

learning experience for both client and nurse. She identifies four actions that must take place between nurse and client:

1. An initial action by the nurse.
2. A reaction response from the client.
3. An interaction in which nurse and client assess client needs and define goals.
4. A transaction in which a reciprocal relationship is finally established to achieve relationship goals.

FACTORS THAT ENHANCE GROWTH IN OTHERS

Rogers (1967) has identified three personal characteristics that aid in the promotion of change and growth in clients: (1) congruence (genuineness), (2) empathy, and (3) positive regard (Rogers and Truax 1967).

Congruence

Rogers uses the word congruence to signify genuineness, or an awareness of one's personal feelings as they arise within the relationship and the ability to communicate them when appropriate. Essentially it is the ability to meet "person to person" in a therapeutic relationship and is conveyed by such actions as not hiding behind the role of nurse, listening to and communicating with others without distorting their messages, and being clear and concrete in communications with clients. Congruence connotes the ability to use therapeutic communication tools in an appropriately spontaneous manner, not rigidly or in a parrot-like fashion (Egan 1982).

Empathy

Empathy is the ability to get inside another person's world and see things from the other person's perspective and to communicate this understanding to the other person (Egan 1982).

Positive Regard

Positive regard implies respect. It is the ability to view another person as being worthy of caring and as someone who has strengths and achievement potential. Respect is usually not communicated directly in words but rather reflects an attitude that is most often communicated by actions.

ATTITUDES. One attitude a nurse might have that conveys respect is willingness to work with a client. That is, the nurse takes herself or himself seriously, takes the client seriously, and takes the relationship seriously. The experience is not viewed as "a job," "part of a course," or "time spent talking" but rather as an opportunity to work with people to develop their own resources and increase their potential in living.

ACTIONS. Some actions that manifest an attitude of respect are attending, suspending value judgments, and helping clients develop their own resources.

Attending. Attending refers to an intensity of presence, or being with the client (Egan 1982). Some nonverbal behaviors that reflect the degree of attending are body posture of the nurse (leaning forward toward the client and arms comfortably at sides), degree of eye contact, and how relaxed the nurse is during the interaction.

Suspending Value Judgments. Nurses should not immediately judge the client's thoughts, feelings, or behaviors using their own value systems. For example, if a client is taking drugs or acting sexually promiscuous, the nurse might recognize that these behaviors are hindering the client from living a more satisfying life or developing satisfying relationships. However, labeling these activities as "bad" or "good" is not useful. Rather, the nurse focuses on exploring the behavior of the client and works toward identifying the thinking and feelings that influence the behavior. Judgmental behavior on the part of the nurse will most likely interfere with further exploration. Egan (1982) cites the following example:

CLIENT: I am really sexually promiscuous. I give in to sexual tendencies whenever they arise and whenever I can find a partner. This has been going on for at least three years.

NURSE: So, letting yourself go sexually is part of the picture also.

In the preceding example, the nurse focuses on the client's behaviors and the possible meaning these behaviors might have to the client. The nurse does not introduce personal value statements or prejudices he or she might hold regarding promiscuous sexual behaviors.

Helping Clients Develop Resources. The nurse becomes aware of the clients' strengths and encourages them to work at their optimum level of functioning. The nurse does not act for clients unless absolutely necessary, and then only as a step toward helping them act on their own.

CLIENT: This medication makes me so dry. Could you get me something to drink?

NURSE: There is juice in the refrigerator. I'll wait here for you until you get back.

CLIENT: Could you ask the doctor to let me have a pass for the weekend?

NURSE: Your doctor will be on the unit this afternoon. I will let him know you want to speak to him.

Consistently encouraging the client to use his or her own resources helps to minimize the client's feelings of helplessness and dependency while also validating his or her potential for change.

PHASES OF THE NURSE-CLIENT RELATIONSHIP

The ability of the nurse to engage in interpersonal interactions in a goal-directed manner for the purpose of assisting clients with their emotional or physical health care needs is the foundation of nursing practice (Hagerty 1984).

The nurse-client relationship is synonymous with that of a professional helping relationship. The behaviors described by Mauksch and David (1972) have relevance to many health care workers, including nurses, and are as follows:

1. *Accountability.* The nurse assumes responsibility for the conduct and consequences of the task. As originator of the tasks, the nurse is fully answerable for them.
2. *Primacy of Client Interest.* The interest of the client, not that of other health care workers or of the institution, is given first consideration. The nurse's role is that of client advocate.
3. *Scientific Competence.* The criteria on which the nurse bases his or her conduct are principles of knowledge and selected appropriateness to the specific situation, as well as the latest knowledge made available from research.
4. *Supervision.* Validation of performance quality is through regularly scheduled supervisory sessions. Supervision is conducted either by a more experienced clinician or through discussion with one's peers in professionally conducted supervisory sessions.

Nurses interact with clients in a variety of settings, such as emergency rooms, medical-surgical units, maternity and pediatric units, clinics, community settings, schools, or client homes. Nurses who are sensitive to a client's needs, have sound assessment skills, and have effective communication skills can have a great impact on the client's present problems and on future choices he or she makes.

Sometimes, the type of relationship that occurs may be informal and not extensive, when the nurse and client meet only for a few sessions. However, even though brief, the relationship may be substantial, useful, and important for the client. This limited relationship is often referred to as a **therapeutic encounter** (Hagerty 1984).

At other times, the encounters may be of longer duration and more formal, such as in in-patient settings, mental health units, crisis centers, and mental health centers. This longer time span allows for the development of a therapeutic nurse-client relationship. The therapeutic nurse-client relationship is the medium through which the nursing process is implemented (Hagerty 1984).

Basically, three distinctive phases of the nurse-client relationship are generally recognized: (1) the orientation phase, (2) the working phase, and (3) the termination phase. Although various phenomena and goals are identified for each stage, they often overlap from phase to phase.

Orientation Phase of the Nurse-Client Relationship

The **orientation phase** can last a few meetings or can extend over a longer period of time, depending upon the client's psychopathology, the complexity of the client's problems, the comfort and experience of the nurse, and other variables.

The first time the nurse and the client meet, they are strangers to each other. When strangers meet, whether or not they know anything about each other, they interact according to their own backgrounds, standards, values, and experiences. This fact—that each person has a unique frame of reference—underlies the need for self-awareness on the part of the nurse. The nurse has a responsibility to identify two phenomena, called **transference** and **countertransference.**

TRANSFERENCE. Transference is a process whereby a client unconsciously and inappropriately displaces (transfers) onto individuals in his or her current life those patterns of behavior and emotional reactions that originated with significant figures from childhood (MacKinnon and Michels 1971). Although the transference phenomenon occurs in all relationships, transference seems to be intensified in relationships with authority (Nicholi 1988). Since the process of transference is accelerated toward a person in authority, physicians, nurses, and social workers are all potential objects of transference. It is important to realize that those thoughts, feelings, and reactions which are realistic and appropriate that a client experiences toward a health care worker are *not* transference phenomena.

Common forms of transference include the desire for affection, respect, and gratification of dependency needs. Other transferential feelings the client might experience are intense feelings of hostility, jealousy, competitiveness, and love. Requests for special favors, e.g., food, cigarettes, water, extra time within the session, are concrete examples of transference phenomena (MacKinnon and Michels 1971).

COUNTERTRANSFERENCE. Countertransference refers to the tendency of the nurse to displace feelings belonging to people in the nurse's past onto the client. If the nurse feels either a very strong positive or strong negative reaction to a client, the feeling may signal a possible countertransferential process in the nurse. A common sign of countertransference in the nurse is overidentification with the client. In other words, the nurse may have difficulty recognizing or understanding problems the client has that are similar to the nurse's own. Other indications of countertransference are when the nurse gets involved in power struggles, competition, or arguing with the client (MacKinnon and Michels 1971). Box 6–1 identifies some common emotional reactions that might signify a nurse's countertransference reaction.

The identification of and working through various transference and countertransference issues is crucial for growth and positive change in the client. These issues are best dealt with in a supervisory capacity either through supervision with a more experienced professional or peer supervision. Regularly scheduled supervision or peer supervision sessions provide the opportunity for increased self-awareness, increased clinical skills, and increased growth on the part of the nurse as well as the client.

ESTABLISHING TRUST. A major emphasis during the first few encounters with the client is providing an atmosphere in which trust can grow. As in any relationship, trust is nurtured by demonstrating congruence, empathy, and positive regard and by offering assistance in alleviating the client's emotional pain and or problems (Hagerty 1984).

During the orientation phase, four important issues need to be addressed: (1) The parameters of the relationship, (2) formal or informal contract, (3) confidentiality, and (4) termination.

1. *The Parameters of the Relationship.* The client needs to know about the nurse, who he or she is, his or her background, and the purpose of the meetings. For example, a student might furnish the following information.

   STUDENT: Hello, Mrs. James. I am Nancy Rivera from Orange Community College. I am in my psychiatric rotation, and I will be coming to York Hospital for the next ten Thursdays. I would like to spend time with you each Thursday if you are still here. We can use that time to discuss areas of your life that are a concern or that you might like to change.

2. *The Formal or Informal Contract.* Contracts emphasize the client's participation and responsibility, since the contract shows that the nurse does something *with* the client rather than *for* the client (Collins 1983, 45). The **contract,** either stated or written, contains the place, time, dates, and duration of the meetings. During the orientation phase, the client may begin to express thoughts and feelings, identify problems, and discuss realistic goals. Therefore, the mutual agreement on goals is also part of the contract. If the goals are met, the client's level of functioning will return to a previous level or at least improve from the present level. If fees are to be paid, the client is told how much they will be and when the payment is due.

   STUDENT: Mrs. James, we will meet at 10:00 A.M. each Thursday in the music room for 45 minutes, from September 15th through November 16th. We can use that time for further discussion of your feelings of loneliness and anger with your husband and to explore some things you could do to make things better for yourself.

3. *Confidentiality.* The client has a right to know who else will know about the information he or she shares with the nurse. The client needs to know that the information may be shared with specific people, for example, a clinical supervisor, the physician, staff, or other students in conference. The client also needs

Box 6–1. POSSIBLE COUNTERTRANSFERENCE REACTIONS

Thoughts wander—feeling detached
Feeling impatient or insensitive to the client
Feeling envy
Sexual or aggressive fantasies about the client
Overconcern for the client between sessions
Power struggling with the client
Dreams about the client
Being intrusive or controlling with the client
Overidentifying with the plight or happiness of the client

to know that the information is **not** shared with the client's relatives, friends, or others outside the treatment team, except in extreme situations. This will usually be done by the physician, according to legal guidelines. (Refer to Chapter 3, p. 53.) The nurse must also be aware of the client's right to **confidentiality** and must not violate that right.

STUDENT: Mrs. James, I will be sharing some of what we discuss with my nursing instructor, and at times I may discuss certain concerns with my peers in conference or the staff. However, I will *not* be sharing this information with your husband or any other members of your family without your permission.

4. *Termination*. Termination begins in the orientation phase. It may be mentioned when appropriate during the working phase as well, if the nature of the relationship is time limited, e.g., ten sessions. The date of the termination phase should be clear in the beginning. In some situations, the nurse-client contract may be renegotiated when the termination date has been reached. In other situations, when the therapeutic nurse-client relationship is an open-ended one, the termination date is not known. Usually, however, for students, the termination date is set by the length of the course and their clinical affiliation, and the termination date is known.

STUDENT: Mrs. James, as I mentioned earlier, our last meeting will be November 16th. We will have nine more meetings after today.

Working Phase of the Nurse-Client Relationship

Moore and Hartman (1988) identify specific tasks of the working phase of the nurse-client relationship. These are to

1. maintain the relationship,
2. gather further data,
3. promote the client's development,
4. facilitate behavioral change,
5. overcome resistance behaviors, and
6. evaluate problems and goals and redefine as necessary.

It is during **the working phase** that the nurse and client together identify and explore areas in the client's life that are causing the client problems in living. Such problems are called *dysfunctional*. Often the client's ways of handling situations stem from earlier ways of coping in order to survive in a chaotic and dysfunctional family environment. Although certain coping methods may have worked for the client at an earlier age, they now interfere with the client's interpersonal relationships and prevent the client from attaining current goals. Since the client's dysfunctional behaviors and basic assumptions about the world are often defensive in nature, and the client is unable to change his or her dysfunctional behavior at will, most of the problem behaviors or thinking continue because of unconscious motivations and needs that are out of the client's conscious awareness.

The nurse can work with the client to identify these unconscious motivations and assumptions which keep the client from finding satisfaction and reaching his or her potential. The describing and often re-experiencing of old conflicts awakens high levels of anxiety in the client. The client may use a variety of defenses against anxiety and displace his or her feelings onto the nurse. Therefore, during the working phase, intense emotions such as anxiety, anger, self-hate, hopelessness, and helplessness may surface. Behaviors such as acting out one's anger inappropriately, withdrawing, intellectualizing, manipulating, denying, and other behaviors are to be expected. During this time strong transferential feelings may appear. The emotional responses and behaviors in the client may also reawaken strong countertransferential feelings in the nurse. *The nurse's awareness of personal feelings and reactions to the client are vital for effective interaction with the client.* Common transferential feelings and reactions that nurses experience in response to different behaviors and situations are dealt with under the planning component of each of the clinical chapters (Chapters 10–25).

The development of a strong working relationship can allow the client to experience increased levels of anxiety and behaviors in a safe setting, as well as try out new and more adaptive coping behaviors.

The nurse, to the best of his or her ability, remains neutral and nondefensive and will work with the client to make connections between inappropriate and dysfunctional behaviors, thinking, and feelings. During this time, the client tries out alternative coping behaviors, increases independent functioning, and takes a more active role in problem solving. Change may begin to occur in the client's self-concept and self-esteem.

Termination Phase of the Nurse-Client Relationship

Termination is discussed during the first interview. During the working stage, the fact of eventual termination may also be raised at appropriate times. Six reasons for terminating the nurse-client relationship have been identified (Campaniello 1980):

1. Symptom relief.
2. Improved social functioning.
3. Greater sense of identity.
4. More adaptive defenses.
5. Accomplishment of goals.
6. Impasse in therapy that the nusre is unable to resolve.

Another reason may be forced termination such as in the completion of a student's course objectives. **Termination** is the final phase of the nurse-client relationship. Important reasons for the student to address the termination phase of the relationship have been identified (Phillips 1968):

1. Termination is a phase of the therapeutic nurse-client relationship, and without it the relationship remains incomplete.
2. Feelings are aroused in both the client and the student regarding the experience they have had; when these feelings are recognized and shared, the client learns that it is acceptable to feel sadness and loss when someone he or she cares about leaves.
3. The client is a partner in the relationship and has a right to see the nurse's needs and feelings regarding their time together and the ensuing separation.
4. Termination can be a learning experience; the client can learn that he or she is important to at least one person.
5. By sharing the termination experience with the client, the nurse demonstrates caring for the client.

Termination often awakens strong feelings in both nurse and client. Termination between the nurse and the client signifies a loss for both, although the intensity and meaning of the termination may be different for each. If a client has unresolved feelings of abandonment or loneliness or feelings of not being wanted or of being rejected by others, these feelings may be reawakened during the termination process. The termination process can be an opportunity for the client to express these feelings, perhaps for the first time.

It is not unusual to see a variety of client behaviors that indicate defensive maneuvers against the anxiety of separation and loss. For example, a client may withdraw from the nurse and not want to meet for the final session. Or, a client may become outwardly hostile and sarcastic, accusing the student nurse of using the client for her "own gains" like a "guinea pig," as a way of deflecting the awakening of anger and pain rooted in past separations. Often, a client will deny that the relationship had any impact or deny that ending the relationship evokes any emotions whatsoever. Regression is another behavioral manifestation that may be seen in increased dependency upon the nurse or an increase in prior symptoms.

It is important for the student to work with the client to bring into awareness the feelings and reactions the client may be experiencing in relationship to separations. If a client denies that the termination is having an effect on him or her (assuming the nurse-client relationship was strong), the student may something like, "Good-byes are difficult for people. Often they remind us of other good-byes. Tell me about another separation in the past." If the client appears to be displacing anger by either withdrawing or displacing overt anger onto the nurse, the nurse may say something like, "People experience anger when saying good-bye. Sometimes they are angry with the person who is leaving. Tell me about how you feel about my leaving." Students need to give thought to their last clinical experience with their client and work with their instructor to facilitate communication during this time.

A common response students have is that of feeling guilty about terminating the experience. This may be manifested in giving the client their telephone number, making plans to get together for coffee after the client is discharged, continuing to see the client afterwards, or exchanging letters. The student needs to understand that such actions may be motivated by the student's sense of guilt or misplaced feelings of responsibility, not by concern for the client. Indeed, part of the termination process may be to explore client plans for the future: where to go for help in the future, which agencies to contact, and which specific resource persons are available, e.g., social workers and job counselors.

During the student affiliation, the nurse-client relationship exists for the duration of the clinical course only. The termination phase is just that. Thoughts and feelings the student may be having about continuing the relationship are best discussed with the instructor or shared in post-conference with peers, since these are common reactions to a student's experience.

The Clinical Interview

The clinical interview is not a random meeting between the nurse and the client. It is a systematic attempt to understand the relation of psychopathology to emotional conflicts (MacKinnon and Michels 1971).

The clinical interview is different from the intake interview, or the assessment interview, which is described in Chapter 7, as part of the nursing process. In most cases, by the time a student meets with a client for the first time, the assessment interview, or intake interview, has already been recorded. In the hospital setting, the intake inerview has often been recorded in the chart by the physician. It is not uncommon, however, that during the clinical rotation, the student obtains important data from the client that can be added to the data base.

The content and the direction of the clinical interview are decided by the client. The client leads. The nurse employs communication skills and active listening (identifying what the client says as well as what the client does not say) to better understand the client's situation. She also observes how congruent the content (what the client says) is with the process (what the client does). During the clinical interview the nurse provides the opportunity for the client to reach the goals mentioned earlier: (1) identify and explore problems relating to others, (2) discuss healthy ways of meeting emotional needs, and (3) experience a satisfying interpersonal relationship (Hays and Larson 1963).

Communication and interviewing techniques are acquired skills. Nurses learn to increase their ability to use communication and interviewing skills through practice and supervision from a more experienced clinician. One method of increasing communication and interviewing skills is through reviewing clinical interactions exactly as they occur. This process offers students the opportunity to identify themes and patterns in their own as well as their client's communication. The student also learns to deal with a variety of situations as they arise in the clinical interview.

Perhaps the best way of reviewing nurse-client interactions is by viewing a video tape, which reveals the nonverbal as well as the verbal communications between both parties. The second best method of capturing the interaction between nurse and client is through an audio tape recording. Unfortunately, these methods are often not possible, for a variety of reasons.

The use of **process recordings** is a popular way to examine the student's and client's communication and to identify patterns. Process recordings have some disadvantages, since they rely on memory and are subject to distortions. However, they can be a useful tool for identifying communication patterns. It is usually best if the student can write verbatim (word for word) notes in a private area immediately after the interaction has taken place. Sometimes, a clinician will takes notes during the interview. This practice also has its disadvantages. For one, it may be distracting for both the interviewer and the client, and some clients (especially one with a paranoid disorder) may resent or misunderstand the nurse's intent. Table 6–4 shows a segment of a process recording. The nurse records her words, the client's words, identifies whether the responses are therapeutic or not, and recalls her emotions at the time.

Students new to the psychiatric setting often say they feel overwhelmed by the severity of some of the client's problems and feel responsible for "doing" something to positively affect the emotional health of their client. It may help you to know that a review of numerous studies positively correlates the strength of the therapist-client relationship as being more important for a successful therapeutic outcome than a variety of other factors (Nicholi 1988). Nicholi further states that recent studies have borne out that the "therapist's ability to convey an intrinsic interest in the patient has been found to be more important than his position, appearance, reputation, clinical experience, training, and technical or theoretical knowledge." This does not deny the importance of clinical training, skill, or experience. It does, however, emphasize the need for the nurse to convey genuine interest in another human being, without being patronizing or condescending (Nicholi 1988).

Anxiety during the first interview is to be expected, as in any meeting between strangers. Clients may be anxious about their problems, the nurse's reaction to them, concerns about their treatment, and so forth. Students may be anxious about the client's reactions to them, their ability to provide help, what the instructor will think of them, and how they will do compared with their peers (MacKinnon and Michels 1971).

Students have many concerns when entering the psychiatric unit for the first time. Two common concerns are (1) how to begin the interview and (2) what to do in response to client behaviors. The following section offers some basic guidelines for the first interview and identifies some common problems in clinical situations and offers possible solutions.

HOW TO BEGIN THE INTERVIEW

SETTING. Effective communication could conceivably take place almost anywhere. Whether in a clinic, ward, or office, the quality of the interaction depends on the degree to which the nurse and client feel safe and secure (Collins 1983, 64). The setting is extremely significant because it can symbolically enhance or diminish the potential of the helping relationship (Collins 1983, 65). A specific location such as a conference room or a quiet part of the unit with relative privacy yet within view of others is ideal.

SEATING. In all settings, chairs need to be placed so that conversation can take place in normal tones of voice and eye contact can be comfortably maintained or avoided (Collins 1983, 65).

INTRODUCTIONS. As previously mentioned, in the orientation phase students tell the client who they are, the name of their school, the purpose of the meetings, and how long and when they will be meeting with the

Table 6–4 • SEGMENT OF A PROCESS NOTE

NURSE	CLIENT	COMMENTS	FEELINGS
"Good Morning Mr. L"	"Who are you and where the devil am I?" Looks around with confused look on face—quickly sits on edge of bed.	*Therapeutic.* Giving recognition. Acknowledging a client by name can enhance esteem and communicates that he is viewed as an individual by nurse.	
"I am Mrs. V. I am a student nurse from X college, and you are at Mt. Sinai Hospital. I would like to spend some time with you today."		*Therapeutic.* Giving information. Informing the client of facts needed to make decisions or come to realistic conclusions. *Therapeutic.* Offering self. Making oneself available to the client.	
	"What am I doing here, how did I get here?" Spoken in a loud, demanding tone.		
"You were brought in by your wife last night after swallowing a bottle of aspirin. You had to have your stomach pumped."		*Therapeutic.* Giving information. Giving needed facts so client can orient himself and better evaluate his situation.	
	"Oh . . . yeah." Silence 2 minutes. Shoulders slump, Mr. L stares at floor and drops head and eyes.		
"You seem upset Mr. L." "What are you thinking about?"		*Therapeutic.* Making observations. He looks sad. *Therapeutic.* Giving broad openings in an attempt to get at his feelings.	
	"Yeah, I just remembered . . . I wanted to kill myself." Said in a low tone almost to self.		
"Oh Mr. L you have so much to live for. You have such a loving family."		*Nontherapeutic.* Defending.	I felt overwhelmed.
		Nontherapeutic. Introducing an unrelated topic.	I didn't know what to say—his talking about killing himself made me nervous. I could have said "You must have been very upset" (verbalizing the implied) or "Tell me more about this" (exploring).
	"What do you know about my life? You want to know about my family . . . my wife is leaving me . . . That's what." Faced nurse with angry expression on face—said in loud angry tones.		
"I didn't know. You must be terribly upset by her leaving."		*Therapeutic.* Reflective. Observes angry tone and content of client's message and reflects back client's feelings.	

client. The issue of confidentiality is also covered at some point during the initial interview. The nurse can then ask the client how he or she would like to be addressed. This question accomplishes several tasks (Shea 1988, 59):

1. It conveys respect.
2. It gives the client direct control over an important ego issue. (Some clients do not like to be called by last names, and others do not like to be called by first names.)
3. One may learn something about the client when his or her preference is revealed.

HOW TO START. Once introductions have been made, the nurse can turn the interview over to the client by using one of a number of open-ended statements (Shea 1988; MacKinnon and Michels 1971):

- *Where should we start?*
- *Tell me a little about what has been going on with you.*
- *What are some of the stresses you have been coping with recently?*
- *Tell me a little about what has been happening in the past couple of weeks.*
- *Perhaps we can begin by letting me know what some of your concerns have been recently.*
- *Tell me about your difficulties.*

The facilitation of communication can be made with the appropriate use of offering leads, e.g., "Go on," statements of acceptance, e.g., "Uh huh," or other conveyances of the nurse's interest (Shea 1988).

TACTICS TO AVOID. Some behaviors the nurse should avoid have been suggested by Wolberg (1977, 445–457) as quoted by Moscato (1988):

- Do not argue with, minimize, or challenge the client.
- Do not praise the client or give false reassurance.
- Do not make false promises.
- Do not interpret to the client or speculate on the dynamics of the client's problem.
- Do not offer the client a diagnosis even if he or she insists on it.
- Do not question the client on sensitive areas.
- Do not try to "sell" the client on accepting treatment.
- Do not join in attacks the client launches on parents, mate, friends, or associates.
- Do not participate in criticism of another nurse or any other staff member.

WHAT TO DO IN RESPONSE TO CLIENT BEHAVIORS

Often students new to the mental health setting are concerned about being in situations that they are unsure of how to handle. These concerns are universal and often arise in the clinical setting. Table 6–5 identifies common client behaviors, such as crying, asking the nurse to keep a secret, or saying he wants to kill himself. The table gives an example of an appropriate response, the rationale for the response, and a possible verbal statement. Read the table, paying particular attention to the **rationale** for responses. Your exact words will

Table 6–5 • WHAT TO DO IF THE CLIENT . . .

POSSIBLE REACTIONS BY NURSE	USEFUL RESPONSES BY NURSE
What To Do If The Client Cries	
Nurse may feel uncomfortable and experience increased anxiety or feel somehow responsible for making the person cry.	Stay with the client; reinforce that it is all right to cry. Often it is at that time that feelings are closest to the surface and can best be identified. "You seem ready to cry." "You still are upset about your brother's death." "What are you thinking right now?" Offer tissues when appropriate.
What To Do If The Client Asks The Nurse To Keep a Secret	
Nurse may feel conflicted by wanting the client to share important information but being unsure about making such a promise.	The nurse canNOT make such a promise. The information may be important to the health or safety of the client or others. "I cannot make that promise. It might be important for me to share it with other staff." The client then decides to share the information or not.

Table 6–5 • WHAT TO DO IF THE CLIENT . . . *Continued*

POSSIBLE REACTIONS BY NURSE	USEFUL RESPONSES BY NURSE
What To Do If The Client Leaves Before The Session Is Over	
Nurse may feel rejected, thinking it was something that he or she did. Nurse may experience increased anxiety or feel abandoned by the client.	Some clients are not able to relate for long periods of time without experiencing an increase in anxiety. On the other hand, the client may be testing the nurse. "I will wait for you here for 15 minutes until our time is up." During this time, the nurse does NOT engage in conversation with any other client or even with the staff. When time is up, approach client, tell him or her your time is up, and restate the day and time you will see him or her again.
What To Do If Another Client Interrupts During Your Time With Your Selected Client	
Nurse may feel a conflict. Does not want to appear "rude." Sometimes tries to engage both in conversation.	The time you have contracted with your selected client is that client's time. Keeping your part of the contract demonstrates that you mean what you say and that you view the sessions as important. "I am with Mr. Rob for the next 20 minutes. At 10 A.M., after our time is up, I can talk to you for 5 minutes."
What To Do If The Client Says He Wants To Kill Himself Or Elope	
Nurse may feel overwhelmed or responsible to "talk the client out of it." Nurse may pick up some of the client's feelings of hopelessness.	The nurse tells the client that this is serious, that the nurse does not want harm to come to the client, and that this information needs to be reported to other staff. "This is very serious, Mrs. Lamb. I do not want any harm to come to you. I will have to report this to other staff. The nurse can then discuss with the client the feelings and circumstances that led up to this decision. (Refer to Chapter 22 for suicide intervention.)
What To Do If The Client Says He Does Not Want To Talk	
The nurse new to this situation may feel rejected or ineffectual.	At first the nurse might say something to this effect: "It's all right. I would like to spend time with you. We don't have to talk." The nurse might spend short, frequent periods of time (e.g., 5 minutes) with the client throughout the day. "Our five minutes is up. I'll be back at 10 A.M. and stay with you five more minutes." This gives the client the opportunity to understand that the nurse means what he or she says and is back on time consistently. This also gives the client time between visits to assess the nurse and perhaps feel less threatened.
What To Do If The Client Seeks To Prolong The Interview	
Sometimes clients will open up dynamic or "juicy" topics right before the interview time is up. This is often done in order to test or manipulate the nurse. Nurse might feel tempted to extend scheduled time or might not want to "hurt" the client's feelings.	The nurse sets limits and restates the original contract—reinforces the original contract. Would use the issues for the next session. "Our time is up now Mr. Jones. This would be a good place to start at our next session, which is on Wednesday at 10 A.M."

depend on the situation, but understanding the rationale will help you apply your learning in the future.

Summary

Communication is a complex, reciprocal process. This chapter dealt with some of those complications by discussing techniques that can enhance or hinder the communication process.

Berlo's communication model was reviewed, and the various components in this model were identified (referent, sender, message, channel, receiver, and feedback). Various personal and environmental factors that can impede accurate transmissions or interpretations of messages were listed, such as emotional factors, physical factors, intellectual factors, and social factors.

During nurse-client interactions there exist verbal and nonverbal levels of communication. Communications also contain a *content* or subject dimension and *process* dimensions. Emphasis was placed on the nurse's ability to be aware of both levels to maximize communication and minimize the continuation of nonproductive behaviors on the part of the client.

Techniques that may enhance or hinder communications were presented. The learner is urged to become familiar with these techniques and to be able to identify personal communication patterns and know when changes in responses may be appropriate.

The nurse-client relationship was discussed. Factors that differentiate a therapeutic relationship from a social relationship and an intimate relationship were outlined. Personal strengths in the nurse that can enhance growth in others, namely genuineness, empathy, and positive regard, were discussed and examples were given.

Phases of the nurse-client relationship were presented, including the orientation phase, the working phase, and the termination phase.

The processes of transference and countertransference were defined. Basic guidelines for the first interview were discussed, and potential clinical situations were identified, with suggestions for nursing action.

References

Berlo DK. The Process of Communication. San Francisco: Reinhart Press, 1960.

Campaniello JA. The process of termination. Journal of Psychiatric Nursing and Mental Health Services, 18:29, 1980.

Collins M. Communication in Health Care: The Human Connection in the Life Cycle, 2nd ed. St. Louis, MO: C.V. Mosby Company, 1983.

Egan G. The Skilled Helper. Monterey, California: Brooks/Cole Publishing Company, 1982.

Gass W. Learning to talk. Seattle, Washington: University Magazine, 1979, p. 21.

Hagerty BK. Psychiatric-Mental Health Assessment. St. Louis, MO: C.V. Mosby Company, 1984.

Hall ET. Excerpts from an interview conducted by Carol Travis. GEO, 25(3):12, 1983.

Haney W. Communication and Organizational Behavior. Chicago: Richard D. Irwin, 1967, p. 88.

Hays JS, Larson KH. Interacting With Patients. New York: Macmillan Publishing Company, 1963.

Johnson B. The relationship between verbal patterns of nursing students and therapeutic effectiveness. Nursing Research, 13:339, 1964.

King IM. Toward a Theory for Nursing. New York: John Wiley & Sons, 1971.

Lego S. Individual therapy. *In* Lego S (ed). The American Handbook Of Psychiatric Nursing. Philadelphia: J.B. Lippincott Company, 1984, pp. 197–205.

MacKinnon RA, Michels R. The Psychiatric Interview in Clinical Practice. Philadelphia: W.B. Saunders Company, 1971

Mauksch G, David M. Prescription for survival. American Journal of Nursing, 72:2189, 1972.

Moore JC, Hartman, CR. Developing a therapeutic relationship. *In* Beck CK, Rawlins RP, Williams SR (eds). Mental Health-Psychiatric Nursing. St. Louis, MO: C.V. Mosby Company, 1988.

Moscato B. The one-to-one relationship. *In* Wilson HS, Kneisl CS (eds). Psychiatric Nursing, 3rd ed. Menlo Park, CA Addison-Wesley Publishing Company, 1988.

Nicholi AM. The Therapist-Patient Relationship. *In* Nicholi AM (ed). The New Harvard Guide to Psychiatry. Cambridge, MA: The Belknap Press of Harvard University, 1988.

Parkinson MH. Therapeutic interaction. *In* Sorensen KC, Luckmann J. Basic Nursing: A Psychophysiologic Approach, 2nd ed. Philadelphia: W.B. Saunders Company, 1986.

Peplau HE. Interpersonal Relations in Nursing. New York: G.P. Putnam & Sons, 1952.

Peplau HE. Interpersonal techniques: the crux of psychiatric nursing. American Journal of Nursing, 62:50, 1962.

Phillips B. Terminating a nurse-patient relationship. American Journal of Nursing, 68(9):1941, 1968.

Richardson S, Dowhrenwend B, Klein D. Interviewing: Its Forms and Functions. New York: Basic Books, 1965, p. 257.

Rogers CR. The Therapeutic Relationship and Its Impact. Madison: University of Wisconsin Press, 1967.

Rogers CR, Truax CB. The therapeutic conditions antecedent to change: A theoretical view. *In* Rogers CR (ed). The Therapeutic Relationship and Its Impact. Madison: University of Wisconsin Press, 1967.

Schulman ED. Intervention in Human Services. St. Louis MO: C.V. Mosby Company, 1974, p. 123.

Shea SC. Psychiatric Interviewing: The Art of Understanding. Philadelphia: W.B. Saunders Company, 1988.

Smitherman C. Nursing Action for Health Promotion. Philadelphia: F.A. Davis Company, 1982.

Ushvendra K. Verbal responses of nurses to patients in emotional-laden situations in public health nursing. Nursing Research, 16:365, 1967.

Wahlous S. Family Communication. New York: Macmillan Publishing Company, 1974, p. 147.

Wolberg L. The Technique of Psychotherapy. New York: Grune and Stratton, 1977, pp. 455–457.

Self-Study Exercises

True or False

1. ________ A referent is the medium by which a message is sent.
2. ________ Feedback can indicate if a message has been correctly interpreted.
3. ________ Communication is a reciprocal process.
4. ________ Emotional factors, intellectual factors, or social factors play no part in accurate transmission or interpreting of communications.

Put a V (verbal) or an N (nonverbal) next to the appropriate communication.

5. ________ Hair is not combed and stringy; clothes have food stains.
6. ________ Person states his body feels heavy.
7. ________ Person licks his lips and grimaces while talking to nurse.
8. ________ Person writes nurse a note before she leaves for the day.

Place a T (therapeutic) or an N (nontherapeutic) next to the appropriate communication, and NAME the response.

9. ________ I know exactly how you feel. RESPONSE________________
10. ________ I am not sure I understand what you mean. RESPONSE________________
11. ________ I noticed you changed into a different dress this evening. RESPONSE________________
12. ________ You should call the doctor and tell him these pills make you dizzy. RESPONSE________________
13. ________ Tell me more about your "bad dream." RESPONSE________________

Place an S (social), an I (intimate), or a T (therapeutic) next to the corresponding behaviors.

14. ________ Initiated primarily for socialization, enjoyment, and friendship.
15. ________ Initiated between two people who have an emotional commitment to each other.
16. ________ Sharing ideas, feelings, and experiences.
17. ________ Focus of the relationship is on the ideas, experiences, and feelings of just one party in the relationship.
18. ________ Content may be superficial; giving advice or meeting certain dependency needs may be appropriate.
19. ________ Evaluation of specific stated goals is ongoing within the life of the relationship.
20. ________ Mutual fantasies and goals that meet mutual needs are an integral part of the relationship.

Place an O (orientation), a W (working), or a T (termination) next to the appropriate phase of the nurse-client relationship.

21. ________ Some regression and mourning may occur, although the client has reached a point of satisfaction, security, and competence in his or her life.
21. ________ The nurse assesses the client's level of psychological functioning, and both begin to identify problems and realistic goals.
23. ________ The client begins to seek connections between actions, thoughts, and feelings, takes a more active role in problem solving, and tries out alternative coping behaviors.

True or False

24. ________ Transference is the attribution of feelings, wishes, and attitudes originally thought and felt regarding significant others in the client's life.
25. ________ It is important for the nurse to be tuned in to personal feelings when working with a client and to use these feelings to understand the client's experience better.
26. ________ Strong and intense (positive or negative) feelings in the nurse toward the client are referred to as countertransference feelings.

Write a short answer to the questions that follow:

27. You are spending time with a young woman who is depressed. She tells you she wants to kill herself. What two actions can you take?

28. You approach a middle-aged man, introduce yourself, tell him your purpose and where you are from. When you mention to him that you would like to spend time with him, he looks down and does not respond. You become anxious. Name three actions you can take.

CHAPTER 7

The Nursing Process in Psychiatric Settings

Elizabeth M. Varcarolis

OUTLINE

KEY TERMS, CONCEPTS, AND PEOPLE

The key terms, concepts, and people listed here also appear in bold where they are defined or discussed in this chapter.

HOLISTIC MODEL

HUMAN NEEDS THEORY—MASLOW

GENERAL SYSTEMS THEORY

ASSESSING BEHAVIOR
Echopraxia
Waxy Flexibility
Akathisia
Dyskinesia

ASSESSING THOUGHT PROCESSES
Tangential
Flights of Ideas
Neologisms
Confabulation
Looseness of Association

OBJECTIVES

After studying this chapter, the student will be able to:

1. Identify the components of each of the five steps in the nursing process.
2. Discuss what is meant by the "process" of psychiatric assessment.
3. Summarize the contents of the *Client History* and the *Mental and Emotional Status* of the psychiatric nursing assessment.
4. Explain five functions of the nursing diagnostic system.
5. Predict when a problem becomes a nursing diagnosis.
6. Illustrate the three components of the nursing diagnosis.
7. Write an effective goal including the three criteria discussed in this chapter.
8. Explain three principles the nurse follows in planning nursing actions to meet goals.
9. Give two examples for each of the six areas of psychiatric nursing intervention as defined by the ANA's *Standards of Psychiatric and Mental Health Nursing Practice*.
10. Outline three areas of concern when validating a plan of care.
11. Discuss two components of the evaluation process.
12. Recognize four possible outcomes after reassessment of the care plan.
13. Discuss three advantages of the problem-oriented record (POR).
14. Write a SOAP note.

The nursing process is an adaptation of the scientific process of problem solving. This problem-solving process is used today by many professions. The problem-solving method encourages clinical care based on scientific and systematic decision making, rather than rote tasks and randomly applied nursing interventions. The use of a scientific and systematic process for planning effective patient care helps to distinguish nursing as a profession, as opposed to a trade comprising technical skills solely (Hagerty 1984).

The terms nursing process and nursing diagnosis first appeared in the nursing literature in the early 1950's. The process of defining and operationalizing these concepts continued to evolve during the 1960's and 1970's through contributions by many nursing scholars (Douglas and Murphy 1981). The first formalized presentation of the nursing process was presented by Yura and Walsh in 1967 and consisted of four steps: assessment, planning, intervention, and evaluation (Yura and Walsh 1983). Later, nursing diagnosis was included as a separate step, apart from assessment, resulting in the five accepted steps used today: assessment, diagnosis, planning, intervention, and evaluation. The components of each step are presented in Figure 7 – 1.

Assessment is done for the purpose of identifying client problems and formulating *nursing diagnoses*. *Planning* includes identifying desired outcome criteria in the format of long- and short-term goals. Goals give direction for effective nursing actions. The nurse determines the *interventions* that will result in the desired outcomes. The process of *evaluating* whether or not the outcome criteria have been obtained is the fifth phase of the process. If the goals have not been met, then reassessment and replanning may be necessary.

The nurse must determine if necessary data are available, if the diagnosis is correct, the goals realistic and obtainable, and the interventions appropriate for meeting the goals.

These five steps help to operationalize the ongoing nursing process. In reality, these steps often overlap. The nurse continually assesses and analyzes data, identifies needs, resets goals, and brings a variety of appro-

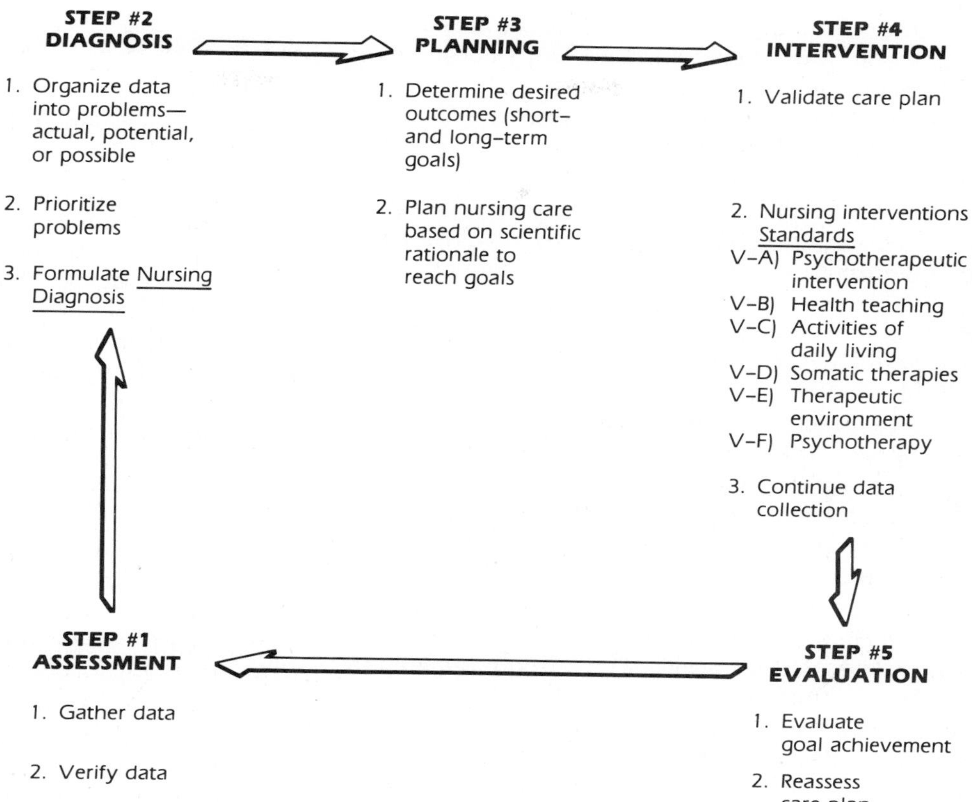

Figure 7–1. *Components of the nursing process.*

priate nursing skills into play. Evaluation of these activities is ongoing.

Today, the nursing process is the basic framework for nursing practice. The nursing process has been used as a basis for the following (Yura and Walsh 1983):

1. *Standards of Nursing Practice*, and *Standards of Psychiatric and Mental Health Nursing Practice* of the American Nurses' Association
2. Criteria for certification
3. Legal definition of nursing, as reflected in many states' *Nurse Practice Acts*
4. NCLEX-RN (the National Council of State Boards of Nursing licensure examination) format since July 1982

The nurse uses the nursing process when evaluating the client at any point on the health-illness continuum. A client may be an individual, a family, a group, or a community. Assessment is made on a variety of levels: physical, social, emotional, intellectual, spiritual, and cultural. Nursing diagnosis and planning of interventions may include primary, secondary, or tertiary interventions, depending on the specific needs and environment of the client.

In order for the nurse to work within the framework of the nursing process, it is important to recognize that the actions of the nurse are based on a number of accepted theoretical frameworks: (1) a holistic model, (2) human needs theory (Maslow), and (3) general systems theory.

The **holistic model** supports the assessment, diagnosis, planning, intervention, and evaluation of care for the total person. The holistic approach considers the client's physical, emotional, social, spiritual, intellectual, and cultural stresses and their impact on the whole individual (Bower 1982).

Human needs theory is most basic to the nursing process. When an individual's ability to meet a need is interrupted, a problem exists. Abraham Maslow has outlined our basic needs in a hierarchy familiar to all nurses (Maslow 1962).

1. Hunger, thirst, sex, and survival
2. Safety, self-preservation, security
3. Belongingness and love
4. Social esteem and self-respect
5. Self-actualization

Recognition of unmet needs is made evident from information the nurse has gathered in the assessment. An unmet need constitutes a problem. The problems nurses are most involved with are in the area of physical and emotional health. Problems are formulated into nursing diagnoses and listed in order of priority. Assessment, planning, interventions, and evaluation are ongoing until an acceptable alternative for dealing with the unmet need or problem is found.

General systems theory recognizes the impact a person's internal and external environments have on personal health. All things belong to a matrix of complex systems. Individuals are constantly being influenced and affected by the systems of which they are a part. External systems include family, community, regional, and national influences. Internal systems include body systems, organs, cells, chemical elements, and atoms (Coombs 1976).

Each level of systems can be seen as composed of subsystems. For example, internal systems, such as the respiratory, digestive, reproductive and immune systems, are all part of the larger system, the human body. Nursing is a subsystem of an external system, the health care system, which is made up of other subsystems such as medicine, dentistry, pharmacology, and social work. Any change in one system or subsystem can have a profound impact on related systems. Therefore, a thorough assessment takes into account both the internal and the external systems of the client. Nursing diagnoses and interventions address both the internal and the external environments for optimum total patient care.

There are many nursing frameworks that may be used as guides when making a nursing assessment, such as those of Rogers (1970), Riehl and Roy (1980), and Orem (1980). However, the holistic approach, Maslow's human needs theory, and general systems theory are inherent to the nursing process.

As previously stated, the *Standards of Psychiatric and Mental Health Nursing Practice* developed by the American Nurses' Association are based on the nursing process. These standards, listed on the inside front cover of the book, are used as a framework for presenting the syndromes discussed in the clinical chapters (10–25) of this book. The relationship between these standards and the nursing process is discussed in this chapter.

The first *Standard of Psychiatric and Mental Health Nursing Practice* addresses the issue of basing nursing judgments and behaviors on an accepted theoretical framework.

Standard I: Theory

All psychopathology will be presented within the framework of the nursing process. The most recent and prevalent theories of etiology will be presented for the clinical syndromes discussed in the clinical chapters (10–25).

Standard II: Data Collection

Although high levels of anxiety and maladaptive behaviors are central to the practice of psychiatric nursing, these phenomena are encountered in all areas in the health care setting. Depression, suicidal thoughts, anger, disorientation, delusions, and hallucinations are frequently encountered on medical-surgical wards and obstetrical and intensive care units, as well as in emergency rooms, clinics, and pediatric settings. The assessment of the client's psychosocial status is a part of any nursing assessment, along with the assessment of the client's physical health.

The nursing process is a cyclical one. Assessment is ongoing and continues throughout the planning, intervention, and evaluation phases. The initial assessment often clarifies the client's immediate needs. As the nurse works further with the client, the data base is enlarged, and other problems may become evident.

Psychiatric nursing assessment is done within the framework of the psychiatric interview. The assessment interview in psychiatric nursing is often done in the psychiatric inpatient units; however, it can be done in a variety of settings: emergency rooms, medical-surgical units, intensive care units, crisis units, community mental health centers, private practice, on home visits, and in schools. The time given for the interview varies depending on the clinical setting and circumstances of the client. During emergencies, immediate intervention is often based on a minimal amount of data. A scheduled psychiatric interview and psychosocial assessment in a more structured setting allows more time for a more elaborate assessment (Hagerty 1984). At other times, completing the assessment process may involve a number of interviews.

The purpose of the psychiatric assessment (Hagerty 1984) is to

1. Assess a person's current level of psychological functioning
2. Establish a trusting rapport
3. Understand how previous modes of coping contributed to the person's psychosocial development.
4. Formulate a plan of care

Although the nurse might obtain a lot of needed data from the physician's assessment, the nurse's *primary source* for data collection is the client. There may be times when the client is unable to assist with the assessment. For example, if the client is severely delusional, mute, comatose, or extremely confused, then secondary sources would be used. *Secondary sources* include members of the family, friends, neighbors, police, other members of the health team, medical records, and laboratory results. Both primary and secondary sources need to be utilized during assessment.

PROCESS OF THE PSYCHIATRIC NURSING ASSESSMENT

If the nursing process is the framework for nursing practice, the therapeutic relationship is the medium through which the nursing process is implemented. Although the client is the focus, the nurse and the client work together to reduce anxiety, relieve pain, satisfy unmet needs, and promote optimum functioning. Assisting a person toward optimum functioning is accomplished through three levels of nursing intervention:

- Preventive (primary intervention)
- Restorative (secondary intervention)
- Rehabilitative (tertiary intervention)

Underlying these three levels of nursing intervention are certain premises (Bower 1982):

1. Individuals have the right to decide their destiny and to be involved in decisions that affect them.
2. Nursing intervention is designed to assist individuals to meet their own needs or to solve their problems.
3. The ultimate goal of all nursing action is to assist individuals to maximize their independent level of functioning.

The development of the therapeutic relationship is a crucial factor in the implementation of the nursing process. As discussed in Chapter 6, the optimum use of communication skills and therapeutic use of self greatly affects all phases of the nursing process (Hagerty 1984). This is especially true during the assessment phase.

When assessment occurs during the initial interview, the nurse and the client are essentially strangers. Both experience anxiety, as in any other meeting between strangers. The interviewer's anxiety may stem from the client's self-perception or the interviewer's ability (or inability) to help the client. If the interviewer is a nursing student, anxiety regarding the instructor's evaluation becomes an added dimension. Clients' anxiety centers on their problem(s), the nurse's view of them, and what is ahead for them in treatment (MacKinnon 1971).

Both client and nurse bring to their relationship their total background experiences. These experiences include cultural beliefs and biases, religious attitudes, educational background, and occupational and life experiences, as well as attitudes regarding sexual roles. These attitudes, beliefs, and values influence the nurse's interactions with clients. It is important for nurses to be aware of their biases and values and not feel compelled to impose personal beliefs on others. Although the nurse shares perceptions and alternatives with the client, the goal is to work with the client so that decisions and actions taken are the right ones for the client. Theoretically, this sounds easy, but often it is not. When beginning practitioners share their perceptions and thoughts with a more experienced nurse, unrecognized biases and value judgments often become evident. Experience and supervision help a nurse separate that which is important to the client from any bias that might impede mutually agreed upon goals.

Although the purpose of the psychiatric assessment is to gather data that will help clarify the client's situation and problem, this is best done in an atmosphere of minimal anxiety. Therefore, if an individual becomes upset, defensive, or embarrassed regarding any topic, the topic should be abandoned. The nurse can acknowledge that this is a subject that makes the client uncomfortable and can suggest that it would best be discussed at a time when the client feels more comfortable. It is important that the nurse not probe, pry, or push for information that is difficult for the client to discuss. The purpose of an assessment is to gather data pertaining to the client's problem, not to collect a lot of data.

CONTENT OF THE PSYCHIATRIC NURSING ASSESSMENT

The actual assessment consists of (1) gathering data and (2) verifying the data.

Gathering Data

The use of a standardized nursing assessment tool facilitates the assessment process. A number of assessment forms are available for use. Most health care systems and schools of nursing have their own assessment tool. Even though an assessment tool is used, it is best to gather information from the client in an informal fashion, with the nurse clarifying, focusing, and exploring pertinent data with the client. This allows clients to state their perceptions in their own words and enables the nurse to observe a wide range of nonverbal behaviors. When the order and the questions on the assessment tool are too rigidly applied, spontaneity is reduced. Assessment is a skill that is learned over a period of time. The development of this skill is enhanced by practice, supervision, and patience. A personal style of interviewing congruent with the nurse's personality develops as comfort and experience increase.

The basic components of the psychiatric nursing assessment include (1) client history and (2) mental/emotional status.

The client's history is the subjective part of the assessment. The focus of the history is the client's perceptions and recollections in three broad areas: presenting problem, current lifestyle, and brief sketch of the client's life (family, friends, education, and work experience) (Eisenman and Dubbert 1978).

The mental/emotional status is the objective part of the assessment. The nurse observes the person's physical behavior and nonverbal communication, appearance, speech patterns, thought content, and cognitive ability.

The assessment covers social, physical, emotional, cultural, cognitive, and spiritual aspects of an individual. It elicits information about the systems in which a person operates. It is assumed the nurse has fundamental knowledge of growth and development and of basic cultural and religious practices, as well as pathophysiology, psychopathology, and pharmacology.

Figure 7–2 (pp. 142–144) is a sample assessment tool. It is presented in outline form. The following information helps to clarify the use of the tool.

1. CLIENT HISTORY

I. General History of Client

Data include the client's age, sex, and culture. Behaviors can be evaluated as to age-appropriate activity for an individual who operates from a specific cultural base. "Age, sex, and culture are inextricably bound to growth and development, and may be assessed simultaneously" (Yura and Walsh 1983).

Who does the client live with? Who is his family? What are the ages of children or siblings? Whom does he trust? Who cares for him? Information regarding the constellation of the client's family helps the nurse determine the client's role in his family. How does his

ASSESSMENT TOOL

1. **Client History**

I. GENERAL HISTORY OF CLIENT

Name ______________________ Age ________ Sex ________
Racial and ethnic data ______________________
Marital status ______________________
Number and ages of children/siblings ______________________
Living arrangements ______________________
Occupation ______________________
Education ______________________
Religious affiliations ______________________

II. PRESENTING PROBLEM

A. Statement in client's own words of why he is hospitalized or seeking help.
____
____
____

B. Recent difficulties/alterations in
1. Relationships
2. Usual level of functioning
3. Behavior
4. Perceptions
5. Cognitive abilities

C. Increased feelings of
1. Depression
2. Anxiety
3. Hopelessness
4. Being overwhelmed
5. Suspiciousness
6. Confusion

D. Somatic changes
1. Constipation
2. Diarrhea
3. Insomnia
4. Lethargy
5. Weight loss or gain
6. Anorexia
7. Palpitations
8. Pruritus
9. Nausea
10. Vomiting
11. Headaches

Continued

ASSESSMENT TOOL *(Continued)*

III. RELEVANT HISTORY—PERSONAL

A. Previous hospitalizations and illness ______

B. Educational background
 1. Highest grade completed ______ 2. Special skills ______

C. Occupational background
 1. If employed, where? ______
 2. Describe job. ______
 3. How long at that job? ______
 4. Previous positions and reasons for leaving. ______

D. Social patterns
 1. Describe friends. ______
 2. What is important in a friend? ______
 3. With whom does the client identify? ______
 4. Describe a usual day. ______

E. Sexual patterns
 1. Sexually active? ______
 2. Sexual orientation ______
 3. Sexual difficulties ______

F. Interests and abilities
 1. What does the client do in his spare time? ______
 2. What is he good at? ______
 3. What gives the client pleasure? ______

G. Substance use and abuse
 1. Does client overeat or undereat? ______
 2. What psychotropic drugs does the client take? ______
 How often? ______ How much? ______
 3. How many drinks of ETOH does the client take per day? ______
 Per week? ______
 4. Does the client identify use of drugs as a problem? ______

H. How does client cope with stress?
 1. What does client do when he gets upset? ______
 2. Whom can he talk to? ______
 3. What usually helps to relieve stress? ______
 4. What did he try this time? ______

IV. RELEVANT HISTORY—FAMILY

A. Childhood
 1. Who was important to client growing up? ______
 2. Who cared for him? ______
 3. Was there physical or sexual abuse? ______
 4. Did parents drink or use drugs? ______
 5. Who was in the home when the client was growing up? ______

B. Adolescence
 1. How would the client describe his feelings in adolescence?
 Depressed ______ Lonely ______ Happy ______
 Confused ______ Adjusted ______ Rebellious ______
 2. Describe peer group at that time. ______

C. Use of drugs
 1. Was there use or abuse of drugs by any family member? ______
 Prescription ______ Street ______ By whom? ______
 2. What was the effect on the family? ______

D. Family physical or mental problems
 1. Who in the family had physical or mental problems? ______
 2. Describe the problems. ______
 3. How did it affect the family? ______

E. Was there an unusual or outstanding event client would like to mention? ______

Continued

ASSESSMENT TOOL *(Continued)*

2. **Mental and Emotional Status**

A. Appearance
Tall ______ Obese ______ Physical handicaps ______
Deformities ______ Dress appropriate ______ Sloppy ______
Bizarre ______ Grooming neat ______ Poor ______
Eye contact held ______ Describe posture ______ Slumped ______ Rigid ______
Face away from interviewer ______

B. Behavior **(See Table 7–1)**
Restless ______ Agitated ______ Lethargic ______
Mannerisms ______ Facial expressions ______ Echopraxia ______
Echolalia ______ Waxy flexibility ______ Akathisia ______
Dyskinesia ______ Other ______

C. Speech
Clear ______ Mumbled ______ Rapid ______ Whispers ______ Monotone ______ Slurred ______
Loud ______ Constant ______ Mute or Silent ______ Barriers to communications ______ (i.e., client has delusions or is confused, withdrawn, or verbose) Specify ______

D. Mood
What mood does the client convey (helpless, fearful, friendly, euphoric, tearful, aggressive, anxious, hostile, sarcastic, apprehensive, depressed)? Describe ______
______

E. Affect
Is the client's affect bland, apathetic, dramatic, bizarre, appropriate? Describe ______

F. Thought process **(See Table 7–2)**
1. Characteristics
Describe the characteristics of the person's responses. Flights of ideas ______ Neologisms ______
Looseness of association ______ Blocking ______ Perseveration ______ Circumstantiality ______
Tangentiality ______ Concrete ______ Confabulation ______
Describe ______
2. Cognitive ability
Proverbs: Concrete ______ Abstract ______
Serial Sevens: How far does client go? ______ Can he do simple math? ______
What seems to be the reason for poor concentration? ______
______

G. Thought content
1. Central theme: What is important to client? ______
Describe ______
2. Self-concept: How does client view himself? ______
Overrates, underrates self? ______ What does he want to change about himself? ______
3. Insight? Does he realistically assess his symptoms? ______
Realistically appraise his situation? ______
Describe ______
4. Suicidal or homicidal ideation? ______ What is suicide potential? ______ Family history of suicide or homicide attempt or successful completion? ______
Explain ______

Preoccupations **(see Table 7–3).** Does the client have hallucinations? ______ Delusions ______
Obsessions ______ Rituals ______ Phobias ______ Grandiosity ______ Religiosity ______ Worthlessness ______ Describe ______
______

H. Reality orientation
Time: Day ______ Month ______ Year ______
Place: Describe location ______
Person: Can name self ______ family ______ nurse ______
Memory: Recent ______ Past ______

I. Level of Anxiety
Mild Data ______
Moderate Data ______
Severe Data ______
Panic Data ______

Figure 7–2.

illness affect the family members? How does the family influence the client? What is the birth order of the client in his family of origin?

What level of education does the client have? Is he working to his full potential? How does he perceive his standard of living? Are his living conditions adequate for physical and emotional health?

Religious beliefs can provide an important source of strength for many clients. What are the specific values and norms with which the individual identifies? What customs or needs does the client have (i.e., special diets, spiritual counseling, mode of dress, restrictions on treatment)?

II. Presenting Problem

A. In the client's own words, what is happening that needs changing? What was the reason for seeking treatment? If the person was brought in by others, what reasons were given for hospitalization? What is the individual's perception of what he was told? Has he experienced any recent traumatic events? Has anything like this experience happened before? What does he think could help his problem?

B. Are there recent difficulties or alterations in relationships? Is the person functioning at his usual level? Has he noticed changes in behavior or perceptions in people and things around him? Is he having difficulty thinking or problem solving?

C. Can the client identify increased feelings of depression, anxiety, suspiciousness, hopelessness? Is the person feeling overwhelmed or confused? How does the person describe what he is feeling at this moment? Some clients will deny feelings such as depression or anxiety and concentrate only on somatic complaints, e.g., lethargy, anorexia, insomnia, palpitations. Others will be so overwhelmed with high anxiety or so immobilized by depression that they deny or cannot attend to real physical needs.

D. What kind of somatic changes has the individual noticed? Changes in bowel patterns, sleep, and eating habits? Has the person gained or lost weight recently? Has the person been bothered with pruritus, nausea, vomiting, headaches? Stress can affect the body physiologically, and somatic symptoms may be a signal for serious psychological problems. Conversely, physical problems can affect an individual's behavior and relationships with others in his environment. This is an important area for the nurse to assess.

III. Relevant History—Personal

A. Previous hospitalizations and illness. What physical and mental problems has the person experienced? Did he need hospitalization? How many times? Did he perceive past medical attention helpful? What prescribed or over-the-counter medications does he take? Does he have any allergies? Does the client have any current health problems? Is the client pregnant?

B. Educational background includes the person's experience with schooling, positive or negative. Did he do well? Did he ever leave school? Does he have any special skills or training?

C. Assessment of occupational background includes the person's present place of employment. How does he describe what he does? Last place of employment and reason for leaving. If the client is not employed, what kind of job would the client prefer? Does the client have any self-taught skills?

D. Who are the client's friends? Does he belong to a subcultural group? With whom does he identify? Describe a usual day. Questions along these lines yield information about the person's lifestyle and social patterns.

E. Sexual patterns. Is the person active sexually? Are there problems or concerns the person has relating to his sexual habits or orientation?

F. What are the person's interests and abilities? What does he do in his spare time? What kinds of activities give him pleasure? What is he good at?

G. Issues of substance use and abuse are of a great importance and relate directly to a person's physical and emotional health. Does the person overeat or undereat? What drugs does the person take? How often? How many drinks (ETOH or alcohol) does the person take per day/per week? At what age did use of drugs begin? Does the client identify any of these habits as problematic?

H. How does the person cope with stress? What does he usually do when upset? Whom can he talk to? What does the client find the most helpful? What has he tried recently that did not work?

IV. Relevant History—Family

A. Who was important to the client during his childhood? Who cared for him? Was there any physical or sexual abuse? Did his parents drink? How much? Who was in the home during his childhood?

B. How does the client describe his adolescence? Was he lonely? Did he have friends? How would he describe himself during this time? Was he angry, happy, rebellious, compliant, confused, adjusted, lonely, or fearful?

C. Was there use or abuse of drugs by family members? Prescription drugs? Street drugs? What were they? Who used them? What was the effect on the family?

D. Who had physical or mental problems in the family? Describe the problems. How did these illnesses affect the client? What changes did it make in how the family functioned?

E. Any unusual or outstanding events the client wishes to mention?

2. MENTAL/EMOTIONAL STATUS

A. Appearance

What does the client look like? Is he tall? Overweight? Does he have any physical handicaps or deformities? How is he dressed? Is his dress appropriate for age, culture, time of year, situation? Is the client well-groomed or are hair and nailbeds dirty? Does he appear neat or disheveled? How does he relate to the interviewer? Does he maintain eye contact? Describe the client's posture. Does he slump in the chair? Lean forward? Face away from the interviewer? Draw a picture in words.

B. Behavior

Describe the motor activity. Is he restless, agitated, lethargic? How does he walk? What kind of mannerisms and facial expressions does he use when talking? When silent? Is he aware of the environment? Does he show signs of **echopraxia, waxy flexibility, akathisia, dyskinesia?** Table 7–1 defines these behaviors.

C. Speech

Is the client's speech intelligible and clear, or does he mumble or speak fast and forcefully? Are there barriers to communications, such as confusion or delusions?

Table 7–1 • ABNORMAL MOTOR BEHAVIORS

DEFINITION	EXAMPLE
Echopraxia	
Mimicking the movements of another person.	Every time the nurse would move or gesture with her hands, the client would copy her gestures.
Echolalia	
Mimicking the speech of another person.	The nurse said to the client, "Tell me your name." The client responded, "Tell me your name, tell me your name."
Waxy Flexibility	
Having one's arms or legs placed in a certain position and holding that same position for hours.	The nurse lifted the client's arm to check the pulse, and the client left his arm extended in the same position.
Parkinson-like Symptoms	
Mask-like faces, drooling, shuffling gait, tremors and muscular rigidity. Seen in people who are on antipsychotic medication, such as phenothiazines.	The nurse noticed that the client's face held no emotion. He walked very stiffly, leaning forward, almost robot-like.
Akathisia	
Regular rhythmic movements usually of lower limbs. Can also see constant pacing. This constant motor restlessness is seen in people taking antipsychotic medication.	The client's leg kept jiggling up and down when he talked to the nurse. When his feet were still, his arm would jiggle constantly during the interview.
Dyskinesia	
Involuntary muscular activity, such as tic, spasm, or myoclonus.	The client had a marked facial tic around his mouth, which was distracting to the nurse during the interview.

D. Mood

What mood does the client convey to the nurse? Hostile? Sarcastic? Tearful? Grandiose? Apathetic? Helpless? Fearful? Friendly? Is the mood appropriate for the topics being discussed?

E. Affect

Describe the client's presenting affect. Is the affect appropriate, bizarre, bland, apathetic, or overly dramatic?

F. Thought Process

1. Describe the characteristics of the person's responses. Does he change the topic often **(tangential)**? Are his responses appropriate to the questions asked? Does he jump from topic to topic so that it is difficult to follow the thought process **(flights of ideas)**? Does he make up words **(neologisms)** or make up events to fill periods of time **(confabulation)**? Is there an illogical stream of thought **(looseness of associations)** or blocking of ideas? Table 7–2 defines these characteristics.
2. Cognitive Ability

   Assessment of language skills and reading and writing abilities can prove helpful in distinguishing between functional psychosis and organic psychosis (Hagerty 1984). Not all clients will require cognitive testing in depth. If, however, a client exhibits disorganized thinking and bizarre behavior, formal testing of cognitive functions is indicated.

   a. Testing Ability to Abstract—Use of Proverbs

   The client's ability to generalize events and understand symbolism can be elicited by asking the client to explain to the nurse the meaning of a proverb. Concrete thinking is often seen in thought disorders and organic mental disorders. For example:

Proverb:	People who live in glass houses shouldn't throw stones.
Concrete Answer:	If you throw stones in the house, you could break a window and shatter the glass.
Abstract:	Don't criticize others for faults you may have yourself.

   b. Testing Concentration—Serial Sevens

   The client is asked to subtract 7 from 100 as far as he is able to go. If the client is unable to subtract by 7's from 100, he is asked to do simpler tasks such as 3 × 7 or 5 × 9. If the client is unable to perform even the simpler tasks, the nurse needs to evaluate the degree to which the client's emotional state is responsible for the difficulty in concentration. For example, if the client is severely depressed or anxious, his impairment in ability to concentrate may be of emotional rather than cognitive origin (Hagerty 1984).

G. Thought Content

1. What are the central themes that are of importance to the client? Does the client have certain preoccupations with any particular subject?
2. Does the client have a good self-concept? How does he view himself? What does he like most about himself? What does he want to change about himself? Does he underrate or overrate his potential?
3. Does the client have insight into his problem? Is he able to assess his symptoms and the importance of his situation realistically? Is he aware of the existing problems or potential problems?
4. Is there suicidal or homicidal ideation? Does the client speak of wanting to harm himself or someone else? If the client has suicidal thoughts, what is his suicide potential (see SAD PERSONS Scale, Chapter 22)? Has he ever attempted suicide in the past? Did anyone in his family commit suicide? If the client is homicidal, have any past attempts been made? Has anyone in his family attempted to, or succeeded in, killing someone?
5. Does his thought content contain any particular preoccupations, such as **hallucinations, delusions, obsessions, rituals, phobias,** religiosity, grandiosity, or worthlessness? (See Table 7–3 for definitions.)

H. Reality Orientation

1. Time

   Can the person tell the nurse the day, the month, and the year? If a person has been hospitalized for an extended period of time, it is not unusual for the client not to know the day or the month. However, not to know the year can be diagnostically significant.
2. Place

   Can the client tell you where he is? If he is in a hospital, have the client name and give the location of the hospital.

Table 7–2 • CHARACTERISTICS OF ABNORMAL THOUGHT PROCESSES

DEFINITION	EXAMPLE
Tangentiality	
An association disturbance in which the speaker goes off the topic. When it happens frequently and the speaker does not return to the topic, interpersonal communication is destroyed.	The nurse asked the client to talk more about his family. The client continuously left the topic and talked about boats, animals, his apartment, and so forth. Each time the nurse tried to help the client to focus, he would go off on another topic.
Neologisms	
Words a person makes up that only have meaning for the person himself, often part of a delusional system.	"I am afraid to go to the hospital because the *norks* are looking for me there."
Looseness of Association	
Thinking is haphazard, illogical, and confused. Connections in thought are interrupted. Seen mostly in schizophrenic disorders.	"Can't go to the zoo, no money, Oh . . . I have a hat, these members make no sense, man . . . What's the problem?"
Flights of Ideas	
Constant flow of speech in which the person jumps from one topic to another in rapid succession. There is a connection between topics, although it is sometimes hard to identify. Characteristically seen in acute manic states.	"Say babe how's it going . . . Going to my sister's to get some money . . . money, honey, you got any bread . . . bread and butter, staff of life, ain't life grand? . . ."
Blocking	
Sudden cessation of a thought in the middle of a sentence. Person is unable to continue his train of thought. Often sudden new thoughts crop up unrelated to the topic. Can be disturbing to the individual.	"I was going to get a new dress for the . . . I forgot what I was going say."
Circumstantiality	
Before getting to the point or answering a question, the person gets caught up in countless details and explanations.	"Where are you going for the weekend, Harry?" "Well I first thought of going to my mother's, but that was before I remembered that she was going to my sister's. My sister is having a picnic. She always has picnics at the beach. The beach that she goes to is large and gets crowded. That's why I don't like that beach. So I decided to go someplace else. I thought of going to my brother's house. He has a large house on a quiet street . . . I finally decided to stay home."
Perseveration	
The involuntary repetition of the same thought, phrase, or motor response to different questions or situations. Associated with brain damage.	N: How are you doing, Harry? H: Fine nurse, just fine. N: Did you go for a walk? H: Fine nurse, just fine. N: Are you going out today? H: Fine nurse, just fine.
Confabulation	
Filling in a memory gap with detailed fantasy believed by the teller. The purpose is to maintain self-esteem and is seen in organic conditions, such as Korsakoff's psychosis.	The nurse asked Harry, who spent the weekend at home, what he did that weekend. "Well, I just came back from California after signing a contract with MGM for a film on the life of Roosevelt. We had the most marvelous tour of the studio . . . went to lunch with the director . . . "
Word Salad	
A mixture of words and phrases that have no meaning.	"I am fine . . . apple pie . . . no sale . . . furniture store . . . take it slow . . . cellar door . . . "

Table 7–3 • PREOCCUPATIONS IN THOUGHT CONTENT

DEFINITION	EXAMPLE
Hallucinations	
A sense perception for which no external stimuli exist. Hallucinations can have an organic or a functional etiology.	
Visual: Seeing things that are not there.	During alcohol withdrawal he kept shouting, "I see snakes on the walls."
Auditory: Hearing voices when none are present.	"I keep hearing my mother's voice telling me I am bad. She died a year ago."
Olfactory: Smelling smells that do not exist.	"I smell my stomach rotting."
Tactile: Feeling touch sensations in the absence of stimuli. (Also referred to as haptic.)	A paranoid man feels electrical impulses "from outer space" entering his body and controlling his mind.
Gustatory: Experiencing taste in the absence of stimuli.	A paranoid woman tastes poison in her food while eating at her son's wedding.
Delusions	
A false belief held to be true even with evidence to the contrary. Three common delusions follow:	
Persecution: The thought that one is being singled out for harm by others.	An intern believes that the chief of staff is plotting to kill him to prevent the intern from becoming too powerful.
Grandeur: The false belief that one is a very powerful and important person.	A newly admitted patient told the nurse that he was God, and he was here to save the world.
Jealousy: The false belief that one's mate is going out with other people. The person may take everyday occurrences for "proof."	Sally "knew" that her husband, Jim, was being unfaithful. Even when Sally's brother swore he and Jim really did play pool Friday nights, Sally declared Jim's not being home then was her "proof."
Obsessions	
An idea, impulse, or emotion that a person cannot put out of his or her consciousness. Can be mild or severe.	A young mother, Jane, told the nurse that she was hounded by constant thoughts that something terrible was going to happen to her baby. She knew that this was crazy, but she could not get the thought to stop.
Rituals	
Repetitive actions that people must do over and over until either they are exhausted or anxiety is decreased. Often done to lessen the anxiety triggered by an obsession.	Jane stated to the nurse the only way she could temporarily get these obsessions to cease was to touch her baby to reassure herself that "nothing terrible was happening."
Phobias	
An intense irrational fear of an object, situation, or place. The fear persists even though the object of the fear is perfectly harmless and the person is aware of the irrationality.	Although aware that cats would not harm her, Mary was deathly afraid of cats and refused to visit her sister and friends who had cats.

3. Memory

Questions such as, Who is the President? or What were you doing last week? are good tests of recent memory. Questions about major news events are also good tests of recent memory. Questions about the client's childhood and events in his adolescence are good indications of remote memory.

I. Level of Anxiety

From the data and observations of the client, the nurse assesses the client's level of anxiety as to mild, moderate, severe, or panic level. An understanding of the level of anxiety facilitates the planning of care and appropriate approaches to intervention (see Chapter 8 for criteria in assessing level of anxiety).

After the nurse has concluded the assessment, it is useful for the nurse to summarize pertinent data with the client briefly. The summary provides the client the reassurance that he has been heard, and it allows him the opportunity to clarify any misinformation (Eisenman and Dubbert 1978). The client should be told what will happen next. For example, if the initial assessment takes place in the hospital, the nurse will tell the client who else he will be seeing. If the initial assessment was by a psychiatric nurse in a mental health clinic, the nurse will let the client know when and how often they will meet to work on the client's problems. If the nurse feels a referral is necessary (psychiatrist, social worker, physician), the nurse will discuss this with the client.

Verifying Data

It is necessary that the nurse verify data with secondary sources. Whenever possible, members of the family should be a part of the assessment. Is there anything going on in the family that is affecting the family? It is important for the nurse to understand how the family views the client. How does the family define the problem? How do the client's problems affect the family? What does the family think might help the client? Who else in the family is having difficulty? Does the client perceive his problems and behavior in the same way the family does?

Friends and neighbors can be important sources of information. They may verify or contradict the client's perception of himself and his actions. They may add information that the client did not think relevant.

Oftentimes, police officers are the ones who bring clients into the psychiatric emergency rooms. It is important for the nurse to know as much as possible about exactly what the client was doing that warranted police intervention. Was the client suicidal, homicidal? Was anyone hurt?

Other members of the health team are important sources of information and data verification. Many members of the health team will have contact with the client on admission to the hospital. The psychiatrist/psychologist, social worker, psychiatric nurse, recreation therapist, therapy aides, and student nurses can add to the nurse's data base. Observations from all health-team members are important for making a thorough assessment. Often the client has been admitted previously. Are the circumstances and symptoms the same as previously, more intense, less intense? Are circumstances totally different on this admission?

Old charts and medical records can help validate information the nurse already has or can add new information. Past medical history can be important for assessing physical losses and stress and can alert the staff to potential medical problems. If the client has been admitted to a psychiatric unit in the past, information relating to his previous level of functioning and behavior gives the nurse a baseline for making clinical judgments. Is the client functioning at a higher level or lower level than previously? Does the client cope with anxiety in similar ways or use different coping skills at present? Is the reason for his present admission similar to that for his past admission(s) or not? What were the previous precipitating events that led up to admission?

Laboratory reports can provide useful information. When the body's chemistry is abnormal, personality changes and violent behaviors can result. For example, abnormal liver enzymes can explain irritability, depression, and lethargy. People who have chronic renal disease often suffer from the same symptoms when their blood urea nitrogen (BUN) and electrolyte levels are abnormal. People with endocrine diseases, like diabetes, can have changes in mood and level of consciousness related to sugar and insulin levels.

Standard III: Diagnosis

Nursing diagnosis is the crucial component in the nursing process. It is the nursing diagnosis that directs nursing actions and provides the focus for evaluating outcomes (Kim 1985).

The development of the concept of "nursing diagnosis" has been controversial and stormy. Nursing authors have written to support and differentiate nursing diagnosis from medical diagnosis from the 1950's through 1979 (Douglas and Murphy1981). The National Group for the Classification of Nursing Diagnosis met for the first time in 1973. The National Group for the Classification of Nursing Diagnosis has been renamed the North American Nursing Diagnosis Association (NANDA), and under this group the development of nursing diagnosis continues. Table 7–4 identifies accepted nursing diagnoses under assessment categories.

WHY A NURSING DIAGNOSTIC SYSTEM?

The use of a unified classification system among nurses helps to identify the nurses' independent functions. There are a number of functions that a formalized diagnostic system can perform for the practice of nursing.

Table 7-4 • NURSING DIAGNOSTIC CATEGORIES

Pattern 1: Exchanging	
Altered Nutrition: More than body requirements	Altered (Specify Type) Tissue Perfusion (Renal, cerebral, cardiopulmonary, gastrointestinal, peripheral)
Altered Nutrition: Less than body requirements	Fluid Volume Excess
Altered Nutrition: Potential for more than body requirements	Fluid Volume Deficit (1)
Potential for Infection	Fluid Volume Deficit (2)
Potential Altered Body Temperature	Potential Fluid Volume Deficit
Hypothermia	Decreased Cardiac Output
Hyperthermia	Impaired Gas Exchange
Ineffective Thermoregulation	Ineffective Airway Clearance
Dysreflexia	Ineffective Breathing Pattern
Constipation	Potential for Injury
Perceived Constipation	Potential for Suffocation
Colonic Constipation	Potential for Poisoning
Diarrhea	Potential for Trauma
Bowel Incontinence	Potential for Aspiration
Altered Patterns of Urinary Elimination	Potential for Disuse Syndrome
Stress Incontinence	Impaired Tissue Integrity
Reflex Incontinence	Altered Oral Mucous Membrane
Urge Incontinence	Impaired Skin Integrity
Functional Incontinence	Potential Impaired Skin Integrity
Total Incontinence	
Urinary Retention	
Pattern 2: Communicating	
Impaired Verbal Communication	
Pattern 3: Relating	
Impaired Social Interaction	Sexual Dysfunction
Social Isolation	Altered Family Processes
Altered Role Performance	Parental Role Conflict
Altered Parenting	Altered Sexuality Patterns
Potential Altered Parenting	
Pattern 4: Valuing	
Spiritual Distress (distress of the human spirit)	
Pattern 5: Choosing	
Ineffective Individual Coping	Ineffective Family Coping: Compromised
Impaired Adjustment	Family Coping: Potential for Growth
Defensive Coping	Noncompliance (Specify)
Ineffective Denial	Decisional Conflict (Specify)
Ineffective Family Coping: Disabling	Health-Seeking Behaviors (Specify)
Pattern 6: Moving	
Impaired Physical Mobility	Feeding Self-Care Deficit
Activity Intolerance	Impaired Swallowing
Fatigue	Ineffective Breastfeeding
Potential Activity Intolerance	Bathing/Hygiene Self-Care Deficit
Sleep Pattern Disturbance	Dressing/Grooming Self-Care Deficit
Diversional Activity Deficit	Toileting Self-Care Deficit
Impaired Home Maintenance Management	Altered Growth and Development
Altered Health Maintenance	
Pattern 7: Perceiving	
Body Image Disturbance	Sensory/Perceptual Alterations (Specify) (Visual, auditory, kinesthetic, gustatory, tactile, olfactory)
Self-Esteem Disturbance	Unilateral Neglect
Chronic Low Self-Esteem	Hopelessness
Situational Low Self-Esteem	Powerlessness
Personal Identity Disturbance	
Pattern 8: Knowing	
Knowledge Deficit (Specify)	Altered Thought Processes

Table continued on following page

Table 7–4 • NURSING DIAGNOSTIC CATEGORIES *Continued*

Pattern 9: Feeling	
Pain	Post Trauma Response
Chronic Pain	Rape-Trauma Syndrome
Dysfunctional Grieving	Rape-Trauma Syndrome: Compound Reaction
Anticipatory Grieving	Rape-Trauma Syndrome: Silent Reaction
Potential for Violence: Self-directed or directed at others	Anxiety
	Fear

From North American Nursing Diagnosis Association. Classifications of nursing diagnosis: Proceedings of the Eighth Conference. Philadelphia: J. B. Lippincott Company, (in press).

Some of the purposes served by nursing diagnoses follow:

1. Help define the practice of nursing
2. Provide nurses with a common frame of reference
3. Improve communications among staff members and between facilities
4. Help define a body of unique nursing knowledge
5. Differentiate nursing from medicine
6. Facilitate intraprofessional as well as interprofessional communications
7. Make nurses more accountable for care
8. Assist educators and students in focusing on nursing phenomena rather than on medical phenomena

WHAT IS A NURSING DIAGNOSIS?

There are a number of definitions for **nursing diagnosis** in the literature. The following three definitions are among those widely accepted:

1. Gordon defines nursing diagnosis as an "actual or potential health problem which nurses, by virtue of their education and experience are capable and licensed to treat" (Gordon 1979).
2. Shoemaker's definition of a nursing diagnosis is "a clinical judgment about an individual, family, or community which is derived through a deliberate, systematic process of data collection and analysis. It provides the basis for prescriptions for definitive therapy for which the nurse is accountable. It is expressed concisely and it includes the etiology of the condition when known" (Shoemaker 1984).
3. Carpenito defines nursing diagnosis as "a statement that describes a health state or an actual or potential alteration in one's life processes (physiological, psychological, socio-cultural, developmental and spiritual). The nurse uses the nursing process to identify and synthesize clinical data and to order nursing interventions to reduce, eliminate, or prevent (health promotion) health alterations which are in the legal and educational domain of nursing" (Carpenito 1987).

Common threads among these definitions are evident. The following seven assumptions can be drawn from these three definitions:

1. Health problems or alterations in a client's life process can be actual or potential.
2. A client can be an individual, a family group, or a community.
3. Health problems can be physiological, psychological, sociocultural, developmental, or spiritual.
4. The health problems are identified through a systematic process of data collection and data analysis.
5. The clinical judgment made from the assessment provides the basis for nursing interventions (primary, secondary, or tertiary).
6. The intervention and treatment are prescribed within the educational and legal domain of nurses, by way of licensure.
7. The statement of the problem is expressed concisely and includes the etiology when known.

A nursing diagnosis has three structural components: problem (unmet need), etiology (probable cause), and signs and symptoms (identifying data) (Gordon 1982).

The problem, or unmet need, describes the state of the client at present. Those problems that are within the nurse's domain to prescribe and treat are termed nursing diagnoses. The nursing diagnostic title states what should change. For example:

Altered Thought Processes

Etiology, or probable cause, is linked to the diagnostic title with the words *related to*. Stating the etiology or probable cause tells what needs to be done to effect the change. The etiology or probable cause identifies causes that the nurse can treat through nursing interventions.

Altered Thought Processes:
Related to Psychological Conflicts

The signs and symptoms, or supporting data, state what the condition is like at present.

Altered Thought Processes:
Related to Psychological Conflicts
Supporting Data Present to Validate Diagnosis

- Client thinking has slowed down.
- Client states he has trouble with his memory.
- Complains of difficulty concentrating.

A nursing diagnosis can reflect an actual, potential, or possible problem.

An actual problem means that the problem has been clinically identified by the supporting data. For example:

Self-esteem Disturbance:
Related to Recent Divorce
Supporting Data Present to Validate Diagnosis

- Signs of weeping and despair.
- Withdrawal from social contacts.
- States "I feel like half a person."

A potential nursing diagnosis suggests a problem that might occur if nursing intervention is not ordered. For example:

Potential for Violence: Related to Aggressive Behaviors
Supporting Data Present to Validate Diagnosis

- Client becomes physically aggressive when drinking.
- States "I know I drink too much . . . but I can't stop."
- Has been arrested twice for disorderly conduct while drinking.

Possible nursing diagnosis is used to alert the nurse that a problem may be present but more data are needed. For example:

Possible Altered Family Processes:
Related to Mother Having to go to Work to Support Children's Education
Supporting Data Present to Validate Diagnosis

- Husband had been against mother working in the past.
- Insufficient finances to support education for two children.
- Need more data.

WHEN IS A PROBLEM A NURSING DIAGNOSIS?

Nursing consists of three levels of nursing functioning determined by the type of problem. These levels of nursing functions are (1) dependent, (2) interdependent, and (3) independent. Carpenito clarifies the dependent dimension as follows (Carpenito 1987): Dependent nursing functions occur when the problem is a clinical medical problem, and the diagnosis and prescription of treatment come under the direct responsibility of the physician. Nursing practices in clinical medical problems are dependent actions prescribed by the physician. Medical problems are not within the legal or educational realm of the nurse to diagnose or to treat.

Information from the following vignette will be used to illustrate the three levels of nursing functions.

Assessment

Mr. Saltzberg is a 47-year-old man, the father of two boys, ages seven and nine. He is admitted to the hospital because of depression. Two months ago his business failed. Mr. Saltzberg states, "I built that business up from nothing; now I am left with nothing." He states he has been feeling depressed and "I just want to be alone."

He has been anorexic and has lost 19 pounds in the past two months. He weighs 140 pounds and is ten pounds under his range for normal body weight, 150–165 pounds. He has no interest in sex or any other activity. Family history reveals that his father suffered from depression and attempted suicide at age 60.

He appears unkempt — clothes are wrinkled, and he has not shaved for three days. He sits slumped in the chair, facing the interviewer but seldom making eye contact, and keeps his head down. His speech is slow, and his mood is depressed. His thinking is slowed down. He states, "I can't think."

He admits that the idea of suicide has occurred to him. His wife states he just sits and stares into space all day, keeping to himself. She states this is the first time she has ever known him to react like this, and his behavior is greatly upsetting the whole family. Mrs. Saltzberg is very upset and states that she feels overwhelmed without his help and support. The children are confused and upset and miss doing things with their father. The family has not gone to temple, the movies, or sports activities for two months — all of which are important events for this family.

Mr. Saltzberg was seen by the psychiatrist on the unit and was given the DSM III-R diagnosis of dysthymic disorder (depressive neurosis).

In this case, a dependent nursing function would be administering medication prescribed by the psychiatrist:

DSM III-R Diagnosis

Dysthymic disorder (depressive neurosis)

Medical Orders
Elavil 75 mg HS
Nursing Interventions
Administer Elavil 75 mg HS (dependent function)

Interdependent nursing functions refer to those problems on which health care professionals collaborate to prescribe and treat. Carpenito describes these problems as *clinical nursing problems*. For example:

DSM III-R Diagnosis
Dysthymic disorder (neurotic depression)
Medical Order
Elavil 75 mg HS
Clinical Nursing Problem
Potential orthostatic hypotension (common side effect of prescribed medication)
Nursing Order
1. Take BP, P on both arms in standing, sitting, and supine positions.
2. Have client dangle legs by side of bed before getting up.

Independent nursing functions involve actual, potential, or possible clinical problems or situations that are the direct responsibility and under the influence of the nurse. Problems or situations that call for independent nursing interventions are termed *nursing diagnoses* (Carpenito 1987). Independent nursing interventions are aimed at preventing, reducing, or alleviating identified problems.

The nurse met with Mr. Saltzberg and made an initial assessment. The nurse spoke with Mrs. Saltzberg and verified and added to the data base. Information is shared with other staff, and the admitting notes by the psychiatrist are read.

The analysis of the data consists of (1) organizing the data into problems (actual, potential, or possible), (2) prioritizing problems, and (3) formulating nursing diagnoses.

After the nurse assessed Mr. Saltzberg, the data were organized into problems and placed in order of priority. Three major problem areas were identified: potential self-harm, inadequate nutrition, and possible disrupted family functioning. From these problem areas, three nursing diagnoses were formulated:

Potential for Self-directed Violence:
Suicide Related to Multiple Losses
Supporting Data Present to Validate Diagnosis
- States, "I have nothing left to live for."
- Has suffered a great loss.
- Father attempted suicide at age 60.
- States he has had vague thoughts of killing himself.

Altered Nutrition:
Less than Body Requirements, Related to Apathy and Poor Self-Concept
Supporting Data Present to Validate Diagnosis
- 19-pound weight loss in two months.
- 10 pounds under his accepted weight range.
- Refuses to eat prepared meals.
- States he has no appetite.

Altered Family Process:
Related to an Ill Family Member
Supporting Data Present to Validate Diagnosis
- Since illness, family has not participated in usual family activities.
- Wife and husband have not shared usual activities involving companionship since illness.
- Wife states she feels overwhelmed without husband's help and support.

Standard IV: Planning

A clearly stated nursing care plan is the most effective means of assuring clients that their needs are heard and their problems are being addressed (Yura and Walsh 1983). When possible, the nurse works with the client to identify problems and plan care. Planning care is also done collaboratively with other health care workers, as well as individually.

In order to design a care plan that is appropriate and workable, it is necessary to have a direction of care. Planning a direction of care consists of deciding in advance what to do, who is to do it, and what is needed to get the job accomplished.

Planning involves (1) determining desired outcomes (short term and long term goals) and (2) identifying appropriate nursing care based on scientific principles or rationales designed to reach stated goals.

DETERMINING THE DESIRED OUTCOMES

For each nursing diagnosis, outcome criteria are established. Outcome criteria are the behaviors or situations hoped for after the implementation of nursing interventions designed to remedy or lessen the problem identified in the nursing diagnosis. Therefore, the nurse sets client-centered goals for nursing care aimed at alleviating the client's problems. Clearly stated goals give direction to needed nursing actions. There are two categories of goals, long term goals and short term goals. Long term goals are the hoped-for outcomes that reflect the maximum level of client health that can be reached realistically by nursing interventions. Short term goals are the intermediate goals that assist the client in achieving the long term goal(s).

Each goal is derived from only one nursing diagnosis. Goals should be realistic and acceptable to the client. An appropriate goal meets the following criteria (Atkinson and Murray 1983):

1. It is stated in observable or measurable terms.
2. It indicates client outcomes.
3. It has a specific time set for achievement.
4. It should be short and specific.
5. It is written in positive terms.

The following is a generally held formula for writing goals (Atkinson and Murray 1983):

Subject + Verb + Criteria of Performance + Conditions = Goal
(if needed)

The subject refers to the client or any part of the client, not the nurse, for example, *the client* or *the client's anxiety level*.

The verb refers to the action the client will perform. For example:

- the client *will state*
- the client *will name*
- the client's anxiety level *will decrease*

The criteria of performance refer to how long, how far, how much, and by when the behavior or situation will be altered. Therefore, the criteria include a measure of performance and a realistic deadline by which the behavior or situation will be altered. For example:

- *by the end of two weeks*, the client will state *three things he values in himself*
- *by* 7/2, the client will name *three alternative actions he can take*
- *by* 8:00 P.M. *tonight*, the client's anxiety level will decrease from *severe to moderate*

The conditions refer to those circumstances under which the behavior or situation will be altered. Not all goals need conditions. For example,

- the client will remain safe while in the hospital *with the help of the staff*
- by 8:00 P.M., the client's anxiety level will decrease from severe to moderate *with the aid of medications*

Referring to the nursing diagnoses formulated for Mr. Saltzberg, the nurse sets long term and short term goals. The long term and short term goals for the second nursing diagnosis are provided here as an example.

Nursing Diagnosis: Altered Nutrition: less than body requirements, related to apathy and poor self-concept

Long Term Goal	Short Term Goal
1. By discharge, client will be within normal body weight range (150–165 pounds).	1. Client will gain two pounds per week while in the hospital. 6/4—Present weight is 140 pounds

IDENTIFYING INTERVENTIONS NECESSARY TO HELP CLIENTS ACHIEVE GOALS

The nurse writes a set of interventions appropriate for reaching each goal. Each stated goal should have a number of nursing interventions. These nursing interventions should be seen as instructions for all people working with the client. These instructions, written in the Kardex, aid in the continuity of care for the client and are points of information for all members of the health team. When the short term goals are reached and charted, as reflected on the Kardex, a picture of the client's progress is evident. There are specific principles the nurse considers when planning care. Nursing interventions planned for meeting a specific goal should include the following principles (Atkinson and Murray 1983):

1. They must be safe for the client.
2. They must be compatible with other therapies as well as with the client's personal goals and cultural values.
3. They should be based on scientific principles.
4. They should be realistic, that is, (1) within the capabilities of the client's age, physical strength, condition, and willingness to change, (2) based on the number of staff available, (3) reflect the level of experience and ability of the staff, and (4) utilize available equipment and resources.

The nurse plans the interventions to meet the goals set for Mr. Saltzberg. For example:

Nursing Diagnosis: Potential for Self-directed Violence: suicide related to multiple losses
Long Term Goal: By discharge, client will state he wants to live.

Short Term Goal	Nursing Intervention
1. Client will remain safe while in the hospital, with the aid of staff.	1a. Remove all possible weapons or potential weapons, i.e., belts, ties, shoelaces, razors, plastic bags. 1b. Assess immediate degree of suicidal risk, and ask client if he is thinking of killing himself. 1c. Check client q 15 minutes, and keep him in view at all times. 1d. Observe for any signs of suicidal indicators: sudden sense of well-being, giving away prized possessions, making out a will. 1e. Spend time with client for 15 minutes, three times a day. 1f. Recognize suicide as realistic option; do not discredit. 1g. Document all assessments, interactions, and interventions.
2. By 6/13, client will name three personal strengths.	2a. Approach client in a positive, open, and nonjudgmental manner. 2b. Assess with client effective coping skills he has used in the past. 2c. Assist client to identify personal strengths.
3. By 6/20, client will name three realistic future job options.	3a. Encourage client to discuss situation and examine alternative actions that may be available. 3b. Reinforce use of problem-solving skills in exploring present situation and where he would like to go from here.
4. By 6/29, client will name three actions he can take if he feels overwhelmed or depressed in the future.	4a. Evaluate with client his social and personal support system. 4b. Involve the family with client in problem-solving actions that can lower feelings of helplessness and feelings of being overwhelmed within the family. 4c. Provide information on local self-help groups and resources for suicide prevention. 4d. Assess relationship with rabbi and encourage involvement in activities that provide a source of support. 4e. Work with the client to set future goals that are meaningful and important to client.

Refer to the working care plan for Mr. Saltzberg (Nursing Care Plan 7 – 1), which includes the rationale behind each nursing intervention.

Standard V: Intervention

Implementation of nursing care includes three basic areas: (1) validating the care plan, (2) giving nursing care, and (3) continued data collection.

VALIDATING THE NURSING CARE PLAN

It is sound practice when writing care plans for less experienced staff members or students to review their care plans briefly with more experienced staff members (team leader, colleague, instructor, head nurse). Often, experienced nurses have parts or all of their care plans reviewed by other professionals. By having the care plan reviewed, quality of care can be maximized. This reviewing process is called validating the care plan. Areas of concern include the following (Atkinson and Murray 1983):

1. Does the plan assure the client's safety?
2. Is the plan based on sound scientific principles?
3. Are the nursing diagnoses supported by the data?
4. Does the goal contain time criteria and client behavior for evaluation?
5. Can the planned nursing action realistically assist the client in achieving the intended goal?
6. Are the client's priorities being considered?

Nursing care plans are often transferred to a Kardex,

Nursing Care Plan 7–1 • A DEPRESSED INDIVIDUAL: Mr. Saltzberg

NURSING DIAGNOSIS

Potential for self-directed violence: suicide related to multiple losses

Supporting Data

- States, "I have nothing left to live for."
- Has suffered a great loss.
- Father attempted suicide at age 60.
- Admits to vague thoughts of killing himself.

Long Term Goal: By discharge, the client will state he wants to live.

Short-Term Goal	*Intervention*	*Rationale*	*Evaluation*
1. Client will remain safe while in the hospital, with the aid of the staff.	1a. Remove all possible weapons, e.g., belts, ties, shoelaces, razors, plastic bags.	1a. Minimize potential for self-harm.	Goal Met. Client states he no longer thinks of killing himself; has been working on plans for the future in business and with his family.
	1b. Assess immediate degree of suicidal risk, and ask client if he is thinking of killing himself.	1b. Evaluation of level of suicidal potential can determine the degree of suicide precautions.	
	1c. Check client q 15 minutes, and keep him in view at all times.	1c. Maximizes client's safety and lets him know he is cared for.	
	1d. Observe for any signs of suicidal indicators: sudden sense of well-being, giving away prized possessions, making out a will.	1d. Nonverbal clues need to be noted in assessing suicidal ideation.	
	1e. Spend time with client for 15 minutes, three times a day.	1e. Provides the opportunity to build rapport and trust with client. Client senses others are concerned and feel he is worthwhile. Forms the foundation for problem solving and sharing.	
	1f. Recognize suicide as realistic option; do not discredit.	1f. Acknowledges that situation is serious; can give client a feeling he is understood.	
	1g. Observe for signs of orthostatic hypotension and dizziness from medication. a. check BP lying and standing b. instruct to dangle feet before getting out of bed	1g. Prevents injury from falls.	
	1h. Document all assessments, interactions, and interventions.	1h. Vital for communication among all health team members and for legal purposes.	
2. By 6/13, client will name three personal strengths.	2a. Approach client in a positive, open, and nonjudgmental manner.	2a. Minimizes guilt, increases hope, and encourages disclosure.	Goal met. On 6/13 client identified three positive strengths: (1) he is conscientious, (2) he is a good observer of people, and (3) he is creative in advertising and marketing.
	2b. Assess with client effective coping skills he has used in the past.	2b. Redirect negative self-assessment to positive skills he has and has used in the past.	
	2c. Assist client to identify personal strengths.	2c. Can raise self-esteem, restore hope, and help client recognize his own resources.	

Continued on following page

Nursing Care Plan 7-1 • A DEPRESSED INDIVIDUAL: Mr. Saltzberg

(Continued)

Short-Term Goal	Intervention	Rationale	Evaluation
3. By 6/20, client will name three realistic future job options.	3a. Encourage client to discuss situation and examine alternative actions that may be available. 3b. Reinforce use of problem-solving skills in exploring present situation and where he would like to go from here.	3a. When depressed, people often have difficulty identifying alternate solutions. 3b. Reinforces client's skills and gives structure to the future.	Goal partially met. Client stated that he could work in his friend's store until he could think of what else he might want to do. He also talked about going to school at night for a real estate license. He admits to hating to sell his business, and he states he needs more time to make a decision in this area.
4. By 6/29, client will name three actions he can take if he feels overwhelmed or depressed in the future.	4a. Evaluate with client his social and personal support system. 4b. Involve the family with client in problem-solving actions. 4c. Provide information on local self-help groups and resources for suicide prevention. 4d. Assess relationship with rabbi and encourage involvement in activities that provide a source of support. 4e. Work with client to set future goals that are meaningful and important to client.	4a. Reinforces the availability of resources and can decrease anxiety and feelings of isolation. 4b. Lowers feelings of isolation and helplessness and gives client sense that he is cared for. 4c. Increases knowledge of resources and options. 4d. Religious ties strong in this family. Reinforce as a source of support. 4e. Projection into the future helps client view himself moving toward a goal and as part of the process of life.	Goal partially met. Client met with family on 6/11, 6/18, and 6/29 and stated he felt relieved that he could talk to them about feelings of failure and doubt and still be loved and supported by them. He also mentioned that he would talk to his rabbi in the future. As for continuing counseling on the outside, he has not decided. "It would mean I am weak." He is aware that he will be taking medication (Elavil) when he goes home, and he hopes it will continue to help.

NURSING DIAGNOSIS

Altered nutrition: less than body requirements, related to apathy and poor self-concept.

Supporting Data

- 19-pound weight loss in two months.
- Refuses to eat prepared meals.
- States he has no appetite.
- 10 pounds under minimum weight for age and height (present weight 140 pounds).

Long Term Goal: By discharge, client will be within normal body weight range (150–165 pounds).

Short Term Goal	Intervention	Rationale	Evaluation
1. Client will gain two pounds per week while in the hospital. Present weight is 140 pounds.	1a. Call dietitian for consultation with client regarding special diets (kosher), food preferences, and high caloric snacks. 1b. Check with doctor to okay wife bringing in foods prepared at home. 1c. Meet with wife and Mr. Saltzberg and plan foods and schedule of foods he finds more appetizing. 1d. Encourage client to take a high-caloric snack during times spent with the nurse.	1a. Various members of the health team are called in whenever appropriate to maximize skilled intervention. 1b. Clear any medical contraindications or conflicts in strategy for obtaining goal. 1c. Client participates in own plan of care whenever possible to increase feelings of control and competence. 1d. Food is often part of social interactions. While not a "social" meeting, sharing activities (games, talking, and eating) can be used therapeutically.	Goal partially met. Client's weight on date of admission (6/4) was 140 pounds. (see weight table below) Appetite has improved and client states he has more interest in food than when first admitted.

		Gained	Total needed to make goal
6/10	141	+1	9
6/17	143	+2	7
6/24	144	+1	6
7/1	147	+3	3

Nursing Care Plan 7–1 • A DEPRESSED INDIVIDUAL: Mr. Saltzberg

(Continued)

NURSING DIAGNOSIS

Altered Family Process related to an ill family member

Supporting Data

- Family has not participated together in usual activities (temple, movies, sports) since illness.
- Wife and husband have not shared usual activities together (sex, walks, private talks) since illness.
- Wife states she feels overwhelmed without the help and support of her husband.

Long-Term Goal: By discharge client and family will discuss and identify three outside supports available to them all.

Short Term Goal	*Intervention*	*Rationale*	*Evaluation*
1. By 6/11, client will meet with family and discuss feelings each member is experiencing related to client's illness.	1a. Nurse will talk to client about meeting together as a family with the nurse to discuss his illness and related matters.	1a. Client participates in planning care to increase feelings of control and participation in own care.	Goal met. Family was able to share with client and each other their own experiences. Client stated he felt very supported and cared for. Wife and children stated they felt relieved to talk about things together again like a family.
	1b. Nurse will suggest to wife that all family members meet together to discuss the feelings she and the children are having regarding her husband's illness.	1b. Reopens channels of communication; decreases feelings of isolation and anxiety.	
	1c. Nurse will suggest to the family to meet once a week with nurse on a regular basis to work on family issues.	1c. As some issues become resolved, underlying concerns are free to surface. Keeping channels of communication open maximizes problem solving and family cohesion.	
2. By 6/21, client and family will plan two family activities they wish to resume.	2. The family will discuss activities they enjoyed together and will choose two or more that they all are eager to resume upon Mr. Saltzberg's discharge.	2. Enjoyable and meaningful memories are reactivated and shared, and focus is on positive events in the near future.	Goal met. Client suggested that he and his wife go to the movies once a week like they had in the past. Client agreed to go with his sons to Little League practice at least three times per month.
2. By 6/28, family will discuss resources and supports they feel are important to the family unit.	3a. The nurse will meet with the family and encourage problem solving of each member's needs and discuss supports to meet these needs.	3a. Each member may have different perceptions of what is going on within the family. Each may be affected differently. All members have a chance to address their needs and concerns.	Goal met. Family states that going to temple and talking to their family rabbi was special to them all. They mentioned certain family friends in whom they could confide and two relatives who were especially close to the family. The wife asked if there was a women's support group in her area. "Now the boys are growing, maybe I'll go back to work. It would be helpful to see how other women manage."
	3b. The nurse will discuss the community resources available (suicide prevention center, family counseling services, individual and group psychotherapy) and explore resources they find useful (temple, family, friends).	3b. Family will problem solve together on resources that are meaningful to them as a family and learn of new resources they might choose to use in the future.	
	3c. The nurse will explain the medication that Mr. Saltzberg is on, the action, the side effects, and when not to use the drug.	3c. Knowledge demystifies the disorder and treatment. Can increase understanding.	
	3d. The family will meet with other members of the health team before discharge to clarify questions and receive information (psychiatrist, social worker, dietitian).	3d. Family is given a chance to clarify questions and misconceptions and gain more knowledge and support.	

although the working nursing care plan (see Nursing Care Plan 7–1) may be condensed. Usually, new plans of care are discussed in team meetings that take place once or twice a week among the staff. Sharing plans of care with other staff members allows for further input and suggestions. This helps to ensure consistency of care and commitment of all staff toward the stated goals.

GIVING NURSING CARE IN THE PSYCHIATRIC SETTING

The *Standards of Psychiatric and Mental Health Nursing Practice* identifies six areas of intervention in psychiatric nursing: psychotherapeutic interventions, health teaching, activities of daily living, somatic therapies, therapeutic environment, and psychotherapy.

Standard V-A: Psychotherapeutic Interventions

Intervention at this level is usually carried out by a nurse minimally prepared as a generalist in psychiatric and mental health nursing. Some of the interventions include reinforcing functional coping patterns, employing problem-solving and communication skills, and utilizing other members of the health team to help in evaluating the outcome of interventions. The dialogue in Box 7–1 illustrates the use of psychotherapeutic interventions.

Standard V-B: Health Teaching

Health teaching includes identifying health education needs of the client and teaching basic principles of

Box 7–1. PSYCHOTHERAPEUTIC INTERVENTIONS

Short Term Goal: Client will name three personal strengths that have worked for him in the past.

	Interaction	Rationale
NURSE:	You mentioned everything coming down on you when your business began to fail.	Nurse places the event in time and sequence, validating the precipitating event.
CLIENT:	Yes . . . everything I had worked for was lost. That business was my whole life. Everything I did was for my business. It was my baby.	
NURSE:	You lost a great deal. You said it was like your baby?	Reflecting/empathy. Restating.
CLIENT:	Yeah, well, I had dreamed of it for years. My brother lent me some money, but it was my idea, and I did most of the work to get it going.	
NURSE:	It seems to me that building up a business from scratch takes a lot of work and know-how.	Pointing out realities and assisting to clarify strengths.
CLIENT:	Oh yes, I was never afraid of hard work. I used to be good at figuring my way out of a tight spot. Now . . . I don't know . . . Ever since that automated shop came in, I couldn't keep up with those prices. Everything caved in . . . It doesn't seem to matter anymore.	
NURSE:	What doesn't seem to matter?	Clarifying.
CLIENT:	Me . . . being a success . . . being somebody. I guess now I'll never be anybody.	

(Continued)

Box 7–1. PSYCHOTHERAPEUTIC INTERVENTIONS *(Continued)*

	Interaction	Rationale
NURSE:	Are you saying that you equate what happens in business with your personal worth?	Validating client's perception.
CLIENT:	Yes . . . I mean . . . no, I just felt so awful when everything caved in . . . I felt so responsible.	
NURSE:	Responsible?	Restating.
CLIENT:	Yeah . . . responsible to my family.	
NURSE:	How did your family react?	Giving broad openings.
CLIENT:	Well . . . I really didn't say too much to them. I didn't want to worry them . . . I guess I was afraid.	
NURSE:	Afraid?	Restating.
CLIENT:	Yeah. That they would think I was no longer a success now that the business was failing.	
NURSE:	You were afraid they would see you as a failure if the business ran into trouble?	Reflecting.
CLIENT:	I don't know . . . the business was such a great success in the beginning.	
NURSE:	What do you think made the shop so successful in the beginning?	Encourages the client to realistically appraise his strengths.
CLIENT:	Well, I worked very hard . . . and I am good at knowing what people want. Everyone always says I have a unique way of marketing and advertising.	
NURSE:	You are conscientious, observant of others, and creative.	Restates what the client has said. At this point the client can agree or clarify what he meant.
CLIENT:	Well . . . yes, but what does it matter now?	
NURSE:	In what other ways could you use these qualities?	The nurse encourages client to problem-solve.
CLIENT:	Huh . . . I hadn't thought about other ways . . . *Silence* Sam Cohn . . . well . . . Sam . . . he always wanted me to come in with him. I always wanted my own place though.	
NURSE:	Well, that is one possibility. We talked this morning about some of your strengths and maybe this afternoon we can talk some more about other ways you can use these strengths in the future.	Summarizes and encourages collaboration in setting future goals.
CLIENT:	Yeah . . . some other possibilities.	

physical and mental health. The following vignette illustrates health teaching:

While working with the client on creating alternatives to his present solution, the nurse noted that family communications seemed to break down when the client was faced with an issue that threatened his self-image. Mr. Saltzberg stated that the family was usually able to talk about personal concerns. However, when the business started to falter, Mr. Saltzberg began to think of himself as a failure. He felt ashamed and impotent, and he isolated himself from his family emotionally, hiding his feelings. Thus, he increased his feelings of isolation and helplessness. As anxiety increases, the ability to solve problems decreases. Eventually, Mr. Saltzberg felt overwhelmed and defeated.

The nurse intervenes to suggest alternative interpersonal communication skills Mr. Saltzberg can use within the family to minimize feelings of hopelessness and helplessness when problems arise. The nurse suggests to Mr. Saltzberg that the family and nurse meet together so that he can "practice" sharing personal feelings. Illness or problems of one family member usually affect all family members. By having the family meet together and work on important issues with some degree of safety and guidance, problems can be minimized. For example, the family may decide to encourage Mr. Saltzberg to talk things out when he seems preoccupied or upset. Discussing problem situations as a family can help put situations into a realistic perspective, provide a variety of alternative actions, and decrease feelings of isolation and helplessness. The family may also identify outside resources that could prove helpful, for example, religious counseling and sympathetic relatives and friends.

Standard V-C: Activities of Daily Living

The activities of daily living include an individual's developmental and intellectual levels, as well as emotional state and physical limitations.

The nursing interventions aimed at increasing Mr. Saltzberg's physical care will center on nutrition. Mr. Saltzberg will gain two pounds per week while in the hospital.

Getting an anorexic person to eat takes creative thinking and patience. In implementing the plan of care for Mr. Saltzberg, the nurse first finds out whether there are any religious dietary restrictions. Mr. Saltzberg states that he eats only kosher foods and that he does have food preferences. These preferences are special dishes his wife makes for him at home. He states he never eats breakfast but usually has his big meal in the middle of the day. At night he likes to eat lightly, but he also admits to snacking on junk food before bedtime.

By working with Mr. Saltzberg and contacting other members of the health team and family, the nurse sets up optimum conditions for increasing Mr. Saltzberg's weight. The doctor is first contacted to okay Mrs. Saltzberg's bringing in foods from home. The dietitian is contacted to visit Mr. Saltzberg. Kosher foods are requested, and food preferences are listed. Nutritious high-caloric snacks are planned with the client. Mrs. Saltzberg is contacted and agrees to make foods her husband especially likes and that she feels will tempt him to eat. The nurse works with Mr. Saltzberg, and it is agreed that during the three times he meets with her each day, he will eat a high-caloric snack.

The importance of follow-up care, community resources, and suicide prevention centers is also a vital part of the nurse's health teaching for Mr. Saltzberg and his family when planning discharge.

Standard V-D: Somatic Therapies

One of the nurse's responsibilities relating to somatic therapies includes the observations and judgments made concerning the effects of drugs and other somatic treatments.

One of the nurse's dependent functions is the administration of medications to clients. There are many nursing responsibilities associated with administering medications to clients. An important responsibility is to observe for the client's reaction to the medication and to observe for known side effects and toxic effects.

Mr. Saltzberg is taking Elavil, and the nurse notes in her care plan to watch for signs of orthostatic hypotension, a common side effect. Her interventions include checking his blood pressure when he is lying down and when he is standing, and instructing him to dangle his feet before getting out of bed.

If medications do not elevate Mr. Saltzberg's mood, other somatic therapies may be tried. Electroconvulsive therapy (ECT) would be a consideration.

The nurse has certain responsibilities when working with a client who is getting ECT. All somatic treatment modalities have guidelines for nursing care and nursing responsibilities.

Standard V-E: Therapeutic Environment

A therapeutic environment is an extremely important consideration in working with a client. The client should feel comfortable and safe and have the feeling that help is available. A positive environment can greatly affect a client's outlook and ability to solve problems. Not all clients at all times can make use of the therapies available to them at a particular time. However, a therapeutic environment can influence the choices a client makes.

A safe therapeutic environment for Mr. Saltzberg was the highest priority when he was first admitted to the unit. A person who is feeling overwhelmed and in a great deal of emotional pain often has difficulty figuring out ways to solve his problems. Sometimes suicide appears to be the only solution at the time. Mr. Saltzberg had suffered a great loss, is a male, and is over 45 years old; his father had attempted suicide at age 60; Mr. Saltzberg is clinically depressed. All of these factors place him at risk.

A safe environment was arranged for by providing Mr. Saltzberg with close observation and setting limits. All potential weapons were removed, and he was put on suicide precautions. Suicide precautions entailed checking the client every 15 minutes and keeping him in view at all times. He was also observed for any behaviors that might indicate thoughts of suicide, such as a sudden sense of well-being, giving away possessions, or making out a will.

Another safety precaution the nurse identified was watching for the possible side effect of his prescribed medication, Elavil. Ongoing evaluation for orthostatic hypotension and dizziness was done to prevent injuries from falls.

These nursing interventions were taken within the framework of building a relationship with Mr. Saltzberg. The nurse sets aside at least 15 minutes three times per day for Mr. Saltzberg. The *content* included sitting, talking, walking, planning, and engaging him in recreational activities — whatever seemed the most useful to Mr. Saltzberg at the time. The *process* is providing the presence of a person who is interested in the client's situation, is willing to work on issues in a nonjudgmental and nonthreatening manner, and is able to provide important resources when needed.

Standard V-F: Psychotherapy

A nurse qualified to work with a client as a psychotherapist is prepared at the master's level or higher. Most nurses who engage in psychotherapy have obtained certification through the American Nurses' Association. Certification entails many hours of supervised clinical work and passing the certification exam, as well as achievement of specific educational credentials (Fickeissen 1985). A nurse may choose adult or child as specialty areas, although many nurses prefer work as family therapists.

If, at the time of discharge, Mr. Saltzberg wanted to explore further his motivations, coping patterns, life goals, and emotional responses that keep him from meeting his goals, referral to a nurse psychotherapist would be appropriate.

CONTINUED DATA COLLECTION

Data collection is an ongoing process throughout all the phases of the nursing process. While observing Mr. Saltzberg, one nurse noted that he had difficulty sharing problems with his family when his self-esteem was threatened. During these times, family communications broke down, and family members became confused and isolated. The added data directed future nursing intervention.

Standard VI: Evaluation

Evaluation is often the most neglected part of the nursing process. Ideally, evaluation should be part of each phase in the nursing process. Evaluation of a plan of care involves two basic steps: (1) evaluation of goal achievement and (2) reassessment of care (Atkinson and Murray 1983).

EVALUATING GOALS ACHIEVED

There are three possible alternatives when evaluating whether a goal has been met: goal met, goal not met, goal partially met. Along with the statement of evaluation, the nurse documents the client's behavior as evidence as to the status of the goal. Diagrammatically, evaluation of goal achievement appears as follows (Atkinson and Murray 1983):

EVALUATION =

Goal Met + Supporting Behaviors
Goal Not Met + Supporting Behaviors
Goal Partially Met + Supporting Behaviors

For example, evaluation of the goals set by the nurse for Mr. Saltzberg's third nursing diagnosis might be:

Nursing Diagnosis: Altered Family Process related to an ill family member
Long Term Goal: By discharge, client and family will discuss and identify three outside supports available to them all.

Short Term Goal	Evaluation
1. 6/4—By 6/11, client will meet with family and discuss feelings each member is experiencing related to client's illness.	1. 6/11—Goal met. Family was able to share with client and each other their own experiences. Client stated he felt very supported and cared for. Wife and children stated they felt relieved to talk about things together again like a family.
2. By 6/21, client and family will plan two family activities they wish to resume.	2. 6/21—Goal met. Client suggested that he and his wife go to the movies once a week, as they had in the past. Client agreed to go with his sons to Little League practice at least three times per month.
3. By 6/28, family will discuss resources and supports they feel are important to the family unit.	3. 6/30—Goal was met. Family states that going to temple and talking to their family rabbi was special to them. They mentioned certain family friends in whom they could confide and two relatives who were especially close to the family. The wife asked if there was a women's support group in her area. "Now the boys are growing, maybe I'll go back to work. It would be helpful to see how other women manage."

REASSESSMENT OF CARE PLAN

The nurse continuously collects data during the planning and implementation of nursing interventions. After evaluating the client-centered goals, it is often necessary to re-evaluate why some goals were not met, and, if some goals were met, whether the nursing diagnoses or goals are still an appropriate focus of nursing care. For example, do the nursing diagnoses still have the same order of priority, or are there new diagnoses and goals that must be set to assure effective, safe, and appropriate nursing interventions?

The following are five possible outcomes after reassessment of the care plan (Atkinson and Murray 1983):

1. Priorities may change, and the order of nursing diagnoses will change.
2. New data may point to the need for new diagnoses, goals, and nursing actions.
3. When a goal is met and the problem no longer exists, a nursing diagnosis is dropped after appropriate documentation on either the client's records or the Kardex or both.
4. At other times, although a goal might be met, the problem still exists. If a number of short term goals need to be set to achieve a long term goal, the nurse would choose another goal reflecting the client's progress and ability.
5. When a goal is not met or is only partially met, reassessment is done to identify and rewrite a more successful plan. The problem with an unsuccessful plan can be an incorrect nursing diagnosis, unrealistic goals, ineffective nursing measures planned to meet goals, or a change in the client's status. Reassessment of a client's care plan with other members of the nursing staff can aid in the creation of a more effective plan.

Documentation—SOAP Format

Today, one of the most popular systems for documenting client problems and progress is called the problem-oriented record (POR). Compared with the more traditional systems, the POR system has many advantages. The problem-oriented record increases communication among the mental health workers. All nurses, doctors, social workers, and activities therapists record their notes chronologically. The POR also helps to avoid duplication of observations by a number of health-team members. New data are added, and the inclusion of extraneous material is minimized. The format of the POR follows most of the steps in the nursing process: subjective and objective data, analysis, and plan. The format for the documentation using the POR system is the acronym SOAP: subjective data, objective data, assessment, and plan.

S SUBJECTIVE DATA are quotes or paraphrases from the client that define his experience regarding a specific problem.
  S = Client states, "I know it is silly, but I am terrified of the dark."

O OBJECTIVE DATA are observations, measurements, and data from secondary sources (charts, laboratory results, other health-team members).
  O = Client constantly around nurses' station, refusing to go into room for the night for four nights. Became irritable when told by therapy aide she had to go to her room. Face is drawn, and she has dark circles under eyes.

A ANALYSIS includes synthesizing the objective and subjective data in the form of the problem statement, often stated as the nursing diagnosis. More information may be included, such as the rationale for the problem and the interpretation of the data.
  A = Sleep pattern disturbance: related to extreme fear of the dark (night phobia).

P PLAN includes the short term goals and nursing actions to be taken.
  P = The client will get at least seven hours of sleep per night.
    1. Move client to single room.
    2. Allow light to be on all night.
    3. Spend five minutes with client each evening.
    4. Record hours of sleep per night until goal has been met for one week.

The procedure for writing progress notes may vary within each institution, depending on its particular needs. Box 7–2 shows how the nurse might document Mr. Saltzberg's progress in the SOAP format on admission and toward the middle of his hospitalization.

Summary

The nursing process is an adaptation of the problem-solving process used by many professions. Inherent in the nursing process are three theoretical frameworks: (1) the holistic model, (2) Maslow's human needs theory, and (3) general systems theory.

The *primary* source of assessment is the client. The psychiatric nursing assessment is done within the psychiatric interview. *Secondary sources* of information are the family, neighbors, friends, police, and other members of the health team. The *process* component of the interview, use of communications skills and therapeutic use of self, have a great impact on the resulting relationship. Both the nurse's and the client's anxiety levels need to be acknowledged, as do personal biases and value judgments. The *content* of the interview includes gathering subjective data (client history) and objective data (mental/emotional status). An assessment tool is provided, and charts defining motor behaviors and thought content are included. Assessment tools are useful and can help the nurse focus the interview. When the nurse develops the skill and becomes more comfortable in this role, the interview becomes less formal without sacrificing important data. The two major components of the assessment process are (1) gathering data and (2) verifying the data. Verifying the data is done by checking with secondary sources of information.

The nursing diagnosis is a crucial phase in the nursing process. The nursing diagnosis performs a number of functions: it defines the practice of nursing, improves communication between staff, assists in accountability for care, differentiates nursing from medicine, and so forth. A nursing diagnosis consists of (1) an unmet need or problem, (2) etiology or probable cause, and (3) supporting data. A problem becomes a nursing diagnosis when it falls under the independent functions of nursing practice—areas the nurse is trained and licensed to treat. A nursing diagnosis can be stated as an actual, potential, or possible problem.

Planning nursing care involves (1) determining desired outcomes and goals and (2) planning nursing actions to reach those goals. A goal should be measurable, indicate desired outcome, have a set time for achievement, and be short and specific. Goals identify the direction for nursing care. Planning nursing action to achieve the goals includes using specific principles. The plan should be safe, based on scientific rationale, realistic, and compatible with other therapies.

The implementation of psychiatric care involves (1) verifying the care plan, (2) giving nursing care, and (3) continuous data collection. Validating the care plan includes specific areas of concern: Is the plan safe? Is it based on scientific principles/rationales? Do the data support the nursing diagnosis? Are priorities correct? Practice in psychiatric nursing encompasses six areas as defined by the ANA *Standards of Psychiatric and Mental Health Nursing Practice*. Data collection continues throughout the nursing process.

The evaluation of care involves (1) evaluation of goal achievement and (2) reassessment of care. The nurse judges the goal to be either met, not met, or partially met. Supporting data are included to clarify the evaluation. Reassessment of the care plan is done periodically. The nurse decides whether priorities in diagnosis need changing, new diagnoses need to be added, new interventions are needed to meet goals, and whether diagnosis, goals, interventions, and plans are currently appropriate.

The most widely used form of documentation is the problem-oriented record (POR). The format for documentation using the POR system is called SOAP. The

Box 7–2. SOAP NOTES ON MR. SALTZBERG

Admission

1. 6/4

S: "I have nothing to live for." Admits to vague thoughts of suicide.

O: Client sits slumped in chair, no eye contact, depressed face. Recent loss; father attempted suicide at age 60.

A: Potential for self-directed violence related to suicidal thoughts and depressed demeanor.

P: Client will not harm himself.
1. Suicide precautions:
   a. take away all potential weapons
   b. check every 15 minutes
   c. know whereabouts at all times.
2. Assess suicide potential.
3. Meet with client three times a day for 15 minutes.
4. Check effect and possible side effects of medication.

2. 6/4

S: "I have no appetite."

O: Client went from 159 to 140 pounds in two months. Ten pounds under minimum weight. Looks drawn, clothes hang on body.

A: Altered nutrition: less than body requirements, related to anorexia and depression.

P: Client will gain two pounds per week.
1. call in dietitian
2. have wife bring food from home
3. encourage high-caloric snacks while with nurse three times a day
4. weigh weekly

3. 6/4

S: "I just want to be left alone."

O: Wife states family has not shared in activities since illness. Wife feels overwhelmed without husband's help and support.

A: Altered family process related to an ill family member.

P: Client and family will meet and discuss feelings.
1. ask client about meeting
2. suggest family meetings to wife
3. nurse will be present to facilitate communication and be supportive to family

During Hospitalization

1. 6/24

S: "I feel much better about things. I feel better about myself and about the future."

O: Client is physically active and participates in all activities. Grooming improved. Socializes with other clients in A.M. and P.M.

A: Potential for self-directed violence diminished. Denies suicidal thoughts and appears sociable and more interested in his surroundings than on admission.

P: Client will name actions he can take if he feels overwhelmed in future.
1. Continue to meet with client three times a day, and meet with family once a week.
2. Assess with client social and personal supports.
3. Give client information or referral as indicated.
4. Continue to work with client in setting future goals.

2. 6/24

S: "I'm getting my appetite back."

O: Eats little at breakfast or lunch. Eats dinner, all food wife brings in, and two to three high-caloric snacks a day. Has gained four pounds.

A: Altered nutrition continues, but client is less anorexic and states he feels depressed.

P: Continue plan as outlined on 6/4.

3. 6/24

S: "My family has been great. I look forward to being with them again."

O: Family openly expresses support of client. Client was able to discuss feelings of failure. Have met twice thus far.

A: Increase in the ability of the family to plan and share together related to an increase in communication.

P: Family will identify resources and available supports.
1. continue meeting with family once a week or more.
2. give information regarding community resources as needed.
3. encourage problem-solving of each member's needs and seeking available supports.

records are organized into subjective and objective data, analysis of the data, and plan of care.

References

American Nurses' Association. Standards of Psychiatric and Mental Health Nursing Practice. Kansas City, MO: American Nurses' Association, 1982.

Atkinson LD, Murray ME. Understanding the Nursing Process, 2nd ed. New York: Macmillan Publishing Company, 1983.

Barry PD. Psychosocial Nursing Assessment and Intervention. Philadelphia: J.B. Lippincott Company, 1984.

Bower FL. The Process of Planning Nursing Care. St. Louis: C.V. Mosby Company, 1982.

Carpenito LJ. Nursing Diagnosis: Application to Clinical Practice. Philadelphia: J.B. Lippincott Company, 1987.

Coombs RA, et al. Perceptual Psychology: A Humanistic Approach to the Study of Persons. New York: Harper & Row, 1976.

Douglas DJ, Murphy EK. Nursing process, nursing diagnosis and emerging taxonomies. *In* McCloskey JC, Grace HK (eds). Current Issues in Nursing. Boston: Blackwell Scientific Publications, 1981.

Eisenman EJP, Dubbert PM. Mental health assessment interview. *In* Backer, et al. (eds). Psychiatric/Mental Health Nursing: Contemporary Readings. New York: D Van Nostrand Company, 1978.

Fickeissen J. Getting certified. American Journal of Nursing, 86:265, 1985.

Field LL. The implication of nursing diagnosis in clinical nursing practice. Clinics of North America, 14:497, 1979.

Geltrust KV, et al. Applied Nursing Diagnosis Guides for Comprehensive Care Planning. New York: John Wiley & Sons, 1985.

Gordon M. The concept of nursing diagnosis. Nursing Clinics of North America, 14:487, 1979.

Gordon M. Historical perspective: The national group for classification of nursing diagnosis. *In* Kim MJ, Moritz DA (eds). Classification of Nursing Diagnoses. New York: McGraw-Hill Book Company, 1982.

Hagerty BK. Psychiatric Mental Health Assessment. St. Louis: C.V. Mosby Company, 1984.

Kim MJ. Without collaboration, what's left? American Journal of Nursing, 85:281, 1985.

Lesse S. Anxiety—Its Components, Development and Treatment. New York: Grune and Stratton, 1970.

Lesse S. The relationship of anxiety to depression. American Journal of Psychotherapy, 36:332, 1982.

MacKinnon RA, Michels R. The Psychiatric Interview in Clinical Practice. Philadelphia: W.B. Saunders Company, 1971.

Maloney EM. The nursing process. *In* Haber, et al. (eds). Comprehensive Psychiatric Nursing, 2nd ed. New York: McGraw-Hill Book Company, 1982.

Maslow AH. Toward a Psychology of Being, 2nd ed. New York: D Van Nostrand Company, 1962.

Newman MA. Nursing diagnosis: Looking at the whole. American Journal of Nursing, 84:1496, 1984.

Orem D. Nursing Concepts of Practice. New York: McGraw-Hill Book Company, 1980.

Riehl J, Roy C (eds). Conceptual Models for Nursing Practice. New York: Appleton-Century-Crofts, 1980.

Rogers M. An Introduction to the Theoretical Basis of Nursing. Philadelphia: F. A. Davis Company, 1970.

Shoemaker J. Essential features of nursing diagnosis. *In* Kim MJ, et al. (eds). Classification of Nursing Diagnoses. Proceedings of the Fifth National Conference. St. Louis: C.V. Mosby Company, 1984.

Tartaglia MJ. Nursing diagnosis: Keystone of your care plan. Nursing 85, 15:34, 1985.

Weber S. Nursing diagnosis in private practice. Nursing Clinics of North America, 14:533, 1979.

Webster M. Psychiatric nursing assessment. *In* Lego S (ed). The American Handbook of Psychiatric Nursing. Philadelphia: J.B. Lippincott Company, 1984.

Yura H, Walsh MB. The Nursing Process—Assessing, Planning, Implementing, Evaluating, 4th ed. Norwalk, CT: Appleton-Century-Crofts, 1983.

Annotated Bibliography

BOOKS

Atkinson LD, Murray ME. Understanding the Nursing Process, 2nd ed. New York: Macmillan Publishing Company, 1983.

This is an excellent reference for students for applying the theories of the nursing process to the clinical setting. The authors break down the nursing steps in the nursing process very concretely. There is frequent use of diagrams and examples to take the student through each step. The instructions make the process very comprehensible and easy to use, minimizing the errors often made when applying the process to the clinical setting.

Geltrust KV, et al. Applied Nursing Diagnosis: Guides for Comprehensive Care Planning. New York: John Wiley & Sons, 1985.

This is an excellent guide for planning care for both the student and the professional nurse. It includes the nursing diagnosis, lists the possible risk factors, and offers guidelines for goals. The unique aspect of this book is that it includes a large spectrum of possible nursing interventions with rationales. The nurse can pick those interventions that specifically meet his or her client's special needs. It is well organized and an extremely useful tool.

Rapp SR, Wilcox SM. Methods of assessment in psychiatric nursing. *In* Backer BA, et al. (eds.) Psychiatric Mental Health Nursing: Contemporary Readings, 2nd ed. Monterey, CA: Wadsworth Health Sciences Division, 1985.

The authors discuss the pros and cons of a structured versus an unstructured interview for the psychiatric nursing assessment. There are helpful clinical guidelines especially in the areas of assessment by direct observation and assessment by indirect observation.

Townsend MC. Nursing Diagnoses in Psychiatric Settings: A Pocket Guide for Care Plan Construction. Philadelphia: F.A. Davis Company, 1988.

Excellent guide for planning nursing interventions, employing many of the nursing diagnoses used in psychiatric settings. Gives a brief, concrete overview of theory.

ARTICLES

Carpenito LJ. Diagnostics: Actual, potential, or possible? American Journal of Nursing, 85:458, 1985.

Clarifies the use of actual, potential, or possible problems and translates that knowledge into nursing diagnosis.

Dettmore D. Spiritual care: Remembering your patients' forgotten needs. Nursing 84, 14:46, 1984.

This short article encourages nurses to assess and intervene in an area of great importance to many clients. It validates how real the need for spiritual care is and emphasizes that nurses are often the only ones who can intervene while the client is hospitalized.

Self-Study Exercises

Name the components for each of the steps in the nursing process.

1. Assessment
   A. ______________________
   B. ______________________
2. Diagnosis
   A. ______________________
   B. ______________________
   C. ______________________
3. Planning
   A. ______________________
   B. ______________________
4. Intervention
   A. ______________________
   B. ______________________
   C. ______________________
5. Evaluation
   A. ______________________
   B. ______________________

Label each of the behaviors described with one of the following parts of the psychiatric interview: P (Process), C-H (Content: history), and C-M/E (Content: mental/emotional).

6. ________ Nurse approaches client, lets him know when the interview will be, how long it will be, and what it will entail.
7. ________ Nurse asks the client to explain what he sees as his problem and what he thinks might help him at this time.
8. ________ Is the client able to assess his symptoms realistically?
9. ________ When assessing the client's sexual orientation, the client becomes defensive, evasive, and anxious. The nurse goes on to another topic.
10. ________ The nurse concludes the client is confabulating, since he says he went to England over the weekend, and he has been hospitalized for a month.
11. ________ The nurse asks the client how he usually copes with stress.
12. ________ The nurse asks the client what he values. Are there religious beliefs that are particularly important to him?
13. ________ When explaining the saying, "Don't put all your eggs in one basket," the client states that if you do that, and the basket drops, you won't have any eggs left.

Situation

Ms. Jamison is a 25-year-old woman who came to the hospital because her voices told her to kill herself, and she became very frightened. She appears tense. Her posture is rigid, her respirations rapid, and she states she has not eaten for three days. When asked what she usually does when she gets upset, she states that she used to talk to her mother, but her mother died a year ago. Since then, she has been extremely lonely. She tells the nurse she does not have any friends and works part-time as a temporary secretary. She says her voices started a week after her mother died. "They used to be friendly voices, but now they want me to die." She has an aunt and a brother but is hesitant to contact them. She states, "They don't really need my problems . . . they have busy lives." She says she is frightened about the voices and is afraid she might obey them. She asks the nurse to help her.

Questions 14 through 19 refer to the preceding situation. The questions are organized according to the steps of the nursing process.

14. There are a number of nursing diagnoses the nurse could choose. Formulate one nursing diagnosis for Ms. Jamison. Include the problem statement, probable etiology, and supporting data.

    A. The diagnostic title: What should change? ______________________
    B. The etiology or possible cause related to: ______________________
    C. Supporting data to validate diagnosis:
       -
       -
       -

15. State at least one long term goal and two short term goals, using all four criteria for setting an effective goal.

    A. *Long Term:* ______________________
    B. *Short Term:* ______________________
    C. *Short Term:* ______________________

16. Write two SOAP notes for Ms. Jamison, one upon admission and one shortly before discharge. Assume your goals were met.

UPON ADMISSION	UPON DISCHARGE
S: ______________________	S: ______________________
O: ______________________	O: ______________________
A: ______________________	A: ______________________
P: ______________________	P: ______________________

17. When planning nursing care for Ms. Jamison, list four principles you would consider.

    A. ______________________ B. ______________________
    C. ______________________ D. ______________________

Ms. Jamison is to be discharged tomorrow. She tells the nurse that the voices no longer tell her to kill herself and do not seem as threatening. She stated that she would like to continue seeing the nurse therapist in the clinic and planned to continue visiting her brother on weekends but did not feel up to trying any other activity at this time, although she completes her self-care. She is able to explain to the nurse the dose and time of the medications and the side effects.

18. For the following goals, state whether the goal was met, not met, or partially met, and give the supporting data.

    Long Term Goal: By discharge, client will state she no longer hears voices.
    A. Goal: ______________________ Supporting Data: ______________________

    Short Term Goal: Within two weeks, the client will be able to name three sources of support (church, community health center, women's group, relatives, neighbors) that she is comfortable using.
    B. Goal: ______________________ Supporting Data: ______________________

    Short Term Goal: Client will complete self-care while in the hospital, with the aid of medication and a daily therapy session with the nurse.
    C. Goal: ______________________ Supporting Data: ______________________

19. Refer to question 15 and evaluate the goals you had for Ms. Jamison.

On reassessment of the care plan shortly before Ms. Jamison's discharge, the staff felt that the long term goal "By discharge, client will state she no longer hears voices" was an unrealistic goal. A more realistic goal would be, "By discharge, client will not hear voices telling her to kill herself."

CHAPTER 8

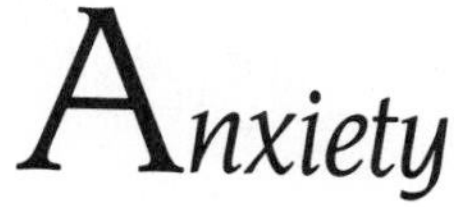

Elizabeth M. Varcarolis

OUTLINE

STANDARD I: THEORY
- Psychodynamic Theory
- Behavioral Theory
- Biological Theory

STANDARD II: DATA COLLECTION
- Assessing Levels of Anxiety
- Assessing Relief Behaviors
  - Interpersonal Relief Behaviors
  - Intrapsychic Relief Behaviors—Defense Mechanisms
- Assessing Circumstances Surrounding Increases in Anxiety

STANDARD III: DIAGNOSIS

STANDARD IV: PLANNING
- Content Level—Planning Goals
- Process Level—Nurses' Reactions and Feelings

STANDARD V: INTERVENTION
- V-A: Psychotherapeutic Intervention
- V-B: Health Teaching
- V-D: Somatic Therapies
- V-F: Psychotherapy

STANDARD VI: EVALUATION

CASE STUDY: WORKING WITH A PERSON IN MODERATE LEVELS OF ANXIETY
- Assessment
- Nursing Diagnosis
- Planning
- Intervention
- Evaluation

CASE STUDY: WORKING WITH A PERSON IN SEVERE LEVELS OF ANXIETY
- Assessment
- Nursing Diagnosis
- Planning
- Intervention
- Evaluation

SUMMARY

KEY TERMS AND CONCEPTS

The key terms and concepts listed here also appear in bold where they are defined or discussed in this chapter.

FEAR

ANXIETY

ACUTE ANXIETY (STATE)

CHRONIC ANXIETY (TRAIT)

MILD-MODERATE-SEVERE-PANIC LEVELS OF ANXIETY

EMPATHY

SELECTIVE INATTENTION

ACTING OUT BEHAVIORS

SOMATIZING

DEFENSE MECHANISMS
- Repression
- Sublimation

Regression
Displacement
Projection
Compensation
Reaction-Formation
Denial
Conversion
Undoing
Rationalization
Identification
Introjection
Suppression

NORMAL ANXIETY
PRIMARY ANXIETY
SECONDARY ANXIETY

OBJECTIVES

After studying this chapter, the student will be able to:

1. Identify one contribution made by each of the following etiological theories of anxiety that can be used in nursing practice:
   A. Psychodynamic theory
   B. Learning theory
   C. Biological theory
2. Compare and contrast the meanings of the following concepts:
   A. Anxiety and fear
   B. Primary and secondary anxiety
   C. Acute and chronic anxiety
3. Discuss what is meant by normal anxiety.
4. Define the term empathy.
5. Name and give an example of each step in the operational definition of anxiety.
6. Select six defense mechanisms and give examples of both adaptive and maladaptive ways they are used.
7. Write three characteristics (perceptual field, ability to learn, or other defining characteristics) for a person in each of the following levels of anxiety:
   A. Mild
   B. Moderate
   C. Severe
   D. Panic
8. Give two examples of basic goals for a person in each of the following levels of anxiety:
   A. Mild to moderate
   B. Severe to panic
9. Discuss various nursing interventions, including rationales for a person in each of the following levels of anxiety:
   A. Mild to moderate
   B. Severe to panic

Anxiety is a universal human experience. It is an everyday component of our lives and a stranger to no one. Anxiety is the most basic of emotions and is part of all emotions. It is the basic ingredient in the most unpleasant emotions, such as grief, jealousy, and anger, as well as in those emotions that lead to our peak experiences, such as love and joy.

Behavior stems from anxiety. A basic principle in psychiatric nursing is, "all behavior is purposeful, meaningful, and can be understood" (Burd 1968). Dysfunctional behavior is often a defense against anxiety. When behavior is recognized as dysfunctional, interventions to reduce anxiety can be initiated by the nurse. As anxiety decreases, dysfunctional behavior will frequently decrease.

Anxiety is experienced on four levels, namely, mild, moderate, severe, and panic. It can be broken down into three categories — normal, acute, and chronic — and it can be operationally defined.

Hildegard Peplau, one of the first nurse theorists, identifies anxiety as one of the most important concepts in psychiatric nursing. Nurses can use the concept of anxiety to explain many clinical observations. Peplau has conceptualized an anxiety model that is useful in the practice of nursing. Conceptualizing anxiety using Peplau's model has led to principles that serve as guides in nursing intervention (Burd 1968). This conceptual basis of anxiety can be used by nurses as a framework to guide approaches to clients inside and outside the hospital setting.

Anxiety can be defined as a state of feeling apprehension, uneasiness, uncertainty, or dread resulting from a real or a perceived threat whose actual source is unknown or unrecognized. Physiological responses to anxiety and fear are similar. However there are important distinctions between anxiety and fear.

First, there is general agreement that **fear** is a reaction to a specific danger, whereas anxiety is a vague sense of dread from an unspecified danger (May 1983). The body reacts in similar ways physiologically, however, to both anxiety and fear.

Second, an important distinction between anxiety and fear is that anxiety attacks us at a deeper level than fear. Anxiety invades the central core of the personality. It erodes the individual feelings of self-esteem and personal worth that contribute to a sense of being fully human (Chapman and Chapman 1980).

Normal anxiety is a healthy life force that is necessary for survival. It provides the energy needed to carry out the tasks in living and striving toward goals. Anxiety motivates people to make and survive change. It prompts constructive behaviors, such as studying for an examination, being on time for job interviews, preparing for a presentation, and working toward a promotion.

Acute anxiety is precipitated by an imminent loss or change that threatens an individual's sense of security. Acute anxiety may be seen in performers before a concert. For example, Barbara Streisand admits to experiencing acute anxiety before live concerts. Patients preparing for surgery often experience acute anxiety. The death of a loved one can stimulate acute anxiety, when there is great disruption in one's life. In general, crisis involves the experience of acute anxiety. Acute anxiety is also referred to as *state anxiety*.

Chronic anxiety is anxiety that the person has lived with for a period of time. Ego psychologists suggest that in a nurturing environment, the developing personality incorporates the positive attributes of the parents. This incorporation of positive values allows the child to tolerate anxiety. When conditions for personality growth are less than adequate, positive values may not be incorporated, and the child may become anxiety-ridden, which often covers up overwhelming, angry, and hostile impulses (Sullivan 1953). A child may demonstrate chronic anxiety by a permanent attitude of apprehension or overreaction to all unexpected environmental stimuli. In the adult, chronic anxiety may take the form of chronic fatigue, insomnia, discomfort in daily activities, and discomfort in personal relationships. Poor concentration may interfere with effective work functioning. When the subjective feelings of anxiety become too overwhelming, anxiety is unconsciously placed out of awareness (repressed) and is expressed in behavioral characteristics or symptoms. *Trait anxiety* is another name for chronic anxiety.

Understanding the types, levels, and defensive patterns used in response to anxiety is basic to psychiatric nursing care. This understanding of anxiety is essential for assessing and planning interventions to lower a client's level of anxiety, as well as one's own, effectively. With practice, one becomes more skilled at identifying levels of anxiety and defenses used, as well as evaluating the possible stressors contributing to increases in a person's level of anxiety.

This chapter deals with basic concepts regarding anxiety used by all nurses in all clinical settings. Common psychotherapeutic interventions are introduced for mild to moderate and severe to panic levels of anxiety. Brief case studies of a person in moderate levels of anxiety and a person in severe levels of anxiety are presented to illustrate the theoretical component through use of the nursing process. Figure 8–1 presents a conceptual framework for anxiety.

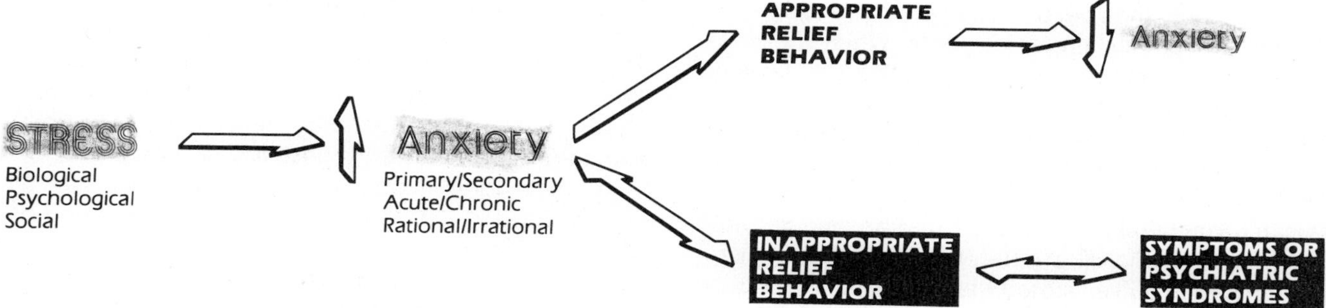

Figure 8–1. *Conceptualization of psychiatric symptoms or syndromes along the anxiety continuum.*

Standard I: Theory

Anxiety is a response to a stressful situation. Stress can be defined as a perceived threat to an expectation, which triggers anxiety. The result is some form of relief behavior (Knowles 1981). Therefore:

STRESS ⇨ ⇕ Anxiety ⇨ RELIEF BEHAVIOR

The stress can be psychological, social, or physical. Anxiety can be an appropriate or inappropriate response, and the relief behaviors can take the form of healthy relief behaviors or psychiatric symptoms (Lesse 1982). Thus, anxiety may be experienced as a (1) *symptom* involving a subjective feeling of apprehension or nervousness, or (2) *syndrome* involving both psychic and somatic symptoms, or (3) *primary disease*, such as generalized anxiety disorder or phobic disorder. As a symptom or syndrome it may be "normal" in certain circumstances. Anxiety may be "abnormal" when its severity is inappropriate or when it occurs in inappropriate circumstances (Cameron 1985).

There is no one etiological theory of anxiety that explains all the clinical and biological data. A variety of theories have made contributions to possible etiological factors in the development of anxiety. Three major theories are (1) psychodynamic, (2) behavioral, and (3) biological.

PSYCHODYNAMIC THEORY

Chapter 2 discusses in detail the major personality theories and therapies. Here we briefly review them in relation to the concept of anxiety.

Freud (1939) proposed that anxiety is the result of *unconscious* psychic conflicts. When these *intrapsychic conflicts* in the form of forbidden impulses (sexual or aggressive) threaten to become conscious, anxiety is experienced. Anxiety then becomes a *signal* to the ego to take defensive action to repress anxiety. When these defense mechanisms are successful, anxiety is lowered and a sense of security returns. However, if the conflict is intense and the anxiety level high, the defense mechanisms might be experienced as symptoms, such as phobias, regression, or ritualistic behaviors.

Harry Stack Sullivan believed that anxiety resulted from *interpersonal conflicts* rather than from an intrapsychic process. Sullivan stated that anxiety is linked with the anxiety experienced in infancy and early childhood. The infant's first experiences with emotional discomfort and acute anxiety become the prototype for future emotional distress. For example, a child reared by hostile and rejecting parents may later react with painful anxiety when treated in a cold or critical manner by another individual. Past experiences leave people vulnerable to anxiety in the present, and specific events or interpersonal exchanges can trigger underlying anxiety (Chapman and Chapman 1980). Two principles basic to nursing practice are based on Sullivan's theory of anxiety.

First, anxiety can be communicated interpersonally. Anxiety is communicated from one person to another via empathy (Sullivan 1953). **Empathy** is the ability to feel for and with another and to understand the other's experience (Kolb and Brodie 1982). Often in mass crisis situations, those in high levels of anxiety need to be dealt with first, to avoid the spread of anxiety which could lead to group panic and confusion.

Second, anxiety is an energy (Peplau 1968). We cannot see anxiety in others. Behavior expresses the anxiety that a person feels. No one wants to experience uncomfortable levels of anxiety. *Relief behaviors* are behaviors that discharge the energy of anxiety. Familiar behaviors such as movement, talking, and meditation are examples of relief behaviors used to lessen the experience of anxiety.

Rollo May (1983) states, "Anxiety is the apprehension cued off by a threat to some value that the individual holds essential to his existence as a personality." These threats comprise threats to biological integrity, for example, food and warmth and threats to psychological existence, such as loss of respect or freedom. A person experiencing an unconscious conflict may become anxious, although the reason for the anxiety may not be known. People modify their relationships with others constantly to keep anxiety as low as possible, thereby maintaining a feeling of emotional security.

Anxiety that is caused by psychological factors (intrapsychic or interpersonal conflicts) is referred to as **primary anxiety** (Rockwell 1982).

BEHAVIORAL THEORY

The success of behavioral therapy techniques in the treatment of phobias and obsessive-compulsive behaviors gives support to the theory that anxiety is a result of a learned conditioned response (Curtis 1985). According to behavioral theory, anxiety results from a system of responses to a particular stimulus. Over a period of time, an individual develops a learned conditioned response to certain stimuli. This assumption has given rise to the concept that anxiety can be learned and unlearned as a result of experience. Some behavioral therapists have regarded Freud's *signal* theory as identical to the learned conditioned response (Curtis 1985). Chapter 16 discusses behavioral interventions used effectively in the treatment of certain anxiety disorders such as phobias.

BIOLOGICAL THEORY

There is an increasing body of knowledge that supports the hypothesis that manifestations of anxiety may be due to physiological abnormalities (Hagerty 1984). Diagnostic decisions need to be made when one is confronted with anxiety symptoms to determine whether the anxiety is (1) secondary to a medical disorder, (2) secondary to a pervasive psychiatric disorder, such as depression, or (3) a primary anxiety disorder, such as phobias (Curtis 1985).

In many cases (5% to 42%), anxiety may be a warning of an underlying physiological process (Hall 1980). That is, the anxiety is caused by a physical disease or abnormality, *not* an emotional conflict. Anxiety secondary to a physical condition is termed **secondary anxiety.** For example, people with certain neurological disorders (multiple sclerosis, brain tumor), endocrine disorders (thyroid, pituitary), circulatory disorders (anemia, coronary insufficiency), and other disorders may experience anxiety due to physiological processes (Rockwell 1982; Hollander et al. 1988).

Recent studies suggest a strong correlation between mitral valve prolapse and panic attacks (Crowe 1985). Also, there seems to be some speculation of genetic and neurophysiological contributions to obsessive-compulsive disorders, although there are no conclusive data at present (Hollander et al. 1988).

Standard II: Data Collection

Assessing the presence of problematic levels of anxiety may or may not be easy. For example, a person in *acute* anxiety may demonstrate obvious signs and symptoms of distress and may be experiencing the anxiety subjectively: "I feel so upset." Or, a person might not be aware of experiencing anxiety. Instead, the anxiety might be repressed from conscious awareness but expressed in some other form of relief behavior. For example, a woman who is unaware of experiencing anxiety related to feelings of inadequacy might be *displacing* her anxiety as anger toward her family. A man who is unaware of experiencing anxiety related to low self-esteem might *compensate* by drinking or taking drugs in order to feel better temporarily. Established patterns of dealing with anxiety may be observed by noting specific relief behaviors a person uses.

The nursing assessment of the anxious client should include information about the (1) level of anxiety, (2) relief behaviors used to minimize the subjective experience of anxiety, and (3) circumstances surrounding increases in anxiety.

ASSESSING LEVELS OF ANXIETY

Levels of anxiety range from mild/moderate to severe/panic. Peplau's (1968) classic delineation of these four levels of anxiety is based on Harry Stack Sullivan's work. Assessment of a client's level of anxiety is basic to therapeutic intervention in any setting—psychiatric, hospital, or community. Determination of specific levels of anxiety can be used as guidelines for intervention (Table 9–1). Anxiety is experienced on a continuum from mild to moderate to severe to panic, and overlapping can and does occur. Use Table 8–1 as a guide.

MILD. Mild anxiety occurs in the normal experience of everyday living. The person's ability to perceive reality is brought into sharp focus. A person sees, hears, and grasps more information, and problem solving becomes more effective. A person might display such physical symptoms as slight discomfort, restlessness, irritability, or mild tension-relieving behaviors, such as nail biting, foot/finger tapping, or fidgeting.

MODERATE. As anxiety escalates, the perceptual field narrows and some details are excluded from observation. The person in moderate anxiety sees, hears, and grasps less information. Individuals may experience selective inattention. **Selective inattention** means that only certain things in the environment are seen or heard unless they are brought to the person's attention. Although the ability to think clearly is hampered, learning and problem solving can still take place, though not at an optimum level. At this level the person's ability to problem solve is greatly enhanced by the supportive presence of another. Physical symptoms include tension, pounding heart, increased pulse and respiration rate, perspiration, and mild somatic symptoms (gastric discomfort, headache, urinary urgency). Voice tremors and shaking might be noticed.

Mild or moderate anxiety levels can be constructive, since anxiety can be viewed as a signal that something in the person's life needs attention (Chapman and Chapman 1980).

SEVERE. The perceptual field of a person experiencing severe anxiety is greatly reduced. A person in severe anxiety may focus on one particular detail or many scattered details. When in severe anxiety, a person has

Table 8–1 • LEVELS OF ANXIETY

MILD	MODERATE	SEVERE	PANIC
		Perceptual Field	
Perceptual field can be heightened Person is alert and can see, hear, and grasp what is happening in the environment. Person can identify things that are disturbing and that are producing anxiety.	Perceptual field narrows. Person grasps less of what is going on. Person can attend to more *if pointed out by another* (selective inattention).	Perceptual field greatly reduced. Focus is on details or one specific detail. Attention is scattered. Complete absorption with self. Person may not be able to attend to events in the environment *even when* pointed out by others.	Person is unable to focus on the environment. Person experiences the utmost state of terror and emotional paralysis. Feels he "ceases to exist." In panic, hallucinations or delusions may take the place of reality.
		In severe and panic levels of anxiety the environment is blocked out. It is as if these events are not occurring.	
		Ability to Learn	
Able to effectively work toward a goal and examine alternatives.	Able to solve problems but not at optimum ability. Benefits from guidance of others.	Inability to see connections between events or details.	May be mute or have extreme psychomotor agitation leading to exhaustion.
Mild and moderate levels of anxiety can alert the person that something is wrong and stimulate appropriate action.		**Severe and panic levels prevent problem solving and finding effective solutions. Unproductive relief behaviors are called into play, thus perpetuating a vicious cycle.**	
		Physical and Other Characteristics	
Slight discomfort Attention seeking behaviors Restlessness Irritability/impatience Mild tension-relieving behavior, such as foot/finger rapping, lip chewing, fidgeting	Voice tremors Change in voice pitch Difficulty concentrating Shakiness Repetitive questioning Somatic complaints, such as urinary frequency and urgency, headache, backache, insomnia Increased respiration rate Increased pulse rate Increased muscle tension More extreme tension relieving behavior, such as pacing and banging hands on table	Ineffective functioning Inability to concentrate May appear confused Purposeless activity Sense of impending doom More intense somatic complaints, such as dizziness, nausea, headache, and sleeplessness Hyperventilation Tachycardia Withdrawal	Experience of terror and dread Immobility or severe hyperactivity Dilated pupils Pallor Unintelligible communication or inability to speak Severe shakiness Sleeplessness Severe withdrawal Hallucinations or delusions likely

Data from Peplau 1968, Chapman and Chapman 1980, McFarland and Wasli 1984.

difficulty noticing what is going on in the environment *even when* pointed out by another. Learning and problem solving are not possible at this level, and the person may be dazed and confused. Behavior is "automatic" and aimed at reducing or relieving anxiety. The person may complain of increased severity in somatic symptoms, (headache, nausea, dizziness, insomnia), trembling, and pounding heart. The person may also experience hyperventilation and a sense of impending doom or dread.

PANIC. Feelings of panic are very painful. Panic is the most extreme form of anxiety and results in marked disturbed behavior. The person is not able to process what is going on in the environment and may lose touch with reality. The behavior that results may be confusion, shouting, screaming, or withdrawal. Hallucinations may be experienced by people in panic levels of anxiety. Hallucinations are false sensory perceptions, such as seeing people or objects that are not present in reality (refer to Chapter 20). Physical behavior may be erratic, uncoordinated, and impulsive (Schwartz and Shockley 1956). Automatic behaviors are used to reduce and relieve anxiety, although efforts may be ineffective. Acute panic may lead to exhaustion. Table 8–1 identifies levels of anxiety in relation to (1) perceptual field, (2) ability to learn, and (3) physical and other defining characteristics.

ASSESSING RELIEF BEHAVIORS

Interpersonal Relief Behaviors

Anxiety and defenses against anxiety are a necessary part of human life. Peplau (1968) has identified four major patterns of reducing and relieving anxiety:

1. Acting out behaviors
2. Somatizing
3. "Freezing to the spot"
4. Learning

ACTING OUT BEHAVIORS. Acting out behaviors refer to behaviors that originate on an unconscious level to reduce anxiety and tension. Anxiety is displaced from one situation to another in the form of observable behavioral responses. Some examples follow:

Anger can be used to conceal thoughts or feelings that threaten to trigger anxiety. Anger distracts an individual from threatening thoughts and feelings. Anger can effectively remove the focus from the self and redirect attention to something or someone in the environment.

Crying can at times be an effective relief from tension and painful feelings. When a person is crying, feelings are close to the surface, thereby enabling a person to identify what he or she is feeling.

Laughter can afford a partial relief of tension. Laughter can express conscious and unconscious psychological meanings and may mask feelings like hostility, fear, despair, or triumph.

Physical and verbal abuse distracts the person from realizations that are threatening. By lashing out at others, personal doubts and insecurities can remain out of awareness.

SOMATIZING. To somatize is to experience an emotional conflict as a physical symptom. When attention is focused on bodily complaints, underlying anxiety and interpersonal difficulties can be kept out of awareness. Physical discomfort can be used to distract one from threatening emotional anguish. Therefore, the energy of anxiety is internalized physiologically (Chapman and Chapman 1980). For example, a person might experience a headache or backache as a distraction from focusing on interpersonal conflicts.

"FREEZING TO THE SPOT." "Freezing to the spot" involves withdrawal and depression. Withdrawal is a reaction in which psychic energy is withdrawn from the environment into the self in response to anxiety. An example of severe withdrawal is seen in the catatonic schizophrenic (Chapter 20). A person with catatonia may sit for days or months without moving or speaking. Investment in the environment is lost while the person is in a withdrawn state.

One theory of depression is that anxiety is stimulated when unconscious aggressive impulses threaten to become conscious. If faulty learning occurred at an early age, angry feelings may be equated with the threat of losing approval and acceptance (Chapman 1976). The client learns to repress aggression and directs the anger toward the self.

LEARNING—PROBLEM SOLVING. Learning takes place when anxiety is recognized and the unconscious unmet need identified. This process is often referred to as "talking it out" and "figuring it out" and involves talking about the anxiety-producing event and figuring out feelings resulting from a threat or an unmet expectation (Peplau 1968). When painful feelings or unsatisfying behaviors can be discussed with a caring person in a counseling situation, alternative and more satisfying solutions can be evaluated.

Intrapsychic Relief Behaviors—Defense Mechanisms

Defense mechanisms are used by everyone. They serve to lower anxiety, maintain ego function, and protect self-esteem. Defense mechanisms can be classified as relief behaviors, since they lessen or relieve anxiety. High levels of anxiety can disturb problem solving and learning as well as perception and functioning. Unconscious defensive maneuvers are mobilized in order that an individual can continue to meet personal and social goals in acceptable ways. All defense mechanisms are mobilized by the ego, with the exception of regression. In regression, the ego itself (personality) is relegated to a less mature, although more comfortable, mode of operation. Most defense mechanisms are mobilized by the ego on an unconscious level. A notable exception is suppression, which uses the conscious mind.

Adaptive use of defense mechanisms helps people lower anxiety to achieve goals in acceptable ways. Maladaptive use of defense mechanisms may lead to distortions in reality and self-deception that can interfere with individual growth and interpersonal satisfaction. Determination of effective use of defense mechanisms is based on frequency, intensity, and duration of use.

A review of some of the most commonly used defense mechanisms is presented subsequently. Refer to Table

8–2 for illustrations of adaptive and maladaptive examples of each.

REPRESSION. Repression is the exclusion of unpleasant or unwanted experiences, emotions, or ideas from conscious awareness. "Forgetting" the name of a former husband and "forgetting" an appointment to discuss poor grades are examples. Repression is considered the cornerstone of the defense mechanisms, and it is the first line of psychological defense against anxiety.

SUBLIMATION. Sublimation is an unconscious process of substituting constructive and socially acceptable activity for strong impulses that are not acceptable in their original form. Usually these impulses are sexual or aggressive in nature. A man with strong hostile feelings becomes a butcher, or he may be involved with rough contact sports. A person who is unable to experience sexual activity may channel this energy into a creative activity, like painting or gardening.

REGRESSION. In regression the ego returns to an earlier, more comforting, although less mature way of behaving. For example, an adult who cannot have his own way pouts and whines and behaves in a manner that got him his own way as a child. When regression is severe, a person may regress to an infantile level and be unable to care for his own needs.

DISPLACEMENT. Transfer of emotions associated with a particular person, object, or situation to another person, object, or situation that is nonthreatening is called displacement. The frequently used example, boss yells at man—man yells at wife—wife yells at child—child kicks the cat, demonstrates a successive use of displaced hostility. The use of displacement is common but not always adaptive. Spouse, child, and elder abuse are often cases of displaced hostility.

PROJECTION. A person unconsciously rejects emotionally unacceptable features and attributes them to other people, objects, or situations through projection. This is the hallmark of "blaming" or "scapegoating," which is the root of prejudice. A person who always feels that others are out to deceive him or do him out of something may be projecting to others those characteristics in himself that he finds distasteful and cannot consciously accept. Projection of anxiety can often be seen in systems (family, hospital, school, and business). In a family in which there are problems, often the child is "scapegoated," and the pain and anxiety within the family are projected onto the child: "the problem is Tommy." In a larger system in which anxiety and conflict are present, the weakest members are scapegoated; "The problem is the nurses' aides, the students, the new salesman" (Miller and Winstead-Fry 1982). When pain and anxiety exist within a system, projection can be an automatic relief behavior. Once the cause of the anxiety is identified, changes in relief behavior can ensue and the system can become more functional and productive (Miller and Winstead-Fry 1982).

COMPENSATION. Making up for deficits in one area by excelling in another area in order to raise or maintain self-esteem is called compensation. An unsuccessful actor becomes a successful playwright, or a student with poor grades becomes outstanding in sports. These are two examples of adaptive compensation.

REACTION-FORMATION. In reaction-formation (also termed **overcompensation**), unacceptable feelings or behaviors are kept out of awareness by developing the opposite behavior or emotion. For example, a man who harbors hostility toward children becomes a boy scout leader.

DENIAL. Denial involves escaping unpleasant realities by ignoring their existence. A man might "deny"

Table 8–2 • EXAMPLES OF DEFENSE MECHANISMS

ADAPTIVE USE	MALADAPTIVE USE
Repression	
Man forgets wife's birthday after a marital fight.	A woman is unable to enjoy sex after having pushed out of awareness a traumatic sexual incident from childhood.
Sublimation	
Woman who is angry with her boss writes a short story about a heroic woman. By definition, use of sublimation is always constructive.	None
Regression	
Four-year-old with new baby brother starts sucking his thumb and wanting a bottle.	Man who loses a promotion starts complaining to others, hands in sloppy work, misses appointments, and comes in late for meetings.

Table 8–2 • EXAMPLES OF DEFENSE MECHANISMS *Continued*

ADAPTIVE USE	MALADAPTIVE USE
Displacement	
Patient criticizes the nurse after his family failed to visit.	Child unable to acknowledge fear of his father becomes fearful of animals.
Projection	
Man who is unconsciously attracted to other women teases his wife about flirting.	A woman who has repressed an attraction toward other women refuses to socialize. She fears another woman will make homosexual advances toward her.
Compensation	
A short man becomes assertively verbal and excels in business.	An individual drinks when self-esteem is low to diffuse discomfort temporarily.
Reaction-Formation	
Recovering alcoholic constantly preaches about the evils of drink.	A mother who has an unconscious hostility toward her daughter is overprotective and hovers over her to protect her from harm.
Denial	
Reaction to news of the death of a loved one: "No, I don't believe you. The doctor said he was fine."	A woman whose husband died three years ago still keeps his clothes in the closet and talks about him in the present tense.
Conversion	
Student is unable to take a final exam because of a terrible headache.	A man becomes blind after seeing his wife flirting with other men.
Undoing	
After flirting with her male secretary, a woman brings her husband tickets to a show.	A man with rigid and moralistic beliefs and repressed sexuality is driven to wash his hands when around attractive women to gain composure.
Rationalization	
"I didn't get the raise because the boss doesn't like me."	Father who thinks his son was fathered by another man excuses his malicious treatment of the boy by saying, "He is lazy and disobedient," when that is not the case.
Identification	
Five-year-old girl dresses in her mother's shoes and dress and meets daddy at the door.	Young boy who thinks a pimp in the neighborhood with money and drugs is someone to look up to.
Introjection	
After his wife's death, a husband has transient complaints of chest pain and difficulty breathing—the symptoms his wife had before she died.	A young child whose parents were overcritical and belittling grows up thinking that she is not any good. She has taken on her parent's evaluation of her as part of her own self-image.
Suppression	
A business man who is preparing to make an important speech that day is told by his wife that morning that she wants a divorce. Although visibly upset, he puts this incident aside until after his speech, when he can give the matter his total concentration.	A woman who feels a lump in her breast shortly before leaving for a three-week vacation puts the information in the back of her mind until after returning from her vacation.

chest pains even though heart attacks run in his family, because of the threat to his self-image as a man. A woman whose health has deteriorated because of alcohol abuse denies she has a problem with alcohol by saying she can stop drinking whenever she wants.

CONVERSION. Transforming anxiety on an unconscious level to a physical symptom that has no organic cause is called conversion. Often the symptom functions to provide for attention or as an excuse. For example, a professor develops laryngitis on the day he or she is scheduled to defend a research proposal to a group of peers.

UNDOING. Undoing makes up for an act or communication. For example, giving a gift to "undo" an argument. A common behavioral example of undoing is compulsive handwashing. This can be viewed as cleansing oneself of a perceived unacceptable act or thought.

RATIONALIZATION. Rationalization is justifying illogical or unreasonable ideas, actions, or feelings by developing acceptable explanations that satisfy the teller as well as the listener. Common examples are, "If I had his brains then I'd get good grades also" or "Everybody cheats, so why shouldn't I?" Rationalization is a form of self-deception.

IDENTIFICATION. Identification is an unconscious mechanism used to protect the person against anxiety and loss by imitation of mannerisms or behaviors of a person or group. By identification with the parent of the same sex the child resolves his Oedipal conflict. Hero worship is a form of identification.

INTROJECTION. Introjection involves intense identification in which a person incorporates or takes into his or her own personality qualities or values of another person or group with whom or with which intense emotional ties exist. The use of introjection is frequently seen in the grieving process and serves to lessen the anxiety of separation temporarily by the mourner. The mourner may take on some of the physical symptoms or behavioral mannerisms of the deceased for a period of time as a way of "holding on" to the deceased.

SUPPRESSION. Suppression is the conscious putting off of awareness of disturbing situations or feelings. A student who has been studying for the State Board Examinations says, "I can't worry about paying my rent until after my exam tomorrow." A more destructive use of suppression would be, "I know my child is having trouble in school, but I just don't want to think about it."

ASSESSING CIRCUMSTANCES SURROUNDING INCREASES IN ANXIETY

The nurse can work with the client to determine what triggered an increase in anxiety if the precipitating stress has not already been identified. Understanding the steps that operationally define the process of anxiety can help both nurse and client identify unmet needs and expectations. People are often not aware of the process of their thinking, especially in emotional areas. Sometimes just figuring out the source of the behavior or feelings is sufficient to lower anxiety effectively. The steps that operationally define anxiety are as follows (Manaser and Warner 1964):

Steps	Examples
1. Expectation/need present (status, recognition, success).	1. Client expects nurse to talk to him after rounds.
2. Expectation/need not met (threat, or precipitating stress).	2. Nurse unable to return to client's room.
3. Feelings of discomfort and uneasiness. Anxiety may be out of the individual's awareness.	3. This step often goes unnoticed. Step 4 follows immediately.
4. Relief behavior mobilized (for example, withdrawal, anger, somatizing, crying).	4. Client accuses nurse of being "no good," lazy, and incompetent.
5. Relief behavior is rationalized but not understood.	5. "Nurses are just doctors' maids. They don't count anyway."

In the preceding example, the client's problem is not competent or incompetent nurses, but rather the threat to the client's need for recognition. The client's expectation was that the nurse would visit to talk to him. When the nurse did not return, the client felt slighted, thinking, "I'm not good enough for her to spend time with me." The "uneasy feeling" stemming from the unmet need for recognition was quickly transferred into relief behavior. In this example, *projection* occurred when the client's feelings of low self-esteem were transferred onto the nurse, for example, "She is no good." Projection lowers the subjective feelings of anxiety, thereby protecting self-esteem, but it does not help the situation. The client's need for recognition is still not met.

At times, nurses react to the relief behavior of clients rather than to the clients' needs. For example, after being told she is lazy, the nurse might get angry with the client. She could choose to spend less time with the client and rationalize her behavior by labeling him as difficult. Or, the nurse might recognize the client's reaction as relief behavior. The nurse could then explore further the "unmet" needs: "You seem so upset. You didn't seem upset at rounds. What happened to upset you?" This response opens the avenue for identifying unmet needs, clarifying misconceptions, and offering alternatives for the clients to meet their own needs. This kind of response also prevents the nurse from personalizing the client's comments and becoming angry.

Thus far in this chapter, several concepts related to anxiety have been introduced:

1. Anxiety can be *primary* (caused by interpersonal or intrapsychic conflicts) or *secondary* (caused by physical disorders or processes).
2. Anxiety is experienced on a continuum from *mild* to *moderate* and *severe* to *panic*. Each level has specific characteristics.
3. Anxiety can be *acute* (state) or *chronic* (trait) in nature.
4. Anxiety can be *operationally defined*. Briefly, a need or an expectation is not met, anxiety results, and relief behaviors are called into play and then rationalized.
5. *Relief behaviors* can be viewed as interpersonal (*acting out, somatizing, withdrawal, or problem solving*) or intrapsychic (*defense mechanisms*).
6. *Anxiety* and *fear* are experienced in similar ways physically, but anxiety is said to be a response to an unknown or unconscious threat, and fear a response to a known or identified threat. Anxiety is more erosive to a person's sense of self than is fear.
7. One way to conceptualize anxiety is shown in Figure 8–1.

Standard III: Diagnosis

Anxiety exists on a continuum from mild to moderate to severe to panic. The nursing diagnosis of anxiety is made when there are supporting physical, emotional, and cognitive signs and symptoms of anxiety (Carpenito 1987). The diagnosis of anxiety is always qualified by the level of anxiety, such as mild, moderate, severe, or panic.

Evaluating perceptual field, ability to learn, and other defining characteristics helps nurses to assess a person's level of anxiety. Equally important to assess are the client's physiological reactions to anxiety. This is especially true on a medical-surgical unit in which high anxiety levels may be physiologically detrimental to a person's health (increased blood pressure, increase in blood glucose, and more). Common physiological responses to anxiety are found in Table 8–1. For more detailed physiological responses to stress and anxiety, refer to Chapter 15.

Without a clear idea of the level of anxiety a client is in, planning effective goals and interventions is minimized. The level of anxiety helps clarify the goal and suggests specific interventions. The "related to" component of the nursing diagnosis guides the formulation of goals and interventions. If the "related to" component has to do with primary anxiety, the goals and interventions might be different than if it has to do with secondary anxiety. Carpenito (1987) identifies three etiological, contributing risk factors that help identify the nursing diagnosis of anxiety:

1. *Situational* (personal/environmental), such as failure, lack of recognition, hospitalization, death, and divorce.
2. *Maturational* (threat to developmental tasks), such as separation, sexual development, pregnancy, and financial problems. Anxiety arising from these areas would be considered primary anxiety, that is, anxiety caused by psychological stress.
3. *Pathophysiological* causes of anxiety include any factors interfering with basic human needs (food, air, comfort). Pathophysiological causes include those factors in which anxiety is caused by a physical disease or abnormality, such as brain tumors, multiple sclerosis, ovarian dysfunctions, chronic infections, and rheumatoid arthritis. Anxiety arising from a physical disease or disorder is called secondary anxiety.

Standard IV: Planning

Planning involves more than just the identification of measurable and attainable goals. Planning should include the identification of personal reactions and feelings the nurse might experience in response to a client's feelings or behaviors. Sometimes, personal responses interfere with effective nursing care. Therefore, planning includes planning on the (1) content level (planning goals) and (2) process level (nurses' reactions and feelings).

CONTENT LEVEL—PLANNING GOALS

Long term and short term goals are often guided by the "related to" component of the nursing diagnosis. When planning long term goals (LTG) and short term goals (STG), the nurse considers both the contributing factors and the data that helped to formulate the actual nursing diagnosis. Since the goals and nursing diagnosis depend on the level of anxiety, it is best to divide goals and interventions into *mild-moderate* and *severe-panic* levels of anxiety.

Essentially, goals for people in mild to moderate levels of anxiety often include preventing further escalation of anxiety, decreasing anxiety levels, and facilitating effective problem solving. For example:

Nursing Diagnosis: Anxiety (Moderate): related to hospitalization, as evidenced by difficulty in concentrating, irritability and stating "I don't know what the devil is going on here."

Long Term Goal	Short Term Goal
1. Client will state he understands need for hospitalization and can describe proposed diagnostic procedures.	1. By 4:00 P.M., client will relate to nurse what doctor has told him regarding his need for hospitalization. 2. By (establish time), client will describe the two tests he is having after health teaching by nurse. 3. Client will name two staff members with whom he can discuss his concerns when questions arise.

Goals for people in severe to panic levels of anxiety may center on physical safety, such as protection from aggressive drives and physical neglect. Lowering levels of anxiety is crucial, although the interventions for lowering anxiety may be different for a person in severe to panic levels of anxiety than for someone in mild to moderate levels of anxiety.

Nursing Diagnosis: Anxiety (Severe): related to loss of spouse, evidenced by 16-pound weight loss, insomnia, and withdrawal

Long Term Goal	Short Term Goal
1. Client will remain physically healthy while going through grieving process.	1. Within two days, client will discuss feelings of grief with one other person. 2. Within one week, client will spend one hour per day with a friend, neighbor, or group in activities (shopping, church, visiting). 3. Client will gain one to two pounds per week until baseline weight is achieved by (establish date). 4. Client will sleep six hours per night by (date). 5. Client will state she has three important support people or groups available while going through the grief process.

PROCESS LEVEL—NURSES' REACTIONS AND FEELINGS

Nurses are constantly working with people in high stress situations resulting in high levels of anxiety. Anxiety can be experienced by clients, clients' families, and health care workers. Mild to moderate anxiety reactions are commonly seen in clients on the medical and surgical units, as well as in the obstetrical and gynecological and pediatric settings. Severe to panic levels of anxiety can also be seen in the general hospital setting, but they are most often observed in the psychiatric setting.

Working with people in high levels of anxiety can be uncomfortable and intimidating at times for all staff members, but especially for students new to the psychiatric setting. Since anxiety is communicated from person to person through the process of empathy (Sullivan 1970), it is expected that some anxiety will be experienced when working with clients in any hospital setting.

At times the nurse may find that before he or she is ready to interact with a client, personal feelings need to be sorted out in order to maximize therapeutic communication between nurse and client. Identifying levels of anxiety in the client and in oneself, and dealing with some strong and sometimes confusing countertransferential feelings triggered by certain client behaviors can be greatly facilitated by working closely with the instructor.

The discussion of feelings and reactions and problem solving is a process that is ongoing in the practice of psychiatric nursing (see Chapter 6). In most hospitals, staff on psychiatric units have regularly scheduled supervisory sessions where client-staff interactions are discussed, along with planning and evaluating intervention strategies. This may take the form of peer group supervision, supervision with a psychiatric clinical nurse specialist, or joint sessions with medical and nursing staff.

Each clinical chapter in this book (Chapters 10–25) will discuss common reactions and countertransferential feelings experienced by health care workers when dealing with specific behaviors.

Standard V: Intervention

Perhaps one of the most helpful and meaningful experiences for a person in uncomfortable levels of anxiety is the presence of a calm and caring human being. The calmness of another helps deflect some of the anxious person's own anxiety. The feeling that someone cares helps lessen the feelings of isolation and "aloneness" and offers a connection to stability.

Specific nursing interventions will always be based on assessment of the client's specific needs, and many of the interventions suggested for people in mild to moderate levels of anxiety are also appropriate for people in other levels of anxiety and vice versa. Guidelines that can be helpful in planning care for anxious clients are provided subsequently.

V-A: PSYCHOTHERAPEUTIC INTERVENTIONS

MILD TO MODERATE ANXIETY LEVELS. A person in mild to moderate levels of anxiety is still able to problem solve; however, the ability to concentrate decreases as anxiety increases. The nurse can help the client to focus and solve problems with the use of specific communication techniques, such as open-ended questions, giving broad openings, and exploring and seeking clarification. These techniques can be useful to a client experiencing mild to moderate anxiety. The nurse is aware of both the content and the process levels in the client's communication. Closing off topics of communication and bringing up irrelevant topics are avoided.

Reducing the anxiety level and preventing escalation of anxiety to more distressing levels can be aided by a calm presence, recognition of the anxious person's distress, and willingness to listen. Evaluation of effective past coping mechanisms is useful.

Often the nurse can assist the client in considering alternatives to problem situations and offer activities

Table 8–3 • PSYCHOTHERAPEUTIC INTERVENTIONS FOR PEOPLE IN MILD TO MODERATE LEVELS OF ANXIETY

INTERVENTION	RATIONALE AND COMMENTS
Help client identify anxiety.	Nurse needs to validate observations with client, name anxiety, and start to work with client to lower anxiety.
Anticipate anxiety-provoking situations.	Prevents escalation of anxiety to more disorganizing levels.
Use nonverbal language to demonstrate interest, e.g., lean forward, maintain eye contact, nod your head.	Verbal and nonverbal messages should be consistent. The presence of an interested person provides a stabilizing focus.
Encourage the client to talk about his or her feelings and concerns.	When concerns are stated out loud, problems can become clearer and less overwhelming, and solutions can be discussed.
Avoid closing off avenues of communication that are important for the client. Stay with the client's concerns.	When staff anxiety increases, "changing the topic" or "offering advice" is common but not useful to the client.
Ask questions to clarify what is being said, for example, "I'm not sure what you mean. Give me an example."	Increased anxiety results in scattering of thoughts. Clarifying helps the client identify thoughts and feelings.
Help the client identify thoughts or feelings prior to the onset of anxiety. "What were you thinking right before you started to feel anxious?"	Help client identify the unmet expectations/needs.
Discuss the client's expectations or needs and the difference between the expectation and the outcome.	When differences between expectation and outcome can be clarified, alternatives for meeting needs can be explored.
Encourage problem solving with the client.	Encouraging clients to explore alternatives increases sense of control and decreases anxiety.
Explore behaviors that have worked to relieve anxiety in the past.	Encourages mobilization of successful coping mechanisms and strengths.
Provide outlets for working off excess energy (walking, ping pong, dancing).	Physical activity can provide relief of built-up tension.
Choose reassurance carefully. NOT "Everything will be all right" BUT "You seem upset, let me stay with you for a while."	False reassurance may increase feelings of alienation or not being understood. Everything may not turn out all right; this blocks communication. Acknowledging concern and offering presence can increase feelings of security and decrease anxiety.

that may temporarily relieve feelings of inner tension.

Table 8–3 offers some concrete examples of appropriate nursing interventions.

SEVERE TO PANIC ANXIETY LEVELS. A person in severe and panic levels of anxiety is unable to solve problems and may have a poor grasp of what is happening in the environment. Unproductive relief behaviors may take over, and the person may not be in control of his or her actions. Extreme regression or running about aimlessly may be the behavior manifestations of the person's intense pain. The nurse is concerned with the client's safety and, at times, the safety of others. Physical needs (e.g., fluids and rest) may have to be met to prevent exhaustion. Anxiety reduction measures may take the form of removing the person to a quiet environment, where there is minimal stimulation, and providing gross motor activities to drain off some of the tension. The use of medications may have to be considered, but both medications and restraints should be used only after other more personal and less restrictive interventions have failed to decrease anxiety to safer levels. Although communications may be scattered and disjointed, themes can often be heard, and the nurse can address these themes. The feeling that one is understood can decrease the sense of isolation and reduce anxiety.

Since the person in severe and panic levels of anxiety is unable to solve problems, communication techniques suggested for the person in mild to moderate levels of anxiety are not always effective. Since the client in severe to panic levels of anxiety is out of control, he needs to know that he is safe from his own impulses. Firm, short, and simple statements are useful. Reinforcing commonalities in the environment and

Table 8–4 • PSYCHOTHERAPEUTIC INTERVENTIONS FOR PEOPLE IN SEVERE TO PANIC LEVELS OF ANXIETY

INTERVENTION	RATIONALE AND COMMENTS
Maintain a calm manner.	Anxiety is communicated interpersonally. The quiet calm of the nurse can serve to calm the client. The presence of anxiety can escalate anxiety in the client.
Always remain with the person experiencing severe to panic levels of anxiety.	Alone with immense anxiety, a person feels abandoned. A caring face may be the only contact with reality when confusion becomes overwhelming.
Minimize environmental stimuli. Move to a quieter setting and stay with the client.	Prevents further escalation of anxiety to self and to others in the setting.
Use clear and simple statements and repetition.	A person has difficulty concentrating and processing information in severe to panic levels of anxiety.
Use a low-pitched voice.	A high-pitched voice can convey anxiety.
Reinforce reality if distortions occur, e.g., seeing objects that are not there or hearing voices when no one is present.	Anxiety can be reduced by focusing in on, and validating, what is going on in the environment.
Listen for themes in communication.	In severe to panic levels of anxiety, verbal communication themes may be the only indication of the client's thoughts or feelings.
Attend to physical needs when necessary, e.g., warmth, fluids, elimination, pain relief, and need for family contact.	High levels of anxiety may obscure client's awareness of physical needs.
When physical limits need to be set, speak in a firm, authoritative voice, "You may not hit anyone here. If you can't control yourself, we will help you."	A person who is out of control is often terrorized. Staff must offer the client and others protection from destructive and self-destructive impulses.
Provide opportunities for exercise, e.g., pacing with nurse, punching bag, ping pong.	Physical activity helps channel and dissipate tension and may temporarily lower anxiety.
When a person is constantly moving or pacing, offer high caloric fluids.	Prevent dehydration and exhaustion.
Assess person's need for medication or seclusion after other interventions are tried.	Prevent exhaustion and/or physical harm to self and others.

pointing out reality when there are distortions can also be useful interventions for the severely anxious person. Table 8–4 suggests basic nursing interventions for the client in severe to panic levels of anxiety.

V-B: HEALTH TEACHING

Examples of health teaching for clients who experience anxiety include teaching relaxation techniques and progressive muscle relaxation (PMR). Nurses at any level of preparation can be trained in these techniques, which can then be taught to the client in any setting. These techniques are taught to clients with the consent of the client's doctor, since there are some contraindications. Refer to Chapter 15 for Benson's relaxation techniques, other relaxation techniques, and precautions.

V-D: SOMATIC THERAPIES

People in acute levels of anxiety may benefit by temporary use of medication in an effort to reduce anxiety. One group of drugs used for this purpose is called the anxiolytic (antianxiety) agents. Diazepam (Valium) and chlordiazepoxide hydrochloride (Librium) are two common drugs effective in relieving symptoms of anxiousness, agitation, and tension. These drugs should always be used with caution and on a short term basis because of their ability to lead to physical dependence. Refer to Chapter 16 for actions, side effects, and toxic effects and Chapter 24 for signs of withdrawal from and intoxication by anxiolytic agents.

People in chronic anxiety who are in severe to panic levels of anxiety may benefit from a neuroleptic (antipsychotic) agent. These drugs are effective in altering thought disorders and reducing psychotic behaviors. For example, haloperidol (Haldol) is an effective drug used to reduce assaultive behavior as well as clear a thought disorder. Refer to Chapter 20 for discussion of the neuroleptic drugs.

Biofeedback is another somatic therapy that is used for people who suffer from disorders of chronic intermittent anxiety. People are taught how to reduce physical reactions to stress by learning to control sympathetic responses (see Chapter 15).

V-F: PSYCHOTHERAPY

Nurses trained at the master's level may use a variety of therapies when working with clients who experience uncomfortable levels of anxiety. Two common modalities of therapy are psychotherapy and behavior therapy. Psychotherapy helps people understand their experience by identifying unconscious conflicts and developing more productive and satisfying coping behaviors.

Behavioral therapists focus on the problematic behavior and work with the client to modify or change the behavior. One very effective behavioral approach for people with high levels of anxiety is called desensitization. An overview of behavior therapy is given in Chapters 2 and 16 for use with the anxiety disorders.

Various modes of group therapy are also effective.

Standard VI: Evaluation

Evaluation is "always considered in terms of how the client responds to the planned nursing intervention" (Yura and Walsh 1983). The nursing diagnosis and the client-centered goals are the framework for the evaluation process. The nurse and client are the main evaluators of the nursing interventions and actions taken, although the client's family, health team members, and others may be involved. Evaluation and reassessment go hand-in-hand.

Since interventions for a person in mild to moderate levels of anxiety often center on decreasing anxiety, prevention of future escalation of anxiety, and facilitating effective problem solving, specific goals set to reach these desired outcomes are evaluated.

Interventions for a person in severe to panic levels of anxiety often center on physical safety, such as protection from aggressive drives and personal neglect. Therefore, evaluation of the specific goals that identify the status of the client's physical safety is needed. Once these goals are met, further goals and interventions focus on reducing anxiety to a more moderate level. Whenever possible, the client works with the nurse to plan future goals and identify potential solutions to problems.

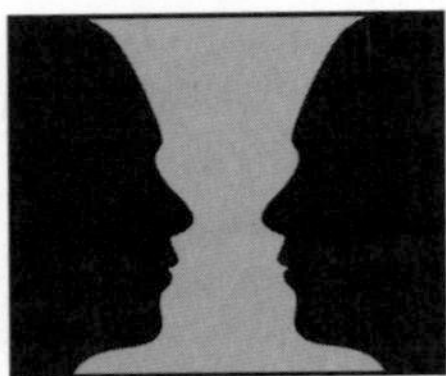

Case Study: Working With a Person in Moderate Levels of Anxiety

Donna James, a 24-year-old, recently married woman, had been brought to the hospital for vaginal bleeding during her fourteenth week of pregnancy. The medical team was unable to save the baby. Donna had learned about the loss of her baby early that morning.

That evening, after dinner trays had been served, Jane Johnson, the evening nurse, went in to check Donna's vital signs. She found the dinner tray untouched and Donna crying. Jane introduced herself and asked Donna what was wrong. Donna started talking rapidly in a high-pitched voice, asking the nurse several times when she could go home. She said, "I didn't know I'd be so upset." Donna's pulse rate was 112, and her respiration rate 26. She stated that she was not hungry and had a terrible headache. The nurse checked Donna for signs of shock and bleeding, but the physical assessment was normal.

Assessment

From her data, the nurse assessed Donna's anxiety level as moderate. Donna had repeatedly asked the same question in a high-pitched voice. She had an increase in pulse and respiration rates; she was crying; and she complained of lack of appetite and a headache. Further assessment and intervention could increase Donna's comfort and prevent her anxiety from escalating. The nurse told Donna that she understood that Donna was very upset. She told Donna that when she was finished taking the vital signs in 15 minutes, she would be back to spend 20 minutes with her.

OBJECTIVE DATA

1. Increase in pulse and respiration rates (P 112, R 26)
2. Change in voice pitch
3. Crying—relief behavior
4. Repetitive questioning

SUBJECTIVE DATA

1. I didn't know I'd be so upset.
2. I have a terrible headache.
3. "I'm not hungry."

Nursing Diagnosis

From her data, Ms. Johnson devised the following nursing diagnosis:

1. *Anxiety (Moderate)* possibly related to termination of pregnancy (situational crisis), as evidenced by crying and somatic complaints.

However, more data would be needed.

Planning

Since general goals center on decreasing anxiety, preventing further escalation of anxiety, and facilitating effective problem solving for a person in a moderate level of anxiety, Ms. Johnson proposed the following short term goal:

1. Client's anxiety level will be mild by 11:00 P.M., with aid of nursing interventions.

The nurse planned to spend time with Donna to assess Donna's concerns further. Donna needed to discuss her feelings and concerns further and mobilize some of her usual coping patterns.

Intervention

When Ms. Johnson returned, she pulled the curtain around the bed. She leaned forward and sat where eye contact was possible. The nurse told Donna she had 20 minutes to spend with her. At first, Donna's talk shifted from topic to topic, and it was difficult for the nurse to identify Donna's feelings.

Dialogue	Therapeutic Tool/Comment
N: I came back Donna, because you looked so upset.	Initially, the nurse provides privacy and decreases the environmental stimuli.

Intervention
(Continued)

D: Yes . . . the baby . . . we wanted the baby, but my husband says we can have more . . . he's quite right, I guess. My mother-in-law blames the whole thing on me . . . says I'm too irresponsible and that we can't afford a family right now. I did want the baby . . . my husband is so worried about all the bills. He just got a job last month, you know. He couldn't come to see me because he is working overtime. My mother-in-law phoned, but I could tell she wanted to get off the phone.	The nurse demonstrates concern for Donna by: A. Making the observation that she understands that Donna is upset. A. Coming back at the time she had indicated C. Letting Donna talk about how she is feeling. She did not assume what Donna was feeling or why. She neither cut Donna off nor offered advice. D. Letting Donna talk, listening for themes.

At first the nurse sat with Donna, nodding and listening carefully to what was being said and listening for themes. The nurse waited until she had more data, then began to redirect and comment on what was being said.

Dialogue	Therapeutic Tool/Comment
N: It sounds as if there is a lot going on, but no one seems available for you now.	The nurse listens to the content of what Donna is saying and tries to focus on the themes.
D: My husband is a good man, he's very concerned with the bills. We were just starting to save some money (begins to cry). N: Tell me what you're feeling right now. D: Lonely . . . I feel so alone.	Crying can be a healthy release of tension. It is an excellent time to identify feelings, since at that time feelings are close to the surface.
N: What usually helps you when you're feeling lonely? D: My husband . . . talking to my husband. He's my best friend.	The nurse assesses past coping mechanisms that have been helpful.
N: Since he's not here now, perhaps it will help if we talk.	Nurse offers her assistance.

The nurse and Donna continued to talk. Donna talked about the lack of support she felt from her mother-in-law and her feelings of being left alone by her husband owing to his new job. They talked together about the possibility of Donna finding a part-time job that would help the financial situation. Donna would have an opportunity to be a part of a social network other than her immediate family if she worked. The nurse felt that the actual loss of the baby was only a part of what was bothering Donna. Donna explained that once the bleeding started, they had prepared themselves for the loss.

After 20 minutes, the nurse said their time was up, but she would come back before the end of the shift at 11:00 P.M., and she would spend ten more minutes with her. The nurse asked Donna about her headache. Donna said that she felt much better and her headache was gone. She appeared more relaxed and her vital signs had returned to baseline. Her voice was softer and more natural, and she was no longer easily distracted. Donna stated she felt she was now able to get some rest.

When the nurse went back at 11:00 P.M., Donna was asleep. When the nurse reported off, she asked that the day shift spend some time with Donna before discharge.

Evaluation

The goal was set that Donna's anxiety level would be reduced to mild by 11:00 P.M. with the aid of nursing intervention. This was an appropriate and realistic goal set within a realistic time frame, and most important, was measurable.

The nurse noted that one of Donna's somatic complaints (headache) was gone, her vital signs were baseline, her speech was no longer rapid and forced, her thoughts were more coherent, and she was now asleep. The nurse evaluated the stated short term goal as met.

Continued on following page

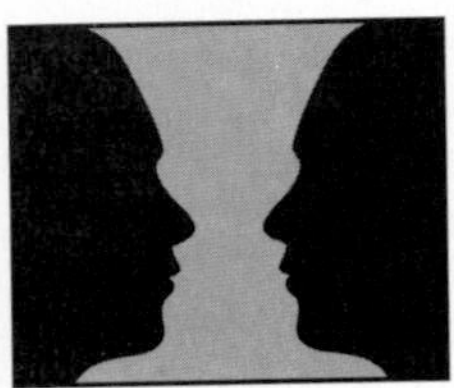

Case Study: Working With a Person in Severe Levels of Anxiety

Tom Michaels, a 63-year-old man, came into the emergency room (ER) with his wife, Anne, who had taken an overdose of sleeping pills and antidepressant medications. Ten years ago, Anne's mother had died, and since that time she had suffered several episodes of severe depression with suicidal attempts. During these episodes she had needed hospitalization. Anne Michaels had just been released from a psychiatric unit two weeks previously for another bout of depression and threatened suicide.

Tom Michaels had long established a routine of giving his wife her antidepressant medications in the morning and her sleeping medication at night and keeping the bottles hidden when he was not at home. Today, he had forgotten to hide the medications before he went to work. His wife had taken the remaining pills from both bottles with large quantities of alcohol. When Tom returned home for lunch, Anne was comatose.

In the ER, Anne suffered a cardiac arrest and was taken to the intensive care unit (ICU).

Mr. Michaels appeared very jittery. He moved about the room aimlessly. He dropped things, such as his hat, medication card, and keys. His hands were trembling, and he looked around the room bewildered. He appeared unable to focus on any one thing. He said over and over in a loud, high-pitched voice, "Why didn't I hide the bottles?" He was wringing his hands, and he began stamping his feet, saying, "It's all my fault. Everything is falling apart."

Other people in the waiting room appeared distracted and alarmed by his behavior. He appeared oblivious to his surroundings.

Assessment

Mr. Brown, the psychiatric nurse clinician working in the ER, came into the waiting room and assessed Mr. Michaels's behavior as at a severe anxiety level. After talking with Mr. Michaels briefly, Mr. Brown felt nursing intervention was indicated.

The nurse based his conclusion on the following assessment of the client:

OBJECTIVE DATA

1. Unable to focus on anything
2. Purposeless activity (walking around aimlessly)
3. Appears oblivious to his surroundings
4. Appears confused and bewildered
5. Unproductive relief behavior (stomping, wringing hands, dropping things)

SUBJECTIVE DATA

1. "Everything is falling apart."
2. "Why didn't I hide the bottles?"

Nursing Diagnosis

Mr. Brown formulated the following nursing diagnosis:

1. *Anxiety* (*Severe*) related to the client's perception of responsibility for his wife's coma and possible death.

Planning

Mr. Brown thought that if he could lower Mr. Michaels's anxiety to a moderate level, Mr. Michaels could work with him to get a clear picture of his situation and place the events in a more realistic perspective. The nurse also thought that Mr. Michaels needed to talk to someone and share some of his pain and confusion and sort out what he was feeling. Mr. Brown identified two short term goals:

1. Client's anxiety will decrease to moderate levels by 4:00 P.M.
2. Client will talk about his feelings and plans by 4:00 P.M.

Intervention

The nurse took Mr. Michaels to a quiet room in the back of the ER. The nurse introduced himself to Mr. Michaels and said he noticed that Mr. Michaels was upset. He said, "I will stay with you." At first, Mr. Michaels found it difficult to sit down, and he continued his pacing around the room. Mr. Brown sat quietly and calmly, listening to Mr. Michaels's self-recriminations. The nurse listened carefully to what Mr. Michaels was saying and what he was not saying, to identify themes.

Intervention
(Continued)

After a while Mr. Michaels became calmer and was able to sit next to the nurse. The nurse offered him orange juice, which he accepted and held tightly.

Mr. Brown spoke calmly, using simple, clear statements. He used communications tools that were helpful to Mr. Michaels in sorting out his feelings and naming them.

Dialogue		Therapeutic Tool/Comment
MR. M.:	Yes . . . yes . . . I forgot to hide the bottles. She usually tells me when she feels bad. Why didn't she tell me?	
N:	You think that if she had told you she wanted to kill herself you would have hidden the pills?	The nurse asks for clarification on Mr. Michaels's thinking.
MR. M.:	Yes, if I had only known, this wouldn't have happened.	
N:	It sounds as if you believe you should have known what your wife was thinking without her telling you.	Here the nurse clarifies Mr. Michaels's expectations that he should be able to read his wife's mind.
MR. M.:	Well . . . yes . . . when you put it that way . . . I just don't know what I'll do if she dies.	

When the nurse thought that Mr. Michaels had discussed his feelings of guilt, he asked Mr. Michaels to clarify his thinking about his wife's behavior. Mr. Michaels was able to place his feelings of guilt in a more realistic perspective. Next Mr. Brown brought up another issue — the question of whether Mr. Michaels's wife would live or die.

Dialogue		Therapeutic Tool/Comment
N:	You stated that if your wife dies, you don't know what you will do.	Reflecting.
MR. M:	Oh God, (*Mr. Michaels begins to cry*) I can't live without her . . . she's all I have in the world. *Silence.*	
N:	She means a great deal to you.	The nurse reflects Mr. Michaels's feelings back to him.
MR. M:	Everything. Since her mother died, we are each other's only family.	
N:	What would it mean to you if your wife died?	The nurse asks Mr. Michaels to evaluate his feelings vis-a-vis his wife.
MR. M:	I couldn't live by myself, alone. I couldn't stand it. *Starts to cry again.*	
N:	It sounds as if being alone is very frightening to you.	The nurse restates in clear tones Mr. Michaels's experience.
MR. M:	Yes . . . I don't know how I'd manage by myself.	
N:	A change like that could take time adjusting to.	The nurse validates that if Mr. Michaels's wife died it would be very painful. At the same time, he implies hope that Mr. Michaels could work through the death, in time.
MR. M.:	Yes . . . it would be very hard.	

Continued on following page

Intervention *(Continued)*

Again, the nurse gave Mr. Michaels a chance to sort out his feelings and fears. The nurse helped him focus on the reality that his wife might die and encouraged him to express fears related to her possible death. After a while, the nurse offered to go up to the ICU with Mr. Michaels to see how his wife was doing. On arrival at the ICU, Mrs. Michaels, although still comatose, was stabilized and breathing on her own.

After arrival at the ICU, Mr. Michaels started to worry about whether he had locked the door at home. The nurse encouraged him to call neighbors and ask them to check the door. At this time, Mr. Michaels was able to focus on everyday things. The nurse made arrangements to see Mr. Michaels the next day when he came in to visit his wife.

The next day, Mrs. Michaels regained consciousness, and she was discharged one week later. At the time of discharge, Mr. and Mrs. Michaels were considering family therapy with the psychiatric nurse clinician once a week in the outpatient department.

Evaluation

The first goal was to lower anxiety from severe to moderate within a given period of time. The nurse could see that Mr. Michaels had become more visibly calm; his trembling, wringing of hands, and stomping of feet had ceased, and he was able to focus on his thoughts and feelings with the aid of the nurse.

The second short term goal set for Mr. Michaels stated that he would talk about his feelings and plans within a given period of time. Mr. Michaels was able to identify and discuss with the nurse feelings of guilt and fear of being left alone in the world if his wife should die. Both these feelings were overwhelming him. He was also able to make tentative plans with the nurse for the future.

Summary

Anxiety is the most basic of all emotions, and it is an integral part of all emotions. Dysfunctional behavior stems from anxiety. As an everyday component of life, anxiety can facilitate learning and attainment of goals. It can also lead to ineffective and unsatisfying behaviors. The outcome depends upon the level of anxiety, the choice of relief behaviors, and the intervention and guidance received. Anxiety is triggered by a threat to biological safety or psychological security (May 1983).

Anxiety is an energy, and it can be communicated interpersonally via empathy from one person to another. Anxiety can be triggered by a psychological conflict (primary anxiety) or a biological cause (secondary anxiety). Anxiety can be experienced on four levels: mild, moderate, severe, and panic. Steps in the operational definition of anxiety follow:

1. Expectation (need) held.
2. Expectation not met and felt as a threat.
3. Uneasiness or anxiety felt.
4. Relief behavior mobilized.
5. Relief behaviors rationalized.

Relief behaviors moderate anxiety through various patterns of behavior and defense mechanisms.

Stress can be psychological, social, or biological. Anxiety can be rational or irrational, and the relief behavior can be adaptive relief behavior or take the form of symptoms or syndromes (see Fig. 8–1).

Physiologically, the body reacts to anxiety and fear by the arousal of the sympathetic nervous system. Specific symptoms include rapid heartbeat, increased blood pressure, increased pulse rate, diaphoresis, peripheral vasoconstriction, restlessness, repetitive questioning, feelings of frustration, and difficulty in concentration.

The nurse learns to assess (1) the level of anxiety, (2) the relief behaviors used, and (3) the circumstances surrounding the escalation of anxiety. For example, anxiety is assessed as mild to moderate or severe to panic. Different levels may indicate the need for different goals and nursing interventions. Relief behaviors can be interpersonal (acting out, somatizing, freezing to the spot, or problem solving) or intrapsychic (defense mechanisms).

Anxiety is not a constant state, but it can be conceptualized on a continuum. People move up and down on the continuum of anxiety. Anxiety follows specific principles, and these principles can be used as guides to planning effective nursing care. Specific nursing interventions are useful to people in moderate levels of anxiety, and other nursing interventions are useful to those experiencing severe to panic levels of anxiety. The ability to evaluate personal levels of and reactions to anxiety is a process that can be learned. The ability to assess personal anxiety, as well as the anxiety of others, enables the nurse to increase his or her effectiveness in interpersonal exchanges with clients, peers, and others. Applying the conceptual model of anxiety while implementing the nursing process was illustrated in two case studies.

References

American Psychiatric Association. Diagnostic and Statistical Manual of Mental Disorders, 3rd ed., revised. Washington DC: American Psychiatric Association, 1987.

Burd SF. Effects of nursing intervention in anxiety of patients. *In* Burd SF, Marshall MA (eds). Some Clinical Approaches to Psychiatric Nursing. New York: MacMillan Publishing Company, 1968.

Bruch H. Eating Disorders: Obesity, Anorexia Nervosa and the Person Within. New York: Basic Books, 1973.

Cameron OG. The differential diagnosis of anxiety: Psychiatric and medical disorders. Psychiatric Clinics of North America: Symposium on Anxiety Disorders, 8(1), March 1985.

Carpenito LJ. Handbook of Nursing Diagnosis, 2nd ed. Philadelphia: J.B. Lippincott, 1987.

Chapman AH. Textbook of Clinical Psychiatry, 2nd ed. Philadelphia: J.B. Lippincott, 1976.

Chapman A, Chapman M. Harry Stack Sullivan's Concepts of Personality Development and Psychiatric Illness. New York: Brunner/Mazel, 1980.

Crowe RR. Mitral valve prolapse and panic disorder. Psychiatric Clinics of North America: Symposium on Anxiety Disorders, 8(1), March 1985.

Curtis CC. Anxiety and anxiety disorders: Toward a conceptual reorientation. Psychiatric Clinics of North America: Symposium on Anxiety Disorders, 8(1), March 1985.

Curtis CC. New findings in anxiety. A synthesis for clinical practice. Psychiatric Clinics of North America: Symposium on Anxiety Disorders, 8(1), March 1985.

Engel GL. A unified concept of health and disease. Perspectives in Biology and Medicine, 3:459, 1960.

Freedman A, Kaplan H, Saddock B. Modern Synopsis of Comprehensive Textbook of Psychiatry, vol. 11. Baltimore: Williams & Wilkins Company, 1976.

Hagerty BK. Psychiatric-Mental Health Assessment. St. Louis: C.V. Mosby Company, 1984.

Hall R. Anxiety. *In* Hall R (ed). Psychiatric Presentations of Medical Illness. Jamaica, NY: Spectrum Publications, 1980.

Jimerson S. Anxiety. *In* Haber J, et al. (eds). Comprehensive Psychiatric Nursing, 2nd ed. New York: McGraw-Hill Book Company, 1982.

Knowles RD. Managing anxiety. American Journal of Nursing, 81(1), 1981.

Kolb LC, Brodie HKH. Modern Clinical Psychiatry, 10th ed. Philadelphia: W.B. Saunders Company, 1982.

Lentz JR. Therapy with clients with organic brain syndromes. *In* Beck, et al. (eds). Mental Health–Psychiatric Nursing: A Holistic Life-Cycle Approach. St. Louis: C.V. Mosby Company, 1984.

Lesse S. Relationship of anxiety to depression. American Journal of Psychotherapy, 36:332, 1982.

Manaser JC, Warner AM. Instruments for the Study of Nurse-Patient Intervention. New York: MacMillan Publishing Company, 1964.

May R. Anxiety and stress. *In* Seyle H (ed). Seyle's Guide to Stress Research, vol. 2. New York: Scientific and Academic Editions, 1983.

May R. The meaning of anxiety. New York: Ronald Press, 1950.

McFarland GK, Wasli EL. Nursing care of patients with psychiatric mental health problems, mild, moderate, severe, panic anxiety. *In* Kim MJ, et al. (eds). Pocket Guide to Nursing Diagnosis. St. Louis: C.V. Mosby Company, 1984.

Miller S, Winstead-Fry P. Family Systems Theory in Nursing Practice. Reston, Virginia: Reston Publishing Company, 1982.

Morris C. Relaxation therapy in a clinic. American Journal of Nursing, 79:1958, 1979.

Morse D, et al. A physiological and subjective evaluation of meditation, hypnosis, and relaxation. Psychosomatic Medicine, 39:305, 1977.

Peck MS. The Road Less Traveled. New York: Simon and Schuster, 1978.

Peplau HE. A working definition of anxiety. *In* Burd S, Marshall M (eds). Some Clinical Approaches to Psychiatric Nursing. New York: Macmillan Publishing Company, 1968.

Programmed instruction, anxiety recognition and intervention. American Journal of Nursing, vol. 65, no. 9, 1965.

Rockwell D. Anxiety and related disorders. *In* Donlon P, Rockwell D (eds). Psychiatric Disorders, Diagnosis and Treatment. Bowie, MD: Robert J. Brady Company, 1982.

Schwartz M, Schockley E. The Nurse and the Mental Patient. New York: John Wiley & Sons, 1956.

Sullivan HS. The Interpersonal Theory of Psychiatry. New York: W.W. Norton & Company, 1953.

Sullivan HS. The Psychiatric Interview. New York: W.W. Norton & Company, 1970.

Yura H, Walsh MB. The Nursing Process. Connecticut: Appleton-Century-Crofts, 1983.

Suggested Readings

Classics

Benson H. The Relaxation Response. New York: The Hearst Corporation, 1975.

Benson demonstrates how the use of the relaxation response can alter the body's physiological reactions to stress. He outlines the simple steps a person can follow to elicit the relaxation response. Benson's scientific work had a marked influence in further stress research and in the therapeutic use of the relaxation response in a variety of physical and behavioral problems, i.e., cancer, HBP, *phobias, alcoholism. The relaxation response is taught by health care professionals to clients routinely in a variety of health care settings and is in common use by laymen as an effective tool to combat stress and increase a person's sense of well-being.*

May R. The Meaning of Anxiety. New York: Ronald Press, 1950.

A book that had tremendous impact on the psychiatric community and is still regarded as a reference as well as a classic. May contributed to the theoretical understanding of anxiety and its experience from cultural, philosophical, biological, and psychological standpoints.

Peplau HE. Working definition of anxiety. *In* Burd S, Marshall M (eds). Some Clinical Approaches to Psychiatric Nursing. New York: Macmillan Publishing Company, 1968.

This classic work by Hildegard Peplau *provides nurses with a clear and meaningful understanding of the components of anxiety (definition, etiology, effects, and levels) and offers a theoretical base for the practice of psychiatric nursing. Peplau is very much influenced by the works of Harry Stack* Sullivan *and has adapted Sullivan's interpersonal approach to the practice of psychiatric nursing.*

MORE ON ANXIETY FOR FURTHER STUDY

Programmed instruction, anxiety recognition and intervention. American Journal of Nursing, vol. 65, no. 9, 1965.

This programmed instruction is a helpful self-study guide for students. It is clear and concrete and covers understanding the experience of anxiety, bodily and emotional responses to anxiety, levels of anxiety, and nursing intervention with people who are experiencing anxiety.

Programmed instruction, understanding defense mechanisms. American Journal of Nursing, vol. 72, no. 9, 1972.

This programmed guide is a helpful self-study tool for students in understanding the role of defense mechanisms and in testing their recognition of various defense mechanisms.

FOR USE IN NURSING PRACTICE

Clark CC. Inner dialogue: A self-healing approach for nurses and clients. American Journal of Nursing, 81:1191, 1981.

The author explores a method using relaxation techniques for eliciting alternative ways of solving problems for nurses and their clients. Its aim when taught to clients is to help the client take an active and responsible role in his or her healing process. Relaxation and visualization are used to help the client tap his or her own inner resources. The goal is to aid the client in understanding the meaning of his or her symptoms and provide a focus away from self-destructive feelings.

Dillon A. Reducing your stress. Nursing Life, 3:17, 1983.

This article discusses the stages of mounting stress that hospital nurses experience and some of the reasons why stress is inherent in hospital nursing. Six experienced health care professionals offer suggestions for dealing with hospital stress.

Dossey B. A wonderful prerequisite. Nursing, 14:42, 1984.

The author's premise is that in order for nurses to teach their clients to relax, they themselves must know how to relax. The author offers step-by-step instructions on muscle relaxation and provides suggestions for teaching clients using the nursing process.

Vissing Y, Burke M. Visualization techniques for health care workers. Journal of Psychosocial Nursing, vol. 22, 1984.

A small study of the effects of the use of visualization on problem solving with health care professionals. The literature review is informative for students interested in the relaxation therapies as a nursing intervention.

Self-Study Exercises

True or False. If false, change the statement to make it true.

1. ________ The concepts that anxiety (1) is an energy and (2) can be communicated interpersonally come from *Psychodynamic Theory*.
2. ________ Secondary anxiety originating from physiological abnormalities or processes is consistent with *Behavioral/Learning Theory*.
3. ________ Anxiety is a learned response, and learned responses to anxiety can be unlearned. This is a basic premise of *Biological Theory*.

Matching

4. ________ A feeling of dread resulting from a threat whose source is unknown.
5. ________ Anxiety precipitated by an imminent loss or change.
6. ________ Anxiety that a person has lived with for a long time and that possibly results from inadequate nurturing.
7. ________ Anxiety triggered by a physiological process or dysfunction.
8. ________ The ability to feel for and with another and understand the other's experience.

A. Fear
B. Primary anxiety
C. Chronic anxiety
D. Empathy
E. Normal anxiety
F. Anxiety
G. Secondary anxiety
H. Acute anxiety

Match the steps in the operational definition of anxiety.

9. ________ Need/expectation exists.
10. ________ Need/expectation not met.
11. ________ Anxiety ensues.
12. ________ Relief behavior.
13. ________ Behavior rationalized.

A. Momentary uneasiness
B. For approval and praise
C. Nurse calls in sick

D. "They don't need me anyway"

E. Head nurse doesn't commend nurse for job well done.

Matching

14. ________	Physical disability with no organic base.	A. Somatizing
15. ________	Self righteous man always finds fault in everyone else, never himself.	B. Displacement
16. ________	Student who is angry at the teacher picks a fight with a friend.	C. Undoing
17. ________	Physical disability in which emotions play a significant role.	D. Conversion
18. ________	When speaking of a bad omen, a woman knocks on wood to prevent an untold event.	E. Projection

Complete the statements by filling in the appropriate information.

19. Jean unconsciously harbors intense feelings of hostility toward her roommate who is always flirting with her dates. However, Jean is always extremely sweet and giving to her roommate in interpersonal exchanges. She is using the defense mechanism of ________________ .

In questions 20 through 25, identify levels of anxiety.

20. Rosa is extremely agitated. She is pacing up and down, complaining of nausea and headache, and is unable to concentrate on anything but her lost cat. She is in ________________ level of anxiety.
21. Neil is having difficulty taking in what is going on around him since he heard his promotion was denied. His heart is pounding, and his hands are diaphoretic. He finds a friend, who helps him look at his situation and figure out his alternatives. He is in ________________ level of anxiety.
22. Gary tells his neighbors that he has been chosen by God to bring peace to the world and that God speaks to him all the time. He is too disorganized to work at a steady job but sometimes helps neighboring farmers harvest their crops. He is in chronic ________________ level of anxiety.
23. Denise is told she has been chosen to compete in the final rounds of the championship spelling bee in her state. She starts planning her strategy by making up study time schedules and lists of words to go over, and she becomes very intent on her goal of doing her best. She is in ________________ level of anxiety.
24. A man who is to have open heart surgery in the morning starts to complain of palpitations and nausea, has difficulty articulating, and his speech jumps from one topic to the next. He can hardly take in what is going on around him unless it is pointed out to him. He is in ________________ level of anxiety. State three interventions that would be useful to this client and give the rationale for each intervention.

   A. ________________________ R ________________________

   ________________________ ________________________

B. ______________________________ R ______________________________

______________________________ ______________________________

C. ______________________________ R ______________________________

______________________________ ______________________________

25. A woman comes into the emergency room after having been beaten by a mugger. She is incoherent, says she feels like she is going to die, vacillates between periods of withdrawal and crying and screaming. She is in acute ______________ level of anxiety. State at least three interventions a nurse could use with a person in this level of anxiety, and give the rationale for each intervention.

A. ______________________________ R ______________________________

______________________________ ______________________________

B. ______________________________ R ______________________________

______________________________ ______________________________

C. ______________________________ R ______________________________

______________________________ ______________________________

CHAPTER 9

The Anxiety Continuum As A Conceptual Framework

Elizabeth M. Varcarolis

OUTLINE

OBJECTIVE

After studying this chapter, the student will be able to:

Visualize a relationship between the different levels of anxiety and selected psychiatric syndromes.

As discussed in Chapter 8, anxiety can be *primary* (caused by interpersonal or intrapsychic conflicts) or *secondary* (caused by physical disorders or processes). Anxiety can be *acute* (as in a crisis situation) or *chronic* (operating over a long period of time and to which a person finds some form of adjustment in either a psychiatric symptom, syndrome, physiologic disorder or organic disorder). Anxiety can also be *appropriate* to a given situation (before an exam) or *inappropriate* (fear of leaving one's apartment or home). Whether anxiety is acute or chronic, primary or secondary, appropriate or inappropriate, anxiety and the client's response to anxiety play a significant role in the nurse's work in a psychiatric setting. Much of the nurse's work is aimed at

STRESS ⇨ ⇅ Anxiety ⇨ EFFECTIVE RELIEF BEHAVIOR ⇨ ⇅ Anxiety

lowering the client's level of anxiety, and figuring out what the anxiety, or dysfunctional behaviors stemming from anxiety, is all about.

Anxiety is not a static state, and the level of anxiety is constantly fluctuating. Anxiety can fluctuate among the different levels (mild, moderate, severe, panic) or even within a single level.

In assessing clinical syndromes, anxiety needs to be evaluated to determine whether the origins of anxiety are primary or secondary. Disorders that are caused by primary anxiety are termed functional. The anxiety disorders such as phobias and obsessive-compulsive disorders are considered by many to be examples of functional psychiatric syndromes.

Secondary anxiety is that which is triggered by organic dysfunctions. The anxiety experienced in alcohol withdrawal delirium, for example, is triggered by physiological dysfunctions secondary to alcohol withdrawal.

Whether anxiety is primary or secondary, acute or chronic, the following chain reaction occurs:

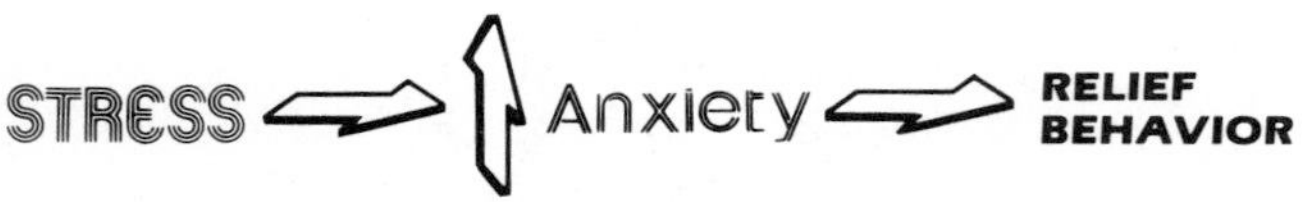

Figure 9–1 further illustrates the process.

Anxiety seems to be the primary clinical response to stress. When a person's anxiety threshold has been reached, secondary defense mechanisms (relief behaviors) are activated.

Psychiatric syndromes are conceptualized along the anxiety continuum (Fig. 9–2). A brief overview of various psychiatric syndromes discussed in the clinical chapters (Chapters 10–25) in this text is presented.

Acute Anxiety (Unit III)

A "normal" or healthy person is able to gain pleasure from work and interpersonal relationships. Commitment to an intimate relationship is possible, and affectionate exchanges within a social network are present. Periods of anxiety and "feeling down" occur with the changes and challenges encountered in the course of living. For the healthy individual, effective relief behaviors can be called upon to stabilize the personality and allow for attainment of goals and prevent serious disruptions in living. Creative accomplishments and a zest for living are familiar events in the life of a healthy individual. The healthy person can be viewed as reacting to an increase in anxiety as shown above.

CRISIS AND CRISIS INTERVENTION (Chapter 10)

When acute anxiety escalates in response to stress, and a person's usual relief behaviors (defense mechanisms) are no longer able to control disorganizing levels of anxiety, a crisis can ensue. A crisis is usually precipitated by an overwhelming event or events in a person's life, and these events can be identified. Crisis intervention increases the likelihood that the person will return to a pre-crisis level of functioning. Without support, a person with severe levels of anxiety may experience confusion and personality disorganization. The anxiety can become chronic if it is not reduced within a short period of time (four to six weeks). A true crisis situation is a psychiatric emergency. People with high levels of chronic anxiety are also susceptible to crisis, and the

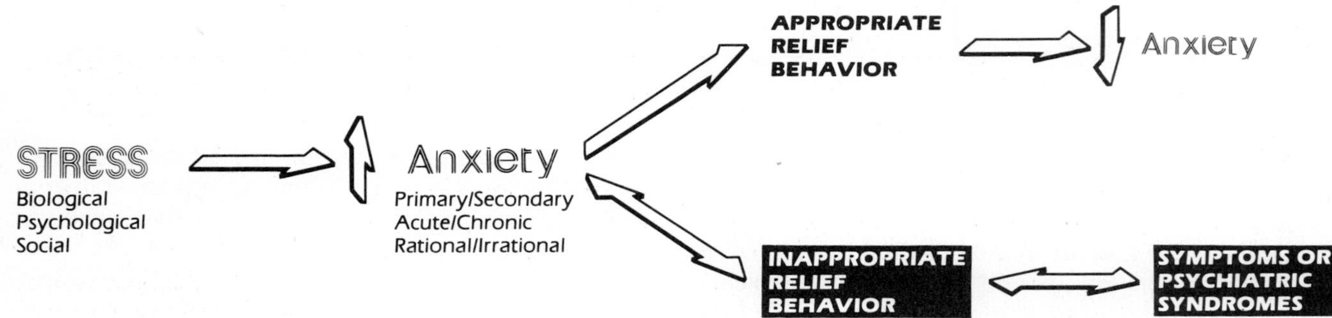

Figure 9–1. *Conceptualization of psychiatric symptoms or syndromes along the anxiety continuum.*

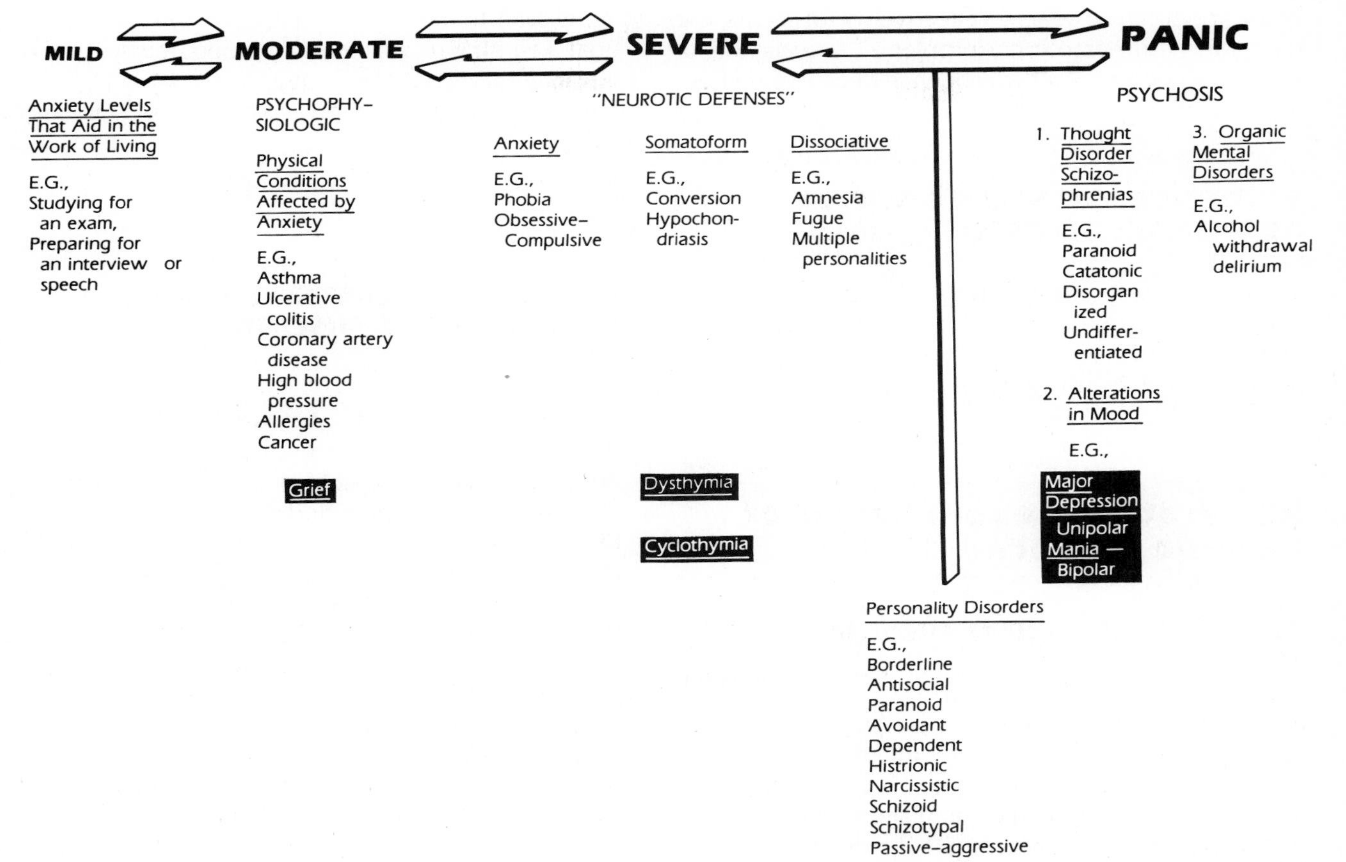

MILD
MODERATE
SEVERE
PANIC
Anxiety Levels That Aid in the Work of Living
E.G., Studying for an exam, Preparing for an interview or speech
PSYCHOPHYSIOLOGIC
Physical Conditions Affected by Anxiety
E.G., Asthma, Ulcerative colitis, Coronary artery disease, High blood pressure, Allergies, Cancer
Grief
"NEUROTIC DEFENSES"
Anxiety
E.G., Phobia, Obsessive–Compulsive
Somatoform
E.G., Conversion, Hypochondriasis
Dissociative
E.G., Amnesia, Fugue, Multiple personalities
Dysthymia
Cyclothymia
PSYCHOSIS
1. Thought Disorder Schizophrenias
E.G., Paranoid, Catatonic, Disorganized, Undifferentiated
2. Alterations in Mood
E.G.,
Major Depression Unipolar
Mania — Bipolar
3. Organic Mental Disorders
E.G., Alcohol withdrawal delirium
Personality Disorders
E.G., Borderline, Antisocial, Paranoid, Avoidant, Dependent, Histrionic, Narcissistic, Schizoid, Schizotypal, Passive-aggressive

Figure 9–2. *Anxiety continuum and psychiatric syndromes.*

STRESS
Anxiety
USUAL COPING MECHANISMS INEFFECTIVE
ADAPTIVE PROBLEM-SOLVING SOLUTIONS
Anxiety
PRE-CRISIS LEVEL FUNCTIONING
TRIAL & ERROR SOLUTIONS
ANXIETY (SEVERE-PANIC)
PERSONALITY DISORGANIZATION

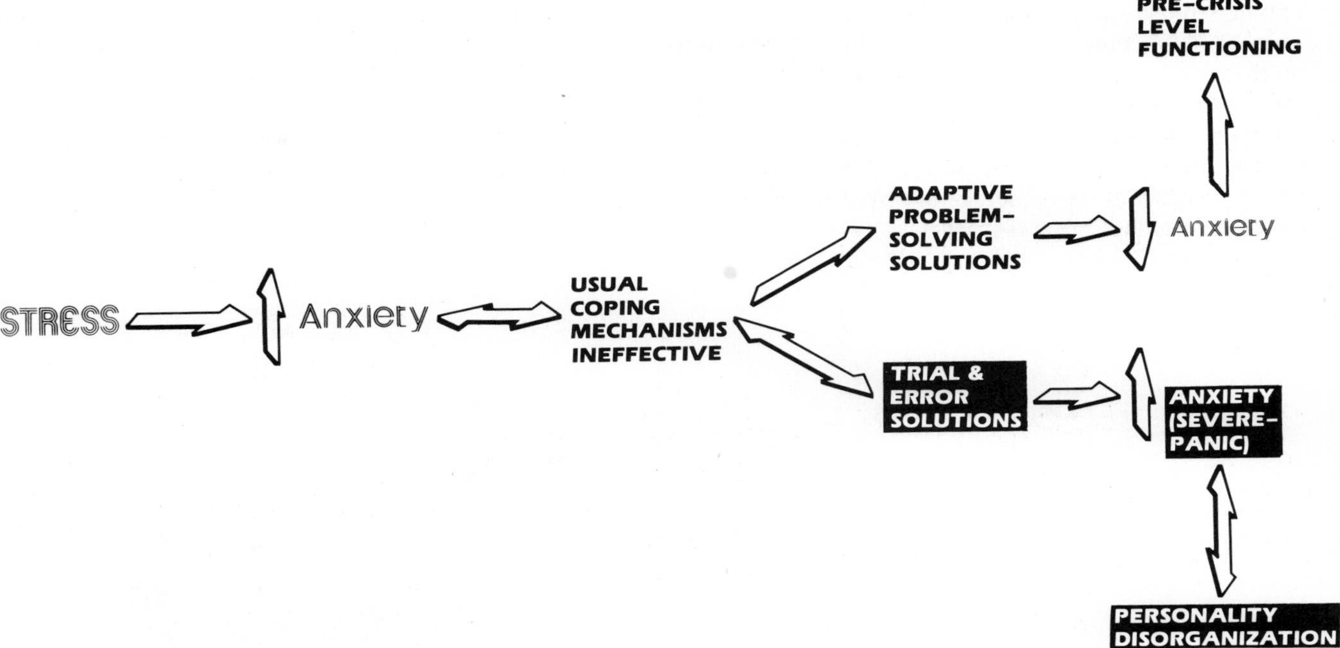

Figure 9–3. *Conceptualization of the phases in the process of crisis.*

crisis model can be adapted effectively with clients who have long term emotional problems. A crisis can be viewed as occurring in the sequence depicted in Figure 9–3.

EVIDENCE OF MALADAPTIVE RESPONSES TO CRISIS (Chapters 11–14)

Maladaptive responses to acute anxiety, such as the automatic response, can be seen in child abuse, spouse abuse, rape, and elder abuse. The diagram in Figure 9–4 illustrates maladaptive responses to crisis.

Moderate to Severe Levels of Chronic Anxiety (Unit IV)

Psychophysiological Disorders (Chapter 15)

Psychophysiological disorders result in part from internalizing chronic anxiety and prolonged stress on a body system or process. When anxiety is internalized, the focus becomes the somatic complaints rather than the distressing life events or emotional conflicts triggering the anxiety. Psychological factors can be an important etiological factor in many physical disease entities. It is usually necessary to consider the precipitating stress (divorce, death, job pressure) as well as the presenting physiological symptoms when planning interventions to decrease anxiety. It must be understood that although stress and resulting anxiety are important etiological considerations, the medical disease itself can be life-threatening. Ulcerative colitis, high blood pressure, and peptic ulcers are examples of physical diseases affected by psychological factors.

Physical homeostasis is imperative as a short term goal. Learning to deal more appropriately with anxiety is a long term goal. The sequence shown in Figure 9–5 illustrates how a psychophysiological disorder may develop.

ANXIETY, SOMATIZING, AND DISSOCIATIVE DISORDERS (Chapter 16)

These syndromes used to be classified as the "neurotic disorder." Defenses seen in these disorders are said to be predominantly *ego-alien* or *ego-dystonic*, that is, the defense is unacceptable and disturbing to the person. For example, a person who has acrophobia (fear of heights) can find this fear annoying, embarrassing, and limiting to his or her lifestyle, yet the person will also feel terrified when the feared object is encountered. The symptom is not a part of the person's self-concept; it is alien to the person's view of him- or herself, and often the person wishes to be free of the symptom.

People who use ego-alien defenses against anxiety are able to function, but not to their optimum levels of creative, intellectual, or social ability. Problems with intimacy and satisfying interpersonal relationships are prevalent. The "neurotic" person applies rigid, repetitive, and inappropriate solutions to problems. General dissatisfaction with life often occurs. These disorders are considered as functional. Hallucinations or delusions are not experienced. Anxiety may be felt keenly or may be partially repressed. Repressed anxiety usually comes out in the form of symptoms. The symptoms of these disorders are said to be symbolic of the unconscious conflict or unmet need. The disorder can be severe, but it may be seen in a range from mild to severe. Phobias, conversion reactions, obsessive-compulsive

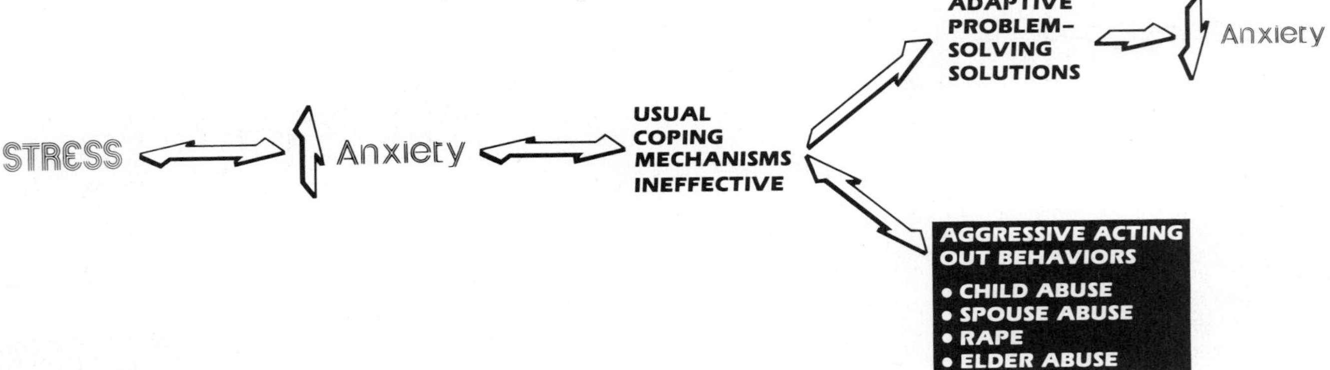

Figure 9–4. *Conceptualization of the phases of aggressive acting-out behaviors in maladaptive responses to crisis.*

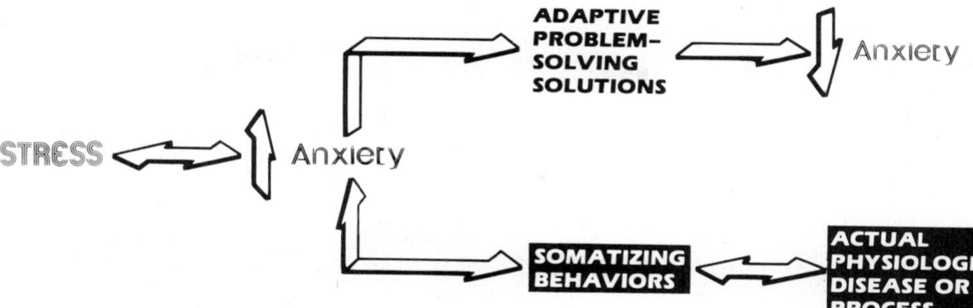

Figure 9–5. *Conceptualization of the process of psychophysiologic disorders.*

disorders, and multiple personality are some examples of the "neurotic disorders." The differences between "neurotic" and psychotic disorders are clarified in Chapter 16. Figure 9–6 identifies the role anxiety plays in development of the "neurotic disorders."

PERSONALITY DISORDERS

(Chapter 17)

Although all of the personality disorders are introduced in this text, the borderline and antisocial personality disorders are the two personality disorders discussed in depth. Nurses are often in situations that call for interventions in antisocial and borderline acting out behaviors. People with either of these disorders can cause constant upheaval and disruption in hospital units by pitting staff against staff, and clients against staff. Often staff members are left confused and angry until the dynamics of the interactions are clarified and team interventions are initiated.

Not all of the personality disorders are severe; however, people with borderline and antisocial personality disorders are more likely to be hospitalized than are people with other personality disorders. "Personality traits are enduring patterns of perceiving, relating to, and thinking about the environment and oneself, and are exhibited in a wide range of important social and personal contexts" (DSM III-R 1987). If these traits are maladaptive and rigid and cause significant impairment in occupational and interpersonal functioning or personal distress, a personality disorder is suspected. Often these characteristics have been present from childhood.

The personality traits of people with personality disorders are *ego-syntonic*, that is, they are part of the person's personality and self-concept and are not experienced as undesirable (Fig. 9–7). For example, a person with an antisocial personality disorder may *not* understand that lying, cheating, stealing, or aggressive sexual behavior is problematic, nor is there a desire to change or relate differently to others. These characteristics are part of the person's integral personality makeup and are accepted by the person as part of his or her self-concept. When those with personality disorders are in conflict with others, they assume others are at fault.

Severe to Panic Levels of Chronic Anxiety (Unit V)

Alterations in Mood (Chapters 18, 19)

The essential feature of the affective disorders is an alteration of mood that dominates the person's life ex-

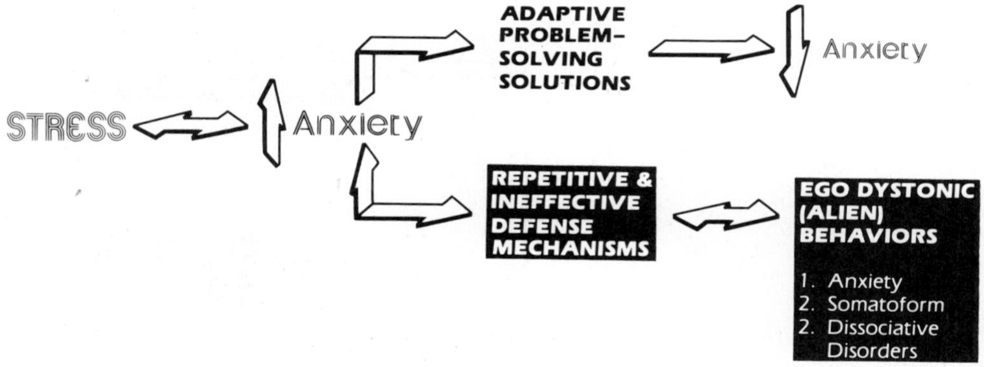

ADAPTIVE PROBLEM-SOLVING SOLUTIONS
Anxiety
STRESS
Anxiety
REPETITIVE & INEFFECTIVE DEFENSE MECHANISMS
EGO DYSTONIC (ALIEN) BEHAVIORS
1. Anxiety
2. Somatoform
2. Dissociative Disorders

Figure 9–6. *Conceptualization of the process of "neurotic defenses."*

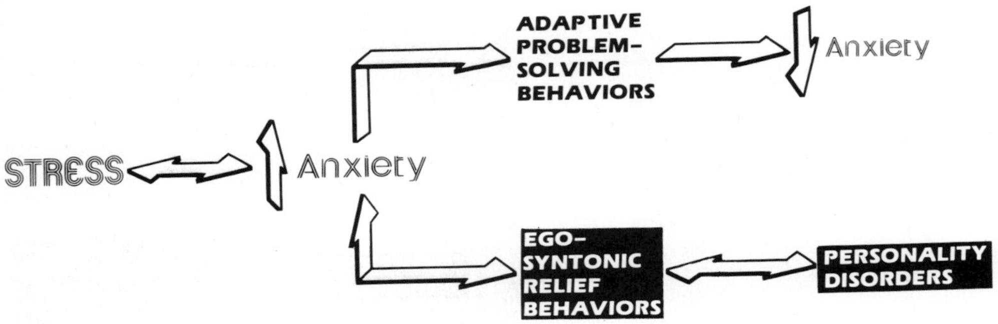

Figure 9–7. *Conceptualization of the process in the development of personality disorders.*

perience. Basically, the moods are those of depression and elation (mania). Depression exists on a continuum from mild to severe. The least severe is the normal depression experienced in grief. Grief is an acute reaction to a significant loss. In dysthymia, a mild to moderate depression, a person can usually function, but not at optimum levels. The major depressions are characterized by severe disturbances in a person's ability to function, and difficulty identifying reality may be present. The disorders of dysthymia and the major depressions (mania and depression) are usually longstanding.

Mania can be seen on a continuum from hypomania to mania to extreme mania. When mania is a feature of a major depressive disorder, it is called bipolar disorder; a person experiences both extremes (poles)—ups (mania) and downs (depression) (Fig. 9–8).

SCHIZOPHRENIC DISORDERS
(Chapter 20)

The primary symptoms of the schizophrenic disorders are the four A's described in Chapter 20: disturbances in affect, autistic thinking, associative looseness, and ambivalence. Many secondary characteristics are inherent in the schizophrenic disorders, and hallucinations and delusions are always present at some stage.

There are four major schizophrenic disorders. First, the paranoid disorder, in which the main defense mechanism is projection. In paranoia, disturbing and conflicting emotions such as aggression and terror are projected outward to the world. Therefore, a person may project personal hostility to others and then say, "They are trying to harm me."

Second, the catatonic disorder, in which the main defense is withdrawal (withdrawal catatonia). In catatonia, when repression fails, the opposite extreme is seen (excited catatonia). Third, the disorganized disorder, in which regression is most pronounced. Fourth, the undifferentiated disorder, in which a mixture of the previously described features is assessed. Projection, withdrawal, and regression are felt to be among the most primitive of the defense mechanisms, since they are the earliest to develop in the process of growth (Fig. 9–9).

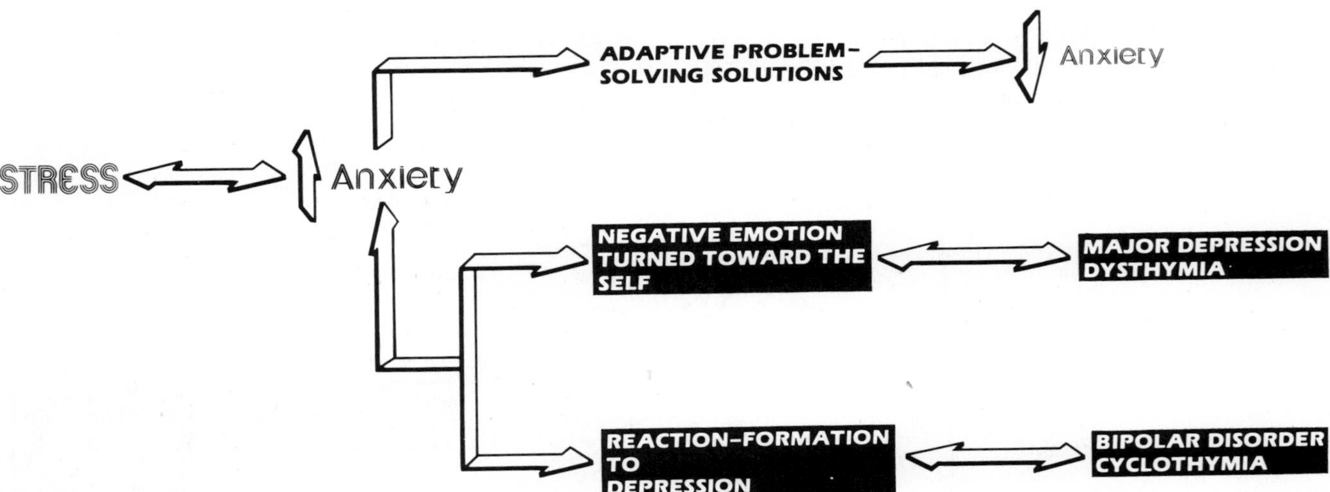

Figure 9–8. *Conceptualization of the process in alteration of moods.*

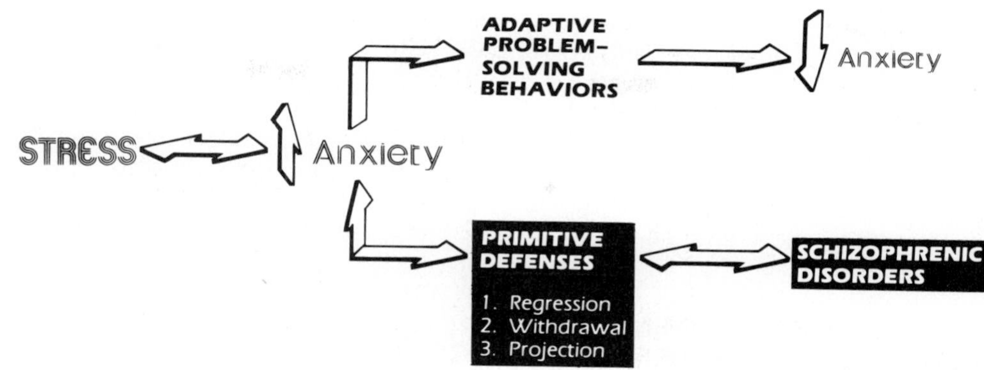

Figure 9–9. *Conceptualization of the process of schizophrenia.*

ORGANIC MENTAL SYNDROMES AND DISORDERS (Chapter 21)

All organic brain dysfunctions affect orientation, memory, intellect, affect, and judgment to some extent, regardless of specific cause and severity. Organic mental disorders include primary dementias (degenerative changes in the brain itself, e.g., Alzheimer's), secondary dementias (those caused by other pathological processes, i.e., trauma, brain tumor), and delirium.

An organizational chart of the DSM III-R (1987) categories of the organic mental disorders is presented. The majority of the substance-induced organic mental disorders are discussed in Chapters 23 and 24.

Alzheimer's disease is discussed under primary dementia, Wernicke-Korsakoff syndrome under secondary dementia, and alcohol withdrawal dilirium under delirium (Fig. 9–10).

Self-Destructive Defenses Against Anxiety (Unit VI)

SUICIDE (Chapter 22)

Suicide is the ultimate act of self-destruction. Suicide is the tenth leading cause of death for adults in the United States and the third leading cause of death for teenagers. It is increasing in our elder population. Nurses need to assess suicide clues in all hospital populations and have guidelines for when and how to intervene.

PEOPLE WHO DEPEND ON ALCOHOL (Chapter 23)

Alcohol is the most widely used and abused drug in the United States. Alcohol dependence and alcohol-related

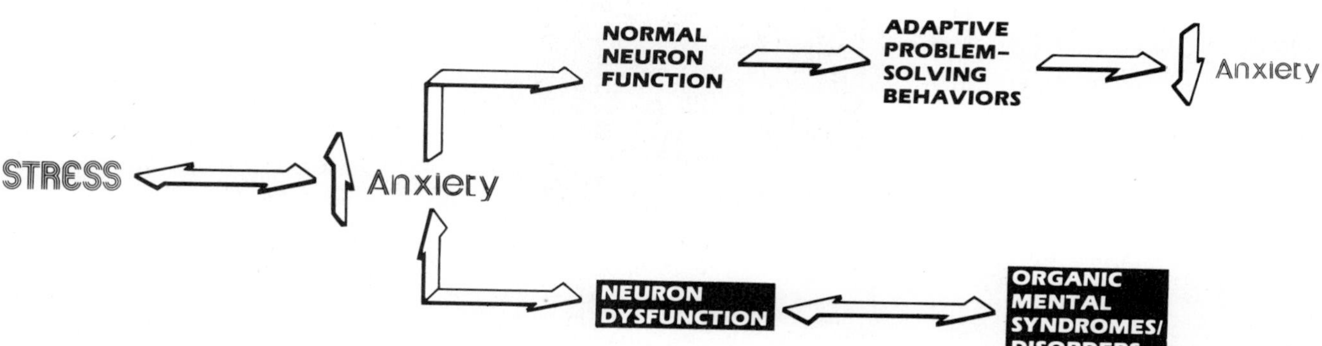

Figure 9–10. *Conceptualization of the process of organic mental syndromes and disorders.*

problems affect a significant percentage of our adolescent, adult, and elder populations. Alcohol-related problems are progressive in nature, so early detection is crucial to ensure a positive prognosis. Nurses need to know about alcohol dependence and alcohol-related problems. Nurses assess and treat people with alcohol dependence and alcohol-related problems in clinics, inpatient units, and even schools.

PEOPLE WHO DEPEND ON DRUGS OTHER THAN ALCOHOL (Chapter 24)

We have evolved into a drug-oriented culture. We use a host of drugs for a variety of purposes: to restore health, to reduce pain, to relieve anxiety, to increase energy, to create feelings of euphoria, to induce sleep, and to enhance alertness. The nurse's role in assessing and treating drug intoxication, overdose, and dependencies for the following groups of drugs is discussed: (1) sedatives and hypnotics, (2) psychostimulants (cocaine), (3) opioids (narcotics), and (4) psychotomimetics (hallucinogens).

DISORDERS IN EATING (Chapter 25)

Anorexia nervosa, bulimia nervosa, and obesity due to compulsive overeating are the eating disorders discussed in this text. Bruch (1973) was the first to propose that all people with eating disorders had difficulty as children identifying and expressing needs. Therefore, food became a response for dealing with anxiety. The incidence of anorexia nervosa and bulimia nervosa has markedly increased since the 1970s. A recent study indicated one severe case of anorexia nervosa in every 200 adolescent women. Nursing assessments and interventions are discussed within the framework of the nursing process.

Figure 9–11 identifies the role that self-destructive relief behaviors play in an attempt to relieve anxiety.

Summary

This chapter presented an overview of the clinical chapters (10–25) to be covered in this text within the framework of the anxiety continuum. The diagrams conceptualize the role of stress (biological, psychological or social) leading to increased levels of anxiety (either primary, secondary, acute or chronic) resulting in either crises, selected disorders, or psychiatric syndromes. The anxiety continuum and the Standards of Psychiatric and Mental Health Nursing Practice are the conceptual models for the presentation of the clinical chapters in this text. It is hoped that these models will be an effective format for students to organize the vast amount of psychiatric mental health material they are given to assimilate in a short time period.

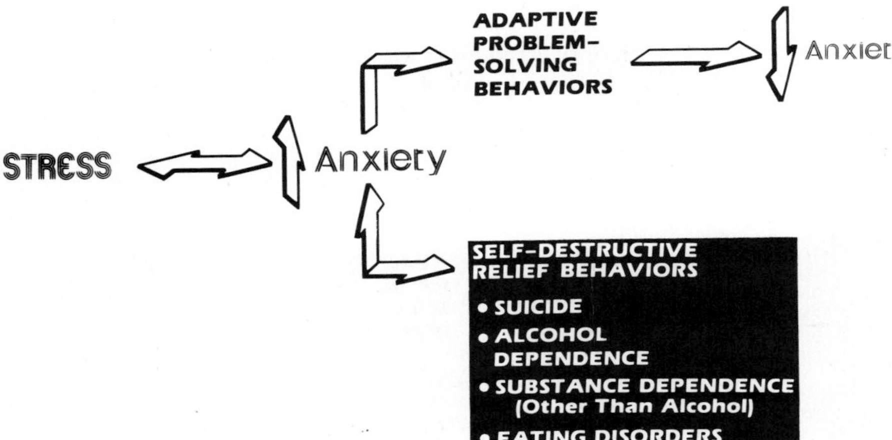

Figure 9–11. *Conceptualization of self-destructive relief behaviors.*

PART TWO

FOUNDATIONS IN PRACTICE: THE ANXIETY CONTINUUM

PEOPLE IN ACUTE ANXIETY

UNIT III

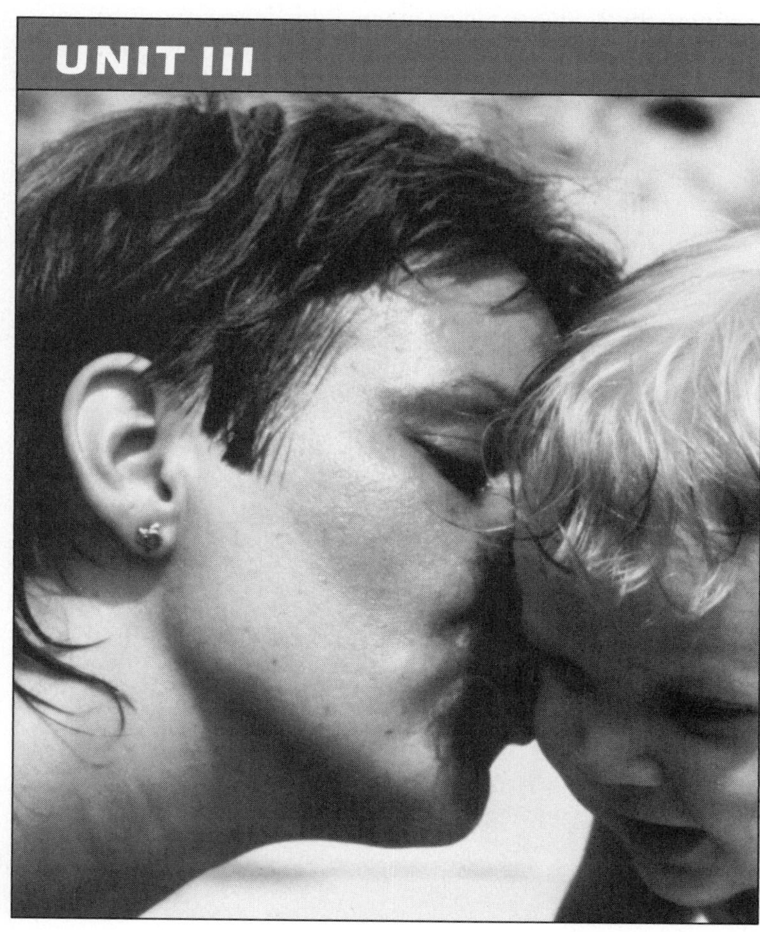

Love cures people— both the ones who give it and the ones who receive it.

DR. KARL MENNINGER

A Nurse Speaks

by Kathleen Smith-DeJulio

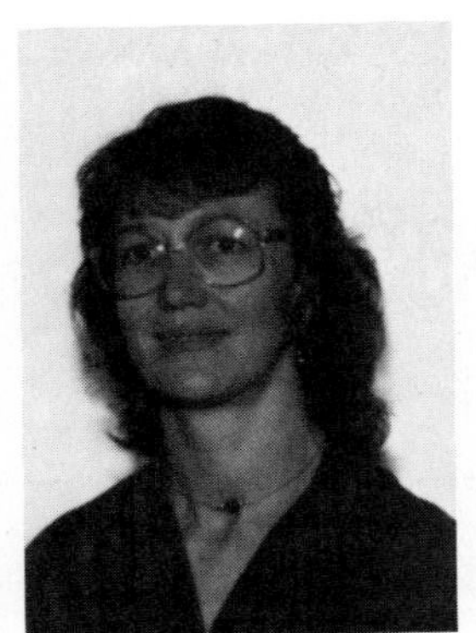

It is another busy night in the emergency room, and patients for the crisis counselor (me!) are lining up. I have a grieving family in one room, a psychotic individual wanting hospitalization in another, a teenager experiencing a cocaine psychosis in the seclusion room, motor vehicle accident victims arriving with their families to arrive soon, and a patient with a panic attack awaiting my intervention in an examination room. I know how she feels!

For a brief moment, I wonder why I do this to myself. Why do I always end up working in such intense situations? Then I remember that nursing—no matter where one practices—is intense. And I do it because I love it! I'm intense. Human needs are intense. Social-emotional-psychological problems are intense. There's no escaping it. So I consciously move into my "practice what I preach" mode. I'm a psychiatric nurse. I know that crisis is not ameliorated by a crisis response. I take a few precious moments to do a body check for muscle tension and to let it go, to reframe the demands facing me by formulating priorities, to tell myself calmly that I will do the best I can do. I will be honest and direct with patients and other staff about what I am doing. I tell myself that "this too will pass." I breathe deeply, sigh, and go forth, intentionally demonstrating contagious calmness, hoping to bring some peace to stressful moments for many people. I want to show them what nurses do and have them be glad we're around. I want to make a difference in people's lives. I care.

CHAPTER 10

Crisis and Crisis Intervention

Elizabeth M. Varcarolis

OUTLINE

KEY TERMS AND CONCEPTS

The key terms and concepts listed here also appear in bold where they are defined or discussed in this chapter.

CRISIS

MATURATIONAL CRISIS

SITUATIONAL CRISIS

ADVENTITIOUS CRISIS

PHASES OF CRISIS
Primary Care—Intervention
Secondary Care—Intervention
Tertiary Care—Intervention

OBJECTIVES

After studying this chapter, the student will be able to:

1. Define the three types of crises and give an example of each.
2. Diagram Caplan's four phases of crisis.
3. State at least six aspects of crisis that have relevance for nurses involved in crisis intervention.
4. Identify three areas to assess during crisis, with two sample questions for each area.
5. List three qualities the nurse can develop that can greatly enhance effective crisis intervention.
6. Identify two out of four common problems health care professionals may have when starting crisis intervention, and discuss at least two interventions for each problem.
7. Compare and contrast the difference between (a) primary, (b) secondary, and (c) tertiary intervention, including appropriate intervention strategies.
8. Identify four situations that can precipitate a crisis in an individual with chronic mental health problems.
9. Name four potential crisis situations common in the hospital setting that a client may face.

Crisis refers to the emotional reaction to an event and not necessarily to the threatening situation or event itself. One person may perceive a stressful event as overwhelming, whereas another person may view the same stressful event as a challenge. For example, one woman on finding that she is pregnant may experience anxiety and depression, whereas another woman will feel joy and excitement. Stress by itself does not constitute a crisis, but it is often a stressful event that precipitates a crisis.

usual defense mechanisms are not able to lower or maintain anxiety, personality disorganization and interferences with daily living may follow. When the ability to cope with specific stresses is hampered, anxiety may rise to severe or panic levels, and this interferes with problem solving. The person in crisis needs immediate help or intervention. Help in this psychiatric emergency is termed crisis intervention. Basic steps in the development of a crisis can be conceptualized as follows:

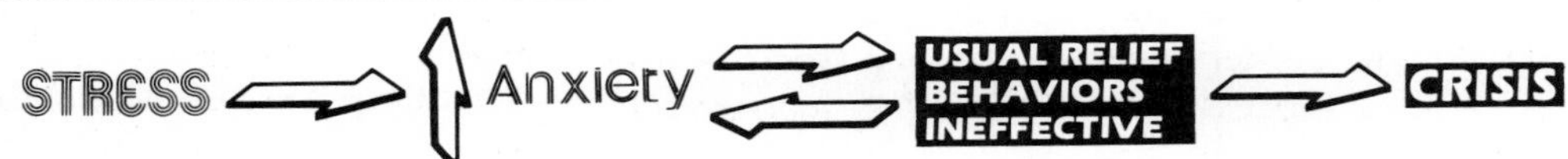

Life events such as marriage, job promotion, death of a spouse, loss of job, can be viewed as potential crises and may lead to psychological or physical illness (Holmes and Masuda 1972). Refer to Figure 10–1 for an assessment tool to measure the stress level of life events. Anxiety usually characterizes the reaction to crisis, but other emotions, such as depression, anger, and fear, may also be involved (Taylor 1986).

The crisis itself is not a pathological state. It is a struggle for equilibrium and adjustment when problems are perceived as insolvable. Crisis presents both a danger to personality organization and a potential opportunity for personality growth. The outcome depends on how the individual deals with the crisis and what outside supports are available at the time the crisis occurs (Ewing 1978).

As anxiety escalates in response to a stressful event, relief behaviors are called into play. When a person's

Essentially, a **crisis** is a temporary state of disequilibrium (high anxiety) in which a person's usual coping mechanisms or problem-solving methods fail. Crisis can result in personality growth or personality disorganization, depending on personal and social supports.

Crisis and crisis intervention have the following features: (1) crisis intervention is short term; (2) it focuses on solving the immediate problem; (3) it aims to re-establish former coping patterns and problem-solving ability; and (4) the crisis is usually limited to a four- to six-week period of time—then an initial resolution will be made (Croushore et al. 1981; Robinson 1973).

Nurses, perhaps more than any other group, deal with people who are experiencing disruption in their lives. People often undergo increased amounts of stress and anxiety in the medical-surgical, pediatric, obstetrical, and emergency room settings, as well as in the formal psychiatric setting. Understanding what constitutes a

LIFE EVENTS AND SOCIAL READJUSTMENT SCALE

DIRECTIONS:
Using yourself or a client as the subject, place a check mark on the line to the left of each event that has occurred in the subject's life during the past year. If the event has occurred more than once, place a check mark for each occurrence, then add up the accumulated points.

	Event	Points
______	1. Death of a spouse	100
______	2. Divorce	73
______	3. Marital separation	65
______	4. Jail term	63
______	5. Death of a close family member	63
______	6. Personal injury or loss	53
______	7. Marriage	50
______	8. Firing from work	47
______	9. Marital reconciliation	45
______	10. Retirement	45
______	11. Change in health of family member	44
______	12. Pregnancy	40
______	13. Sexual difficulties	39
______	14. Gain of new family member	39
______	15. Business readjustment	39
______	16. Change in financial state	38
______	17. Death of a close friend	37
______	18. Change to different line of work	36
______	19. Change in number of arguments with spouse	35
______	20. Mortgage over $10,000	31
______	21. Foreclosure of mortgage or loan	30
______	22. Change in responsibilities at work	29
______	23. Son or daughter leaving home	29
______	24. Trouble with in-laws	29
______	25. Outstanding personal achievement	28
______	26. Spouse beginning or stopping work	26
______	27. Beginning or ending school	26
______	28. Change in living conditions	25
______	29. Revision of personal habits	24
______	30. Trouble with boss	23
______	31. Change in work hours or conditions	20
______	32. Change in residence	20
______	33. Change in schools	20
______	34. Change in recreation	19
______	35. Change in church activities	19
______	36. Change in social activities	18
______	37. Mortgage or loan less than $10,000	17
______	38. Change in sleeping habits	16
______	39. Change in number of family get-togethers	15
______	40. Change in eating habits	15
______	41. Vacation	13
______	42. Christmas	12
______	43. Minor violations of the law	11

SUBJECT'S TOTAL ______________

FIND THE SUBJECT'S LIFE CRISIS LEVEL AMONG THE FOLLOWING:

150–199	Mild risk
200–299	Moderate risk
300 or more	Major risk

Figure 10–1. *Life events and social readjustment scale.* (*Adapted from* Holmes TH, Masuda M. *Psychosomatic syndrome. Psychology Today*, April 1972, *p.* 71.)

crisis and possessing a basic knowledge of crisis intervention enable the nurse to cope effectively with potential and actual crisis situations. The ability to recognize a crisis and intervene in a timely manner can influence the quality and course of another person's life.

Standard I: Theory

Crisis theory came about in the early 1940's from a classic study of the grief reactions of close relatives of victims in the Coconut Grove nightclub fire. Erich Lindemann's Coconut Grove study formed the foundation of crisis theory and clinical intervention in human crisis. Lindemann observed that "acute grief was the normal reaction to a distressing situation" (Ewing 1978). He showed that preventive intervention in crisis situations could eliminate or decrease serious personality disorganization and devastating psychological consequences from sustained effects of severe anxiety (Hoff 1989).

Gerald Caplan, in the early 1960's, defined crisis theory and outlined crisis intervention. Since that time, our understanding of crisis and effective intervention has been refined and enhanced by competent clinicians and theorists.

In 1961, a report from the Joint Commission on Mental Illness and Mental Health spoke about the need for community mental health centers throughout the country (Levenson 1974). This report stimulated the establishment of crisis services, which are now an important part of mental health services in hospitals and communities.

Health care workers who engage in crisis intervention base their assessment on theory drawn from both Lindemann and Caplan, as well as from developmental theory, life events theory, and other sources.

In all areas of nursing practice, a solid base of knowledge is needed in each specific area before the nursing process can be applied. The areas discussed subsequently are derived from established crisis theory and constitute a sound knowledge base for the application of the nursing process when intervening in a crisis. Understanding of these three areas of crisis theory provides the knowledge base for application of the nursing process. These areas are (1) types of crises, (2) phases of crisis, and (3) aspects of crisis that have relevance for nurses.

TYPES OF CRISES

Three basic types of crisis situations have been identified:

1. Maturational
2. Situational
3. Adventitious

MATURATIONAL CRISIS. A process of maturation occurs throughout the life cycle. Erikson identified eight stages of growth and development in which specific maturational tasks must be mastered. Each of these stages constitutes a crisis in personal growth and development. The eight stages and their tasks as defined by Erikson are reviewed in Table 10–1 (Erikson 1963). (Refer to Chapter 2 for more developmental theory.)

Each stage can be referred to as a **maturational crisis.** When a person arrives at a new stage, the old coping styles are no longer appropriate and new coping mechanisms have yet to be developed. For a period of time, the person is without effective defenses. This often leads to increased anxiety, which may be seen in variations of the person's normal behavior. Temporary disequilibrium may affect interpersonal relationships, body image, and social and work roles (Hoff 1989). Successful resolution of these tasks leads to development of basic human qualities. Erikson believes that how these crises are solved at one stage affects the ability to pass subsequent stages, since each crisis provides the starting point for moving to the next stage. If a person lacks support systems and adequate role models, successful resolution may be difficult or may not occur. Unresolved problems in the past and inadequate coping mechanisms can adversely affect what is learned in each developmental stage. When a person is experiencing severe difficulty during a maturational crisis, professional intervention may be indicated.

SITUATIONAL CRISIS. Situational crises arise from external sources as opposed to internal sources. Examples of external situations that could precipitate a crisis include loss of a job, death of a loved one, abortion, change of job, change in financial status, divorce, additional family members, pregnancy, and severe physical illness. Holmes and Masuda (1972) referred to these situations as life events. Each event is assigned stress points, which, when added, may predict the risk for illness. A high point count can act as a predictor of physical or psychological illness. This *Life Events and Social Readjustment Scale* (Fig. 10–1) can be a useful tool for evaluating potential crisis situations and for planning primary intervention. Some authors refer to these events as critical life problems, since these problems are encountered by most people to some extent during the course of their lives. Whether or not these events precipitate a crisis depends upon such factors as the degree of support available from caring friends and family members, one's general emotional status, and ability to

Table 10–1 • ERIKSON'S EIGHT STAGES AND THEIR MATURATIONAL TASKS

STAGE	AGE	PSYCHOLOGICAL TASK
1. Infancy	0–1	Trust versus mistrust
2. Late infancy	1–3	Autonomy versus shame and doubt
3. Early childhood	4–5	Initiative versus guilt
4. Middle childhood	6–11	Industry versus inferiority
5. Puberty and adolescence	12–20	Ego identity versus role confusion
6. Early adulthood	20–30	Intimacy versus isolation
7. Middle adulthood	30–50	Generativity versus stagnation
8. Late adulthood	50+	Ego integrity versus despair

understand and cope with the meaning of the stressful event.

As in all crises or potential crisis situations, the stressful event involves a loss that threatens a person's self-concept and self-esteem. To varying degrees, successful resolution of a crisis is contingent upon resolution of the grief associated with the loss that has occurred.

ADVENTITIOUS CRISIS (CRISIS OF DISASTER). **Adventitious crises** are not a part of everyday life; they are unplanned and accidental. Adventitious crises come under the following headings: (1) natural disasters (floods, fires, earthquakes), (2) national disasters (wars, riots, concentration camps), and (3) crimes of violence (rape, murder, spouse and child abuse).

PHASES OF CRISIS

Caplan has identified four distinct **phases of crisis** (Caplan 1964):

1. A person confronted by a conflict or problem that threatens the self-concept responds with increased feelings of anxiety. The increase in anxiety stimulates the use of usual problem-solving techniques and defense mechanisms in an effort to solve the problem and lower anxiety.
2. If the usual defensive response fails, and if the threat persists, anxiety continues to rise, which produces feelings of extreme discomfort. Individual functioning becomes disorganized. Trial-and-error attempts at solving the problem and restoring a normal balance are begun.
3. If the trial-and-error attempts fail, anxiety can escalate to severe and panic levels, mobilizing automatic relief behaviors such as withdrawal and flight. Some form of resolution may be made in this stage by either compromising needs or redefining the situation to make an acceptable solution.
4. If the problem is not solved, anxiety can overwhelm the person and lead to serious personality disorganization (Ewing 1978). This can take the form of yelling, confusion, running about aimlessly, immobilization with fear, violence against others, or suicidal behavior (Robinson 1973; Hoff 1989).

Figure 10–2 is a diagram of the phases of crisis.

ASPECTS OF CRISIS THAT HAVE RELEVANCE FOR NURSES

The specific aspects of crisis theory that are basic to crisis intervention follow:

1. A crisis is self-limiting and is usually resolved within a period of four to six weeks (Aguilera and Messick 1986; Croushore et al. 1981).
2. The resolution of a crisis results in one of three different functional levels. The person will emerge at (a) a higher level of functioning, (b) the same level of functioning, or (c) a lower level of functioning.
3. The goal of crisis intervention is to maintain the pre-crisis level of functioning (Aguilera and Messick 1986).
4. The form of the resolution of the crisis is dependent upon the actions of the subject and the intervention of others (Ewing 1978).

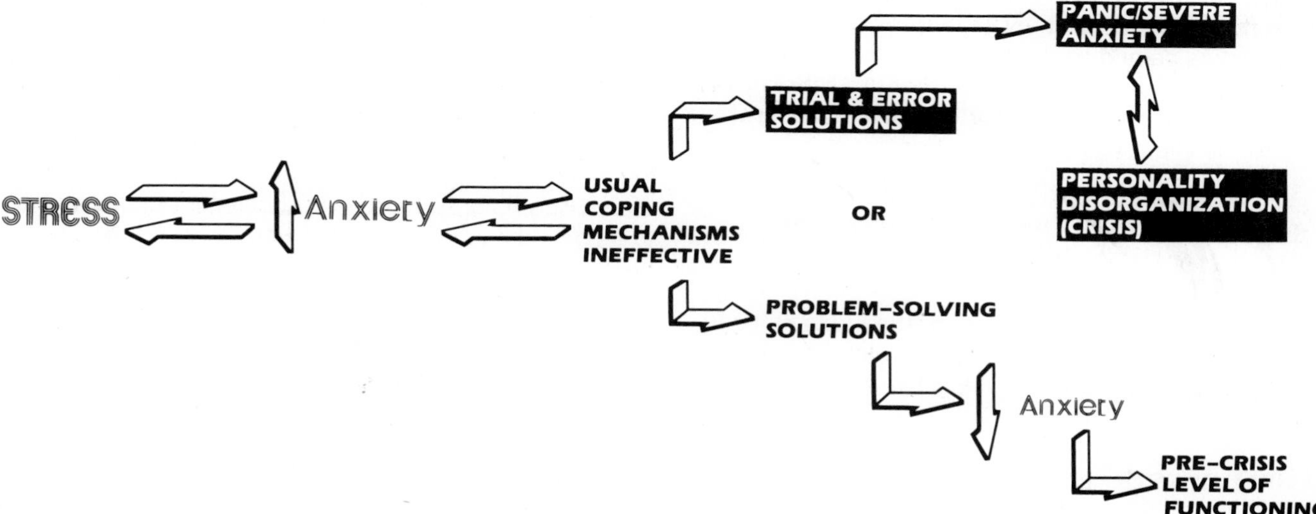

Figure 10–2. *Phases in the process of crisis.*

5. During a crisis, the individual is more open to outside intervention than at times of stable functioning (Ewing 1978). With intervention, the person can learn adaptive means of problem solving to correct inadequate solutions.
6. An assumption is made that the person in a crisis situation is mentally healthy and has functioned well in the past *but* is presently in a state of disequilibrium.
7. Crisis intervention deals with the person's present problem and resolution of the immediate crisis only (Aguilera and Messick 1986). Dealing with material not directly related to the crisis can take place at a later time. Crisis intervention deals with the "here and now."
8. The *nurse* must be willing to take an active, even directive role in intervention. This is in direct contrast to conventional therapeutic intervention techniques, which stress a more passive and nondirective role (Aguilera and Messick 1986).
9. Early intervention probably increases the chances for a better prognosis.
10. The client is encouraged to set realistic goals and plan intervention focused on the realities of the current situation.

Standard II: Data Collection

A person's equilibrium may be adversely affected by one or more of the following: (1) an unrealistic perception of the precipitating event, (2) inadequate situational supports, or (3) inadequate coping mechanisms (Aguilera and Messick 1986; Ewing 1978). It is crucial to assess these factors when evaluating a crisis situation, because data gained from the assessment are used as guides for both the nurse and the client to set realistic and meaningful goals, as well as to plan possible solutions to the client's problem situation.

ASSESSING THE PERCEPTION OF THE PRECIPITATING EVENT

The initial task is the assessment of the individual and the problem. The more clearly the problem can be defined, the better the chance an effective solution will be found.

SAMPLE QUESTIONS TO ASK (Croushore et al. 1981; King 1971)

1. Has anything particularly upsetting happened to you within the past few days or weeks?
2. What was happening in your life before you started to feel this way?
3. What leads you to seek help now?
4. Describe how you are feeling right now.
5. How does this problem affect your life?
6. How do you see this problem affecting your future?

Laura, a 15-year-old girl, was brought to the emergency room (ER) after slashing her wrists. She was found by her mother, who had returned home early from a date. Her mother called the police and they rushed Laura to the hospital. After Laura had been seen by the medical personnel, she was interviewed by the psychiatric nurse working in the ER. The nurse spoke calmly. She introduced herself and told Laura she would like to spend some time with her. The nurse stated that she could see that Laura was upset. She made the observation that things must be very bad if she wanted to kill herself. Laura sat slumped in a chair with her hands in her lap and her head hanging down. There were tears in her eyes.

Example: Assessing Laura's Perception of the Precipitating Event

NURSE: Laura, tell me what has happened to make you feel like killing yourself.

LAURA: I can't . . . I can't go home . . . no one cares or believes me . . . I can't go through it again.

NURSE: Tell me what you can't go through again, Laura.
Laura starts to cry, shaking with sobs. The nurse sat quietly for a while, offered Laura some tissues, then spoke:
Laura tell me what is so terrible. Let's look at it together.

After a while, Laura started telling the nurse that when she was nine, her mother had a boyfriend. When her mother was out of the house, the boyfriend would touch her and eventually forced her to have sex with him. He threatened Laura that if she told, he would kill her. When she was 11, the boyfriend moved south. Two weeks ago, Laura's mother told her the old boyfriend was coming back to live with them. Laura, terrified, told her mother what had happened years ago, but her mother refused to believe her and called her a liar. Her mother said that if it came to a choice between Laura and the boyfriend, the mother would take the boyfriend.

ASSESSING SITUATIONAL SUPPORTS

The client's support systems are assessed to determine the available resources surrounding the person. Does the stressful event involve important people in the support system? Is there isolation from others or are there family and friends who can provide the vital support? Family and friends may be called upon to aid the individual by offering material or emotional supports, for example, lending money, offering services, or being available to give affection and understanding. If these resources are not available, the therapist acts as a temporary support system while relationships with individuals or groups in the community are established.

SAMPLE QUESTIONS TO ASK (Aguilera and Messick 1986)

1. With whom do you live?
2. To whom do you talk when you feel upset?
3. Whom can you trust?
4. Who is available to help you?
5. Where do you go to church/school/other community-based activities?

Assessing Laura's Situational Supports

NURSE: Laura, who can you go to, do you have any other family?

LAURA: No. My dad left when I was six. We stay pretty much alone. My mom doesn't allow my brother and me to play with other kids.

NURSE: Do you have anyone you can talk to?

LAURA: No, I really don't have any friends. All the other kids think I'm stuck-up. I don't fit in too well, I guess. My mom would never let me go out anyway; there's always things to do at home.

NURSE: What about church, or your teachers at school?

LAURA: The teachers are nice and all, but I can't tell them things like this. They wouldn't believe me either.

ASSESSING PERSONAL COPING SKILLS

In crisis situations, it is important to evaluate the person's level of anxiety. Common coping mechanisms may be overeating, drinking, smoking, withdrawal, seeking out someone to talk to, yelling, fighting, or physical activity (Croushore et al. 1981). The potential for suicide or homicide must be assessed. If the patient is suicidal, homicidal, or unable to take care of personal needs, hospitalization should be considered (Aguilera and Messick 1986).

SAMPLE QUESTIONS TO ASK

1. What do you usually do to feel better?
2. Did you try it this time? If so, why do you think it didn't work?
3. Have you thought of killing yourself or someone else?
4. Has anything like this ever happened before?
5. What do you think might happen now?

Example: Assessing Laura's Personal Coping Style

The nurse learned that Laura did very well in school, especially in math. Laura explained that when she studied, she could forget her problems and get lost in other worlds. Getting good grades also had another reward: it was the only time her mother said anything nice about her. Her mother would boast to her boyfriends about how bright her daughter was.

NURSE: What would you think would help your situation?

LAURA: I don't want to die . . . I just don't know where to turn.

The nurse told Laura that she wanted to work with her to find a solution, and that she was concerned for Laura's safety and well-being.

Standard III: Diagnosis

A person in crisis may exhibit a variety of behaviors that may indicate a number of human problems. For example, when a person is in crisis, the nursing diagnosis *ineffective individual coping* is often evident. Since anxiety levels may escalate to moderate or severe levels, the ability to solve problems is usually impaired, if present at all. Ineffective individual coping may be evidenced by inability to meet basic needs, inability to meet role expectations, alteration in social participation, use of inappropriate defense mechanisms, or impairment of usual patterns of communication. Possible "related to's" for ineffective individual coping could include situational crises, inadequate support systems, maturational crises, multiple life changes, inadequate coping methods, unrealistic perceptions, and unmet expectations (Doenges and Moorehouse 1988).

Altered thought processes may be noted as evidenced by altered attention span, distractibility, or disorientation to time, place, person, circumstance, and events. Altered thought processes in a crisis situation could be "related to" psychological conflicts or impaired judgment.

Since change in one member of a family most always affects all members of a family, *altered family process* is probable. Altered family process can be "related to" situational crisis or developmental crisis of one or more members. Altered family process may be evidenced by subjective data regarding confusion or objective data identified by the nurse. For example, the family may no longer be able to help each other or the member in crisis in meeting physical or emotional needs. The family may have difficulty being able to adapt or respond to the changes or traumatic experience of the member in crisis. The family's ability to make decisions or accomplish developmental tasks may be impaired. Communications may become confused and inability to express feelings may be evident.

Anxiety (moderate/severe/panic) is always present, and the nurse works with the client to lower the anxiety to a level at which the client is able to start problem solving and making effective plans for dealing with the crisis situation. Anxiety can be "related to" a variety of etiologies such as situational or maturational crises, threat to self-concept, threat to or change in health status (role functioning or socioeconomic status), and physiological factors (hyperthyroidism or use of some medications) (see Chapter 9).

Example: Nursing Diagnosis — Laura

The assessment of Laura's (1) perception of the precipitating event, (2) situational supports, and (3) personal coping skills gave the nurse enough data to formulate two diagnoses and to work with Laura in setting goals and planning interventions.

The nurse formulated the following goals:

1. *Anxiety (Moderate/Severe):* related to rape trauma syndrome as evidenced by ineffectual problem solving and feelings of impending doom.
2. *Ineffective Family Coping:* compromised, related to inadequate understanding by Laura's mother.

Standard IV: Planning

Planning involves planning on the (1) content level and (2) process level. Planning on the content level includes setting realistic goals and identifying actions that will meet these goals. Planning on the process level involves identifying personal feelings or behaviors that would diminish effective interventions.

CONTENT LEVEL — PLANNING GOALS

Planning realistic goals is done with the client. Goals are made to fit the person's cultural and personal values. Without the client's involvement, the goals may be irrelevant to what would be acceptable solutions to the crisis. For example, the nurse who suggests to a woman to leave her husband because he beats her may find that the woman has different goals. The basic goal in all potential crisis situations is to resolve the presenting problem and to support the person in crisis in an attempt to regain a normal level of functioning (Finkelman 1977). Defining realistic goals gives the client a sense of control, which can decrease the impact of the crisis. The nurse and the client plan together acceptable means of meeting these goals.

The client — not the nurse — solves the problem. The nurse helps the client refocus to gain new perspectives on the situation. The nurse supports the client during the process of finding constructive ways to solve or cope with the problem. The client is involved in setting both the long term and the short term goals, as well as in planning intervention.

PROCESS LEVEL — NURSES' FEELINGS AND REACTIONS

All types of people may be involved in helping individuals in crisis. For example, people from various professional backgrounds are trained in crisis intervention — police, teachers, welfare workers, clergy, social workers, psychologists, as well as nurses. Crisis intervention is often practiced unwittingly by people without formal training, such as bartenders, concerned bystanders, friends, and neighbors. People can play a crucial role in the successful resolution of a crisis by responding spontaneously with concern and caring.

Beginning practitioners in crisis intervention often face common problems that must be worked through before they become comfortable and competent in the role of a crisis counselor. Four of the more common problems are (1) the counselor's need to be needed, (2) setting unrealistic goals for clients, (3) difficulty dealing with the issue of suicide, and (4) difficulty terminating. Refer to Table 10 – 2 for examples and results of these problems, appropriate interventions, and desired outcomes. It is crucial in beginning crisis intervention that supervision be made available as an integral part of the training process. The supervisor should be an experienced professional who could be a peer, teacher, or supervisor.

Table 10–2 • COMMON PROBLEMS FACED BY BEGINNING PRACTITIONERS

PROBLEM 1. *Counselor needs to feel needed.* Feels total reponsibility to "care for" or "cure" client's problems.

EXAMPLES	RESULT	INTERVENTIONS	OUTCOME
The nurse • Allows excessive phone calls between sessions. • Gives direct advice without sufficient knowledge of client's situation. • Attempts to influence lifestyle of client on a judgmental basis.	Client becomes more dependent on nurse and relies less on own abilities. Nurse reacts to client's not getting "cured" or taking advice by projecting feelings of frustration and anger onto the client.	The nurse • Evaluates with an experienced professional her needs versus client's needs. • Discourages dependency by the client. • Encourages goal setting and problem solving by the client. • Takes control only if suicide or homicide is a possibility.	Client is free to grow and problem solve own life crises. Nurse's skills and effectiveness grow as comfort with role and own goals are clarified.

PROBLEM 2. *Setting unrealistic goals for clients.* Goals become nurse's goals and not mutually determined goals for the client.

EXAMPLES	RESULT	INTERVENTIONS	OUTCOME
The nurse • Expects physically abused woman to leave battering partner. • Expects man who abuses alcohol to stop drinking when loss of family or job is imminent.	Nurse feels anxious and responsible when expectations are not met. Anxiety resulting from feelings of inadequacy are projected onto the client in the form of frustration and anger.	The nurse • Examines with an experienced professional realistic expectations of self and client. • Re-evaluates client's level of functioning and works with the client on his level. • Encourages setting of goals by client.	Nurse's ability to assess and problem solve increases as anger and frustration decrease. Client feels less alienated and a working relationship can ensue.

PROBLEM 3. *Difficulty dealing with suicidal client.*

EXAMPLES	RESULT	INTERVENTIONS	OUTCOME
Nurse selectively inattends by • Denying possible clues. • Neglecting to follow up on clues. • Changing topic to less threatening subject.	Client is robbed of opportunity to share feelings and find alternatives to intolerable situation. Client remains suicidal. Nurse's crisis intervention ceases to be effective.	The nurse • Assesses her own feelings and anxieties with the help of an experienced professional. • Evaluates all clues or slight suspicions and acts upon them, for example, "Are you thinking of killing yourself?" If yes, the nurse assesses a. Suicide potential. b. Need for hospitalization.	Client experiences relief in sharing feelings and evaluating alternatives. Suicide potential can be minimized. Nurse becomes more adept at picking up clues and minimizing suicide potential.

PROBLEM 4. *Difficulty terminating* after crisis has resolved.

EXAMPLES	RESULT	INTERVENTIONS	OUTCOME
Nurse tempted to work on other problems in the client's life.	Nurse steps into territory of traditional therapy without proper training or experience.	The nurse • Works with an experienced professional to a. Explore own feelings regarding separations and termination. b. Reinforce crisis model. Crisis intervention is a preventive tool, not psychotherapy.	Nurse becomes better able to help client with his feelings when own feelings are recognized. Client is free to go back to his life situation or request appropriate referral to work on other issues of importance to him.

Data from Finkelman 1977; Wallace and Morley 1970.

Personal Qualities That Enhance Nursing Effectiveness

Nurses need to monitor personal feelings and thoughts constantly when dealing with a person in crisis. It is important to recognize one's own level of anxiety to prevent closing off the expression of painful feelings by the client. Since at times, a client's situation or anxiety level may trigger uncomfortable levels of anxiety in the nurse, there is a tendency to repress such feelings to maintain personal comfort. When the nurse is not aware of personal feelings and reactions, the nurse may unconsciously prevent the expression of the painful feelings in the client that are precipitating the nurse's own discomfort. Thus, closing off feelings in the client can render the nurse ineffective. However, specific personal attributes in the nurse can contribute favorably to the outcome of an individual in crisis (Donlon and Rockwell 1982).

CARING. The caring nurse has profound respect for the human condition and believes that the person in crisis should have the opportunity to ease his or her pain and to alter his or her situation. A cold and technical approach will have little success with a person in crisis.

LISTENING. This specifically refers to (Donlon and Rockwell 1982):

1. Hearing what the client says and leaves out in the conversation.
2. Monitoring what goes on in the interaction between the client and the nurse.
3. Identifying one's own feelings during the interaction with the client.

Listening is facilitated by looking at the person who speaks. Feedback can be given by clarifying what the person is saying. This is done by repeating a short summary to the patient, who agrees with or corrects the nurse's impression. Refrain from judging or moralizing, but try to understand the other person's experience. The importance of having someone to listen during a difficult time is described in the poem "Listening" (Box 10–1).

CREATIVITY AND FLEXIBILITY. A helping person must be able to look at another person's crisis situation from a variety of angles and work with the client to find possible solutions. Each individual is unique, and one's perception of the situation is filtered through cultural, family, and personal traditions and beliefs. The possible alternatives must be compatible with these traditions and beliefs. What is helpful for one person is often not appropriate for another. There are no simple solutions for people in crisis. The nurse must be able to view the

Box 10–1. LISTENING

When I ask you to listen to me
and you start giving me advice,
you have not done what I asked.

When I ask you to listen to me
and you begin to tell me why I shouldn't feel that way,
you are trampling on my feelings.

When I ask you to listen to me
and you feel you have to solve my problems,
you have failed me, strange as that may seem.

Listen! All I asked was that you listen . . .
not talk or do—just hear me.
Advice is cheap; 10 cents will get you both Dear Abby and
Billy Graham in the same newspaper.
And I can do for myself; I'm not helpless.
Maybe discouraged and faltering, but not helpless.

When you do something for me that I can and need to do
for myself, you contribute to my fear and weakness.
But, when you accept as a simple fact that I do feel what I feel
no matter how irrational, then I can quit trying to convince
you and get about the business of understanding what's
behind this irrational feeling.
And when that's clear, the answers are obvious and I don't
need advice.

Irrational feelings make sense when we understand what's
behind them.
Perhaps that's why prayer works, sometimes, for some people
because God is mute, and he doesn't give advice or
try to fix things. He just listens and lets you work it out for yourself.

So please listen and just hear me. And, if you want to talk,
wait a minute for your turn; and I'll listen to you.

ANONYMOUS

situation from the client's perspective (have empathy) and work with the client to identify alternatives that will be effective in lowering anxiety and facilitating normal functioning.

Example: Planning Intervention With Laura

A social worker was called. The three met together—Laura, the nurse, and the social worker. All agreed that Laura should not be in the home if the boyfriend returned. The nurse then met with Laura and her mother; however, Laura's mother continued to berate Laura for lying. She stated she did not care what Laura said, she had her own life to live. She said if Laura didn't like it, she could move out. The nurse and Laura set three goals together:

1. A safe environment will be found for Laura before the boyfriend comes to live with the mother.
2. At least two support systems will be made available to Laura within 24 hours.
3. Continued evaluation and support will be available until the immediate crisis is over (six to eight weeks).

After talking with the nurse and the social worker, Laura seemed open to the possibility of going to a foster home. She also agreed to talk to a counselor at her school. The nurse set up an appointment when she, Laura, and the counselor could meet. The nurse would continue to see Laura twice a week.

Standard V: Intervention

Crisis intervention has two basic thrusts. First, external controls may be applied for protection of the person in crisis. Second, anxiety reduction techniques are used, so inner resources can be put into effect.

During the initial interview, the person in crisis first needs to gain a feeling of safety. Solutions to the crisis may be offered, so there is an awareness of other options. Feelings of support and hope will temporarily diminish anxiety. The nurse needs to play an active role by indicating that help is available. Help is conveyed by the competent use of crisis skills and genuine interest and support. It is *not* conveyed by the use of false reassurances and platitudes, such as "everything will be all right."

Crisis intervention requires a creative and flexible approach by the use of traditional and nontraditional therapeutic roles. The nurse may act as educator, adviser, and model.

V-A: PSYCHOTHERAPEUTIC INTERVENTIONS

There are three levels of nursing care in crisis intervention. Psychotherapeutic nursing interventions in crisis are directed toward these three levels of care: (1) primary, (2) secondary, and (3) tertiary (Hoff 1989).

PRIMARY CARE. Primary care promotes mental health and reduces mental illness in order to decrease the incidence of crisis. On this level the nurse can:

1. Work with an individual to recognize potential problems by evaluating the stressful life events the person is experiencing.
2. Teach specific coping skills to handle stressful events, such as decision-making, problem-solving, and assertiveness skills, and mediation and relaxation skills.
3. Assist individuals to evaluate the timing or reduction of life changes in order to decrease the negative effects of stress as much as possible. This may involve working with a client to plan environmental changes, make important interpersonal decisions, and rethink changes in occupational roles.

SECONDARY CARE. Secondary care establishes intervention during an acute crisis to prevent prolonged anxiety from diminishing personal effectiveness and personality organization. The nurse works with the client to assess the client's problem, support systems, and coping styles. Desired goals are explored, and interventions are planned. Secondary care lessens the time a person is mentally disabled during a crisis. Secondary level care occurs in hospital units, emergency rooms, clinics, or in mental health centers, usually during the day hours.

TERTIARY CARE. Tertiary care provides support for those who have experienced and are now recovering from a disabling mental state. Social and community facilities that offer tertiary intervention include rehabilitation centers, sheltered workshops, day hospitals, and outpatient clinics. Primary goals are aimed at facilitating optimum levels of functioning and preventing further emotional disruptions. People with chronic mental problems are often extremely susceptible to crisis, and community facilities provide the structured environment that can help prevent problem situations.

Example: Secondary Crisis Intervention With Laura

The nurse met with Laura twice weekly during the next four weeks. Laura was motivated to work with the social worker and the nurse to find another place to live. The nurse suggested several times that she start to see a counselor in the outpatient clinic after the crisis was over, where she could talk about some of her pain. Laura was not interested, however, and said she would talk to the school counselor if she needed to talk.

Three weeks after the attempted suicide, foster placement was found for Laura. The couple seemed very interested in Laura, and Laura appeared happy about the attention she was receiving.

Standard VI: Evaluation

Goals are compared with the outcomes for the effectiveness of the crisis intervention. This is usually done from four to eight weeks after the initial interview, although it can be done in a shorter time frame. If the intervention has been successful, the person's level of anxiety and ability to function should be at pre-crisis levels. Often a person chooses to follow up additional areas of concern, and referral to other agencies for more long term work is made. Crisis intervention often serves to prepare a person for further treatment (Ewing 1978).

Example: Evaluation of Laura's Crisis

After six weeks, Laura and the nurse decided that the crisis was over. Laura remained aloof and distant. The nurse evaluated Laura as being in a moderate amount of emotional pain. Laura felt she was doing well, however, and she felt more secure and accepted. She was satisfied with the way things were, and again stated that if she was having any problems she would see her school counselor.

Postscript

Two years later, Laura was continuing to do well in school and was planning to go to a local community college for computer programming. Laura got along well with her foster parents, and plans were being made for adoption. Laura remained aloof. She had no close friends and continued to throw her energy into her studies. For the present, she was getting pleasure from her academic accomplishments, and she had security and warm attention in her new home environment. If, at a later date, she decided there were other things for her to work out, she knew the resources in the community.

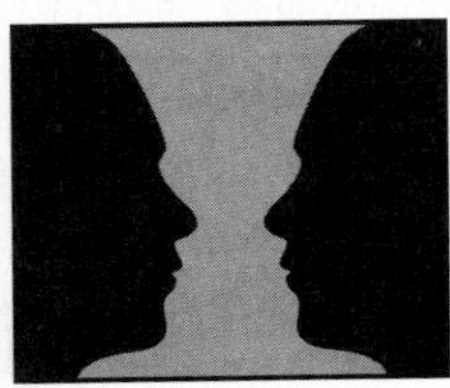

Case Study: Working With a Person In Crisis

Ms. Greg, the psychiatric nurse consultant, was called to the neurological unit. Ms. Greg was told that Mr. Raymond, a 43-year-old man with Guillain-Barré syndrome, was presenting a serious nursing problem, and the staff requested a consult.

The head nurse said Mr. Raymond was hostile and sexually abusive to the nursing staff. His abusive language, demeaning attitude, and angry outbursts were having an adverse effect on the unit as a whole. The nurses stated they felt ineffective and angry, saying they had tried to be patient and understanding; however, nothing seemed to get through to him. The situation had affected the morale of the staff, and the nurses felt the quality of their care was affected.

Mr. Raymond, an American Indian descendant, was employed as a taxicab driver. Six months before his admission to the hospital he had given up drinking after years of episodic alcohol abuse. He was engaged to a woman who visited him every day.

He needed a great deal of assistance with every aspect of his activities of daily living (ADL). His muscle weakness had progressed, so that he was essentially paralyzed. At the time the consult was made he could breathe on his own, but he had to be turned and positioned every two hours. He was fed through a gastrostomy tube.

Assessment

Ms. Greg gathered data from Mr. Raymond and the nursing staff and spoke with Mr. Raymond's fiancee.

MR. RAYMOND'S PERCEPTION OF THE PRECIPITATING EVENTS

During the initial interview, Mr. Raymond spoke to Ms. Greg angrily, using profanity and making lewd, sexual suggestions. He also talked with anger about needing a nurse to "scratch my head and help me blow my nose." He still could not figure out how his illness suddenly developed. He said the doctors told him it was too early to know for sure if he would recover completely. They told him the prognosis was good.

MR. RAYMOND'S SUPPORT SYSTEM

Ms. Greg spoke with Mr. Raymond's fiancee. Mr. Raymond's relationships with his fiancee and with his Indian culture group were strong. With minimal ties outside this group, both Mr. Raymond and his fiancee had little knowledge of outside supportive agencies.

MR. RAYMOND'S DEFENSE SYSTEM

Mr. Raymond came from a male-dominated society in which the man was expected to be a strong leader. His ability to be independent with the power to affect the direction of his life was central to his definition of being acceptable as a man.

Mr. Raymond felt powerless, out of control, and enraged. He was handling his anxiety by displacing these feelings onto the environment, namely, the staff and his fiancee. The redirection of anger temporarily lowered his anxiety, and it distracted him from painful feelings. When he intimidated others through sexual profanity and hostility, he felt temporarily in control, experiencing an illusion of power. He used displacement to relieve his painful levels of anxiety when he felt threatened.

Mr. Raymond's use of displacement was not adaptive, since the issues causing his distress were not being resolved. His anxiety continued to escalate. The effect his behavior was having on others caused them to move away from him. This withdrawal further increased his sense of isolation and helplessness.

Nursing Diagnosis

Based on her assessment, Ms. Greg formulated the following nursing diagnosis:

1. *Ineffective Individual Coping* related to inadequate coping methods, as evidenced by inappropriate use of defense mechanism (displacement)
   - Anger directed to staff and fiancee.
   - Profanity and crude sexual remarks aimed at staff.
   - Frustration and withdrawal on the part of the staff.
   - Anxiety continued to escalate.
2. *Powerlessness* related to health care environment, as evidenced by frustration over inability to perform previous tasks
   - Angry over nurses having to "scratch my head and blow my nose."
   - Minimal awareness of available supports in larger community.
3. *Ineffective Staff Coping* related to exhaustion of staff supportive capacity toward client, as evidenced by staff withdrawal and limited personal communication with client
   - Staff felt ineffective.
   - Morale of staff poor.
   - Nurses believed the quality of their care to be adversely affected.

Planning

Ms. Greg spoke to Mr. Raymond and told him she would like to spend time with him for 15 minutes every morning and talk about his concerns. She suggested that there might be alternative ways he could handle his feelings and community resources she could suggest to him. Mr. Raymond gruffly agreed, "You can visit me, if it will make you feel better." They made arrangements to meet at 7:30 A.M. for 15 minutes each morning.

For each nursing diagnosis the following short term goals were set:

Nursing Diagnosis	Short Term Goal
1. *Ineffective Individual Coping* related to inadequate coping methods, as evidenced by inappropriate use of defense mechanisms (displacement)	1. Mr. Raymond will be able to name and discuss at least two feelings regarding his illness and lack of mobility (by the end of the week).
2. *Powerlessness* related to health care environment, as evidenced by frustration over inability to perform previous tasks	2. Mr. Raymond will be able to name two community organizations that could offer him information and support (by the end of two weeks).

Continued on following page

Planning (Continued)

3. *Ineffective Staff Coping* related to exhaustion of staff supportive capacity toward client, as evidenced by staff withdrawal and limited personal communication	3. Staff and nurse will discuss reactions and alternative nursing responses to Mr. Raymond's behavior (two times within the next seven days).

Ms. Greg made out a nursing care plan (Nursing Care Plan 10–1) and shared it with the staff.

Intervention

The following morning Ms. Greg went into Mr. Raymond's room at 7:30 A.M. and sat by his bedside. At first, Mr. Raymond's comments were hostile.

Dialogue		Therapeutic Tool/Comment
N:	Mr. Raymond, I'm here as we discussed. I'll be spending 15 minutes with you every morning. We could use this time to talk about some of your concerns.	Nurse offers herself, gives information, and clarifies her role and client expectations. Night was the most difficult time for Mr. Raymond. In early morning he would be the most vulnerable and open for therapeutic intervention and support.
Mr. R.:	Listen sweetheart, my only concern is how to get a little sexual relief, get it?	
N:	Being hospitalized and partially paralyzed can be overwhelming for anyone. Perhaps you wish you could find some relief from your situation.	Nurse focuses on the process "need for relief" and not the sexual content. Encourages discussion of feelings.
Mr. R.:	What do you know, Ms. Know-it-all? I can't even scratch my nose without getting one of those fools to do it for me . . . and half the time those bitches aren't even around.	
N:	It must be difficult to have to ask people to do everything for you.	Nurse restates what client says in terms of client's feelings. Continues to refocus away from the environment back to the client.
Mr. R.:	Yeah . . . the other night a fly got into the room and landed on my face. I had to shout for five minutes before one of those bitches came in . . . just to take the fly out of the room.	
N:	Having to rely on others for everything can be a terrifying experience for anyone. It sounds extremely frustrating to you.	Acknowledges that frustration and anger would be a normal and healthy response for anyone in this situation. Encourages client to talk about these feelings instead of acting them out.
Mr. R.:	Yeah . . . it's a bitch . . . like a living hell.	

Ms. Greg continued to spend time with Mr. Raymond in the mornings. He was gradually able to talk more about his feelings of anger and frustration and was less apt to act with hostility toward the staff. As he began to feel more in control, he became less defensive about others caring for him.

After two weeks, Ms. Greg cut her visits down to two times a week. Mr. Raymond was beginning to get gross motor movements back but was not walking yet. He still displaced much of his frustration and lack of control on the environment, but he was better able to acknowledge the reality of his situation. He could identify what he was feeling and talk about those feelings briefly.

Dialogue		Therapeutic Tool/Comment
N:	You seem upset this morning, Mr. Raymond.	Observes client's clenched fists, rigid posture, and tense facial expression.
Mr. R.:	I had to wait ten minutes for a bedpan last night.	
N:	And you're angry about that.	Verbalizes the implied.
Mr. R.:	Well, there were only two nurses on for 30 people, and the aide was on her break . . . You can't expect them to be everywhere . . . but still . . .	
N:	It's hard to accept that people can't be there all the time for you.	Validates the difficulty of accepting situations one does not like when one is powerless to make changes.
Mr. R.:	Well . . . that's the way it is in this place.	

Ms. Greg met with the staff twice. The staff discussed their feelings of helplessness and lack of control, since they felt rejected by Mr. Raymond. They talked about their anger with Mr. Raymond's demeaning behavior, and their frustration in the situation. Ms. Greg pointed out to the staff that Mr. Raymond's feelings of helplessness, lack of control, and anger at his situation were the same feelings the staff was experiencing. Displacement of the helplessness and frustration by intimidating the staff gave Mr. Raymond briefly the feeling of control. It also distracted him from feelings of helplessness.

The nurses had become more understanding of the motivation for the behavior Mr. Raymond employed to cope with moderate to severe levels of anxiety. The staff focused more on the client, and less on personal reactions. The staff decided together on two approaches they could try as a group. First, they would not take Mr. Raymond's behavior personally. Second, Mr. Raymond's feelings that were displaced would be refocused back to him.

Evaluation

After six weeks, Mr. Raymond was able to get around with assistance, and his ability to care for his ADL was increasing. Although Mr. Raymond was still angry, and he felt overwhelmed at times, he was able to identify more of his feelings. He did not need to act them out so often. He was able to talk to his fiancee about his feelings, and he lashed out at her less. He was looking forward to going home, and his boss was holding his old job.

Mr. Raymond contacted the Guillain-Barré Society, and they made arrangements for a meeting with him. He was still thinking about A.A., but thought he could handle this problem himself.

The staff felt more comfortable and competent in their relationships with Mr. Raymond. The goals had been met. Mr. Raymond and Ms. Greg both felt the crisis was over, and the visits were terminated. Mr. Raymond was given the number of the crisis unit. He was encouraged to call if he had questions or felt the need to talk.

Nursing Care Plan 10–1 • A PERSON IN CRISIS: Mr. Raymond

NURSING DIAGNOSIS

Ineffective individual coping related to inadequate coping methods, as evidenced by inappropriate use of defense mechanisms (displacement)

Supporting Data

- Anger directed at staff and fiancee.
- Profanity and crude sexual remarks aimed at staff.
- Isolation related to staff withdrawal.
- Anxiety continues to escalate.

Long Term Goal: By discharge, Mr. Raymond will state he feels more comfortable discussing difficult feelings.

Short Term Goal	*Intervention*	*Rationale*	*Evaluation*
1. Mr. Raymond will be able to name and discuss at least	1a. Nurse will meet with client for 15 minutes at 7:30 A.M.	1a. Night was usually the most frightening for the client; in	Goal met Within seven days, Mr.

Continued on following page

Nursing Care Plan 10–1 • A PERSON IN CRISIS: Mr. Raymond *(Continued)*

Short Term Goal	Intervention	Rationale	Evaluation
two feelings about his illness and lack of mobility (by the end of the week).	each day for a week.	early morning, feelings are closer to the surface.	Raymond was able to speak to nurse more openly about feelings of anger and frustration.
	1b. When client lashes out with verbal abuse, nurse will remain calm.	1b. Client perceives that nurse is in control of her feelings. This can be reassuring to client and increase client's sense of security.	
	1c. Nurse will consistently redirect and refocus anger from environment back to the client, e.g., "It must be difficult to be in this situation."	1c. Refocusing feelings offers the client the opportunity to cope effectively with his anxiety and decreases the need to act out toward staff and fiancee.	
	1d. Nurse will come on time each day and stay for allotted time.	1d. Reinforces that client's anger will not drive nurse away. Consistency sets the stage for trust.	

NURSING DIAGNOSIS

Powerlessness related to health care environment, as evidenced by frustration over inability to perform previous tasks

Supporting Data

- Angry over nurses having to "scratch my head and help me blow my nose."
- Minimal awareness of available supports in larger community.

Long Term Goal: By discharge, Mr. Raymond will have contacted at least one outside community support.

Short Term Goal	Intervention	Rationale	Evaluation
1. By the end of two weeks, Mr. Raymond will be able to name at least two community organizations that can offer information and support.	1a. Nurse will spend time with the client and his fiancee. The role of specific agencies and how they may be of use will be discussed.	1a. Both client and fiancee will have the opportunity to ask questions with nurse present.	Goal met By end of ten days, Mr. Raymond and his fiancee could name two community resources that they were interested in.
	1b. The nurse will introduce one agency at a time.	1b. Allows time for information to sink in and minimizes feeling of being pressured or overwhelmed.	At the end of six weeks, Mr. Raymond had contacted the Guillain-Barré Society.
	1c. The nurse will follow up but not push or persuade client to contact any of the agencies.	1c. Client is able to make own decisions once he has appropriate information.	

NURSING DIAGNOSIS

Ineffective staff coping related to exhaustion of staff supporting capacity, as evidenced by staff withdrawal and limited personal communication

Supporting Data

- Staff state they feel ineffective.
- Morale of staff poor.
- Nurses state the quality of their care is adversely affected.

Long Term Goal: By the end of three weeks, staff will state interactions with Mr. Raymond are comfortable and effective.

Short Term Goal	Intervention	Rationale	Evaluation
1. Staff and nurse will meet for 15 minutes twice by the end of the week to discuss reactions and alternative nursing responses to Mr. Raymond's behavior.	1a. Specific time for staff meeting is set aside and participation is encouraged.	1a. Message that meeting is serious and input from entire staff is needed to plan effective intervention.	Goal met By the end of seven days, staff had met twice to discuss feelings and reactions toward Mr. Raymond.

Nursing Care Plan 10–1 • A PERSON IN CRISIS: Mr. Raymond *(Continued)*

Short Term Goal	*Intervention*	*Rationale*	*Evaluation*
	1b. Staff is encouraged to identify commonalities in their feelings and how these feelings are affecting their level of care.	1b. Sharing can minimize feelings of isolation and guilt over angry feelings. Examining reactions to client behaviors and possible client motivation for behavior can facilitate staff problem solving.	Staff planned to redirect feelings back to client.
	1c. The nurse will support group planning of effective nursing actions.	1c. When anxiety is lowered, staff is able to discuss as a unit the aspects of the client's behavior they view as a problem. Interventions then can be carried out with consistency and mutual support.	Staff planned to make an effort to remember Mr. Raymond's remarks were a defensive reaction. By the end of six weeks, staff stated they felt more comfortable and competent in their care of Mr. Raymond.

Crisis Intervention With the Chronically Mentally Ill Client

The client with chronic mental health problems also experiences crisis. The incidence of crisis may be increased in this population owing to the nature of chronic mental illness. Crisis theory and intervention can be adapted successfully with clients who have long term mental illness. Five characteristics of people with chronic mental illness have been identified (Finkelman 1977):

1. Inadequate problem-solving ability.
2. Inadequate communication skills.
3. Low self-esteem.
4. Poor success with endeavors such as work, school, family, and social relationships.
5. Inpatient or outpatient treatment for at least two years.

Although the client's illness is in the chronic state, there are healthy and unhealthy aspects of the client's personality. It is important to stress the healthy aspects of the client's personality, rather than the pathological aspects, during assessment of this client. Some of the major differences between the person who has chronic and severe difficulties in living and the mentally healthy person are outlined in Table 10–3.

POTENTIAL CRISIS SITUATION FOR A PERSON WITH CHRONIC MENTAL HEALTH PROBLEMS

People usually have a number of coping responses they can utilize when there are stresses in their everyday world. Any kind of change in our routines or lives constitutes some degree of stress (see Fig. 10–1). For the person with limited abilities, even slight change might constitute the potential for a full-blown crisis. Four specific areas that are common potential crisis situations for the chronic patient have been identified (Finkelman 1977):

1. Change in treatment approaches, such as change in routine of treatment, therapist's absence due to vacation or illness, or change in appointment time.
2. Problems or changes at work, school, or with the family, and anniversaries of significant or traumatic events in the person's life.
3. Lack of money, inadequate transportation, and problems meeting basic needs.
4. Sexual relationships for someone who is unsure about his or her own sexual identity are always a source of anxiety. This can be compounded in the chronic client if there are other complications, for example, pregnancy or impotence.

ADAPTING THE CRISIS MODEL TO MEET THE NEEDS OF A PERSON WITH CHRONIC MENTAL HEALTH PROBLEMS

Traditionally, crisis intervention refers to disequilibrium in the functioning of otherwise mentally healthy persons. The goal is to prevent temporary difficulty in functioning from progressing to severe personality disorganization. Intervention and support can aid the person in finding the way back to his or her previous level of functioning. People with chronic mental health problems, however, are readily susceptible to crisis. It is important for the nurse to be able to adapt the crisis model

Table 10-3 • MENTALLY HEALTHY VERSUS CHRONICALLY MENTALLY ILL PERSON IN CRISIS

MENTALLY HEALTHY PERSON	LONG TERM MENTALLY ILL PERSON
1. Has realistic perception of potential crisis event.	1. Because of chronic high anxiety state, potential crisis event is usually distorted by minimizing or maximizing the event.
2. Has healthy ego boundaries, good problem-solving abilities.	2. Inadequate ego functioning assumes inadequate problem-solving abilities; nurse becomes more active in assisting the person with this task.
3. Healthy persons usually have adequate situational supports.	3. Often the person has no family or friends and may be living an isolated existence.
4. Healthy persons usually have adequate coping mechanisms. Defense mechanisms can be used as support to lower anxiety.	4. Since ego functioning in the chronic patient is poor, coping mechanisms are usually inadequate or poorly utilized.

Data from Finkelman AW. The nurse therapist: Outpatient crisis intervention with the chronic psychiatric patient. Journal of Psychosocial Nursing and Mental Health Services, 8:27, 1977.

to this group. These adaptations include focusing on the person's strengths, modifying and setting realistic goals with the client, taking a more active role in the problem-solving process, and direct interventions, such as making arrangements the person would ordinarily be able to make.

Summary

A crisis is not a pathological state but rather a struggle for emotional balance. A crisis can offer the opportunity for emotional growth, as well as possible personality disorganization. Early intervention during a time of crisis greatly increases the possibility for a successful outcome. There are three types of crises: maturational, situational, and adventitious, as well as specific phases in the development of a crisis. Crisis and crisis intervention are built upon certain assumptions:

1. A crisis is usually resolved within a period of four to six weeks.
2. Crisis intervention therapy is short term, from one to six weeks, and focuses on the present problem only.
3. Resolution of a crisis takes three forms. A person comes out at a higher level, pre-crisis level, or lower level of functioning.
4. Social support and intervention maximize successful resolution.
5. Crisis therapists take an active and directive approach with the client in crisis.
6. The client takes an active role in setting goals and planning possible solutions.

Traditionally, crisis intervention is aimed at the mentally healthy person who is functioning well but is temporarily overwhelmed and unable to function. However, people who have chronic mental problems are also susceptible to crisis, and the crisis model can be adapted for their needs as well.

The steps in crisis intervention are consistent with the nursing process (assessment, nursing diagnosis, planning, intervention, and evaluation). Each has specific goals and tasks.

Specific qualities in the nurse that can facilitate effective intervention are a caring attitude, flexibility in planning care, and an ability to listen.

The nurse's ability to be aware of his or her feelings and thoughts is crucial in working with a person in crisis. The availability of peer supports and supervision to discuss the questions that normally arise is essential for the beginning crisis counselor. Learning crisis intervention is a process, and there are certain problems all health care professionals must deal with in order to improve their skills.

The basic goals of crisis intervention are to reduce the individual's anxiety level and to support the effort to return to a normal level of functioning.

References

Aguilera DC, Messick JM. Crisis Intervention Theory and Methodology, 5th ed. St. Louis: C.V. Mosby Company, 1986.

Barry PD. Psychosocial Nursing Assessment and Intervention. Philadelphia: J.B. Lippincott, 1984.

Caplan G. Symptoms of Preventive Psychiatry. New York: Basic Books, 1964.

Croushore T, et al. Using crisis intervention wisely. Philadelphia: Nursing 81 Books, Intermed Communications, 1981.

Doenges M, Moorehouse M. Nurse's Pocket Guide: Nursing Diagnoses With Interventions, 2nd ed. Philadelphia: F.A. Davis, 1988.

Donlon PT, Rockwell DA. Psychiatric Disorders, Diagnosis and Treatment. Bowie, Maryland: Robert J. Brady Company, A Prentice-Hall Publishing and Communications Company, 1982.

Erikson E. Childhood and Society, 2nd ed. New York: Norton, 1963.
Ewing CP. Crisis Intervention as Psychotherapy. New York: Oxford University Press, 1978.
Finkelman AW. The nurse therapist: Outpatient crisis intervention with the chronic patient. Journal of Psychosocial Nursing and Mental Health Services, 8:27, 1977.
Hoff LA. People in Crisis: Understanding and Helping, 3rd ed. Menlo Park, CA: Addison-Wesley, 1989.
Holmes TH, Masuda M. Psychosomatic syndrome. Psychology Today, p 72, April 1972.
King JM. The initial interview: Basis for assessment in crisis intervention. Perspectives in Psychiatric Care, 6:247, 1971.
Levenson AI. A review of the Federal Community Mental Health Centers Program. *In* Arieti S, Caplan G (eds). American Handbook of Psychiatry, vol II, 2nd ed. New York: Basic Books, 1974.
Robinson L. Psychiatric emergencies. Nursing, 73, 7:43, 1973.
Taylor CM. Mereness' Essentials of Psychiatric Nursing, 12th ed. St. Louis: C.V. Mosby Company, 1986.
Wallace MA, Morley WE. Teaching crisis intervention. American Journal of Nursing, 7:1484, 1970.

Suggested Readings

CLASSICS

Caplan G. Principles of Preventive Psychiatry. New York: Basic Books, 1964.

Drawing from the work of Lindemann, his own experience, and that of others, Caplan lays down the theoretical basis for crisis that is in current practice today. Caplan identifies four distinctive phases of crisis. He maintains that crisis is not a pathological state but a predictable reaction of a person overwhelmed by problems that appear insolvable. He also identifies a number of aspects of crisis that have relevance for therapeutic intervention and are integral to the present-day practice of crisis intervention.

Lindemann E. Symptomatology and management of acute grief. American Journal of Psychiatry, 101:141, 1944.

Lindemann's classic study of the grief reactions of 101 persons, victims and relatives of those lost in the infamous Coconut Grove nightclub fire. The results of this study provide the foundation of crisis theory and crisis intervention. Lindemann identified grief as "the normal reaction to a distressing situation," and identified uniform and predictable stages in the grief reaction. He proposed that appropriate intervention in an acute grief reaction (crisis) would minimize subsequent mental problems.

MORE ON CRISIS FOR FURTHER STUDY

Aguilera DC, Messick JM. Crisis Intervention: Theory and Methodology, 5th ed. St. Louis: C.V. Mosby Company, 1986.

An important reference for all health professionals dealing with people in crisis. Now in its fifth edition, this text provides a comprehensive overview of crisis theory and intervention techniques by individuals and groups. The authors discuss the sociocultural factors that influence interventions, and outline in detail the problem-solving approach to intervention. A variety of situational crises are discussed and case examples are given, for example, rape, divorce, suicide, death, and grieving. Maturational crises from infancy to old age are well presented with helpful case studies. A chapter is also provided on the burn-out syndrome.

Flax JW. Crisis intervention with the young adult chronic patient. *In* Pepper B, Rygkewicz H (eds). New Dimensions for Mental Health Services: The Young Adult Chronic Patient. San Francisco, CA: Jossey-Bass, June 1982.

The young adult chronic client is increasingly coming to the attention of mental health care workers. This population appears to be growing and using more and more of the community health care facilities. Flax states that assessment of these clients can be difficult, since they present many problems. He outlines an assessment model including prerequisites for outpatient treatment. He presents a case study to illustrate his model of assessment and intervention. The article provides useful guidelines to a population that nurses will be dealing with in all areas of practice.

Murphy SA. After Mount St. Helens: Disaster stress research. Journal of Psychosocial Nursing and Mental Health Services, 22(7), 1984.

The author studied the adventitious crisis of the eruption of Mount St. Helens in terms of (1) the relationship between illness and presumed death of a loved one, (2) the effects of social supports and self-efficacy as influencing positive or negative outcomes of health, and (3) the perceived effects of the media on coping with the loss following a disaster. This nurse-author's research project is well written and points out important guidelines for psychiatric mental health workers in mass crisis situations.

Swanson AR. Crisis intervention. *In* Lego S (ed). The American Handbook of Psychiatric Nursing. Philadelphia: J.B. Lippincott, 1984.

A concise and thorough overview of crisis, including the basic concepts, facts and misperceptions, characteristics of crisis intervention, assumptions about people in crisis, developmental and situational crisis, and general and specific guidelines in crisis intervention. A helpful, quick reference with useful charts and tables.

Self-Study Exercises

Match the situation with the type of actual or potential crisis.

1. ________ New baby in the household
2. ________ Rape
3. ________ Man celebrates 50th birthday
4. ________ House burned down
5. ________ Battered child/spouse
6. ________ Girl becomes a teenager

A. Maturational

B. Situational

C. Adventitious

Place a T (True) or F (False) next to each statement. Correct the false statements.

7. ________ A crisis situation can last up to four months before it is resolved.
8. ________ The goal of crisis therapy is to have the person obtain a higher level of functioning.

9. ________ Crisis therapy deals with the person in his present situation and his immediate presenting problems.
10. ________ A person in crisis has always had problems and does not cope well in his or her usual life situations.
11. ________ A crisis situation can offer the opportunity for personality growth as well as the potential for personality deterioration.
12. ________ Intervention rarely has any effect in the resolution of a crisis.
13. ________ The nurse counselor must take a firm and direct approach with a person in crisis.
14. ________ It is necessary for the nurse counselor to do all the planning and make all the decisions for the person in crisis, since the person is often too disorganized.

Write a short paragraph in response to the following:

15. After determining whether a person is homicidal or suicidal, identify the three important areas in the assessment. Give examples of two questions in each area that need to be answered before planning can take place.

Complete the statements by filling in the appropriate information.

16. Three personal qualities that can enhance a nurse's effectiveness in a crisis are
   A. ________
   B. ________
   C. ________

17. Three ways you can demonstrate concern and show that you are listening are
   A. ________
   B. ________
   C. ________

18. Identify two self-interventions a nurse can use if problems arise when starting crisis counseling.

The Problem	*Intervention*
A. Need to feel needed	1. ________
	2. ________
B. Setting unrealistic goals	1. ________
	2. ________

Match the appropriate intervention to the appropriate level of intervention.

19. ________ Teach problem solving
20. ________ Rehabilitation center
21. ________ Assess precipitating events
22. ________ Teach assertiveness training

A. Primary

B. Secondary

C. Tertiary

Complete the statements by filling in the appropriate information.

23. Four experiences that could potentiate a crisis in a person with a chronic mental problem are
    A. ____________________
    B. ____________________
    C. ____________________
    D. ____________________

24. Four common crisis situations that a nurse may encounter in a general hospital are
    A. ____________________
    B. ____________________
    C. ____________________
    D. ____________________

CHAPTER 11

Evidence of Maladaptive Responses to Crisis: Child Abuse

Kathleen Smith-DiJulio

OUTLINE

KEY TERMS AND CONCEPTS

The key terms and concepts listed here also appear in bold where they are defined or discussed in this chapter.

ABUSE-PRONE PARENT
VULNERABLE CHILD
CRISIS SITUATION
PHYSICAL BATTERING
PHYSICAL ENDANGERMENT
SEXUAL ABUSE
NEGLECT
EMOTIONAL ABUSE

LEGAL RESPONSIBILITY TO REPORT SUSPECTED ABUSE
CHILD'S MEDICAL/NURSING RECORD
PRIMARY PREVENTION
SECONDARY PREVENTION
TERTIARY PREVENTION

OBJECTIVES

After studying this chapter, the student will be able to:

1. Name three factors that can signal conditions for child abuse.
2. List seven characteristics of abusing parents.
3. Describe three characteristics of a vulnerable child.
4. Describe three types of neglect.
5. List three each physical and behavioral indicators of physical abuse.
6. List three each physical and behavioral indicators of sexual abuse.
7. List two each physical and behavioral indicators of neglect.
8. List two each physical and behavioral indicators of emotional abuse.
9. List four forms of emotional abuse.
10. Compare and discuss primary, secondary, and tertiary levels of intervention, giving two examples of intervention for each level.
11. Describe five factors to assess to elicit signs and symptoms of child abuse when making a home visit to any family.
12. Identify three specific interventions for the abused child.
13. Identify three specific interventions for the parent(s) of abused children.
14. Discuss two common emotional responses by health personnel when faced with situations of child abuse.

History is full of examples of abuse, brutality, and inhumanity toward children. Historically, children were considered property of their parents, with obligations, but no rights. Infanticide was practiced in civilized societies from Ancient Greece to China to eliminate unwanted babies. The story of Moses is well known. Less known, however, is that it was the custom during that time to send unwanted babies down the Nile (McKittrick 1981). During Roman times unwanted children were often mutilated to arouse pity and increase their value as beggars (Radbill 1980). Charles Dickens, in *Oliver Twist*, chronicled the exploitation of children made to toil long hours in sweat shops during the industrial revolution. The Puritan ethic "spare the rod and spoil the child" supported the earlier belief that physical abuse builds character. Child abuse is not new; however, research on child abuse is relatively recent.

In 1946, Caffey was credited with the medical discovery of child abuse. His research, coupled with research of colleagues, on fractures in children of "unspecific origin" led to the belief that these injuries were "deliberately inflicted" (Snyder et al. 1983). In 1962, Kempe and associates published a paper describing the "battered child syndrome" (Kempe et al. 1962). By providing this diagnostic label, Kempe and his associates paved the way for physicians and health care workers to become involved in treating complex family and social problems (Snyder et al. 1983).

It took until 1967 for all states to enact laws against child abuse. Statutes against child abuse vary from state to state. Each state, however, emphasizes protection of children through identification of abuse and provision of services to stabilize conditions for troubled families (Kreitzer 1981). For the first time in history, child abuse was not an acceptable practice in this country.

Awareness and public concern have grown. Increasingly, parents, other significant caretakers, and society in general have been mandated to provide a milieu responsive to children's needs. Reporting of child abuse cases is encouraged by all states providing immunity from legal liability for those persons filing abuse reports. Not only are persons protected by immunity and encouraged to report suspected cases of child abuse or neglect, but *failure to report cases of abuse and neglect may result in civil or criminal penalties* (Kreitzer 1981).

Laws and awareness are, unfortunately, not enough to decrease the incidence of child abuse in the United States. As long as families live in crises and social changes are not forthcoming, the conditions for abuse are ripe. One child in four under the age of six lives in poverty; 25% of the children living in the richest nation on earth do not have their basic needs met (Gabinet

1983). Parents rearing children in poverty are unlikely to have the skills to teach their children to function more effectively as adults than they themselves function (Gabinet 1983). Social realities often lead to family stress. For example, fathers of children living in poverty situations often cannot support their families because they are chronically unemployed. Or, fathers cannot be permanent family members without jeopardizing their families' welfare payments, so they cannot maintain their role as responsible adults (Gabinet 1983).

In addition to the poverty issues, the subject of violence in the United States must be addressed if we are to make long-lasting changes in the treatment of children. Child abuse is only one form of violence. We declare that violence against children is wrong but maintain that violence is acceptable on television, in movies, and even in schools. Role models are critically important in child development, and mixed messages lead to developmental confusion (Whitworth 1985).

Child abuse occurs if the caretaker of that child allows or causes the child to suffer (1) physical harm, (2) mental ill-health, or (3) sexual molestation (Ghent et al. 1985). Today the reported incidence of child abuse is increasing rapidly in all levels of society. *Child abuse occurs in all socioeconomic, racial, cultural, and religious groups.* The number of reported cases in the United States is currently one million per year. It is estimated that only 10–25% of abuse cases are reported. Abuse of infants is one of the leading causes of postneonatal mortality (Fischler 1984).

The effects of abuse last a lifetime. Psychiatric studies have shown that abuse is common in childhood histories of juvenile delinquents, runaways, violent criminals, prostitutes, and parents who, in turn, abuse their children (Fischler 1984). Abuse in childhood can lead to later social and mental maladjustment for the individual. Studies indicate that abused adolescents report more psychopathology, poorer coping skills, higher incidence of multiple personality disorder, and poorer impulse control than nonabused adolescents. Differences are also found in orientation to future vocational and educational goals, as well as peer relationships (Hjorth and Ostrov 1982; Kluft 1987). Child abuse as a maladaptive response to crisis can be conceptualized as illustrated in Figure 11–1.

Standard I: Theory

When working with families of child abuse, it is important to have an understanding of (1) conditions for abuse and (2) types of abuse.

CONDITIONS FOR ABUSE

The phenomenon of child abuse is present in all segments of American society. Theoretically, however, it is thought that one, two, or a combination of three specific factors signal conditions for abuse (Helfer and Kempe 1976). These factors are (1) **abuse-prone parents,** (2) **vulnerable child,** and (3) a crisis situation.

ABUSE-PRONE PARENTS. Parents involved in child abuse situations vary in intelligence and educational background and come from all socioeconomic levels. Abusive parents reflect a cross section of the population and represent all ethnic backgrounds and religious affiliations (Warner 1981).

Specific characteristics, however, have been found either singly or in combination among parents who abuse their children (Warner 1981). Box 11–1 lists some of these characteristics. The abusing parent is most often the mother. Often, the abuser is a stepparent who projects his or her hostility toward the new mate onto the child. At other times, the abuser may be a friend of the parent. Abusive parents are described as socially isolated and suspicious. Often there is little contact with the outside world.

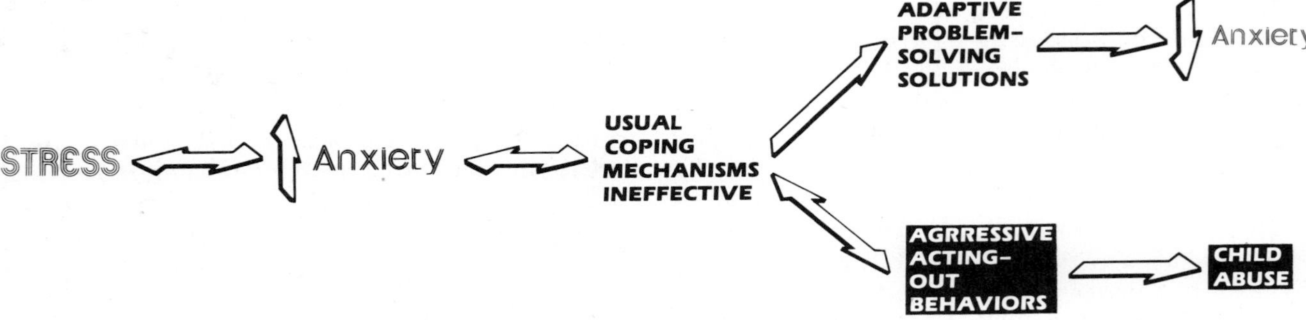

Figure 11–1. *Conceptualization of the process of aggressive acting-out behaviors in the development of child abuse.*

Box 11–1. CHARACTERISTICS OF ABUSING PARENTS

A history of abuse, neglect, or emotional deprivation as a child.
Family authoritarianism—raises children as was raised by own parents.
Low self-esteem, feelings of worthlessness, depression.
Poor coping skills.
Social isolation (may be suspicious of others)—few or no friends, little or no involvement in social or community activities.
Involved in a crisis situation—unemployment, divorce, financial difficulties.
Rigid, unrealistic expectations of child's behavior.
Frequently uses harsh punishment.
History of severe mental illness, such as schizophrenia.
Violent temper outbursts.
Look to child for satisfaction of needs for love, support, and reassurance (often unmet due to parenting deficits in family of origin).
Projects blame onto the child for their "troubles," e.g., stepparent may project hostility toward new mate onto a child.
Lack of effective parenting skills.
Inability to seek help from others.
Perceive the child as bad or evil.
History of drug/alcohol abuse.
Feel little or no control over life.
Low tolerance for frustration.
Poor impulse control.

Data from Warner CG (ed). Conflict Intervention in Social and Domestic Violence. Bowie, MD: Robert J Brady Company, 1981.

Most abusive parents are emotionally isolated and cannot provide for their own emotional needs. They often look to the child to meet their needs and fill an emotional void. The child, requiring nurturing, respect, and affectionate physical care to survive, is unable to meet the parents' enormous emotional needs. The child then becomes the projection of the parents' unhappiness, feelings of rejection, and low self-esteem. The abuse cycle can be operationally defined as follows:

1. A person is brought up in an atmosphere devoid of love, affection, and security.
2. A sense of being valued and cared for never develops.
3. Person is left with tremendous needs for love and security.
4. This person looks to the child to fill the void for love and acceptance.
5. When the child is unable to meet these unrealistic demands, feelings of rejection and anger are mobilized in the parent.
6. Rage and helplessness, coupled with poor impulse control, lead to projection onto the child.

VULNERABLE CHILD. At times, one child in the family is singled out as the recipient of all parental hostility. All the other children may receive adequate parenting. The "scapegoated" child may be the one the parent most identifies with, or the one who reminds him or her of a hated parent or former spouse (Warner 1981). Sometimes the child is different from the other children. The vulnerable child might look different, have a deformity, or be mentally retarded or gifted. Interference with emotional bonding between parents and child has also been found to increase the risk of possible future abuse.

Factors that place a child at risk have been studied (Warner 1981):

1. A child who is a product of an *unwanted pregnancy*, an older child who comes too soon after the marriage, or an unplanned late child.
2. *Early prolonged parent-child separation* as with a premature birth or prolonged illness requiring hospitalization.
3. *Low birth weight baby.*
4. *Child that is difficult to care for*: sickly, hyperactive, colicky, deformed, or retarded.

CRISIS SITUATION. A perfectly normal child may be at risk for abuse in a situation that puts stress and strain in a family with an abuse-prone parent. Stressful life events can tax the abuse-prone parent's coping skills, leaving the parent incapable of dealing with periods of increased stress. Overwhelming life situations tax any person's coping skills. Refer to the Holmes and Masuda stress scale in Chapter 10. A *person with good impulse control who can solve problems and has a healthy support system is less likely to resort to abusive behavior*. A person who projects anger and frustration onto the environment in times of stress is at high risk for an abusive situation.

TYPES OF ABUSE

Four specific types of abuse have been identified: (1) physical abuse, (2) sexual abuse, (3) neglect, and (4) emotional abuse.

PHYSICAL ABUSE. Physical battering and **physical endangerment** are two seriously harmful parental behaviors. **Physical battering** refers to physical assaults such as hitting, kicking, biting, throwing, or burning (Besharov 1983). Parental abuse can occur at any age; however, approximately 32% of victims are under 5 years of age (Fontana 1985). **Physical endangerment** is reckless behavior toward a child that could lead to the child's serious physical injury, such as leaving a young child alone, or placing a child in a hazardous environment.

SEXUAL ABUSE. Sexual abuse is now reported in such numbers that it may well be the most common form of abuse of children. Father-daughter incest exists on a large scale. Father-daughter incest is a violation of law in all 50 states. Incest is usually defined as "sexual intercourse" between "near relatives." Near relatives may be natural or stepchildren (de Chesnay 1984). Sexual intercourse may be described as penis penetration, penetration of inanimate objects, oral sex, and genital fondling (de Chesnay 1984). Included in the definition of incest by the National Center on Child Abuse are those "acts designated to stimulate the child sexually, or use a child for sexual stimulation, either of the perpetrator or of another person" (Sideleau 1982). See Box 11-2 for forms of sexual abuse of children.

Box 11-2. FORMS OF SEXUAL ABUSE OF CHILDREN

Touching, fondling, and physically exploring child's genitalia.
Masturbation by male abuser against child's perineum, buttocks, abdomen, or thighs.
Manual masturbation of abuser by child.
All combinations of oral-genital contact between children of either sex and adults of either sex.
Actual or attempted anal intercourse with child of either sex.
Actual or attempted vaginal intercourse (without force).
Forceful attempt at vaginal intercourse, with local or general trauma.
Exhibitionism.
Voyeurism.
Exploitation of children in preparation of sexually suggestive or pornographic visual materials.

Data from Ghent WR, DaSylva NP, Farren ME. Family violence: Guidelines for recognition and management. Canadian Medical Association Journal, 132(5):545, 1985.

Sexual abuse is thought to happen most often to girls and most frequently between the ages of two and six, when children are most trusting and vulnerable, and again between 12 and 16 years as they develop sexually. As many as one of five girls and one of ten boys may experience some form of sexual abuse during their childhood (Thomas and Rogers 1981). Sexual abuse often goes unreported, since many incest victims are afraid to report incest and families collude to keep the secret (de Chesnay 1984). Another factor in the underreporting of child sexual abuse cases is the problem of denial by professionals (Snyder 1983). The abuser is generally normal in appearance and behavior and usually known to the victim.

There are many nurses today involved in "abuse work." One pioneer in the field of abuse is Ann Burgess. Ann Burgess, D.N.Sc., R.N., a psychiatric nurse, educator, and researcher, began studying the victims of rape in the early 1970's at Boston City Hospital's emergency room. She is now well known as a victimologist and works with victims of incest and other types of sexual violence. She has worked closely with the F.B.I. in closing child sex rings and is a member of the United States Attorney General's Task Force on Family Violence.

NEGLECT. Neglect can be physical, developmental, or educational (Besharov 1983). *Physical neglect* is failure to provide the medical, dental, or psychiatric care needed to prevent or treat physical or emotional illnesses. *Developmental neglect* is failure to provide emotional nurturing and the physical and cognitive stimulation needed to ensure freedom from developmental deficits. *Educational neglect* occurs when a child's caretakers deprive the child of the education provided in accordance with the state's education law (Besharov 1983).

EMOTIONAL ABUSE. Emotional abuse can be difficult to define. Although it does not literally kill the child, it can kill the child's spirit. What dies is the child's ability to succeed later in life, to feel deeply, and to make emotional contact with others. Emotional abuse causes unseen inner changes in a child's mind and personality that permanently alter the child's perception of reality and ability to interact with others (Fortin and Reed 1984). Essentially, emotional abuse and neglect deprive the child of a nurturing atmosphere in which a child can thrive, learn, and develop. Emotional abuse can take the form of:

- terrorizing the child,
- demeaning the child's worth,
- blatant or subtle hostility and hate directed toward the child,
- constantly ignoring the child and his or her needs,
- consistent belittling and criticisms,
- withholding warmth or affection.

Standard II: Data Collection

When a nurse deals with abuse situations, in particular those situations dealing with child abuse, considerations must first be given to (1) the nurse's feelings and (2) the process and setting of the interview. After these considerations have been made, (3) actual assessment for physical and behavioral indicators of abuse is made.

In all other sections and chapters, the feelings and reactions of the nurse are discussed as part of the process of planning nursing care. Certain behaviors and personality characteristics in patients often elicit specific feelings and behaviors on the part of nurses and other health care professionals. These feelings may be either conscious or unconscious. Whatever these feelings are, they most decidedly influence the quality and effectiveness of care given to the patient. Therefore, identifying common feelings and reactions to specific behaviors and situations can help alert the nurse to those feelings and reactions that may be influencing personal attitudes and reactions toward the clients. Dealing with negative or uncomfortable emotions in oneself can maximize successful and effective nursing measures.

However, perhaps more than in any other situation, intense and overwhelming feelings may be aroused when working with a family involved in child abuse. It is for this reason that the feelings and reactions of the nurse are discussed when studying the assessment aspect of nursing care. For it is in the assessment phase of the nursing process that personal prejudices and intense reactions often occur, before interaction with the family has even taken place.

ASSESSING THE NURSE'S FEELINGS

In all areas of psychiatric nursing and counseling, personal emotions and thoughts should be consciously available to the nurse. Strong negative feelings can cloud one's judgment and interfere with intervention no matter how well the nurse or health care professional tries to deny or cover his or her feelings. Common reactions include (1) intense protective feelings and sympathy for the child and (2) anger and outrage toward the abusive parent.

1. Intense feelings of sympathy and protectiveness triggered by the child's pain and vulnerability may lead to "rescue fantasies" in the nurse. When this happens, the nurse projects personal emotional needs onto the child, and the tendency is to exclude the parent(s) and to be the "one to save the child." When the rescue contract is not fulfilled, the child is left more isolated than ever (Sideleau 1982).
2. Outrage and anger toward the parent(s) may lead to removing and keeping the child out of the home until an adequate assessment of the family situation is made. A nurse's rejection of the parents also leads to ignoring the parents' needs. Without the parents' support and involvement in a treatment plan, hope for cessation of abuse is slim.

Interdisciplinary team conferences can be especially helpful in clarifying reactions and neutralizing intense emotions. Information from pediatricians, psychologists, nurses, and social workers can make positive steps in refocusing efforts to work constructively with a family in crisis. Sharing perceptions and feelings with other disciplines can also help reduce feelings of isolation for nurses and lessen the feelings of responsibility for the child.

Nurses come from a cross section of the population. Many are mothers or fathers; some may have been victims of abuse as children; most come from a variety of cultures and hold various ethical beliefs regarding child rearing and what constitutes abuse. Health care professionals should evaluate their own attitudes toward violence. Is nonviolence a lifestyle that the nurse actively advocates and models?

Whatever beliefs or feelings a nurse holds, *nurses have a legal responsibility to report suspected or actual cases of child abuse.* A nurse who suspects child abuse is still **legally responsible for reporting suspicions,** even if the attending physician disagrees with the suspicion.

THE PROCESS AND SETTING OF THE INTERVIEW

Important and relevant information about the family situation can be gathered from the conversations with the parent(s) and the child. A great deal of tact, understanding, and thought needs to go into planning an interview with the suspected abusive parent and the child. A parent who feels judged or accused of wrongdoing will most likely become defensive, and any attempts at changing coping strategies in the family will be thwarted. Important guidelines for interviewing parents in abusive or suspected abusive situations have been set (Table 11 – 1) (Heindl et al. 1979).

Ideally, a relationship built on concern and carried out in an atmosphere that is nonjudgmental is best. Statements such as, "It must be difficult to care for three small children when there is little food in the house," or "Being responsible for two children without the help of family or friends must be hard on you," are more apt to elicit important data that will help the nurse and parent

Table 11–1 • INTERVIEW WITH THE PARENT OF AN ABUSED CHILD OR A CHILD SUSPECTED OF BEING ABUSED

DO	DON'T
1. Conduct the interview in private.	1. Do NOT try to "prove" abuse by accusations or demands.
2. Be direct, honest, and professional.	2. Do NOT display horror, anger, or disapproval of parent(s) or situation.
3. Be understanding.	3. Do NOT place blame or make judgments about the parent(s) or child.
4. Be attentive.	
5. Inform them if you must make a referral to Child Protective Services and explain the process.	

plan more effective alternatives and coping strategies. When the parent is informed that Child Protective Services must be contacted, it should be emphasized that the referral is not punishment, but an attempt to safeguard the child and obtain help for the family. The nurse should also tell the parent(s) that the child has been assured that there will be no punishment for telling the medical personnel about the situation (Heindl et al. 1979).

Questions that are open-ended and require a descriptive response can be less threatening and elicit more relevant information than questions that are direct or can be answered yes or no. Some examples follow:

- *What arrangements do you make when you have to leave your child alone?*
- *How do you punish your child?*
- *When your infant cries for a long time, how do you get him to stop?*
- *What does your child do that makes you cry?*

Openness and directness about the child's situation strengthen the relationship with the parent(s), rather than the reverse. Important suggestions for talking with a child who has been or is suspected of having been abused are listed in Table 11–2 (Heindl et al. 1979).

While interviewing the child, a calm and relaxed attitude is extremely important to lower the anxiety in the child. The nurse should sit near the child, not behind a desk, and the interview should be private and uninterrupted. Spend some time establishing a rapport with the child before focusing in on the details of the abuse experience. Use terminology that the child will understand. Reassure the child that he will not be punished or hurt and that he did not do anything wrong. Children should not feel pressured to talk about topics they are unwilling or unable to discuss. The experience should be nonthreatening and supportive and not resemble a trial or inquisition. Preschoolers may be better able to express their experiences through playing out the incident with dolls or with drawings (Kelly 1984). Open-ended questions are best. Questions that may be asked include the following:

- *How did this happen to you?*
- *Who takes care of you?*
- *What do you do after school?*
- *Who are your friends?*
- *What happens when you do something wrong?*

ASSESSING PHYSICAL AND BEHAVIORAL INDICATORS OF ABUSE

PHYSICAL ABUSE. Nonspecific bruising in older children is common. Any bruises on an infant less than six months old should be considered with suspicion. A specific type of physical abuse to which young children are more susceptible is shaking. They are more vulnerable because of their relatively large head size and weight, weak neck muscles, thin, friable central nervous system vasculature, and soft, less myelinated brain tissue. The baby who has been shaken may often present respiratory problems. If the pulmonary exam is normal, the possibility of rigorous shaking must be considered. Full, bulging fontanelles and a head circumference greater than the 90th percentile are also suspicious. Shaking can cause intracranial hemorrhage leading to cerebral edema and death (Ludwig 1984). Table 11–3 lists the physical and behavioral indicators of all types of physical abuse.

Along with recognition of the indicators of physical child abuse, nurses should note the alleged method of injury. Inconsistent explanations serve as a warning that further investigation is necessary. Vague explanations such as "the child fell from a chair, a lap, down the stairs; the child was running away; the hot water was turned on by mistake" should alert the nurse to possible abuse (Ghent et al. 1985).

Table 11-2 • INTERVIEW WITH THE CHILD WHO HAS BEEN ABUSED OR IS SUSPECTED OF HAVING BEEN ABUSED

DO	DON'T
1. Conduct the interview in private.	1. Do NOT allow the child to feel "in trouble" or "at fault."
2. Sit next to the child, not across the table or desk.	2. Do NOT suggest answers to the child.
3. Tell the child that the interview is confidential.	3. Do NOT probe or press for answers the child is not willing to give.
4. Use language the child understands.	4. Do NOT display shock or disapproval of parents, child, or situation.
5. Ask the child to clarify words that you do not understand.	5. Do NOT force the child to remove clothing.
6. Tell the child if any future action will be required.	6. Do NOT conduct the interview with a group of interviewers.

SEXUAL ABUSE. The increasing evidence of sexual abuse of children, e.g., father-daughter incest and sexual abuse of young children in day care centers, Boy Scouts, and church groups, has been receiving more attention and concern. Unfortunately, there is a drastic lack of documentation by health care professionals of medical and social data in cases of sexual abuse (Orr 1978; Finkelhor 1984). Nurses and other health care professionals need to be familiar with the physical and behavioral indicators of sexual abuse as presented in Table 11-4. Once these indicators have been identified, and the possibility of sexual abuse is suspected,

Table 11-3 • PHYSICAL AND BEHAVIORAL INDICATORS OF PHYSICAL ABUSE

PHYSICAL INDICATORS	BEHAVIORAL INDICATORS
Unexplained bruises and welts of varying age: • on face, lips, mouth • on torso, back, buttocks, thighs • in various stages of healing • clustered forming regular patterns • reflecting shape of article used to inflict (e.g., electrical cord, belt buckle) • on several different surface areas • regular appearance after absence, weekend, or vacation • human bites • fingernail indentations Unexplained burns: • small, circular burns—cigar or cigarette burns, especially on soles, palms, back, or buttocks • immersion burns, socklike, glovelike • patterned like electrical burner, iron, etc. • rope burns on arms, legs, neck, or torso Unexplained fractures or dislocations (especially in children under one year): • to skull, nose, facial structure • in various stages of healing • multiple spiral fractures • dislocation of shoulder or hip Unexplained lacerations or abrasions of varying age: • to mouth, lips, gums, eyes • to external genitalia Other: • bald patches on the scalp • subdural hematoma in a child under two years • retinal hemorrhage	Wary of adult contacts Apprehensive when other children cry Behavioral extremes: • aggressiveness or • withdrawal Frightened of parents or constant effort to please parents Afraid to go home Reports injury by parents Monosyllabic speech Ability to withstand examination and painful procedures with little movement or crying Indiscriminate seeking of affection Goes to extremes (including misbehaving) to call attention to self

Data from Heindl C, et al. The nurse's role in the presentation and treatment of child abuse and neglect. (Pub. 79-30202.) Washington DC: U.S. Department of Health, Education and Welfare, August, 1979.

Table 11–4 • PHYSICAL AND BEHAVIORAL INDICATORS OF SEXUAL ABUSE

PHYSICAL INDICATORS	BEHAVIORAL INDICATORS
Difficulty in walking or sitting Vulvovaginitis Torn, stained, or bloody underclothing Pain or itching in genital area Bruises or bleeding in external genitalia, vaginal, or anal areas Venereal disease, especially in pre-teens Pregnancy Evidence of physical manipulation of the vagina Evidence of foreign body in the vagina In boys, pain on urination or penile swelling or discharge	Unwilling to change for gym or participate in physical education class Seductive behavior Withdrawal, fantasy, or infantile behavior (regression) Bizarre, sophisticated, or unusual sexual behavior or knowledge Phobias: • fear of the dark, men, strangers, leaving the house Poor peer relationships Delinquent or runaway—severe acting out Profound personality change: • depression, aggression, decline in school performance Reports sexual assault by caretaker Self-destructive behavior: • alcohol/drug abuse • attempted suicide

Data from Heindl C, et al. The nurse's role in the presentation and treatment of child abuse and neglect. (Pub. 79-30202.) Washington DC: U.S. Department of Health, Education & Welfare, August, 1979.

appropriate action must be taken to protect the child from further devastating emotional and physical effects of sexual abuse.

NEGLECT. Neglect of a child may stem from a number of different sources. Lack of coordination between a parent's actions and the cues of the child can result in neglect of a child's needs. When a parent does not know what to do or what an infant wants or a child needs, the neglect is benign. When the parent is well intentioned, response to educational efforts is healthy and constructive. Education combined with support is sufficient to create positive change. However, neglect may also stem from hostility of a parent toward the child, signaling a serious disturbance in the parent-child relationship. In such a case, education is not sufficient, and more rigorous interventions are needed to safeguard the child from permanent physical and emotional handicaps. Neglected children often appear undernourished, dirty, and poorly clothed. Neglect is also manifested by inadequate medical care, e.g., lack of immunizations or untreated ear infections. Specific physical and behavioral indicators of neglect are listed in Table 11–5.

EMOTIONAL ABUSE. Any child who is neglected or physically or sexually abused is most certainly emotionally abused as well. Emotional abuse leaves tremendous scars throughout the person's adult life. Emotional abuse robs the child of the potential for living a full and meaningful life unless interventions are made along the way to bolster self-esteem and heal the anguish and isolation instilled in the place of love and acceptance. Table 11–6 lists the physical and emotional indicators of emotional abuse.

Table 11–5 • PHYSICAL AND BEHAVIORAL INDICATORS OF NEGLECT

PHYSICAL INDICATORS	BEHAVIORAL INDICATORS
Consistent hunger, poor hygiene, inappropriate dress (for weather conditions) Consistent lack of supervision, especially in dangerous activities or for long periods Unattended physical problems or medical or dental needs Abandonment Poor growth patterns: underweight, failure to thrive	Begging, stealing food Extended stays at school (early arrival and late departure) Constant fatigue, listlessness, or falling asleep in class; dull, inactive (in infants also) Alcohol or drug abuse Psychosomatic complaints Delinquency (e.g., thefts) Assumes adult responsibilities States there is no caretaker

Data from Heindl C, et al. The nurse's role in the presentation and treatment of child abuse and neglect. (Pub. 79-30202.) Washington DC: U.S. Department of Health, Education & Welfare, August, 1979.

Table 11–6 • PHYSICAL AND BEHAVIORAL INDICATORS OF EMOTIONAL ABUSE

PHYSICAL INDICATORS	BEHAVIORAL INDICATORS
Speech disorders Lag in physical development	Habit disorders (sucking, biting, rocking, head banging, feeding problems) Conduct disorder (antisocial, destructive, etc.) Difficulty in learning and living up to full potential Neurotic trait (sleep disorders, inhibition of play, unusual fearfulness) Psychoneurotic reaction (hysteria, obsession, compulsion, phobias, hypochondriasis) Behavior extremes: • compliant, passive • aggressive, demanding Overly adaptive behavior • inappropriately adult or inappropriately infantile • "on guard"—trying to please everyone Developmental lag (mental, emotional) Suicide attempt

Data from Heindl C, et al. The nurse's role in the presentation and treatment of child abuse and neglect. (Pub. 79-30202.) Washington DC: U.S. Department of Health, Education & Welfare, August, 1979.

MAINTAINING ACCURATE RECORDS

Because of the possibility of legal action, it is essential that the **medical/nursing record** contain an accurate and detailed description of the child's medical history, the psychosocial history of the family, and observations of the family interactions during the interviews. Especially important in documenting findings from initial assessment are (1) verbatim statements of both child and parent(s), (2) a body map to indicate areas and types of injuries, and (3) physical evidence, when possible, of sexual abuse.

If the abuse occurred recently, or the child is in distress, an immediate extended interview by a child protective worker may be required. Hospitalization or foster home placement may be considered. Hospitalization may be preferred because it is not as threatening to parents. It allows for thorough medical investigation, complete assessment of the child's emotional development, and observation of the parent-child interaction. It is often easier subsequently for the child protective worker to establish rapport with the parents, to identify the major problems, and to begin to plan for ongoing treatment with other members of the health team (Ghent et al. 1985).

Standard III: Diagnosis

In cases of child abuse, there will most likely be a number of areas of concern and problems resulting from the abuse as well as the actual issue of the child's immediate safety. Initially, the focus may be on the child, especially if there is imminent threat to physical safety; however, the problem is a problem of a system in crisis. Nursing diagnoses should reflect the concern for the child's immediate safety and welfare as well as the concerns that reflect focus on support and interventions for the family. Most child abuse situations will warrant at least one of the following possible nursing diagnoses.

The most immediate concern is for the child's safety. *Potential for injury* related to violent parent/neglect/sexual assault/constant ridicule/confinement needs to be explored first. *Pain* related to physical injury or trauma would most certainly take high priority and would need immediate attention. *Panic* or *severe levels of anxiety* related to fear of retaliation/fear of doing something wrong/confusion or isolation/fear of separation from parents may also be a nursing diagnosis that would need immediate intervention. A clear understanding of the child's perspective and experience is important in planning, and high levels of anxiety in the nurse can distort the nurse's assessment and understanding. *Altered nutrition, less than body requirements*, related to neglect/poverty/educational deficit may also be an area of intervention. *Disturbance in self-esteem* would most definitely be an area that would necessitate interventions and should be ongoing, especially after the immediate crisis has subsided.

The nursing diagnosis *altered parenting* must be included. This diagnosis could be related to physical/psychosocial abuse of the nurturing figure, unmet social and emotional maturational needs of parenting figures, or mental or physical illness, to name but a few (Kim

1989). Whatever the related area, interventions and support must be made available if positive change in the family system is to occur. *Altered family process* related to situational or maturational crisis may apply. Situational crisis may be divorce, loss of a loved one, financial problems, illness, or loss of employment. Maturational crises may occur with adolescence, aging, pregnancy, or retirement.

Standard IV: Planning

Planning interventions always includes planning on both the (1) content level and the (2) process level. The content level is the actual setting up of client-centered goals and designing nursing interventions that facilitate meeting the goals. The process level of planning care involves the recognition of common reactions and emotions that may be evoked in health professionals by specific client behaviors. Awareness of how to deal effectively with strong feelings and reactions is important in maximizing patient care. Intense feelings, either positive or negative, can interfere with judgment, attitudes, and reactions to our patients whether on a conscious or an unconscious level. As previously mentioned, awareness on the part of the nurse of common reactions experienced by other health care workers can aid the nurse in identifying those personal feelings in him- or herself that could both affect the experience of the interactions as well as interfere with the effectiveness of the nurse. Intense unexamined feelings toward patients can lead to power struggles, mutual lowering of self-esteem, and mutual withdrawal.

CONTENT LEVEL—PLANNING GOALS

Appropriate interventions for families in abusive situations are directly dependent upon the goals set for the family unit. The specific goals will depend upon the nursing diagnosis and specifically that aspect of the nursing diagnosis as formulated in the assessment. For example, the goals for *altered nutrition, less than body requirements, related to neglect* would not be the same as for *altered nutrition related to educational deficits*. Goals for a child who is in a violent, physically abusive situation that could include fear of retaliation from parent(s) would be different from those for a child in *severe levels of anxiety* related to fear of separation from parents. Goals devised for a child in a dangerous physically abusive situation could include the following:

1. Actual injury related to violent parent.
   - Child will be safe until adequate home and family assessment is made by (state the date).
   - Child will be treated by physician and receive medical care for injuries within one hour.
   - Child will participate with therapist (nurse, social worker, counselor) for the purpose of therapy and emotional support (art, play, group, or other) within 24 hours.
   - Child will know what plans are made for his or her protection and will state them to the nurse after decision is made by health team.

Goals for a parent in family crises involving child abuse could include the following

1. Altered family process related to illness of one parent and difficulty with finances.
   - Within 24 hours, parent(s) will be able to name and call three agencies that can help financially during the crises.
   - By the end of the first interview, parent(s) will be able to name two places to contact to discuss feelings of rage and helplessness.
   - Within two weeks, parent(s) will be able to name three alternative actions to take when feelings of helplessness and rage start to surface.
   - By (state the date) parent(s) will state that group meetings with other parents who have battered are useful.
   - Parent(s) and child will share in two planned pleasurable activities twice a day, when child returns to the home.

PROCESS LEVEL—NURSES' REACTIONS AND FEELINGS

The intense emotions and reactions evoked in health care professionals have been discussed in this chapter under *Standard II: Data Collection*. Ideally, other members of the health team are available to assess, evaluate, and plan intervention for what is often a complex and multiproblem family in crisis. Recognizing, expressing, and working through many of the feelings aroused in situations of family violence facilitate planning and interventions for the interdisciplinary team. Ideally, there should be a pediatrician, a nurse, a psychiatrist, a social worker, and an attorney available to the family or child.

Standard V: Intervention

When child abuse is suspected, a report should be made to the appropriate child protective agency designated by each state. Reports can be filed by health professionals, social service personnel, law enforcement personnel, educators, and any other professional person working with children (Kreitzer 1981). The appropriate state agency may be the state or county child welfare agency, law enforcement agency, juvenile court, or county health department.

Each state has specific guidelines for reporting. **However, each state mandates that a report must be filed when "suspected" abuse or neglect is encountered.** State guidelines include whether the report can be oral or written or both, time allowed to elapse after suspicion of abuse or neglect (stat, 24, or 48 hours), and statements as to protection from legal liability for persons filing an abuse report "in good faith" (Kreitzer 1981).

Determining the degree of pathology in a given case of child abuse is essential before specific interventions are mobilized. The degree of pathology can be measured by

- the severity of the child's condition at the time of diagnosis,
- the degree of hostility in the parent-child interaction, and
- the specific psychological conflicts or social stresses interfering with successful caregiving.

Studies have shown that a more positive prognosis correlates with (1) early diagnosis, (2) relative lack of hostility in the parent-child interaction, and (3) the quality of the parent's experiences of nurturance as a child (Haynes et al. 1984). Selecting the appropriate treatment, maintaining compliance, coordinating the various disciplines, and evaluating results are essential for attainment of goals (Fischler 1984).

Certain axioms of management have been identified in the literature (Snyder 1983) and can be used as guides for implementing care:

1. Once diagnosed, abused children are at great risk for reinjury or neglect.
2. When the child is reinjured, parents often go to a different medical facility.
3. If the child is at major risk, hospitalization is appropriate to allow for interdisciplinary assessment.
4. Protection of the child is the principal goal of intervention; however, protection must go hand-in-hand with a family-oriented service plan.
5. Frequent multidisciplinary follow-up is key to encouraging healthy child development and monitoring family stress.
6. Simply reporting a case to a public agency may not be sufficient to protect an abused child or to help the family.

Primary prevention in cases of child abuse are those measures that are taken to prevent or reduce the occurrence of abusive situations. The aim of the interventions in primary prevention is to prevent maladaptive behaviors or disease by promoting optimum help. Identifying people in high risk categories, providing health teaching, and coordinating supportive services to prevent crises are examples of primary prevention.

Secondary prevention involves early intervention in abusive situations to minimize their disabling or long term effects. Nurses providing secondary prevention work with families and other members of the health team to help these abusive families find alternative ways to deal with stress. Community resources are mobilized (schools, clinics, homemaker agencies, and more) to relieve overwhelming stress and to offer alternative outlets for emotions. Secondary prevention is often carried out in an outpatient setting.

Tertiary prevention involves interventions aimed at maintaining or reducing the severity of mental illness or handicaps resulting from chronic abusive trauma. Examples of settings for tertiary care are psychiatric inpatient units, day care hospitals, and group homes.

V-A: PSYCHOTHERAPEUTIC INTERVENTIONS

Inpatient Setting—Secondary Prevention

CHILD. When physical injury from suspected child abuse warrants or when further assessment is needed by a multidisciplinary team to further evaluate suspected child abuse, the child should be hospitalized.

Failure to provide an abused child with psychological rehabilitation can result in serious emotional and cognitive deficits in the future. Objectives for working with the hospitalized abused or neglected child include the following (Smith 1981):

1. An environment that fosters trust, e.g., consistency on the part of staff and clear explanations of all routines and procedures.
2. Warmth and affection coupled with reasonable limits.

3. Socialization with age-mates and adults. Organized play and school-promoted socialization.
4. Encouragement of maintenance of the child-parent relationship.
5. Promotion of the child's physical recovery through physical care, adequate nutrition, and treatments.
6. Encouragement of the expression of feelings either verbally or through play or art modalities.

ABUSIVE PARENT. An abusive parent usually requires treatment over long periods of time and the involvement of a number of people and groups (Smith 1981). The relationship the abusive parent establishes with the nurse and other members of the health team is predictive of continued family involvement in treatment. Efforts to decrease the family's defensiveness and increase family participation in resolving their crisis are necessary steps before more ambitious goals can be met. Some initial objectives that can lessen parents' guilt and anxiety while the child is hospitalized are listed here (Smith 1981).

1. Provide information in neutral and supportive terms of what is being planned for them and their child. Parents need to be oriented to the hospital routines.
2. Encourage identification and evaluation of parental strengths; give recognition for positive efforts toward change.
3. Encourage parent-child interactions, i.e., feeding, bathing, or socializing.
4. Support parents while encouraging their acceptance of assistance from nurses, physicians, and social workers on the child abuse team.
5. Provide role models that encourage alternative ways of handling feelings, dealing with children, and interacting with others.

Careful documentation of the child, parent, and the parent-child interactions need to be made available to the other health care personnel involved with the child's case (Smith 1981).

V-B: HEALTH TEACHING

Health teaching is one of the most important aspects of primary prevention. The first line of intervention is prevention through health education. Family education in maternity and well-baby clinics, day care centers, and schools can go a long way in preventing abusive situations. Childbirth classes as well as parenting classes directed to all levels of child development should be readily available.

Nurses can be invaluable during a family pregnancy. Encouraging the couple to discuss their feelings and expectations for the baby and assessing areas of strength and areas that could be problematic for the couple should be done (Ghent et al. 1985). Emotional support for the mother during pregnancy and a shared birth experience have been linked to the amount of emotional support a mother will provide to her baby later in infancy (Lally 1984). Once the child is born, positive emotional connections between parents and children can be stimulated by maximizing the opportunity for emotional bonding at birth and during the first few days of life. To achieve this end, parents should be allowed privacy with their infants for 30–60 minutes after birth. The infant should remain undressed. Skin contact and touch should be maximized (Lally 1984). Rooming-in for the baby while the mother is in the hospital is very important for bonding. At this time, parents should be given maximal support, encouragement, and teaching by nurses.

Recognition of an abuse-prone parent before abuse takes place is possible. Nurses who work on a maternity unit are often in a position to spot potential abusive situations in new mothers and to initiate appropriate interventions including education about effective parenting techniques. Mothers who stand out for special attention include

1. New mothers whose behavior toward the infant is rejecting, hostile, or indifferent.
2. Teenage mothers—most are children themselves and require special help and guidance in handling the baby and discussing their expectations of the baby and their support system.
3. Retarded mothers—careful, explicit, and repeated instructions on caring for the child and recognizing the infant's needs are indicated.
4. Mothers who were abused as children or abused by a spouse—women who were abused as children, or women in abusive situations are more likely to abuse their child than a person who has lived without physical and emotional violence.

Nurses who work in maternity and in the nursery can also recognize the vulnerable child. Knowing that specific children are at risk, referrals to community resources are in order. These may include emergency child care facilities, emergency telephone numbers, numbers of 24-hour crisis centers or hotlines, and respite programs, where volunteers take the child for an occasional weekend so that parents can get some relief. Public health nurses can make home visits. Home visits allow for assessment of potential abuse situations in the crucial first few months of life. This early period is when the style of parent-child interactions is set for later life. Nurses in clinical and public health settings make such observations, which are fundamental in casefinding and evaluation (Snyder 1983). Important factors the public health nurse can assess are noted in Box 11–3.

V-E: THERAPEUTIC ENVIRONMENT

All children need reassurance, emotional warmth, and validation. Children who have been abused are especially in need of warmth and acceptance. Specific treatments such as play therapy or stimulation are indicated for these children. Unfortunately, facilities for these specialized interventions are meager. At best, children are offered day care, time away from home in a nurturing setting. Usually, however, children are placed in foster care.

Foster care is often very disruptive for children. Placement in foster care often involves substantial risk to the child's health and emotional development. The usual purpose of foster care is to provide a temporary home-like environment where safety and nurturance can take place. The stated purpose is to provide the child an environment in which injuries can heal and normal development can take place while parents seek treatment. Ideally, foster care should be therapeutic for children and should prepare them to return home or to be adopted (Fischler 1984).

Unfortunately, foster parents receive no special training on how to interact effectively with a troubled child. Consequently, if a child acts out, foster parents often request that the child be removed from the home. The child then goes to another home, then another, and becomes part of a revolving door pattern of repeated foster home placements. The constant experience of separation further reinforces the child's insecurity, poor self-concept, and negative behaviors.

In order to maintain a therapeutic environment when the child is out of the home and under foster care, supervision is necessary. Periodic review of all children in foster care should be conducted routinely to ensure that proper planning is ongoing.

Whenever possible, the goal of intervention is to keep the family together. Interventions are geared toward stabilizing the home situation and maintaining a violence-free environment. Ideally, interventions offered would leave options for growth, increase in self-esteem, and a higher quality of life for all family members.

Providing and maintaining a therapeutic environment in the home involves three levels of help for abusing families (Taskinen 1984):

1. Provide the family with economic support and social services, such as family service agencies.
2. Arrange social support in the form of a public health nurse, lay home visitor, day care teacher, school teacher, social worker, or any other potential contact person with a good relationship with the family or child.
3. Therapy for the family and, where necessary, hospital care for the child.

Day care centers for small children can help relieve the caregiver and offer her a few hours to herself. Homemakers, brought into the home to help with direct household assistance, can reduce feelings of being overwhelmed. Some communities offer parent-aid programs. Nonprofessionals are trained to work with and relate closely with abusing and neglecting parents.

Failures in interventions with abusive families are

Box 11–3. FACTORS TO ASSESS DURING A HOME VISIT

Responsiveness to infant crying.
Responsiveness to infant signals related to feeding.
Caregiver facial expressions in response to infant.
Holding of the child.
Playfulness of caregiver with infant.
Type of physical contact during feeding.
Temperament of the infant: average, quiet, or active.
Parent's attitudes signaling possible warnings:

- complaints of inadequacy as a parent
- complaints of inadequacy of the child
- fear of "doing something wrong"
- attribution of badness to the newborn
- history of a destructive childhood
- misdirected anger
- continued evidence of isolation, apathy, anger, frustration, projection
- adult conflict

Environmental conditions:

- sleeping arrangements
- child management
- home management
- use of supports (formal and informal)

Need for immediate services for situational (economics, child care), emotional, or educational information, i.e.,

- sharing information about hotlines, babysitters, homemakers, parent groups
- sharing information about child development
- child care and home management

Data from Ghent et al. 1985; Lally 1984; and Pawl 1984.

often not due to our lack or theirs, but to deficits in the social, economic, and political systems in which we live (Lally 1984). Our society needs to believe that "being a parent is not only a right but a privilege, and that being valued and protected as a child is not merely a privilege but a right." Often our institutions demonstrate the opposite (Pawl 1984).

V-F: PSYCHOTHERAPY

CHILD. Psychotherapy is practiced by persons with advanced training: psychiatric nurses, psychiatric social workers, psychologists, and psychiatrists. Therapeutic experiences permit the child to explore his or her feelings and make corrective changes. A child crippled by ambivalent, negative, and confused feelings is unable to grow into a happy, confident, and fulfilled adult (Drake 1984).

Since children often have difficulty identifying or discussing painful feelings, alternative modes of therapy are often successful. Play therapy and art therapy are frequently used modalities to help children explore their feelings. For children, especially those children who have been sexually abused, expression through art, in contrast to verbalization, is often a less threatening way to communicate confusing and painful emotions (Kelly 1984).

ABUSIVE PARENTS. Since violence begets violence, many parents who abuse their children were themselves abused. Parents who have been abused themselves have tremendous unmet needs and feelings of low self-esteem and tend to project blame for their actions on others. Often distrustful of others, abusive families are often isolated and poorly socialized in their community. Refer to Box 11-1 for characteristics of abusive parents. Therapeutic efforts are long term, and a multidisciplinary approach as well as community services are needed to be successful. Useful therapies include (1) individual, (2) family, and (3) group therapy.

Individual Therapy. Individual therapy is often indicated, particularly when individual psychopathology is identified and sexual abuse has occurred. For example, a parent who is identified as psychotic, borderline, drug dependent, or depressed usually needs immediate and rigorous medical and psychiatric follow-up.

Family Therapy. Therapy, however, should always involve the whole family. Since family violence is a symptom of a family in crisis, each part of the family system needs attention. Since change in one member of the family system effects change in the whole system, support and understanding are needed by all members.

Group Therapy. Group therapy for parent(s) who abuse children can offer isolated and suspicious parents the opportunity to identify with others. Sharing with others who have similar problems can help minimize feelings of isolation and allow mutual problem solving for handling overwhelming feelings.

Self-help groups such as Parents Anonymous and Parents United serve a vital function for abusive parents. Hotlines, such as Childline Hotline, provide emergency resources when parents feel overwhelmed and enraged.

Standard VI: Evaluation

Evaluation should be done by all members of the health team on an ongoing basis. Since child abuse is a symptom of a family in distress, diagnosis, interventions, and evaluation should be carried out by a multidisciplinary team. Ideally, a team would include a pediatrician, a nurse, a social worker, a psychiatrist, and an attorney. Unfortunately, conditions are not always ideal.

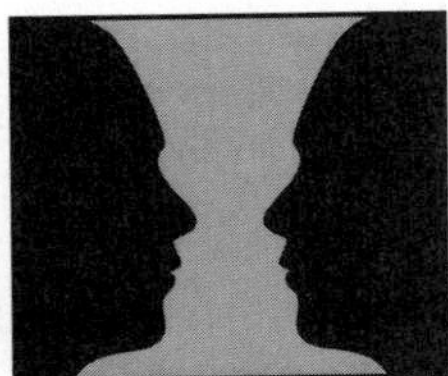

Case Study: Working With a Family Involved With Child Abuse

Billy John, four years old, was brought into the emergency room with second-degree burns on his right hand. Mary frequently babysits for Billy and for his younger brother Jimmy, two, and older brother Tom, six. Mary appeared apprehensive and stated she was very concerned. Mary told the nurse, Ms. Douglas, that the children have told her in the past that Billy's mother has threatened the children with burning if they did not behave. Billy told her that once his mother had held his hands on a cold stove and told him if he was bad, she would burn him. Mary was shocked that Billy's mother would do such a thing, but at the same time, she mentioned she felt guilty for "telling on Mrs. John." Mary also stated that the older brother, six-year-old Tom, told Mary what had happened but was afraid that if his mother found out she would burn him also. Mary stated that she is aware that the mother hits the children, but she didn't believe that anyone could burn her own child.

Ms. Douglas reported what had happened to the physician, and the mother was called and asked to come to the clinic.

Assessment

Billy appeared frightened and in pain. The nurse, Ms. Douglas, asked Mary to come with Billy while she examined him.

NURSE: Tell me about your hand, Billy.
Billy looked down and started to cry
NURSE: It's O.K. if you don't want to talk about it, Billy.
BILLY: *Not looking at the nurse, he says softly,* My mommy burned my hand on the stove.
NURSE: Tell me what happened before that happened.
BILLY: Mommy was mad because I didn't put my toys away.
NURSE: What does your mommy usually do when she gets mad?
BILLY: She yells mostly, sometimes she hits us. Mommy is going to be so mad at Tommy for telling.
NURSE: Tell me about the hitting.
BILLY: Mommy hits us a lot since daddy left us.
Billy starts to cry to himself.

Upon examination the nurse notices a ringed pattern of burns across Billy's right palm like those of a burner of an electric stove. There are blisters on the fingers. Billy appears well nourished and properly dressed. Billy is at his approximate developmental age except for some language delay.

Ms. Douglas divided the data into objective and subjective components.

OBJECTIVE DATA

1 Second-degree burns across right palm, like those of an electric burner
2 Child is well nourished
3 Child is properly clothed
4 Child is up to developmental level

SUBJECTIVE DATA

1 "Mommy burned my hand on the stove."
2 Brother afraid of retaliation for telling Mary what happened
3 Mother threatened children with burning if they "don't behave"
4 Mother often hits children when "mad"
5 Recent separation in the family unit
6 Physical abuse seems to have escalated since father left the family

Nursing Diagnosis

Based on the data, the nurse made the following diagnoses:

1. *Actual Injury* related to poor impulse control of parent, as evidenced by burn on right palm and history of hitting
   - Second-degree burns on right hand.
   - "Mommy burned my hand on the stove."
   - Reports of being hit by mother in the past.
   - Mother often hits children when "mad."
2. *Altered Family Process* related to actual physical abuse and change in the family unit.
   - Father recently left family unit.
   - Physical abuse seems to have escalated since separation.
   - Mother often hits children when "mad."
3. *Fear* related to retaliation from mother as evidenced by feelings of dread in children
   - Children threatened with burning "if they don't behave."
   - Brother afraid he will be punished for "telling" on mother.
   - Mother often hits children when "mad."

Planning

CONTENT LEVEL — PLANNING GOALS

Because of the physical evidence and history, there was a strong suspicion of child abuse. Children's Protective Service was notified by the clinical nurse. The Children's Protective Service requested an evaluation of the family situation for possible placement of Billy in protective custody. In Washington state, the evaluation is done by a local police officer. The officer interviewed the clinical nurse, the child, and the mother. His initial evaluation was that there was no indication of serious potential harm to the child, and Billy should return home.

Continued on following page

Planning *(Continued)*

Ms. Douglas found Billy's mother to be defensive and very angry when she initially tried to talk to her. Shortly, however, Billy's mother started to cry, stating that she can't cope with being alone and doesn't know where to turn.

The nurse devised a plan of care for the family based on her initial nursing diagnoses.

Nursing Diagnosis	Long Term Goals	Short Term Goals
1. *Actual Injury* related to poor impulse control of parent, as evidenced by burn on right palm and history of hitting	Complete healing of burns by (state date).	1. Billy's wounds will show signs of healing by third day after being dressed. 2. Mother will state she is comfortable changing the dressing at home by the end of the first visit.
2. *Altered Family Process* related to actual physical abuse and change in family unit	Mother will use two new appropriate disciplinary techniques by (state date).	1. By end of initial interview, mother will state she wants support to help her channel frustration more appropriately. 2. Mother will state she feels more support in parenting role by next appointment. 3. Mother will name three actions she can take when feeling overwhelmed in the future by (state the date). 4. Mother will begin to practice alternative discipline techniques based on natural consequences within three weeks.
3. *Fear* related to retaliation from mother as evidenced by feelings of dread in children	Children will state and show by behavior feelings of safety and comfort around mother.	1. Tom and mother will spend 15 minutes twice a day talking or engaged in play activity.

PROCESS LEVEL—NURSES' REACTIONS AND FEELINGS

Ms. Douglas has been working with abusive families for five years. She has worked through many of her own feelings of initial anger at parents and rage at the brutality inflicted onto young children by others in the household. Most often her first reaction would be to want the child out of the home and to find a "proper and good" home for the child. She still becomes upset at times and angry toward parents. Her anger now is usually lessened by talking to other members of the health team where interventions are focused onto the family unit. She realizes now that each member of the health team has had similar feelings and thoughts, and sharing these is vital to prevent burnout and to gain a sense of validation and support. Ms. Douglas remembers a time when she was thinking of asking for a transfer. At that time she didn't think she could handle her intense feelings of anger.

Intervention

The local police officer and the health team thought that the degree of pathology in this case was mild. The mother seemed to care for her children but appeared overwhelmed by the separation from the father and the degree of isolation from others in her community. The children seemed to be well nourished and properly clothed and were at or near their developmental level. Planning was focused on (1) Billy's immediate health needs, (2) finding a number of supports for the mother to facilitate her being able to cope with the crises, (3) helping the mother to identify

Intervention *(Continued)*

other means of expressing her anger and interacting with her children, and (4) increasing feelings of security in the children. Specific interventions are identified in the Nursing Care Plan for a Family Involved With Child Abuse (Nursing Care Plan 11–1).

Evaluation

Mrs. John, Billy's mother, kept the clinic appointment one week later. Ms. Douglas examined Billy's hand, and the burn seemed to be healing well. Mrs. John, the mother, seemed more relaxed and asked what to do about her son Tom's cold.

Mrs. John stated that she had called the day care center number the nurse had given her and was planning to put the two younger boys in for two mornings a week. She also stated that she was thinking of joining a parents group.

She stated that the father of the children had called and was not planning to come home at this time but would send money for the children. At this point she started to cry. Mrs. John stated that she felt lonely and overwhelmed and was thinking of having her sister come and stay for a while. She admitted that the burning incident scared her, and she didn't want that to happen again. Ms. Douglas and the mother discussed the mother's feelings and the alternatives she could take. She gave her support for the positive aspects of the children's care, and empathized with the family's situation. Ms. Douglas gave the mother alternative techniques for disciplining the children and offered other community resources she might want to use in the future, like Parents Without Partners.

Tommy told the nurse that he and his mom had spent time together most every day, and that "Mommy still gets mad, but hits us less than before Billy's burn." The mother admitted she still loses control but does feel more supported than before.

On the next clinic appointment, three weeks later, the mother appeared much more relaxed. She smiled at Tommy twice, held the two-year-old gently in her arms, and praised Billy when he returned the nurse's pen to the desk. She admitted feeling depressed and overwhelmed by the father's absence; however, she stated she felt fewer stresses on the days the younger boys went to the day care center. She also went to the parents group once and was planning to go again. She mentioned that she was thinking of going to work again but wasn't ready to make that decision now. She stated that she did feel better knowing there were places to turn to for support.

Ms. Douglas gave the mother another appointment and briefly mentioned other possibilities they could discuss on the next visit if the mother was interested.

Nursing Care Plan 11–1 • A FAMILY INVOLVED WITH CHILD ABUSE: Billy

NURSING DIAGNOSIS

Actual injury related to poor impulse control by parent, as evidenced by burn on right palm and history of hitting

Supporting Data

- Second-degree burns on right hand.
- "Mommy burned my hand on the stove."
- Reports of threats of burning and hitting in the past.
- Mother hits children when "mad."

Long Term Goal: Billy's hand will be healed of burns by (state date).

Short Term Goal	*Intervention*	*Rationale*	*Evaluation*
1. Wound will show signs of healing by third day after being dressed.	1. Assess wound and care for wound per orders.	1. Promote healing and prevent infection.	Goal met By next visit, wound healing well.
2. Mother will state she is comfortable changing dressing at home by end of first visit.	2a. Arrange with M.D. for visiting nurse in home to supervise dressing change.	2a. Allows for health teaching and further family assessment.	Mother states that she felt comfortable changing the dressing after return demonstration.

Continued on following page

Nursing Care Plan 11–1 • A FAMILY INVOLVED WITH CHILD ABUSE: Billy *Continued*

Short Term Goal	*Intervention*	*Rationale*	*Evaluation*
	2b. Demonstrate to mother changing the dressing and ask for a return demonstration.	2b. Provides opportunity for questions and concern.	
	2c. Give mother telephone number of clinic to talk to nurse if questions arise.	2c. Reduces feelings of isolation and offers support.	

NURSING DIAGNOSIS

Altered family process related to actual physical abuse and change in family unit.

Supporting Data

- Father recently left family unit.
- Physical abuse appears to have escalated since separation.
- Mother often hits children when "mad."

Long Term Goal: Mother will use two new appropriate discipline techniques by (state date).

Short Term Goal	*Intervention*	*Rationale*	*Evaluation*
1. Mother will state she wants support to help channel frustration more appropriately by end of initial interview.	1a. Discuss with mother medical findings and indicate abuse in nonthreatening and supportive manner.	1a. When parent feels supported, family change is more likely.	Goal met Mother states she felt overwhelmed and wanted support.
	1b. Explain need to report situation to appropriate state agency.	1b. Parent needs to be aware of decisions made in child's behalf.	
2. Mother will state she feels more support in parenting role by next appointment.	2a. Give positive feedback about how mother is doing, e.g., children look well fed, are clean. Point out strengths and accomplishments.	2a. Raises self-esteem, restores hope, and helps mother recognize her own resources.	Goal met Mother less defensive and more relaxed.
	2b. Inform about options for low-cost day care to give mother occasional time to herself.	2b. Involvement in support agencies and groups may help reduce anxiety and promote positive change.	States children are in day care twice a week.
	2c. Give appointment for one week follow-up.	2c. Evaluate healing and family progress.	
	2d. Document in detail history and observations. Draw detailed diagram of hand with burn.	2d. Documentation needed for both legal and medical purposes.	
3. By (state the date) mother will name three actions she can take when feeling overwhelmed in the future.	3a. Refer to support agencies, hotlines, counseling groups.	3a. Availability of resources lowers feelings of helplessness.	Goal partially met Mother states she is thinking of joining a parents group
	3b. Work with mother to set future goals for herself and her relationships with her children.	3b. Projection toward the future helps visualize movement and growth. Each day is a part of the process.	
4. Within three weeks, mother will begin to practice alternative discipline techniques based on natural consequences.	4. Educate about effective discipline techniques geared toward child's developmental stages.	4. Knowledge is the first step toward changing behavior.	Goal met Mother states she is hitting the children less and is finding alternative methods effective.

NURSING DIAGNOSIS

Fear related to retaliation from mother, as evidenced by feelings of dread in children

Supporting Data

- Children threatened with burning "if they don't behave."
- Brother afraid he will be punished for "telling on mother."
- Mother often hits children when "mad."

Long Term Goal: Children will state and show by behavior more feelings of safety and comfort around mother by (state date).

Short Term Goal	*Intervention*	*Rationale*	*Evaluation*
1. Oldest boy (Tom) and mother will spend 15 minutes twice a day talking or engaged in play activity.	1a. Talk about resolving children's fear with both mother and oldest brother.	1a. Minimize potential for abuse directed at oldest brother. Communicating openly about feelings assists in their resolution.	Goal met Tom states most days he and mother spend time together.
	1b. Reassure brother that his actions were correct and he did nothing wrong by telling.	1b. Children need to know that nothing they do causes them to be abused.	Mother gets "mad" still "but doesn't hit so much." Mother appears more relaxed with children, smiling and putting arm around Tom twice.

Summary

Child abuse is a long-standing phenomenon, which only recently is being viewed as unacceptable. Abuse occurs across all age groups of people but can be predicted to occur with some accuracy by examining characteristics of parents who abuse, children who are vulnerable to abuse, and situations in which abuse is more likely to occur. Abuse can be physical, sexual, emotional, or caused by neglect. Emotional abuse can occur in isolation, but where other types of abuse occur, emotional abuse also occurs. Child abuse leads to disorders in physical health and in cognitive and emotional development.

When assessing for child abuse the nurse needs to evaluate the parents' emotional and physical needs and their level of maturity, the child's needs, and the stress factors impinging on the family. Suspicion or actual evidence of abuse *must* be carefully documented and then reported to the appropriate authorities.

Intervention occurs at primary, secondary, and tertiary levels. Primary intervention aims at preventing child abuse. Providing expectant and new parents with maximal support, encouragement, and education in addition to sustained early contact with their baby minimizes risk. Early recognition and secondary intervention in cases where child abuse has already occurred but is not an ingrained habit can greatly reduce the subsequent incidence of child abuse. Tertiary intervention occurs as a last resort, in the worst cases of abuse, and when previous intervention techniques have failed.

Evaluation and follow-up of interventions are vital to promote family growth and child safety. The well-being of children cannot be secured if left to chance or half-hearted attempts at change, hoping that "things will work out."

References

Besharov DJ. Protecting abused and neglected children: Can law help social work? Child Abuse and Neglect 7(4):421, 1983.

de Chesnay M. Father-daughter incest: Issues in treatment and research. Journal of Psychiatric Nursing, 22(9):9, 1984.

Drake VK. Therapy with victims of abuse. *In* Beck et al. (eds). Mental Health-Psychiatric Nursing. St. Louis: C.V. Mosby Company, 1984.

Feinfeld L. The nature of child abuse and its treatment. *In* Laurel, MD (ed). Treatment of Emotional Disorders in Children and Adolescents. New York: Spectrum Publications, 1980.

Finkelhor D. Child Sexual Abuse: New Theory and Research, New York: Free Press, 1984.

Fischler RS. Child abuse treatment and follow-up: Can the pediatrician help improve outcome? Child Abuse and Neglect, 8(3):361, 1984.

Fontana VJ. Child maltreatment and battered child syndromes. *In* Kaplan HI, Sadock BJ (eds). Comprehensive Textbook of Psychiatry/IV, 4th ed. Baltimore, MD: Williams & Wilkins, 1985.

Fortin PJ, Reed SR. Diagnosing and responding to emotional abuse within the helping system. Child Abuse and Neglect, 8(1):117, 1984.

Gabinet L. Child abuse treatment failures reveal need for redefinition of the problem. Child Abuse and Neglect, 7(4):395, 1983.

Ghent WR, DaSylva NP, Farren ME. Family violence: Guidelines for recognition and management. Canadian Medical Association Journal, 132(5):541, 1985.

Haynes CF, Cutler C, Gray G, Kempe RS. Hospitalized cases of nonorganic failure to thrive: The scope of the problem and short-term lay health visitor intervention. Child Abuse and Neglect, 8(2):229, 1984.

Heap KK. Families with abused children: A follow-up study of post-crisis support. Child Abuse and Neglect, 8(4):467, 1984.

Heindl C, et al. The nurse's role in the prevention and treatment of child abuse. (Publication No. 79-30202.) Washington, DC: U.S. Department of Health, Education and Welfare, August, 1979.

Helfer RE, Kempe CH (eds). Child Abuse and Neglect: The Family and the Community. Cambridge, MA: Bollinger Publishing Company, 1976.

Hjorth CW, Ostrov E. The self-image of physically abused adolescents. Journal of Youth and Adolescence, 55(2):71, 1982.

Kelly SJ. The use of art therapy with sexually abused children. Journal of Psychosocial Nursing, 22(12):12, 1984.

Kempe CH, Silverman FN, Steele BF, et al. The battered child syndrome. Journal of American Medical Association, 181(1):17, 1962.
Kim MJ, McFarland GK, McLane AM (eds). Pocket Guide to Nursing Diagnosis, 3rd ed. St. Louis: C.V. Mosby Company, 1989.
Kluft RP. Multiple personality disorder: an update. Hospital and Community Psychiatry, 38:363, 1987.
Kreitzer M. Legal aspects of child abuse: guidelines for the nurse. Nursing Clinics of North America, 16(1):149, 1981.
Lally JR. Three views of child neglect: Expanding visions of preventive intervention. Child Abuse and Neglect, 8(2):243, 1984.
Ludwig S. Shaken baby syndrome: A review of 20 cases. Annals of Emergency Medicine, 13(2):104, 1984.
McKittrick CA. Child abuse: Recognition and reporting by health professionals. Nursing Clinics of North America, 16(1):103, 1981.
Orr DP. Limitations of emergency room evaluations of sexually abused children. American Journal of Diseases of Children, 132:873, 1978.
Pawl JH. Strategies for intervention. Child Abuse and Neglect, 8(2):261, 1984.
Radbill SX. A history of child abuse and infanticide. *In* Helfer RE, Kempe CH (eds). The Battered Child, 3rd ed. Chicago: University of Chicago Press, 1980.
Sideleau BF. Abusive families. *In* Haber, et al. (eds). Comprehensive Psychiatric Nursing, 2nd ed. New York: McGraw-Hill Book Company, 1982.
Smith J. Care of the hospitalized abused child and family: A framework for nursing intervention. Nursing Clinics of North America, 16(1):127, 1981.
Snyder JC. Family dysfunction: violence, neglect, and sexual misuse. *In* Devine MD, et al (eds). Developmental-Behavioral Pediatrics. Philadelphia: W.B. Saunders Company, 1983.
Taskinen S. The Finnish approach to helping personnel deal with child abuse and neglect. Child Abuse and Neglect, 8(1):113, 1984.
Thomas JN, Rogers CM. Sexual abuse of children: Case finding and clinical management. Nursing Clinics of North America, 16(1):179, 1981.
Warner CG. Conflict Intervention in Social and Domestic Violence. Bowie, MD: Robert J. Brady Company, 1981.
Whitworth JM. Child abuse: Old problem, new perspectives. Journal of the Florida Medical Association, 72(7):495, 1985.

Bibliography

Gilbert M. Sexual abuse and group therapy. Journal of Psychosocial Nursing, 26(5):19, 1988.
Heindl C, et al. The nurse's role in the prevention and treatment of child abuse and neglect. (DHEW, Pub. No. (OHDS) 79-30202.) Washington DC: U.S. Government Printing Office, 1979.
Jacoby LE, Jones SL. The psychiatric clinical specialist in the emergency room. Journal of Psychosocial Nursing, 22(5):8, 1984.
Sloan MP, Meier JH. Typology for parents of abused children. Child Abuse and Neglect 7(4):443, 1983.
Warner CG (ed). Conflict Intervention in Social and Domestic Violence. Bowie, MD: Robert J. Brady Company, 1981.
Wharton R, et al. Violence on television and imitative behavior: Impact on parenting practices. Pediatrics, 75(6):1120, 1985.

Self-Study Exercises

Choose the answer that most accurately completes the statement.

1. Which answer is NOT an example of the three factors that can signal conditions for abuse:

   A. a family illness
   B. a parent who has a drinking problem
   C. a child who is highly gifted in an "average-to-below-average" household
   D. a parent who comes from another country

2. All of the following are common characteristics of abusing parents EXCEPT

   A. unrealistic expectations of child's behavior
   B. lack of effective parenting skills
   C. male
   D. poor coping skills
   E. alcoholic

3. Any of the following are examples of children vulnerable to abuse EXCEPT

   A. premature infant
   B. child with congenital anomalies
   C. low birth weight infant
   D. hyperactive child
   E. child of foreign descent

Match the example on the left with the type of abuse listed in the right column

4. ________ "You no good slut. I wish you were never born."
5. ________ SB says children don't know how to behave unless you give them good healthy spankings.
6. ________ CS says life is the best teacher. His children don't need schools.
7. ________ As KS ate her lunch at the park, she noticed a man near her with his penis sticking out of his pants.
8. ________ WB refused to get his child counseling even though it had been recommended by his child's teacher, the principal, and concerned friends.
9. ________ The playground equipment in PD's backyard was in a dangerous state of disrepair. Yet his eight children and neighbor children continued to play on it. "They'll survive" was his attitude.
10. ________ When PC misbehaved, she would get locked in her closet for hours at a time.
11. ________ FD never played with her baby and rarely touched him, feeling that he could do just fine for himself.

A. Physical battering
B. Physical endangerment
C. Sexual abuse
D. Physical neglect
E. Developmental neglect
F. Educational neglect
G. Emotional abuse

Match the symptom listed in the left column with the type of abuse it indicates in the right column.

12. ________ Apprehensive when other children cry.
13. ________ Profound personality change.
14. ________ Unusual fearfulness.
15. ________ Constant fatigue.
16. ________ Pain in genital area.
17. ________ Always begging kids at school for food. Never seems to bring own lunch.
18. ________ Bald patches on scalp.
19. ________ Always careful of behavior; wants to please.

A. Physical abuse
B. Sexual abuse
C. Neglect
D. Emotional abuse

Choose the most appropriate answer.

20. To assess whether a child's safety or security needs are being met, which question would be appropriate to ask parents?
   A. What do you do when you get angry with your child?
   B. Did you graduate from high school?
   C. How did this happen?
   D. Describe your marriage.

21. When interviewing the child about the abuse episode, which question should be included?

    A. Do you like school?
    B. What happens when you do something wrong at home?
    C. Do you have any brothers or sisters?
    D. What is your favorite TV program?

22. Questioning the acceptance of violence in America and modeling nonviolent problem-solving strategies are examples of what level of intervention?

    A. Primary intervention
    B. Secondary intervention
    C. Tertiary intervention

Place a T (True) or F (False) next to each statement.

23. ________ "Shared parenting" gives parents of vulnerable infants time away for themselves.
24. ________ It is not only a right but a privilege to be a parent.
25. ________ It is not only a privilege but a right to be valued and protected as a child.
26. ________ Parenting comes naturally and requires no special education, learning, or resources.
27. ________ Foster care is ideally designed to be therapeutic for children and to prepare them to return home or to be adopted.

CHAPTER 12

Evidence of Maladaptive Responses to Crisis: Spouse Abuse

Kathleen Smith-DiJulio

OUTLINE

KEY TERMS AND CONCEPTS

The key terms and concepts listed here also appear in bold where they are defined or discussed in this chapter.

SPOUSE ABUSE

MEN WHO BATTER

COPING MECHANISMS OF BATTERED WOMEN

CYCLE THEORY OF VIOLENCE
- Tension-Building Stage
- Acute Battering Stage
- Honeymoon Stage

TWO STAGES OF TREATMENT
Crisis Stage
Stage of Internal Change and Rebuilding
SHELTERS/SAFE HOUSES
SAFETY PLAN
TITLE XX OF THE 1974 SOCIAL SECURITY ACT
ACCURATE RECORDS

OBJECTIVES

After studying this chapter, the student will be able to:

1. Name two characteristics of battering families.
2. Name two characteristics of men who batter.
3. Name two characteristics of the abused woman.
4. Briefly name and discuss three stages in the process of the cycle of violence that results in spouse abuse.
5. List four areas of assessment when interviewing an abused woman.
6. Identify four nursing diagnoses that apply to families of spouse abuse.
7. Name four reactions the nurse may have when working with an abused woman, and discuss personal thoughts and feelings regarding these reactions.
8. Name and discuss three areas of intervention in the crisis stage of counseling an abused woman.
9. Name and discuss three psychotherapeutic modalities that are useful for families of spouse abuse.
10. Discuss the evaluation process.
11. Name three areas of evaluation when working with families of spouse abuse.

Spouse abuse has been described as a transcultural phenomenon with roots in respected and sometimes legal traditions found in patriarchal societies (Martin 1978). The battered spouse syndrome is a symptom complex of physical and psychological abuse of a woman by her husband (or any male with whom she has an intimate relationship) (Swanson 1984).

Many of our current beliefs regarding spouse abuse have been handed down since antiquity and subsequently have reflected Judeo-Christian patriarchy. Married women have been considered necessary and inseparable possessions of their husbands. Until recently, the husband has had the legal, social, and religious authority to chastise his wife and "keep her in line." And women, as the mainstays of the relationships, have been expected to "kiss and make up" after an episode of domestic violence. People have been socialized to accept female passivity and male dominance.

For a long time, society has tolerated and ignored the battering of women. The women's movement has been instrumental in stimulating changes of attitude toward abuse of both women and children. Women are no longer considered property to be used or abused by others. In conjunction with changes in attitude came changes in social institutions as well. For example, in 1978, 12 women sued the New York City Police Department for refusing them protection by not arresting their abusive husbands (Greany 1984). Consequently, in most communities, battered women can expect to be somewhat protected. Unfortunately, most battered women do not know their rights.

It is estimated that five million wives are assaulted by their husbands each year (DeLorto and LaViolette 1980). The F.B.I. considers spouse abuse America's most underreported crime (DeLorto and LaViolette 1980). The family is the most frequent focus for intrapersonal abuse ranging from verbal threats to murder (Hilberman 1980). It has been estimated that one half of all Americans have experienced violence in their families. Of all murders in the United States, 20–50% occur within families (Hilberman 1980). Yet violence within families is seldom recognized by outsiders, including nurses.

Spouse abuse, dangerous and potentially life-threatening, is a health care issue. The secondary effects of abuse, such as anxiety, depression, and suicide attempts, are also health care issues. A majority of battered women seek out health care at some point in the abuse cycle. The nurse is often a first point of contact for the woman after an incident of abuse. The information the woman receives may be a key factor in helping her act decisively to end the abuse (Delgaty 1985).

The nurse's support and respect for the woman's situation and safety may be the first indication to her that the battering is serious and is not her fault. This attitude will often help her consider alternatives (Ghent et al. 1985). The time and energy spent with an abused woman may have future, rather than immediate, impact. The abused woman is terrified of her husband, afraid of her surroundings, and too numb to help herself (Greany 1984). The valuable time that the nurse takes to tell her that she can live in peace may one day save her life.

Spouse abuse as a maladaptive response to acute anxiety can be conceptualized as shown in Figure 12–1.

Standard I: Theory

Martin (1978) describes **spouse abuse** as "an act carried out with the intention of, or perceived intention of, physically injuring one's spouse." Any person who has suffered physical violence at the hand of their mate is also suffering from mental cruelty and the mental consequences of physical violence (Sanchez-Dicks 1979). Spouse abuse includes not only physical battering, but sexual abuse, social isolation, home imprisonment, economic deprivation, or verbal harassment (Germain 1984).

Although the estimation for women who have been abused by their mates is five million per year, there are no reliable estimates for the number of men who are battered per year (Martin 1978; Morton 1984). This chapter deals more directly with women who are abused by their mates.

In this section, characteristics of (1) battered families, (2) the men who batter, (3) the abused woman, and (4) the cycle of violence are discussed.

BATTERED FAMILIES

Perhaps the most disconcerting aspect of spouse abuse is that it is multigenerational. Family histories of both the abused and the abuser often contain accounts of violence. In many cases, women with violent histories will accept violence in their intimate relationships as "normal" interaction between a man and a woman (DeLorto and LaViolette 1980). And children of violent families will grow up believing violence is "normal" and accepting it as a problem-solving technique.

Violence often does not occur until after the legal marriage of couples who have lived together or dated for a long time (Gemmill 1982). Perhaps this reflects the notion of women as property legally bound to the husband by virtue of the marriage ceremony.

Pregnancy serves to increase violence even further. One reason may be that the husband resents the added responsibility that a baby requires. Or he may resent the relationship that the baby will have with his mate. Violence also escalates when the wife makes moves toward independence such as visiting friends "without permission," getting a job, or going back to school.

Most abuse takes place in the evenings or on weekends, when most traditional resource agencies (e.g., doctors' offices, clinics) are closed. Holidays are more stressful times, and violence may occur more frequently then.

Marriages in which abuse is a norm have been described as intense, with both partners investing a great deal of emotional energy into each other (Gemmill 1982). Displays of jealousy and possessiveness by the male may be construed by the woman to be "proof" that she is really loved. In general, the marriage (and family) is dysfunctional. These families are characterized as being isolated from neighbors, having different religious backgrounds, and arguing about sex.

MEN WHO BATTER

Spouse abusers are found in all socioeconomic, educational, age, and racial groups. They usually do not break the laws in other ways. The violence is learned behavior, which they use to control the woman. **Men who batter**

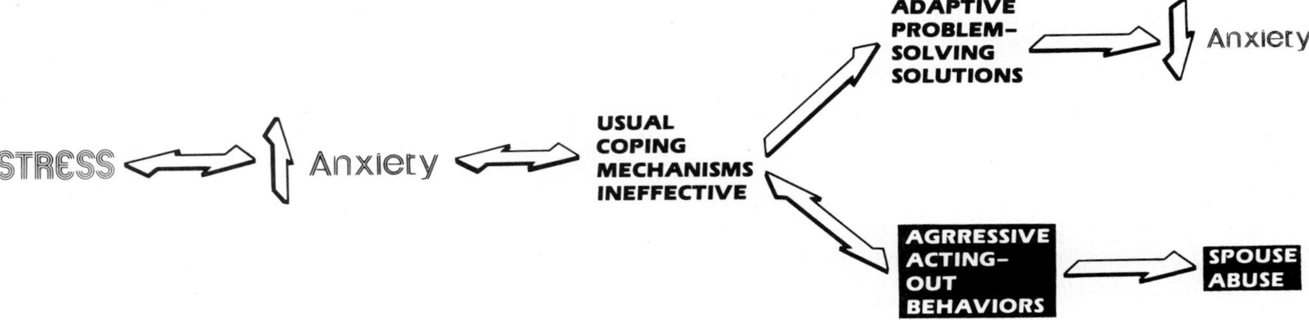

Figure 12–1. *Conceptualization of the process of aggressive acting-out behaviors in the development of spouse abuse.*

believe in male supremacy, being in charge and dominant. They act out these stereotyped sex roles within the family because it has traditionally been a safe place to do so. Acting out physically makes them feel more in control, masculine, and powerful, which attests to their low self-esteem and insecurity. Regardless of how well adjusted they may appear externally, both partners report dissatisfaction with themselves. Interestingly, both partners frequently appear *very* successful to the outside world (Boyd and Klingbeil 1977).

Men who batter cannot control their aggression and have no guilt about expressing it, nor do they believe it should have negative consequences. They are usually impulsive, immature, or inarticulate about their feelings and have not learned to deal with their anger (Greany 1984).

Extreme pathological jealousy is characteristic of batterers. Many refuse to let their wives work. Others have her work in the same place they do so that they can monitor her activities and friendships. Many accompany their wives to and from all activities and forbid them to have personal friends or to participate in recreational activities outside the home. Even with such restrictions, these men accuse their wives of infidelity. Many batterers maintain their possessiveness by controlling the family finances to the extent that there is barely enough money for daily living.

Individuals are more likely to engage in family violence when intoxicated. Spouse abuse seems to be a characteristic mode of interaction for some couples, and intoxication seems to increase the possibility of abuse occurring (Corenblum 1983). The batterer may initially drink excessively to avoid the issue of violence (Flanzer 1985). Unfortunately, the consumption of alcohol and drugs is often used as a rationalization by the battered woman, e.g., "He was drunk; he didn't know what he was doing." Rationalization such as this helps to maintain denial. The fact is that when drugs and alcohol use are reduced or eliminated, family violence still escalates (Walker-Hooper 1981a; Delgaty 1985).

The batterer perceives himself as having poor social skills. He describes his relationship with his mate as being the closest he has ever known. He lacks supportive relationships outside of the marriage and has only superficial interactions with those outside the family unit.

When not being abusive, spouse abusers have been described as childlike, remorseful, and yearning to be nurtured (Swanson 1984). This picture of fragility is confirmed by occasional reports of a husband's suicidal or psychotic behavior when his wife threatens to end the relationship. In these instances, the marriage often becomes a life sentence for the wife (Swanson 1984).

THE ABUSED WOMAN

Popular myths that women who are battered are masochistic, poor, and uneducated have been shown to be false. Theorists and practitioners are in agreement that women who are battered are not masochists. They do not enjoy being beaten, nor do they ask to be beaten (Gemmill 1982). Women who are battered come from a variety of socioeconomic, educational, ethnic, racial, and age groups (Boyd and Klingbeil 1977; DeLorto and LaViolette 1980).

There does seem to be, however, a positive correlation between women who witnessed their mothers being beaten and those women who later become victims of spouse abuse (Walker 1979, Gemmill 1982). Since abused women are often the subject of extreme and irrational jealousy, isolation, and verbal as well as physical abuse, feelings of powerlessness and low self-esteem are common. After years of being told she is no good, stupid, or incompetent, a woman is so psychologically destroyed that she believes her mate (Langly and Levy 1977).

Health care professionals often find it difficult to understand why women stay in these violent relationships. The process of change takes a long time. There may be many reasons why a woman doesn't leave her situation. One of the strongest motives for staying in a violent relationship is fear of being killed if found by the batterer. Abused women are often isolated from family, friends, or neighbors, have no other source of financial support, and often cannot leave because they have no way of supporting themselves and their children. Fear of being alone is another reason women give for not leaving their situation.

The **coping mechanisms many battered women employ** to live in violent and terrifying situations often prevent the dissolution of the marriages. These coping mechanisms are in the form of beliefs or myths that reinforce the denial and protect the marriage (Walker-Hooper 1981a; Gemmill 1982).

1. She stays for "the sake of the children."
2. She can't survive without him.
3. He will change.
4. She deserved the beating because she was "bad" or provocative.
5. If she doesn't do anything "wrong," he won't beat her again.

See Table 12–1 by Boyd and Klingbeil, which compares and contrasts the behavioral characteristics of the batterer, the battered mate, and the children raised in violent homes.

Table 12–1 • BEHAVIORAL CHARACTERISTICS OF DOMESTIC VIOLENCE

BATTERERS	BATTERED MATES	CHILDREN
Batterers are found in all socioeconomic, educational, ethnic, racial, and age groups.	Battered mates are found in all socioeconomic, educational, ethnic, racial, and age groups.	Battered children are found in all socioeconomic, educational, ethnic, racial, and age groups.
. . . use psychological, verbal, and physical abuse including sexual abuse.	. . . are psychologically, verbally, and physically abused. Are frequently sexually abused.	. . . are psychologically abused and may be verbally, physically, and sexually abused.
. . . engage in excessive minimization and denial.	. . . engage in excessive minimization and denial.	. . . engage in excessive minimization and denial.
The Batterer Is Characterized By	**The Battered Mate Is Characterized By**	**Children In Violent Homes Are Characterized By**
. . . poor impulse control—limited tolerance for frustration, explosive temper—rage. Constantly demonstrating, but often successfully masking, anger.	. . . long-suffering, martyrlike endurance of frustration, passive acceptance, internalizing anger.	. . . a combination of limited tolerance for frustration, poor impulse control, and martyrlike long-suffering—they externalize/internalize anger.
. . . stress disorders and psychosomatic complaints; sophistication of symptoms and success at masking dysfunction vary with social and educational levels.	. . . stress disorders and psychosomatic complaints.	. . . sadness, depression, stress disorders, and psychosomatic complaints; absences from school, pre-delinquent and delinquent behavior.
. . . emotional dependency—subject to secret depressions known only to family.	. . . economic and emotional dependency; subject to depression, high risk for secret drugs and alcohol, home accidents.	. . . economic and emotional dependency, high risk for alcohol/drugs, sexual acting out, running away, isolation, loneliness, and fear.
. . . limited capacity for delayed reinforcement—very "now" oriented.	. . . unlimited patience for discovery of "magic combination" in solving marital and abusive problems—"travels miles" on tiny bits of reinforcement.	. . . combination of poor impulse control and continual hopefulness that situation will improve.
. . . insatiable ego needs and qualities of childlike narcissism (not generally detectable to people outside family group).	. . . being unsure of own ego needs, defining self in terms of partner, children, family, job.	. . . very shaky definition of self—grappling with childlike responses of parents for modeling; poor definition of self and/or defines self in parenting role (role reversal).
. . . low self-esteem; perceived unachieved ideals and goals for self, disappointment in career, even if successful by others' standards.	. . . low self-esteem, continued faith and hope that battering mate will get "lucky" break.	. . . low self-esteem, seeing self and siblings with few options or expectations to succeed.
. . . qualities that suggest great potential for change and improvement; i.e., makes frequent "promises" for the future.	. . . unrealistic hope that change is imminent, belief in "promises."	. . . mixture of hope/depression that there is no way out; peer group can be most important contact, if available.
. . . perception of self as having poor social skills; describing relationship with mate as closest he has ever known; remaining in contact with his own family.	. . . gradually increasing social isolation, including loss of contact with own family and friends.	. . . increased social isolation, increased peer isolation *or* complete identification with peers. Poor social skills.
. . . accusations against mate, jealousy, voicing great fear of abandonment or "being cheated on," possessive, controlling, hovering.	. . . inability to convince partner of loyalty, futilely guarding against accusations of "seductive" behavior toward others; compliant, helpless, and powerless.	. . . bargaining behavior with parents; attempts to prove self; compliant, but may run away. Feelings of powerlessness.
. . . fearfulness that partner and/or children will abandon, fear of being alone.	. . . constant fear, which gradually becomes cumulative and oppressive with time.	. . . constant fear and terror for their lives as well as parents'; confusion and insecurity.

Table continued on following page

Table 12–1 • BEHAVIORAL CHARACTERISTICS OF DOMESTIC VIOLENCE *Continued*

The Batterer Is Characterized By	The Battered Mate Is Characterized By	Children In Violent Homes Are Characterized By
. . . containment of mate and employment of espionage tactics against her (e.g., checks mileage/times errands); cleverness depends on level of sophistication.	. . . helplessly allowing containment or confinement/restriction by mate mistakenly interpreted as sign that partner "cares."	. . . increasing deceptiveness: lying, excuses for outings, stealing, cheating.
. . . violating others' personal boundaries; accepts no blame for failures (marital, familial, or occupational) or for violent acts.	. . . gradually losing sight of personal boundaries for self and children (unable to assess danger accurately), accepts all blame.	. . . poor definition of personal boundaries, violation of others' personal boundaries, accepting blame or projecting blame.
. . . belief that forcible behavior is aimed at securing the family nucleus ("for the good of the family").	. . . belief that transient acceptance of violent behavior will ultimately lead to long term resolution of family problems.	. . . little or no understanding of the dynamics of violence; often assumes violence to be the norm.
. . . absence of guilt on an emotional level even after intellectual recognition.	. . . emotional acceptance of guilt for mate's behavior, thinking mate "can't help it," considering own behavior as provocative.	. . . self-blame (depending on age) for family feuding, separations, divorce, and internal conflicts.
. . . generational history of abuse.	. . . generational history of witnessing abuse in family and/or being abused.	. . . continuation of abuse pattern in adult life.
. . . frequently participating in pecking order battering.	. . . occasionally participating in pecking order battering.	. . . frequently participating in pecking order battering (maim or kill animals, batter siblings); often batters parents in later years.
. . . assaultive skills that improve with age and experience (increase in danger potential and lethality risks to family members over time).	. . . "creative" behavior that either diverts or precipitates mate's violence; but level of carelessness increases (judgment of lethality potential deteriorates) over time.	. . . poor problem-solving skills: may use violence as problem-solving technique in school, with peers, with family (appears as early as pre-school), demonstrates aggression or passivity.
. . . demanding and often assaultive role in sexual activities: sometimes punishes w/abstinence, at times experiences impotence.	. . . poor sexual self-image, assuming that role is total acceptance of partner's sexual behavior. Attempts at abstinence result in further abuse.	. . . poor sexual image, uncertainty about appropriate behavior, confused model identification, immaturity in peer relationships.
. . . increasingly assaultive behavior when mate is pregnant—pregnancy often marks the first assault.	. . . being at high risk for assaults during pregnancy.	. . . being at higher risk for assaults (either as witnesses or victims) during mother's pregnancy.
. . . exerting control over mate by threatening homicide and/or suicide . . . often attempts one or both when partners separate—known to complete either or both.	. . . frequent contemplation of suicide—history of minor attempts, occasionally completing suicide or becoming a homicide victim, frequently wishing partner dead. Occasionally completes homicide in self-defense.	. . . heightened suicide risks and attempts—increased thoughts of suicide and/or murdering parents, prone to negligence and carelessness.
. . . frequently using children as "pawns" and exerting power and control through custody issues . . . may kidnap children or hold them hostage.	. . . feeling powerless in custody issues, living in fear children will be "kidnapped," struggling to maintain rights of children.	. . . feeling used and powerless in all decisions (age specific) regarding custody issues.

THE CYCLE OF VIOLENCE

Walker's **cycle theory of violence** was developed from a study of 400 women in violent families (Walker 1979, Ghent et al. 1985; Morton 1984; Billy 1983). The theory consists of three stages: the tension-building stage, the acute battering stage, and the honeymoon stage.

TENSION-BUILDING STAGE. The **tension building stage** is characterized by minor incidents such as pushing, shoving, and verbal abuse. During this time, the woman does *not* state that the abuse is unacceptable, for fear more severe abuse will follow. The abuser then rationalizes that his abusive behavior is acceptable.

As the tension escalates, both spouses may try to reduce the tension. The batterer may try to reduce the tension with the use of alcohol or drugs. The woman may try to reduce the tension by minimizing the importance of the incidents, i.e., "I should have had the house neater . . . the children fed." The woman may also try to reduce the tension by somatizing, thus perpetuating the "poor-me image."

ACUTE BATTERING STAGE. During the **acute battering stage,** the batterer releases the built-up tension by brutal and uncontrollable beatings. The batterer is unable to control his blind rage or the degree of destructiveness inflicted upon the woman. The woman may suffer severe injuries. The batterer usually has complete amnesia and will not remember what happened during the battering. The woman usually will depersonalize the incident and will be able to remember the beatings in detail.

After the beatings, both are in shock. At this time, the woman may contemplate leaving or initiating legal action.

HONEYMOON STAGE. The **honeymoon stage** is characterized by kindness and loving behaviors. The man feels remorseful and is apologetic. He may bring the woman presents, make promises, and tell the woman he loves her and needs her. The woman believes the promises and feels needed and loved. She then drops legal proceedings or her plans to leave. The victimization is now complete. Unfortunately, without intervention, the cycle will repeat itself. The honeymoon stage will fade away as tension starts to build. *Violence never diminishes. Violence always escalates in frequency and intensity.* Usually with each repeat of the cycle the beatings become more severe, and the woman's self-esteem more and more eroded. The woman either believes she deserved the beatings or puts the blame on herself. This leads to feelings of depression, hopelessness, and immobilization.

Standard II: Data Collection

Battered women present in nearly every health care setting. Examples include outpatient clinics, emergency rooms, and obstetric-gynecologic units. Complaints may be of physical injuries or vague symptoms such as sleep disorders, abdominal pain, or menstrual problems. Sensitivity on the part of the nurse is required in suspecting the possibility of spouse abuse. Refer to Box 12–1 for types of presenting injuries dealt with in the emergency room versus the clinical setting.

Greany (1984) divides the process of identifying the signals of a battered woman into three phases: ingress, contact, and processing.

INGRESS. In this first phase, the abused woman voluntarily seeks help, although she may not describe abuse as her presenting problem. Complaints of abdominal pain are probably second only to headaches as a presenting problem (Swanson 1984). Other presenting complaints may include symptoms of chronic stress

Box 12–1. TYPES OF PRESENTING INJURIES DEALT WITH IN THE EMERGENCY ROOM VERSUS THE CLINICAL SETTING

In the Emergency Room

- Bleeding injuries, especially to the head and face.
- Internal injuries, concussions, perforated ear drums, abdominal injuries, severe bruising, eye injuries, and strangulation marks on the neck.
- Back injuries.
- Broken or fractured jaws, arms, pelvis, ribs, clavicle, and legs.
- Burns from cigarettes, appliances, scalding liquids, and acids.
- Psychological trauma, anxiety, attacks of hyperventilation, heart palpitations, severe crying spells, and suicidal tendencies.
- Miscarriages.

In the Office, Clinic

- Perforated ear drums, twisted or stiff neck and shoulder muscles, headache.
- Depression, stress-related conditions (e.g., insomnia, violent nightmares, anxiety, extreme fatigue, eczema, loss of hair).
- Talk of having "problems" with her husband, describing him as very jealous, impulsive, and/or an alcohol/drug abuser.
- Repeated visits with new complaints.

In Both Settings

- Observe children for signs of stress due to family violence: emotional, behavioral, school, or sleep problems, and/or increased aggressive behavior.

such as insomnia, a choking sensation, hyperventilation, anxiety, chest pain, and back pain (Swanson 1984). Most of these women have several encounters with health care professionals before the problem is discovered, if it is discovered at all. Chief complaints and presenting problems that may indicate spouse abuse are presented in Box 12–2.

CONTACT. This phase consists of conducting a nursing history and a physical examination. As the woman still may not admit abuse, empathy and a nonjudgmental attitude are important. When battering is a possibility, the nurse asks the woman directly if she is abused. If she denies physical abuse at this time, the chart should be flagged (Morton 1984).

It is best to interview the woman in private. Addressing her by title (Ms./Mrs.) can help bolster her self-esteem. Be purposeful. Encourage her to recognize her situation and needs. If she *does* admit to being abused, the nurse should be aware that often the details of the incident(s) may be raw and shocking. It is very important at this point that the nurse not register dismay that the woman has not left such a horrible situation. This kind of reaction will only reinforce the woman's sense of guilt, shame, and low self-esteem (Gemmill 1982).

Box 12–2. PHYSICAL SYMPTOMS INDICATING POSSIBLE SPOUSE ABUSE

Chief Complaints Without Physical Cause

- Headache
- Abdominal pain
- Insomnia
- Choking sensation
- Chest pain
- Back pain
- Dizziness
- "Accidents"

Presenting Problems (Signs of High Anxiety and Chronic Stress)

- Agitation
- Hyperventilation
- Panic attack
- Gastrointestinal disturbances
- Hypertension
- Physical injuries (listed in Box 12–1)

Data from Swanson RW. Battered wife syndrome. Canadian Medical Association Journal, 130(6):709, 1984.

PROCESSING. This is the time to pull information together to determine needs for further help. In doing so the nurse assesses (1) the level of anxiety and coping responses, (2) support systems, (3) actual physical abuse, (4) suicide potential, and (5) drug and alcohol abuse.

ASSESSING LEVEL OF ANXIETY AND COPING RESPONSES

Nonverbal responses to history-taking can be indicative of the woman's anxiety level. The identification of anxiety levels is described in Chapter 8. Hesitation, lack of eye contact, and vague statements, such as "it's been rough lately," indicate that the woman is dealing with a problem that is difficult for her to talk about. She may appear hesitant, shy, frightened, passive, or evasive or may be screaming or crying (Swanson 1984). Agitation and anxiety bordering on panic are almost always present. These women may be apprehensive of imminent doom, with good reason, as their husbands threaten violence, death, or mutilation. Because they live in terror, battered women remain vigilant, unable to relax or sleep. When they do sleep, they may have nightmares of danger and violence (Swanson 1984). Signs of the effect of living with chronic stress and severe levels of anxiety may be present, such as hypertension, irritability, or gastrointestinal disturbances.

Because of their feelings of confusion, shame, despair, and powerlessness, these women may withdraw from interaction with others. As a result, their self-esteem plummets further and they lose the sense that they have any control over their lives. Self-blame is used as a temporary coping device. In an attempt to retain a sense of control, the woman thinks that if she had done something different she would not have been beaten. So she tries to be the perfect wife and mother. Eventually, all efforts fail, and a profound sense of powerlessness results. She begins to feel that she deserves the abuse and sees no options for escape, even if alternatives are present. A pattern of learned helplessness develops. Since solutions to the problem have failed in the past, she stops trying.

ASSESSING SUPPORT SYSTEMS

Women are often trapped in abusive situations because they are economically dependent, culturally or religiously constrained, socially isolated, or have no alternative home (Germain 1984). Their husbands may have been jealously restricting their contacts with families and friends, causing the women to feel so unconnected that they cease to think of these groups as helpful and supportive. Or they may feel that they are so unworthy that no one else could possibly want anything to do with them, a reflection of their low self-esteem. Feelings of shame and disgrace also prevent them from talking to others, including social agency supports or the criminal justice system. Decreasing the isolation of these women is a major task, yet crucial to effecting change in their lives.

ASSESSING ACTUAL PHYSICAL ABUSE

A series of minor complaints such as headaches, dizziness, and "accidents," especially falls, may be indicative of abuse. Signs of battering include bruises, scars, burns, and other wounds in various stages of healing, particularly around the head, face, chest, arms, abdomen, and genitalia (Brown and Lewis 1985; Wilcoxen 1981) (See Box 12–2). Injuries seen in emergency rooms and offices that should arouse the nurse's suspicion are included in Box 12–1. A doctor's office or clinic may be one of the few places a battered woman is allowed to go by her husband. If the explanation does not match the injury seen or if the patient minimizes the seriousness of the injury, spouse abuse may be suspected.

Ask directly, but in a nonthreatening manner, whether she has been injured by her husband or boyfriend. Observe the nonverbal response, such as hesitation or lack of eye contact, as well as the verbal response. Then ask specific questions, such as "When was the last time it happened?" "How often does it happen?" "In what ways are you hurt?" *Always ask about the abuse of children* (Swanson 1984).

Once the history of abuse has been ascertained, carefully document verbal statements as well as physical findings. Sketch a body map and draw areas of injury with accompanying explanation. If the woman consents, take Polaroid photos. If she has just been beaten, ask her to return in a day or two for more photos, as bruises may be more evident at that time.

ASSESSING SUICIDE POTENTIAL

An abused woman may feel so trapped in a detrimental relationship yet be so desperate to get out that she may attempt suicide. A suicide attempt may be the presenting symptom in the emergency room. With sensitive questioning conducted in a caring manner, the nurse can elicit the abuse history. Often the woman will have overdosed on a combination of alcohol and other central nervous system (CNS) depressants, tranquilizers, or sleeping medications that have been prescribed for her in previous visits to doctors' offices, clinics, or emergency rooms.

When the crisis of the immediate suicide attempt has resolved, the woman must be questioned carefully to determine her lethality (see Chapter 22, Suicide Assessment). If, for example, she still feels that life is not worth living and has some pills stashed away that she says she may use, admission to an inpatient psychiatric unit must be considered. If, on the other hand, she has future plans and ways to live "for the sake of the children," then outpatient referrals may be given and the patient can be discharged. Each situation is dealt with individually, depending upon individual circumstances and marital state.

ASSESSING DRUG AND ALCOHOL USE

A battered spouse may self-medicate with alcohol or other drugs as a way to escape a dreadful situation. The drugs are usually CNS depressants, such as benzodiazepines, prescribed by physicians in response to the battered woman's presentation with "vague" complaints. Alcohol/drug use also obviates a woman's responsibility in the battering situation: "I was intoxicated, I couldn't defend myself," or "I couldn't think clearly."

The level of intoxication can be determined by history, physical examination, and blood alcohol level. If the woman is intoxicated, allow her to sober up in the emergency room before instituting referral. Referral information will not be understood or assimilated if she is intoxicated. She should not be discharged with her husband.

The abused woman may have a chronic alcohol or drug problem. This needs to be assessed (refer to Chapters 23 and 24), and appropriate treatment referrals provided. Again, choices for treatment can include both inpatient and outpatient options.

Standard III: Diagnosis

Nursing diagnoses can be many and varied for the woman who is abused. Some, but not all, possibilities are suggested (Kim 1984).

Spouse abuse is a situational crisis with attendant

threats to the woman's physical, emotional, and psychological health, and, ultimately, even her life. *Potential for violence*, *anxiety*, and *fear* are three diagnoses that apply. *Ineffective individual coping* is an expected diagnosis related to feelings of powerlessness and vulnerability. Often the abused spouse feels trapped. As a result, *powerlessness* is a diagnosis that can be applied to abused women.

Battered women often think they have no control or influence over what happens to them. Feelings of helplessness, hopelessness, and powerlessness contribute to the diagnosis of *body image disturbances* and *self-esteem disturbances*. Since the abused woman is so often without friends or extended family, *social isolation* is a nursing diagnosis that merits special attention. For the nuclear family, the crisis of violence precipitates *altered family process* as the family system becomes less and less able to meet the emotional, physical, or security needs of its members.

Standard IV: Planning

The nurse plans nursing care for a family in an abusive situation on both the (1) content level (planning long term and short term goals) and the (2) process level (awareness of personal reactions to family violence).

CONTENT LEVEL—PLANNING GOALS

Long term and short term goals are set for each nursing diagnosis. Each woman will have special needs and personal goals. It is vital to understand that these goals are the woman's goals. If the woman decides to go back to the abusing situation, the nurse will support her decision. The nurse, however, continues to affirm that no one has the right to abuse another human being and no one deserves to be abused by another, no matter what the relationship might be.

For the nursing diagnosis *potential for violence* related to rage reaction and poor impulse control of mate, the following goals may apply:

Long Term Goals

- Within three weeks, client will state that she believes that she does not deserve to be beaten.
- Within three weeks, client will state that she has joined a woman's support group/family counseling.
- Client will state that her living conditions are now safe from spouse abuse or
- Within two months, client will state that she has found safe housing for herself and the children.

Short Term Goals

- After initial interview, client will name four community resources she can contact.
- After initial interview, client will describe a safety plan to be used in future violent situations.
- Client will state her rights to live in a safe environment.
- Client will state the dangers to her and her children in her home situation.

Goals for the *self-esteem disturbance* related to chronic battering and belittling may include the following:

Long Term Goals

- Within two months, client will state that she feels more competent and in charge of her life.
- Within four months, client will name three things she has been able to change.
- Within three months, client will name one action taken to become more independent (job/home change/new friends, etc.).

Short Term Goals

- Client will state she feels better about herself after talking to the nurse.
- Client will name three myths about spouse abuse that she has incorporated into her life.
- Client will be able to discuss the reality of living with a violent mate.
- Client will name three things she would like to change in her life.

Spouse abuse is a symptom of a dysfunctional family. If the woman chooses to stay with her mate, which is often the case, planning needs to include the family. *Ineffective family coping* related to relationship problems may be applicable. Goals to be considered include the following:

Long Term Goals

- The batterer will state that he realizes that he must change in order to stay with his family.
- The batterer will join and attend group for spouses who batter.
- Within three months, the couple will state that they want to join a couples therapy group.
- The couple will be able to name three possible effects that family violence may have on their children.

- Within six months, the couple will state that the battering has ceased.

Short Term Goals

- Client will state she is interested in knowing about family treatment modalities.
- Client will state that she no longer chooses to live in a situation with violence.
- Client will name three places she can call to receive counseling for herself, family, or batterer.

It is important that the goals set are realistic and not too ambitious. It often takes an abused spouse a long time to make changes. Unfortunately, many take no action at all. This is usually very frustrating to health care professionals. This is particularly true for nurses who are often task oriented and trained to "fix things up." The nurse provides information and options and can make suggestions as to possible goals and outcomes. However, the final decision is the client's. She is the one who must live with the consequences.

PROCESS LEVEL—NURSES' REACTIONS AND FEELINGS

The more thought the nurse gives to the issue of spouse abuse prior to ever encountering the abuse victim, the more effective will be the subsequent interaction with the victim. Acknowledging accepted myths is the first step in at least putting them aside when working with a battered spouse and eventually allows for counteracting them with facts. Myths have served to perpetuate acceptance of spouse abuse. Some myths regarding spouse abuse and facts that counter them are found in Table 12–2.

Awareness of personal feelings in response to the battered woman stimulates examination of personal views toward violence and the status of women. Understanding the dynamics of battering is crucial to effective nursing intervention. It is helpful, as well as advisable, for nurses working with people involved in family violence to review their cases with other professionals in peer supervision or with a clinical supervisor. Issues involving abuse usually evoke irrational feelings. Nurses need to sort out their own strong feelings before they can work effectively with their clients.

Nurses are members of society and have been socialized to live within the social norms that contribute to women being treated as second-class citizens. Some nurses may still believe that it is acceptable for men to physically beat women; others will not. American society is violent, and some nurses may accept violence as a way of life; others will not. A nurse reacts to an abused female patient in large measure as a result of the way the

Table 12–2 • SPOUSE ABUSE: MYTH AND FACT

MYTH	FACT
1. The woman's behavior often causes the man to strike out at her.	1. The woman's behavior is NOT the cause of spouse abuse.
2. Men have the right to keep their wives in line.	2. No one has the right to beat or hurt another person.
3. Battered women are masochistic and like to be beaten.	3. Women do not like, ask for, or deserve to be abused.
4. Battered women come from poor working class backgrounds and are usually poorly educated.	4. Studies show that battered women and batterers come from all socioeconomic, religious, and educational backgrounds.
5. The family is sacred and should be allowed to take care of its own problems.	5. Intervention in family violence is justified since it always escalates in frequency and intensity, can end in death, and is passed on to future generations.
6. Women who are abused are crazy.	6. Women who are abused are not different from the rest of the population except that most grew up with violence in their homes. After years of abuse, self-esteem is devastated.
7. Myths abused women believe: "I can't live without him." "If I didn't do . . . , it wouldn't have happened." "He will change." "I will stay for the sake of the children." "His jealousy and possessiveness prove he really loves me."	7. These myths are coping mechanisms women use to allay panic in a situation of random and brutal violence. They give the illusion of control and rationality.

Data from Billy 1983; Gemmill 1982; Walker-Hooper 1981b.

nurse has been socialized. Some nurses have grown up in abusing households. Awareness of individual feelings and reactions facilitates caregiving in that the nurse can consciously and deliberately respond to the victim rather than get sidetracked into having to deal with personal reactions. Common responses of health care professionals to spouse abuse are listed in Table 12–3 (Delgaty 1985; Greany 1984). These feelings need to be recognized when they arise and dealt with in supervision in order to maximize therapeutic intervention.

Standard V: Intervention

Although a large number of women who are seen in the emergency room will admit to being abused, few come for treatment (Rounsaville 1979). This is unfortunate because it is almost impossible for a woman to cope with a violent mate without psychological and moral support (Strauss 1977). When women do come for treatment **two stages of treatment** appear most helpful, (1) the crisis stage and (2) the stage of internal change and rebuilding (Weingourt 1985).

The **crisis stage** includes (Houghton 1981)

1. Providing a safe atmosphere for reducing post-traumatic injury.
2. Encouraging decision making.
3. Providing referral information.
4. Maintaining concise, accurate records.

The **stage of internal change and rebuilding** includes focusing on rebuilding lives so destructive ways of relating are eliminated and self-esteem is elevated (Weingourt 1985).

It must be re-emphasized that throughout the process of working with a woman who has been battered, nurses must monitor their feelings and be aware of their own bias. The ability to accept what the woman says in a nonjudgmental atmosphere can help her regain self-esteem and restore self-confidence (Billy 1983). The woman's decision to stay in the battering situation or leave it must be supported by the nurse.

V-A: PSYCHOTHERAPEUTIC INTERVENTIONS

A woman who has been battered is in a state of crisis. If there is time to listen, encourage catharsis. Do not do so if you have to leave mid-sentence, as this will likely increase feelings of rejection. This may be the first time the woman has discussed the abuse, and merely doing that will be helpful to her. Explain that she is not alone. Tell her that this is a problem seen regularly and that it can happen to anyone. Such information will help diminish her feelings of isolation. Reassure her that she is safe. Use reflective communication techniques when she expresses shame or guilt about the abuse.

Psychotherapeutic interventions include crisis intervention and the promotion of growth. Crisis intervention refers here to the crisis stage.

PROVIDING A SAFE ATMOSPHERE FOR REDUCING POST-TRAUMATIC INJURY. If physical abuse is severe and the woman consents, a safe environment needs to be found. Battered women are more successful

Table 12–3 • COMMON RESPONSES OF HEALTHCARE PROFESSIONALS TO SPOUSE ABUSE

FEELING	SOURCE
Anger	At the man who did it; at the woman who allowed it to happen; at society for condoning its occurrence through attitudes, traditions, laws.
Embarrassed	The battered woman is a symbol of something close to home—the stress and strain of family life unleashed as uncontrolled anger.
Confused	The battered woman challenges our cherished view of the family as a haven of safety and privacy.
Afraid	A small percentage of batterers are dangerous to others.
Anguished	The nurse may have experienced family violence as a victim or a relative of a victim.
Helpless	Wanting to do more, to eliminate the problem, to cure.
Discouraged	If the woman chooses not to prosecute, not to leave.

at reversing their helplessness when they leave their husbands than when they remain and try to change their relationship (Swanson 1984).

If the woman has no other alternatives within her own support system, **shelters** or **safe houses** for battered women are available in many communities. They are open 24 hours a day and can be accessed through hotline information, hospital emergency rooms, YWCAs, or the local office of the National Organization for Women (NOW). The address of the house is usually kept secret to protect the women from attack by their mates. Besides protection, many of these safe shelters provide important education and consciousness-raising functions (Strauss 1977). The woman should be given the number of the nearest available shelter, even if she decides for the present to stay with her husband.

If the woman chooses to stay, the next best approach is to help her develop a **safety plan,** a plan for a fast escape if violence recurs. Ask her to identify the signs of escalation of violence and to pick a particular sign that will tell her in the future — "Now is the time to leave." If she plans ahead, she may be able to leave before the violence occurs. She should plan where she is going to go and how she will get there. Suggest that she have a bag already packed for herself and her children — a few articles of clothing, essential toiletry items, money for cab fare or a phone call, identification cards, insurance information, and a list of referral sources with their telephone numbers. If children are present, they can all agree on a code word that, when spoken by the mother, means "It is time to go."

ENCOURAGING DECISION MAKING. When discussing the future, the battered woman may have difficulty imagining options. She should be encouraged to realize that she has a right to live without fear of violence or physical harm, without fear of assault. In fact, she has the option of charging her husband with assault. The nurse can offer to call the police. A restraining order can be obtained. This makes it illegal for the husband to go near his wife. The role of the nurse is to support the woman, whatever she decides to do. By listening, giving support, discussing options, and encouraging her to imagine other ways of living, the nurse has initiated an awareness of other possibilities (Billy 1983).

PROVIDING REFERRAL INFORMATION. Resources for battered women include emergency shelters, crisis intervention teams, the police, battered women's support groups, task forces for battered wives, hotlines, and feminist groups (Ghent et al. 1985). The battered woman should be provided with a wealth of referral information. While she may not be able to use the services immediately, she will have the information for future reference. Most communities have a 24-hour telephone number provided by the Domestic Abuse Warning Network (DAWN). People who answer the phone have information on the services available for battered women, from shelters to legal assistance, and can help women find alternatives. Referral phone numbers may be kept for years before the decision is made to call. Having the number all that time contributes to thinking about options.

Battered women should also be given referrals to parenting resources that enable them to explore alternative approaches to discipline, i.e., no hitting, slapping, or other expressions of violence. It is disconcerting to see women in shelters use these methods with their children. Such behavior perpetuates the idea that violence solves problems and passes the problem of violence on to the next generation.

Individual counseling referrals and referrals for group therapy may also be given when available. Evaluating the need for referrals for the children may also be indicated if the children are in danger. Refer to Table 12–1 for the effects on children in homes where battering occurs.

Vocational counseling is another referral that may be appropriate. A list of programs for both men and women should be available to the client when indicated.

Specific referrals regarding emergency money and legal counseling should be made available to each woman. Emergency money is available through **Title XX of the 1974 Social Security Amendment Act** (Morton 1984). These monies cover one month's rent and utilities, food for one month, emergency clothing, and emergency furniture.

Legal counseling can be helpful. Strauss (1977) recommends the assistance of a feminist-oriented lawyer (male or female), since the judicial system often focuses on "preserving the family." Legal assistance can take the form of an injunction, a civil suit, or criminal charges.

MAINTAINING CONCISE, ACCURATE RECORDS. The importance of keeping **accurate records** of the woman's medical injuries and verbatim accounts of her emotional status cannot be stressed enough. The woman may have to depend on these in the future during litigation. The injuries should be described in detail and a body map drawn. When possible, and with consent, photographs should be taken (Billy 1983).

V-F: PSYCHOTHERAPY

Psychotherapy is carried out by a nurse who is educated at the master's level in psychiatric nursing and certified or eligible for certification (Morton 1984).

Therapy is most effective after crisis intervention,

when the life of the woman is less chaotic (Weingourt, 1985). A variety of therapeutic modalities are available for a woman/couple/family living in a violent family. Therapies for individuals, couples, and groups are discussed subsequently.

INDIVIDUAL THERAPY. The goals of individual therapy with a battered woman center on helping the woman recognize feelings about being battered, about herself, and about her options regarding the battering (Morton 1984). Expected outcomes include an increase in the woman's self-esteem, affirmation that she does not deserve to be beaten, and a sense that she has control over the decisions in her life.

COUPLES THERAPY. In about 10% of the cases, husbands will be motivated to change their behavior, and the couple will undergo therapy together (Gemmill 1982). One of the goals of couples therapy is to decrease the frequency and intensity of the battering (Morton 1984). Expected outcomes are that the husband will recognize inner states of anger and learn alternative ways of dealing with anger. The couple will be able to open communication and learn to listen to each other (Gemmill 1982).

GROUP THERAPY. A variety of groups are available to abused women. Therapy groups provide assurances that one is not alone and positive change is possible. Since many of these women have been isolated over a period of time, they have been deprived of validation and positive feedback from others. Working in a group can help diminish feelings of isolation, strengthen feelings of self-esteem and self-worth, and increase the potential for realistic problem solving in a supportive atmosphere.

Self-help groups serve an important function. Some women may feel more comfortable in an informal setting among women with common problems, especially if they have been socially and psychologically isolated over a period of time. Often a woman will have a sponsor, and information as well as emotional support is offered.

Feminist groups, even if not specifically concerned with abuse, can be immensely important in helping women to regain the psychological and moral initiative necessary to change their lives (Strauss 1977).

Niksaitis (1985) states that the real problem in a violent relationship is the batterer. The abused woman is the symptom of the problem. In the groups for men that batter, the men are taught to recognize signs of escalating anger and learn ways to channel their anger nonviolently. Men who have never discussed problems with anyone before learn that it is all right to have feelings.

Standard VI: Evaluation

Evaluating goals within the time period specified is done frequently throughout the process of intervention. Generally, if the woman and children are living in a family where battering has ceased, the most important immediate goals have been met. Other important goals would be met if there was an increase in self-esteem by both partners, a decrease in physical symptoms, a decrease in alcohol and drug abuse, and an increase in satisfaction within the relationship (Morton 1984).

If the batterer refuses to become involved with working toward change (group, individual, family therapy), the goal of living in a violence-free setting would be met only if the woman and children left the situation. Since, often, the woman is not ready to leave a violent mate, the goal might be to anticipate escalating anger and to have a number of viable safety plans available. In cases of spouse abuse, change often takes a long time, and the nurse has to learn to be comfortable with the goals the woman is able to meet, although they may not be the goals the nurse wants for the client.

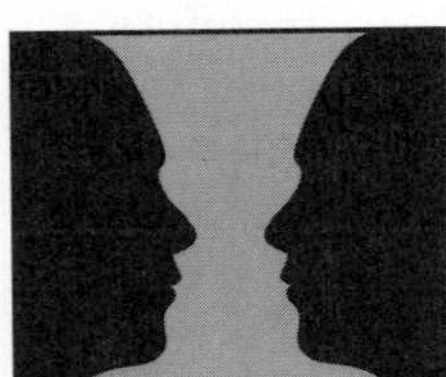

Case Study: Working With a Family Involved in Spouse Abuse

Darnell Peters is a 42-year-old married woman in a relationship she states "has been bad for a long time. We don't communicate." She was brought to the emergency room by ambulance with lacerations to her face and swollen, blackened eyes, lips, and nose. She told the nurse that her husband had been in bed asleep for hours before she joined him. Upon getting into bed, she attempted to redistribute the bed covers. Suddenly, the husband leaped from the bed, started punching her in the face, and began to throw her against the wall. She called for her 11-year-old son to call the police. After her husband finished beating her, he went back to sleep. The police arrived, called an ambulance, and took Mr. Peters to jail.

Mrs. Peters stated their relationship was always stormy. "He always was putting me down and yelling at me." He started hitting her five years ago when she became pregnant with her second and last child. The beatings have increased in intensity over the past year, and this emergency room visit was the fifth this year. Tonight was the first time she ever called the police.

Mrs. Peters was visibly upset. Periods of crying alternated with periods of silence. She appeared apathetic and depressed. The nurse remained calm and objective. After Mrs. Peters had finished talking, the nurse explored alternatives.

Assessment

NURSE:	Have you thought of you and your children living a life without violence?
MRS. PETERS:	Yes . . . I have been thinking about divorce for two years now. I even went to an attorney. I am the one supporting my family, and the attorney told me I would need evidence to support this claim. I can't get it; he controls everything.
NURSE:	Yes . . .
MRS. PETERS:	My husband keeps all the bank statements, check stubs, and other financial data under lock and key. Once I had access to the check stubs, but I became so frightened of what he would do to me if he found out that I put them back. Now I am afraid I am going to lose my job; I have lost so much time with injuries.
NURSE:	Is there someone who can help you?
MRS. PETERS:	I don't have any friends anymore . . . our neighbors kind of stay away because of my husband's gruffness and jealousy. My brother-in-law told me once that I could stay with his family if my husband ever abused me. You see, my husband was married before and he beat his first wife also.
NURSE:	What about the children, are they abused in the home?
MRS. PETERS:	Well . . . no. Lately I haven't had much time for them, and I notice I am yelling at them over nothing.

Mrs. Peters and the nurse discussed safety issues, devised a safety plan, and considered legal options, including a restraining order. Mrs. Peters left the emergency room with referral information, including the number of a safe house.

One week later Mrs. Peters returned to the emergency room; again she was beaten. She asked for referrals and said she needed help to leave him, because she was afraid that he was going to kill her: "I don't know what to do."

The nurse organized her data into subjective and objective components.

OBJECTIVE DATA

1. Beatings escalating in frequency and severity over past year
2. Husband has been jailed for abuse once
3. Husband had beaten his first wife
4. Husband controls all bank statements and records
5. One brother-in-law willing to help wife
6. Two children in the home exposed to abuse
7. Woman is able to support herself and children
8. Physical injuries due to current episode of abuse

SUBJECTIVE DATA

1. "He controls everything."
2. "I am afraid he will kill me."
3. Appears depressed and overwhelmed
4. Fears losing job because of missed time from beatings

Nursing Diagnosis

The nurse devised the following nursing diagnoses:

1. *Violence* related to home violence, as evidenced by verbalization of abuse by spouse
   - Physical injuries due to current episode of abuse
   - History of past abuse

Continued on following page

Nursing Diagnosis *(Continued)*

- Husband beat first wife
- Husband jailed once for inflicting abuse
- Beatings escalating in intensity and frequency over past year
- "I'm afraid he will kill me"

2. *Powerlessness* related to marital violence, as evidenced by inability to make decisions
   - "He controls everything."
   - "I'm afraid he will kill me."
   - Fears losing job because of missed time from beatings
   - "I don't know what to do."

Planning

Mrs. Peters talked to the nurse about what things she would like to change. Since she had already decided on divorce, she was ready to move out as long as she could feel that she and her children would be safe. Mrs. Peters agreed to see the nurse once a week and to be in contact with her by telephone until the crisis was resolved. She stated, "I know I need help to get out of this nightmare." The nurse and Mrs. Peters set the following long term and short term goals:

Nursing Diagnosis	Long Term Goals	Short Term Goals
1. *Violence* related to home violence, as evidenced by verbalization of abuse by spouse	Mrs. Peters will state that she and her children live in a safe environment in four weeks.	1. Before leaving emergency room client will name two agencies she will contact. 2. Client will have safe place to stay within 24 hours. 3. Client will have legal protection by end of week.
2. *Powerlessness* related to marital violence, as evidenced by inability to make decisions	Within two months Mrs. Peters will state that she feels more in control and has made two major changes in her life.	1. Mrs. Peters will make one decision about her life while in the emergency room. 2. Within two weeks Mrs. Peters will state she does not deserve to be abused. 3. Mrs. Peters will set two goals for the future within three weeks.

Intervention

The nurse and Mrs. Peters plan to meet at least once a week. Interventions are planned to help meet the long term and short term goals (Nursing Care Plan 12–1). Mrs. Peters seemed to respond well to support, and once legal restraints were taken, she felt less anxiety and fear for herself and the children.

Evaluation

Mrs. Peters was able to make arrangements with the shelter to take her and her two children in until after she had secured a restraining order. She called her brother-in-law, and he stated that he would go to the house with her while she packed and got the children. He told her that she and the children could stay with them, but she wanted to wait until she had a restraining order. She was terrified of what her husband would do if he found her, and she stated she would feel safer if she had police protection.

She continued to see the nurse once a week and called her frequently in between for information and direction. As time went on she joined a women's support group, which proved extremely supportive and informative, giving her hope and increasing her self-esteem. She was worried about her youngest, and she also agreed with the nurse that both children should have an evaluation and possible short term counseling during the crisis.

Mrs. Peters had a lot of strengths, had a means of earning a living, and had an important outside support system (brother-in-law). Since she already planned on divorce, leaving her husband was an easier decision for her to make than for many women in her situation.

Nursing Care Plan 12–1 • A FAMILY INVOLVED WITH SPOUSE ABUSE: Mrs. Peters

NURSING DIAGNOSIS

Violence related to home violence, as evidenced by verbalization of abuse by spouse

Supporting Data

- Physical injuries due to current episodes of abuse.
- History of past abuse.
- Husband beat first wife.
- Husband jailed once for inflicting abuse.
- Beatings escalating in intensity and frequency over past year.
- "I'm afraid he will kill me."

Long Term Goal: Within four weeks Mrs. Peters will state that she and her children live in a safe environment.

Short Term Goal	*Intervention*	*Rationale*	*Evaluation*
1. Before leaving the emergency room client will name two agencies she will contact.	1a. Provide information on shelters, legal services, self-help groups, etc.	1a. Educates as to services available. Reinforces the availability of help and lessens isolation.	Goal met On first visit Mrs. Peters called a shelter and made an appointment with an attorney.
	1b. Explore alternatives with Mrs. Peters.	1b. Verbalizing options aids decision making. Anticipatory planning helps mobilize energy for action.	
	1c. Be supportive of decisions Mrs. Peters makes, affirming that no person deserves to be abused.	1c. Mrs. Peters can do only what she is ready to do at this time. Reaffirmation of right to live without violence puts situation in perspective, aids decision making.	
2. Client will be in a safe place within 24 hours.	2. Explore options with Mrs. Peters, i.e., shelter versus brother-in-law.	2. Client makes decisions based on options and what is best for her regarding safety.	Goal partially met Mrs. Peters decided to go to a shelter until she had a restraining order; then brother-in-law would take her in.
3. Client will have legal protection within one week.	3. Explain to Mrs. Peters where she can get legal counseling and the types of help she can receive.	3. Anxiety will decrease when fear of retaliation is diminished.	Goal met Appointment was kept and Mrs. Peters got a restraining order within five days (date).

NURSING DIAGNOSIS

Powerlessness related to marital violence, as evidenced by inability to make decisions

Supporting Data

- "He controls everything."
- "I'm afraid he will kill me."
- Fear of losing job because of missed time due to beatings.
- "I don't know what to do."

Long Term Goals: Within two months, Mrs. Peters will state that she feels more in control and has made two major changes in her life.

Short Term Goals	*Intervention*	*Rationale*	*Evaluation*
1. Mrs. Peters will take one action toward making desired changes before she leaves the emergency room.	1a. Actively listen while Mrs. Peters talks.	1a. Concern and respect bolster self-esteem and reduce feelings of alienation.	Goal met Called brother-in-law to take her to the house while she packed and took the children to the shelter.
	1b. Demonstrate concern for her feelings and safety.	1b. Lowers anxiety, validates life is valuable.	
	1c. Discuss actions she feels ready to take now.	1c. Prioritizing goals can help mobilize actions.	

Continued on following page

Nursing Care Plan 12–1 • A FAMILY INVOLVED WITH SPOUSE ABUSE: Mrs. Peters *(Continued)*

Short Term Goal	*Intervention*	*Rationale*	*Evaluation*
	1d. Support decision and offer ways she can carry out action ONLY when she asks for advice.	1d. Supporting decisions and encouraging problem solving helps person function at more optimum level and encourages forward movement.	
2. Within two weeks Mrs. Peters will state she does not deserve to be abused.	2a. Explain she is not alone.	2a. Can motivate examination of situation.	Goal met For a long time Mrs. Peters was fearful for her life. Now she no longer chooses to stay in her present circumstances.
	2b. Explain others have learned to live in safety and have fuller and more meaningful lives.	2b. Decreases feelings of helplessness and offers hope.	
	2c. Discuss women's groups that are supportive and deal with issues of abuse.	2c. Encourages an increase in social contacts and expanding support system.	
	2d. Discuss effects of living in abusive environment on children.	2d. Growing up in abusive homes can result in cognitive and behavioral problems for children.	
3. Mrs. Peters will set two future goals within three weeks.	3. While meeting short term goals, help Mrs. Peters project herself into the future.	3. Continuing the momentum of positive change and movement minimizes feelings of helplessness and powerlessness.	Goal met Plans to join a women's group and file for divorce.

Summary

The practice of spouse abuse is a transcultural phenomenon, which is minimized by myths and supported, until recently, by legal sanctions. Nurses can use the data gleaned from clinical observations and research findings on characteristics of the battered family, the batterer, and the abused woman to plan effective nursing interventions. The cycle of violence follows predictable stages, and unless interventions are applied, violence will grow in frequency and intensity. Assessment includes identifying levels of anxiety, coping mechanisms, and the woman's support system, the actual physical abuse, suicide potential, as well as drug abuse. Nursing diagnoses of potential for violence, powerlessness, self-esteem disturbance, isolation, and altered family process often apply to these situations.

In planning care, the nurse must be sure the goals set are the goals that reflect the woman's wishes at that time. Strong and irrational responses by health care professionals are common when working with abused women. Knowing about these reactions and how to reduce intense feelings increases the nurse's therapeutic effectiveness. Interventions are planned in terms of whether the woman/family is currently in crisis or whether more corrective changes are possible when the anxiety has lessened within the family system.

Evaluation is based on the stated goals; however, certain indications of successful outcomes are universal. Cessation of the battering, increase in self-esteem, increase in family communication and satisfaction, and evidence of nonviolent coping strategies are all indications of effective interventions.

References

Billy BJ. Life patterns and emergency care of battered women. Journal of Emergency Nursing, 9(5):251, 1983.

Boyd VD, Klingbeil KS. Battered women: The everyday crime. Paper presented at the National Meeting of the American Psychological Association, Panel on Domestic Violence, August, 1977.

Brown M, Lewis DJ. Battered women: How nurses can help. RNABC News, 17(2):16, 1985.

Campbell J. A survivor group for battered women. Advances in Nursing Science, 8(2):13, 1986.

Corenblum B. Reactions to alcohol-related marital violence. Journal of Studies on Alcohol, 44(4):665, 1983.

Delgaty K. Battered women: The issues for nursing. The Canadian Nurse, 81(2):21, 1985.

DeLorto DO, LaViolette AD. Spouse abuse. Occupational Health Nursing, 28(8):17, 1980.

Flanzer J. Alcoholism is a key in many family abuse cases. Paper presented at the Seventh National Conference on Child Abuse and Neglect, Chicago: November, 1985.

Gemmill FB. A family approach to the battered woman. Journal of Psychosocial Nursing and Mental Health Services 20(9):22, 1982.

Germain CP. Sheltering abused women: A nursing perspective. Journal of Psychosocial Nursing 22(9):24, 1984.

Ghent WR, DaSylva NP, Farren ME. Family violence: Guidelines for recognition and management. Canadian Medical Association Journal, 132:541, 1985.

Greany GD. Is she a battered woman? A guide for emergency response. American Journal of Nursing, 85(6):724, 1984.

Hilberman E. Overview: The "wife beater's wife" reconsidered. American Journal of Psychiatry, 137:1336, 1980.

Houghton B. Domestic violence training: Treatment of adult victims of family violence. Journal of New York State Nurses Association, 12:25, 1981.

Kim MJ, McFarland GK, McLane AM (eds). Pocket Guide to Nursing Diagnoses. St. Louis: C.V. Mosby, 1984.

Langly R, Levy R. Wife Beating. The Silent Crisis. New York: E.P. Dutton, 1977.

Martin D. Overview: Scope of the problem. *In* U.S. Commission on Civil Rights, Battered Women: Issues of Public Policy. 1978, pp. 3–19.

Morton T. The client who has been battered. *In* Lego S (ed). The American Handbook of Psychiatric Nursing. Philadelphia: J.B. Lippincott, 1984.

Niksaitis G. Therapy for men who batter: Interview. Journal of Psychosocial Nursing, 23:33, July 1985.

Rounsaville B. Battered Women. New York: Harper & Row, 1979.

Sanchez-Dirks R. Reflection on family violence. Alcohol Health and Research, Fall:12,1979.

Strauss MA. A sociological perspective on the prevention and treatment of wifebeating. *In* Roy M (ed). Battered Women: A Psychosociological Study of Domestic Violence. New York: Van Nostrand Reinhold Company, 1977.

Swanson RW. Battered wife syndrome. Canadian Medical Association Journal 130(6):709, 1984.

Walker L. The Battered Woman. New York: Harper & Row, 1979.

Walker-Hooper A. Domestic violence: Assessing the problem. *In* Warner CG (ed). Conflict Intervention in Social and Domestic Violence. Bowie, MD: Robert J Brady, 1981a.

Walker-Hooper A. Responding to victim's needs. *In* Warner CG (ed). Conflict Intervention in Social and Domestic Violence. Bowie, MD: Robert J Brady, 1981b.

Weingourt R. Never to be alone: Existential therapy with battered women. Journal of Psychosocial Nursing, 23:24, March, 1985.

Wilcoxen M. Assaulted Women: A handbook for health professionals. Toronto: Support Services for Assaulted Women, 1981, pp. 6–11.

Self-Study Exercises

Place T (True) or F (False) next to each statement.

1. ________ Most spouse abuse takes place on weekdays.
2. ________ Men who batter are usually sociopaths or psychotic.
3. ________ Women usually stay in abusive relationships because they are masochistic.
4. ________ Headaches, palpitations, stomach ache, back aches, and other somatic complaints are *not* signals that a woman may be abused at home.
5. ________ Low self-esteem is characteristic of the abused woman, not the abusive mate.
6. ________ Children from violent homes often use violence later in life to cope with stress.
7. ________ Anxiety, depression, and suicidal thoughts/attempts are often seen in abused women.
8. ________ You can usually tell if people are in abusive situations by the way they present themselves to the world.
9. ________ Men often do not remember clearly their acts of violence and use denial and rationalization as coping mechanisms.
10. ________ Promises, gifts, and loving behavior are characteristic of the honeymoon stage of the cycle theory of violence.

Choose the letter that best answers the following questions.

11. Which of the following is NOT a myth a woman may believe that keeps her locked into an abusive relationship?

    A. She stays "for the sake of the children."
    B. "He will change."
    C. She deserves the beatings once in a while.
    D. No one has the right to harm or beat another.

12. Which of the following is NOT a coping device women use who are abused?

    A. Self-blame
    B. Rationalization
    C. Somatization
    D. Assertiveness

13. Of the following, which area is the LEAST important to assess for a woman presenting with spouse abuse?

    A. Suicide potential
    B. Use of drugs/alcohol
    C. Woman's support system
    D. Ethnic background

Write brief responses in answer to the following:

14. List two possible nursing diagnoses for a victim of spouse abuse and one goal for each.
    1. ND: ____________________
       GOAL: ____________________
    2. ND: ____________________
       GOAL: ____________________

15. List three common responses nurses have when working with a woman who is abused that would warrant peer supervision or clinical supervision.
    1. ____________________
    2. ____________________
    3. ____________________

16. Identify three areas to assess in order to evaluate the effectiveness of intervention in a spouse abuse family.
    1. ____________________
    2. ____________________
    3. ____________________

State whether the following interventions are part of the crisis (C) stage or are more apt to be carried out during the stage of internal change (I).

17. __________ Encourage catharsis, explaining she is not alone and reassuring her that she is safe in the emergency room.
18. __________ Devise with her a safety plan.
19. __________ Explore options and encourage decision making.
20. __________ Start couples therapy with both husband and wife.
21. __________ Have children evaluated for emotional and cognitive effects of violent environment.
22. __________ Make referrals.
23. __________ Refer husband to groups for men that batter.

CHAPTER 13

Evidence of Maladaptive Responses to Crisis: Rape

Kathleen Smith-DiJulio

OUTLINE

KEY TERMS AND CONCEPTS

The key terms and concepts listed here also appear in bold where they are defined or discussed in this chapter.

RAPE-TRAUMA SYNDROME
Acute Phase
Long Term Reorganization Phase
CONTROLLED STYLE OF COPING
EXPRESSED STYLE OF COPING
COMPOUND REACTION
SILENT REACTION
BEHAVIORAL SELF-BLAME

OBJECTIVES

After studying this chapter, the student will be able to:

1. Discuss and define the meaning of a sexual assault.
2. Name two reasons why rapes often go unreported.
3. List three common reactions to the first phase—acute phase—of the rape-trauma syndrome.
4. List three common reactions to the second phase—long term reorganization—of the rape-trauma syndrome.
5. List five areas to assess when working with a person who has been sexually assaulted.
6. List two long term goals and two short term goals for the nursing diagnosis rape-trauma syndrome.
7. Discuss five myths popularly believed about rape and its victims.
8. Discuss five psychotherapeutic techniques that are useful when working with a person who has been sexually assaulted.
9. Briefly discuss the nurse's role during the physical examination.
10. Briefly discuss the responsibilities of the nurse when discharging a rape victim from the emergency room, and three specific referrals.
11. Briefly discuss the nurse's role when staffing a rape-crisis hotline.
12. Name three outcomes that would signify successful interventions with a victim of sexual assault.

Rape can be one of the most devastating experiences a person lives through—if he or she lives. It is one of the most traumatic of the adventitious crises. The violent act of rape escalates anxiety to severe and panic levels and engulfs its victims in fear, the fear of death. The rape victim carries the additional burden of shame, guilt, and embarrassment. Rape is an act of violence, and sex is the weapon used by the aggressor on the victim (Burgess and Holstrom 1974).

Rape is generally understood as being *forced* and *violent* (without consent) vaginal or anal penetration against the victim's will and *without* the victim's consent. The legal definition of rape varies from state to state and, in addition to penetration, can include any type of forced genital contact, such as oral-genital contact. The term "sexual assault" more accurately describes what constitutes rape and is increasingly used in place of the word "rape."

Partly because definition varies, the incidence of rape is very difficult to determine. According to the President's Task Force on Victims of Crime (1982), there were 77,000 cases of reported rapes in 1982. In actuality, those figures must be doubled, since it is estimated that 50% of the cases go unreported (Pres. Task Force 1982). In some locales, rape is the fastest growing crime (Bradford 1983). It has been estimated that one in six women will be raped in her lifetime (Nelson 1980).

It is men who rape. It is extremely uncommon for a woman to rape another person. The vast majority of rape victims are women. Males are raped less frequently and are usually raped by heterosexual males. Although men are susceptible to rape, this chapter will use the female pronoun throughout. The principles are the same for all victims of rape.

It has been mentioned that rape often goes unreported. One major reason for the underreporting of rape is that the victim, as well as the rapist, goes on trial. Rape is the only crime in which the victim is required to prove innocence. Women victims have historically been held responsible for the occurrence of rape. It was believed that if the victim had not, for example, been so careless, been drinking, been dressed so provocatively, or been out too late, she would not have been raped. Additionally, women have usually been required to show evidence of having attempted to resist rape.

Another reason that rapes go unreported is because of social taboos against talking about sex—especially forced, violent sex crimes. And men who are raped are less likely to report than women because of the general lack of social acceptance of sex between two men. It can be seen that victims of rape are victimized not only by the crime itself but also by society's reactions. Personal anguish and grief also keep the person from seeking emergency medical care and reporting the crime (Warner 1980).

Recent changes in awareness of what rape is and laws governing sexual assault are largely due to the women's movement. Feminists have done a great deal to raise the consciousness of individuals and American society as a whole to allow acceptance of the concept that women are people, not property, and are to be accorded the same rights and privileges as men. Women are now also seen as equals in the marriage relationship, so laws are changing to allow a wife to bring rape charges against her husband. Formerly it was believed that a man was entitled to sex in a relationship, no matter how he got it. Thanks to the women's movement, gradual change is occurring.

Sexual assault as a maladaptive response to crisis can be conceptualized as shown in Figure 13–1.

Standard I: Theory

Sexual assault may occur within the context of a social relationship that goes too far, by a neighbor or relative, or by a total stranger. The assailant may use weapons, restraints, direct physical force, threats of physical harm, or other types of intimidation. Regardless of the methods employed to force the victim, the victim usually fears death (Abarbanel 1980). Most victims of rape suffer severe and long-lasting emotional trauma. Five features of the assault experience that contribute to psychological trauma have been identified by Abarbanel (1980):

1. The assault experience is sudden and arbitrary.
2. The assault experience is perceived as life threatening.
3. The main purpose of an assault is to violate the victim's physical integrity and render her helpless.
4. The assault experience forces the victim to participate in the crime.
5. The assault experience renders the victim helpless to prevent or control the assailant, once normal coping strategies fail. She becomes the victim of someone else's rage and aggression.

Based on a landmark study of 92 rape victims, Burgess and Holstrom (1974) documented the existence of the **rape-trauma syndrome.** The rape-trauma syndrome comprises (1) acute phase and (2) the long term reorganization process that occurs following an actual or attempted sexual assault. Each phase has its separate symptoms.

ACUTE PHASE OF RAPE-TRAUMA SYNDROME

The **acute phase** occurs immediately following the assault and may last for a couple of weeks. This is the stage seen by hospital personnel in the emergency room. Nurses are most involved in dealing with these initial reactions. During this phase there is a great deal of disorganization in the person's lifestyle, and somatic symptoms are common. Burgess (1985) describes this disorganization in terms of impact reactions, somatic reactions, and emotional reactions. Refer to Table 13–1 for identifying symptoms for each reaction.

The most common initial reaction is shock, numbness, and disbelief. Outwardly the person may appear self-contained and calm. Frequent remarks include, "It doesn't seem real," "I don't believe this really happened to me." The person may also appear extremely confused, have difficulty concentrating, and have difficulty with decision making. Or, the person may become hysterical, restless, cry, or even smile. These are typical reactions to crisis and reflect cognitive, affective, and behavioral disruptions (Warner 1980).

People who have experienced an emotionally overwhelming event may need to deny the event. Denial in this case is an adaptive and protective reaction and gives the person time to prepare for the reality (Abarbanel 1980). Examples of denials may be found in such statements as "I don't want to talk about it," "I just want to forget what happened."

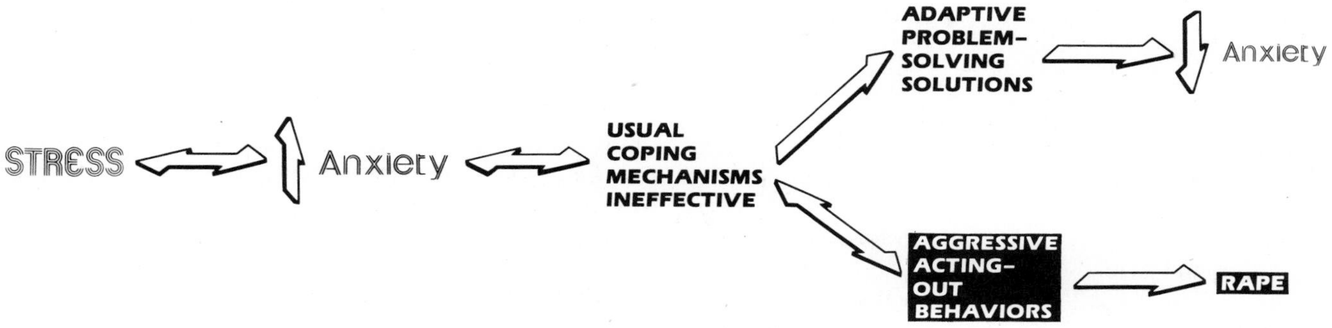

Figure 13–1. *Conceptualization of the process of aggressive acting-out behaviors in the development of rape-trauma syndrome.*

Table 13–1 • ACUTE PHASE OF RAPE-TRAUMA SYNDROME

IMPACT REACTION	SOMATIC REACTION	EMOTIONAL REACTION
1. **EXPRESSED STYLE** Overt Behaviors such as • Crying, sobbing • Smiling • Restlessness, agitation, hysteria • Volatility, anger • Hysteria • Tenseness 2. **CONTROLLED STYLE** Reactions more covert • Masked facies • Appears calm, subdued • May appear shocked, numb, confused, disbelieving • Easily distracted, difficulty making decisions	Evidenced within the first several weeks following a rape **PHYSICAL TRAUMA** • Bruises (breasts, throat, back) • Soreness **SKELETAL MUSCLE TENSION** • Headaches • Sleep disturbances • Grimaces, twitches **GASTROINTESTINAL** • Stomach pains • Nausea • Poor appetite • Diarrhea **GENITOURINARY** • Vaginal itching • Vaginal discharge • Pain, discomfort	• Fear of physical violence and death • Denial • Anxiety • Shock • Humiliation • Fatigue • Embarrassment • Desire for revenge • Self-blame • Lowered self-esteem • Shame • Guilt

Data from Abarbanel 1980; Burgess 1985; Burgess and Holstrom 1974.

LONG TERM REORGANIZATION PHASE OF RAPE-TRAUMA SYNDROME

The **long term reorganization phase** occurs two or more weeks following the rape. Nurses who initially care for the victim can help victims anticipate and prepare for the reactions they are likely to experience. Reactions include the following (Abarbanel 1980; Burgess 1985; Burgess and Holstrom 1974):

1. Intrusive thoughts of the rape break into the victim's conscious mind during the day and during sleep. These thoughts include anger and violence toward the assailant. Flashbacks, dreams with violent content, and insomnia are common.
2. Increased motor activity follows, i.e., moving, taking trips, changing telephone numbers, and frequent visits to old friends. This activity stems from fear that the assailant will come back. Anxiety, mood swings, crying spells, and feelings related to depression are likely to be observed.
3. Fears and phobias develop as a defensive reaction to the rape. Typical phobias include
   - Fear of the indoors — if the rape occurred indoors.
   - Fear of the outdoors — if the rape occurred outdoors.
   - Fear of being alone — common for most women after an assault.
   - Fear of crowds — "Any person there might be a rapist."
   - Fear of sexual encounters and activities — many women experience acute disruption of their sex life with husbands or boyfriends. Rape is especially upsetting for those with no prior sexual experience.

Standard II: Data Collection

Once at the emergency department, the attention the rape victim receives depends upon the protocol of the particular hospital. Lederle et al. (1985) suggest the following:

1. Provide immediate care and privacy.
2. Provide quality collection of evidence.
3. Conduct a physical examination.
4. Offer follow-up care.

The nurse talks with the victim, family or friends who accompany the victim, and the police to gather as much data as possible for assessing the crisis.

The nurse assesses the (1) level of anxiety, (2) coping mechanisms used, (3) support systems available, (4) signs and symptoms of emotional trauma, and (5) signs and symptoms of physical trauma. Information obtained from assessment is then analyzed and nursing diagnoses are formulated.

ASSESSING LEVEL OF ANXIETY

Assessing, understanding, and evaluating the reactions and feelings of the victim following a rape are essential nursing skills. Because of the personal threat to the victim's sense of safety and security, it can be surmised that the victim experiences acute anxiety. If nurses are sensitive to this fact they will take their time with the patient. Support, reassurance, and appropriate therapeutic techniques can help diminish anxiety.

Depending on the individual's intrapersonal and interpersonal resources, the anxiety level may be moderate to panic. (These levels are discussed in Chapter 8.) It is important to take cues from the patient. Do *not* initiate touching, as this may further increase the victim's anxiety level. If the victim reaches out and makes the first contact, then touch is acceptable.

The presence of a supportive, helpful person can assist in diminishing anxiety caused by the rape. If the victim is with a third party, obtain the victim's permission before history-taking in front of someone else. The third party should be there only for support, not to answer questions. If the third party interferes with the history-taking process or seems to make the victim uncomfortable, he or she should be asked to wait in another area.

ASSESSING COPING MECHANISMS USED

Everyone has ways of dealing with stressful situations. The same coping skills that have helped the victim through other difficult problems will be used in adjusting to rape. In addition, new ways of getting through difficult times may be developed — for both the short term and the long term.

Behavioral mechanisms can be seen and therefore fairly easily assessed. Examples include crying, withdrawing, smoking, wanting to talk about the event, hysteria, confusion, disorientation, incoherence, and even laughing or joking.

Cognitive coping mechanisms are the thoughts people have that help them deal with high anxiety levels. If the victim is able to verbalize thoughts, the nurse will know what the victim is thinking. If not, the nurse can ask questions, e.g., "What do you think might help now?" or "What can I do to help you in this difficult situation?"

ASSESSING SUPPORT SYSTEMS AVAILABLE

The *availability, size,* and *utility* of a victim's social support system need to be addressed. The nurse asks the victim if there are family or friends with whom she feels safe and in whom she can confide. They can be used as a means to strengthen self-confidence and to assist her in resuming a normal style of living. However, nurses need to be aware that family, neighbors, and friends, generally the people considered as valuable support, are the people most often involved in perpetrating the unwanted sexual experience(s) (Mims and Chang 1984). Pay careful attention to verbal and nonverbal cues the victim may be communicating regarding persons in her social network. For example, someone the victim knows may suggest that they have a spare room and the victim can spend the night there so she won't be alone, yet the victim seems hesitant. Be certain the source of the hesitancy is privately explored before railroading her into doing something that might be detrimental. The hesitancy could be due to increased anxiety and decreased ability to make decisions — or it could be due to fear of finding herself in another sexual assault situation. The following vignette illustrates this point:

Joyce, an 18-year-old, was brought to the emergency room by a concerned neighbor. She was wandering aimlessly outside her house, sobbing and muttering, "He had no right to do that to me." Because of Joyce's distraught appearance and her statement, the triage nurse suspected sexual assault and brought the victim to the office of the psychiatric nurse, Ms. Webster. Ms. Webster introduced herself, explained her role, and stated that she was there to help. Ms. Webster then asked Joyce what had happened. With careful, sensitive, nonthreatening questioning, Joyce divulged that she had been out with her boyfriend, who had raped her and then dropped her off at her house. Because no one else was at home and she was so upset and afraid, she did not go inside, and the neighbor, Mrs. Green, had seen her outside.

After the entire history and examination were completed, plans for discharge were being discussed. Joyce stated no one would be home until Sunday night, two days away, and she did not feel comfortable calling any friends because she did not want them to know what had happened. The neighbor, Mrs. Green, had told the nurse earlier that Joyce could stay with her family.

NURSE: Earlier, your neighbor, Mrs. Green, told me that you were welcome to spend the weekend with her family.

JOYCE: *(Loudly, sharply with eyes wide)* Oh, no, I couldn't do that.

NURSE: You don't seem to like that idea.

JOYCE: Oh, I just wouldn't want to bother them.

NURSE: Mrs. Green seems quite concerned about your welfare.

JOYCE: Oh, yes, she's very nice. *(Pause)*

NURSE: But not someone you would want to spend the weekend with.

JOYCE: Her children are too noisy. I've got homework to do.

NURSE: You might not get the quiet you need to study. *(Pause)* Yet you also do not want to be alone.

JOYCE: *(Wringing a tissue in her hands, head hanging, soft voice)* I can't go in that house anymore.

NURSE: Something about being in that house disturbs you.

JOYCE: Mr. Green *(deep sigh, pause)* used to . . . uh . . . take advantage of me when I used to babysit his children.

NURSE: Take advantage?

JOYCE: Yes . . . *(sobbing)* he used to force me to have sex with him. He said he'd blame it on me if I told anyone.

NURSE: What a frightening experience that must have been for you.

JOYCE: Yes.

NURSE: I can see why you would not want to spend the night there. Let's continue to explore other options.

A suitable place to stay was finally arranged. Joyce was given counseling referrals that would help her deal with the process of reorganization from the current rape experience as well as begin to explore her feelings about past sexual abuse she suffered at the hands of her neighbor.

ASSESSING SIGNS AND SYMPTOMS OF EMOTIONAL TRAUMA

Nurses work most frequently with rape victims in the emergency room soon after the rape has occurred. When the rape victim comes to the emergency room, the triage nurse makes the initial assessment. A special waiting area, separate from the general lobby, should be provided. The victim should be admitted to the emergency room ahead of all patients except those with life-threatening emergencies. However, when extreme emotional or physical trauma is present, the victim is immediately escorted to the treatment area. This kind of focused supportive attention helps the rape victim to begin to feel safe and at ease.

The extent of the psychological and emotional trauma sustained by the victim may not be readily apparent from the victim's behavior (Antognoli-Toland 1985). If the person uses the **controlled style** during the acute phase of the rape trauma (see Table 13–1), ill-informed staff may wonder whether the person was really raped. That skepticism may be communicated to the victim, serving to increase anxiety and lower self-esteem. It is important to remember that despite the person's apparent response, *there is always psychological and emotional trauma experienced by a victim during and after an assault*. Nurses are *never* in the position of judging the validity of a rape.

It is important that a nursing history be conducted and properly recorded. When obtaining a history, the nurse needs to determine only the details of the assault that will be helpful in addressing the immediate physical and psychological needs of the victim.

Allow the person to talk at a comfortable pace. Pose questions in nonjudgmental, descriptive terms. Do not ask "why." To relate the events of the rape most likely will be traumatic and embarrassing for the victim. Besides assessing the time, place, and circumstances of the rape, the *type of assault* is important. What occurred?

Fondling?
Oral penetration or attempted penetration?
Vaginal penetration or attempted penetration?
Rectal penetration or attempted penetration?
Ejaculation—Where? On or in the body?

ASSESSING SIGNS AND SYMPTOMS OF PHYSICAL TRAUMA

Most medical-legal evidence that must be collected is designed to document trauma, determine the presence or absence of sperm or semen, and help identify the assailant. The most characteristic physical signs of sexual assault are face/head/neck and extremity injury; vaginal/perineal injury is absent in the vast majority of sexual assault victims. Most victims will have no evidence of sperm upon physical examination, and they will have no evidence of trauma (Tintinalli 1985). Medical evidence, per se, does not prove rape. It is only supportive evidence. Rape is a legal decision, not a medical diagnosis.

A brief gynecological history is taken, including date of last menstrual period, the likelihood of current pregnancy, and history of venereal disease. It should *not* be assumed that the victim has had a pelvic examination prior to this event (Lederle et al. 1985). Many women have never had a pelvic examination. If the victim has not, the steps of the examination will need to be explained.

The victim has the right to refuse either a legal or a medical exam. Consent must be signed for photographs, pelvic examination, and whatever other procedures might be needed to collect evidence and treat the victim. During the pelvic examination, the nurse plays a crucial role in giving support to the victim and minimizing the trauma of the exam. A water-moistened speculum is used to preserve all evidence.

Cultures of the urethra, vagina, and anus for gonorrhea (GC) are obtained. A serological test is done for syphilis (serum VDRL). Usually prophylactic treatment is given for venereal disease. Many hospitals suggest procaine penicillin G intramuscularly or ampicillin orally when appropriate (i.e., for the woman *not* allergic to penicillin). There is some controversy over routinely giving antibiotics, as there is evidence that the gonococcus is becoming resistant to penicillin. Some experts suggest that venereal disease should not be treated until it occurs.

More controversial is the routine of using DES (diethylstilbestrol) for postcoital contraception (except in cases of women already pregnant). The absolute effectiveness of postcoital contraception has not been determined. Statistics show that only 3–5% of women who are raped become pregnant as a result (Lederle et al. 1985). If the victim is likely to seek aftercare, she may want to wait to initiate intervention until results of a pregnancy test are obtained or until her next period is due to begin. If DES is administered, close follow-up care should be provided to anticipate or eliminate complications, especially those associated with inadvertent pregnancy (Tintinalli 1985). When a rape counseling center is available, it is suggested that the unit assume close and direct responsibility for directing patients for medical follow-up, regardless of emergency room treatment (Tintinalli 1985).

If possible, a shower and fresh clothing should be available for the victim immediately after the examination.

Although the medical examination helps determine whether any injury occurred and also is used to collect evidence for identification and prosecution of the rapist, the victim may feel as if it is another violation of her body. Recognizing this, the nurse can explain the examination procedure in a way that will be reassuring and supportive to the victim. Allowing the victim to participate in all decisions affecting care helps her regain a sense of control over her life.

All data should be carefully documented. Documentation includes verbatim statements by the victim, detailed observations of emotional and physical status, and all results from the physical examination. All laboratory tests done should be noted, and findings should be recorded as soon as they are available.

Standard III: Diagnosis

Rape-trauma syndrome is the nursing diagnosis that applies to the physical and psychological effects resulting from an episode of rape. It includes an acute phase of disorganization of the victim's lifestyle and a long term reorganization. The diagnosis has application regardless of the setting in which the victim is encountered. This syndrome comprises the following three subcomponents with defining characteristics (Kim et al, 1989).

Rape-Trauma Syndrome. Rape-trauma syndrome can be divided into two phases.

- Acute Phase: See Table 13–1.
- Long Term Phase: See planning section, rape-trauma syndrome: long term **reorganization** phase.

Rape-Trauma Syndrome: Compound Reaction. Compound reaction refers to victims who have had previous or current physical, emotional, or social difficulties and are suffering rape-trauma syndrome. Symptoms include the following:

- All symptoms listed under *Rape-Trauma Syndrome*
- Reliance on alcohol or other drugs
- Reactivated symptoms of previous conditions such as physical illness or psychiatric illness

Rape-Trauma Syndrome: Silent Reaction. Silent reaction is a complex stress reaction to rape, in which an individual is unable to describe or discuss the rape. Symptoms include the following:

- Abrupt changes in relationships with men
- Increase in nightmares
- Increasing anxiety during the interview, i.e., blocking of associations, long periods of silence, minor stuttering, physical distress
- Marked changes in sexual behavior
- Sudden onset of phobic reactions
- No verbalization of the occurrence of rape

Standard IV: Planning

Planning care for a person who has been the victim of a sexual assault includes planning on the (1) *content level* (planning goals) and the (2) *process level* (nurses' reactions and feelings)

CONTENT LEVEL—PLANNING GOALS

Client-centered goals for alleviating the victim's discomfort and distress grow out of the nursing diagnosis applied. The goals are both short term and long term. Short term goals are those that the nurse and the victim can achieve while they are working together to relieve the symptoms exhibited during the acute phase of the rape-trauma syndrome. Long term goals are those that will allow the victim to begin to reorganize her life after the immediate crisis.

Examples of short term goals could be:

1. Rape-trauma syndrome: acute phase.
   - Victim will begin to express reactions and feelings about the assault before leaving the emergency room.
   - Victim will have short term plan for handling immediate situational needs.
   - Victim will list common physical, social, and emotional reactions that often follow a sexual assault before leaving the emergency room.
   - Victim will speak to community-based rape-victim advocate in emergency room.
   - Victim will be able to state the results of the physical examination completed in the emergency department.
   - Victim will state she will keep follow-up appointment with nurse/rape-victim advocate/social worker on (date).
2. Rape-Trauma syndrome: long term reorganization phase.
   - By (state the date) victim will discuss need for follow-up crisis counseling and other supports.
   - Within three to five months, victim will state memory of the rape is less vivid and less frightening.
   - Within three to five months, victim will state that the physical symptoms (sleep disturbances, poor appetite, physical trauma, etc.) have subsided.

PROCESS LEVEL—NURSES' REACTIONS AND FEELINGS

As members of society, nurses have been exposed to the various myths and judgments that exist about the event of rape and the victim of rape. Nurses' attitudes influence the physical and psychological care administered to rape victims, and knowing the myths and facts surrounding rape can increase nurses' awareness of their personal beliefs and feelings regarding rape. Nurses must examine these personal feelings and reactions prior to encountering a rape victim to minimize interference in caregiving. The nurse has her own reality and values to explore concerning rape before she can be objective in dealing with the reality of others.

Belief in myths is presumed to be associated with denial and minimization of perceived injury and with blaming the victim for her own victimization. Acceptance of myths has been shown to go along with beliefs that women's social roles and rights should be more restricted than those of men (Costin 1985). Table 13–2 compares rape myths and facts.

Standard V: Intervention

The experience of rape can be the most devastating experience in a woman's life and constitutes an *acute situational crisis*. It is a total violation of the person's body and will and can be perceived as an annihilation of the self. Typical crisis reactions reflect cognitive, affective, and behavioral disruptions. In order for the victim to return to her previous level of functioning it is necessary for her to mourn her losses, experience anger, and work through her terrifying fears.

V-A: PSYCHOTHERAPEUTIC INTERVENTIONS

Nurses usually work with rape victims in the emergency room. However, many times a person is too traumatized, ashamed, or afraid to come to the hospital. For that reason, most communities provide telephone "hotlines" on a 24-hour basis. A discussion of psychotherapeutic interventions (1) in the emergency room and (2) on crisis hotlines follows.

Psychotherapeutic Interventions in the Emergency Room

Nurses' attitudes can have an important therapeutic impact on the victim's trauma. The most effective approach is to *maintain neutral behavior* with victims. This means that displays of shock, horror, disgust, surprise, disbelief, or any other emotion are not appropriate. *Provide nonjudgmental care* as well as *maximum emotional support* to the victim. Crisis management of the rape victim is actually the practice of primary prevention of psychiatric disorders (Burgess and Holstrom 1973). *Confidentiality* is, of course, crucial in rape cases. Without the patient's consent, sexual assault cases are not to be discussed except with medical personnel involved.

The most helpful things the nurse can do are to *listen* and to *let the victim talk*. When the nurse listens carefully, the distress of the victim can be heard. A woman who feels understood is no longer alone; she then feels more in control of her situation. "A special dimension of listening and understanding is to help people bear the feelings they are trying to express. Sharing the pain is an emotionally strengthening experience for a person" (Burgess and Holstrom 1973).

Allowing the person to express negative affect and "*behavioral self-blame*" has been recognized as helpful. **Behavioral self-blame** represents an adaptive, func-

Table 13–2 • RAPE: MYTH AND FACT

MYTH	FACT
1. Many women really want to be raped.	1. No women ask to be raped—no matter how they are dressed, what their behavior, or where they are at any given time. No one asks to be hurt.
2. Most rapists are oversexed.	2. Sex is used as an instrument of violence in rape. Rape is an act of aggression, anger, or power.
3. Most women are raped by strangers.	3. 50% are raped by someone they know and who are a part of their extended family.
4. No healthy adult female who resists vigorously can be raped by an unarmed man.	4. Most men can overpower most women because of differences in body build. Also the victim may panic, making her actions less effective than usual.
5. Most charges of rape are unfounded.	5. There is NO evidence to show that there are more false reports for rape than for other crimes. Most rape victims do not even report the rape.
6. Rapes usually occur in dark alleys.	6. More than one half of all rapes occur in the home.
7. Rape is usually an impulsive act.	7. Most rapes are planned; over 50% involve a weapon.
8. Nice girls don't get raped.	8. ANY woman is a potential rape victim. Victims range in age from 6 months to 90 years old.
9. There was not enough time for a rape to occur.	9. There is no minimum time limit that characterizes rape. It can happen very quickly.
10. Don't fight or try to get away because you will just get hurt.	10. There are no verifiable data to substantiate that a victim will be injured if she tries to get away.
11. Only females are raped.	11. There is a growing number of male rape victims—not necessarily just men in prisons or in the homosexual community.
12. Rape is a sexual act.	12. Rape is a violent expression of aggression, anger, or need for power.

Data from Berkow 1982; Costin 1985; Helen 1984.

tional response to the psychological needs of rape victims (Damrosch 1985). The implication is not that the victim perceives herself to be the cause of the crime but that the person needs to restore control. Efforts to restore control are a positive response to victimization. Behavioral self-blame functions to help the person restore a sense of control.

Self-blame helps preserve one's belief in a just world in which people generally get what they deserve. Attributions to one's behavior (which is controllable) allows the victim to believe that similar experiences can be avoided in the future. Therefore, within this framework, self-blame serves to explain events that are otherwise incomprehensible.

When nurses fail to recognize the function of behavioral self-blame, they may try to dissuade the rape victim from beliefs that are helpful. Using reflective communication techniques (see Chapter 6) to respond to the psychological themes expressed is more helpful than discounting the victim's role. Examples of helpful and unhelpful responses follow:

Woman states, "I am so mad at myself. I should have never gone out tonight."

Helpful Response	**Unhelpful Response**
You believe if you had made a different decision earlier this evening, this wouldn't have happened.	Your actions had nothing to do with what happened.

Awareness that the expression of negative affect and behavioral self-blame may be quite helpful to the rape victim will enable nurses to avoid committing acts of *secondary victimization* (the process by which victims are victimized once again by others' reactions, including awkward or ineffective efforts to help) (Damrosch 1985).

When desirable, involve the victim's support system, family or friends, and discuss with them the nature and trauma of sexual assault and possible delayed reactions the victim may experience. Unfortunately, significant relationships frequently deteriorate as a result of the crisis of rape. Reactions on the part of the significant other range from indignation, to denial, to focusing blame on the victim. For this reason and because of the long term process of reorganization, follow-up care for the victim is strongly encouraged. Table 13–3 summarizes the main psychotherapeutic techniques used by the nurse working with a victim of rape.

When preparing the victim to go home, discuss follow-up procedures, and give all referral information in writing. Referral to ongoing professional counseling resources as well as community support groups, e.g., rape crisis services, should be offered routinely. The victim's emotional state and other psychological needs should be reassessed 24–48 hours after discharge from the hospital. This may be done by phone or personal contact. During this time, repeat referrals are made for needed resources or support services. *Effective crisis intervention and continuity of care requires outreach activities and services beyond the emergency medical setting.*

A repeat GC culture, VDRL, and gynecological exam is recommended in one to two weeks and again at eight weeks. Legal referrals can also be given, e.g., names of attorneys who specialize in rape cases and options for low-cost legal assistance.

As described, crisis resolution involves several tasks that can only be initiated in the emergency department. Effectiveness of the interventions can be measured by certain observable outcomes, the achievement of goals.

Psychotherapeutic Intervention on the Crisis Hotline

Nearly all communities provide 24-hour-a-day crisis telephone service. Some provide 24-hour-a-day hotlines for rape victims (e.g., Rape Relief in Seattle, Washington). The hotline may be for information, referral, or as a prelude to a personal contact for future telephone counseling.

The phone counselor talks briefly with the person to determine where she is, what has happened, and what kind of help she needs. The counselor provides empathic listening, and the victim is further encouraged to go to the hospital and is advised *not to wash, change clothes, douche, brush teeth, or eat or drink anything,* all of which might destroy evidence. The victim is urged to call the police. The police and rape advocate can meet the victim at the emergency department. Over the phone, the counselor also can encourage the victim to make necessary decisions about communications with family and friends and give information about what to expect from the hospital and the police. However, all this is better done in person, if possible. The main focus of the telephone contact is on the immediate steps the victim may take. The counselor provides the necessary information for the victim to make decisions. Unfortunately, the victim frequently remains anonymous. Some do not want any immediate or follow-up counseling (Brodyaga et al. 1975).

Table 13–3 • KEY THERAPEUTIC TECHNIQUES USED WITH VICTIMS OF RAPE

INTERVENTION	RATIONALE
1. Do not leave person alone.	1. Prevents increase in isolation, escalation of anxiety.
2. Maintain neutral behavior.	2. Decreases emotional burden.
3. Provide nonjudgmental care.	3. Lessens feelings of shame and embarrassment
4. Maximize emotional support: • stay with victim • show concern for victim's needs • encourage problem solving whenever possible	4. Prevents further disorganization: • decreases potential for escalation of anxiety • validates worth of person • increases person's sense of control
5. Assure confidentiality.	5. Encourages sharing event and protects a person's self-concept and sense of control.
6. Encourage person to talk.	6. Helps person sort out thoughts and feelings. Lowers anxiety by lowering feelings of isolation.
7. Allow negative expression of affect and "behavioral self-blame."	7. Helps person gain a sense of control.
8. Engage support system (family, friends) when appropriate.	8. Provides warmth and feelings of safety when shock wears off and acute disorganization phase begins.
9. Emphasize that the person did the right thing in order to save her life.	9. Helps reduce guilt and maintain self-esteem.

Data from Burgess and Holstrom 1973; Damrosch 1985.

V-F: PSYCHOTHERAPY

Some people who are victimized by rape may be susceptible to a psychotic episode or an emotional disturbance so severe that hospitalization is required. Others whose emotional life may be so overburdened with multiple internal and external pressures may require individual psychotherapy. Most people, however, after supportive services and crisis counseling, are eventually able to resume their previous lives. However, many of these victims of sexual assault carry with them a constant emotional trauma: flashbacks, nightmares, constant fear, phobias, and other symptoms associated with the post-traumatic stress reaction (refer to Chapter 16).

Often family and friends of victims of rape are unable or unwilling to be supportive. The long-standing cultural myth that women are the property of men still prevents family and friends from empathizing with the woman's severe psychic injury. She is, instead, often thought of as "devalued goods" (Rose 1986).

Some clinicians are now offering other forms of therapy after the immediate crisis is lessened, because the intrapsychic impact of the rape experience is so profound and can leave such devastating scars. One such therapy, psychodynamic psychotherapy (once considered not appropriate for rape victims), is being re-evaluated (Rose 1986).

Group therapy with other victims of rape has been very healing for many people. Group therapy can make the difference between a person coming out of the crisis at a lower level of functioning or gradually adapting to her experience with an increase in coping skills (Gallese and Treuting 1981).

Standard VI: Evaluation

Completion of the process of reorganization after a rape crisis can be evaluated by assessing sleeping and eating patterns, presence or absence of phobias, motor behavior, relations, self-esteem, and presence or absence of somatic reactions (DiVastro 1985). The victim is recovered if she is

1. sleeping well with only very few episodic nightmares or broken sleep.
2. eating as was her pattern before the rape.
3. calm and relaxed or only mildly suspicious or restless.
4. getting support from family and friends. Some strain might still be present in relationships, but it should be minimal.
5. generally positive about self. On occasion doubts about self-worth may occur.
6. free from somatic reactions. If mild symptoms persist and minor discomfort is reported, the victim should be able to talk about it and feel in control of the symptoms.

In general, the closer the victim's lifestyle is to the pattern that was present before the rape, the more complete the recovery has been.

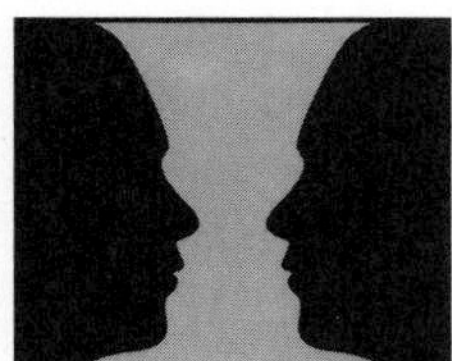

Case Study: Working With a Person Who Has Been Raped

Carol Smith, a 36-year-old single mother of two, went out one evening with some friends. Her children were at a slumber party and, "I needed to get away and have a little rest and relaxation." She and her friends had gone bowling. Later in the evening, Carol was tired and ready to go home. One of the men who had joined the group offered to take Carol home. She had seen the man at the bowling alley before but did not know much about him. Not in the habit of going home alone with men she did not know, she hesitated. One of her friends, whom she trusted, told her it was OK to go with Jim because he was a nice man.

Jim drove Carol home. He then asked her if he could come into her house to use the bathroom before he drove the long distance to his house. Carol reluctantly agreed and sat on the living room couch. After using the bathroom, Jim sat next to Carol and began to kiss her and fondle her breasts. As Carol protested Jim became more forceful in his advances. Carol was confused and frightened. She managed to get away from him briefly, but he began grabbing, squeezing, and biting her. He told her gruffly, "If you don't do what I say I'll break your neck." She screamed, but he proceeded to rape her. Jim became nervous that the noise would alert the neighbors and raced out of the house. A neighbor did in fact arrive just after Jim fled. The neighbor called the police and then brought Carol to the local hospital emergency room for a physical exam, crisis intervention, and support.

In the emergency room Carol was visibly shaken. She kept saying over and over, "I

Continued on following page

Case Study: Working With a Person Who Has Been Raped *(Continued)*

shouldn't have gone home with him, I should have fought harder, I shouldn't have let him do this."

The nurse took Carol to a quiet cubicle. She didn't want Carol to stay alone, and asked the neighbor to stay with Carol. The nurse then notified the doctor and the rape-victim advocate. When the nurse came back, she told Carol she would like to talk to her before the doctor came. Carol looked at her neighbor and then down. The nurse asked the neighbor to wait outside for awhile, and would call her later.

CAROL: It was horrible. I feel so dirty.
NURSE: You have had a terrible experience. Do you want to talk about It?
CAROL: I feel so ashamed, I should have never let that man take me home.
NURSE: You think that if you hadn't gone home with a stranger this wouldn't have happened?
CAROL: Yes . . . I shouldn't have let him do it to me anyway, I shouldn't have let him rape me.
NURSE: You mentioned that he said he would break your neck if you didn't do as he said.
CAROL: Yes, he said that . . . he was going to kill me, it was awful.
NURSE: It seems you did the right thing in order to stay alive.

As the nurse continued to talk with Carol, Carol's anxiety level seemed to lessen. The nurse talked to Carol about the kinds of experiences rape victims often have and collected necessary information. She explained that the doctor would want to examine her and explained the procedure to her. She then asked Carol to sign a consent. While preparing Carol for examination, the nurse noticed bite marks and bruises on both breasts. She also remarked on Carol's lower lip, which was cut and bleeding. After the examination, Carol was given clean clothes and a place to shower.

Assessment

The nurse organized her data into subjective and objective components.

OBJECTIVE DATA

1. Crying and sobbing
2. Bruises and bite marks on each breast
3. Lip cut and bleeding
4. Reported rape to the police

SUBJECTIVE DATA

1. "He was going to kill me."
2. "It was horrible . . . I feel so dirty."
3. "I shouldn't have let him rape me."

Nursing Diagnosis

The nurse formulated the following diagnosis:

1. Rape-Trauma Syndrome
   - "I shouldn't have let him rape me."
   - "He was going to kill me."
   - Crying and sobbing
   - Bruises and bites on both breasts
   - Reported rape to the police
   - "It was horrible . . . I feel so dirty."

Planning

CONTENT LEVEL—PLANNING GOALS

The nurse devised a plan of care for Carol based on the nursing diagnosis and the nurse's training as a crisis counselor.

Nursing Diagnosis	Long Term Goals	Short Term Goals
1. *Rape-Trauma Syndrome*	Within three months Carol will state she thinks less about the rape, is sleeping better, feels safer, and is functioning at previous level.	1a. Carol will begin to express emotional reactions and feelings before she leaves the emergency room. 1b. Carol will be able to list possible socio-emotional reactions following sexual assault. 1c. Carol will have written referrals for legal, medical, and crisis counseling before she leaves the emergency room. 1d. Carol will have a follow-up appointment with the GYN clinic and the rape advocate-counselor for weekly meetings before she leaves the emergency room. 1e. Carol's anxiety level will go from severe to moderate before she leaves the emergency room.

PROCESS LEVEL — NURSES' REACTIONS AND FEELINGS

The nurse had worked with victims of rape before and had helped plan the hospital protocol. It had taken a while to be able to remain neutral as well as responsive, since initially her own anger at the assailant would get in the way. She also remembers a time when a woman came in stating she was raped, but was so calm, smiling, and polite, that the nurse initially did not believe her story. She hadn't, at that point, examined her own feelings or dealt with the popular societal myths regarding rape. It was only later, when talking to more experienced health care personnel, that she learned that crisis reactions can seem bizarre, confusing, and contradictory.

The nurse learned that staying with the victim, encouraging the victim to express her reactions and feelings, and listening went a long way to reduce feelings of anxiety. Once the nurse learned to let go of her personal anger at the attacker and ambivalence with the victim, her care and effectiveness improved greatly. All this took time and support from more experienced nurses and other members of the health team.

Intervention

Carol stated she felt more comfortable after taking a shower and talking to the nurse. She seemed less confused, better able to concentrate, and began to discuss what she would tell her children. Specific interventions are found in Nursing Care Plan 13-1.

It was decided that Carol's neighbor would stay with her overnight. Carol had an appointment the following week with the rape-victim advocate and with a gynecologist in the clinic. Carol was also given written information about legal counseling, crisis groups, and other community follow-up services for victims of rape.

The nurse documented Carol's physical and emotional status including verbatim responses, as well as the results of the physical examination and tests. The nurse called Carol the next morning and encouraged Carol to call her if she had any further questions.

Continued on following page

Evaluation

Carol kept her appointment with the rape-victim advocate for counseling, as well as with the gynecologist at the clinic. She continued with the counseling for several months. For a period of time, she experienced acute anxiety attacks when she went out at night and had new locks put on all the windows and doors. After three months, she expressed interest in a group that was forming in the next town for women who had been raped; however, she stated she didn't know if she could go, since it started at 6:00 P.M. The counselor told her that arrangements could be made for a volunteer to take her there and back until she felt safer going out at night.

After four months, Carol stated she did feel safer and had been out at night twice in the past week. She was not comfortable yet, but stated she was making progress. She told the counselor she was not ready to date. The group had been a great help to her. She continued to call the nurse about once every two weeks and report on her progress. She told the counselor that the nurse had really "saved her life" and she wasn't ready to let that support go.

She was functioning well as a mother and in her job. After five months, the flashbacks ceased and she started sleeping throughout the night without nightmares.

Nursing Care Plan 13-1 • A VICTIM OF SEXUAL ASSAULT: Carol

NURSING DIAGNOSIS

Rape-trauma syndrome

Supporting Data

- "I shouldn't have let him rape me."
- "He was going to kill me."
- Sobbing and crying.
- Bruises and bites on both breasts.
- Reported rape to the police.
- "It was horrible, I feel so dirty."

Long Term Goal: Within five months Carol will state that she thinks less about the rape, is sleeping better, feels safer, and is functioning at previous level.

Short Term Goal	*Intervention*	*Rationale*	*Evaluation*
1. Carol will begin to express emotional reactions and feelings before she leaves emergency room.	1a. Nurse remains neutral, nonjudgmental, and assures Carol of confidentiality.	1a. Lessens feelings of shame and guilt and encourages sharing of painful feelings.	Goal met Carol discussed feelings of shame, self-blame, and fear. Continues counseling with rape-victim advocate.
	1b. Does not leave Carol alone.	1b. Deters feelings of isolation and escalation of anxiety.	
	1c. Allows negative expressions and "behavioral self-blame"—uses reflective techniques.	1c. Fosters feeling of control.	
	1d. Assures Carol she did the right thing to save her life.	1d. Decreases the burden of guilt and shame.	
	1e. When anxiety level is down to moderate, encourages problem solving.	1e. Increases feeling of control in own life (when in severe and panic levels a person cannot problem solve).	
2. Carol will be able to list possible socio-emotional reactions following sexual assault.	2. Tell Carol of common reactions experienced by people in the long term reorganization phase, i.e., phobias, flashbacks, insomnia, increased motor activity, etc.	2. Helps Carol anticipate reactions and understand them as part of the recovery process.	Goal met Was able to state five possible future reactions.

3. Carol will state she will keep a follow-up appointment with the GYN clinic and rape advocate/counselor before leaving emergency room.	3a. Explain ER procedure to Carol.	3a. Lowers anticipatory anxiety.	Kept appointments with GYN clinic and rape advocate.
	3b. Explain to Carol about the physical examination.	3b. Allows for questions and concerns; may be too traumatized and refuse.	
	3c. Have consent signed.	3c. Legal protocol.	
	3d. Nurse (or female rape-victim advocate) stays with Carol during examination.	3d. Often presence decreases isolation and anxiety.	
	3e. Role of rape-victim advocate explained.	3e. Awareness of supports and why needed.	
	3f. Results of GYN and physical examination given to Carol.	3f. Enables Carol to participate in decisions, to understand need for follow-up care.	
	3g. Nurse documents all physical and emotional data (with verbatim remarks) and lists laboratory tests.	3g. Not only for medical follow-up but legal as well.	
4. Carol's anxiety level will go from severe to moderate before she leaves emergency room.	4a. Written referrals for legal, medical, and crisis counseling given.	4a. Increase in anxiety level is minimal.	Goal met Carol was able to start making future plans, stated she felt less anxious.
	4b. Inform Carol you will call her tomorrow A.M.	4b. Validates concern for her feelings and safety.	
	4c. Plans are made so Carol is not alone for a few days.	4c. Helps decrease anxiety and increase feelings of safety.	Carol called nurse to "check in." Nurse plans to have conferences with Carol.

Summary

In recent years rape victims have begun to receive the attention they deserve from the health care system—and the empathy and support they need. A rape victim experiences a wide range of feelings, which may or may not be exhibited. Feelings of fear, degradation, anger and rage, helplessness, and nervousness are common. Long term sequelae such as sleep disturbances, disturbed relationships, and somatic complaints are common.

For the victim, the circumstances of the initial medical evaluation may be frightening and stressful. Police interrogation, repeated questioning by health professionals, and the physical examination itself all have the potential to add to the trauma of the sexual assault. Nurses, in the role of case managers, can serve to minimize repetition and support the victim as she goes through the entire ordeal. Following resolution of the immediate crisis, victims require follow-up and often counseling in an effort to minimize the long term effects of the rape and to assist in an early return to a normal living pattern.

Although community resources may vary considerably, most metropolitan areas now have special programs to assist rape victims. Such assistance usually includes advice as to the management of the acute crisis, as well as guidelines for the collection of evidence and preparation for trial should legal action follow.

References

Abarbanel G. Roles of the clinical social worker. *In* Warner CG (ed). Rape and Sexual Assault. Germantown, MD: Aspen Systems Corporation, 1980.

Antognoli-Toland P. Comprehensive program for examination of sexual assault victims by nurses: A hospital-based project in Texas. Journal of Emergency Nursing, 11(3):132, 1985.

Berkow R. (ed). The Merck Manual of Diagnosis and Therapy, 14th ed. Rahway, NJ: Merck Sharp & Dohme Research Laboratories, 1982.

Bradford JM. Research on sex offenders. Psychiatric Clinics of North America, 6(4):715, 1983.

Brodyaga L. Rape and its victims: A report for citizens, health facilities, and criminal justice agencies. Washington DC: National Institute of Law Enforcement and Criminal Justice, Law Enforcement Assistance Administration, U.S. Department of Justice, 1975.

Burgess AW. Rape trauma syndrome: A nursing diagnosis. Occupational Health Nursing, 33(8):405, 1985.

Burgess AW, Holstrom LL. The rape victim in the ER. American Journal of Nursing, 73(10):1740, 1973.

Burgess AW, Holstrom LL. Rape trauma syndrome. American Journal of Psychiatry, 131:981, 1974.

Costin F. Beliefs about rape and women's social roles. Archives of Sexual Behavior, 14(4):319, 1985.

Damrosch SP. Nursing students' assessments of behaviorally self-blaming rape victims. Nursing Research, 34(4):221, 1985.

DiVastro P. Measuring the aftermath of rape. Journal of Psychosocial Nursing, 23(2):33, 1985.
Gallese LE, Treuting EG. Help for rape victims through group therapy. Journal of Psychosocial Nursing and Mental Health Services, 19:20, 1981.
Helen M. Rape: Some facts, myths and responses. The Australian Nurses Journal, 13(8):42, 1984.
Kim MJ, McFarland GK, McLane AM (eds). Pocket Guide to Nursing Diagnoses. St. Louis: C.V. Mosby, 1984.
Lederle DJ, DiGirolamo J, Poskins P. Rape crisis services. Illinois Medical Journal, 167(4):305, 1985.
Mims FH, Chang AS. Unwanted sexual experiences of young women. Journal of Psychosocial Nursing, 22(6):7, 1984.
Nelson C. Victims of rape: who are they? *In* Warner CG (ed). Rape and Sexual Assault. Germantown, MD: Aspen Systems Corporation, 1980, pp. 9–26.
President's Task Force on Victims of Crimes. Washington DC: Government Printing Office #82-24146, 1982.
Rose DS. "Worse than death": Psychodynamics of rape victims and need for psychotherapy. American Journal of Psychiatry, 143:817, 1986.
Ruch LO, Chandler. Sexual assault trauma and trauma change. Women and Health, 8(4):5, 1983.
Tintinalli JE. Clinical findings and legal resolution in sexual assault. Annals of Emergency Medicine, 14(5):447, 1985.
Warner CG. Rape and Sexual Assault. Germantown, MD: Aspen Systems Corporation, 1980.

Self-Study Exercises

Place T (True) or F (False) next to each statement.

The definition of rape:

1. ________ Is forced and violent vaginal or anal penetration.
2. ________ Can include forced genital contact, i.e., oral-genital contact.
3. ________ CANNOT be used between husband and wife.
4. ________ Is increasingly used against women raping men.

The truth regarding rape:

5. ________ Most rapists are oversexed.
6. ________ Don't fight or try to get away, for you will just get hurt.
7. ________ Most women who are raped "asked" for it.
8. ________ Rape is usually an impulsive act.

Place an A (Acute Phase) or an LT (Long Term Reorganization Phase) next to the symptoms most likely found in that phase.

9. ________ Skeletal muscle tension, i.e., headaches, twitches, grimaces.
10. ________ Intrusive thoughts of the rape the woman is unable to control.
11. ________ May have a controlled style of handling trauma, i.e., calm and subdued or numb and shocked.
12. ________ Phobias develop, i.e., fear of strangers, being alone, of someone behind her, of going out, etc.
13. ________ May present with self-blame, shame, guilt.
14. ________ Increased motor activity, takes trips, changes phone number, moves to new location.
15. ________ May have expressed style of handling trauma, i.e., crying, hysteria, tense, smiling, sobbing, etc.

Choose the letter that best answers the following questions:

16. When assessing a person who has been sexually assaulted, all the following are important considerations. Which of the following is NOT appropriate during the assessment in the emergency room:

    A. Do not touch the person, unless she reaches out for tactile support.
    B. Do not leave the person alone.

C. If the person is extremely anxious, remove her to the treatment room/private place right away.
D. The victim should not be seen until the emergency room is almost empty.

17. When helping with the physical part of the assessment, the nurse should be aware of all of the following EXCEPT:

A. The victim has the right to refuse a medical examination.
B. The absence of sperm proves the absence of a rape.
C. The physical examination should be carefully explained to the victim, and a nurse should stay with the person.
D. Fresh clothes and a shower should be made available after the examination.

18. Choose the goal that is NOT a short term goal formulated for rape-trauma syndrome.

A. Victim will experience reduction of anxiety before leaving the emergency room.
B. Victim will state short term plan for handling immediate situation.
C. Victim will begin to express reactions and feelings before leaving emergency room.
D. Victim will state that physical symptoms (sleep disturbances, poor appetite, etc.) have subsided.

19. Choose the intervention that is NOT a therapeutic technique when working with a victim of sexual assault.

A. Never leave the woman alone.
B. Allow negative expression and "behavioral self-blame."
C. Emphasize that the person did the right thing in order to save her life.
D. Initiate touching the victim as a means of emotional support.

20. The main focus of the telephone contact in a rape crisis hotline is to

A. Get the victim to prosecute her assailant.
B. Find out where she is and get the police.
C. Insist she come to the hospital emergency room for further treatment.
D. Provide information to facilitate the victim's decision making and help plan the next steps.

21. Which of the following is NOT a reason many rapes go unreported?

A. The rape victim goes on trial as well as the rapist.
B. Men are less likely to report rape because of strong reactions from society.
C. Fear and anguish prevent people from seeking medical help and reporting the crime.
D. Rape is not a crime.

Write brief responses in answer to the following:

22. Name four areas that the nurse carefully documents in the victim's chart.

A. ____________________
B. ____________________
C. ____________________
D. ____________________

23. Name four nursing responsibilities the nurse takes with a victim of rape during a physical examination.

    A. ______________________________
    B. ______________________________
    C. ______________________________
    D. ______________________________

CHAPTER 14

Evidence of Maladaptive Responses to Crisis: Elder Abuse

Sally Kennedy Holzapfel

OUTLINE

KEY TERMS AND CONCEPTS

The key terms and concepts listed here also appear in bold where they are defined or discussed in this chapter.

FINDINGS OF UNITED STATES CONGRESS (1980's) ON ELDER ABUSE

PHYSICAL INDICATIONS OF ABUSE

PSYCHOLOGICAL ABUSE AND NEGLECT

CLIENT COMPETENCY

OBJECTIVES

After studying this chapter, the student will be able to:

1. Briefly discuss changes in family structure that increase anxiety within families and the possibility of abuse to the elderly.
2. Discuss the epidemiological theory of elder abuse in terms of stresses on the (1) caregiver, (2) elder, and (3) environment, which could escalate anxiety to the point at which violence becomes the relief behavior.
3. Name three signs and symptoms of physical abuse to the elderly.
4. Name three signs and symptoms of psychological abuse to the elderly.
5. List seven conditions that can contribute to family abuse.
6. Identify pertinent nursing diagnoses for the abused elderly and list supporting data from the assessment.
7. Identify pertinent nursing diagnoses for the abuser of the elderly and list supporting data from the assessment.
8. Formulate two short term goals for each, the abused elder and the abuser.
9. State three interventions that would be appropriate in dealing with (1) the elderly abused and (2) the abuser.
10. Briefly discuss the legal issues that are relevant when working with a family with an abused elderly member.

Elder abuse, which, by definition, includes neglect, is a crime occurring with increasing regularity. The number of victims exceeds 500,000 annually and has been as high as 1,200,000 (Hamilton 1989; Giordano and Giordano 1984; Rathbone-McCuan and Hashimi 1982). Abuse can be found in rural as well as urban areas and is spread throughout the United States.

Abuse has been defined as "an act committed or omitted, that jeopardizes the well-being or safety of the individual and if observed by a third party would lead to negative judgments" (Stannard 1973). Phrases such as "granny bashing" and the "battered elderly syndrome" have been used to describe the disturbed interactions between the older adult and his or her caregiver (Galbraith 1986). Elder abuse may be considered a consequence of the caregiver's attempt to cope with a stressful situation (Burnside 1988).

In the legal sense, abuse is the "willful infliction of physical injury or mental anguish and the deprivation by the caregiver of essential services. The neglected individual is defined by law as one who is unable to provide for himself and is not receiving the services from his caregivers" (Verwoerdt 1976).

There are two major types of abuse: physical and psychological. Abuse can take place in a variety of settings, such as an institution, a home, or a hospital. Much abuse toward the elderly appears to occur in the home (Anderson and Thobaben 1984). More than one in ten elderly persons living with a family member are abused each year (Giordano and Giordano 1984). Eighty-four percent of such abuses at home are committed by family members (Rathbone-McCuan and Hashimi 1982).

An increase in abuse of our aging population appears to parallel the changes in the basic structure of the family unit from the nineteenth century through the present time. With these changes, family violence has increased. Understanding family changes from a historical perspective is important. The increased stress, feelings of alienation, and personal isolation that appear to be prevalent in our modern age are related to the changes in family structure.

In the nineteenth century, social and economic changes affected perceptions of "old age." The population increased considerably, accompanied by an increase in the number of elderly. The Industrial Revolution encouraged a movement of the population from the countryside to urban areas and brought forth the emergence of the working class, changes that resulted in increasingly negative views of the older adult. They were viewed as nonproductive, became unemployed, and often fell into extreme poverty. Their grown-up children had difficulty providing sustenance for their parents: they had to choose "between feeding their own children or wasting food on useless mouths who could not contribute to the household" (Eastman 1984). As a consequence some were forced into asylums even though most were kept at home by their children.

The second half of the twentieth century brought concerns about continued growth of the population.

Increasing life expectancy, smaller family units, working mothers, and one-parent households changed the character of the family structure. The larger families in earlier generations allowed sons and daughters to divide responsibilities for their parents among a broad base of support. This meant that, on the average, one married couple could plan on caring for only one of their parents in old age. Today, the same couple would need to allocate their resources between three of their four parents (Olsen and Cahn 1980).

By the year 2040, the population over age 85 in the United States will have grown from the present 2.2 million to nearly 13 million. It is projected that the number of Americans over 65 will have then increased to over 66 million. The prospect for our society is that of an aging population in which the old will care for the very old "with all the emotional and financial strains that it implies" (Gelman et al. 1985).

Elder abuse as a maladaptive response to acute anxiety can be conceptualized as shown in Figure 14–1.

Standard I: Theory

Theories on the etiology of family violence abound. The epidemiological theories of abuse are the broadest. Essentially, as discussed in the chapter on child abuse, there are three essential areas that can be problematic. These are (1) the agent (abuser), (2) the host (victim), and (3) the environment (social and psychological stressors) within a given cultural process (Foley 1983). A general discussion of these three areas as pertaining to elder abuse are presented, along with recent research findings.

In the early **1980's the United States Congress** held hearings on the subject of elder abuse. It found that the most likely victim was an elderly Caucasian female (70 or older) with a moderate to average degree of physical or mental impairment. The abuser most often resided in the same household as the victim (Anderson 1984; Rathbone-McCuan and Hashimi 1982). Financial difficulties, chronic medical problems, a history of alcoholism, drug use, or child abuse (real or perceived) are also frequently present in these families. The abuser often has difficulty communicating, which strains his relationship with the elder and others (Falconi 1982).

Most abused elders depended on their care providers for transportation, assistance with everyday activities, and companionship. Many, though, were financially independent. If the abuser was dependent on his victim for financial support, the abuse was more apt to be physical or involved the misuse of the older adult's monetary resources or possessions. On the other hand, if the victim relied strongly on the abuser for assistance because of severe physical or mental impairments, the abuse was more likely to be psychological (Tallying risks 1986).

Frequently it is the "young-old" children who take care of their "old-old" parents. This situation can be stressful, since both generations are faced with separate though similar adjustments to old age (Olsen and Cahn 1980). This period of dependency is apt to fall on a "sandwich generation of adult children who are still coping with the demands of their own growing offspring or just beginning to savor some long-awaited respite from them" (Gelman et al. 1985).

The Industrial Revolution has left the family with two major functions: procreation and socialization of the offspring. As a result, the nuclear family has fewer roles to perform, leaving the elderly person essentially roleless. If the older adult is no longer able to live independently because of age or ill health, conflict may occur if she is taken into the family. Competition may occur between the young-old and the old-old for the existing family roles (Johnson 1979).

Too often our culture assigns the older person a childlike status. Individuals who, because of illness, loss of income, or other physical or mental infirmities, are

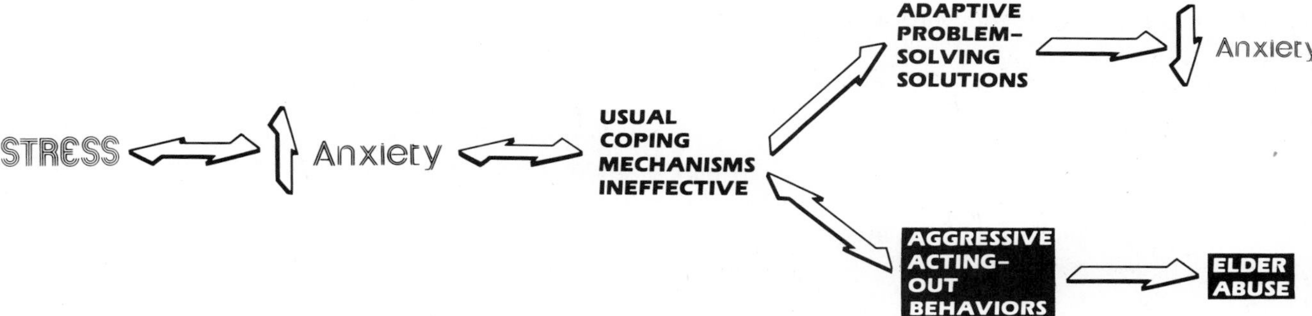

Figure 14–1. *Conceptualization of the process of aggressive acting-out behaviors in the development of elder abuse.*

incapable of meeting some of their needs will often be considered incapable of meeting any. A role reversal then is likely to occur between grown children and elderly parents. The children will assume the role of authority; it may or may not be justified by the elderly parent's condition (Johnson 1979).

Dealing with problems of aged parents can be very stressful for adult children. In addition, the stresses of our modern life have been known to generate violent behavior in individuals (Fulmer and Cahill 1984). Numerous sources form the basis of the confronting problems: financial, physical, psychological, family relationships, social, and housing. The introduction of an elderly parent, particularly when the parent is viewed as dependent, roleless, or noncontributing, into the nuclear family creates additional stress within the family and can, in some cases, lead to neglect and abuse of the elderly (Johnson 1979).

Standard II: Data Collection

The nurse identifies nursing diagnoses based on the assessment of (1) physical indications of abuse, (2) psychological indications of abuse, (3) coping mechanisms used by the victim, (4) support systems available, and (5) family coping patterns.

ASSESSING THE PHYSICAL INDICATIONS OF ABUSE

The **physical indications of abuse** range from simple bruises and welts to serious lacerations, puncture wounds, and fractures. More common, however, are clusters of symptoms. Look for two or more of the following: bruises, welts, lacerations, punctures, malnutrition, dehydration, fractures, symptoms of overmedication, burns, poor hygiene, or lack of needed medication (Eastman 1984; Fulmer and Cahill 1984; Galbraith 1986). Determine whether there are any signs of sexual assault.

Abuse may require a physician's attention. Only a careful check may reveal that the affliction was intentional. Repeated visits for the same or related injury often are an indication of abuse.

When making home visits, look for signs of crowding, lack of home maintenance, inadequate heating, cooling, or ventilation, and unhygienic conditions (Phillips 1983).

Neglect is a form of physical abuse. It manifests itself frequently in situations in which the caregiver does not provide, or withholds, necessary assistance, e.g., he or she does not make arrangements for the elder to have necessary medical or nursing care, does not administer needed medications, or fails to supervise a confused adult adequately.

If the elderly client is bed bound or lacking mobility, poor care might result in untreated sores or other skin injuries (such as decubitus ulcers and excoriated perineum), poor grooming, and poor hygiene. The elder may also have muscle contractures caused by immobilization or physical restraints (Ferguson and Beck 1983).

In the assessment process, the nurse should have a basic knowledge of the aging process to understand and differentiate the normal aspects of aging from the abnormal pathological states in the older adult.

ASSESSING THE PSYCHOLOGICAL INDICATIONS OF ABUSE

Psychological abuse and neglect are often less obvious and thus more difficult to assess than physical abuse. Psychological abuse and neglect often takes the form of insults, ridicule, or humiliation (Milt 1982); and includes verbal assaults and threats, provocation of fear, and isolation of the older person either physically or emotionally (Beck and Ferguson 1981).

Threats may be used to make the older adult conform to the wishes of the caregiver or the caregiver's family. Intimidation or threats may be used to keep the victim from revealing his or her plight, causing the victim to react to the nurse's visit with passivity, withdrawal, or denial (Milt 1982).

If the relationship between the caregiver and the aged adult is strained and burdened with shouting, harsh orders, or even a total breakdown in any positive communication, anxiety in the elder escalates. Along with other signs and symptoms of increased anxiety, added stress can trigger in the elderly behaviors such as incontinence, screaming, or the repetition of the same phrase (Eastman 1984).

A poor relationship usually exists if the caregiver perceives the elderly as "negatively dependent," i.e., the elderly person is not doing what he or she could or should be doing (Eastman 1984). Other factors may affect the caregiver's relationship: he or she (1) does not understand the significance of losses experienced by the elder (such as physical changes, loss of a job, death in family); (2) does not acknowledge older adults' social needs and treats them like children, including the denial of their sexuality (Beck and Ferguson 1981).

The reactions of older persons to such losses are often misunderstood or ignored. Their feelings of despair and helplessness, which are in themselves normal reactions to loss, may be viewed by the caregiver as burdensome. If the caregiver fails to understand their significance, he or she may degrade the reaction they evoke in the elderly. Not understanding the elder's behavior, or worse, considering it troublesome, may become a stimulus for abuse (Simos 1973).

Treating the aged as dependent children is another form of psychological abuse. This attitude fosters the creation of regressive traits in the elderly. Feelings of dependency, decreased self-reliance, and helplessness emerge, all of which undermine any remaining sense of strength or dignity (Beck and Ferguson 1981).

Last, psychological abuse can involve material abuse, which includes theft or misuse of money or property. At times money may serve as a motive for keeping the older adult at home, even if institutionalization is recommended. If the elderly are no longer able to care for their funds, the family may use some for their own personal purposes, thus restricting the older adult or not allowing the elder to meet his or her basic needs. In a case in which the elder is compelled to use all personal resources in return for care, the elder clearly is a victim of abuse (Beck and Ferguson 1981; Fulmer and Cahill 1984).

In cases of abuse or potential abuse of the elderly, the behavioral patterns frequently show a combination of factors of both physical and psychological abuse. Such clusters of behavior are evidence that a family is at risk of abuse. The nurse must differentiate a potential for abuse from actual abuse and then intervene accordingly.

When the caregiver is present during the interview, notice the interaction between the two. If there is a family relationship (which prevails in over 80% of abuse cases) such as parent-child, observe whether or not the usual expectations of affection are present. Is there eye-to-eye contact? Does the caregiver touch, look, listen, and talk to the aged parent? Notice whether the parent's response is fear, anger, withdrawal, or passivity. Posture (relaxed or rigid) can also be indicative of the type of relationship (Ferguson and Beck 1983).

During the assessment, the nurse must remain cognizant of the normal changes occurring with age in order to evaluate if other factors are present and what they signify. Were there losses in roles, resources, and independence facing the older adult that resulted in possible reactions of "fear, depression or a possible sense of disorientation and concern"?

The nurse needs to acknowledge that most abused elders are reluctant to report abuse by their relatives. Abused elders may experience shame or guilt that they have children who could abuse them or feel that they have failed as parents. Other reasons include "fear of retaliation, exposure of their sons or daughters to the community censure, or legal punishment, and fear of potential removal from the only home they know" (Anderson and Thobaben 1984). This apprehension is not without basis, since well-meaning professionals often recommend removal. In the more unusual case, if the elder elects separation, he or she often may be in no position to carry out personal wishes (Rathbone-McCuan and Hashimi 1982).

ASSESSING THE COPING MECHANISMS USED BY THE VICTIM

Through observation and obtaining the client's history, the nurse assesses the day-to-day living situation and the family's method and level of functioning. Having the client relate the events of an average day can supply essential information about how he or she is coping. Have the elder enumerate daily activities, relationships, and socialization within the family. Knowledge so obtained can be helpful for the appraisal of the elder's mental status (Anderson and Thobaben 1984).

When there is concern about abuse, part of the interview with the client should be conducted without the caregiver or other family members being present. This is particularly important when questions are asked about the actions of the client's family members and when the client displays a reluctance to speak about them.

ASSESSING SUPPORT SYSTEMS AVAILABLE

The victim of abuse is often in a dependent position, relying on his or her caregiver—most likely a family member—for supportive care. In such a situation, the dependent elder may be or feel isolated from others. The elder's contacts to the outside are controlled by the family (Rathbone-McCuan and Hashimi 1982). Here it is necessary to assess the client's support system to ascertain what resources are available. Are there other members of the family nearby? What about grown grandchildren? Could friends or neighbors be called on for some supportive activities? If the client has a religious affiliation, support by the church or the religious group might be available. Does the community provide services, e.g., Friendly Visitors, Meals on Wheels, Visiting Homemaker Service? Based on the availability of these resources, a plan should be worked out to get the elder more involved.

ASSESSING FAMILY COPING PATTERNS

In assessing abuse in a family situation, the nurse must use great skill in questioning about the subject of potential abuse, since the caregiver may react with indifference or anger to such questions. The nurse should show a willingness to listen and avoid any censuring tone during the interview. Questioning the caregiver about memories of early family relationships should help provide additional information about attitudes in the home. Find out about the caregiver and his family's educational level, occupation, general income level, and religious and cultural beliefs (Anderson and Thobaben 1984).

Attitudes about aging and the roles and duties of the elder should be considered further. If the caregiver views old age in a negative light and adds his or her own unrecognized fears of aging, the caregiver often will tend to deny the aging process and its consequences for his or her parents (Rathbone-McCuan and Hashimi 1982).

When older adults can no longer provide for themselves, they will become dependent on the family. The caregiver will then need to assume the role of "parent" to the older adult. Such a change often occurs at "some tangible personal costs" (Rathbone-McCuan and Hashimi 1982).

The caregiver's sense of duty toward aged parents varies with the adult child's sex, birth order, experience during childhood, and present life situation. Caring for an ill aged parent is particularly difficult, since it requires the almost constant presence of a family member in the house.

In our society, responsibility for care for the elderly usually falls on the woman. If there are disputes, she is generally expected to mediate between the needs of her spouse and those of the elderly person. This burden may be difficult to bear physically and emotionally. The problem is compounded if the husband refuses to share in the responsibility while expecting his wife to provide care for his parents or other elderly persons for whom he feels accountable (Rathbone-McCuan and Hashimi 1982).

If there is a decrease in the living standards because of the older adult's presence in the home, the aged adult is at risk for abuse if he or she (1) has money but refuses to spend it, (2) uses the money to control the caregiver, or (3) is without funds but does not apply for needed financial aid (Ferguson and Beck 1983).

Living with an older adult in the same household or being responsible for his or her care can cause anger, frustration, and stress. Abusive behavior is linked to reactions by the family to such a situation. Violence and abuse are among the possible coping behaviors of the family that arise in such situations.

When the caregiver first assumes the caring responsibility, he or she may be unprepared for future changes and demands. The elder may display a sufficient independence that makes the caregiver's task easier. However, circumstances may change drastically. Once the elder has exhausted personal and financial resources and is faced with a decrease in activities due to declining health, the caregiver's responsibilities, and thereby the stress of providing care, are intensified (Rathbone-McCuan and Hashimi 1982).

Standard III: Diagnosis

Formulating a nursing diagnosis is dependent on an assessment of both the victim and the abuser. *Potential for injury* should be considered first, since it deals with the client's physical safety. If the abuse results in rape, the nursing diagnosis would be *rape - trauma syndrome* or *sexual dysfunction*.

If the client's judgment and perception of the present situation are disturbed, *altered thought processes* would be the corresponding nursing diagnosis. If the victim is withdrawn or agitated or has difficulty dealing with the situation, this could be a demonstration of *ineffective individual coping*.

The victim is often in a dependent position, relying on the abuser to meet personal physical and emotional needs. The victim's feelings of helplessness and hopelessness would make *powerlessness* an appropriate diagnosis. If the client is afraid or is uneasy about discussing the abusive situation with the nurse or others because of fear of retaliation by the caregiver, the diagnoses of *fear* and *anxiety* may be indicated.

With aging, the older adult may be experiencing losses, e.g., changing body image, role in the family, social relationships, death of a spouse. *Grieving* about these losses or changes should be considered. The elder can also be experiencing *self-esteem disturbance* related to the losses or to the abuse.

In cases of abuse, victims are often without support systems or social contacts. They may be cut off from any community or religious supports. They may be experiencing *social isolation* or *spiritual distress*.

Three nursing diagnoses can be made with regard to the abuser and the general family situation: *potential for violence*, *ineffective family coping*, and *altered family processes*.

Standard IV: Planning

In developing a nursing care plan for the abused client, two levels need be considered content, which includes long term and short term goals, and process, which includes the nurse's awareness of reactions to client's and abuser's behavior.

CONTENT LEVEL—PLANNING GOALS

With each nursing diagnosis, long term and short term goals are identified. They are directed toward the client and the abuser in specific circumstances. The diagnoses with their possible goals are listed subsequently.

Possible Goals for the Abused Elder

1. Potential for injury.
   - Client will be free of physical signs of abuse by (state the date).
   - Client will state that he or she feels safer and more comfortable by (state the date). OR
   - Client will ask to be removed from abusive situation by (state the date).
   - Client will name one person he or she can call for needed help by (state the date).
   - Client will state that the caregiver has provided adequate food, clothing, housing, and medical care by (state the date).
2. Rape-trauma syndrome or sexual dysfunction.
   - Client will state sexual abuse has ceased by (state the date).
   - Client will identify abuser by (state the date).
   - If sexual abuse continues, client will initiate actions (with aid of health care workers) to remove self from present situation by (state the date).
   - Client will verbalize feelings about sexual abuse by (state the date).
3. Altered thought processes and ineffective individual coping.
   - Client will state the environment she is in is not safe by (state the date).
   - Client will make one decision about the future with assistance of nursing counsel by (state the date).
   - Client will name a person he or she will call in case of further abuse by (state the date).
   - Client will take two actions to improve the present situation by (state the date).
   - Client will make one suggestion for change of the present condition by (state the date).
4. Powerlessness.
   - Client will state that he or she is being abused or experiencing neglect by the caregiver by (state the date).
   - Client will have demonstrated a new coping skill he or she has used by (state the date).
   - If abuse continues, client will notify nurse or other significant person by (state the date).
   - Client will state that he or she feels more supported by family to make personal decisions by (state the date).
   - Client will state an action that he or she will take if she is verbally abused or neglected by (state the date).
   - Client will express desire to change living situation by (state the date).
   - Client will carry out one action to change the present situation by (state the date).
5. Grieving.
   - Client will state acceptance of changes in body image by (state the date).
   - Client will express feelings of loss by naming two losses experienced by (state the date).
   - Client will name two actions to be taken to overcome feelings of loss by (state the date).
6. Social isolation.
   - Client will name one person available to meet with by (state the date).
   - Client will telephone an old acquaintance by (state the date).
   - Client will attend one social activity in the community by (state the date).
   - Client will have a nonfamily visitor by (state the date).
7. Spiritual distress.
   - Minister or religious person will visit with the client by (state the date).
   - Client will attend one religious service by (state the date).
   - Client will have a visit by another person in his or her parish or religious organization by (state the date).

Possible Goals for the Caregiver/Family

1. Potential for violence directed at others.
   - Caregiver will state that physical abuse of elder has ceased by next visit.
   - Caregiver will state that yelling and controlling the

elder's behaviors and actions has ceased by (state the date).
- Caregiver will seek counseling to help with control of behavior by (state the date).
- Caregiver will meet with counselor at least once a week by (state the date).
- Caregiver will discuss three positive reasons for joining a self-help group by (state the date).

2. Ineffective family coping and altered family process.
   - Family members will meet together and discuss alternative ways of dealing with elderly client by (state the date).
   - Family members will name two strategies to avoid physical or emotional abuse of the client by (state the date).
   - Family members will name two support services to whom they can turn for help by (state the date).
   - Family members will seek counseling for behaviors by (state the date).
   - Family members will state they will meet with the nurse on a weekly basis for counseling starting (state the date).
   - Abuser will meet with other family members and discuss feelings on care of elderly by (state the date).
   - One other family member will spend time with the elder and relieve abuser of care by (state the date).
   - Family members will meet together and discuss alternatives to care of the elderly by (state the date).
   - Client and family will meet together and discuss resources and supports that they feel are important to them by (state the date).

PROCESS LEVEL—NURSES' REACTIONS AND FEELINGS

Decisions about abuse of the elderly are not easy to make. Abuse is an uncomfortable subject for many to deal with, for it can arouse great feelings of repugnance and disdain toward the abuser. The nurse must be prepared to deal with the consequences of the intervention. Interventions may trigger events for which the nurse is unprepared, i.e., threats of bodily harm from the caregivers or the client's refusal to accept assistance. The nurse must evaluate whether it would be better to end an abusive situation and place the client (consenting) with another family member or institution, or whether the client should be left in a compromising situation. These thoughts and feelings should be shared in conference with other members of the health team, e.g., the social worker and doctor, to maximize effective decision making.

Standard V: Intervention

Nurses are in a special position to identify, and intervene in, cases of elder abuse because of their frequent, often daily, contact with the elderly.

Obtaining a complete picture of the client's situation is not always easy. The nurse should realize that the elderly are often reluctant to admit to any problem in their own families. They may refrain from acknowledging to others the abusive behavior of their children and may remain silent in fear of retaliation or abandonment (Anderson 1981).

The nurse should be cognizant of the legal constraints for reporting abuse and planning interventions. Laws vary from state to state. Unlike the situation with child abuse, not all states have laws that protect the abused older person. In fact, there are few states that mandate reporting suspected cases of elder abuse. Moreover, most states have no provisions to protect health professionals against libel if suspected elder abuse is reported. In most cases the elder victim must file criminal charges (Sanders and Plummer 1983). Since the caregiver is often a family member, the elder, often dependent upon the caregiver and often frail and frightened, is put in an impossible situation.

Client competency is another area of nursing consideration when intervening in an elder abuse situation. Unless incompetency has been established legally, elders have the right to self-determination and may refuse necessary or appropriate medical care (Fulmer and Cahill 1984). Intervention then is not possible without their consent. This may apply even when the client's life is endangered.

If the client rejects help in a life-threatening situation, the nurse should seek legal counsel to determine whether the law of the state allows the elder to refuse intervention in such an acute situation. Should the law of the state not provide for intervention, the nurse should then see whether the client's competency could be challenged through legal action.

Some institutions and health-care agencies have developed guidelines on how to deal with actual or suspected abuse situations. These protocols list possible behaviors or conditions of the elderly, and the most appropriate intervention. The establishment of such protocols is highly recommended, because it gives support to the nurse's actions.

V-A: PSYCHOTHERAPEUTIC INTERVENTIONS

Intervention carried out by the nurse at this level is geared toward assisting the client and the family to recover, or improve on, their ability to deal with the abusive and stressful situation facing them.

The nurse would assist the abused client to improve his or her relationship with the caregiver and other family members and work with the family members to communicate more effectively with one another in support of the client. Lack of communication in the family is one of the most frequent problems. It is particularly true for multigenerational (children, parents, and grandparents) families (Lund et al. 1985). Under the nurse's direction, problem-solving skills are developed to improve the family's handling of stress and abuse. The nurse can help the family to identify and engage available resources within the family and from health-care providers and the community.

V-B: HEALTH TEACHING

Health teaching includes meeting with both the client and the family and discussing risk factors associated with abuse. In particular the nurse attempts to teach the abuser nonviolent coping behaviors. The client, caregiver, and family should learn to recognize behaviors and situations that might trigger abuse.

The normal aging changes should be explained to enable the family members to gain a more positive view of the older adult; this will help them avoid the often negative stereotyping of the elderly. In gaining a more complete understanding of the aging process, the family members can better comprehend their own parents as individuals. They may then begin to anticipate new stress situations and thus be able to prepare for them before a crisis occurs (Olsen and Cahn 1980).

Besides understanding aging changes, the family should be taught how losses affect and are being manifested in the aging adult. "Losses of mobility, eyesight or hearing may be just as painful as the loss of a loved one" (Anderson and Thobaben 1984). With this knowledge, the family members can broaden their insight and thus increase their compassion.

Educating family members to analyze their respective roles and to develop suggestions for realignment or redistribution of responsibilities is important for effecting change in an abusive situation. Ferguson and Beck (1983) suggest "the process would include assessing the need for role changes in all family members, identifying role conflicts, clarifying expectations, and strengthening the ability of family members to perform their own role, that is, support of the older members by identifying some new function for him or her."

V-E: THERAPEUTIC ENVIRONMENT

By getting involved with the client and the family, the nurse tries to create a more secure setting. The nurse should acknowledge the family's contribution to the elder's care and suggest services that would aid the family members in their caregiving role (Giordano and Giordano 1984). Such services include the Visiting Homemaker Service, Meals on Wheels, Friendly Visitors, respite and day care, and chore and transportation services. The nurse should also explore community support groups for caregivers of physically and mentally impaired relatives. When working with the family, the nurse should provide a therapeutic environment through an open, supportive, and nonthreatening relationship.

Standard VI: Evaluation

Assessment and evaluation are an ongoing process. Evaluating the set goals can lead to new goals when old ones are reached or to changes in intervention if set goals have not been met.

Evaluation in elder abuse would primarily be appraisal of the goals set to change family interactions and to influence positively the incidence of abuse in the family. The nurse would assess for signs of changes. Changes would be noted in evidence of physical abuse, psychological abuse, in the coping patterns used by the victim, change in support systems available, or changes in the family coping patterns. When these changes are positive, the nurse may continue to work with the family as a resource person or facilitator. When changes are not noted or are negative, the nurse works with the family to re-evaluate the goals and the interventions originally set for their attainment.

As in the case of child abuse, careful and frequent documentation must be kept. Documentation should include descriptive body drawings, written descriptions, and verbatim statements made by the victim, caregivers, and family members.

Text continued on page 301

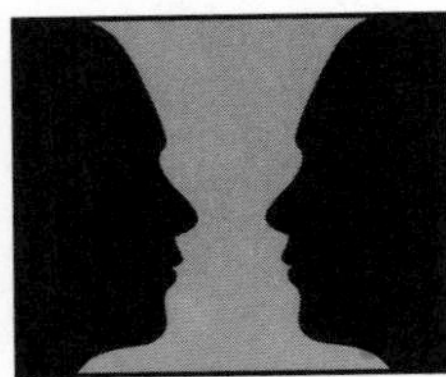

Case Study: Working With a Family Involved With Elder Abuse

Mrs. Rob, an 84-year-old recently widowed woman, moved to her son's apartment three months ago. She had been living alone in her third-floor walk-up in the city. Because of her declining health, crime in the neighborhood, and three flights of stairs to climb, and with her son John's encouragement, she went to live with him. He and his wife, Judy, who have been married for almost 20 years, have five children, ages 6 to 18, all living in a rather cramped three-bedroom apartment.

Mrs. Rob was being cared for by the visiting nurse to monitor her blood pressure and adjust her medication. Over a series of visits, the nurse, Ms. Green, noticed that Mrs. Rob was looking noticeably unkempt, pale, and withdrawn. While taking her blood pressure, the nurse observed bruises on Mrs. Rob's arms and neck. When questioned about the bruises, Mrs. Rob appeared anxious and nervous. She said that she had slipped in the bathroom. Mrs. Rob became increasingly apprehensive and stiffened up in her chair when her daughter-in-law, Judy, came into the room asking when the next visit was. The nurse noticed that Judy avoided eye contact with Mrs. Rob.

When the injuries were brought to Judy's attention, she responded by becoming angry and agitated, blaming Mrs. Rob for causing so many problems. She would not explain the reason for the change in Mrs. Rob's behavior nor the origin of the bruises to the nurse. She merely commented, "I have had to give up my job since my mother-in-law came here. . . . It has been difficult and crowded ever since *she* moved in. The kids are complaining. We are having trouble making ends meet since I gave up my job. And my husband is not being any help at all."

Assessment

Ms. Green suspected that Mrs. Rob was in an abusive situation and spoke of the case with her team back at the visiting nurse center. The nurse identified objective and subjective data that supported suspected elder abuse.

OBJECTIVE DATA

1. Physical symptoms of abuse, i.e., bruises, unkempt appearance, withdrawn attitude
2. Stressful, crowded living conditions
3. No eye contact between elder and daughter-in-law
4. Economic hardships leading to stress
5. No support for the daughter-in-law from rest of family for care of Mrs. Rob
6. Elder unable to make decisions

SUBJECTIVE DATA

1. Mrs. Rob states she "slipped in the bathroom," but physical findings don't support explanation
2. Daughter-in-law states, "It's been difficult and crowded ever since *she* moved in."
3. Mrs. Rob exhibits withdrawn and apprehensive behavior

Nursing Diagnosis

Based on the data, the nurse formulated the following nursing diagnoses:

1. *Potential for Injury* related to increase in family stress, as evidenced by signs of abuse
   - Mrs. Rob states she slipped in the bathroom, but physical findings don't support that explanation
   - Physical symptoms of abuse present (bruises, unkempt appearance, withdrawn attitude)
   - Stressful, crowded living conditions
2. *Ineffective Individual Coping* related to helplessness, as evidenced by inability to meet role expectations
   - Mrs. Rob appears unkempt, anxious, depressed
   - Mrs. Rob exhibits withdrawn and apprehensive behavior
   - Mrs. Rob is unable to make decisions

3. *Potential for Violence* related to increased stressors within a short period, as evidenced by probable elder abuse and feelings of helplessness
   - Judy states, "It's been difficult and crowded ever since *she* moved in."
   - No eye contact between Judy and Mrs. Rob
   - Signs and symptoms of physical abuse on elder
   - "My husband is no help at all."
4. *Ineffective Family Coping* related to unmet psychosocial needs of elder by son and daughter-in-law
   - Family not helping with care of mother-in-law, burden of care on Judy
   - Economic hardships leading to stress when Judy gave up job to care for Mrs. Rob

Planning

CONTENT LEVEL—PLANNING GOALS

The nurse discussed several possible goals with members of her team, giving attention to the priority of goals and to whether they are realistic in this situation.

Nursing Diagnosis	Long Term Goal	Short Term Goal
1. *Potential for Injury* related to increase in family stress, as evidenced by signs of abuse	Mrs. Rob will be well nourished and free from signs of physical abuse by (state the date).	1. Mrs. Rob will name two persons she can call in case of further abuse in one week (date).
2. *Ineffective Individual Coping* related to helplessness, as evidenced by inability to meet role expectations	Mrs. Rob will have definite alternative plans for living situation by one month (state the date).	2a. Mrs. Rob will identify three personal strengths in one week (date). 2b. Mrs. Rob will make one decision about her future in two weeks (date). 2c. In three weeks Mrs. Rob will state two behavioral changes she will make (date).
3. *Potential for Violence* by abuser related to increased stressors within a short period of time, as evidenced by probable elder abuse and feelings of helplessness	Judy will state she has control of feelings and is no longer abusing Mrs. Rob by one month (state the date).	3a. Judy will name three conditions that led to her loss of control with elder in one week (date). 3b. Judy will use three new coping behaviors within three weeks (date). 3c. Judy will seek counseling in three weeks (date). 3d. Judy will name three support services she can call in one week (date).
4. *Ineffective Family Coping* related to unmet psychosocial needs of elder by son and daughter-in-law	Mrs. Rob and family will meet together and discuss mutual expectations and actions they wish to share.	4a. Family members will meet with nurse on regular basis starting in one week (date). 4b. Family will identify supports and resources they feel are important to them in one week.

Continued on following page

Planning (Continued)

4c. One other family member will spend one-half day per week with Mrs. Rob.

PROCESS LEVEL—NURSES' REACTIONS AND FEELINGS

Ms. Green has been in a number of situations with abusive families, but this was the first time she encountered elder abuse. She discussed her reactions with the other team members. She was especially angry at Judy, although she was able to understand the daughter-in-law's frustration. The team concurred with Ms. Green that there seemed to be a lot of potential for positive change with this family. If abuse does not abate, more drastic measures will need to be taken, and legal services contracted.

Intervention

Elder abuse is a signal of a family in crisis. Ms. Green knew she had to address the needs of the whole family to effect change within the family system. She focused on Mrs. Rob's physical safety first, then on Mrs. Rob's strengths to work within the family system. It was evident that Judy was overwhelmed with multiple stressors, and interventions for her and the rest of the family were vital for effective change.

Ms. Green continued to meet with the family on a weekly basis. Interventions were mapped out, with input from the family. Although it was difficult at first to get the husband involved, he became more active when his feelings of helplessness and guilt began to fade. Ms. Green encouraged the children to participate, and many useful suggestions came from their observations and ideas.

This family seemed motivated to change their circumstances, since all members were feeling overwhelmed and helpless. Although initially suggestions regarding outside services were met with some resistance, other services were contacted. Judy stated that she found weekly counseling a great help. The Friendly Visitors Service allowed Judy some time to herself each week. Refer to Nursing Care Plan 14–1 for specific interventions for this family.

Evaluation

Eight weeks after the nurse's initial visit, Mrs. Rob appeared well-groomed, friendly, and more spontaneous in her conversation. She commented, "things are better with my daughter-in-law." No bruises or other signs of physical abuse were noticeable. She was considerably more outgoing and even took the initiative to contact an old friend. She had talked openly with her son and daughter-in-law about stress in the family. When her daughter-in-law, Judy, appeared tense, Mrs. Rob went out for a walk and returned to find the tension had lessened. Neither Mrs. Rob nor her family had initiated plans for alternative housing.

As a further result of the nurse's intervention, Judy was more in control of her emotions. Although she did on occasion yell at her mother-in-law, she felt this was no longer the same uncontrolled explosive anger. Verbalizing her feelings to her husband helped alleviate her frustrations. Judy was seeing a counselor at the hospital and was planning to look for a part-time job to "get out of the house."

Gradually, the family members began to communicate with one another. Mrs. Rob's other son and his family were contacted for assistance. Although this son had not yet offered to share some of the responsibility for taking care of his mother, he did agree to give some financial support. The family continued to meet with the nurse.

Nursing Care Plan 14–1 • A FAMILY INVOLVED WITH ELDER ABUSE: Mrs. Rob

NURSING DIAGNOSIS

Potential for injury related to increase in family stress, as evidenced by signs of abuse

Supporting Data

- States that she slipped in the bathroom.
- Physical symptoms of abuse, i.e., bruises, unkempt appearance, withdrawn attitude.
- Stressful, crowded living conditions.

Long Term Goal: Mrs. Rob will be well nourished and free from signs of physical abuse by (date).

Short Term Goal	*Intervention*	*Rationale*	*Evaluation*
1. Client will state the abuse is decreased by (date).	1a. Assess severity of signs and symptoms of abuse and potential for further injury on weekly visits.	1a. Determine need for further intervention.	Goal met Client says she is no longer abused in family situation.
	1b. Discuss with client factors leading to abuse and concern for physical safety.	1b. Validates situation is serious and increases client's knowledge base.	
2. In one week client will name two persons she can call in case of further abuse.	2. Discuss with client support services such as hotlines and crisis units to call in case of emergency situation.	2. Maximizes client's safety through use of support systems.	

NURSING DIAGNOSIS

Ineffective individual coping related to helplessness, as evidenced by inability to meet role expectations

Supporting Data

- Appears unkempt, anxious, depressed.
- Exhibits withdrawn and apprehensive behavior.
- Unable to make decisions.

Long Term Goal: Client will have definite plans for alternatives to present living situation within one month.

Short Term Goal	*Intervention*	*Rationale*	*Evaluation*
1. Client will identify three personal strengths by (state the date).	1a. Approach client in positive, nonjudgmental manner.	1a. Encourages disclosure and development of relationship.	Goal partially met Client has identified personal strengths and made two behavioral changes. She has not made any definite plans for a change in living situation. She says she is feeling a little better about living with son's family.
	1b. Assist client to develop effective coping skills.	1b. Redirects self-assessment to positive skills.	
	1c. Assist client to identify personal assets.	1c. Can help increase self-esteem.	
2. Client will make one decision about the future by (state the date).	2a. Encourage client to examine situation and alternatives.	2a. When in a dependent situation, individuals may have difficulties making decisions.	
	2b. Reinforce client's use of problem-solving skills.	2b. Encourages client to function at optimum level.	
3. Client will state two behavioral changes to be carried out by (state the date).	3a. Explore with client ways to make changes.	3a. Directs assessment to positive areas.	
	3b. Assist client in making decisions for action for future.	3b. Can help improve self-esteem.	

NURSING DIAGNOSIS

Potential for violence by abuser related to increased stressors within a short period of time, as evidenced by aggressive behaviors

Supporting Data

- States "It's been difficult and crowded ever since *she* moved in."
- No eye contact with Mrs. Rob.
- Signs and symptoms of physical abuse on mother-in-law.

Continued on following page

Nursing Care Plan 14-1 • A FAMILY INVOLVED WITH ELDER ABUSE: Mrs. Rob *(Continued)*

NURSING DIAGNOSIS

Long Term Goal: By (state the date), abuser will state that she has control over her feelings and is not abusing Mrs. Rob.

Short Term Goal	*Intervention*	*Rationale*	*Evaluation*
1. Abuser will name three conditions that contribute to her loss of control with Mrs. Rob by (state the date).	1. Nurse will meet with abuser and encourage problem-solving approach.	1. Develops abuser's abilities.	Goal met Abuser has not abused Mrs. Rob. Daughter-in-law states, "I feel better about dealing with stressful situations."
2. Abuser will have used three new coping behaviors with Mrs. Rob by (state the date).	2a. Encourage abuser to verbalize feelings about Mrs. Rob and understand what conditions lead to stress so that they can be avoided.	2a. Positive approach to deal with stress.	
	2b. Encourage development of alternative behaviors.	2b. Acceptable manner of dealing with stress.	
	2c. Reinforce positive approaches suggested by abuser.	2c. Increases abilities to deal with stress.	
3. Abuser will seek counseling by (state the date).	3a. Encourage abuser's use of counseling, reinforcing benefits and needs gained from such a regular intervention.	3a. Increases coping abilities	
4. Abuser will name three support services she can call on and will have utilized one by (state the date).	4a. Explore with abuser available support services. Encourage utilization.	4a. Increases knowledge of resources.	
	4b. Initiate referrals for support services.	4b. Provides needed support.	

NURSING DIAGNOSIS

Ineffective family coping related to unmet psychosocial needs of elder by son and daughter-in-law

Supporting Data

- Family not helping with care of mother-in-law. It is being left to daughter-in-law, who states, "My husband is not being any help at all."
- Economic hardships leading to stress when wife gave up job to care for elder.

Long Term Goal: Client and family members will meet together and discuss mutual expectations and actions they wish to share by (state the date).

Short Term Goal	*Intervention*	*Rationale*	*Evaluation*
1. Family members will meet for counseling with nurse on a regular basis by (state the date).	1a. Nurse will meet with family members and encourage problem solving of present situation.	1a. Family members have opportunity to verbalize their feelings about present situation, offering different perspectives.	Goal met Family members are meeting regularly.
	1b. Nurse will suggest that family members meet together on regular basis for problem solving and support.	1b. Family will solve problems together.	

Long Term Goal: Family members will share the responsibilities of caring for Mrs. Rob by (state the date).

Short Term Goal	*Intervention*	*Rationale*	*Evaluation*
1. Family will identify supports and resources they feel are important to them by (state the date).	1a. Nurse will assist family in identifying support services available, then select appropriate services. 1b. Nurse will contact suggested services for family when requested.	1a. Support services can provide assistance to the family. 1b. Nurse can provide needed support and expertise.	Goal partially met No other outside family member is providing the half-day respite for Mrs. Rob's immediate family. The family has identified support services and contacted one agency.
2. One other family member will spend one-half day per week with Mrs. Rob by (state the date).	2. Family will meet together and discuss responsibility for care of Mrs. Rob and make suggestions for more support by family members. Nurse will act as facilitator in discussion, if necessary.	2. Family will problem-solve and explore avenues for needed assistance.	

Summary

The elderly are vulnerable to physical and emotional abuse and neglect. Nurses have the responsibility to provide accurate assessment, relevant planning, and quick intervention to protect their elderly clients in suspected and actual cases of abuse. Abuse is not always obvious. Therefore, early and continuous assessment of families at risk is important to prevent and reduce abuse of the older adult's physical, emotional, and material rights.

References

Anderson C. Abuse and neglect among the elderly. Journal of Gerontological Nursing, 7(2):77, 1981.

Anderson L, Thobaben M. Clients in crisis. Journal of Gerontological Nursing, 10(12):7, 1984.

Beck C, Ferguson D. Aged abuse. Journal of Gerontological Nursing, 7(6):333, 1981.

Burnside I. Nursing and the Aged: A Self-Care Approach, 4th ed. New York: McGraw Hill, 1988.

Eastman M. Abusing the elderly. Nursing Mirror, 159(15):19, 1984.

Falconi D. Assessing the abused elderly. Journal of Gerontological Nursing, 8:208, 1982.

Ferguson D, Beck C. H.A.L.F.—A tool to assess elder abuse within the family. Geriatric Nursing, 4(5):301, 1983.

Foley TS. Nursing intervention in family abuse and violence. *In* Stuart GW, Sundeen SJ. (eds). Principles and Practice of Psychiatric Nursing, 2nd ed. St Louis: C.V. Mosby Company, 1983.

Fulmer T, Cahill V. Assessing elder abuse. Journal of Gerontological Nursing, 10(12):16, 1984.

Galbraith M (ed). Elder Abuse: Perspectives on an Emerging Crisis, vol 3. Kansas City, KS: Mid-American Congress on Aging, 1986.

Gelman D, Hanger M, et al. Who's taking care of our parents? Newsweek, May 6, 1985, pp. 61–68.

Giordano N, Giordano J. Elder abuse: Review of the literature. Social Work, 29:232, 1984.

Hamilton G. Prevent elder abuse using a family systems approach. Journal of Gerontological Nursing, 15(3):21–31, 1989.

Johnson D. Abuse and neglect—Not for children only! Journal of Gerontological Nursing, 5(4):11, 1979.

Lund D, Feinhaurer L, et al. Living together: Grandparents and children tell their problems. Journal of Gerontological Nursing, 11(11):29, 1985.

Milt H. Family neglect and abuse of the aged: A growing concern. New York: Public Affairs Committee, 1982.

Olsen J, Cahn B. Helping families cope with elderly parents. Journal of Gerontological Nursing, 6(3):152, 1980.

Phillips L. Elder abuse—What is it? Who says so? Geriatric Nursing, 4(3):167, 1983.

Rathbone-McCuan E, Hashimi J. Isolated Elders. Rockville, MD: Aspen Systems, 1982.

Sanders FV, Plummer EM. Assault on the aged: Is your patient a secret victim? RN, :21(July), 1983.

Simos B. Adult children and their aging parents. Social Work, 18(3):79, 1973.

Stannard C. Old folks and dirty work: The social conditions for patient abuse in nursing home. Social Problems 20:329, 1973.

Tallying risks for elder abuse. Medical World News, January 23, 1986, pp. 72–73.

Verwoerdt A. Clinical Geropsychiatry. Baltimore: Williams & Wilkins, 1976.

Annotated Bibliography

Anderson C. Abuse and neglect among the elderly. Journal of Gerontological Nursing, 7:77, 1981.

Anderson defines and discusses types of abuse and neglect and gives brief case histories to highlight and explain her observations.

Beck C, Ferguson D. Aged abuse. Journal of Gerontological Nursing, 7:333, 1981.

The authors define and explore types of elder abuse with particular emphasis on psychological abuse. They discuss three theoretical frameworks stressing family systems theory.

Douglas R. Domestic Mistreatment of the Elderly—Towards Prevention. Washington DC: American Association of Retired Persons, 1987.

Handbook concentrating on definitions and examples of abuse. Focus is also on prevention by the older adult and the community as a key to the problem of abuse. Methods of early planning are considered.

Falconi D. Assessing the abused elderly. Journal of Gerontological Nursing, 8:208, 1982.

This article is of particular significance on the subject of abuse. Falconi gives a brief review of the literature on abuse. She defines possible causes of abuse and discusses the characteristics of the abused and the abuser. The author presents a complete assessment guide for an elderly client who might be abused. Falconi expertly explains how to obtain key information on abuse through a thorough history taking and physical assessment.

Ferguson D, Beck, C. H.A.L.F.—A tool to assess elder abuse within the family. Geriatric Nursing, 4:301, 1983.

The authors have developed a tool to help the nurse assess abuse within the family. The tool concentrates on family dynamics, which is considered a key aspect of the assessment. Examples demonstrate how to use this tool.

Galbraith M (ed). Elder Abuse: Perspectives on an Emerging Crisis, vol 3. Kansas City, KS: Mid-American Congress on Aging, 1986.

Galbraith presents an extensive overview of current literature on the subject of violence toward older adults, providing a helpful outline for practitioners, researchers, and educators. Besides providing a review of current assessment tools, techniques and strategies for interventions by health care providers are discussed. The role of inpatient geropsychiatry in the network of elder abuse services is explored. Older adult volunteers and their potential for identifying and treating elder abuse are discussed.

Johnson T, et al. Elder Neglect and Abuse: An Annotated Bibliography. Westport, CT: Greenwood Press, 1985.

This book offers a comprehensive review of literature on elder abuse in the United States and England since 1975. References are drawn from eight disciplines: journalism, law, medicine, psychiatry, psychology, public health, social work, and sociology. The annotations deal with abuse in family settings only. The work is well organized. A directory is provided of national and state organizations, including agencies that can help in the protection of the elderly.

Self-Study Exercises

Choose the answer that most accurately completes the statement.

1. Changes during the 19th and 20th centuries that have increased stress and escalated anxiety within the family system include all of the following EXCEPT

   A. The Industrial Revolution
   B. Longer life span and smaller family units
   C. One-parent families and older children caring for parents
   D. Plentiful resources in the community available to stressed families

Identify physical abuse with an X and psychological abuse with an O.

2. __________ Overmedication or lack of needed medication in the home
3. __________ Elder subjected to ridicule and humiliation
4. __________ Screaming at elder because of irritation over elder's grieving physical and other losses
5. __________ Decubitus ulcers, contractures, and forced immobilization
6. __________ Misuse or theft of elder's money
7. __________ Treating the aged as a dependent child

8. Circle the conditions that can exacerbate family abuse.

   A. Lack of finances
   B. Negative attitudes toward aging on the part of the caretaker
   C. Lack of knowledge of the aging process
   D. Close family ties
   E. A physically or mentally dependent elder
   F. Use of alcohol or drugs or physical illness within the family system
   G. Good friends and involved extended family members
   H. Inadequate living conditions
   I. Fond family memories
   J. The caregiver being abused as a child

Situation

Mr. and Mrs. Samuels are an 85-year-old married couple living in their own home. They both appear frail, underweight, and fragile. In December, when the visiting nurse came in for an initial assessment visit, he found their home in poor repair, without heat or food. The couple said they were waiting for their 65-year-old son to bring over the food for the day. When questioned further, they said they had been waiting almost two days for him. They then said, "Please, don't bother our son. He will get so angry. He doesn't want outsiders in here. He has so many problems. . . . Don't call him or he won't come at all."

Questions 9 through 13 refer to the preceding situation.

9. Identify one nursing diagnosis for the abused couple and list supporting data.
   ND: ______________________________
   -
   -
   -

10. Identify one nursing diagnosis for the abusive son and list supporting data.
    ND: ______________________________
    -
    -
    -

11. Name and briefly discuss the type of abuse evident in this example.
12. For each of the nursing diagnoses previously identified, state one short-term goal.
13. For each goal, plan three interventions that would be appropriate for meeting your goals.

Short Answer and Discussion

14. Name three community agencies that can lower stress for the caregiver in cases of suspected or actual abuse.
    -
    -
    -

15. Briefly discuss the legal issues involved in cases of elder abuse.

Place T (True) or F (False) next to each statement. Correct the false statements.

16. ________ More than 80% of abuse of the elderly is committed by a family member.
17. ________ The most likely victim of elder abuse is a male.
18. ________ The victim usually resides in the household of the abuser.
19. ________ Abuse occurs only on the person of the afflicted individual.
20. ________ Psychological abuse is more easy to identify than physical abuse.
21. ________ The elderly will readily admit to being abused by a family member.
22. ________ One form of psychological abuse is treating the aged as dependent children.
23. ________ Responsibility for the care of the elderly falls on the family breadwinner regardless of sex.

24. __________ Rape-trauma syndrome and sexual dysfunction are two possible nursing diagnoses in cases of abuse.
25. __________ Increased anxiety in the elder can result in incontinence, screaming, or repeating the same word over and over.
26. __________ The abuser might verbally or physically attack the nurse or the elder when abuse is discovered.
27. __________ All states have laws to protect health care professionals against libel suits from caregivers when elder abuse is reported.

PEOPLE IN MODERATE TO SEVERE LEVELS OF CHRONIC ANXIETY

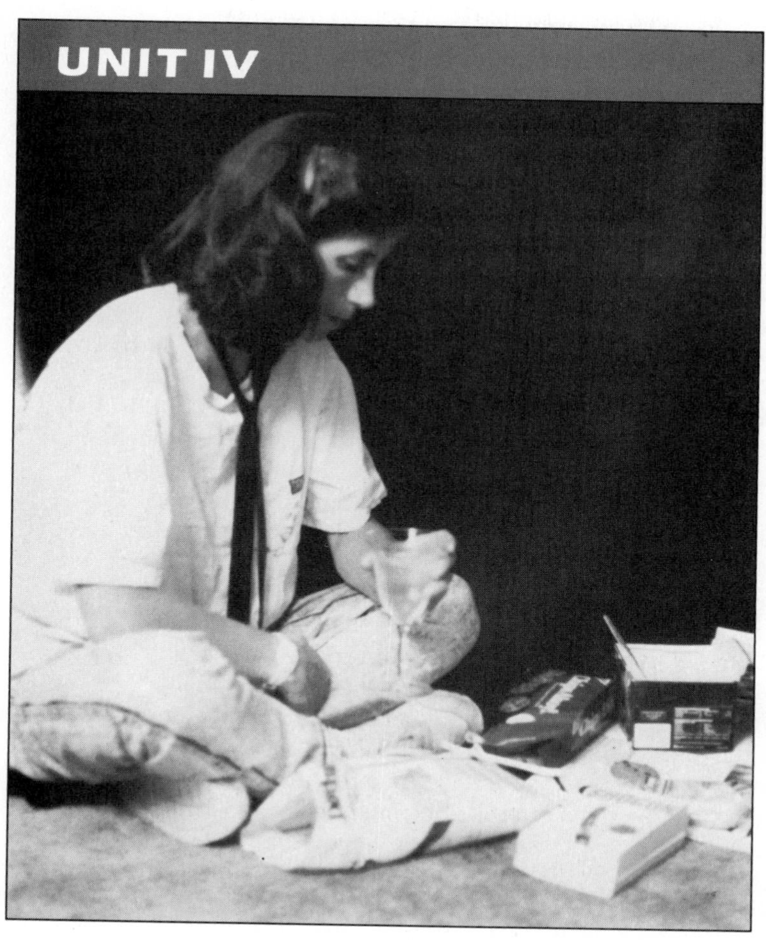

No matter how good things get, my capacity to make myself unhappy is always equal to it.

HUGH PRATHER

A Nurse Speaks

by L. Sharon Shisler

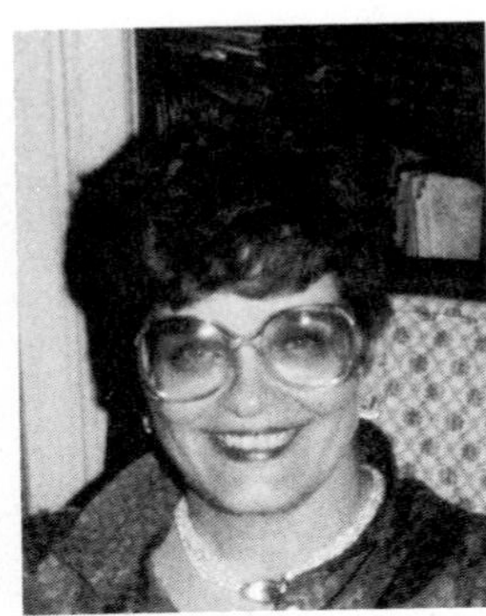

My entrance into private practice in psychiatric nursing occurred when three adult psychiatric nurses asked me to join them in a group practice that they were forming. At the time, I was working full-time as an instructor in continuing education and was seeing one patient weekly for supportive psychotherapy. I had had 20 years of experience in the mental health field, had earned a master of arts degree ten years earlier, and had been certified by the American Nurses' Association as a Child and Adolescent Clinical Specialist.

One of the biggest questions in starting and maintaining a private practice is: "How do you get referrals?" I wondered, "Would other mental health professionals see us as taking their 'bread and butter' in the competitive market place?" "Would professionals and the consumers see us as adequate for the task?" "Would we be seen as qualified?" "Would insurance companies reimburse our charges?" "Would patients and families respond positively to seeing a nurse?"

These fears vanished when one family, who had seen me previously when I co-led a parent-child psychotherapeutic group, was simultaneously referred to me by three professionals and the family, itself. The psychiatrist currently seeing the mother and six-year-old daughter was moving to another state. She asked the family to decide whom they would like to continue to see in family therapy to work on various problems that had been dealt with by various professionals over a five-year period. They selected me, a nurse.

This family illustrates one of the surprises that occur in private practice but are not addressed in books. I saw the family for about ten months, twice a week, with either all members present or various subsets of the family present. As the total family's functioning increased and symptoms subsided, the mother unexpectedly started having major anxiety attacks. Although more than one health professional had done a thorough assessment and taken a history, the mother had not revealed these anxiety attacks to anyone. The attacks started when she was around two years of age and recurred at major transitions in her life.

These attacks were successfully treated with behavioral modification, relaxation techniques, and visualization techniques. Exploring with the mother the family dynamics in her family of origin and observing how these dynamics were being repeated in her present family proved extremely valuable. Although a medication consultation was obtained, the attacks subsided without medication through the use of relaxation techniques.

The mother was able to use relaxation techniques and visualization techniques to minimize her anxiety attacks. She responded positively to the use of a small special thermometer taped to her finger that measured her skin temperature and gave her feedback during the initiation of the relaxation response.

A few weeks later, the oldest daughter brought into the therapy session, unbeknownst to her mother, a large mercurial oral thermometer so that she could learn relaxation techniques "just like her mother." The daughter proved an excellent candidate for relaxation techniques and also opted to try some visualization techniques. During an exercise in which she visualized going up a flight of stairs, she was encouraged to feel herself getting lighter and lighter with each step. She was then instructed to visualize a favorite place and see, smell, feel, and hear all the sensory stimuli she usually experienced in that place. As she responded to the directions, she appeared very calm and passive while lying on the couch with the large thermometer taped to her finger. Then, tears slowly rolled down her cheeks.

After her return to a more alert state, she described seeing a pasture and fence, hearing bees buzzing around her, feeling the hot sun on her skin, and spotting "Lightning." Lightning was a favorite horse briefly mentioned many months earlier on the first anniversary of the horse's death. She continued in a very open and poignant way, sharing her grief and sadness, and she told of the nightly crying spells she had had over the loss of her companion. The experience appeared to be a turning point in the therapeutic alliance with me. Her ability to describe the significance of the loss, grieve the loss, and share this experience served as a positive model when a favored clergyman died. It also helped her understand a frightening experience she had had of seeing her uncle lose control and punch his fist into a wall after the loss of his mother.

Thus, through continued family treatment, positive changes were made over time. Many nurses are functioning effectively in private practice and are thought of highly by other health professionals, as well as their clients.

CHAPTER 15

PSYCHOPHYSIOLOGICAL DISORDERS

Ardis R. Swanson

OUTLINE

KEY TERMS AND CONCEPTS

The key terms and concepts listed here also appear in bold where they are defined or discussed in this chapter.

PSYCHOSOMATIC

PSYCHOPHYSIOLOGICAL

PSYCHOGENIC

FIGHT OR FLIGHT RESPONSE (Sympathetic Response)

RELAXATION RESPONSE (Parasympathetic Response)

GENERAL ADAPTATION SYNDROME (GAS)

TYPE A PERSONALITY

SOMATIZING

PRIMARY GAIN

SECONDARY GAIN

OBJECTIVES

After studying this chapter, the student will be able to:

1. Discuss the difference between psychosomatic and psychophysiological.
2. List nine internal and external factors that may contribute to a psychophysiological disorder.
3. Discuss the body's physiological response to stress as it relates to the autonomic nervous system (fight or flight response) and the general adaptation syndrome (GAS).
4. Explain the roles that biological influences (autoimmune, genetic), personality traits, and environmental influences play in the disease process.
5. Discuss the importance of assessing each of the following in a person with a psychophysiological disorder:
   A. Levels of anxiety.
   B. Sources of stress—internal and external.
   C. Resources for dealing with stress—internal and external.
   D. Presence of secondary gains.
6. Identify two long term and two short term goals that would be appropriate for most persons with a psychophysiological disorder.
7. Name four client behaviors that elicit unhelpful responses in nurses. Give an intervention for each.
8. Summarize four important therapeutic approaches a nurse can use when working with a client with a psychophysiological disorder.
9. Compare and contrast four treatment modalities that have proved effective in a person with a psychophysiological disorder.
10. Name two classifications of drugs that may be used with any number of psychophysiological disorders.

It has long been recognized that psychological and sociocultural stresses play a role in the predisposition, onset, course, and response to treatment of certain medical illnesses (Thompson 1988). It is also true that physiological stresses can affect mental functioning. In 1952 the American Psychiatric Association used the term **psychosomatic** in the DSM I to identify specific body system diseases (e.g., peptic ulcers, asthma, rheumatoid arthritis) thought to be caused by psychological factors. The term psychosomatic describes the interaction of the *mind* (*psyche*) and the *body* (*soma*). In 1968, the term **psychophysiological** (DSM II) was adopted. **Psychophysiological** referred to all physical symptoms in which psychic elements played a significant role in initiating or maintaining chemical, physiological, or structural alterations responsible for the client's complaint. The DSM III (1980) and the DSM III-R (1987) now refer to physical conditions affected by psychological factors as those disorders that are to some extent **psychogenic,** that is, psychologically induced or maintained, and places them on Axis III. Therefore, physical disorders with psychogenic components are "any physical conditions to which psychological factors are judged contributory" (DSM III-R 1987). Essentially,

1. The initiation or exacerbation of a specific physical condition or disorder can be related to specific stimuli that are psychologically meaningful to an individual (separation, death, loss of job).
2. There is actual organ pathology (e.g., ulcers) or a known pathophysiological process (e.g., migraine headache).
3. A somatoform disorder is ruled out (see Chapter 16).

Table 15–1 gives an example of a physical condition in which psychological factors are judged contributory, using the DSM III-R Axis System (refer to Chapter 1 for the DSM III-R Multiaxial System of Evaluation).

The list of conditions thought to have psychogenic components grows day by day, and changes in vocabulary reflect a field of knowledge that is still young and controversial. A partial list of disorders classified as having psychogenic components is found in Table 15–2.

In the earlier half of this century the specific disorders that were first classified as "psychosomatic" were ulcerative colitis, rheumatoid arthritis, hyperthyroidism, hypertension, peptic ulcer, bronchial asthma, and neurodermatitis. These are known as Alexander's Seven,

Table 15-1 • DSM III-R AXIS SYSTEM

CATEGORY	EXAMPLE
Axis I	
Clinical syndrome	None
Axis II	
Personality disorder or specific developmental disorder	Compulsive personality disorder
Axis III	
Physical disorders & conditions	Ulcerative colitis
Axis IV	
Severity of psychosocial stressors (scale 1-6)	Code 3—moderate marital separations
Axis V	
Global assessment of functioning (GAF)	Goal—minimal symptoms Current GAF—80 Highest GAF past year—88

after the clinician who studied these disorders and identified emotional components for each. Today, many more conditions are recognized as having psychogenic components. A modern text in this subject is likely to include such conditions as pain, menstrual disorder, insomnia, sexual dysfunction, obesity, and cancer. These disorders can be placed on the anxiety continuum (Fig. 15-1). The development of these disorders can be conceptualized as shown in Figure 15-2.

Standard I: Theory

EARLY MIND-BODY CONNECTIONS

In 1775 Franz Mesmer found he could modify or change the course of physical symptoms through "animal mag-

Table 15-2 • PARTIAL LIST OF PHYSICAL DISORDERS WITH PSYCHOGENIC COMPONENTS

BODY SYSTEM	DISORDERS
Gastrointestinal	Esophageal reflux/spasms, peptic ulcer, Crohn's disease, irritable bowel, colitis, chronic diarrhea, ulcerative colitis, nausea and vomiting, belching, heartburn, gastritis
Respiratory	Asthma
Circulatory	Palpitation, hypertension. cardiac arrhythmias, myocardial infarction, coronary artery disease
Neuromuscular-skeletal	Migraine, lower back pain, rheumatoid arthritis, chronic pain
Integumentary	Skin rashes, itching, pruritus, alopecia
Hormonal	Hypothyroidism, premenstrual syndrome (PMS), Addison's disease, Cushing's syndrome

Cancer, sexual dysfunction (Chapter 28), and eating disorders (Chapter 25) also are thought to have a strong psychological component.
Data from Kaplan, HI. Psychological factors affecting physical conditions (psychosomatic disorders). *In* Kaplan HI, Sadock BJ (eds). Comprehensive Textbook of Psychiatry, 4th ed. Baltimore: Williams & Wilkins, 1985.

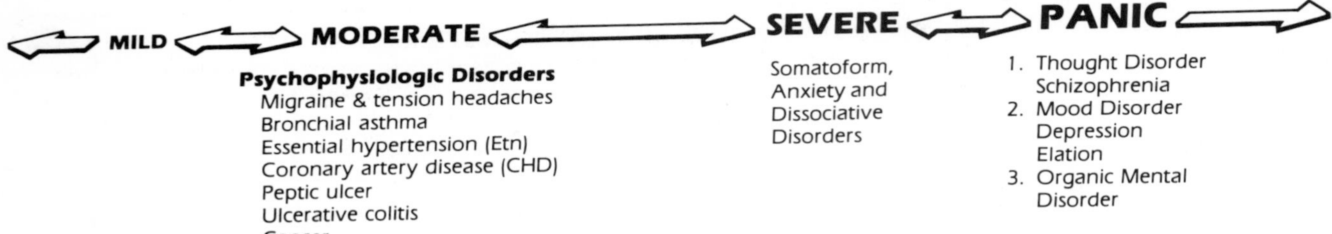

Figure 15–1. *The anxiety continuum and conditions recognized to have psychogenic components.*

netism." With the work of Jean Charcot (1880's), hypnosis gained medical acceptance (see Chapter 1). For example, Charcot demonstrated in people with conversion disorders (hysteria neurosis) the emergence and disappearance of physical symptoms through the use of hypnosis. Freud, very much influenced by Charcot, elaborated on unconscious processes influencing psychophysiological phenomena. Freud's work involving the psychodynamics of "conversion" symptoms (1894–1905) hypothesized that many physically expressed symptoms are defenses against "hidden impulses" (sexual + aggression) (Sheelan and Hackett 1980). Later the work of Pavlov, Cannon, and Selye would clarify the neurophysiological link between emotions and the physiological process.

EMOTIONS—STRESS AND PHYSIOLOGICAL RESPONSES

Walter Cannon emphasized that emotions can affect bodily changes. Emotions serve as energizers. For example, in response to fear or rage, the body prepares for flight or aggression **(fight or flight response).** Cannon, in 1932, identified stress as an actual cause of disorders. Emotional arousal triggers the **sympathetic branch of the autonomic nervous system** (fight or flight response), as well as the endocrine system.

Whereas behavioral responses to stress and anxiety are variously affected by age, sex, culture, and lifestyle, the physiological response is more predictable (Lesse 1982). The physiological response to stress is the same whether the stress is physical, psychological, or social. The fight or flight response may be useful in emergencies, but when this response is sustained, pathophysiological changes may ensue, for example, high blood pressure, ulcers, cancer, and cardiac problems (Luckmann and Sorensen 1987).

The opposite of the fight or flight response is the **relaxation response** identified by Herbert Benson (1975). The relaxation response is synonymous with the functioning of the **parasympathetic branch of the nervous system.** The relaxation response has a stabilizing effect on the nervous system and that is directly opposite the disordering effects of the fight or flight response (Aron and Aron 1980).

The objective, behavioral, and subjective experiences of the fight or flight response and the relaxation response are compared in Table 15–3.

In 1936, Hans Selye further demonstrated the body's organized response to stress. His focus was more on the pituitary adrenocortical system's response to stress and the role of adrenocorticotropic hormones (ACTH) as the mediators (Sheelan and Hackett 1980). He called his theory the **general adaptation syndrome (GAS).** The GAS progresses through three stages: (1) stage of alarm, (2) stage of resistance, (3) stage of exhaustion.

The *alarm stage* is the immediate life-preserving reaction of the sympathetic branch of the autonomic nervous system. During this stage, the fight or flight

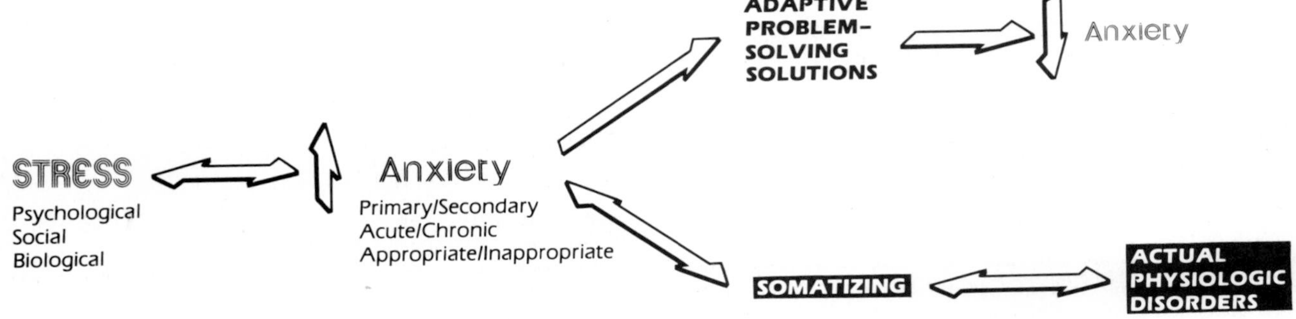

Figure 15–2. *Conceptualization of the process of psychophysiological disorders.*

Table 15–3 • FIGHT OR FLIGHT RESPONSE VERSUS THE RELAXATION RESPONSE

FIGHT OR FLIGHT RESPONSE (Sympathetic Branch—Epinephrine/Norepinephrine)	RELAXATION RESPONSE (Parasympathetic Branch—Acetylcholine)
Objective Findings	
1. Increased heart rate	1. Decreased heart rate
2. Increased blood pressure	2. Decreased blood pressure
3. Increase in O_2 consumption	3. Decrease in O_2 consumption
4. Peripheral vasoconstriction	4. Peripheral vasodilation
5. Sweat gland stimulated (hands, feet, axillae)	5. None
6. Pupils dilate	6. Pupils normal or constricted
7. No release of endorphins	7. Increase in endorphin levels (body's natural opiate)
8. Minimal or absent slow alpha waves on electroencephalogram (EEG); no theta waves	8. Increase in slow alpha and theta waves on EEG (associated with feelings of well-being)
9. Increase in blood lactate levels (associated with high anxiety)	9. Decrease in blood lactate levels (associated with lowered anxiety)
10. Increase in blood glucose, free fatty acid, and cholesterol levels	10. Sufficient blood glucose, free fatty acid, and cholesterol levels for normal body functioning
Some Behavioral Manifestations	
Frequent urination, restlessness, sleeplessness, hostility, motor incoordination, repetitive questioning, disorganized speech, scattered thoughts	Comfortable posture, speech clear, thinking process intact, behavior effective and purposeful
Some Subjective States	
Tense, fearful, frustrated, difficulty concentrating, "pressured," shaky, jittery, confused, wanting to flee, butterflies in stomach, nausea, irritable, depressed, pounding heart	Increased sense of well-being, greater ability to cope with stress, refreshed, more energy, increased concentration

Adapted from Benson 1975; Gellhorn and Kiely 1972; Snyder 1977; Varcarolis 1984.

response is activated, increasing secretions of epinephrine and norepinephrine.

The *resistance stage* occurs when the body adapts through changes in the adrenocortical response in order to sustain the body's fight for preservation. If the person then adapts psychologically, physiologically, or behaviorally or the stressors have diminished, the body returns to normal. However, if the biological, social, or psychological stressors continue unrelieved over a period of time, a stage of exhaustion is reached.

When a person's physical, emotional, and social resources are depleted (*stage of exhaustion*), physical or emotional disorders will ensue, even to the point of death. Refer to Table 15–4 for the physical and psychological changes during each stage of the general adaptation syndrome (GAS).

PSYCHOLOGICAL CONTRIBUTORS

Flanders Dunbar in 1947, was the first to propose specific personality profiles for specific organic diseases. It was during this time that psychosomatic medicine became a distinct branch of medicine.

Franz Alexander (1948), like Freud and others, believed that unconscious neurotic conflict could result in specific organ disease. As mentioned, Alexander's Seven included ulcerative colitis, rheumatoid arthritis, hyperthyroidism, neurodermatitis, hypertension, peptic ulcer, and asthma.

Some studies have indicated that people with profound unmet yearnings for affection and strong needs to be dependent on others are candidates for peptic ulcers. However, a person's outward behaviors often obscure these conflicts with a facade of energetic self-sufficiency and a drive to succeed in social and vocational activities (Chapman 1976). Other studies using a different socioeconomic population found many people with ulcers were not ambitious and independent-acting, and many were even overly dependent and regressed (Oken 1985).

Presently, however, it is recognized that peptic ulcers represent a group of disorders with different subgroups demonstrating different physiological and genetic

Table 15–4 • THE GENERAL ADAPTATION SYNDROME

STAGE	PHYSICAL CHANGE	PSYCHOLOGICAL CHANGE
Stage I: **Alarm Reaction** (mobilization of the body's defense forces and activation of the fight or flight mechanism)	Release of norepinephrine and epinephrine, causing vasoconstriction, increased blood pressure, and increased rate and force of cardiac contraction Increased hormone levels Enlargement of adrenal cortex Marked loss of body weight Shrinkage of the thymus, spleen, and lymph nodes Irritation of the gastric mucosa	Increased level of alertness Increased level of anxiety Task-oriented, defense-oriented, inefficient, or maladaptive behavior may occur
Stage II: **Stage of Resistance** (optimal adaptation to stress within the person's capabilities)	Hormone levels readjust Reduction in activity and size of adrenal cortex Lymph glands return to normal size Weight returns to normal	Increased and intensified use of coping mechanisms Tendency to rely on defense-oriented behavior
Stage III: **Stage of Exhaustion** (loss of ability to resist stress because of depletion of body resources)	Decreased immune response with suppression of T cells and atrophy of thymus Depletion of adrenal glands and hormone production Weight loss Enlargement of the lymph nodes and dysfunction of lymphatic system If exposure to the stressor continues, cardiac failure, renal failure, or death may occur	Defense-oriented behaviors become exaggerated Disorganization of thinking Disorganization of personality Sensory stimuli may be misperceived with appearance of illusion Reality contact may be reduced with appearance of delusions or hallucinations If exposure to the stressor continues, stupor or violence may occur

Kneisl CR, Ames SW. Adult Health Nursing: A Biopsychosocial Approach. Menlo Park, CA: Addison-Wesley Publishing Company, 1986, p. 20.

characteristics (Oken 1985). A more recent study hypothesizes that some individuals are genetically more prone to developing ulcers than are others. An inherited autosomal recessive trait has been linked with elevated levels of pepsinogen (Oken 1985).

There is no doubt, however, that emotions can stimulate gastric secretions (as well as other functions) and that psychological factors associated with emotional arousal can increase gastric functioning.

Studies indicate that people experience ulcers in times of anxiety associated with social tension and upheaval and increased life stress. Generally, studies associating psychological conflicts and personality disorders with peptic ulcers or any other psychophysiological disorder are conflicting and inconclusive, and some appear to have flaws in methodology. For example, some studies include only men, high socioeconomic samples, low socioeconomic samples, whites, blacks, and other skewed populations. Other studies may include too few subjects or subjects from one geographic region, making generalization impossible.

Since Alexander's Seven, the list of psychophysiological disorders has expanded (see Table 15–2) and so has interest in identifying personality traits and unconscious conflicts that may be contributing factors. One of the most widely received personality correlates was that of the **type A personality** proposed by Friedman and Rosenman (circa 1969). By 1978, type A behavior was officially recognized as an independent risk factor for heart disease by a National Institutes of Health panel. Type A's were essentially viewed as hostile, hurried, competitive, and driven. Now it seems that more recent studies are failing to find a correlation between type A and heart disease (Fischman 1987). Some researchers are now examining certain components of the type A personality, such as hostility, to correlate with coronary heart disease (Wood 1986). For example, some studies indicate that people who are hostile have a higher rate of coronary heart disease than people who are not hostile (Fischman 1987). Now even Rosenman states: "Type A behavior is not an illness . . . only type A's who are truly coronary prone should be treated" (Fischman 1987). Table 15–5 identifies personality traits, genetic and biological correlates, and stress-related findings of some common physical dis-

Table 15–5 • ETIOLOGIC CONSIDERATIONS FOR SOME PSYCHOPHYSIOLOGICAL DISORDERS

ASSOCIATED PERSONALITY TRAITS	INCIDENCE	GENETIC & BIOLOGICAL CORRELATES	COMMON PRECIPITATING FACTORS	USEFUL THERAPIES OTHER THAN MEDICAL MANAGEMENT
Migraine—Vascular Headaches				
Obsessive personalities, overly controlled, perfectionistic, suppress anger	15–20% men, 20–30% women between puberty and menopause Begins in mornings or on weekends Lasts a few hours to a few days	Two thirds have family history	Can be brought on by foods (e.g., monosodium glutamate, tyramine, chocolate), fluctuating levels of estrogen Often in unilateral, temporal, or frontal areas. May include prodromata (nausea, vomiting, photophobia)	Prodromal stage treated most effectively with ergotamine or analgesics
Tension Headache—Muscular Contractions				
People with type A characteristics, such as being tense, high-strung, or competitive, are especially prone to these headaches	Occur in 80% of population when under stress Begins end of work day or early evening		Anxiety and depression are associated with these headaches Begins suboccipitally; usually bilateral	Psychotherapy usual prescription for chronic tension headaches Learning to cope or avoiding tension-creating situations or people Relaxation techniques helpful for some
Respiratory—Bronchial Asthma				
No one personality type identified Some asthmatic children have poor impulse control, are babyish, are overly polite, and are emotionally explosive; boys—passively dependent, timid, immature; girls—try to be self-sufficient, often are chronically depressed	Usually occurs in younger children Usually occurs in people 40 and over	**Extrinsic**—usually in 30–50% of younger children, immunoglobin E (IgE) type antibody formation to specific antibodies as a predisposition 1. Runs in families 2. Occurrence is seasonal 3. Allergens play a part **Intrinsic**—often marked by sensitivity to drugs, intense emotions, exercise, or weather changes	Social/Environmental—actual or anticipated separation or loss in about 50% of attacks in all ages Often follows a viral infection of the lungs	Children—removal from home can radically alter attacks in some children Others—need for steroids is lessened when removed from home environment Others—have attacks in home environment only, not in schools, for example

Table continued on following page

Table 15-5 • ETIOLOGIC CONSIDERATIONS FOR SOME PSYCHOPHYSIOLOGICAL DISORDERS *Continued*

ASSOCIATED PERSONALITY TRAITS	INCIDENCE	GENETIC & BIOLOGICAL CORRELATES	COMMON PRECIPITATING FACTORS	USEFUL THERAPIES OTHER THAN MEDICAL MANAGEMENT
Cardiovascular—Essential Hypertension (ETN)*				
Anecdotal Accounts—compliant and congenial, longs for approval, superficially easygoing, suppresses rage and suspicion	Higher in males until age 60	Family history of cardiac disease and hypertension	Life changes & traumatic life events Related to stressful jobs, e.g., air traffic controller Hypothesized to be found more in areas of social stress and conflict	Behavioral—biofeedback, stress reduction techniques, meditation, yoga, hypnosis. However, *pharmacological treatment is considered primary*
Cardiovascular—Coronary Heart Disease (CHD)*				
Type A personalities Time Urgency—difficulty doing nothing, always on time, harried Excessive Competitiveness and Hostility—always plays to win, general distrust of others' motives (e.g., altruism), irritation, authoritarian	Higher in males until age 60 Higher in white population than in black population	Family history of cardiac disease is a risk factor Other Risk Factors—HBP, increased serum lipids, obesity, sedentary lifestyle, cigarette smoking	Often myocardial infarction (MI) occurs after sudden stress preceded by a period of losses, frustration, and disappointments	Progressive relaxation, autohypnosis, meditation, biofeedback; behavior modification; support groups for type A personalities; prescribed program of physical exercise (prophylaxis against post MI depression) When indicated—anxiolytics (benzodiazepines), antidepressants
Gastrointestinal—Peptic Ulcer				
Ambitious, independent Regressive, overly dependent Inconclusive—not supportive of male findings	12% men, 6% women (More prevalent in "civilized" society)	Elevated pepsinogen level identified as an autosomal recessive trait Both peptic ulcers & duodenal ulcers cluster in families, but separately from each other	Periods of social tension; increased life stress After losses—often after menopause	Biofeedback can alter gastric acidity; behavioral approaches are used to reduce stress
Gastrointestinal—Ulcerative Colitis				
Compulsive personality traits; neatness, orderliness, cleanliness; punctuality; hyperintellectualism; obstinancy; humorlessness;	Occurs equally in men and women Develops in second and third decades of life and around age 50	Possible autoimmune response Runs in families; no genetic markers found	Centered on losses, especially key relationships Narcissistic Loss—thinks has failed, feels hurt or humiliated, unable	Psychotherapy—issues of separation, loss, rejection, dependency

Table 15-5 • ETIOLOGIC CONSIDERATIONS FOR SOME PSYCHOPHYSIOLOGICAL DISORDERS *Continued*

ASSOCIATED PERSONALITY TRAITS	INCIDENCE	GENETIC & BIOLOGICAL CORRELATES	COMMON PRECIPITATING FACTORS	USEFUL THERAPIES OTHER THAN MEDICAL MANAGEMENT
		Gastrointestinal—Ulcerative Colitis *(Continued)*		
timidity; inhibition of feelings (especially anger); very sensitive to real or imagined hurts	High in Jewish population Higher in whites than in blacks		to please others he or she depends on	
		Cancer		
Suppression of emotions, e.g., anger; easy to please and unaggressive; stoic, self-sacrificing; inhibited; self-effacement; rigid; may appear strong, puts others' needs in front of own, conscientious	Men—most common in lung, prostate, colon/rectum Women—most common in breast, uterus, colon/rectum Death rates higher in males (especially black males) than in women	Genetic evidence suggests dysfunction of cellular profusion Familial Patterns—breast cancer, colorectal cancer, ovarian cancer, stomach cancer, melanoma	Prolonged and intensive stress Stressful life events, e.g., separation from or loss of significant other 2 years before diagnosis Feelings of helplessness, hopelessness, and despair (depression) may precede diagnosis of cancer	Relaxation, e.g., meditation, autogenic training, self-hypnosis Visualization Psychological counseling

* Hypertension (ETN) and coronary disease (CHD) are the primary causes of death in the United States.
Data from Kaplan HI, Sadock BJ (eds). Comprehensive Textbook of Psychiatry, 4th ed. Baltimore: Williams & Wilkins, 1985, and Kneisl CK, Ames SW (eds). Adult Health Nursing: A Biopsychosocial Approach. Menlo Park, CA: Addison-Wesley Publishing Company, 1986.

orders with psychogenic components. The psychophysiological disorders examined are those disorders nurses are most likely to encounter in the hospital or clinical settings. Other disorders that have strong psychogenic correlates include the eating disorders (anorexia, bulimia, obesity), which are discussed in Chapter 25, and psychogenic pain, which is discussed in Chapter 26.

BIOLOGICAL INFLUENCES ON PSYCHOPHYSIOLOGICAL DISORDERS

FACTORS THAT AFFECT IMMUNE RESPONSE. Autoimmune diseases result when a person's immunological system attacks its own normal cellular components. Three psychophysiological disorders thought to have autoimmune involvement include ulcerative colitis, rheumatoid arthritis, and gastritis (Ames and Kneisl 1986). Other studies link psychosocial stress with immune dysfunction (Achterberg et al. 1976; Stein et al. 1985). Psychological stress by way of the general adaptation syndrome (GAS) can lead to overproduction of cortisone and depression in the immune system, leaving a person more vulnerable to cancer. Many studies have been done and are as yet inconclusive; however, severe emotional factors thought to be associated with cancer have been identified (e.g., powerlessness, anxiety, loss of a significant other, and frustration).

GENETIC FACTORS. Influences of genetic transmission of specific diseases are as yet unclear, although certain relationships have been found to exist. Knapp (1985) states that there does seem to be a genetic overlap between some disease groups (ulcerative colitis, some forms of arthritis, and Crohn's disease). Also, asthma, hay fever, neurodermatitis, and some forms of urticaria occur in family clusters.

One way of looking at the influence of genetic factors is that although a specific factor might exist, manifestation of a physiological disease may depend upon a variety of personal or environmental conditions (e.g., coping styles, family interactions, and social conditions).

THE NONSPECIFIC HYPOTHESIS

This theory states that there are four varieties of reactions to stress (Kaplan 1985):

1. *Healthy-Normal*: Anxiety is followed by an effective action or defense mechanism.
2. *Neurotic*: Alert signal of anxiety is so great that ego defenses fail.
3. *Psychotic*: Anxiety may be misperceived or ignored.
4. *Psychophysiological*: Ego defenses become ineffective, and anxiety is translated into somatic systems, causing changes in body structure.

Figure 15–3 conceptualizes this model.

It appears that there is, as yet, no one etiological factor in the development of a psychophysiological disorder. It is a fact that environmental, interpersonal, and psychological stress play a large part in the occurrence or maintenance of many physical disorders. How a person responds to stress emotionally (personality traits) can be an important factor. A person's genetic and biological predisposition, constitutional strengths, and physiological response to stress are other important factors.

Standard II: Data Collection

Nurses function with and without the availability of medical diagnostic services. When a medical diagnosis is available—often the case in a hospital setting—it provides the nurse with some clues for making a ***nursing*** assessment. For example, a provisional diagnosis of psychogenic pain will alert the nurse to be observant for possible stressors in the client's life, as well as to observe carefully the person's present experience of pain. Whatever the situation, nurses are responsible for using their own knowledge and skill to establish a relationship wherein a nursing assessment can be made.

How does one go about establishing a relationship that is conducive to obtaining relevant data for making a nursing diagnosis with a person who has a psychophysiological disorder?

The nurse who has considerable self-knowledge and acceptance of self is more free to be comfortable, aware, perceptive, and nonjudgmental of another. This nurse is more able to be attentive. In that attention the nurse focuses on communication—both verbal and nonverbal. The relationship established by the nurse who exhibits these characteristics carries the potential of facilitating change in another. Although these are general statements applicable to all nurse-patient relationships, they are highly relevant to persons who have physical symptoms related to psychological factors.

The nurse acknowledges that the client is experienc-

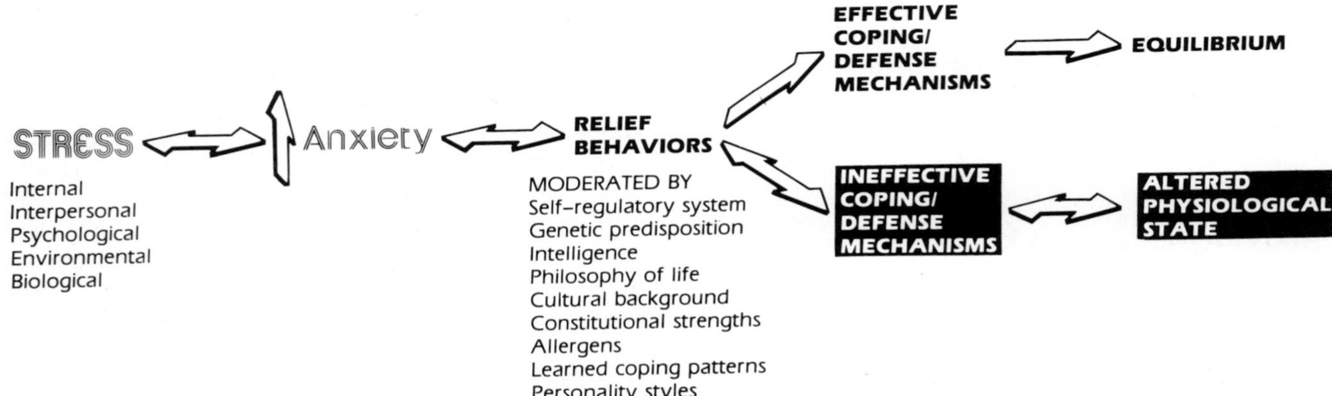

Figure 15–3. *Nonspecific stress response.*

ing physical alterations or very genuine discomforts. It is best to begin data gathering with what the client wishes to tell you, without responding with interpretations or judgments. The person's perception of his or her illness is usually described entirely in physical terms, possibly without any reference to stressors or anxiety or what they fear is about to come. The nurse listens to the overt statements and, with a "third ear," listens for the less obvious or covert information, including the stressors and anxieties in the life of the person. The nurse assesses (1) levels of anxiety, (2) sources of stress, (3) resources for dealing with stress, and (4) the presence of secondary gains.

ASSESSING LEVELS OF ANXIETY

Anxiety does not manifest itself overtly in most psychophysiological conditions. It is mostly disguised or transformed into physical symptoms by somatizing. **Somatizing** is the conversion of emotional feelings or experiences into physical symptoms when direct expression of such feelings or experiences is blocked. Therefore, anxiety may not be easily recognized initially. The nurse is alert for signs of it nevertheless. See Chapter 8 for a discussion on manifestations and levels of anxiety.

Many clients with a psychophysiological disorder will deny the role of anxiety, fear, or anger as a stimulus for their physical symptoms. However, physical symptoms betraying the existence of anxiety may be more readily acknowledged, e.g., tension, insomnia, anorexia, fatigue, nightmares, or sexual disturbances (MacKinnon and Michels 1971). When a client acknowledges such symptoms, the nurse might ask questions such as:

- What kinds of situations make you tense?
- When do you experience the most fatigue?
- When do your nightmares seem to occur?
- When did you start having difficulty sleeping? Not feeling hungry?

The nurse can also be alert for specific physiological or motor clues that might signal the presence of anxiety. For example, a client may appear restless, perspire, blush, or repeat the same statement or question.

The nurse can help the person by subtly diverting the focus from the person's somatic symptoms to the circumstances of the person's present and recent life. The initial perception of the person's illness is noteworthy, and an expanding awareness of his or her present experience may be a step toward change.

When a behavior is noticed that suggests anxiety, the nurse can bring it into the client's awareness. This may help the client acknowledge the link between anxiety and health, and eventually to find a more effective way to deal with certain stressors that evoke the anxiety. A sample dialogue follows:

NURSE: I notice that as we talk you are shifting about in your chair a great deal. Are you feeling anxious?
CLIENT A: No. This is not a comfortable chair.

The nurse does not challenge but will be alert to other signs and will speak of them in a manner similar to that previously illustrated. Alternatively, if the client acknowledges the anxiety, the nurse invites speculation as to what the anxiety might be about. For example, after the nurse's observation as above:

CLIENT B: Oh? I don't think so. Well, maybe a little.
NURSE: Do you have any idea what you might be anxious about?

The nurse is aware that "acute" episodes of anxiety do occur; anxiety fluctuates. An acute episode, such as a severe asthmatic "attack," is viewed as a medical emergency. Life-threatening situations are typically accompanied by very high anxiety. An acute episode of a psychophysiological disorder may occur when there is a threat to survival. It is imperative at those times that emergency medical and nursing measures be taken. When life sustenance is threatened, immediate *action* is the only appropriate response.

ASSESSING SOURCES OF STRESS

A full assessment requires identifying possible sources of stress in the person's life. Sources of stress fall into two broad categories based on whether the stress comes from within (*internal*) or is *external* to the individual. For example, internal stressors include direct physical stress, such as infections, or psychological stress, such as conflicts regarding dependency or powerlessness. External stressors include both interpersonal and socioeconomic conditions. Interpersonal factors that may be sources of stress include marriage, loss of a loved one, incompatibilities at work, and many others. Socioeconomic factors that may be sources of stress include inadequate housing, high noise level at place of work, or language barriers. A partial list of internal and external stressors is provided in Table 15–6. These categories are somewhat arbitrary in that one event may evoke stress and anxiety in more than one area. For example, poor housing is a socioeconomic matter but at the same time is likely to be an interpersonal stressor as well. The actual source is not as important as how the event is perceived by the individual. The table is intended to provide the reader with an overview of differ-

Table 15–6 • STRESSORS: SOURCES AND EXAMPLES

SOURCES	EXAMPLES
Internal Stressors	
Physical	Overexertion or other imposed strains on body system; infections or allergens; physical trauma, e.g., surgery, accident; nutritional deficiency
Psychological	
Intrapsychic conflict	Feeling angry while fearing the consequences of expressing it
Perception of threat from events	Observing an angry person; illness of a loved one
Feelings of inadequacy, dependency, helplessness, powerlessness	Belief that life is impossible without the help and love of a significant other
Boredom	Isolated from friends and/or gratifying life experiences
External Stressors	
Conflictual relations	Marital conflict; incompatibility at work
Loss of relationship	Death of a loved one
Inability to relate, or so perceived	Language barrier
Socioeconomic	
Economic inadequacies	Unemployment, poor diet, poor housing, little recreation
Climatic extremes	Rain, clouds, little sun
Noxious stimuli	Noise, odors
Sensory deprivation	Isolation from things, people
Political climate	Repressive social system
Ethnic, religious, or national difference	Prejudice based on nationality, race, or creed

ent events, any one of which could be relevant data for making the nursing assessment.

Some questions that might help the client and the nurse identify particular sources of stress, if not already obvious (e.g., divorce, death, loss of job), might include

- Tell me about a typical day.
- Describe the events of the last week before the symptoms started.
- What do you like least about your job? What do you like most about it?
- What is one thing you would like to change about your job, home, relationship?
- What kinds of situations upset you the most?
- What do you think would make life better for you?

It has been proposed that what causes the most stress is the amount of change that an event requires of a person. Two researchers, Holmes and Masuda, have developed a list of life events that require the person experiencing the event to change (see Chapter 10, Figure 10–1, for a list of life events). They have established a point system for how much stress a person experiences with each event. The list acts as a tool for measuring the amount of change required of a person in recent months. The tool has been used extensively as a way of indicating the amount of stress a person is experiencing.

ASSESSING RESOURCES FOR DEALING WITH STRESS

Essentially people rely on the following aids in handling stress: (1) internal resources (self-regulation and ego defenses) and (2) external resources (environmental supports).

Internal Resources—Self-Regulation and Ego Defenses

Mild to moderate anxiety is remarkably purposeful and self-regulatory. Even ordinary experiences in life set into motion subsystems to protect the human being and to equip the person for similar events in the future. Individuals may have countless experiences from infancy on, through which they acquire "habits" of a sort —habitual physiological responses and psychological ways of coping. For example, the thought of a quiz may set into motion an interactive process between the perceptual and autonomic nervous systems such that the person is alert, with muscles in readiness for fight or flight. Drawing upon multiple past experiences of the same sort, a student may learn ways to deal directly and effectively with the encounter, forming a study group or attending review sessions. Or, the person may develop a less effective *flight* response for dealing with the stress of the exam, such as using an ego-defense mechanism, rationalizing "there is no way to study this stuff" or developing a physical symptom that detracts from the threat and provides some artificial security, e.g., "I had such a headache, I couldn't possibly study." Subsequently, these types of responses may be triggered in that person in future situations requiring preparation for achievement. Therefore, in this example, the stress (exam) triggers initially a *physiological response* (autonomic nervous system or fight or flight response). Depending upon the person's physiological and psychological learning experiences and defense mechanisms, usual coping patterns are put into play.

To cope is to struggle or contend, with some degree of success. On the surface, a physical symptom does not look like success. But underneath, psychophysiological responses are ways of struggling and contending with an adverse condition and with success of a sort. Some ways of coping with stresses are more socially acceptable than others. For example, to many Americans, coping with economic hardship by working two jobs is acceptable, but coping with economic hardship by getting ill and having to go on public assistance is not. Still, becoming ill is a kind of solution. If the person could succeed by alternatives, however, he or she might surely choose one of them. The problem is that these procedures are not within the conscious awareness, choice, and control.

Other internal resources for dealing with stress effectively include genetic endowments such as intelligence and constitutional strengths, acquired resources for coping such as knowledge and skills that equip a person for gainful employment, and a developed philosophy of life—perhaps from a satisfying religious orientation.

Less effective "resources" are the use or overuse of unproductive defense mechanisms or somatic symptoms. Some defense mechanisms go hand-in-hand with somatic symptoms (e.g., denial, a primitive defense in which unpleasant realities or internal perceptions of a painful nature are disavowed).

Some questions that can help the nurse and the client identify physical and emotional coping patterns include

- What is your usual emotional reaction to stressful situations?
- What do you do that helps relieve feelings of stress or anxiety?
- Do you notice any physical reactions you have when you are feeling stress (e.g., headache, stomach ache, palpitations, back ache)?
- How much alcohol do you ingest per day?
- What medications or drugs do you take to relieve stress (e.g., marijuana, Valium, cocaine, others)? How often? How much?
- How many cigarettes do you smoke a day?
- Does your work often interfere with social and leisure activities?
- What do you think would help make your life better?
- What kinds of things in life give you the most pleasure?
- What do you like most about yourself?
- What would you like to change?

External Resources—Environmental Supports

Just as there are internal resources to help deal with stress, so are there external resources to deal with stress.

External resources include agencies and personal social networks. These resources vary in the support they provide according to the state of the home and community. Potentially there are many supports in the home and community. Human beings require first and foremost that their basic needs for survival be met. The most basic need in life is a home in which survival needs can be met, where safety exists and a sense of security can develop. Educational opportunity and employment availability are important. Agencies in society that are potentially supportive include health facilities and protective services. The absence or lack of quality of these agencies can add stress. High-quality community agencies can alleviate stress and promote healthy development for families and individuals.

External human resources for a person are referred to as a person's "social support" system. The mere presence of a family and many other people in one's life does not necessarily mean support. The nature of these human systems and the kind of relationship that exists with them determine the quality of the support.

As is well known, families vary from supportive to abusive. There is evidence that the way a family functions internally has much to do with the health and illness of its members. Salvadore Minuchin, family theorist and practitioner, in working with many families in which a member had a psychophysiological disorder, noted an association between a particular family structure and psychophysiological illness. He calls the families "psychosomatic." The family factors for the development of psychophysiological disorders in children Minuchin has conceptualized as (1) enmeshed, by which he means an overcloseness of the members, (2) overprotective, (3) rigid, by which he means resistant to change, (4) overinvolved with the child, and (5) experiencing a high degree of family conflict. (Refer to Chapter 25 for Minuchin's theory as it relates to people with eating disorders.)

Nurse researchers Baillie, Norbeck, and Barnes (1988) have devised an instrument for measuring social support. The questionnaire asks first for a listing of the "important" persons in the life of the person answering the questionnaire. The list may include family members, relatives, friends, work or school associates, neighbors, health providers, counselors, minister/rabbi/priest, and others. Second, nine questions are asked about each person on the list. For example, the first question is, "How much does this person make you feel liked or loved?"; the sixth question is, "If you were confined to bed for several weeks, how much could this person help you?" The developed instrument is being used quite extensively where social support is a concept of interest. Although its use is mainly in nursing research, the questions offer relevant suggestions for the nurse clinician assessing a client's social support system. Research reports using this instrument are beginning to show the role of social support in preventing illness and in promoting health.

Questions that may help to identify a person's social support system include

- Who are the people you consider most important in your life?
- Whom do you talk to when you are upset?
- Whom do you trust?
- How many close friends do you have?
- Do you have important relationships from any outside activities (e.g., church, community organizations, work)?
- How would you describe your relationships with others?
- How much time do you spend alone? When?
- How much time do you spend with others? When?

ASSESSING THE PRESENCE OF SECONDARY GAINS

The primary reason a person employs defense mechanisms or relief behaviors is to reduce anxiety. Primary gain refers to a person's efforts to cope with a conflicting or anxiety-producing situation, thought, or relationship. Therefore, the **primary gain** refers to the use of a symptom in order to decrease anxiety. The symptom may be physical or emotional unconsciously employed initially and primarily to reduce anxiety. A **secondary gain** refers to those advantages a person realizes from whatever symptoms or relief behaviors he or she employs. Secondary gains usually provide

- increased attention from others,
- a way of getting out of expected responsibilities and chores, and
- a means of manipulating others in the environment.

The more satisfying and rewarding the secondary gains become, the more difficult it is for a person to give up maladaptive physical and emotional symptoms or relief behavior.

Secondary gains usually play a part in all mental disorders (e.g., depression, the "neurotic" disorders [anxiety, somatization, dissociative diseases], and others). Nurses need to be aware of the secondary gains a person is receiving. Much of a nurse's intervention strategy is aimed at minimizing secondary gains and working with clients to get their needs met in more appropriate and satisfying ways (see Chapter 16).

To illustrate, a hospitalized client with a psychophysiological disorder may act passively, taking little responsibility for self-care. The nursing staff would then try to minimize the secondary gains from this behavior by (1) minimizing the attention the client gets through his symptoms, (2) refraining from performing self-care responsibilities that the client is able to do, and (3) reducing the manipulation of the staff's time and skills. The staff might decide to decrease the secondary gains by giving the client recognition when he does things for himself and rewarding him with short periods of socialization. Questions the nurse might ask that may elicit the presence of secondary gains are

- What would you be doing if you were well that you are not able to do right now?
- How has this illness changed your usual level of functioning?
- How does this illness affect your husband/wife/children/friends?

Standard III: Diagnosis

Nursing diagnosis for a person with a psychophysiological disorder may initially focus on physical concerns that require immediate skilled nursing care. For example, a person just admitted with ulcerative colitis may initially require a nursing diagnosis of *diarrhea* related to inflammation, or *fluid volume deficit* related to diarrhea. A person who is admitted in staticus asthmaticus would warrant a nursing diagnosis of *impaired gas exchange* related to loss of lung elasticity (e.g., bronchospasms).

Psychophysiological disorders can be life-threatening and do involve actual organ changes. Often when people are admitted to a hospital unit with a disorder classified as psychophysiological, medical and skilled nursing care take priority in stabilizing a life-threatening condition. Therefore, nursing interventions in collaboration with medical treatment may take initial priority.

Since the psychophysiological disorder does have a psychological component, more than just the physical disorder is involved. It is not uncommon to note that some clients have a history of failure to follow treatment regimes when it comes to their physical health. Therefore, *altered health maintenance* related to inadequate health practices or poor self-esteem may be appropriate. The following discussion will deal with the nursing diagnoses that focus on the psychological component of the psychophysiological disorder.

Most people believe that a person with a psychophysiological disorder is often unaware of the presence of distressing conflicts and disturbing feelings. Instead there is a tendency to somatize feelings. These conflicts and the resulting anxiety are thought to be "acted out" through "organ language." Therefore, *moderate or severe anxiety* related to unconscious conflict is almost always present.

Since there may not be an awareness of personal feelings, the ability to communicate feelings and thoughts to others is diminished. Often it is through talking with others and trusting others with painful emotions that viable alternatives for stressful situations and feelings can be found. Therefore, *impaired verbal communication* related to psychological barriers (e.g., fear) may be appropriate.

A person with a psychophysiological disorder may have limited coping skills when dealing with anxiety. Somatizing may be a major defense used. Therefore, whenever the person encounters a stressful situation or conflict, the distress is evidenced in the "organ language" of the client, for example, in the respiratory system or the gastrointestinal system. The nurse may find that *ineffective individual coping* related to inadequate psychological resources (e.g., helplessness, poor self-esteem) is appropriate.

These are a small sample of some of the nursing diagnoses that the nurse would consider when working with a patient with a psychophysiological disorder.

Standard IV: Planning

As with all disorders discussed in this text, planning includes two levels. One is the content level of planning care, which includes setting concrete, realistic, and measurable goals. Second is the process level of planning nursing care. Process level planning includes awareness of common emotional reactions of health care workers that arise when dealing with certain client behaviors.

CONTENT LEVEL—PLANNING GOALS

During the acute stage of a somatic illness, medical and nursing management focuses on stabilizing the client's physical condition. As the illness progresses to a chronic state, long term psychotherapeutic measures may help lessen the frequency or intensity of future episodes of physical symptoms.

Clients with psychogenically determined chronic disorders usually do not show overt anxiety and are convinced that their illness is primarily organic. Therefore, motivation to explore emotional problems or interpersonal difficulties is often limited.

Once clients are able to relate certain life events with exacerbation of their illness and realize that emotional stress may affect their physical condition, therapeutic intervention is possible (Kaplan 1985).

Therefore, *clients must participate with the nurse in planning goals* and agree upon interventions that have the potential of improving their life situation. No matter how ambitious or elaborate the plan, if the client does not perceive personal benefits, compliance will be nil.

Since anxiety, stress, self-regulation, and coping are central concepts of this text and chapter, the planning of goals and interventions discussed will focus on these. This choice in no way is meant to ignore, or render to a secondary position, the physiological management by physicians and nurses. What is intended in the sections on planning goals and interventions is a focus on goals and interventions that have applicability to nearly all the conditions of a psychophysiological nature. People with psychophysiological disorders often use somatic patterns of dealing with stress in their interpersonal relations. Since these patterns of responding to stress are unconscious, it is helpful to point out these patterns. New and healthier patterns or coping styles can then be introduced (Kaplan 1985). Therefore, *ineffective individual coping* is almost always an appropriate nursing diagnosis.

When planning specific goals, the nurse makes careful note of the "related to" component of the nursing diagnosis. For example, the following nursing diagnoses are the same, although the "related to" components differ. Therefore, the goals differ.

1. Ineffective individual coping related to inadequate psychological resources—*helplessness* may include the following goals:
   - By (state the date) client will be able to identify thoughts and feelings surrounding an episode of physical discomfort (e.g., migraine, stomach ache, difficulty breathing).
   - By (state the date) client will be able to identify one situation that precipitates somatic distress.
   - By (state the date) client will be able to identify one feeling surrounding the events that precipitate somatic distress.
   - Within (state the date) client will be able to verbalize angry and upsetting feelings more directly.
   - By (state the date) client will be able to link stressful events and emotions with somatic distress.
   - By (state the date) client will be able to name and demonstrate, with the aid of the nurse, one new way of dealing with upsetting feelings (e.g., exercise, talking with confidant, increased assertiveness).
   - By (state the date) client will state that somatic symptoms have decreased since employing new coping method.
2. Ineffective individual coping related to inadequate psychological resources—*inability to relax* would include a different set of goals.
   - By (state the date) client will be able to recognize difficulties and issues surrounding inability to relax (e.g., fear of losing control, fear of being viewed as weak).
   - By (state the date) client will name one relaxation technique he or she will learn to use to aid in reduction of tension (e.g., recreational activity, physical exercise, breathing exercises, meditation, progressive muscle relaxation [PMR]).
   - By (state the date) client will be able to demonstrate the use of one relaxation technique he or she can use to diminish stress and physical tension.
   - By (state the date) client will state that he or she is able to use this relaxation technique every day on a regular basis.
   - By (state the date) client will state that he or she has experienced less somatic distress since the use of the relaxation technique.

Anxiety related to unconscious conflict is most always present whether the behaviors related to anxiety are observable or not. The symptoms are a means of controlling anxiety and maintaining ego integrity. It is important, as in the goals previously mentioned, to assist the patient to explore some of the precipitating situations and feelings surrounding the onset of somatic distress.

The ability of the client to identify and explore upsetting or unacceptable feelings regarding some environmental or interpersonal situations may be deficient. This inability to identify and explore with others one's personal concerns could be a result of *impaired social interactions* related to psychological factors. The nurse will want to evaluate and plan around the client's personal supports, whom the client trusts and talks to, and other interpersonal supports available to the client.

Secondary gains may help account for the tenacity of the symptoms and perhaps play a part in a person's failure to carry out adequate health practices. The function the symptoms serve is an issue the nurse needs to address when setting goals. For example, a person who places a high value on independence may find that the symptoms allow him or her to be "legitimately" dependent on others.

The nurse and client might also realize that when the client is sick, it is the only time he or she feels cared for or gets attention. Therefore, *powerlessness* and *disturbance in self-esteem* could be used. Goals for powerlessness would stress helping the client become more assertive in getting needs met and would provide steps for increasing feelings of control. Goals for disturbance in self-esteem could focus on acceptable and satisfying ways of getting recognition and attention.

PROCESS LEVEL—NURSES' REACTIONS AND FEELINGS

Nurses are accustomed to having clients tell of physical discomforts and other signs and symptoms that suggest organic disorders. These symptoms are assessed, and diagnostic procedures help establish a medical diagnosis. The diagnosis may be clear, and the treatment specific. Nursing diagnoses and a plan of care complement the total plan. When the client's progress is excellent, everyone feels satisfied and competent.

This is not always the case when working with someone who has a physical disorder in which psychological factors play a significant role. When unconscious conflicts interfere with patient compliance or medical progress, things become more complicated. For instance, a client with a physiological disorder may experience increased anxiety in certain situations, which may intensify physical symptoms or interfere with ability to follow a specific medical regime. Nurses and physicians may feel frustration and experience a threat to their own feelings of competence. Worse yet, health care professionals may feel annoyed at the client who has taken their time and energy and does not feel motivated to get well, e.g., "Why should I care if they don't?"

Even with a more enlightened staff, certain behaviors exhibited by clients with a psychophysiological disorder can evoke unhelpful responses from staff. Awareness of common automatic responses can help the nurse respond in a more efficient manner. Table 15–7 identifies four common client behaviors that can be troublesome for nurses. These behaviors include (1) constant complaining of physical symptoms, (2) constant need for sympathy and help, (3) somatizations that are resistant to change, and (4) client's hostility toward staff. Nurses' automatic responses are listed, and alternative responses are suggested.

Standard V: Intervention

Any psychophysiological disorder can become a medical emergency. Examples include the acute severe asthmatic episode, a perforated ulcer, or a cardiac arrythmia. Unless one has been trained for medical emergencies, one's response is to signal the need for assistance immediately, to obtain the specialist, or to transport the patient safely to an emergency facility. Initial medical and nursing interventions usually focus on stabilizing the client's physical condition.

After the client's physical condition is stable, interventions relating to therapeutic approaches and specific areas of teaching and counseling can be useful to help prevent exacerbation and to help the client find alternative ways of dealing with stress.

V-A: PSYCHOTHERAPEUTIC INTERVENTIONS

All nurses at all levels should have a solid understanding of basic therapeutic approaches to general patient care. There are behaviors on the part of the nurse that are useful to clients regardless of their state of health or illness; however, the interventions in Table 15–8 have been selected for emphasis. Although some may seem general, they are at the same time uniquely important for persons who have a physical disorder with psychogenic components.

When a client's personality characteristics are consistent with various research studies (see Table 15–5), specific psychological supportive measures may be useful. Table 15–9 identifies some of the more common psychophysiological conditions, reviews possible client behaviors, gives a clinical example, and offers suggestions for nursing intervention. Use the clinical example to identify the personality traits often associated with each disorder, the possible stressor involved, and interventions that could be psychologically supportive.

Table 15–7 • AUTOMATIC NURSE RESPONSES AND SUGGESTED ALTERNATIVES

PATIENT BEHAVIORS	NURSES' AUTOMATIC RESPONSES	NURSES' ALTERNATIVE RESPONSES	EXAMPLES
1. The patient elaborates in detail the discomforts that nurse has heard before.	Annoyance, boredom, argumentative	Use the patient's focus as starting point for eliciting the circumstances that surround the client's experience.	"What was happening at home/with your job when this first started?"
2. The patient asks for sympathy and help (overtly or covertly).	Annoyed, burdened, or possibly overprotective	Compassion as for clients generally. Maintain clear boundaries of self vis-à-vis patient.	"I can see that you are feeling particularly vulnerable now. Let's look at what *you* can do to feel less upset."
3. Patient's somatization is resistant to change.	Impatience, unrealistic expectations of change	Consistency of availability (within professional structures).	"I know these migraines can be painful. I have 5 minutes to talk about your thoughts or feelings of concern to you."
4. Patients manifest anger/hostility toward staff	Fear, avoidance	Help patient note the difference between effects and action. Accept person having feelings of anger.	"You seem so angry this morning. Let's try and figure out what's going on."

Table 15–8 • BASIC THERAPEUTIC INTERVENTIONS

INTERVENTION	RATIONALE
1. Nonjudgmental listening without premature interpretations.	1. The somatic experience of the client is very real.
2. Provide care without fostering dependency.	2. Working with the client for meeting real needs can enhance a sense of security.
3. Give recognition for client's strength—work with strengths to diminish long term dependencies.	3. Client experiences recognition and attention for healthy aspects of self. Works to undermine sick role as method of dealing with conflict. Minimize secondary gains.
4. Assist client to identify alternative methods of coping to reduce stress.	4. Alternative methods of dealing with stress reduce incidence of internalizing anxiety (anger, depression, etc.) onto body organs.
5. Work with client to identify those situations that increase anxiety/stress.	5. Often client is unaware of unconscious conflicts that trigger anxiety (e.g., difficulty expressing, dependency, hostility, need for recognition).
6. Assist client to identify potential support systems, and work on developing these.	6. Client's resources may be limited or ineffectual. New resources may increase emotional support as well as self-esteem.
7. Examine with client self-imposed demands.	7. Unrealistic demands on self increase experience of anxiety, which may in turn be internalized onto body organs through "body language."
8. Refer or teach client alternative methods of relaxation (e.g., imaging, meditation, PMR, exercising, biofeedback).	8. Body learns alternative ways of channeling stress (other than somatizing).

V-B: HEALTH TEACHING

Nurses are playing a larger and larger role in teaching patients alternative methods of handling stress. By using these techniques, patients can positively affect the course or severity of some physical disorders. Herbert Benson (1975) outlined specific techniques that enable most people to elicit what he referred to as the "relaxation response." Essentially, these techniques teach the client how to switch from the sympathetic mode (fight or flight) of the autonomic nervous system to a state of relaxation (the parasympathetic mode) (Box 15–1). For those who are unable to use these techniques, biofeedback can bring about the same results.

Reducing the chronic sympathetic fight or flight response of the sympathetic nervous system can

1. Alter the course of certain medical conditions (e.g., high blood pressure, arrythmias, migraine headaches) (Kolb and Brodie 1982).
2. Decrease the need for certain medications (e.g., analgesics, antihypertensives) (Morris 1979).
3. Diminish or eliminate unhealthy behaviors (e.g., drug addictions, insomnia, overeating) (Aron and Aron 1980).
4. Increase cognitive functions like concentration and learning ability (Morse 1977).

Benson's relaxation technique has been used successfully in conjunction with meditation and visual imagery in a variety of disorders, e.g., diabetes, high blood pressure, migraines, cancer, and peptic ulcers.

Nurses who teach relaxation techniques need special training. Any client who is to be taught relaxation techniques should have the knowledge and consent of his or her physician. Snyder (1984) cautions against the use of relaxation techniques with certain clients. For example:

1. Depressed persons may experience further withdrawal.
2. Hallucinating and delusional patients may lose contact with reality altogether.
3. The toxic effects of some medication may be enhanced.
4. Some patients in pain may have a heightened experience of pain with increase in body awareness.

Other techniques to induce relaxation have been developed. Some have an inward focus. These include meditation, visual imaging, hypnosis, and therapeutic touch. Others have an external focus. These include (1) progressive muscular relaxation (PMR) and (2) biofeedback.

PROGRESSIVE MUSCULAR RELAXATION (PMR). PMR was first developed by a man named Jacobson who discovered that feelings of deep relaxation can be achieved when muscle concentration is almost com-

Table 15–9 • PSYCHOLOGICAL SUPPORTIVE MEASURES FOR SPECIFIC PERSONALITY PROFILES

CONFLICTS	POSSIBLE BEHAVIORS	CLINICAL EXAMPLES	PSYCHOLOGICAL SUPPORTIVE MEASURES
Gastrointestinal — Peptic Ulcers			
Intense dependency needs associated with underlying hostility. May use reaction-formation as a defense.	Very aggressive, overly independent or demanding. Difficulty trusting or asking others for support. May see regressive behavior. Worry.	Mr. Stubbs, 42, was a hard-driving man who was vice-president of a local insurance company. He prided himself on his self-sufficiency. When the work piled up, he was unable to admit to his boss he needed assistance. After three weeks of working until 11:00 P.M. and popping ASA for stomach pain, he was admitted to the emergency room with a massive gastrointestinal bleed.	1. Meet needs but do not foster or reinforce dependency. 2. Foster activities for self-care. 3. Combine health teaching with psychological support. 4. Work with client to reduce environmental stress. 5. Encourage person to share thoughts and feelings directly.
Gastrointestinal — Ulcerative Colitis			
Issues of control. Strong need for approval. Difficulty with dependency issues and sensitivity to loss.	Rumination, indecision, passive compliance, moral rigidity, perfectionism, conformity, orderliness (obsessive-compulsive trait), passive-aggressive tendencies.	Ms. Lions, a 24-year-old computer operator, was prized by her boss for her efficiency, attention to detail, and handing her work in on time. Although she did not seem to have a sense of humor, she complied with demands and never bothered anyone. Ms. Lions always thought her boss did not appreciate her enough. Three weeks after she broke up with her boyfriend, she noticed blood and mucus in her now frequent watery stools.	1. Encourage person's sense of control. 2. Simplify choices. 3. Work with the person to set realistic goals. 4. Encourage productive activities that will increase self-esteem and decrease self-rumination.
Cardiovascular — High Blood Pressure (HBP)			
Between dependent and aggressive drives.	Often observed to be outwardly pleasant and calm. Use of reaction-formation to repress rage and suspicion.	Tom Sharp, 52, lived most of his life with his invalid mother. Everyone said what a wonderful son he was to devote his life to his mother. He gave up a promotion involving moving to another state to stay with and care for his mother. The mother refused to let anyone but her son care for her and was sharply critical of any woman Tom wanted to date. Three month's after his mother's death Tom complained of dizziness and was found to have a BP of 210/140 on a routine examination.	1. Combine psychological support with health teaching. 2. Evaluate and assess unwanted side effects from antihypertensives, which could affect compliance (e.g., impotence, loss of sexual drive). 3. Teach relaxation techniques. 4. Evaluate situational, environmental, and interpersonal stressors.

Table continued on following page

Table 15-9 • PSYCHOLOGICAL SUPPORTIVE MEASURES FOR SPECIFIC PERSONALITY PROFILES *Continued*

CONFLICTS	POSSIBLE BEHAVIORS	CLINICAL EXAMPLES	PSYCHOLOGICAL SUPPORTIVE MEASURES
Cardiovascular—Coronary Artery Disease			
Around dependency issues.	Type A personality. Highly competitive, sense of time urgency, hard working, aggressive, inability to relax, hostility. Doesn't adhere to medical regime. Use of denial.	Max Bender, 46, started a construction company the year he finished high school. He prided himself on "being a man," that is, tough, lucky with women, and always on top of things. The fact that his business was the most successful in the area was not an accident. Max worked long hours, took charge of everything, and worked his men hard. He smoked, drank, and often overate. One year after his wife died from cancer and two months after an important client defaulted on his payments and went bankrupt, Max was admitted to the emergency room with a massive myocardial infarction.	1. Emotional support with health teaching. 2. Counseling directed toward reducing competitiveness and time urgency and creating lifestyle changes. 3. Teach relaxation training. 4. Sexual counseling where indicated. 5. Marital counseling where needed to decrease family stress. 6. Referral and supervision for prescribed exercise regime.
Respiratory—Asthma			
High dependency needs. Extreme vulnerability regarding issues of separation.	May be overly dependent. Clinging behaviors (e.g., behaviors that indicate a strong need for protection and security). Use reaction-formation. Behavior that rejects need for protection or security (e.g., highly competitive).	Telly Long's dad had left the family when Telly was 3 years old. Her mother was forced to go back to work as a nurse when Telly was 6 years old. When Telly's mom decided to go away for a week's vacation with a friend, Telly started having a serious asthma attack. Telly was brought to the emergency room and given epinephrine. Telly's mom canceled her vacation plans. As the years progressed, Telly continued to have attacks, especially when Telly's mom planned extended time away from home.	1. Explore events and situations that precede an attack. 2. Encourage verbalization of thoughts and feelings to lessen somatic expression of conflict. 3. Maintain a balance between overprotectiveness and denial of disorder. 4. Encourage outside supports (e.g., self-help groups). 5. Emphasize person's strengths, abilities, and accomplishments.

pletely eliminated. He devised a program of instruction wherein systematic tensing and releasing of various muscles and learning to discriminate between sensations of tension and relaxation occur. The technique has been shortened and refined by Bernstein and Borkovec (1973) to one that can be learned and practiced in hospitals for patients with a variety of conditions.

Usually a number of training sessions are needed for mastery (Snyder 1984). As mentioned, for best results the student should receive live instruction and proceed only with the approval of a physician.

BIOFEEDBACK. Relaxation using biofeedback is achieved by learning to control physiological mechanisms that are ordinarily outside one's awareness and control. Awareness and control are accomplished by monitoring body processes, such as muscle tone, heart rate, and brain waves, with mechanical devices. During this time, the client is presented with signal lights that intensify with tension and dim with relaxation. The client learns to use the signals to produce a relaxed state. With practice, an individual can invoke the relaxation state at will.

Box 15–1. BENSON'S RELAXATION TECHNIQUES

Practicing this exercise for 15 to 20 minutes once or twice daily can produce desired results. It may take a number of weeks or a few months before positive benefits are noticed. The essential ingredients for triggering the parasympathetic response (relaxation response) are

1. A quiet environment—External distractions can inhibit relaxation.
2. An object to dwell on—Mediators use a mental device to help them elicit deep stages of relaxation. Such a mental device can be a word, for example, ohm, peace, love, repeated silently over and over. A mental device helps distract the mind from logical thought and prepare for deeper levels of relaxation and "letting go." When distracting thoughts occur, and they will initially, the person is told to push them aside gently. The advice is given, "Tell each thought you will take care of it later, and go back to the mental device or sound."
3. Passive attitude—This can be extremely difficult for people in our culture. Many feel they should be accomplishing some task and may initially view sitting quietly as a waste of time. Once benefits are forthcoming, however, many people regard achieving the relaxation response as one of their most important accomplishments.
4. A comfortable position—A sitting position with hands resting on thighs is suggested. Lying down may lead to sleep. Sitting cross-legged can interfere with circulation, and if position is uncomfortable, the discomfort will distract from the process of relaxation.

Sometimes this exercise is referred to as centering. Many nurses, as well as other health care professionals, are finding this a useful tool in dealing with job stress.

V-D: SOMATIC THERAPIES

Medications play a large role in the treatment of most psychophysiological disorders, since there are actual organ changes or body alterations associated with these disorders. Examples include antihypertensives for high blood pressure, anticholinergics/antispasmodics for peptic ulcers and ulcerative colitis, and bronchodilators for asthmatic conditions. Alerting the patient to the indications, dose, therapeutic effects, and possible side effects comes within the scope of nursing practice.

Since emotional experiences such as anxiety and depression can precipitate psychophysiological disorders, anxiolytic agents, antidepressants, and sedatives may be ordered. Refer to Chapter 16 for a discussion of the antianxiety agents and to Chapter 18 for more on the antidepressant medications.

V-F: PSYCHOTHERAPY

A number of treatment modalities described in Chapter 2 may be used for psychophysiological conditions. Professionals trained in individual psychotherapy, group therapy, family therapy, psychoanalysis, behavior modification, or transactional analysis may use one of these effectively. Many nurses obtained special training to use one or more of these modalities (often at the master's level). However, nurses in all settings are being trained in special techniques such as relaxation, PMR, and biofeedback. Refer to Table 15–5 to see which therapeutic modalities have been found especially useful in specific disorders.

Standard VI: Evaluation

The initial goal of medical and nursing intervention is directed toward alleviation of the client's physical symptoms. The nurse evaluates the client's receptiveness to the planned medical regime as well as the client's awareness of stressors or situations that precede the onset of physical symptoms. Most importantly, the nurse assesses the client's ability and willingness to use alternative ways of dealing with stress. Finally, the nurse evaluates the client's ability to manipulate the environment in order to reduce stress. When these conditions are satisfied, most long term goals will have been met.

The meeting of these long range goals assumes that many of the short term goals leading to this end point have also been met. Therefore, the evaluation of each of the client-centered short term goals is extremely important. Is the client aware of what kinds of situations and environments increase stress? Can the person identify and practice alternative methods of handling stress? Is the client able to accept the limitations of his or her medical disorder? Is the client able to identify changes in his or her life patterns, diet, and medical routines that will maximize his or her health? With realistic and clearly measurable short term goals, the nurse and the client can work together on effecting change in the intensity, frequency, and duration of future episodes of psychophysiological illness.

Text continued on page 336

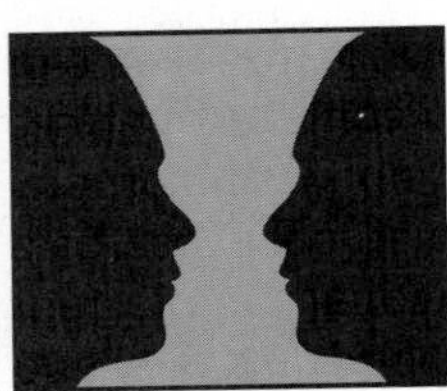

Case Study: Working With a Person Who Has a Psychophysiological Disorder

Mr. Hammond, 45, was brought to the emergency room after having a myocardial infarction (MI). He had no history of coronary disease, although both his father and mother died of heart disease before the age of 65. Mr. Hammond is an executive in a large advertising firm, and according to his wife, he works many evenings and weekends to "beat the competition." Physical assessment reveals a blood pressure of 230/110 and a high serum cholesterol level of 290 mg/100 ml. He is considerably overweight and told the doctor that he has no time for exercise.

After five days in cardiac intensive care Mr. Hammond was sent down to a medical unit. When Mr. Garcia, Mr. Hammond's primary nurse, went to visit, Mr. Hammond appeared restless, hostile, and demanding. Mrs. Hammond was in the room when the nurse arrived, and seemed to be hovering over her husband's bed. Mrs. Hammond appeared greatly distressed, tired, and dejected. After Mrs. Hammond left, Mr. Garcia spent some time with Mr. Hammond. A sample of their interaction is provided subsequently.

Assessment

NURSE:	Your wife seems concerned about you.
MR. HAMMOND:	What does she know. She is treating me like a baby at a time I should be closing the Ford account. How much longer do I have to stay in this place?
NURSE:	You have had a serious heart attack, and your body needs time to heal. You seem to have difficulty relaxing.
MR. HAMMOND:	Relaxing . . . I never have time for relaxing. The minute you look away, someone gets in there ahead of you. Where is my phone? . . . I told them upstairs I needed a phone to make up for all this lost time.
NURSE:	The doctor does not want you to have a phone at present. Your body needs the rest. Is there someone at the job who is taking over for you?
MR. HAMMOND:	Are you kidding? Harry louses everything up. The only way to get anything done right is to do it yourself. If I could get out of here, I'd handle things myself. There is nothing wrong with me!
NURSE:	It does sound like this has been very upsetting for you. We can talk about some of the things that are bothering you. Right now the doctor wants you to relax and has ordered Valium for you.
MR. HAMMOND:	I don't need anything to relax. I don't need anything or anybody. I am not a baby, and I don't need to be treated like one. Leave me alone. I've got a lot of good years ahead of me . . . I'm still the man I was . . . Get out of here!
NURSE:	I can understand you are upset. I will be back in 15 minutes with your medication, and perhaps then we can talk about some of your concerns.

Mr. Garcia divided his data into objective and subjective components.

OBJECTIVE DATA

1. Serum cholesterol level of 290 mg/100 ml
2. Overweight
3. Restless and agitated
4. Male in his 40's
5. Both parents died of heart trouble in their early 60's
6. Blood pressure 230/110

SUBJECTIVE DATA

1. Highly competitive
2. Has strong sense of time urgency
3. Has high performance standards
4. Appears angry and hostile
5. "I don't need anything or anybody."
6. "I'm not a baby and won't be treated like one."
7. "The only way to get things done is to do them yourself."
8. "There is nothing wrong with me."
9. "I never have time for relaxing."
10. "I'm still the man I was."

Nursing Diagnosis

Mr. Garcia realized Mr. Hammond would need a lot of health teaching. At the same time, Mr. Garcia realized that Mr. Hammond had to accept the fact that he had a real medical problem and that certain changes in his diet and lifestyle could greatly increase the length and quality of his life. At the moment, Mr. Hammond did not appear receptive to health teaching. For a man who was accustomed to being in charge and productive, his heart attack appeared to be a great threat. Mr. Garcia thought that besides the threat to his role in business, Mr. Hammond might also be threatened in his role as a sexual partner.

Based on the initial data, Mr. Garcia made the following nursing diagnoses:

1. *Moderate to Severe Anxiety* related to threat to biological integrity as evidenced by denial and irritability
   - "There is nothing wrong with me."
   - "I am still a man."
   - "I don't need anything or anyone."
   - "I am not a baby and won't be treated like one."
2. *Knowledge Deficit* related to new diagnosis
   - "There is nothing wrong with me."
   - "I am still the man I was."
   - "I don't need anything to relax."
   - Overweight
   - High cholesterol level
   - Both parents died of coronary artery disease in early 60's
   - High blood pressure
3. *Ineffective Individual Coping* related to inadequate relaxation
   - "I never have time for relaxing."
   - "The only way to get things done is to do them yourself."
   - "The minute you look away, someone gets in there ahead of you."
   - Has a strong sense of time urgency
   - Highly competitive

Planning

CONTENT LEVEL — PLANNING GOALS

Mr. Garcia thought that once Mr. Hammond felt less threatened and was better able to accept his illness, he would be more open to making positive change. Mr. Garcia realized that until a person recognizes that there is a problem and is motivated to make changes, medical compliance can be difficult. Only goals that a person thinks of as desirable will motivate taking the time and energy needed for change. Therefore, Mr. Garcia planned to work closely with Mr. Hammond in planning nursing care.

Nursing Diagnosis	Long Term Goal	Short Term Goals
1. *Moderate to Severe Anxiety* related to threat to biologic integrity as evidenced by denial and irritability	By (state the date) Mr. Hammond will be able to acknowledge he has a cardiac problem.	1a. By (state the date) Mr. Hammond will discuss concerns of how his cardiac status might affect his work.

Continued on following page

Planning
(Continued)

Nursing Diagnosis	Long-Term Goal	Short-Term Goals
		1b. By (state the date) Mr. Hammond will discuss concerns of how his cardiac status might affect his sexual activity.
2. *Knowledge Deficit* related to new diagnosis	Mr. Hammond will be able to discuss how diet, stress, and medication can influence the course of his disease.	2a. Mr. Hammond will be able to identify foods high in cholesterol and sodium and to name healthy foods he is willing to eat.
		2b. Mr. Hammond will lose two pounds per week for 20 weeks.
		2c. By (state the date) Mr. Hammond will state four changes in his work routine that can reduce stress.
		2d. By (state the date) Mr. Hammond will be able to name his medications, state their purpose, and discuss the side effects of each.
3. *Ineffective Individual Coping* related to inadequate relaxation	By (state the date) Mr. Hammond will state he feels less driven after following relaxation regime.	3a. By (state the date) Mr. Hammond will state he understands benefits of relaxation both medically and emotionally.
		3b. Mr. Hammond will discuss with nurse various relaxation techniques by (state the date).
		3c. By (state the date) Mr. Hammond will choose one technique that he is willing to learn.

PROCESS LEVEL — NURSES' REACTIONS AND FEELINGS

Mr. Garcia had seen denial in men with coronary artery disease before. Initially, Mr. Garcia found this defense very annoying, since it diminished the effectiveness of his health teaching. When he began to understand denial as a defense against anxiety, fear, and helplessness, Mr. Garcia became more understanding. Mr. Garcia now attempts to explore some of the client's thoughts, feelings, and concerns regarding how the disease will affect his or her life. He finds that this often opens up avenues of discussion. Open communication channels pave the way for crucial and needed health teaching. Eventually, Mr. Garcia will discuss with Mr. Hammond acceptable changes in his lifestyle that can minimize stress and add to his quality of life.

Mr. Garcia is aware, however, that each person makes his or her own choices. The nurse can support, teach, and effect a variety of referrals in the least threatening manner possible. Clients will choose those measures or suggestions they are at that time willing or able to follow.

Mr. Garcia no longer takes it personally or becomes angry with clients if they have difficulty accepting or following prescribed medical regimes. For some people it takes a long time before defensive barriers break down, allowing major changes in health practices to take place.

Intervention

Initially, Mr. Garcia worked with Mr. Hammond to lower his anxiety and assist him in feeling more secure and in control (see Nursing Care Plan 15–1). As Mr. Hammond's anxiety began to decrease, he was able to share some of his concerns. After a while, Mr. Hammond was more amenable to health teaching and more motivated to learn about how this heart attack would affect his life.

Mr. Garcia thought that a relaxation exercise might be useful for Mr. Hammond. Mr. Hammond's doctor agreed. After discussing some relaxation techniques, Mr. Hammond stated that he would be willing to try biofeedback; "That meditation mumbo-jumbo is not for me." Mr. Garcia agreed that Mr. Hammond would do better with a relaxation technique that had an external focus.

As Mr. Hammond became less tense and anxious, his wife appeared to relax. The nurse was concerned with the change Mr. Hammond's coronary status would make on the whole family system. Mrs. Hammond seemed relieved when Mr. Garcia suggested that a visiting nurse come after discharge to check on medication, diet, and general progress. The nurse explained to Mrs. Hammond that illness could be a crisis for the whole family. Mr. Garcia explained to the couple that post-infarction despondency is an almost universal response to a heart attack (Kaplan 1985). Counseling during this time could be useful if the depression became severe. The nurse suggested that perhaps Mr. and Mrs. Hammond might speak with the social worker before discharge to acquaint themselves with the resources in their community. Refer to Mr. Hammond's nursing care plan (Nursing Care Plan 15–1).

Evaluation

By discharge, Mr. Hammond appeared to have a basic understanding of his illness and the risk factors. He seemed concerned regarding his cholesterol level and blood pressure, and he admitted he was too heavy. He had worked out a diet with the dietitian, and his wife had been present at one of the meetings. He seemed pleased about the four pounds he had lost while in the hospital.

He was well versed in his medications by discharge, and he shared the information with his wife two days before discharge.

Mr. Hammond still had some questions in regard to the safety of future sexual activity. Both he and his wife decided to make a joint appointment with the doctor to discuss this further. Mr. Hammond was willing to make some changes in his work habits, although he knew this would be hard for him to do.

An appointment was made for Mr. Hammond to start biofeedback training after discharge. He said he would drop by and let Mr. Garcia know how everything was going.

Nursing Care Plan 15–1 • A PERSON WITH A PSYCHOPHYSIOLOGICAL DISORDER: MR. HAMMOND

NURSING DIAGNOSIS

Moderate to severe anxiety related to threat to biological integrity as evidenced by denial and irritability

Supporting Data

- "There is nothing wrong with me."
- "I am still the man I was."
- "I don't need anyone or anything."
- "I am not a baby and won't be treated like one."

Long Term Goal: By (state the date) Mr. Hammond will acknowledge he has a cardiac problem.

Short Term Goal	*Intervention*	*Rationale*	*Evaluation*
1. By (state the date) Mr. Hammond will discuss concerns of how his cardiac status will affect his work.	1a. Reflect back to client feelings when client is hostile or demanding, e.g., "You sound angry . . . "	1a. Not taking client's anger/irritability personally allows client to perceive nurse as safe. Reflecting back feelings allows client to explore real issues of concern.	Goal met Mr. Hammond was able to admit that "this whole business" had him upset.

Continued on following page

Nursing Care Plan 15–1 • A PERSON WITH A PSYCHOPHYSIOLOGICAL DISORDER: MR. HAMMOND *(Continued)*

Short Term Goal	*Intervention*	*Rationale*	*Evaluation*
	1b. Share observance of client's strengths, e.g., "You seem to involve logical thinking and knowledge when making decisions."	1b. Highlighting a person's strengths can help in increasing self-esteem and feelings of control. Helps nurse evaluate strengths to use in planning future care and fostering compliance to health care teaching.	Mr. Hammond stated that he was a good problem solver and had handled many crises with competence in the past.
	1c. Encourage client to voice concerns regarding how his MI will affect his work.	1c. Once fear and concerns are expressed, they can be looked at, evaluated realistically, and dealt with.	Mr. Hammond stated he was afraid that a heart attack would mean he could no longer work. M.D. explained he could return to work and suggested ways to reduce work-related tension.
2. Mr. Hammond will discuss concerns of how his cardiac status could affect his sexual life.	2. Encourage client to discuss concerns regarding future sexual activity.	2a. Many male clients equate ability to perform sexually with "being a man." 2b. Sharing fear and concerns can reduce anxiety. 2c. Once concerns are clarified, specific questions can be answered.	Client stated he felt much better after being told by the M.D. that he could resume normal sexual activity after two months. However, he admitted to still having concerns in this area.

NURSING DIAGNOSIS

Knowledge deficit related to new diagnosis

Supporting Data

- "There is nothing wrong with me."
- "I don't need anything to relax."
- Overweight.
- High cholesterol — 290 mg/100 ml.
- High blood pressure — 210/110.
- Both parents died of coronary artery disease in their early 60's.

Long Term Goal: Mr. Hammond will be able to discuss how heredity, diet, and stress can influence the course of his disease.

Short Term Goal	*Intervention*	*Rationale*	*Evaluation*
1. By (state the date) client will be able to identify foods high in cholesterol and sodium and name healthy foods to eat.	1a. Evaluate client's receptiveness for teaching.	1a. If client is not interested or motivated, learning is less likely to take place.	Goal met Dietitian visited twice. Wife was present second time. Client seemed knowledgeable about information. Questions if he can "stick" to such a diet.
	1b. Ask dietitian to instruct client on prescribed diet.	1b. According to policy in this hospital, the dietitian instructs patients, provides materials, and visits periodically.	
	1c. Suggest wife visit while dietitian is present.	1c. Strengthens teaching. Allows for questions concerning shopping and preparation (if that is wife's role) to be answered.	
	1d. Review diet teaching with client periodically.	1d. Allows for feedback and may raise new questions.	

Short Term Goal	Intervention	Rationale	Evaluation
2. Mr. Hammond will lose two lbs per week for 20 weeks.	2a. Discuss client's thoughts and feelings regarding dieting.	2a. If client is opposed to dieting, any weight lost in the hospital will be regained.	Client admits to needing to lose weight but "never got around to it." Has lost four lbs after three weeks.
		2b. May open up new areas of health teaching.	
3. By (state the date) Mr. Hammond will state four changes in work routine that can reduce stress.	3a. Encourage client to identify work habits he would like to change.	3a. Behaviors a person recognizes as increasing stress are ones he or she will more likely work on changing.	Client had no difficulty in identifying certain behaviors (e.g., working late, working on weekends, not trusting others to do work delegated) but didn't know how he could change all at once.
	3b. Suggest meeting with social worker now or after discharge to discuss changes further.	3b. Type A behavior can take a long time to modify and is best done with support and feedback.	
4. By (state the date) Mr. Hammond will be able to name his medications, state their purpose, and discuss their side effects.	4a. When administering medication, name and briefly describe function of each.	4a. Acquaint client with names and functions of medication ordered.	By discharge, Mr. Hammond was able to identify drugs, dosage, and side effects and was given a number to call if questions arose.
	4b. Encourage client to discuss medication with M.D.	4b. Client should have a good basic understanding of medications, e.g., need, function, and side effects.	
	4c. Review medications with client periodically and at discharge.	4c. Repetition encourages recall. Offers opportunity to ask questions.	
	4d. Discuss with M.D. possibility of sending visiting nurse after discharge to check medication, diet, and general progress.	4d. Ensure continuity of care and further health teaching.	

NURSING DIAGNOSIS

Ineffective individual coping related to inadequate relaxation

Supporting Data

- I never have time for relaxing.
- I don't need anything to relax.
- The minute you look away, someone gets in there ahead of you.
- Has a strong sense of time urgency.
- Highly competitive.

Long Term Goal: By (state the date) Mr. Hammond will state he feels less driven after following relaxation regime.

Short Term Goal	*Intervention*	*Rationale*	*Evaluation*
1. By (state the date) Mr. Hammond will state he understands benefits of relaxation both medically and emotionally.	1. Teach client about body's fight or flight response versus the relaxation response (use charts, etc.).	1. Basic understanding of bodily responses can increase compliance and feeling of control.	Goal met (Fill in date goal was met.)
2. By (state the date) Mr. Hammond will discuss with nurse various relaxation responses.	2a. Describe various techniques that will increase the parasympathetic mode (relaxation response) (e.g., medication, self-hypnosis, PMR, biofeedback, visualization).	2. Gives client choices.	(Fill in date goal was met.)
3. By (state the date) Mr. Hammond will choose one technique that he is willing to learn.			On (fill in date goal was met) Mr. Hammond stated he would be willing to learn biofeedback after discharge.

Summary

Research has repeatedly correlated mental and emotional processes with physical health and physical disease. In fact, there is probably no major health organ system or somatic defense that is not subject to the influence of interactions between the psychological and physiological.

The term psychosomatic (DSM I 1952), referring to the interaction of the mind (psyche) and body (soma), gave way to the term psychophysiological in 1968 (DSM II). Psychophysiological referred to all physical symptoms in which psychic elements played a significant role. The DSM III (1980) and the DSM III-R (1987) presently refer to disorders that are psychogenic as "any physical condition to which psychological factors are judged contributory." The terms psychosomatic and psychophysiologic are still used by many clinicians, although the symptoms and disorders are now identified on Axis III (see Chapter 1).

Alexander (circa 1934) first identified seven physical disorders that correlated with specific psychological conflicts. Alexander's Seven consisted of peptic ulcer, ulcerative colitis, rheumatoid arthritis, hyperthyroidism, high blood pressure, asthma, and neurodermatitis. Today, it is believed a great variety of physical disorders are psychologically induced or maintained. For example, headaches, pain, insomnia, sexual dysfunctions, arrthymias, eating disorders, and cancer are some that are now associated with emotional conflicts and ineffective coping styles.

As yet, there is no one universally accepted model to explain the etiology of psychophysiological disease. It is believed that there are a variety of contributing factors predisposing a person to a psychophysiological disorder. For example, personality profiles, genetic predisposition, environmental conditions, internal and external stressors, personal coping styles, as well as cultural background, are all thought to play an important role. Table 15–5 lists some common psychophysiological disorders, outlining personality traits, biological and genetic correlates, environmental factors, and effective therapeutic approaches.

Assessing a person with a psychophysiological disorder includes a thorough nursing assessment of body functions. Vital psychosocial areas to assess include

1. levels of anxiety,
2. sources of stress (internal and external),
3. resources for dealing with stress (internal and external), and
4. presence of secondary gains.

Planning goals is the crux of a competent nursing care plan and is most effective when planned and evaluated by both nurse and client.

Interventions for people with psychophysiological disorders initially involve nursing skills aimed at saving life and maintaining optimum health. Eventually, psychologically supportive interventions can help in maintaining health and minimizing future exacerbation. Psychotherapeutic measures include helping the client recognize possible internal or external stressors that may exacerbate the client's symptoms. Finding alternate ways of dealing with internal or external stress is the next step. Rechanneling anxiety and stress can be accomplished through a variety of methods. For example, physical exercise, meditation, visualization, biofeedback, and PMR are some techniques nurses with special training can teach their clients. Nurses educated at the master's level may also work with people using a variety of treatment modalities (e.g., individual, group, and family therapy, behavior modification, and transactional analysis).

Long range goals are considered met when the client's physical condition is in remission and the frequency, intensity, and duration of future exacerbations are greatly reduced. Short term goals are tailored to the specific individual and to the individual's circumstances. Frequent evaluation of short term goals and revision of goals made with the client are ongoing processes.

References

Achterberg J, Simonton OC, Matthew-Simonton S. Stress, psychological factors, and cancer. New Medicine, 1976.

American Psychiatric Association. Desk Reference to the Diagnostic Criteria From the Diagnostic and Statistical Manual of Mental Disorders, 3rd ed. Washington DC: American Psychiatric Association, 1982.

American Psychiatric Association: Diagnostic and Statistical Manual of Mental Disorders, 3rd ed. revised. Washington DC: American Psychiatric Association, 1987.

Ames SW, Kneisl CR. How illness develops. *In* Kneisl CR, Ames SW (eds). Adult Health Nursing: A Biopsychosocial Approach. Menlo Park, CA: Addison-Wesley Publishing Company, 1986.

Aron A, Aron E. The transcendental meditation program's effect on addictive behaviors. Addictive Behaviors, 5:(5), 1980.

Baillie V, Norbeck JS, Barnes LEA. Stress, social support, and psychological distress of family caregivers of the elderly. Nursing Research, 37(4):217, 1988.

Benson H. The Relaxation Response. New York: William Morrow & Company, 1975.

Bernstein D, Borkovec T. Progressive relaxation training. Champaign, Ill: Research Press, 1973.

Bulechek G, McCloskey J (ed). Nursing Interventions: Treatments for Nursing Diagnoses. Philadelphia: W.B. Saunders Company, 1985.

Chapman AH. Textbook of Clinical Psychiatry: An Interpersonal Approach. Philadelphia: J.B. Lippincott Company, 1976.

Fischman J. Type A on trial. Psychology Today, 21(2):42, 1987.

Gallon RL. The Psychosomatic Approach to Illness. New York: Elsevier Biomedical, 1982.

Gellhorn E, Kiely W. Mystical states of consciousness: Neurophysical and clinical aspects. Journal of Nervous and Mental Disease, 154:399, 1972.
Hackett TP, et al. Cardiovascular disorders. *In* Kaplan HI, Sadock BJ (eds). Comprehensive Textbook of Psychiatry, 4th ed. Baltimore: Williams & Wilkins, 1985.
Jacobson E. Progressive relaxation. New York: McGraw-Hill Book Company, 1938.
Kaplan HI. History of psychosomatic medicine. *In* Kaplan HI, Sadock BJ (eds). Comprehensive Textbook of Psychiatry, 4th ed. Baltimore: Williams & Wilkins, 1985.
Kaplan HI. Treatment of psychosomatic disorders. *In* Kaplan HI, Sadock BJ (eds). Comprehensive Textbook of Psychiatry, 4th ed. Baltimore: Williams & Wilkins, 1985.
Knapp PH. Current theoretical concepts in psychosomatic medicine. *In* Kaplan HI, Sadock BJ (eds). Comprehensive Textbook of Psychiatry, 4th ed. Baltimore: Williams & Wilkins, 1985.
Kolb LC, Brodie HKH. Modern Clinical Psychiatry, 10th ed. Philadelphia: W.B. Saunders Company, 1982.
Krakowski AJ, Kimball CP. Psychosomatic medicine: Theoretical, clinical and transcultural aspects. New York: Plenum Press, 1983.
Kritek PB. Diagnostics: The struggle to classify our diagnoses. American Journal of Nursing, 86:722, 1986.
Lesse S. Relationship of anxiety to depression. American Journal of Psychotherapy, 36:332, 1982.
Locke S, Colligan D. The Healer Within: The New Medicine of Mind and Body. New York: E.P. Dutton, 1986.
Luckmann J, Sorensen KC. Medical-Surgical Nursing: A Psychophysiologic Approach, 3rd ed. Philadelphia: W.B. Saunders Company, 1987.
MacKinnon RA, Michels R. The Psychiatric Interview in Clinical Practice. Philadelphia: W.B. Saunders Company, 1971.
Minuchin S, Rosman BL, Baker L. Psychosomatic Families. Cambridge, MA: Harvard University Press, 1978.
Morris C. Relaxation therapy in a clinic. American Journal of Nursing, 79:1958, 1979.
Morse D, et al. A psychological and subjective evaluation of meditation, hypnosis and relaxation. Psychosomatic Medicine, 39:305, 1977.
Newman M. Looking at the whole. American Journal of Nursing, 84:1496, 1984.
Oken D. Gastrointestinal disorders. *In* Kaplan HI, Sadock BJ (eds). Comprehensive Textbook of Psychiatry, 4th ed. Baltimore: Williams & Wilkins, 1985.
Pancheri P, et al. Life stress events and state-trait anxiety in psychiatric and psychosomatic patients. Issues in Mental Health Nursing, 7:367, 1985.
Pelletier K. Mind as a Healer, Mind as a Slayer. New York: Dell, 1977.
Sheelan DV, Hackett TP. Psychosomatic disorders. *In* Nicholi AM (ed). The Harvard Guide to Modern Psychiatry. Cambridge, MA: The Belknap Press of the Harvard University Press, 1980.
Snyder M. Progressive relaxation as a nursing intervention: An analysis. Advances in Nursing Science, 6:47, 1984.
Snyder SH. Opiate receptors and internal opiates. Scientific American, 236:44, 1977.
Stein M, et al. Immune disorders. *In* Kaplan HI, Sadock BJ (eds). Comprehensive Textbook of Psychiatry, 4th ed. Baltimore: Williams & Wilkins, 1985.
Thompson TL. Headache. *In* Kaplan HI, Sadock BJ (eds). Comprehensive Textbook of Psychiatry, 4th Ed. Baltimore: Williams & Wilkins, 1985.
Thompson TL. Psychosomatic disorders. *In* Talbott JA, Hales RE, Yudofsky SC (eds). Textbook of Psychiatry, 4th ed. Washington DC: American Psychiatric Press, 1988.
Varcarolis EM. Relaxation. *In* Lego S (ed). American Handbook of Psychiatric Nursing. Philadelphia: J.B. Lippincott Company, 1984.
Weiner H. Respiratory disorders. *In* Kaplan HI, Sadock BJ (eds). Comprehensive Textbook of Psychiatry, 4th ed. Baltimore: Williams & Wilkins, 1985.
Wilder JF, Plutchik R. Stress and psychiatry. *In* Kaplan HI, Sadock BJ (eds). Comprehensive Textbook of Psychiatry, 4th ed. Baltimore: Williams & Wilkins, 1985.
Wood C. The hostile heart. Psychology Today, 20:10, 1986.

Self-Study Exercises

Match the word with the correct definition.

1. ________ Describes the interrelationship between psyche (mind) and soma (body).
2. ________ The conversion of emotions into physical symptoms.
3. ________ Physical symptoms that are psychologically induced or maintained.
4. ________ Those gains a person receives from an emotional or physical symptom that results in attention, ease in manipulating one's environment, or getting out of required responsibilities.
5. ________ The body's organized system response to stress, consisting of three stages: (a) alarm, (b) resistance, and (c) exhaustion.

A. Primary gain
B. Psychogenic
C. Secondary gain
D. Somatize
E. Psychsomatic
F. GAS
G. Fight or flight response
H. Denial

True or false. Correct the false statements.

6. ________ People with a psychophysiological disorder often do not experience a great deal of subjective anxiety.
7. ________ Denial, repression, and somatizing are predominant coping styles among people with psychophysiological disorders.
8. ________ Disorders considered psychophysiological are not serious in nature because they are "all in the head."
9. ________ External stressors include interpersonal relationships, financial security, and job satisfaction.
10. ________ The number of life changes is thought to have little to do with the onset or severity of a psychophysiological condition.
11. ________ Psychological and physical ways of coping learned early in life play an important part in how a person will manifest stress as an adult.
12. ________ Intelligence, knowledge, and religious beliefs can alter the way a person's body responds to stress.
13. ________ Environmental supports have no correlation to outcome of a psychophysiological disorder.

Complete the statements by filling in the appropriate information.

14. When Mrs. Hennies's ulcerative colitis forced her to stop working, she found she received a great deal of attention from friends and neighbors. This could be seen as a ________________ gain from her illness.
15. A young woman of 40 has a great deal of difficulty recognizing and dealing with her aggression. Each time she is in a situation in which she experiences disrespect or hostility from others, she gets terrible migraine headaches.

    A. State one possible nursing diagnosis.

    ____

    B. Identify two possible short term goals.

    ____

    ____

Short Answer

16. For the following patient remarks (1) identify a negative reaction that a nurse might experience and (2) compose a useful response.

    A. "Oh I just don't know what to do . . . I can't seem to do anything without feeling pain . . . Do you have any idea how awful it is to be in pain when nobody seems to care?"

    B. "First it started in my left arm . . . then my right arm . . . now the rash has spread all over my body . . . (time goes on), and then I tried this new lotion . . . "

17. Name four relaxation techniques that nurses can learn to teach their clients.
18. Name two classifications of drugs that can alter stress in a person with a psychophysiological disorder.
19. Name three therapeutic modalities that a nurse at the master's level might practice on a client with a psychophysiological disorder.

CHAPTER 16

Repetitive and Ineffective "Neurotic Defenses"

Helene S. Charron

OUTLINE

KEY TERMS AND CONCEPTS

The key terms and concepts listed here also appear in bold where they are defined or discussed in this chapter.

PHOBIAS
OBSESSIONS
EGO-ALIEN/EGO-DYSTONIC
EGO-SYNTONIC
PRIMARY GAIN
SECONDARY GAIN

ANTIANXIETY DRUGS
ANXIOLYTIC
AGORAPHOBIA
SOCIAL PHOBIA
SIMPLE PHOBIA
OBSESSIONS
COMPULSIONS
SOMATIZATION
MALINGERING
"LA BELLE INDIFFERENCE"
DISSOCIATIVE DISORDERS
DISSOCIATION
DEPERSONALIZATION
PSYCHOGENIC AMNESIA
FUGUE
MULTIPLE PERSONALITY

OBJECTIVES

After studying this chapter, the student will be able to:

1. Identify various theories associated with the anxiety, somatoform, and dissociative disorders.
2. Formulate appropriate nursing diagnoses that can be useful when working with a person with anxiety, somatoform, or dissociative disorder.
3. Propose realistic and measurable long term and short term goals for clients with anxiety, somatoform, and dissociative disorders.
4. Discuss interventions that (a) reduce anxiety and support client during ongoing therapy and (b) assist client to use more effective coping strategies.
5. Evaluate the effectiveness of care based on established outcome criteria.
6. Compare and contrast characteristics of psychotic and "neurotic disorders."
7. Identify examples of primary and secondary gain.
8. Analyze the value of ego-dystonic symptoms to the client.
9. Describe the clinical manifestations of the anxiety disorder, the somatoform disorder, and the dissociative disorder.
10. Identify the ego defense mechanisms commonly associated with each of the clinical disorders discussed in this chapter.
11. Identify psychiatric treatment modalities useful for each of the clinical disorders.
12. Describe the nursing roles associated with each of the appropriate treatments.
13. Recognize negative feelings commonly experienced by nurses assigned to clients manifesting ego-dystonic symptoms.
14. Contrast malingering with ego-dystonic behavior.

As discussed in Chapter 8, ego defense mechanisms are unconsciously used by everyone as buffers against anxiety. This chapter focuses on a group of disorders that result when anxiety is not relieved by ordinary use of defense mechanisms. In these disorders, the individual resorts to the use of multiple defense mechanisms resulting in repetitive and ineffective behaviors. These disorders are

1. Anxiety Disorders
2. Somatoform Disorders
3. Dissociative Disorders

Placement of these disorders on the anxiety continuum can be seen in Figure 16–1.

Historically, these disorders were classified as neurotic disorders. This nomenclature created confusion because its meaning and the characteristics of the disorders were not consistently interpreted by therapists. The DSM III-R (1987) now classifies the old "neurotic disorders" into three groups according to behaviors and symptoms. These groups are the anxiety disorders, the somatoform disorders, and the dissociative disorders. Figure 16–2 provides an overview of these disorders.

Common behaviors and symptoms observed in these disorders include the following:

- **Overt anxiety** with its attendant physical, psychological, and cognitive symptoms (see Chapter 8).
- **Phobias:** excessive, irrational fears causing the individual to avoid the feared object or situation.
- **Obsessions:** persistent and intrusive thoughts that cannot be dismissed.

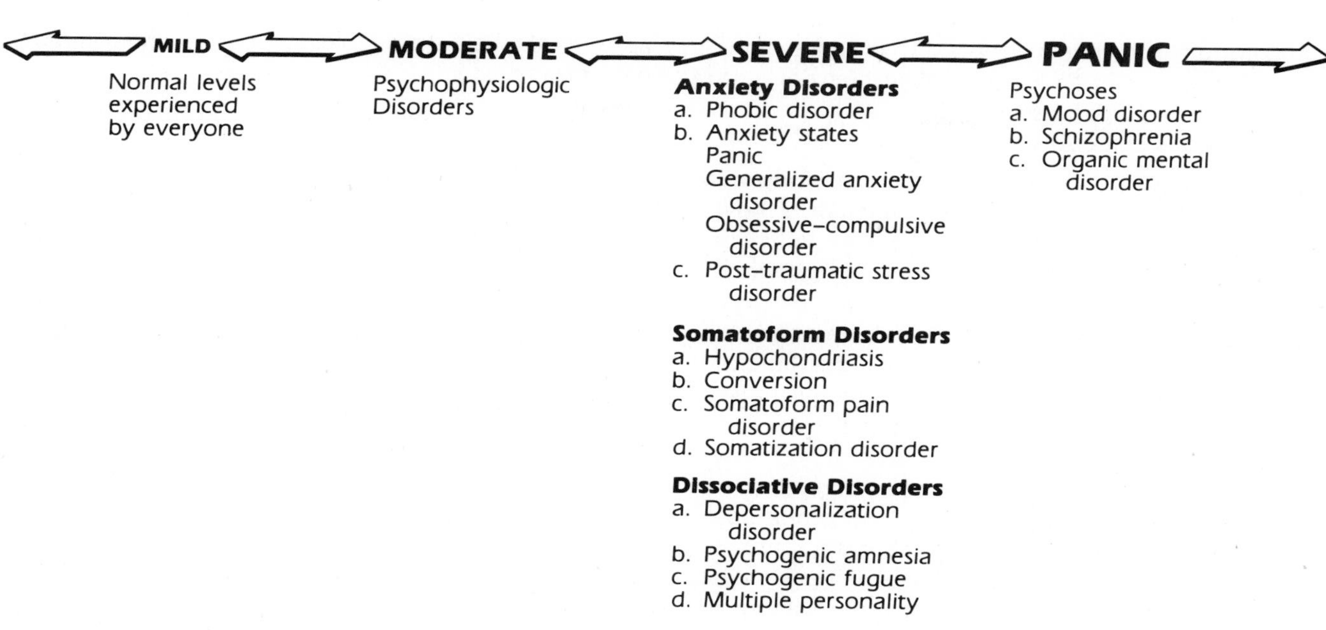

Figure 16–1. *The anxiety continuum.*

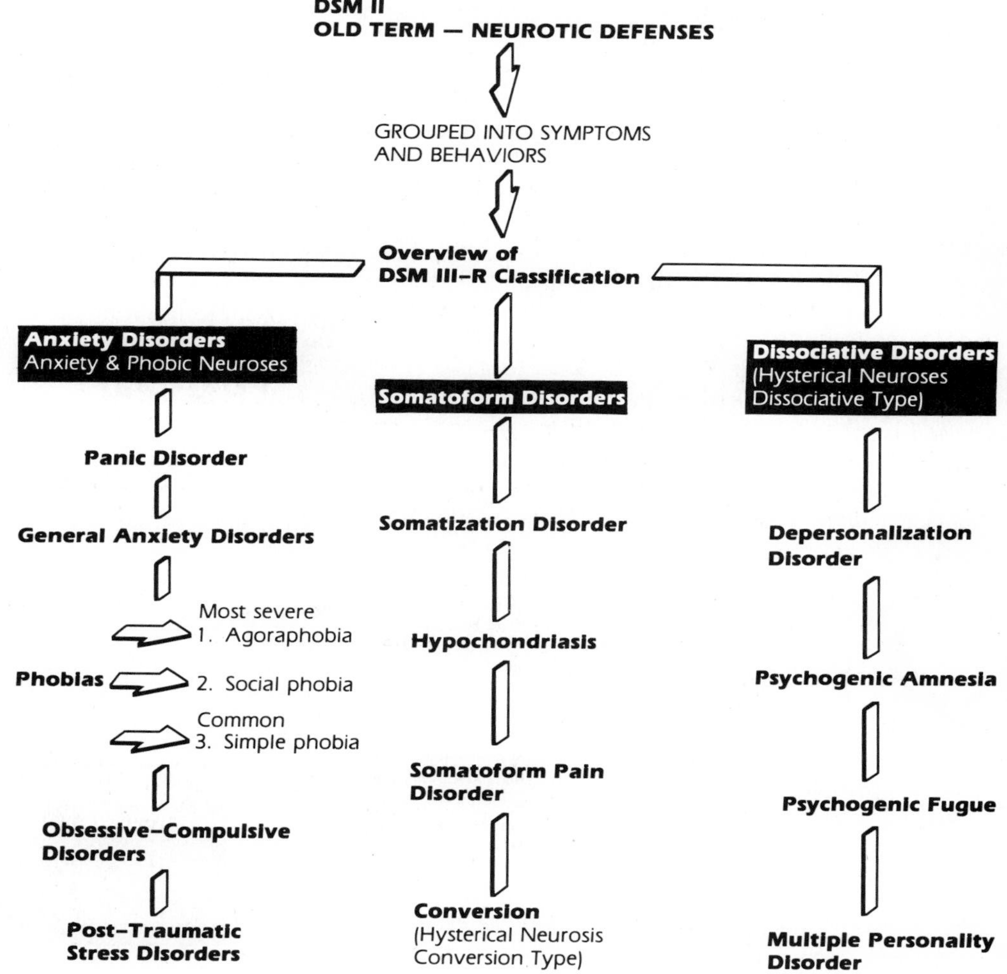

Figure 16–2. *Overview of anxiety, somatoform, and dissociative disorders.*

- **Compulsions:** rituals designed to produce or prevent some event and thereby relieve anxiety.
- Changes in consciousness.
- Alterations in identity.

The symptoms observed in anxiety, somatoform, and dissociative disorders are termed ego-alien or ego-dystonic and are often recognized by the individual displaying them as strange or "silly" and not wholly adaptive. The individual experiences feelings of dissatisfaction, unhappiness, and low self-esteem as a result of their expression. **Ego-alien** and **ego-dystonic** are synonymous terms used to describe symptoms that are unacceptable to the person who has them and not compatible with the person's view of self (e.g., a phobia for cats). **Ego-syntonic** symptoms, on the other hand, are behaviors or beliefs with which clients are comfortable. Clients experience ego-syntonic symptoms as compatible with their personal ideas or impulses. For example, a man who is paranoid (suspicious) might believe the FBI plans to kill him. He does *not* experience this belief as silly or strange. The belief that others wish to harm him is compatible with his suspicious nature and with his view of the world. (See Chapters 17 and 20 for people who display ego-syntonic symptoms.)

Although aware of the "oddness" of ego-dystonic symptoms, individuals who use them feel powerless to change them. Because these behaviors initially produce anxiety relief, they are self-reinforcing and are used again when anxiety occurs. Unfortunately for the individual, most ego-dystonic behaviors are effective in reducing anxiety for only a short time. When anxiety recurs, the behavior must be repeated. By repeating the same behavior in response to anxiety, the individual never learns to cope with the original stress. This process is conceptualized in Figure 16–3.

As time goes by, the person develops *rigid and repetitive behavioral patterns*. Individuals employing ego-dystonic behaviors have no energy to devote to personal growth or to developing mutually satisfying relationships with others. These individuals usually develop inflexible patterns of relating to people. Two of the more common patterns are

1. Exhibiting excessive dependence upon others.
2. Using tactics to distance self from others.

Behaviors associated with these two patterns of relating are described in Table 16–1.

The course of these disorders can be complicated by the development of secondary gains. In the course of these disorders the nurse can usually identify both primary and secondary gains resulting from the use of the symptom(s). The term **primary gain** refers to the anxiety relief resulting from the use of defense mechanisms and symptom formation. **Secondary gain** is defined as any benefit the individual obtains as a result of the symptoms, e.g., financial gain, getting attention, being able to avoid responsibility, or being able to get one's own way. Individuals who experience ego-dystonic symptoms experience primary gains and often secondary gains as a result of their symptoms. The more satisfying and entrenched the secondary gains, the more difficult it is for the individuals to give up their symptoms, maladaptive as the symptoms may be.

Standard I: Theory

Although it is understandable how ego-dystonic symptoms come to be adopted as methods of dealing with anxiety, less is known about the underlying causes. It is helpful to consider (1) biochemical, (2) genetic, (3) psychosocial, and (4) sociocultural factors involved in symptom formation.

BIOCHEMICAL

Researchers are currently exploring possible biochemical causes for anxiety. Andreasen (1984) discusses several interesting research findings.

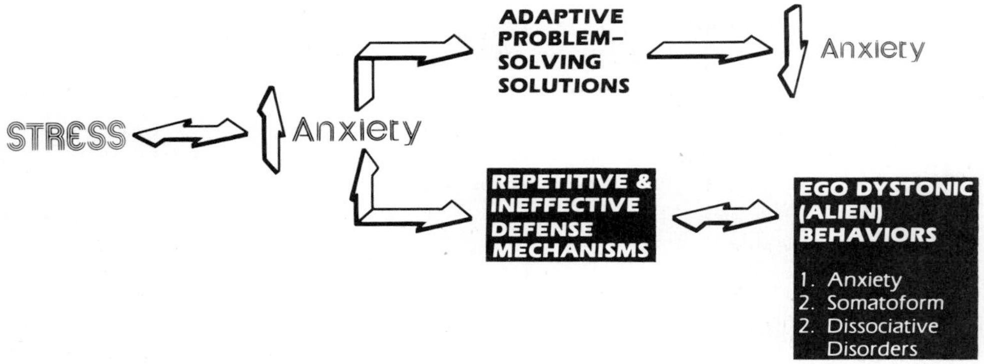

Figure 16–3. *Conceptualization of the process of "neurotic defenses."*

Table 16–1 • BEHAVIORS NOTED AMONG INDIVIDUALS DEMONSTRATING EGO-DYSTONIC DEFENSES AGAINST ANXIETY

PATTERNS OF RELATIONSHIPS	CHARACTERISTIC BEHAVIORS
Dependence on Others	1. Acts helpless. 2. Treats others as superior to self, is self-deprecatory. 3. Adopts others' opinions. 4. Indecisive. 5. Seeks advice. 6. Submits or defers to others. 7. Seeks attention and approval. 8. Tolerates criticism poorly.
Distances Self From Others	1. Believes others are hostile. 2. Takes control of situations. 3. Displays anger when authority/opinions are questioned. 4. Employs manipulation. 5. Is demanding. 6. Rarely admits feelings. 7. Finds fault/blames others. 8. Rejects help. 9. Wants to be left alone. 10. Aloof. 11. Withdraws/rebels when placed in dependent role. 12. Rejects advice. 13. Assumes moral superiority. 14. Treats others as inferior.

1. The brain's gamma-aminobutyric acid (GABA) system is believed to exert a "braking effect" by slowing down other brain systems that produce excitation, arousal, or anxiety.
2. The brain contains receptor or binding sites for antianxiety drugs. Possible substances produced by anxiety-prone individuals may interfere with the function of these binding sites (Hollander et al. 1988).
3. Individuals who have panic attacks tend to have higher levels of norepinephrine, suggesting some abnormality in the catecholamine system.
4. In about 90% of panic-prone individuals, panic attacks can be induced by infusing sodium lactate.
5. Panic-prone clients who are treated with imipramine, a tricyclic antidepressant, report fewer or no panic attacks.
6. Obsessional thinking can be reduced with the tricyclic clomipramine (Anafranil), which reduces serotonergic activity (Hollander et al. 1988). This drug is soon to be released in this country.

These findings indicate that anxiety may be, at least in part, a biochemical event that can be controlled or modified with neuroregulation. Research on the effect of stress and anxiety on neurotransmitters and neuroregulatory systems is likely to produce new and relevant information.

GENETIC

Andreasen (1984) indicates that data from family and twin studies seem to support the premise that a predisposition to develop anxiety disorders may be partially hereditary. One study by Crowe and associates (1983) found a 24.7% incidence of panic disorders among relatives of clients with panic disorders compared with a 2.3% incidence in a normal control group.

PSYCHOSOCIAL

Many theorists and clinicians believe many of these disorders are caused by psychosocial factors such as the following:

- Disturbed family patterns and interpersonal relationships.
- Faulty use of defense mechanisms.
- Faulty learning.
- Threats to one's physical and emotional integrity.

For example, individuals with multiple personalities, almost without exception, have experienced abuse or trauma in early childhood. Amnesia begins suddenly, usually during or after a severe psychosocial stress. Many individuals with somatization disorders were raised by parents who were overly concerned with bodily functions and learned to be overly concerned themselves. Phobias, too, may be the result of faulty learning. Vignettes illustrating evidence of psychosocial factors in causation can be seen in Box 16–1.

From a growth and development perspective, many theorists believe the anxiety, somatoform, and dissociative disorders may stem from difficulty in family relationships occurring before the age of five. Ritualistic behavior (exaggerated in obsessive-compulsive disorders), for example, is often attributed to problems occurring during the stage of toilet training (two to three years). Individuals with somatization disorders often demonstrate dependence and the need to be protected. A child may learn that in his or her family, the only way to receive parental response in times of emotional stress is through "illness behaviors." Both dependence and the need to be protected are traits related to the early years of life. Underlying conflicts with sexual themes can often be traced to experiences and perceptions of the child between the ages of three and five, the time of the family triangle.

SOCIOCULTURAL

According to Colby and McGuire (1981), it can be estimated that 15% to 20% of the population of the United States suffers from some form of "neurotic disorder." Coleman, Butcher, and Carson (1980) state that little reliable data on the incidence of these disorders exist in other cultures. Kidson and Jones (1968) note that among Australian aborigines, somatic complaints become more common with exposure to contemporary civilization, and Coleman, Butcher, and Carson (1980) suggest that anxiety disorders and ritualistic behaviors

Box 16–1. VIGNETTES ILLUSTRATING PSYCHOSOCIAL CAUSATION

Difficulty Handling Dangerous Impulses

Barbara, a 21-year-old student, became severely anxious whenever she heard a siren. She felt afraid that a disaster involving her family had occurred. Therapy uncovered the fact that she had been the butt of many family jokes. She had repressed her hostile feelings, but when repression failed, projections of hostility were seen in her anxiety over the imaginary disasters.

Difficulty Coping With Loss

Martha, deserted by her mother at age three, was raised by her very strict father who put her through beautician's school before he remarried. She performed well for her first boss, but when she transferred to a new site where the boss was exacting and critical, Martha developed severe anxiety. Martha's loss of relationships and self-esteem were central to her anxiety.

Difficulty Meeting High Goals

Andora, 42, returned to college after her children married. She had been described as the "perfect mother" but was very dependent on her husband. While in college, she became very anxious before each examination. Her history revealed that her parents had set high goals for her from childhood and that she had come to fear failure.

Modeling by Significant Others

Pete's mother and father were both described as tense, anxious people. From childhood Pete has felt tense and anxious and now seeks therapy to learn a more relaxed lifestyle.

Anna's mother frequently went to bed because of "sick headaches." Anna and her father waited on her mother to cure and prevent the headaches. Later, Anna used headaches to avoid stress and communicate feelings and needs.

Physical Abuse

Jeanne was three when her stepfather began to abuse her. She describes learning to concentrate hard, clear her mind, and imagine she was another child, an animal, or an adult who was unafraid. Jeanne is host to five distinct personalities.

Table 16–2 • PHYSICAL ASSESSMENT STRATEGIES

PHYSICAL ASSESSMENT	DATA GATHERING STRATEGIES
Presence of anxiety Potential to flee/fight	"Tell me about what you are experiencing." "What are your concerns about your state of health?" Observe appearance, behavior, posture, gait, expression.
Impact of anxiety on physical functioning	Monitor pulse, respirations, sleep patterns, elimination, appetite, energy level.

See Chapter 8 for specific physical symptoms of anxiety.

Table 16–3 • PSYCHOLOGICAL ASSESSMENT STRATEGIES

PSYCHOLOGICAL ASSESSMENT	DATA GATHERING STRATEGIES
Understanding of illness	"What problem brings you here?" "Did this problem occur suddenly or over a period of time?"
Mood	"Describe how you are feeling." Observe affect.
Self-esteem	"How do you feel about yourself?" "What you do you like/dislike about yourself?" "What do you believe you should be doing?"
Normal coping ability	"When you experience stress, what do you do to decrease it?" "What do you do to handle a very distressing situation?"
Defense mechanisms used	Observe/listen during interview.
Orientation	"What is your name?" "What is the name of this place?"
Memory	"Tell me about the events of the past 24 hours." "What are the names of two of your former teachers?"
Attention/concentration	"Subtract 7 from 100 and keep subtracting 7 from the answer you get each time." Note distractibility, vigilance.
Thought content/process	Note circumstantiality (many digressions before eventually concluding a thought), blocking (sudden stopping of speech due to anxiety). "Are you preoccupied with any idea?" "Does one thought repeatedly force itself into awareness?" "Do you have any especially strong fears?"
Potential for suicide	If client indicates feelings of hopelessness, helplessness, or worthlessness, investigate whether he or she has considered suicide.

are more common in societies with high technology. With regard to geography, Dohrenwend and Dohrenwend (1974) found neurotic disorders to occur more frequently among urban dwellers than among rural populations. In general, we can infer that when a society undergoes rapid changes, the stress induced by the changes places the group at risk for the development of these disorders.

Standard II: Data Collection

Assessment should be concerned with the collection of data from the physical, psychological, and social spheres. Specific symptoms manifested by the client should be noted, along with the statements made by the client about his or her subjective distress. The nurse must use clinical judgment to determine the level of anxiety the client is experiencing. (Objective and subjective data associated with each level can be reviewed in Chapter 8.) External and internal stressors should be identified if possible, and the degree to which the client's life is disrupted should be evaluated. Since clients with these disorders usually remain in contact with reality, they are often able to collaborate to some extent with the nurse during the assessment process. Suggestions for the kinds of questions the nurse can ask during the assessment of physical, psychological, and social data are presented in Tables 16–2, 16–3, and 16–4.

People who are experiencing an anxiety, somatoform, or dissociative disorder usually use a limited number of defense mechanisms. The defense mechanisms being employed and the purpose they serve should be determined. Table 16–5 lists commonly used defense mechanisms, behaviors associated with the defense mechanisms, and the purposes served. Although it is difficult to pose specific questions to assess use of defense mechanisms, their use may become apparent to the nurse during the course of the interview.

Although violence is exhibited by only a small number of clients, the nurse must be aware that high levels of anxiety may evoke the need for "fight or flight." The nurse must assess for potential aggression as a defense against high anxiety levels. The potential for suicide must also be assessed. Suicide is a possibility when a person's self-esteem is very low, and the distress related to his or her inability to control ego-dystonic symptoms is high.

Data are collected from clients exhibiting anxiety or ego-dystonic behaviors (anxiety, somatoform, or dissociative disorders) and from clients who have psychotic symptoms. Table 16–6 compares and contrasts ego-alien behaviors with psychotic behaviors.

Table 16–4 • SOCIAL ASSESSMENT STRATEGIES

SOCIAL ASSESSMENT	DATA GATHERING STRATEGIES
Characteristic patterns of relationships	"Describe your relationship with family/friends/peers."
Identification of stressors or threats to self-concept, role, values, social status, support system	"What do you think might be causing this problem?"
	"What do you think might be influencing the way you feel?"
	"What changes have occurred in your life during the past year?"
Ability to function	"How is this problem interfering with your life?"
	Investigate effects on work, school, church, hobbies, social activities, sexual functioning.
Degree of strain in relationships	"Has this problem placed a strain on relationships with others?"
	"Describe how you feel when you are around others."
Secondary gains	Note benefits to client as result of symptoms.
Diversional activity	"What do you like to do for fun/recreation?"

Table 16-5 • DEFENSE MECHANISMS COMMONLY USED BY CLIENTS WITH ANXIETY, SOMATOFORM, AND DISSOCIATIVE DISORDERS

BEHAVIOR	EXAMPLE	PURPOSE SERVED
	Conversion	
Loss or alteration in body function; though the loss or alteration is physical, it actually expresses emotional conflict.	Woman sees husband kissing another woman and suddenly becomes blind.	Physical symptom resolves the anxiety-producing conflict. Loss of vision prevents "seeing" or acknowledging her husband's involvement with another woman.
	Denial	
An aspect of reality is not acknowledged.	Client cannot see the relationship between his or her physical symptoms and the psychological conflict, so he or she maintains the illness is of physical origin even though diagnostic tests do not substantiate this.	Lack of acknowledgment keeps the conflict out of awareness, thus reducing anxiety.
	Displacement	
Shift of emotion associated with anxiety-producing person, object, or situation to a less threatening object.	Client has abnormal fear of cats. In therapy it is discovered that client is sexually attracted to sister-in-law.	In phobias, anxiety is reduced when strong feelings about the original object are directed at a less threatening object, and that object is avoided.
	Dissociation	
Separating a group of mental processes from consciousness or identity.	Amnesic client cannot remember own identity, address, or facts about self. Client with multiple personality alternately displays self as "Ann," "Timmy," "the snake lady," and "Bad Bertha."	Anxiety is reduced when reality is avoided. Each individual personality functions without anxiety.
	Isolation	
Facts associated with an event remain conscious, but associated feelings are separated from the experience.	In conversion disorder, client loses use of arm and discusses this without affect.	Anxiety-producing feelings are kept out of awareness.
	Intellectualization	
Excessive use of reasoning, logic, or words usually without experiencing associated feelings.	Obsessive-compulsive client discusses details of situation rather than feelings about it.	Anxiety is reduced when feelings do not have to be acknowledged or felt.
	Rationalization	
Giving a socially acceptable reason for a behavior rather than acknowledging the "true" reason.	Clients with somatoform disorders often use their physical symptom as the "reason" for needing to be dependent.	Anxiety is reduced when the "true" reason does not have to be acknowledged
	Reaction-Formation	
Showing evidence of conscious attitudes or behaviors that are the opposite of the unconscious feelings.	Obsessions and compulsions often result. Client has strong aggressive feelings toward significant other and repeatedly thinks, "I love him with all my heart," or uses excessive, exaggerated loving behavior toward person. Hostile impulses are also countered by excessive shows of concern and checking behaviors designed to protect a person from a perceived harmful event or object.	Anxiety-producing unacceptable thought or feeling is kept out of awareness by the opposite feeling or idea.

Table continued on following page

Table 16-5 • DEFENSE MECHANISMS COMMONLY USED BY CLIENTS WITH ANXIETY, SOMATOFORM, AND DISSOCIATIVE DISORDERS *Continued*

BEHAVIOR	EXAMPLE	PURPOSE SERVED
	Regression	
Demonstrating behaviors that were appropriate at an earlier stage of development.	Client develops somatic symptoms that require others to care for him or her as for an infant.	Anxiety-producing conflict over dependence; independence is reduced.
	Client with conversion disorder behaves in a little-girlish way and husband responds in a fatherly fashion.	Conflicts about sexuality and dependence are reduced, lowering anxiety.
	Repression	
Unconsciously pushing an anxiety-producing idea or feeling out of awareness.	Is used in association with other defense mechanisms that keep anxiety-producing ideas and feelings out of awareness.	Lowers anxiety.
	Substitution	
An unacceptable thought or emotion is replaced by an acceptable one.	For an obsessive-compulsive client, counting various objects in the environment keep obscene thoughts out of awareness.	When troublesome thoughts are kept out of awareness, anxiety is reduced.
	In hypochondriasis, focusing on illness may deflect guilt, sexual, aggressive, or dependent thoughts.	Guilt and low self-esteem associated with unacceptable drives are kept out of awareness.
	Undoing	
Performing an act that cancels out an already performed and unacceptable act or idea.	Compulsive rituals such as handwashing, cleaning, checking.	Symbolic activity neutralizes the original unacceptable act or idea.

Standard III: Diagnosis

Several nursing diagnoses should be considered for clients experiencing anxiety and ego-dystonic behaviors associated with anxiety reduction. The nursing diagnosis *anxiety* is an obvious choice, but the individualized etiology statement may be more difficult to determine. Possible etiologies include (but are not limited to) the following:

- Exposure to phobic object.
- Threat to self-concept.
- Actual or perceived loss of significant other.
- Actual or perceived change in socioeconomic status.
- Change in status and prestige.
- Threat to or change in health status.
- Lack of recognition from others.

Ineffective individual coping related to overdependence on others or related to distancing oneself from others may be relevant if the client has been assessed as using dysfunctional interpersonal patterns. Other possible etiologies might include

- Physiological manifestations of persistent stress and anxiety.
- Excessive negative beliefs about self.
- Inadequate psychological resources.
- Changes in physical environment.
- Childhood abuse.
- Unsatisfactory support system.

Disturbance in self-esteem is nearly always an actual diagnosis. It may be related to inability to control ego-dystonic symptoms or to other individualized etiologies. A diagnosis of *altered role performance* is possible when assessment of the social domain reveals inability to assume responsibilities associated with the usual roles. Disturbance in self-esteem may be related to threat to physical safety or threat to self-concept, especially if the client displays amnesia, fugue, or multiple personality.

Table 16–6 • EGO-ALIEN BEHAVIORS VERSUS PSYCHOTIC BEHAVIORS

EGO-ALIEN (DYSTONIC) BEHAVIOR	PSYCHOTIC BEHAVIOR
Appearance	
Usually unremarkable except for tension and autonomic symptoms.	May look atypical, bizarre. Grooming may be poor.
Mood/Affect	
Usually appropriate to thought content. Anxiety and depression common.	May be excessive, blunted, or inappropriate to thought content.
Perceptions	
Usually intact except in panic episodes.	Altered, illusions and hallucinations common.
Thinking (cognition)	
Preoccupied with problems, somatic symptoms, may experience depersonalization, phobias, obsessions, indecisiveness, poor concentration, sense of doom. Able to abstract, perform math calculations except in severe anxiety.	Decreased reality testing, delusions, concrete thinking, loose associations.
Orientation	
Intact.	Often impaired.
Memory	
Usually intact except in panic, amnesia, and fugue.	Often impaired.
Insight	
Blames self for psychological problems.	Denies illness, blames others for problems.

Disturbance in *body image* could be related to negative feelings about body image if the client has a somatoform disorder, such as pain or body dysmorphic disorder.

Altered thought processes related to moderate, severe, or panic level anxiety must be considered as a possible diagnosis. The specific thought disorder that is manifested should be specified, e.g., phobia, obsession, inability to concentrate.

Diversional activity deficit is another nursing diagnosis often appropriate for clients with these disorders. The lives of these individuals are so focused on anxiety control that they rarely indulge in pleasurable activity. Many do not know the rules for simple games or do not have the skills to join common activities, such as bowling. If self-esteem is poor, the client may not believe he or she deserves enjoyment. Embarrassment over the "odd" behaviors may prevent the individual from participating with others.

Other nursing diagnoses that should be considered in light of assessment data include the following:

- *Altered family processes* related to an ill family member.
- *Social isolation* related to emotional handicaps (phobias, panic anxiety).
- *Potential for violence* related to sensory-perceptual alterations secondary to severe/panic level anxiety.
- *Spiritual distress* related to lack of hope.
- *Sensory-perceptual alteration*: specify blindness, deafness or other, related to repression of severe anxiety.
- *Impaired skin integrity* related to rituals of excessive washing or excessive picking at skin.

- *Altered nutrition: less than body requirements*, related to inability to stop performance of rituals long enough to eat or related to fear of germs.
- *Ineffective breathing pattern: hyperventilation*, related to severe anxiety.
- *Self-care deficit* related to specify (paralysis of body part; conversion symptom of blindness, deafness; pain; indecisiveness; performance of rituals; or others).
- *Fear* related to phobic object or situation — specify.

Standard IV: Planning

Planning occurs on two levels: (1) the content level — planning goals — and (2) the process level — nurses' reactions and feelings.

CONTENT LEVEL — PLANNING GOALS

Content planning involves establishing goals, outcome criteria, and interventions for a client. The client should actively participate in the process of goal setting whenever possible. By sharing decision making with the client, the nurse increases the potential for goal attainment. Shared planning is appropriate when working with the client with mild or moderate anxiety, but planning remains with the nurse when the client displays severe or panic level anxiety. Sample goals and outcome criteria for several of the relevant nursing diagnoses can be seen in Table 16–7.

Nursing interventions for assisting the client who is experiencing one of the levels of anxiety from mild to panic are discussed in depth in Chapter 8. Although interventions must be individualized to meet each client's unique situation, the planned strategies are geared toward the following objectives:

- Relieving the client's immediate distress.
- Helping the client feel understood.
- Assisting the client in identifying the source of the anxiety.
- Identifying the client's strengths, coping skills, and resources and supporting healthy aspects of the client's personality.
- Supporting the client while new coping measures are learned.
- Assisting the client in applying what is learned during therapy to his or her life situation.
- Assisting the family in changing behavioral patterns that support the client's dysfunctional behaviors.

PROCESS LEVEL — NURSES' REACTIONS AND FEELINGS

When the nurse has contact with an anxious client or with a client who uses ego-dystonic defense to cope with anxiety, the nurse may experience strong feelings. Often the anxiety originating in the client is experienced by the nurse empathically (see Chapter 8). Self-monitoring is vital in order to identify those feelings originating in the nurse and those transferred to the nurse from the client. Without self-monitoring, peer supervision, or other interventions, the following pattern may develop:

Client anxiety is transmitted to the nurse.
↓
The nurse develops feelings of anxiety.
↓
The nurse's anxiety is communicated to the client.
↓
The client's anxiety increases.

Table 16–7 • SAMPLE GOALS FOR NURSING DIAGNOSES FOR CLIENTS WITH ANXIETY, SOMATOFORM, OR DISSOCIATIVE DISORDERS

NURSING DIAGNOSIS	POSSIBLE GOAL AND OUTCOME
Anxiety	Client will demonstrate psychological and physiological comfort by (state the date), as evidenced by • pulse and respiration within normal parameters, • absence of symptoms associated with autonomic stimulation, • statement that anxiety has decreased.

Table 16–7 • SAMPLE GOALS FOR NURSING DIAGNOSES FOR CLIENTS WITH ANXIETY, SOMATOFORM, OR DISSOCIATIVE DISORDERS *Continued*

NURSING DIAGNOSIS	POSSIBLE GOAL AND OUTCOME
Ineffective Individual Coping	Client will employ alternative coping resources to establish and maintain effective interpersonal relationships by (state the date), as evidenced by • appropriate balancing of dependence on and distancing from others, • controlled expression of feelings, • successful use of problem-solving skills, • verbalization of ability to cope.
Disturbance in Self-Esteem	Client will demonstrate improved self-esteem by (state the date) as evidenced by • identifying two personal strengths, • making three positive statements about self, • stating that it is okay not to be perfect.
Disturbance in Self-Esteem Related to Change in Role Performance	Client will demonstrate ability to perform in usual roles at premorbid level by (state the date), as evidenced by • performing usual work and social activities and hobbies, • interacting with significant others in mutually supportive ways.
Disturbance in Self-Esteem Related to Problems With Personal Identity	Client will demonstrate ability to cope with stress without using dissociation or depersonalization by (state the date), as evidenced by • explaining relationship among symptoms, anxiety, and defenses, • recognizing existence of more than one personality, if client has multiple personalities, • maintenance of personal identity in times of high stress.
Altered Thought Processes	Client will demonstrate ability to concentrate by (state the date). Client will report absence of obsessive thoughts by (state the date). Client will report experiencing, and will exhibit, mild to moderate anxiety in presence of phobic object by (state the date).
Diversional Activity Deficit	Client will use leisure time constructively by (state the date), as evidenced by • listing diversional activities of interest, • participating in one diversional activity each day.
Social Isolation	Client will increase interaction with others by (state the date), as evidenced by • interacting with a significant other or peer daily for 20 minutes, • participating in two group activities each week.
Powerlessness	Client will report feeling in control over current situation by (state the date).
Potential for Violence: Self-Directed	Client will remain safe during span of time agreed upon with therapist by (state the date). Client will maintain control.
Knowledge Deficit	Client will state relationship between anxiety and the developing of his or her symptoms by (state the date).

As the process continues, the result is an upward spiraling of anxiety in both the nurse and the client.

The nurse may experience feelings of frustration or anger or both while working with these clients. For example, the rituals of the obsessive-compulsive client may frustrate the nurse's need to accomplish certain tasks within a given time. In caring for the phobic client, the nurse may become frustrated after realizing that both the client and the nurse regard the fear as exaggerated and unrealistic, but that the client is unable to overcome the avoidant behavior. Clients with somatoform disorders tend to cling to their unrealistic beliefs about their physical symptoms long after health care workers have established a lack of physical findings. Nurses may feel frustration or anger over the secondary gains the client receives from family or others.

It is important to remember that behavioral change is often accomplished very slowly. The process of recovery is very different from that seen in a client with an infection who is given antibiotics and begins to demonstrate improvement within 24 to 48 hours. Nurses tend to become impatient with the anxious client and feel frustration and anger when the client does not make rapid progress. Negative feelings are easily transmitted to the client, who then feels increasingly anxious.

The nurse who feels anger or frustration may withdraw from the client both emotionally and physically. This does not go unnoticed by the client. The result is that the client feels greater anxiety. Setting small attainable goals can help prevent the nurse from feeling overwhelmed by negative feelings toward the client.

It is not uncommon for the nurse to experience feelings of fear when confronted by the client in panic. Also, the rapid shifts in personality seen when caring for clients with multiple personalities can be frightening. The team approach to intervention minimizes the fear nurses may experience.

At the very least, the nurse often experiences an increase in tension and fatigue that is related to mental strain associated with working with clients whose needs never seem to be satisfied. Because the anxiety of these clients is controlled for only a short time by the ego-dystonic behaviors, client anxiety recurs and the nurse is called upon to intervene again and again. Unlike the client whose dressing needs to be changed twice a day, this client requires emotional bandaging many times a day.

It may be helpful for the nurse to consider the level of regression displayed by the client. If the client's behavior can be seen as regressive rather than perverse, staff can cope more easily. For example, dependence, excessive demands, and frequent reassurance-seeking are behaviors associated with unmet needs of infancy. Clients with somatoform disorders often demonstrate these behaviors. Excessive neatness, rituals, obsessions, and "pickiness" are behaviors related to the period of toilet training. Attention seeking, overly dramatic behaviors, problems with authority figures of the same sex, and behaviors that seem "adolescent" indicate problems associated with the family triangle. Clients demonstrating conversion disorder often display these behaviors.

It helps to remember that these behaviors help us identify needs that must be met before the client can go on to develop more mature behaviors. By examining personal feelings, the nurse is better able to identify what brought them about and act constructively.

Standard V: Intervention

The nurse may encounter clients manifesting anxiety or ego-dystonic behaviors associated with anxiety in a variety of settings. Such clients may be seen on a medical-surgical unit, where the primary diagnosis will be associated with physical illness. A holistic approach necessitates consideration of psychological as well as physical needs. If the client's needs are difficult to meet or a large amount of staff time is taken by the client, it may be wise to seek the assistance of the psychiatric liaison team (see Chapter 26).

Clients demonstrating anxiety and ego-dystonic symptoms may be encountered in the psychiatric inpatient and outpatient settings, as well as in the home. Community health nurses and community mental health nurses often implement substantial portions of the long term treatment plan.

V-A: PSYCHOTHERAPEUTIC INTERVENTIONS

Table 16–8 identifies general nursing interventions for clients with anxiety, somatoform, and dissociative disorders.

V-B: HEALTH TEACHING

Clients with anxiety, somatoform, and dissociative disorders often had early childhood experiences that fostered inaccurate conclusions about themselves and their abilities. An important part of therapy involves teaching interpersonal and social skills and providing opportunities for clients to try new behaviors in a nonthreatening environment.

Table 16–8 • GENERAL NURSING INTERVENTIONS

INTERVENTION	RATIONALE
Relieve Client's Immediate Distress	
1. Stay with client.	1. Conveys acceptance, ability to give help.
2. Acknowledge the anxiety.	2. Assists client in identifying feelings.
3. Speak slowly, calmly.	3. Conveys calm, promotes security.
4. Use short, simple sentences.	4. Promotes comprehension.
5. Assure client that you are in control and can assist him or her.	5. Severe anxiety gives feeling of loss of control.
6. Give brief direction.	6. Reduces indecision. Conveys belief that client can respond in healthy manner.
7. Decrease excessive stimuli.	7. Reduces need to focus on diverse stimuli. Promotes ability to concentrate.
8. Walk with pacing client.	8. Gives support while client uses anxiety-generated energy.
9. Increase level of supervision for acutely anxious client.	9. Minimizes self injury and/or loss of control.
10. Allow client to use defenses as long as physical well-being is not seriously jeopardized.	10. Challenging defenses when client is acutely anxious causes further anxiety and may lead to panic.
11. After assessing level of anxiety, administer appropriate dose of anxiolytic agent, if warranted.	11. Reduction of anxiety allows client to use coping skills.
12. Monitor and control own feelings.	12. Anxiety is transmissible. Displays of negative emotion cause client anxiety.
Help Client Feel Understood	
1. Listen.	1. Conveys interest. Fosters trust. Provides tension relief. Permits data gathering. Identifies defenses.
2. Use empathy.	2. Conveys concern. Helps client identify and accept feelings.
3. Focus on reality of present discomfort but not on ego-dystonic symptoms.	3. Acknowledges client's distress but does not reinforce maladaptive behavior.
4. Encourage description of feelings.	4. Facilitates identification of feelings.
5. Help client recognize anxiety.	5. Overcomes denial, resistance.
Assist Client in Identifying Source of Anxiety	
1. Encourage to discuss preceding events.	1. Identification of stressors promotes future change.
2. Link client behavior and feelings.	2. Promotes self-awareness.
Identify Strengths/Coping Skills and Support Healthy Behavior	
1. Identify what has provided relief in the past.	1. Provides awareness of self as individual with some ability to cope.
2. Give positive reinforcement for use of healthy behavior.	2. Positively reinforced behavior tends to be repeated.
Support Client While New Coping Measures Are Learned	
1. Accept client's feelings, especially anger, fear, guilt, or shame.	1. Promotes understanding of universality of these feelings.

Table continued on following page

Table 16–8 • GENERAL NURSING INTERVENTIONS *Continued*

INTERVENTION	RATIONALE
Support Client While New Coping Measures Are Learned *Continued*	
2. Assist with practice of relaxation technique.	2. Relaxation response is enhanced by frequent use. Competence in use increases self-esteem and feelings of being able to control symptoms.
3. Promote sleep with warm bath, warm milk, or sitting with client.	3. Provides alternative to and prevents overuse of anxiolytics.
4. Provide full schedule of activities, especially familiar ones client has enjoyed in the past.	4. Expends anxiety-generated energy constructively. Decreases self-preoccupation. Increases self-esteem by providing success experiences.
5. Give positive feedback for capabilities, competence.	5. Enhances self-esteem.
Assist Client in Applying What's Learned During Therapy To Life Situation	
1. Provide opportunities to engage in normal (healthy) role behaviors.	1. Strengthens role taking and self-esteem.
2. Provide behavioral rehearsals for anticipated stressful situations.	2. Predetermination of coping strategy and practice increases potential for success.
3. Discuss coping strategies client successfully employs.	3. Reinforces use of healthy coping strategies.
Assist Family in Changing Behavioral Patterns That Have Been Supportive of Dysfunctional Behavior	
1. Teach family to give reinforcement for use of healthy behaviors.	1. Positively reinforced behavior tends to be repeated.
2. Teach family not to take over roles normally reserved for client.	2. Minimizes secondary gain.
3. Teach family to give attention to client, not to client's symptoms.	3. Minimizes secondary gain.

Clients often lack accurate knowledge about the effect of stress on the body and about the physiological components of anxiety. This information may be given separately or in conjunction with the teaching of relaxation techniques.

If clients are to receive anxiety-relieving medication, they will need to learn about the desired effect and possible side effects of the drug. Many antianxiety, (anxiolytic) drugs are central nervous system depressants. The importance of strict adherence to prescribed dosage must be taught, since the potential for dependence is high. Specific instructions to the client are discussed under V-D: *Somatic Therapies*.

V-C: ACTIVITIES OF DAILY LIVING

The client's ability to meet basic physical needs is often impaired by anxiety or the use of ego-dystonic defenses against anxiety. Areas often affected are discussed subsequently.

NUTRITION AND FLUID INTAKE. Some anxious clients eat little. Ritualistic clients may be too involved with rituals to eat. Phobic clients may be too afraid of "germs" to eat. On the other hand, some anxious clients seem hungry almost constantly. Nutritious snacks need to be provided. Weighing the client daily and keeping a record of food and fluid intake may be useful assessment tools. The nursing diagnosis *altered nutrition*: specify type, related to severe anxiety should be considered.

PERSONAL HYGIENE AND GROOMING. Some clients are excessively neat and demonstrate time-consuming rituals associated with bathing and dressing. Sometimes the rituals are repeated so often that the client does not leave the bathroom. Maintenance of skin integrity may become a problem when rituals involve excessive washing. The nursing diagnosis *impaired skin integrity* should be considered for these clients.

Some clients are indecisive about bathing and what clothing to wear. For the latter, limiting choices to two outfits would be helpful. In severe indecisiveness, simply presenting the client with the clothing to be worn may be necessary. Some clients have somatic complaints that would seem to prevent them from attending to personal hygiene, e.g., paralysis or blindness. The nursing diagnosis *self-care deficit* may be appropriate in these instances. Matter-of-fact support to assist the client in performing as much of the task as possible is effective. Clients should be encouraged to express thoughts and feelings about self-care. This can provide a basis for later health teaching or for ongoing dialogue about clients' abilities.

ELIMINATION. Obsessive-compulsive clients may be so involved with the performance of rituals that they may suppress the urge to void and defecate. Constipation and urinary tract infections may result. Data analysis for these clients will reflect the need to include nursing diagnoses such as *altered bowel elimination* or *altered urinary elimination* in the care plan.

SLEEP. Anxious clients frequently have difficulty sleeping, and ritualistic clients may perform their rituals to the exclusion of resting and sleeping. Physical exhaustion is a very real possibility for many clients. One nursing diagnosis to consider is *sleep pattern disturbance.* Monitoring sleep and keeping a sleep record may be useful in establishing this diagnosis and evaluating progress.

Ongoing assessment of the client's ability to perform self-care activities is important, as is the establishment of attainable goals.

V-D: SOMATIC THERAPIES

Antianxiety drugs, or more recently referred to as the **anxiolytics,** are used to treat the somatic and psychological symptoms of anxiety. Their use is a valuable adjunct to other therapies. When moderate to severe anxiety is reduced, clients are better able to participate in therapies directed at removing underlying problems. Table 16–9 lists commonly prescribed anxiolytics and gives information about their actions and indications for use.

Drugs classified as benzodiazepines, propranediols, and acetylinic alcohols should be used only on a short term basis owing to their potential to promote psychological and physical dependence. Buspirone, a new anxiolytic agent, does not appear to produce dependence. However, it cannot be used to treat acute anxiety attacks, since it must be given over a several week period before its anxiolytic effects become apparent. Propranolol (Inderal), a beta blocker, is rarely thought of as an antianxiety drug. However, it has been found to be highly effective in blocking the physical symptoms of anxiety experienced by individuals who become anxious before performing or speaking in public. Propranolol does not appear to produce dependence.

The emphasis on treatment for the panic disorders is to block the panic attacks with the aid of medication. The most widely used antipanic drugs are the tricyclic

Table 16–9 • MEDICATIONS USED IN TREATMENT OF ANXIETY DISORDERS

GENERIC NAME	TRADE NAME	ACTION/ INDICATIONS
	Benzodiazepines	
alprazolam	Xanax	Increases GABA release and receptor binding at synapses. Shows preferential effect on limbic system. (GABA is an inhibitory transmitter and slows turnover of other neurotransmitters.) Useful for short term treatment of anxiety; 3–4 months maximum, as dependence and tolerance can develop.
chlordiazepoxide	Librium	
clorazepate	Tranxene	
diazepam	Valium	
halazepam	Paxipam	
lorazepam	Ativan	
oxazepam	Serax	
prazepam	Centrax	
	Propranediols	
meprobamate	Equanil Miltown	Anxiety relief. Considered a sedative-hypnotic. Tolerance and addiction develop quickly, making serious withdrawal reactions and overdose real possibilities.

Table continued on following page

Table 16–9 • MEDICATIONS USED IN TREATMENT OF ANXIETY DISORDERS *Continued*

GENERIC NAME	TRADE NAME	ACTION/INDICATIONS
	Acetylinic Alcohol	
ethchlorvynol	Placidyl	Anxiety relief. Considered a sedative-hypnotic. Tolerance and addiction develop quickly, making serious withdrawal reactions and overdose real possibilities.
	Diphenylmethane Antihistamines	
hydroxyzine HCL hydroxyzine pamoate	Atarax Vistaril	Depresses subcortical centers. Produces no dependence, tolerance, or intoxication. Can be used for anxiety relief for indefinite periods.
	Anxiolytic	
buspirone hydrochloride	Buspar	New drug. Alleviates anxiety. Less sedative than benzodiazepines. Does not appear to produce physical or psychological dependence. Requires up to 3 weeks to be effective.
	Beta-adrenergic Blocker	
propranolol	Inderal	Used to relieve physical symptoms of anxiety, as in stage fright. Acts by attaching to sensors that detect arousal messages.
	Tricyclic Antidepressant	
imipramine	Tofranil	Used to prevent panic attacks. Acts by regulating brain's reactions to serotonin. No abuse or addiction potential.

Table 16–10 • SIDE EFFECTS OF BENZODIAZEPINES

CENTRAL NERVOUS SYSTEM	CARDIOVASCULAR	BLOOD	GASTROINTESTINAL	OTHER
Drowsiness	Hypotension	Agranulocytosis, sore throat, fever	Dry mouth	Skin rash
Clumsiness	Palpitations	Thrombocytopenia, unusual bruising	Nausea, vomiting	Pain at injection site
Blurred vision	Tachycardia		Abdominal discomfort	Urinary retention
Slurred speech	Dizziness			Aggravation of narrow angle glaucoma
Headache	Fainting			Menstrual irregularity
Mental confusion				
Disorientation				
Nystagmus				
Ataxia				
Agitation				
Sleep disturbance				
Psychological dependence				
Physical tolerance				

antidepressant drugs (imipramine, desipramine, and amitriptyline). When clients do not respond to the tricyclics, the monoamine oxidase inhibitors have been found to be effective antipanic drugs (Hollander et al. 1988). See Chapter 18 for discussion of the tricyclic and monoamine oxidase inhibitors.

Clients receiving anxiolytics should be assessed on an ongoing basis for anxiety level and side effects or untoward effects of the medication. Benzodiazepines have an extensive list of side effects with which the nurse must be familiar. The more common ones are listed by body system in Table 16–10.

Box 16–2 outlines specified nursing implications associated with anxiolytic drug therapy.

V-E: THERAPEUTIC ENVIRONMENT

Most clients who demonstrate anxiety or use ego-dystonic defenses against anxiety can be treated successfully as outpatients. Severe anxiety or symptoms that interfere with the individual's life may cause the client to be hospitalized on a short term basis.

When hospitalization is necessary, certain features of the therapeutic environment can be especially helpful to the client. These include the following:

1. Structuring the daily routine to offer predictability and reduce anxiety over the unknown.
2. Providing daily activities to prevent constant focus on anxiety or symptoms.
3. Providing therapeutic interactions.
4. Evaluating and communicating the effects of the environment on the client to facilitate nursing care planning.

V-F: PSYCHOTHERAPY

Box 16–3 provides a brief overview of the aim of various therapies the nurse psychotherapist might choose to employ with selected clients who have anxiety, somatoform, or dissociative disorders.

Professional accountability dictates that the nurse psychotherapist establish both a mechanism for peer review and a regular relationship with a professional colleague for the purpose of supervision and consultation. These actions help to ensure a high quality of care. Of particular importance is the need for the therapist to recognize and work through countertransferences that develop.

Standard VI: Evaluation

Evaluation includes careful ongoing assessment of the client by the nurse for the purpose of monitoring progress toward goal attainment. Identified client care goals serve as the basis for evaluation. Whenever goals are not attained, the nurse should identify reasons for nonattainment. If new facts about the client come to light, the data base may be changed and new nursing diagnoses may be established. Interventions, too, may change as a result of the evaluation. When problems are resolved, the plan must also reflect this progress.

In general, evaluation of goal attainment for clients with anxiety, somatoform, and dissociative disorders deals with questions such as the following:

- *Is the client experiencing a reduced level of anxiety?*
- *Does the client recognize his or her anxiety?*
- *Can the client identify stressors?*
- *Have healthy coping strategies been mobilized for use?*
- *Are new coping strategies effectively used?*
- *Does the client exhibit behaviors associated with adequate self-esteem?*
- *Is the client able to engage in more satisfying interpersonal relationships?*
- *Do significant others promote functional behavior by the client, rather than dysfunctional behavior?*

Anxiety Disorders

The anxiety disorders are thought to be the most common of the psychiatric illnesses and cause for a great deal of functional impairment and subjective distress (Hollander et al. 1988). The anxiety experienced by a client with an anxiety disorder is considered pathological because it occurs in response to stressors with which the average individual can usually cope. The clinical picture of anxiety disorders either involves anxiety experienced and overtly displayed or reflects the individual's efforts to avoid or defend against anxiety. Figure 16–4 identifies the syndromes in this group and describes the associated behaviors.

THE CLINICAL PICTURE OF PANIC DISORDER

The panic level, or severest level, of anxiety was described fully in Chapter 8. An overview of diagnostic

Box 16–2. NURSING IMPLICATIONS FOR ANTIANXIETY DRUG THERAPY

Assessment

- Identify other medications/drugs the client is taking.
- Assess frequency of client requests for medication (many anxiolytics are Schedule IV controlled substances).
- Observe for indications that client is exceeding recommended dosage: ataxia, mental confusion, dizziness, slurred speech, and other symptoms of intoxication.
- Observe for paradoxical excitation: restlessness, rage, agitation. More common in elderly.
- Observe for sleep disturbance: nightmares, vivid dreams may occur related to Stage IV sleep suppression.
- Assess change in urinary frequency, odor, or color, as urinary retention may occur.
- Prior to initiating medication, record presence or absence of skin rash, flu-like symptoms, bruising.
- Obtain information about baseline sexual functioning, as changes in libido/functioning may occur, causing client to discontinue medication without discussing with therapist.
- Obtain information about menstrual regularity, as irregularity may occur.

Teaching

- Caution client not to increase dose or frequency of ingestion without prior approval of therapist.
- Caution client that these medications reduce ability to handle mechanical equipment such as cars, saws, machinery.
- Caution client not to drink alcoholic beverages or take other antianxiety drugs because depressant effects of both will be potentiated.
- Caution client to avoid drinking beverages containing caffeine because it decreases desired effects of drug.
- Caution women to avoid becoming pregnant, as taking benzodiazepines increases risk of congenital anomalies.
- Caution new mothers taking benzodiazepines not to breast-feed, as the drug is excreted in the milk and will have adverse effects on infant.

Other

- Abrupt stoppage of benzodiazepines after 3 to 4 months' daily use may cause withdrawal symptoms: insomnia, irritability, nervousness, dry mouth, tremors, convulsions, or confusion.
- Remain with client until medication is swallowed.
- Take with, or shortly after, meals or snacks to reduce gastrointestinal discomfort.
- Be alert for possible drug interactions:
  - Antacids may delay absorption.
  - Cimetidine interferes with metabolism of benzodiazepines, causing increased sedation.
  - Central nervous system depressants such as alcohol and barbiturates cause increased sedation.
  - Pheytoin serum concentration may build up owing to decreased metabolism.
- Lower doses should be considered for elderly clients.
- Read drug literature carefully regarding reconstitution, storage, and administration of parenteral drug.
  - Some drugs, such as Vistaril and Valium, produce irritation at intramuscular injection sites.
  - Valium and Librium require slow intravenous injection.
  - Do not use if solution is cloudy or discolored.
  - Some drugs must be stored away from light.
- When intramuscular injection is ordered, administer deeply and slowly into large muscle to minimize irritation and discomfort.
- After intramuscular or intravenous administration, client should remain recumbent to minimize orthostatic hypotension.
- Note contraindications of administration of individual drugs: e.g., many benzodiazepines should not be given to clients in shock, clients with narrow angle glaucoma, or clients with hepatic or renal disease.
- Investigate complaints of sore throat or fever as possible symptoms of agranulocytosis.
- Adopt positive attitude that medication will be effective.

Box 16–3. PSYCHOTHERAPIES USED IN ANXIETY, SOMATOFORM, AND DISSOCIATIVE DISORDERS

Psychoanalytic Therapy

Assists client in uncovering and analyzing unconscious conflicts and current interpersonal conflicts.

Supportive Psychotherapy

Bolsters the client's existing healthy coping strategies and strengths.

Cognitive Therapy

Helps client reconsider stressors and discriminate real from imagined dangers and identify faulty thinking and beliefs.

Family Therapy

Views the client's disorder as evidence of family system dysfunction. Assists family, rather than the individual, in resolving conflicts. Assesses ways family unwittingly contributes to client's dysfunctional behaviors and seeks resolution.

Behavioral Therapy

Focuses on removing specific symptoms and dysfunctional behaviors and on changing factors in environment that reinforce dysfunctional behaviors.

Relaxation Therapy

Clients are taught to reduce stress and anxiety by using the relaxation response, a protective mechanism that lowers pulse, respiration, and metabolism. Provides consciously induced reciprocal inhibition of anxiety. Techniques may include use of visual imagery, meditation, biofeedback, and self-hypnosis.

Desensitization Therapy

Phobic clients are exposed to a predetermined sequence of real or imaginary anxiety-provoking situations or objects arranged on a continuum from least to most anxiety producing. Relaxation techniques are used at each step to reduce the anxiety response and its symptoms via reciprocal inhibition.

Hypnosis

Useful in identifying the source of anxiety responsible for amnesia and fugue and in establishing contact with multiple personalities.

criteria for panic disorder can be seen in Figure 16–4. The feelings of terror present during a panic attack are so severe that normal function is suspended. The perceptual field is severely limited, and misinterpretation of reality may occur. Severe personality disorganization is evident.

Typically, panic attacks are short. They come on suddenly, increase in intensity, and subside within a few minutes. People experiencing a panic attack for the first time believe they are either losing their mind or having a heart attack. They feel dizzy, lightheaded, their heart begins to pound, and they cannot catch their breath (Hollander et al. 1988). Attacks are so intense that the individual is not able to tolerate the experience for a prolonged period. He or she typically pleads for help or may use massive projection to gain relief from the anxiety.

Clinical Vignette: A Client With Panic Disorder

Dora Mars, a 28-year-old pharmacist, lived at home and cared for her mother. Dora's father left home when Dora was four years old. Dora's mother was cold and cruel to Dora during her childhood. Following her mother's death, Dora admitted feeling tense and irritable and having trouble sleeping.

One night Dora awakened gasping for breath. Her heart was pounding and she felt a tight sensation, like a band around her chest. Her pulse was 110, and she was dizzy. She feared she was going to die. She telephoned

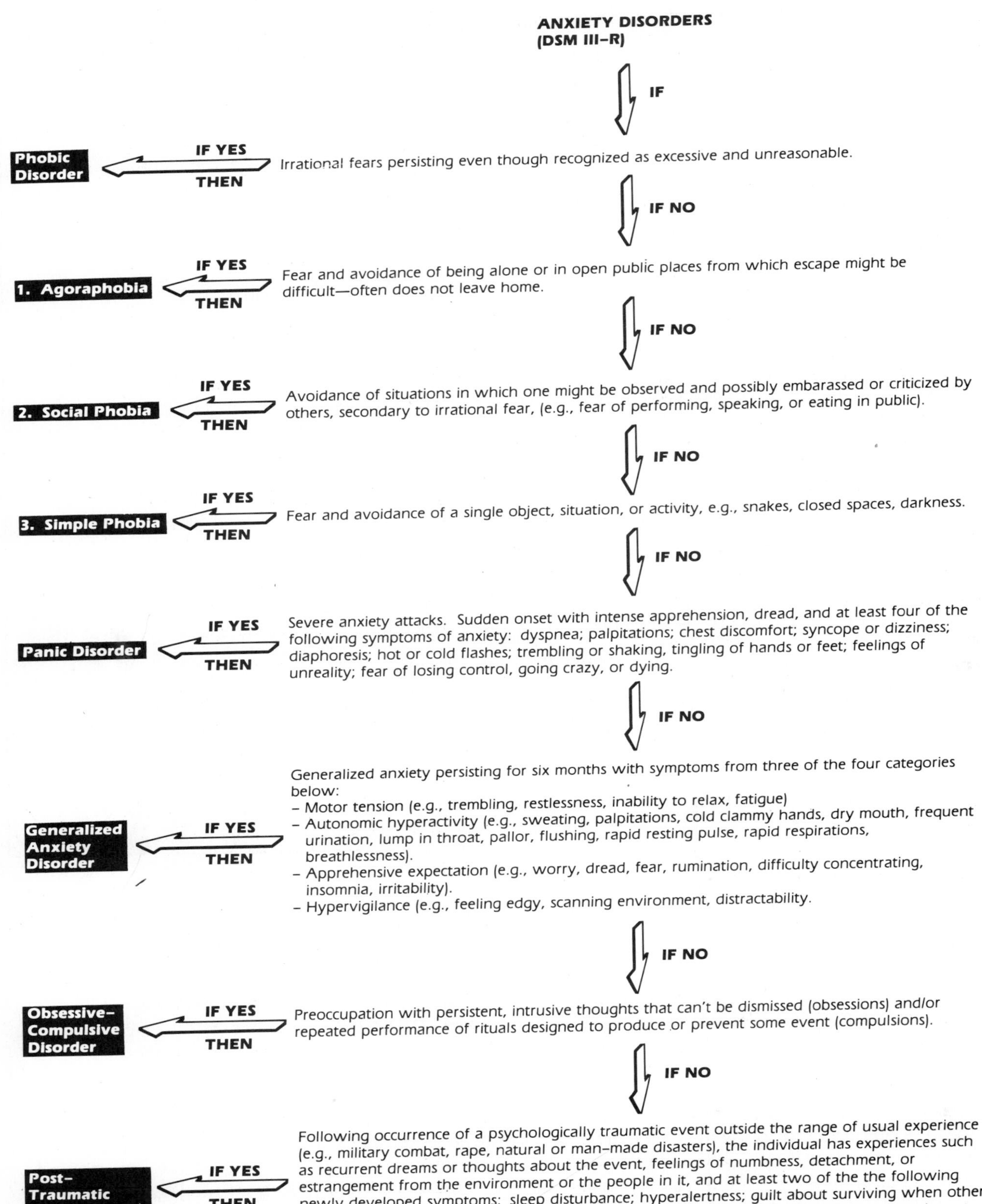

Figure 16–4. *Decision tree for the anxiety disorders.* (Adapted from Janicak PG, Andriukaitis SN. DSM III: *Seeing the forest through the trees.* Psychiatric Annals, 10(8):19, 1980, and *Diagnostic and Statistical Manual of Mental Disorders* [DSM III-R], 3d ed., revised. Washington, DC: American Psychiatric Association, 1987.)

her best friend, who found her pacing, wringing her hands, and moaning. She seemed totally disorganized. The friend took Dora to the emergency room. After a thorough cardiac workup, Dora was kept overnight for observation. All diagnostic tests were normal, and she was discharged the next day. Over the course of the next three weeks, Dora had six attacks. The doctor suggested that since there was no apparent organic basis for these episodes, it was likely they were caused by anxiety.

Imipramine was prescribed to block the panic attacks. In outpatient therapy Dora became aware of intense anger toward her mother that had been repressed. She acknowledged longing for the warmth she had never received from her mother. The immediate stressors were found to be her mother's death and the impending retirement of a coworker of whom she was very fond. Dora was able to discuss and accept her loss, ambivalence, and anger. She was offered a choice of learning self-hypnosis, meditation, or progressive muscle relaxation techniques to help reduce anxiety and tension. She chose to use progressive muscle relaxation exercises and reported ability to monitor her anxiety level and use relaxation effectively. Imipramine was discontinued without recurrence of the attacks.

THE CLINICAL PICTURE OF GENERALIZED ANXIETY DISORDER

The DSM III-R (1987) criteria used for diagnosing generalized anxiety disorder can be reviewed in Figure 16–4. The individual suffering from generalized anxiety disorder lives in a constant state of worry, usually over trivial matters. Decision making is difficult owing to poor concentration and dread of making a mistake. Worry over the physical symptoms being experienced is common, as is worry about inadequacies in interpersonal relationships. Initiating sleep is delayed while the individual worries about the day's events and real or imagined mistakes, reviews past problems, and anticipates future difficulties. During sleep, nightmares of disastrous situations often occur. The individual may dream of being shot, being chased and being unable to run, of falling from high places, or of being choked.

Clinical Vignette: A Client With Generalized Anxiety Disorder

Cameron, a 43-year-old pilot, sought admission to the hospital, stating that for a month he had been unable to sleep without having a nightmare about a plane crash. These began shortly after he was passed over for promotion. After several nightmares, he began to worry during his waking hours about the possibility of being involved in a crash. He experienced so much dread about flying that he grounded himself. He complained of constant fatigue. At interview, he had shaky hands and sat tensely on the edge of the chair. His hands were cold, but facial perspiration was evident. Resting pulse was 100. As he described his nightmares, he began to hyperventilate. Admission for short term therapy was arranged.

Antianxiety medication was not prescribed, as nursing measures were sufficient to intervene and reduce Cameron's anxiety to moderate levels during his first days on the unit. As a result of therapy, Cameron was able to see the loss of the promotion as an assault on self-esteem. He discussed incidents in his childhood during which his father criticized him and told him he would never amount to anything. Loss of the promotion reactivated this conflict, and he again felt incompetent and anxious. Cameron was provided with information about the symptoms of anxiety and taught to time his attacks. Helping him direct his focus from the symptoms (an internal frame of reference) to the time frame of the attacks (an external frame of reference) proved useful in shortening the attacks. Cameron had learned the technique of meditation in college and began to use it again for relaxation. By discharge he had reevaluated his self-concept and was able to state positive self-attributes.

THE CLINICAL PICTURE OF PHOBIAS

Characteristically, phobic individuals experience overwhelming and crippling anxiety when faced with the object of their phobia. Phobic people go to great lengths to avoid the feared object, situation, or activity. A phobic individual may not even be able to think about or visualize the object or situation without becoming severely anxious. The individual becomes more isolated, and his or her life becomes more restricted as activities are given up in order to avoid contact with the feared object or situation.

The three classes of phobias are explained in Figure 16–4. Agoraphobia is the most common phobia for which people seek treatment. **Agoraphobia** is fear and avoidance of being alone or being in open spaces from which escape might be difficult. Although agoraphobic clients may think they are going "crazy," they do not exhibit psychotic symptoms. Agoraphobia can be most debilitating and life constricting. Severely agoraphobic individuals may be unable to leave their homes. Panic attacks are commonly associated with this disorder. Social phobia can cause considerable inconvenience and may result in substance abuse if the individual turns

Table 16–11 • SOME COMMON PHOBIAS

FEAR	CLINICAL NAME
Heights	Acrophobia
Open spaces	Agoraphobia
Electrical storms	Astraphobia
Closed spaces	Claustrophobia
Talking	Glossophobia
Blood	Hematophobia
Water	Hydrophobia
Being alone	Monophobia
Germs, dirt	Mysophobia
Fire	Pyrophobia
Animals	Zoophobia

to alcohol or other drugs for anxiety reduction. Examples of **social phobias** include fear of public speaking, fear of eating with others present, and fear of writing or performing in public. Social phobias may involve general fears of saying foolish things or not being able to answer questions in public. **Simple phobias** involve fear and avoidance of a single object, situation, or activity. Simple phobias usually do not cause the individual as much difficulty, since one can usually avoid a single object, e.g., snakes, closed spaces, darkness, cats. Simple phobias are common in the general public.

It is acceptable to describe phobias in everyday lan-

Table 16–12 • USEFUL TREATMENTS FOR PEOPLE WITH ANXIETY DISORDERS

DISORDER	TREATMENT(S)*
Phobic disorder	Desensitization therapy Short term use of antianxiety medication Psychotherapy Cognitive therapy Relaxation therapy Family therapy Propranolol for stage fright
Panic disorder	Imipramine to prevent attacks Psychotherapy Relaxation therapy
Obsessive-compulsive disorder (OCD)	Psychotherapy Short term use of antianxiety medication Cognitive therapy Relaxation therapy Behavior therapy Family therapy
Generalized anxiety disorder	Psychotherapy Relaxation therapy Short term use of antianxiety medication
Post-traumatic stress disorder	Psychotherapy Short term use of antianxiety medication Relaxation therapy Family therapy Self-help groups

*Treatments may be used singly or in combination.

Box 16–4. FANTASY VERSUS IN VIVO DESENSITIZATION

When *fantasy desensitization* is used, the client is instructed to imagine the anxiety-producing situation or object, beginning with exposure to a situation that produces minimal anxiety or places the feared object at a great distance. As the client gains mastery over anxiety, the intensity of the stimulus is gradually increased, e.g., the client imagines first a small dog, then a larger dog, or the feared object is moved closer and closer.

In vivo desensitization may progress the same way but with the client actually being faced with the feared object rather than imagining it. The technique of implosion, or flooding, involves the client's facing the object without gradual increases.

Muscle relaxation techniques may be used in conjunction with desensitization, with the client being taught to replace the anxiety response with the relaxation response.

guage; however, specific terminology does exist. The list in Table 16–11 gives examples. Useful treatment modalities helpful for people with anxiety disorders are identified in Table 16–12. For clarification, in vivo and fantasy desensitization methods are contrasted in Box 16–4. Specific nursing interventions for people with phobic disorders are described in Table 16–13.

Clinical Vignette: A Client With Phobia

Tim Hansen, age 22, a music theater major, sought treatment for social phobia. He describes himself as a failure because for the past two months he has been fearful of performing on stage. He has suffered severe anxiety attacks whenever scheduled to appear in a student production. Recently, he has suffered from severe anxiety whenever faced with classroom readings or singing solo in music class.

During therapy Tim was able to discuss the fact that his father had strongly objected to a theater career for Tim, saying he would be contaminated by contact with homosexuals. About a month before becoming phobic, Tim was propositioned by a homosexual classmate whose advances he rejected. His phobia seemed to be based on the fear that an audience would identify him as a homosexual and scorn his performance. Therapy focused on exploration of values and sexual role identity, relieving guilt feelings about ignoring his father's wishes, and raising self-esteem.

Tim was offered propranolol (Inderal) but stated he preferred to master the symptoms rather than depend on medication. Systematic desensitization and relaxation techniques were used to help Tim perform gradually. Small doses of Valium were administered before each session. Initially, Tim was able to stand silently on stage, then to sing and recite in an empty theater, and after one month, to perform before an audience.

THE CLINICAL PICTURE OF OBSESSIVE-COMPULSIVE DISORDER (OCD)

An **obsession** is a persistent intrusive thought or image that seems senseless to the individual. An obsession (thought/image) is impossible to put out of one's mind. In true obsessions the person considers the painful rumination of certain ideas or thoughts to be ego-dystonic, as opposed to the person who may persistently brood or ruminate over unpleasant thoughts that are

Table 16–13 • SPECIFIC NURSING INTERVENTIONS: CLIENTS WITH PHOBIC DISORDERS

INTERVENTION	RATIONALE
1. Accept client's fear matter-of-factly.	1. Ego-dystonic symptoms are coping strategies. Use of logic, ridicule, or urging to use self-control increases anxiety and may cause panic.
2. Do not agree with client's assessment that phobia is silly.	2. Acknowledging that behavior serves a purpose helps promote insight.
3. Do not force the client to face phobic object or situation.	3. Panic may result. Gradual desensitization is more successful.

Refer to Table 16–8 for General Interventions.

regarded as meaningful (Hollander et al. 1988). **Compulsions** are repetitive purposeless-seeming behaviors performed according to certain rules known to the client, which seem necessary to produce or prevent some event. The individual usually realizes the behavior is not connected in a realistic way with what it is designed to accomplish. At times, people engage in certain activities excessively, e.g., eating, sexual behavior, gambling, or drinking, and may be labeled by others as "compulsive." These situations are different from true compulsions, since the activity is experienced as pleasurable (although the consequences might not be) (Hollander et al. 1988). Both obsessions and compulsions are ego-dystonic symptoms, because the user recognizes their senselessness. Attempts to resist either the obsession or the compulsion cause the individual to feel increasingly anxious. Performing the action (compulsion) results in temporary anxiety relief; therefore, the *primary gain is anxiety reduction*. Obsessions can occur without compulsions, but often the two symptoms are seen together.

Everyone has had the experience of having a persistent tune run through his or her mind, despite attempts to push it away (obsessions). Also commonly experienced is a nagging doubt as to whether one has locked the door or turned off the stove (obsessions). These nagging doubts or obsessions often cannot be put to rest until the person goes back to check the door or stove. The *action* of going back to check is the compulsion. Obsessions that lead an individual into psychiatric care usually are more troublesome than these, and usually center on issues of sexuality, violence, germs and dirt, or illness and death. People with mild obsessions think of themselves as worriers, whereas people with profound obsessions are deeply affected by them to the point of interpersonal, social, and economic dysfunction (Chapman 1976).

Compulsions also exist on a continuum from mildly annoying to intricate, time-consuming rituals that interfere with the individual's ability to function. Minor compulsions include behaviors such as "knocking on wood," crossing oneself when hearing bad news, or touching a lucky charm. Mild compulsions can be useful. Timeliness, orderliness, and reliability are valued traits in our society. Several of the most common compulsions carried to excess are seen in Table 16–14.

The obsessive-compulsive person is a perfectionist who finds it extremely difficult to admit to making a mistake or to human failings. This need for perfection has its basis in the need to control self and others. At the extreme, such a person cannot make a decision for fear of being wrong. This doubting can be seen, for example, in the constant checking that the stove is turned off, the counting and recounting of a row of figures, or buttoning a button over and over to make sure it is buttoned "correctly."

Phobias, anxiety, and depression frequently accompany obsessive-compulsive disorders and may complicate treatment. Psychoanalytic psychotherapy may be ineffective because it is able to accomplish only half the task. It often promotes an intellectual understanding of the illness but is unable to assist the client in experiencing more appropriate emotions. The client's use of intellectualization as a defense seems to be strengthened in psychoanalytic psychotherapy. Some clients are better helped by psychotherapy with a therapist who is active and energetic and who intervenes whenever communication becomes confused or rambling (Chapman and Chapman 1980; Salzman 1966). The therapist helps the client accomplish the following:

- Discriminate between thought and action.
- Accept "forbidden" desires and "bad" thoughts as common to most people.
- Discriminate between real and imagined danger and act accordingly.

Table 16–14 • COMMON COMPULSIONS

COMPULSION	EXAMPLE
Counting	A person counting each step he or she takes.
Touching	Touching each door knob one sees.
Checking	Repeatedly checking to make sure an appliance is turned off.
Washing/cleaning	Scrubbing one's hands repeatedly.
Avoidance	Taking pains not to come in contact with anything dirty.
Doing-undoing	Walking forward, then backward, or arranging and rearranging items.
Symmetry	Lining up objects.

Behavior therapy has been proved useful in some instances. Nonritualistic behavior can be rewarded and the use of appropriate behaviors supported until rituals become less necessary. Some clients are able to interrupt obsessive thinking by snapping a rubber band worn on the wrist when the obsessive thought begins.

Antianxiety medication may be used to treat recurrent high levels of anxiety. Short term (three to four months) or as needed use is preferable, since the potential for dependence is high. Success with tricyclic antidepressants has been limited; however, it is possible that new serotonin-regulating medications, such as clomipramine (Anafranil), may be useful. Specific nursing interventions for clients demonstrating obsessive-compulsive symptoms can be reviewed in Table 16–15.

Clinical Vignette: A Client With Obsessive-Compulsive Disorder

Tina Jayne, a 32-year-old single parent, sought treatment for obsessive-compulsive disorder. Tina was born 12 years after her sister to parents who were aloof, perfectionistic, and morally strict. Tina often felt she was an unwanted child.

Tina, like her sister, majored in Business Administration in college. During her senior year she became pregnant. She did not seek an abortion because she believed

Table 16–15 • SPECIFIC NURSING INTERVENTIONS: CLIENTS WITH OBSESSIVE-COMPULSIVE DISORDERS

INTERVENTION	RATIONALE
1. Anticipate and meet client's needs: administer medications on time. Give simple explanations before client needs to ask, be on time for appointments, etc.	1. Increases feelings of security by reducing worry and supporting client worth. Early intervention can reduce anxiety and the need for rituals.
2. Permit time for rituals.	2. If rituals are delayed or prevented, client anxiety may reach panic level proportions.
3. Avoid hurrying the client.	3. Hurrying increases anxiety, thus the need for rituals.
4. Do not call attention to rituals.	4. Client already believes them to be "silly."
5. Protect from ridicule.	5. Lowers self-esteem, thus increases anxiety.
6. Institute measures to reduce threats to physical well-being caused by rituals, e.g., between-meal snacks, special skin care, etc.	6. Physiological and safety needs are of high priority.
7. Gradually limit amount of time permitted for rituals as client becomes comfortable and involved with unit activities.	7. Anxiety can be reduced when rituals are replaced by adaptive substitutes.
8. Help client identify situations that create anxiety and prompt rituals.	8. Recognition of anxiety-provoking events is basic to teaching client to interrupt the anxiety cycle.
9. Teach ways to interrupt ritualistic patterns of behavior, e.g., snapping rubber bands on wrist to banish obsessive thoughts.	9. Anxiety can be reduced when other behaviors are gradually substituted for rituals.
10. Help client speak concisely.	10. Reduces circumstantiality (giving tedious unnecessary details).
11. Give positive reinforcement for *nonritualistic* behavior.	11. Positive reinforcement encourages repetition of adaptive behavior and can increase self-esteem.
12. Let client know it is okay to make mistakes.	12. Decreases striving for perfection.
13. Avoid power struggles.	13. These create anxiety in client, frustration in staff.

Refer to Table 16–8 for General Interventions.

it "an act of murder." The father of the baby became so anxious that he left the area. Tina, too embarrassed to go back home, quit school to support herself and the child. She worked as a secretary, took courses at night, and presently holds a job in a prominent law firm.

Recently, Tina started to have intrusive thoughts that some harm would come to her daughter. Even though she knew this was irrational, the thought (obsession) persisted. The only way Tina could reduce her anxiety was to check her daughter's safety (compulsion). She called school hourly. She did not allow her daughter to play sports; she screened her daughter's friends; she monitored her activities and generally tried to control her daughter's every move. Her daughter felt embarrassed because her mother "had to check on her daughter."

Tina got to the point where she hardly ate. She would sleep very little at night because of the need to go to her daughter's room to "check that she is safe." Tina stated that she thought she was stupid for not being able to manage her life as well as her sister and for not being able to get rid of her senseless worries. Tina was admitted for short term intensive therapy. Tina's nursing care plan was written shortly after admission to the unit (Nursing Care Plan 16–1).

During her hospital stay, as noted on the nursing care plan, Tina was able to identify the precipitating stressor. She was able to acknowledge that hostility toward her daughter might be transformed to excessive concern (reaction-formation) and result in checking behaviors. However, she was unable to get in touch with or discuss negative feelings toward her daughter or her parents. Other progress is noted in the nursing care plan.

Nursing Care Plan 16–1 • PERSON WITH OBSESSIVE COMPULSIVE DISORDER: Tina

NURSING DIAGNOSIS

Ineffective individual coping related to unresolved conflict.

Supporting Data

- Reported obsessive thoughts that daughter will be harmed.
- Compulsive checking designed to ensure daughter's safety.

Long Term Goal: Client will demonstrate ability to cope effectively without use of obsessive compulsive behavior.

Short Term Goal	*Intervention*	*Rationale*	*Evaluation*
1. By (state the date) client will experience decrease in incidence of obsessive thinking and compulsive behavior, as evidenced by (a) normal food and fluid intake, (b) six hours of sleep per night, and no more than two calls to school per day.	1a. Anticipate need for information about unit; orient before client must ask.	1a. Increases feelings of security.	Goal met Client states she likes the idea that staff explains things to her; she states that she worries less.
	1b. Focus on client, rather than on symptoms.	1b. Reinforces self-worth.	Client is able to adhere to schedule.
	1c. Permit client to call school six times per day for two days, then four times per day for four days, and twice daily thereafter.	1c. Allowing performance of ritual prevents panic.	Client states it is hard to sit through meals when she feels she should check on her daughter. Eats snacks willingly. Two-lb weight gain in one week.
	1d. Firmly encourage client to attend and eat meals. Offer nutritious snacks between meals.	1d. Limits must be placed on behaviors that threaten health.	Client initiates sleep within 45 minutes but awakens more than 6 times nightly. She refuses sedation because it makes her feel groggy the next day.
	1e. Give warm milk and back rub h.s.	1e–f. Promotes relaxation and sleep.	
	1f. Offer sedation if client has not initiated sleep by midnight.		
2. By (state the date) client will state she is able to dismiss obsessive thoughts and will acknowledge that compulsion is not acted upon.	2a. Teach to interrupt obsessive thoughts by snapping rubber band on wrist.	2a–b. Gives control over obsessive thinking and compulsive rituals.	By the sixth day, client stated, "It's getting easier to ignore my obsessive thoughts."
	2b. Give positive reinforcement for nonritualistic behavior.		

3. Client will state relationship between anxiety and symptoms by (state the date).	3. Support efforts to explore what purpose the behavior serves.	3. Recognition fosters change.	Stated her symptoms worsened when she learned a new secretary had been hired for the office. Was able to see that the new secretary could be seen as a competitor, much as she viewed her sister.

NURSING DIAGNOSIS

Disturbance in self-esteem related to lack of perceived strengths.

Supporting Data

- Verbalization of stupidity associated with not being able to manage life as well as sister.
- Statement that she is "stupid" for not being able to get rid of worrisome ideas.

Long Term Goal: Client will verbalize positive self-perception by (state the date).

Short Term Goal	*Intervention*	*Rationale*	*Evaluation*
1. Client will list five good things about self by (state the date).	1. Encourage client to identify strengths.	1. Fosters realistic self-concept.	Goal met On seventh day client talked with nurse about list of strengths.
2. Client will make realistic positive statements about self by (state the date).	2. Arrange for activities at which she can succeed. Give merited praise.	2. Raises self-esteem.	Stated she sees that she coped well under difficult conditions as a single parent.
3. Self deprecatory statements will be absent by (state the date).	3. Avoid power struggles. Expect cooperation.	3. Power struggles increase anxiety. When client loses power struggle, esteem is lowered. When staff loses, anger is generated.	Skilled negotiation by nurse avoided power struggles.

NURSING DIAGNOSIS

Diversional activity deficit related to preoccupation with performance of rituals

Supporting Data

- Giving up all social activities.

Long Term Goal: Client will balance work and pleasurable activity by (state the date).

Short Term Goal	*Intervention*	*Rationale*	*Evaluation*
1. Client will make list of things she used to enjoy by (state the date).	1. Encourage to survey activities at which she was proficient and activities she enjoyed.	1. Reduces preoccupation with rituals. Provides anxiety relief. Fosters awareness that enjoyment is deserved.	Goal met Listed activities she would enjoy. Attended activities as required but without enjoyment during first week. Now shows enjoyment. Plans to take ceramics class after discharge and to attend single parents social group.
2. Client will engage in one activity per day as assigned by (state the date).	2. Expect participation.	2. Relieves guilt over attendance.	
3. Client will choose daily activities and participate by (state the date).	3. Encourage helping others during activities.	3. Lowers anxiety.	

Continued on following page

Nursing Care Plan 16–1 • PERSON WITH OBSESSIVE COMPULSIVE DISORDER: Tina *(Continued)*

NURSING DIAGNOSIS

Altered family process related to client dominating daughter

Supporting Data

- Not allowing daughter to play sports.
- Screening daughter's friends.
- Monitoring daughter's activities to the point of calling school several times daily.

Long Term Goal: Client will relate to daughter in parental fashion without excessive domination by (state the date).

Short Term Goal	*Intervention*	*Rationale*	*Evaluation*
1. Client will allow daughter appropriate social contacts and school activities.	1. Using cognitive therapy techniques, evaluate "dangers" she imagines for her daughter.	1. Promotes reality.	Goal met Client states she understands that the dangers were more in her own mind than actual. Signed permission for daughter to play intramural sports. Allowed daughter to attend peer group party.

THE CLINICAL PICTURE OF POST-TRAUMATIC STRESS DISORDER

Post-traumatic stress disorder (PTSD) has two subtypes, acute and chronic. The *acute disorder* is diagnosed when symptoms occur within six months of the trauma. The *delayed or chronic* type is diagnosed when the onset of symptoms is delayed at least six months or the symptoms have persisted for at least six months. Post-traumatic stress disorder may occur following any psychologically traumatic event that is outside the range of usual experiences, e.g., assault or rape, military combat, natural disasters (flood, earthquake), and manmade disasters (vehicular accidents, airplane crashes, bombings, torture, death camps).

PTSD has been commonly experienced by veterans of the Viet Nam War. In order to resume a normal civilian lifestyle after combat, a person must come to terms with the experience of war. If some kind of resolution does not occur, PTSD results. The symptoms of the disorder are not as well defined as those of other anxiety disorders, so it may go undiagnosed. The individual may seek some other form of relief by developing additional symptoms such as physiological complaints (headaches, ulcers, hypertension), phobias, or chemical dependence and abuse. Suicide attempts and intermittent psychotic episodes may occur, and problems existing before the traumatic event, such as impulsiveness or antisocial tendencies, may be intensified.

Difficulty in interpersonal relationships often occurs. The PTSD victim frequently states that he or she has turned off feelings and feels empty inside. This psychic numbing protects the client from feelings associated with intense stress. For example, avoiding emotional attachment can become a learned response to protect a veteran from experiencing compound losses in an environment in which death is a common occurrence. Thrill-seeking behavior may allow feelings to surface and can mobilize aggression. Spouse and child abuse can occur. Struggles with bosses, family, and coworkers are frequent themes. Difficulty in trusting authority figures may stem from the traumatic event(s) and contributes to problems in the workplace.

Nurses are in a strategic position to assess post-traumatic stress disorder and make appropriate referrals. The important component of therapy, whether group or individual, is encouraging the expression of stored up bitterness, pain, and resentment. Terror-filled memories need to be shared and let go, enabling the person to engage in relationships with meaning and stability. For war-associated disorders, the Veterans' Administration program Operation Outreach is a nationwide network using rap groups and peer counseling to foster social reintegration, personal growth, and individual comfort. Rape crisis centers serve the same purpose for rape victims.

Clinical Vignette: A Client With Post-Traumatic Stress Disorder

Jim Cash was 21 when he returned home from combat in Viet Nam and was discharged without a reorientation period. He experienced feelings of alienation, indifference, and anger as he faced a society whose attitudes and moods he did not know. He became withdrawn and distrustful and described feeling dead inside. He was jumpy and irritable and often threw himself on the ground when he heard a loud noise. He began drinking heavily, stating it helped him relax and sleep, but nothing stopped his nightmares. When his wife suggested that they have a baby, Jim became violent. He beat her and went on a three-day drinking spree. When he quit his third job in three months, his wife left him. He attempted suicide and was sent to a Veterans' Administration Hospital.

Jim joined a rap group of veterans who had been in combat situations. It was then that he felt understood for the first time since his discharge. He revealed to the group that his two best friends had been killed when one of them held a booby-trapped baby. He slowly began to display appropriate emotions and feelings of concern for, and involvement with, the group members. Use of relaxation techniques helped him promote resumption of sleep after the nightmares. Eventually, the nightmares stopped altogether. After accepting referral for job counseling, Jim began the process of reconciliation with his wife.

Somatoform Disorders

"Soma" is the Greek word for body. Somatoform disorders are a group of conditions characterized by complaints of physical symptoms that suggest a physiological problem but for which no organic basis can be found. Symptoms of these disorders cannot be explained by physical findings but can be linked to psychological factors, such as stress at the time of onset and secondary gain. **Somatization** can be defined as the expression of psychological stress through physical symptoms (Stoudemire 1988).

In somatoform disorders, anxiety is transformed into physical symptoms that often involve sensory and motor function. *The physical symptoms are the primary gain*, since they provide temporary relief from anxiety. In some cases, the physical symptoms are symbolically related to the conflict causing the anxiety. The *physical symptoms are experienced as real and are not under the voluntary control of the individual*. Figure 16–5 outlines the disorders classified as somatoform.

The symptoms of somatoform disorders must be differentiated from malingering. **Malingering** is a *conscious* effort to deceive others, usually for financial gain, by pretending physical symptoms. Malingerers deceive others, but not themselves, about the symptoms. By contrast, individuals with somatoform disorders are deceived by the symptoms, whereas others can see the relationship between symptom and conflict. The transformation of anxiety into physical symptoms occurs at the unconscious level; the individual believes the symptoms are real. It is important to note that both the individual who is malingering and the individual with a somatoform disorder may receive secondary gains from the symptoms.

A tendency to be dramatic is sometimes noted in clients with somatoform disorders, particularly those with a conversion disorder. These individuals often describe symptoms in graphic language or in exaggerated terms and with great emotion: "The pain was searing, like a hot sword drawn across my forehead" or "My symptoms are so rare that I've stumped thousands of doctors." Because such individuals tend to be suggestible, their illness patterns may be influenced by things they observe, such as seeing a seizure and later having convulsive movements during a time of high stress. Nursing interventions and rationales specific to clients with somatoform disorders are presented in Table 16–16. General approaches to treatment are found in Table 16–17.

THE CLINICAL PICTURE OF SOMATIZATION DISORDER

It is not uncommon for the medical record of a client with a somatization disorder to reveal the presence of 15 or more symptoms presented over time. The symptoms must have caused the client to take medicine other than aspirin, have caused alteration in life pattern, or have necessitated seeing a physician. None of the symptoms could have been explained as resulting from physical illness, injury, or drug use. After consulting with numerous doctors, submitting to examinations, diagnostic tests, and exploratory surgery, the client is invariably told that no organic basis can be found. These clients are difficult to convince to seek psychiatric help. Initial contacts with psychiatrists are usually related to complaints of depression or suicidal ideation. Substance abuse is often associated with a somatoform disorder.

Clinical Vignette: A Client With Somatization Disorder

Susanne Barron, a 26-year-old beautician, was admitted to the hospital following an overdose of sedatives. She stated she was sick of not being able to get help from anyone. In describing herself, she mentioned not being well since age 14. She has had seizures, fainting spells, and occasional weakness of the left leg. One year ago she developed abdominal pain, nausea, and diarrhea. Exploratory surgery revealed no significant pathology. The symptoms are better but recur "sometimes." She

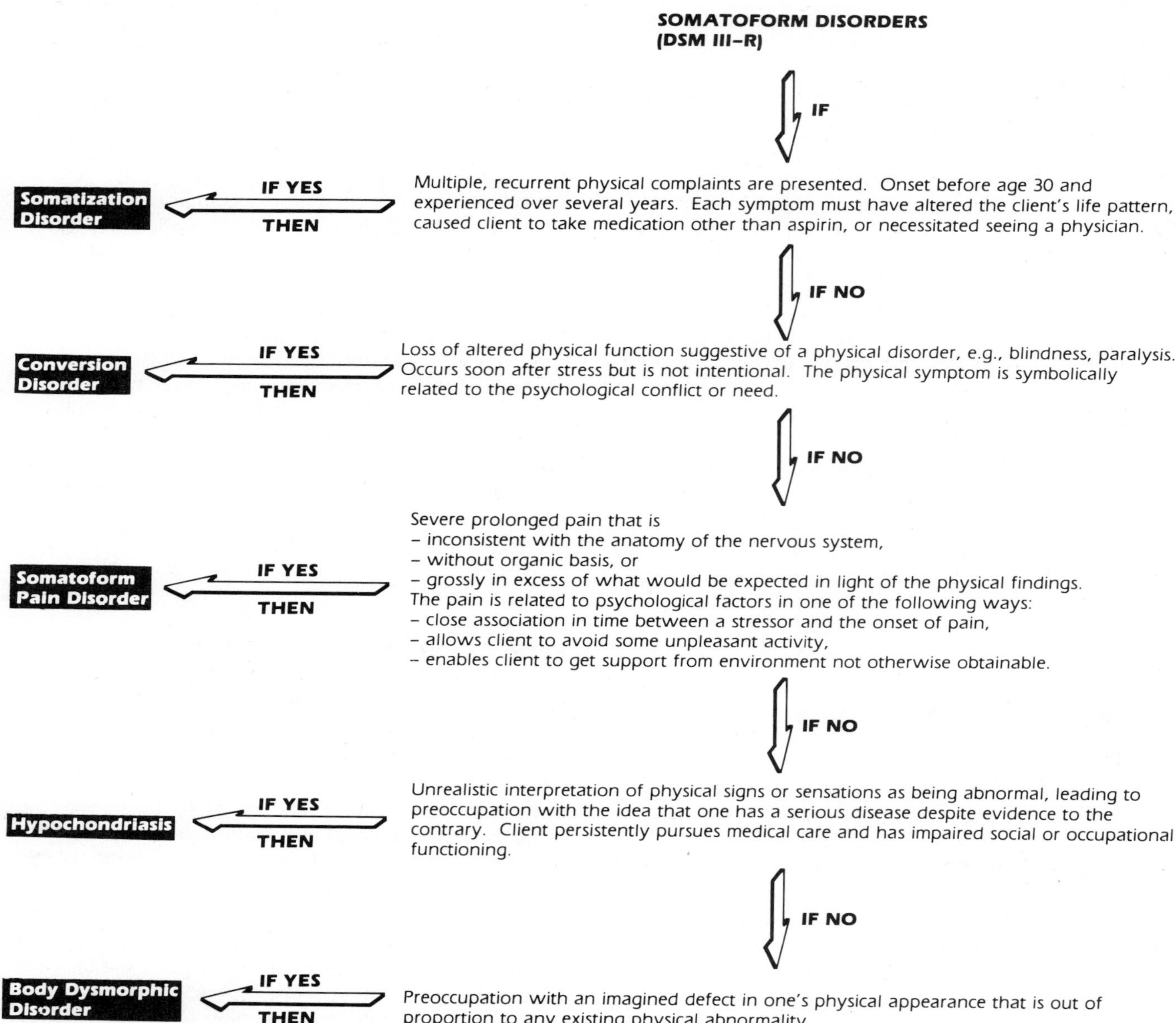

Figure 16–5. *Decision tree for the somatoform disorders.* (*Adapted from* Janicak PG, Andriukaitis SN. DSM III: *Seeing the forest through the trees.* Psychiatric Annals, 10(8):19, 1980, *and* Diagnostic and Statistical Manual of Mental Disorders [DSM III-R], *3d ed., revised.* Washington, DC: American Psychiatric Association, 1987.)

also mentioned experiencing painful menstruation and excessive bleeding over a period of several years. Recently, she has experienced palpitations and tightness of her chest after emotionally trying events. Susanne lived at home until six months ago, when she married a man 15 years her senior. She stated she is "turned off by sex" because it is painful for her, and she stated that her husband is upset by her constant illness. He is considering divorce. A short admission was advised.

Although antidepressant therapy may be used to treat severe depression, Susanne did not require it. In individual therapy Susanne was able to relate her physical symptoms to her parents' concern with health and illness themes. Her father was an invalid due to mitral valve disease, and all her mother's attention had been focused on him, except for times when Susanne had been ill. Susanne's father died when she was 13, and Susanne's "illnesses" began soon after. In group therapy Susanne was able to gain an understanding of how her use of physical symptoms controlled others, and she was encouraged to try new assertive behaviors. Marital therapy was begun to explore the negative effects of Su-

Table 16–16 • SPECIFIC NURSING INTERVENTIONS: CLIENTS WITH SOMATOFORM DISORDERS

INTERVENTION	RATIONALE
1. Offer explanations and support during diagnostic testing.	1. Reduces anxiety while ruling out organic illness.
2. After physical complaints have been investigated, avoid further reinforcement, e.g., do not take vital signs each time client complains of palpitations.	2. Directs focus away from physical symptoms.
3. Spend time with client in 1 : 1 relationship.	3. Builds trust.
4. Observe and record frequency/intensity of somatic symptoms; notify physician of persistent symptoms.	4. Permits evaluation of effectiveness of intervention; prevents overlooking physical illness.
5. Recognize that client experiences symptoms as real. Acknowledge client's concern about state of health.	5. Acceptance promotes relief.
6. Do not imply that symptoms are not real.	6. Symptoms are real to the client even though causation is psychological rather than physical.
7. Shift focus on discussion from physical symptoms to client as a person, or to feelings, or to neutral topics.	7. Provides anxiety relief; conveys interest in client rather than in client's symptoms.
8. Encourage client to assume responsibility for own physical care.	8. Minimizes secondary gain. Fosters independence and self-esteem.
9. Initiate health care teaching to explain role of anxiety in producing physical symptoms. Help client associate occurrence of symptoms with stress.	9. Establishes causation. Increases recognition of own responses to anxiety.
10. Teach assertiveness techniques.	10. Provides positive means of getting needs met; can decrease need for secondary gains.
11. Encourage client to discuss feelings regarding symptoms, dependency created, and effect of client's physical symptoms on interpersonal relationships.	11. Clarifies issues. Reduces need to gain attention via symptoms.
12. Provide client with full schedule of daily activities; require participation.	12. Decreases time spent focusing on symptoms.
13. Teach client stress reduction techniques.	13. Provides healthy method of anxiety relief.

Refer to Table 16–8 for General Interventions.

Table 16–17 • USEFUL TREATMENTS FOR PEOPLE WITH SOMATOFORM DISORDERS

DISORDER	TREATMENT(S)*
Hypochondriasis	Psychotherapy Family therapy Relaxation therapy Behavior therapy
Conversion disorder	Psychotherapy Family therapy Relaxation therapy Behavior therapy Hypnosis
Somatoform pain disorder	Psychotherapy Family therapy Relaxation therapy Self-hypnosis

*Treatments may be used singly or in combination.

sanne's method of coping via physical symptoms and to find ways of minimizing the secondary gains. By discharge Susanne's mood was stable at baseline, she focused less on physical symptoms, and she agreed to return to her job and to continue marital counseling.

THE CLINICAL PICTURE OF HYPOCHONDRIASIS

Hypochondriasis is a disorder in which the individual is preoccupied with the belief that he or she has a serious disease, despite medical evidence to the contrary. The individual unrealistically interprets physical signs or sensations as abnormal and persistently seeks medical care. The client's symptoms are often vague and generalized, e.g., sweating, or they may be specific, e.g., a skin lesion on the neck. Commonly voiced preoccupations include cancer, bowel dysfunction, cardiac abnormality, venereal disease, and vague neurological symptoms. Although medical personnel reassure the client that there is no disease present, the individual cannot permanently accept this "nondiagnosis." Other medical and nonmedical opinions are sought.

Since the symptoms of this disorder serve the purpose of controlling anxiety and maintaining ego integrity (primary gain), and the mental maneuvers required to control the anxiety go on at an unconscious level, it is not difficult to see why a client may cling to the belief that he or she has an illness. Nemiah (1980) provides more specific information about the unconscious emotional forces, stating that hypochondriasis can be understood in one of two ways; as an alternate channel deflecting sexual, aggressive, or oral drives, or as an ego defense against the anxiety created by guilt or low self-esteem.

Impaired social or occupational functioning is always present. Some clients manage to work by setting aside their preoccupation during working hours, whereas others have frequent absences from work to keep appointments with physicians or for diagnostic testing. Still others adopt an invalid role.

Clients with hypochondriasis are commonly seen in medical practice. These clients are so offended at the suggestion that their beliefs about their illnesses are unrealistic that they usually refuse referral to mental health caregivers. In psychiatric treatment, individual or group therapy may be used, but the client rarely puts aside the preoccupation permanently. Teaching significant others to support the client without reinforcing the use of physical symptoms may be the most effective approach in the long run.

Clinical Vignette: A Client With Hypochondriasis

Anthony Estada, age 54, was referred to the mental health center outpatient clinic from the venereal disease (VD) clinic. Mr. Estada has visited the VD clinic almost weekly for two years, asking for diagnostic tests for various venereal diseases. He was always told that he had no illness. Most recently, his preoccupation has centered on AIDS.

Anthony, a widower whose wife died of cancer three years ago, is a self-employed plumber. He has few social contacts other than his two daughters. Since the onset of his wife's illness and his own preoccupation with illness, the daughters have visited at least weekly.

The client was brought up in a strict religious environment, joined the Navy at age 17, and married shortly after discharge. He appeared worried as he discussed his concern over VD with the nurse therapist and shared the story of his unsuccessful search for accurate diagnosis and treatment. The therapist decided it was not realistic to think that Mr. Estada could be "cured" of his preoccupation. Instead, the therapist decided to help Mr. Estada focus less on his symptoms and to assist his significant others in better coping with the situation.

During therapy Mr. Estada revealed that despite his religious upbringing, he had several encounters with prostitutes while he was in the Navy. When his wife's illness was diagnosed, he began to wonder if he had acquired a "disease" and passed it on to her. Cognitive therapy helped him gain an intellectual understanding that this fear was unrealistic. He continued to fail to understand how his family could be frustrated by his behavior and maintained that it was the duty of his daughters to visit him. He agreed not to visit the VD clinic without first calling his therapist but questioned the therapist at each session about the correctness of the last tests performed to rule out venereal disease. At discharge Mr. Estada was evaluated as being somewhat less anxious and much less preoccupied with the idea of having VD. He agreed to have diagnostic tests for VD performed only on a yearly basis.

THE CLINICAL PICTURE OF SOMATOFORM PAIN DISORDER

One of the most common subjective symptoms is pain. Acute pain usually has organic basis and protects us by signaling that something is wrong in the body. Certain illnesses, such as arthritis and angina, produce chronic pain. When pain does not have a physiological explanation or persists despite analgesics, biofeedback, or other medical interventions, psychological origin must be suspected.

Somatoform pain disorder has as its chief symptom severe and prolonged pain that is related to psychological factors. Refer to Figure 16–5 for DSM III-R (1987) diagnostic criteria. Although the pain is of psychogenic origin, it is important to remember that the client experiences the pain as very real. Secondary gain is often evident in the clinical cases of clients with somatoform pain disorder.

Clinical Vignette: A Client With Somatoform Pain Disorder

Robert Priest, age 36, is referred to the outpatient mental health clinic by his private physician. He has suffered from chronic back pain for two years, during which he has been unable to work as a longshoreman. He leans heavily on a cane and moves slowly and deliberately when he walks. Mr. Priest states that he has had myelograms that showed no basis for his pain, he uses a variety of analgesics that afford him no relief, and he has never been free of severe pain.

His back pain began after playing baseball at a picnic celebrating his wife's graduation from a community college nursing program. She had returned to school against his wishes when their youngest child entered high school. When she completed the program he grudgingly agreed to her acceptance of a part-time job, but she chose full-time employment. Now, he states, "It's a good thing she went against me, because she's the breadwinner and has to take care of me, now that I can't work."

During therapy Mr. Priest was taught relaxation techniques and self-hypnosis. He reported that he was helped most by self-hypnosis. He stated that being in control of his body helped him feel like a man rather than a whimpering baby. Individual counseling gave him support, but he was intensely resistant to uncovering material relevant to the underlying conflict. Job counseling enabled him to obtain a job as a dispatcher for a taxi company.

THE CLINICAL PICTURE OF CONVERSION DISORDER

One of the following psychological factors must always be present if a diagnosis of conversion disorder is made:

1. A close relationship in time between the onset of the symptoms and the occurrence of a conflict-producing event.
2. The presence of the symptom allows the individual to avoid some activity that is personally unpleasant.
3. The symptom enables the client to get support from the environment.

The individual achieves *primary gain* by keeping an internal conflict or need out of awareness, thus reducing the experience of anxiety. *Secondary gain* is achieved by avoidance of the unpleasant activity as well as by the support from the environment. The affect of **la belle indifference,** an attitude of *unconcern* about the symptom, is frequently noted. This lack of concern is thought to be a sign that primary gain has been achieved.

It is important to note that conversion symptoms are not under voluntary control. A conversion symptom often suggests neurological disease, such as paralysis, loss of voice, seizures, coordination disturbance, blindness, tunnel vision, loss of feeling or numbness, and tingling of a body part. A possible conversion reaction is suspected when the symptoms do not conform to an appropriate anatomical or physiological pattern, or if the symptom changes with suggestion or during repeated examinations. The symptom is both symbolic of, and a solution to, the underlying conflict.

An example of how a symptom can be both symbolic of, and a solution to, a conflict can be observed in the case of Anita, age 18, who lived with her mother and stepfather. The stepfather had been physically abusive to Anita for many years. Anita hated him but was dependent upon him for financial support. One day as the family stepped off the curb to cross a busy street, the father was hit by a speeding auto. Anita attempted to shout at her stepfather to warn him, but no sound came out. She suffered aphonia (loss of voice) that lasted until psychotherapy helped her regain her ability to speak.

One can see that the conflict for Anita was whether to warn her physically abusive and hated stepfather. The loss of her voice solved the problem and made it impossible to save him.

Conversion disorder often affects the individual's ability to go about life normally. When paralysis occurs as a result of conversion, it is possible for muscle atrophy and contractures to occur. Physical therapy should be ordered as a preventive measure. It is interesting to note that conversion symptoms may be removed under hypnosis but will return unless other treatment is given.

Although conversion disorder is the rarest of the somatoform disorders, it is well known that clients with conversion disorder can be among the most distressing to staff. In the following vignette, special attention has been paid to the interpersonal process concerns.

Clinical Vignette: A Client With Conversion Disorder

Pat Norris, a 30-year-old fashion model, was admitted to the neurological unit on the eve of her birthday with sudden onset of convulsions. She is an extremely attractive woman whose manner with the male nursing staff and physicians was coy and flirtatious. The first seizure recorded after hospitalization happened during morning rounds. During this time Pat arched her back and thrashed her arms about on the bed. There was no loss of consciousness. She was not incontinent nor did she bite her tongue. Afterward, she was alert and well oriented. The second "seizure" occurred in the afternoon during a visit from her mother and father. This episode lasted five minutes. It began with an outcry of obscenities that brought nurses running. This time she exhibited a generalized muscular rigidity, with heavy thrashing of her legs. Again there was no biting of the tongue, incontinence, period of lethargy, or confusion following the attack.

During her hospital stay for a neurological workup, Pat remained relatively unconcerned about her convulsions (la belle indifference) and their potential impact on her career. She seemed to enjoy the attention of the male staff, who responded to her attractiveness and vivacious interactions. When she was told that her electroencephalogram and all other tests were negative, she shrugged and agreed to transfer to the mental health unit "if all the boys (meaning medical staff) could come over" to see her.

Her seizures continued once to twice daily but always occurred in the presence of others, never with incontinence or self-injury, and always included sensual body movements. Initially, Pat refused to come out of her room for fear of an "attack." During this time, helpless dependent behavior was very noticeable. Visits from her parents seemed to support this, as her father called her his "little girl" or "princess," and her mother frequently pleaded with the nurses to take care of her daughter.

From the early days of admission, the staff discussed having negative feelings about Pat, especially the female staff. She made them feel as though they were being used as maids. Many of the staff admitted wanting to avoid her. Male staff reported feeling uncomfortable with her seductiveness, and all staff felt annoyed with her flirtatiousness and dependence.

A nursing care plan for Pat was developed on the mental health unit (Nursing Care Plan 16–2).

Dissociative Disorders

Dissociative disorders, like somatoform disorders, are illnesses that provide the individual with a way of

Nursing Care Plan 16–2 • A PERSON WITH CONVERSION DISORDER: Pat

NURSING DIAGNOSIS

Ineffective individual coping (use of conversion symptoms [seizures]), related to repressed anxiety associated with unresolved conflicts.

Supporting Data

- Seizures of varying patterns, including limb thrashing, muscular rigidity, and seductive pelvic movements.
- No incontinence. No injury. Seizures occur only in presence of others.
- La belle indifference.

Long Term Goal: Client will cope effectively with life stress without using conversion.

Short Term Goal	*Intervention*	*Rationale*	*Evaluation*
1. Client will adjust to unit routine by (state the date).	1. Explain routine. Establish expectations regarding unit routines, e.g., do not allow special privileges. Expect client to eat in dining room, perform ADLs, attend activities.	1. Reduces anxiety. Reduces secondary gain and manipulation.	Goal met Initially refused to leave room for meals. Missed one meal. Went to dining room thereafter. Performs all ADLs with special attention to applying make-up.
2. Client will develop trusting relationship with nurse by (state the date).	2. Be consistent.	2. Enhances trust. Reduces manipulation.	Relationship superficial through day 5, when sincere expression of feelings began.
3. Client will remain safe.	3. Provide safety measures during seizures but limit attention and discussion about seizure afterwards. Monitor physical condition unobtrusively.	3. Prevents harm. Reduces secondary gain. Minimizes secondary gain while assessing condition.	Client has not sustained injury during seizure. Has stated, "I guess my seizures don't interest staff. No one will talk to me about them." No seizures after day 6 on psychiatric unit.

4. Client will identify stressor.	4. Encourage client to discuss life, work, significant others, goals, etc.	4. Uncovers stress, conflict, strengths.	Repeatedly mentions that 30th birthday means she's over the hill as a model.
5. Client will express feelings about the conflict.	5. Use empathy; encourage exploration of feelings.	5. Conveys understanding.	States she's scared of losing her glamorous appearance and her job. Demonstrated appropriate affect.
6. Client will identify relationship between stressor, conflict, and symptom.	6. Reflect on anxiety and stress as they relate to use of physical symptoms. Provide opportunity to consider how the relationship might be valid in client's case.	6. Establishes probable causal relationship.	Client noted during session that first seizure occurred on 30th birthday.
7. Client will evaluate possible solutions to the problem.	7. Focus on alternatives available to her to earn a living when modeling is no longer an option.	7. Teaches problem solving.	Client showed fashion sketches to nurse and revealed she had once thought she might be a good designer. With encouragement decided to explore evening classes in illustration/ design to prepare for second career.
8. Client will discuss ways to cope with stress in future by (state the date).	8. Encourage use of alternate anxiety reduction techniques. Encourage client to select and learn a method.	8. Develops skill in use of a healthy technique.	Client chose to use jogging and progressive muscle relaxation and attended teaching sessions on each. Thinks each is helpful and plans to continue their use.

NURSING DIAGNOSIS

Chronic low self-esteem related to not seeing self as a capable adult.

Supporting Data

- Helpless, dependent behavior.
- Seductive, flirtatious behavior.
- Manipulative behavior such as playing one staff member against another and seeking special privileges.

Long Term Goal: Client will demonstrate adequate self-esteem by relating in age-appropriate ways.

Short Term Goal	*Intervention*	*Rationale*	*Evaluation*
1. Client will identify maladaptive behaviors of excessive dependence, seductiveness, and manipulation by (state the date).	1a. Set limits. Use consistent team approach.	1a. Minimizes maladaptive behaviors.	<u>Goal partially met</u>
	1b. Be nonjudgmental, accepting.	1b. When one is accepted by others, self-acceptance is fostered.	Client has not named any of the cited interpersonal problems, but incidence of behaviors has decreased to less than one per day.
	1c. When negative countertransference occurs, seek supervision.	1c. Supervision helps keep relationship in perspective.	Client often states, "If you think I can do it, perhaps I should reconsider and try it."
	1d. Affirm to client that symptoms can improve.	1d. Conveys hope.	Client admits that it is nice to be pampered by her parents but decided this might not be congruent with a mature role.
	1e. Express confidence in client's ability to function independently.	1e. Reinforces strengths.	Reports she never realized people would meet her requests when she asked in an assertive way. Enjoys using the techniques.
	1f. Reflect on father's choice of nickname. Assist client in assessing role behaviors that might perpetuate the infantile image.	1f. Fosters mature role-taking.	
	1g. Encourage to attend assertiveness training to learn to ask directly for what she needs.	1g. Decreases manipulation.	

avoiding anxiety while at the same time permitting certain needs to be met. **Dissociative disorders** involve sudden temporary disturbances or loss of one's normal ability to integrate identity or motor behavior. When the ability to integrate consciousness is impaired, the individual is unable to remember. When the ability to integrate identity is affected, the individual loses the sense of who he or she is. When failure to integrate motor behavior occurs, the individual wanders from home during the time the ability to integrate consciousness or identity is impaired. An overview of the dissociative disorders is seen in Figure 16–6.

Dissociation is an unconscious defense that protects the person against the disorganizing effects of severe anxiety by splitting off from awareness the idea, emotion, or experience that is too upsetting to handle. The anxiety-producing material is then repressed. Material that has been dissociated remains in the unconscious, where it has a life of its own, separate from what is known to the individual.

It is possible to see the pattern of avoidance when an individual deals with an unpleasant event by not thinking about it, e.g., "tuning out" in class relieves stress. The more anxiety-producing the event, the greater the need not to think about it. It seems, the more dissociation is used, the more likely it is to become automatic. When stress is intolerable and ego disintegration is threatened, the individual may unconsciously use dissociation to force an offending personality segment or memory out of awareness.

Abused individuals may use dissociation to defend against feeling pain and to avoid remembering. If the event is remembered, it has the quality of unreality about it, as though it happened to another person.

Each of us has many conflicting tendencies. They sometimes cause us to behave in surprising ways. Have

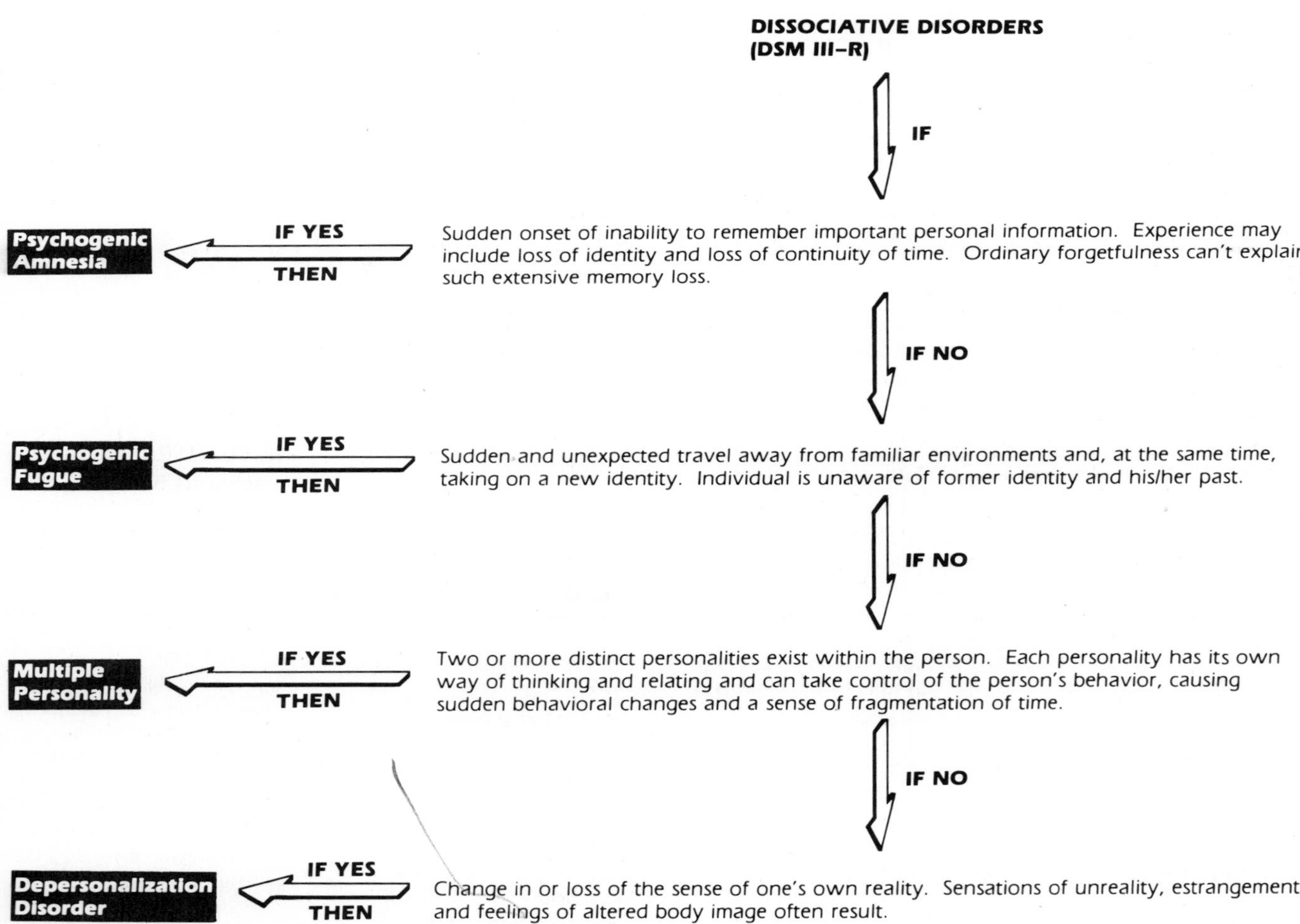

Figure 16–6. *Decision tree for the dissociative disorders.* (*Adapted from* Janicak PG, Andriukaitis SN. DSM III: *Seeing the forest through the trees.* Psychiatric Annals, 10(8):19, 1980, *and* Diagnostic and Statistical Manual of Mental Disorders [DSM III-R], *3d ed., revised.* Washington, DC: American Psychiatric Association, 1987.)

Table 16–18 • SPECIFIC NURSING INTERVENTIONS: CLIENTS WITH DISSOCIATIVE DISORDERS

INTERVENTION	RATIONALE
1. Ensure client safety by providing safe, protected environment and frequent observation.	1. Sense of bewilderment may lead to inattention to safety needs. Some personalities of the "multiple" may be thrill seeking, violent, or careless of personal safety.
2. Provide nondemanding simple routine.	2. Reduces anxiety.
3. Confirm identity of client and orientation to time and place.	3. Supports reality; promotes ego integrity.
4. Encourage client to do things for self and make decisions about the here and now of daily living.	4. Builds ego strength; enhances self-esteem by reducing sense of powerlessness; reduces secondary gain associated with dependence.
5. Assist with other decision making until memory returns.	5. Lowers stress; prevents having to live with the consequences of unwise decisions.
6. Support client during exploration of feelings surrounding the stressful event.	6. Support helps lower the defense of dissociation used by the client to block awareness of the stressful event.
7. Allow client to progress at own pace as memory is recovered.	7. Urging too rapid progress creates anxiety and resistance.
8. Help client see consequences of using dissociation to cope with stress.	8. Increases insight; helps client understand own role in choosing behaviors.
9. Accept client expressions of negative feelings.	9. Conveys permission to have negative/unacceptable feelings.
10. Teach stress reduction methods.	10. Provides alternatives for anxiety relief.
11. If client does not remember significant others, work with involved parties to reestablish relationships.	11. Helps client experience satisfaction; relieves sense of isolation.

you ever said to yourself, "I don't know why I did that" or wondered, "How could he or she do that; it's so out of character." When the conflict is very deep, the only resolution for the individual may be to separate the warring parts and let each function as a separate personality system. Each of the individual parts can function without anxiety or guilt that would be felt if the separation had not occurred. Specific nursing interventions and rationales specific to clients with dissociative disorders are presented in Table 16–18. General approaches to treatment are found in Table 16–19.

Table 16–19 • USEFUL TREATMENTS FOR PEOPLE WITH DISSOCIATIVE DISORDERS

DISORDER	TREATMENT(S)*
Psychogenic amnesia	Hypnosis Psychotherapy Relaxation therapy
Psychogenic fugue	Hypnosis Psychotherapy Relaxation therapy
Multiple personality	Hypnosis, Amytal Sodium interview Psychotherapy Relaxation therapy
Depersonalization disorder	Psychotherapy

*Treatments may be used singly or in combination.

THE CLINICAL PICTURE OF DEPERSONALIZATION DISORDER

Depersonalization disorder involves one or more episodes of experiencing change in, or loss of, the sense of one's own reality. **Depersonalization** is described as an ego-dystonic sensation of unreality or self-estrangement, a feeling that one's extremities have changed, a feeling of seeing oneself from a distance, or a feeling of functioning mechanically or of being in a dream. Depersonalization disorder is diagnosed when there is social or occupational disturbance from the episodes and when the episodes cannot be blamed on another disorder, such as schizophrenia, affective disorder, or epilepsy.

Therapy, either individual or group, aims to assist the client (1) in recognizing anxiety and the role dissociation plays in its avoidance and (2) in developing new effective coping strategies to deal with chronic and acute anxiety. Hospitalization is rarely necessary.

Clinical Vignette: A Client With Depersonalization Disorder

Tim Smith, age 14, came to the mental health clinic with the chief complaint, "I feel like a mechanical boy." He described "going through the motions" at school but feeling that it was "all unreal." He was an "A" student in middle school but has found high school more difficult. He reports that the depersonalization episodes occur only at school. Psychological testing and physical workup revealed no underlying illness, so the diagnosis of depersonalization disorder was made.

During therapy Tim was able to discuss his need to achieve high grades in order to compete with his older brother, a mechanical engineering student. Tim revealed that a few weeks before the symptom began, he told his brother of an embarrassing incident at school when a teacher had asked him a question and he had not known the answer. The teacher, who had known his brother, commented that his brother would never miss an easy question like that. His brother had ruffled Tim's hair and said, "They can't expect someone who's 'out to lunch' to know all the answers." Tim was able to explore the differences between himself and his brother and to see that it was okay to have different abilities and strengths.

THE CLINICAL PICTURE OF PSYCHOGENIC AMNESIA

The individual with psychogenic amnesia is unable to remember important personal information. **Psychogenic amnesia** is different from ordinary forgetfulness because the extent of the disturbance is greater. In *localized amnesia* there is inability to remember all events of a circumscribed period of time, e.g., the hours following the death of a loved one. *Selective amnesia* involves the ability to remember some events during a period, but not others. *Generalized amnesia*, the inability to remember any portion of one's life, is the most dramatic but least common form of amnesia. *Continuous amnesia* is the inability to remember events from a specific event in time to the present.

The stressor responsible for the amnesia is viewed by the individual as a horrible event. Amnesia is most likely to occur during a time of great disorganization, such as war or a natural or manmade disaster in which the threat of physical injury or death is present. Other stressors severe enough to produce psychogenic amnesia include the loss of a loved one and the stress of having to face the unacceptability of certain impulses or acts, such as an extramarital affair.

The individual with amnesia usually appears normal in all areas except memory. Mental functioning seems intact. A sense of calm and lack of concern for the loss of memory are often seen. Because amnesia is adaptive and affords the individual primary gain (relief from anxiety), "la belle indifference" is noted. Occasionally, during an episode of amnesia, the individual may seem perplexed and disoriented and engage in purposeless wandering.

Memory may be regained under hypnosis or with intravenous administration of sodium thiopental (Pentothal), but amnesia recurs when the client returns to a normal state of consciousness. Occasionally, posthypnotic suggestion may be effective in promoting memory return. Hypnosis gives the therapist information about the event that triggered the memory loss and about underlying conflict. This can be useful in choosing the direction for therapy. When hypnosis is not used, the therapist focuses on trust-building and supporting the client until memory returns and conflicts can be explored. Brief therapy is usually all that is required to resolve the problem of amnesia, since memory often returns as abruptly as it was lost. There is little need for medication, since subjective anxiety is not a problem. Recovery is usually complete, and recurrences are rare.

Clinical Vignette: A Client with Psychogenic Amnesia

Joan Moore, an office worker, was abducted on her way to work. She was taken to an abandoned house, bound and gagged, and placed in a room with several other women. The captor periodically tortured the other captives. Joan was left helpless and unable to move for three days. During this time she was terrified that she would be noticed and tortured. Instead, she was rescued by the police. Although very tired and extremely hungry, Joan appeared cheerful and unconcerned. She remembered none of what happened during the ordeal. She was referred to the psychiatrist, who described her as friendly and casual but showing memory loss about where she had spent the past three days. A diagnosis of psychogenic amnesia was made.

Joan was given supportive therapy at the hospital for several days. Then, the memory of the three days returned. She was able to describe feelings of terror and her sense of helplessness. She was left shaken and depressed and decided to enter outpatient therapy. There, she received therapy for post-traumatic stress disorder, and her life eventually returned to normal.

THE CLINICAL PICTURE OF FUGUE DISORDER

Fugue and psychogenic amnesia both involve memory loss triggered by an overwhelming stressful event, but in **fugue** the individual suddenly and unexpectedly travels away from home or usual work locale and assumes a new identity. Extreme cases involve taking on a new personality—often more social, uninhibited, and fun-loving than the former personality. The individual may not seem to have any suggestion of mental disorder. In the majority of cases, the fugue consists of what seems to be purposeful travel, with only minimal contact with others. A new identity is present but not complete. Recovery from fugue leaves the individual able to remember his or her former life but not the time spent in the fugue.

Brief psychotherapy aimed at uncovering the conflict and developing more effective ways to cope is generally all that is needed. Little time is spent focusing on the events that occurred during the fugue period. There is usually no need for antianxiety medication.

Clinical Vignette: A Client With Fugue Disorder

A young, attractive woman awakened one morning and noticed snow outside the window swirling around unfamiliar buildings and streets. The radio told her it was December. She was perplexed to find herself in a residential hotel in Chicago with no idea of how she had gotten there. She felt confused and shaken. As she left the hotel, she was surprised to have strangers recognize her and say, "Good morning, Sally." The name Sally did not seem right, but she could not remember her true identity. She found her way to a hospital, where she was admitted to the mental health unit. Nursing Care Plan 16–3 was developed for "Sally." In the evaluation column you will learn more about her as her memory returns.

THE CLINICAL PICTURE MULTIPLE PERSONALITY DISORDER

Anderson (1988) states that multiple personality disorder **(MPD)**, although still considered somewhat rare, dates back to the late 1800's. Kluft, as reported in *Psychiatric News*, states that the prevalence of **MPD** is one case per 10,000 population (1988a) and has seen a considerable increase in reported cases since 1970. Whether the increase is due to an actual increase in cases, an increase in therapists' reporting of cases, or more accurate diagnosis is still uncertain. Multiple personality disorder is usually seen in early adulthood, although childhood cases have been reported (Kolb and Brodie 1982). Most of the documented cases have been women.

There seems to be no doubt that physical and emotional abuse and sexual trauma during childhood are common in most cases (Boor 1982; Greenberg 1982; Jorn 1982). The steps in the development of dissociated personalities are thought to be as follows:

1. A young child is confronted with an intolerable terror-producing event at a time when defenses are inadequate to handle the intense anxiety.
2. The child *dissociates* the event and the feelings associated with the event. The dissociated material is split off from the memory of the primary personality.
3. The dissociated part of the personality takes on a personality of its own, becoming a subpersonality.
4. The subpersonality learns to deal with feelings and emotions that would overwhelm the primary personality (Greenberg 1982).
5. This process may occur once or several times, creating one or several subpersonalities.
6. When faced with an anxiety-producing situation, one of the subpersonalities takes over to protect the primary personality from disorganization and disintegration.

The essential feature of **multiple personality** is the existence within an individual of two or more distinct personalities, each of whom is dominant at a particular time (DSM III-R 1987). Each personality is a fully integrated and complex unit with its own memories, behavior patterns, and social relationships that dictate how the person will act when that personality is dominant. Often the original or primary personality is religious and moralistic, and the subpersonalities are quite different: aggressive, pleasure seeking, nonconforming, sexually promiscuous. Subpersonalities may exhibit signs of emotional disturbance (Abrams 1983).

The primary personality is usually not aware of the subpersonalities but may be aware of lost time and

Nursing Care Plan 16–3 • A PERSON WITH PSYCHOGENIC FUGUE DISORDER: Sally

NURSING DIAGNOSIS

Ineffective individual coping related to severe anxiety and use of dissociation.

Supporting Data

- Inability to remember identity (residents call her "Sally" but this does not feel right).
- Sensing current surroundings are strange.

Long Term Goal: By (state the date) client will cope with stress without experiencing memory loss.

Short Term Goal	*Intervention*	*Rationale*	*Evaluation*
1. Client will maintain biological integrity.	1. Provide nourishing diet, help establish healthful rest/activity cycle, monitor elimination and safety.	1. Memory loss may create sense of bewilderment requiring guidance.	Goal met Becoming familiar with the unit took two days. Thereafter, all biological functions were normal.
2. Client will perform all ADLs.	2. Provide orientation to routine; make necessary items available. Convey positive expectation that client can take this responsibility.	2. Fosters ego strength, sense of mastery.	Performed ADLs adequately from day of admission.
3. Client will remember own identity and recall life's events by (state the date).	3a. Provide supportive nondemanding environment.	3a. Reduces anxiety.	After three days in hospital, Sally remembered a phone number. Her sister answered, establishing Sally's identity as Mary Hunt of New York. Her sister flew to Chicago to be with Mary.
	3b. Confirm identity.	3b. Supports reality.	After two days Mary stopped asking, "Are you sure that's who I am?"
	3c. Do not push client to remember. Allow client to set the pace.	3c. Symptoms help prevent ego disorientation.	On day 10 Mary recalled an evening when her husband returned to their apartment and asked for a divorce.
4. Client will state feelings about stressful event.	4. Encourage discussion of thoughts/feelings. Show acceptance. Use empathy.	4. Conveying acceptance fosters self-acceptance. Sympathy fosters self-pity. Empathy fosters client acceptance of positive and negative feelings.	Mary stated she felt disbelief and helplessness when her husband asked for a divorce and remembered a fleeting wish that she could run away and hide.
5. Client will state relationship between memory loss and stress by (state the date).	5. Give support as client develops awareness of dynamics of unconscious choice of dissociation.	5. Fosters development of insight.	Mary stated she seems to have acted on her fleeting wish by leaving New York, forgetting who she was, and taking up life in Chicago as Sally.
6. Client will demonstrate ability to use a selected stress reduction technique.	6. Teach progressive relaxation.	6. Provides an appropriate outlet for anxiety reduction.	Mary uses progressive relaxation daily and reported less tension during past week.

NURSING DIAGNOSIS

Social isolation related to inability to remember.

Supporting Data

- Inability to remember sister.
- Inability to feel closeness with sister.

Long Term Goal: Client will reestablish satisfying relations with significant other by (state the date).

Short Term Goal	*Intervention*	*Rationale*	*Evaluation*
1. Client will interact socially with sister by (state the date).	1a. Provide pleasant, neutral environment.	1a. Assists in reducing stress.	Goal met
	1b. Assist sister in understanding Mary's symptom as response to stress.	1b. Fosters acceptance and empathy.	Two days after sister arrived, Mary stated her sister is a "pleasant person who is nice to get to know."
2. Client will share feelings with sister by (state the date).	2. Discuss with client the progress being made in rebuilding the relationship. Encourage risk taking to share feelings to deepen relationship.	2. Self revelation fosters intimacy.	After two weeks Mary and her sister reported a sense of closeness. Mary reports not feeling lonely or estranged anymore.

NURSING DIAGNOSIS

Disturbance in self-esteem, related to rejection by husband and feelings of ineffectiveness.

Supporting Data

- Stating she does not know how to cope.
- Stating she does not know how to get what she wants from others.
- Husband planning to divorce client.

Long Term Goal: Client will state she feels "good" about herself by (state the date).

Short Term Goal	*Intervention*	*Rationale*	*Evaluation*
1. Client will assess her strengths and weaknesses realistically by (state the date).	1. Help client focus on self-assessment, including positive aspects.	1. Helps bolster self-esteem.	Goal met On the seventh hospital day, Mary created a list with shortcomings and five strengths.
2. Client will learn assertiveness techniques by (state the date).	2. Teach client how to ask for what she needs and to say "no" assertively.	2. Assertiveness protects own rights while not violating rights of others.	At discharge, Mary rehearsed telling her husband how she felt about the divorce, using assertiveness techniques. Mary reports feeling prepared to find a job and work on a divorce settlement.

unexplained events, such as finding unfamiliar clothing in the closet, being called by different names, or waking up in strange surroundings (Thigpen and Cleckley 1957). When two or more subpersonalities exist, each is aware of the others to some degree. Some may even interact with each other. Subpersonalities may "listen in on" whatever personality is dominant at the time. It is not unusual for subpersonalities to report being a different race, age, or sex from the original personality. Each behaves according to its stated characteristics.

Transition from one personality to another often occurs during times of stress and is usually a dramatic event. Some clients experience the transition when awakening. Shifts from personality to personality last from minutes to months, although shorter periods are more common (Coleman et al. 1980).

Hypnosis is often used to explore the existence and characteristics of the various subpersonalities. The aim of therapy is to integrate or join the subpersonalities together once they are aware of each other. Integration of the personalities with the primary personality can take place only if the subpersonalities are willing to integrate. Amnesic barriers can then be broken down gradually (Anderson 1988). Total integration is rarely possible during a short term hospital stay. Integration can take up to two or more years (Anderson 1988). Successful achievement includes the combination of psychodynamic psychotherapy with the use of hypnosis and/or sodium amytal interviews (Kluft 1988b).

Clinical Vignette: A Client with Multiple Personalities

Andrea, a 28-year-old fashionable yet conservative engineer, is the primary personality. Four other personalities called subpersonalities coexist with Andrea and vie for supremacy.

Michele is a four-year-old who is sometimes playful and sometimes angry. She speaks with a slight lisp and with the facial expressions, voice inflections, and vocabulary of a precocious 4-year-old. She likes to play on swings, draw with a crayon, and eat ice cream. She likes to cuddle a teddy bear and occasionally sucks her thumb. Her favorite outfit is a Mickey Mouse sweatshirt and a pair of jeans.

Kurt is a calm, deep-voiced man who says he is 26. He is learning to be a chef and is annoyed when he is not allowed to become dominant and take over Andrea's body in order to attend his classes. He pleads he is getting behind in his studies. He recently discovered he needs glasses.

Bridget is near Andrea's age, although she says a lady never tells her age. She dresses seductively in bright colors, wears her hair tousled, and likes to frequent discos and stay out late. She often drinks to excess and has several male admirers.

Ann is an accomplished ballet dancer. She is shy but firm about needing time to practice and perform. When she is dominant, she likes to wear white and fixes her hair in a severe, pulled back style. She does little but dance when she is "out," or in control.

Andrea does not drink, hates ice cream, and sees herself as somewhat awkward in her movements and as not dancing well. She, however, is a paid soprano soloist in a church choir. Andrea takes public transportation, but Kurt and Bridget have driver's licenses. She goes to bed and arises early, but Bridget and Michele like to stay up late.

Andrea sought treatment when she found herself behind the wheel of a moving car and realized she did not know how to drive. She had been concerned for some time because she found strange clothes in her closet—some of them men's. She had also received phone calls from men who insisted she had flirted with them in bars. She sometimes missed appointments and could not account for periods of time but did not understand why. Although she went to bed early, she often was unaccountably tired in the morning.

Because her therapist was familiar with multiple personality, hypnosis was used to confirm the presence of the subpersonalities and to gather data about them. Therapy usually necessitates several years. The goal of therapy is to integrate various components of the subpersonalities into the primary personality.

Summary

Individuals suffering from anxiety disorders, somatoform disorders, and dissociative disorders have several things in common:

- They do not have clearly defined organic bases, rather, an unresolved psychological conflict is often found.
- Many have sustained trauma early in life or have been exposed to anxious, overconcerned adults.
- Although usually in touch with reality, the individual is usually not in touch with his or her real self.
- Great amounts of energy and multiple defense mechanisms are used to deal with anxiety. The defense mechanisms are rarely able to accomplish the goal of permanent anxiety reduction.
- *Rigid behavior patterns* tend to be *repeated* whenever the individual is faced with stress and anxiety.
- Sufferers tend to recognize that their symptoms are odd or strange, i.e., *their symptoms are ego-dystonic.*
- There is a lack of awareness of the relationship among symptoms, anxiety, and underlying conflict.
- Care is usually sought to relieve the distressing effects of anxiety.
- Self-esteem and self-acceptance tend to be low.
- Altered patterns of relatedness, especially domination of others, are characteristic.
- These individuals tend to incite predictable negative feelings in the staff who provide treatment. These feelings make it necessary for nurses to practice self-assessment and be willing to accept supervision from another professional.

Several treatment modalities are useful. Individual therapy, group therapy, behavior therapy, cognitive therapy, and pharmacotherapy may be undertaken. Unfortunately, complete "cure" is rare, but clients can be helped to make more satisfactory adjustments.

The nurse therapist caring for the client with ego-dystonic symptoms will have an opportunity to function in the dynamic and rewarding roles of caregiver, teacher, communicator, and manager and will use the nursing process to provide comprehensive care for the client and the family by doing the following:

- Systematically collecting assessment data about the client's physical and psychosocial status.
- Analyzing this data and selecting relevant nursing diagnoses.
- Establishing a nursing care plan with individualized measurable goals and specific nursing interventions.
- Intervening to reduce anxiety; using psychotherapeutic methods to improve coping skills, providing health teaching, and promoting self-care.
- Collaborating with the health team.
- Evaluating client responses to nursing actions.

References

Abrams S. The multiple personality: A legal defense. American Journal of Clinical Hypnosis, 25(4):225, 1983.

Anderson G. Understanding multiple personality disorder. Journal of Psychiatric Nursing, 26(7):26, 1988.

Andreasen N. The Broken Brain. New York: Harper and Row, 1984.

Boor M. The multiple personality epidemic. Journal of Nervous and Mental Disease, 170(5):302, 1982.

Chapman AH. Textbook of Clinical Psychiatry: An Interpersonal Approach, 2nd ed. Philadelphia: J.B. Lippincott Company, 1976.

Chapman AH, Chapman M. Harry Stack Sullivan's Concepts of Personality Development and Psychiatric Illnesses. New York: Brunner-Mazel Publishers, 1980.

Colby KM, McGuire MT. Signs and symptoms: Zeroing in on a better classification of neuroses. The Sciences, 21–24, Nov. 1981.

Coleman JC, Butcher JN, Carson RC. Abnormal Psychology and Modern Life, 6th ed. Glenview, IL: Scott, Foresman & Company, 1980.

Crowe RR, Noyes R, Pauls DL, et al. A family study of panic disorders. Archives of General Psychiatry, 40:1065, 1983.

Diagnostic and Statistical Manual of Mental Disorders (DSM III-R), 3d ed., revised. Washington DC: American Psychiatric Association, 1987.

Dohrenwend BP, Dohrenwend BS. Psychiatric disorders in urban setting. *In* Arieti S (ed). American Handbook of Psychiatry, 2nd ed. Vol. 2. New York: Basic Books, 1974.

Gray M. Neuroses: A Comprehensive and Critical View. New York: Van Nostrand Reinhold Company, 1978.

Greenberg WC. The multiple personality. Perspectives in Psychiatric Care, 20(3):100, 1982.

Hollander Z, Liebowitz MR, Gorman JM. Anxiety disorders. *In* Talbott JA, Hales RE, Yudofsky SC (eds). Textbook of Psychiatry. Washington, DC: American Psychiatric Press, 1988.

Jorn N. Repression in a case of multiple personality disorder. Perspectives in Psychiatric Care, 20(3):105, 1982.

Kidson MA, Jones IH. Psychiatric disorders among aborigines of the Australian western desert. Archives of General Psychiatry, 19(4):413, 1968.

Kluft RP. Psychiatrists debate multiple personality: Discrete entity or just a symptom? Psychiatric News, 23(11):7, 1988a.

Kluft RP. The dissociative disorders. *In* Talbott JA, Hales RE, Yudofsky SC (eds). Textbook of Psychiatry. Washington DC: American Psychiatric Press, 1988b.

Kolb LC, Brodie HK. Modern Clinical Psychiatry, 10th ed. Philadelphia: W.B. Saunders Company, 1982.

Nemiah JC. Somatization disorder. *In* Kaplan HI, Freedman Am, Saddock BJ (eds). Comprehensive Textbook of Psychiatry, vol 2. Baltimore: Williams & Wilkins Company, 1980.

Salzman L. Therapy of obsessional states. American Journal of Psychiatry, 122(10):1139, 1966.

Stoudemire GA. Somatoform disorders, factitious disorders and malingering. *In* Talbott JA, Hales RE, Yudofsky SC (eds). Textbook of Psychiatry. Washington DC: American Psychiatric Press, 1988.

Thigpen C, Checkley H. The Three Faces of Eve. Kingsport, TN: Kingsport Press, Inc., 1957.

Self-Study Exercises

Place the letter of the item from the right column next to the appropriate phrase in the left column.

1. ______ Showing lack of appropriate concern about one's symptom(s)
2. ______ Interpersonal benefits the individual derives from illness
3. ______ Recurrent, intrusive thought
4. ______ Irrational fear
5. ______ Helpful in treatment of phobias and panic
6. ______ Psychiatric condition resulting from rape, war, or disaster not usually experienced by an individual
7. ______ Splitting off from consciousness of painful feelings
8. ______ Repetitive act that helps lower anxiety
9. ______ Symptoms with which the ego is uncomfortable
10. ______ Preoccupation with the idea that one has a serious disease
11. ______ Involves assumption of a new identity in a distant locale

A. Primary gain
B. Ego-syntonic
C. Secondary gain
D. Post-traumatic stress disorder
E. Dissociation
F. Obsession
G. Compulsion
H. Ego-dystonic
I. Amnesia
J. Antidepressants
K. La belle indifference
L. Fugue
M. Hypochondriasis
N. Phobia

Match the disorder listed in the right column with the nursing diagnosis that might be most appropriate for a client with that condition.

12. ______ Social isolation related to preoccupation with physical symptoms
13. ______ Potential for violence related to sensory-perceptual alteration secondary to severe anxiety
14. ______ Anxiety: severe, related to exposure to heights
15. ______ Disturbance in self-concept: personal identity, related to dissociation of anxiety-producing event

A. Amnesia
B. Somatization
C. Panic
D. Phobia
E. Obsessive-compulsive disorder

Match the disorder listed in the right column with the nursing intervention that might be most appropriate for a client with that condition.

16. ______ Focus on the person, feelings, or a neutral topic to avoid reinforcing physical symptom
17. ______ Examine idea that object has actual power to harm client
18. ______ Have client time length of each attack
19. ______ Allow time for performance of ritual
20. ______ Encourage discussion of adventitious crisis

A. Conversion disorder
B. Phobia
C. Generalized anxiety disorder
D. Multiple personality
E. Obsessive-compulsive disorder
F. Post-traumatic stress disorder

CHAPTER 17

Personality Disorders—Antisocial and Borderline

Kem B. Louie • *Antisocial Personality Disorders*
Suzanne Lego • *Borderline Personality Disorders*

OUTLINE

KEY TERMS AND CONCEPTS

The key terms and concepts listed here also appear in bold where they are defined or discussed in this chapter.

EGO-SYNTONIC
ANTISOCIAL, SOCIOPATH, PSYCHOPATH
MANIPULATION
MALADAPTIVE USE OF MANIPULATION
The Seducer
The Passive-Aggressor
Keep the Ball in the Air
Help Me If You Can
FIVE STEPS IN SETTING LIMITS
IMPULSIVENESS
AGGRESSION
DETACHMENT
MODELING
SPLITTING
PROJECTIVE IDENTIFICATION

An individual's personality encompasses more or less enduring and consistent attitudes, beliefs, desires, values, and patterns of behavior. Personality has also been referred to as an evolving pattern of thinking, perceiving, and experiencing. Personality patterns determine how an individual is liked and judged by others and what a person's goals and accomplishments are in life. To a certain extent, these patterns are acquired at birth through the influence of the parents' genes. For the most part, many believe that it is the influence of the early interactions with the infant that determines the behaviors or personality (Kolb and Brodie 1982).

The American Psychiatric Association (1987) states a person has a personality disorder "when personality traits are inflexible and maladaptive and significantly impair social or occupational functioning." The ability to achieve developmental tasks such as trust, autonomy, independence, and meaningful relationships is limited for individuals diagnosed with personality disorders.

According to the DSM III-R, personality disorders are grouped into three categories. *First*, those that appear *odd* or *eccentric*: the paranoid, schizoid, and schizotypal personality disorders. *Second*, individuals who are *dramatic* or *emotional*: the histrionic, narcissistic, antisocial, and borderline personality disorders. *Third*, those who are *anxious* and *fearful*: the avoidant, dependent, compulsive, and passive-aggressive personality disorders. Tables 17–1, 17–2, and 17–3 provide characteristics and examples of each of these personality disorders. In the DSM III-R multiaxial classification system, the disorders are listed and diagnosed under Axis II.

Axis I	Clinical Syndromes
*Axis II	Personality Disorders
	Specific Developmental Disorders
Axis III	Physical Disorders and Conditions
Axis IV	Severity of Psychosocial Stressors
Axis V	Highest Level of Adaptive Functioning Past Year

The personality disorders can be conceptualized as shown in Figure 17–1.

People with these personality disorders are perhaps the group of patients psychiatrists least like to treat. People with personality disorders are most likely to be clinic dropouts and treatment failures. They also make up a large percentage of the jailed population (Vaillant and Perry 1985). Since symptoms in personality disorders are **ego-syntonic,** they do not seem to bother the owner. In other words, the symptoms "feel right" to the person who possesses them (Millon 1981). To observers, the paranoia and hostility and the passive-aggressive and manipulative behaviors are viewed as deviant, distasteful, deceitful, and infuriating.

Table 17–1 • PERSONALITY DISORDERS DESCRIBED AS ODD OR ECCENTRIC

CHARACTERISTICS	EXAMPLES
Paranoid	
Pervasive and unwarranted suspiciousness—mistrust of people displayed as jealously, envy, and guardedness. Hypersensitivity to others; feels mistreated or misjudged. Displays restricted affect as lack of humor and lack of tender feelings.	Ronald is a successful businessman. He is meticulous and has an intense drive for achievement. He is often described by his business associates as lacking a sense of humor and is perceived as sarcastic, derogatory, and resentful. When his positions or points of view are questioned, he argues and defends them relentlessly, believing others are jealous of him. He has been heard on several occasions belittling and criticizing others. He has no close friends.
Schizoid	
Inability to form social relationships; absence of warm and tender feelings toward others. Indifference to praise, criticism, and feelings of others. Exhibits little or no desire for social involvement. Has few friends. Generally is reserved, withdrawn, and seclusive. Pursues solitary interest or hobbies. Has dull or flat affect; appears cold and aloof.	Juanita is a college graduate who has been working as a librarian for five years. She is very shy and withdrawn but readily assists you when you are looking for a book. When speaking to her, you notice that her speech is monotone, and her appearance very dull. You've heard her tell a coworker that she is not interested in dating and enjoys her time alone.
Schizotypal	
Exhibits various oddities of thought, perception, speech, and behavior that are not severe enough to be diagnosed as schizophrenia. No dominant characteristic is present. May demonstrate magical thinking, ideas of reference, paranoid ideation, illusions, depersonalization, and speech peculiarities. Socially isolated; has inappropriate affect.	Wallace lives over a grocery store down the street. Every day you have noticed Wallace going into an empty lot looking for pieces of glass or scraps of metal. He is never seen talking to anyone and is usually alone. Wallace was seen arguing and laughing by himself in front of the store one evening. He was discussing how the voices in the faucet were talking to him. The conversation had lasted ten minutes when the owner asked Wallace to leave.

Data from American Psychiatric Association. Diagnostic and Statistical Manual of Mental Disorders (DSM III-R), 3d ed., revised. Washington DC: American Psychiatric Association, 1987.

All the personality disorders have four characteristics in common (Vaillant and Perry 1985): (1) an inflexible and maladaptive response to stress, (2) disability in working and loving, (3) ability to evoke interpersonal conflict, and (4) capacity to "get under the skin" of others.

1. *An inflexible and maladaptive response to stress.* Personality patterns are deeply ingrained into the personality structure and persist, unmodified, over long periods of time (Millon 1981). At times, these personality patterns and traits may be compatible and acceptable with societal norms and are valued by the culture or occupation. For instance, an engineer or administrator needs to possess some compulsive traits, such as the ability to organize complex details and meet deadlines. At other times, these same compulsive traits, when too rigid and limited, may interfere with personal, occupational, or social functioning.
2. *Disability in working and loving, which is generally more serious and pervasive than the similar disability found in neurosis.* On the mental health continuum, personality disorders fall between neurosis and psychosis. Certain characteristics observed in people with personality disorders are similar to those characteristics seen in affective and schizophrenic disorders, such as withdrawn behaviors and grandiosity. The difference is that individuals with personality disorders, for the most part, have normal ego functioning and reality testing. There are, however, great disturbances in their ability to love and work.
3. *Ability to evoke interpersonal conflict.* Interpersonal relationships, at best, are marked by intense upheavals and hostility within a precarious interpersonal context. People with personality disorders lack the ability to see themselves objectively. Therefore, the need or desire to alter aspects of their behaviors in order to enrich or maintain important interpersonal relationships is lacking. Thus, annoying and distanc-

Table 17–2 • PERSONALITY DISORDERS DESCRIBED AS DRAMATIC AND EMOTIONAL

CHARACTERISTICS	EXAMPLES
Histrionic	
Behaviors are dramatic and attention seeking; prone to exaggeration; overreacts to situations with irrational, angry outbursts or tantrums. Forms interpersonal friendships quickly but becomes demanding, egocentric, and inconsiderate. Is perceived as shallow and lacking genuineness, although appears charming and appealing. Generally, attractive and seductive; attempts to control the opposite sex or enter into a dependent relationship.	Kelly has many boyfriends. She is attractive, witty, fun to be around, and superficial. She is generally seen and heard with groups of people, particularly men who are athletic and well dressed. Kelly states she does not have any close girlfriends because "they are jealous of me and that is their problem." She is usually heard telling her coworkers what a fabulous and terrific weekend she had with her boyfriends.
Narcissistic	
Exaggerated sense of self-importance as exhibited in extreme self-centeredness and self-involvement; preoccupied with fantasies of unrealistic goals involving power, wealth, success, beauty, or love; need for constant admiration and attention, with interpersonal manipulation of others. Inability to empathize with others.	Laura is a junior executive, married, with two children. She prides herself in being able to care for her husband and children and have a career. Her husband complains that she is cold and aloof. Everything done at home must be approved by her, including vacations, social affairs, and school activities. At work, she is competitive with the other executives. She even used her femininity once to obtain a promotion. Since she has potential, she has attracted several offers for a position as vice president.
Antisocial	
History of continuous and chronic antisocial behaviors against society, such as vandalism, fighting, delinquency, thefts, and truancy. Inability to maintain meaningful employment or relationships; impulsive, reckless, lying, or conning others for personal gain. Unable to maintain intimacy with a sexual partner.	Joseph's father died of a drug overdose when he was six weeks old. His mother had difficulty caring for him, so he was placed in foster care. Until the age of ten, Joey had five foster parents and ran away three times. At the age of 11, Joey joined a group of boys much older than he. This is when he began stealing. Being bright and attractive, Joey was able to "talk to the ladies." With older women, he would act lost and ask to use the phone. When their backs were turned, he would take the purse out of their pocketbooks. Staying out late at night and absence from school led Joey to drop out of school. At age 16, he traveled across the country, where he began fighting and was recently arrested for assault.
Borderline	
Instability is exhibited in interpersonal behavior, where relationships are intense and unstable, marked by impulsive and unpredictable behavior; marked shifts in mood and temper at times inappropriate. Profound disturbance in identity related to self image, gender, values, and future goals.	Rachel was admitted to the hospital for a suicide attempt. She threatened to jump out of a six-story window. When asked how long she felt depressed, she responded "forever." On the unit, Rachel acted helpless—unable to decide what to wear and whether she should continue her medication. At other times, she would demand and threaten to leave the hospital. She was fond of Marvin, her primary nurse, and spent much of her free time with him. For his birthday she even bought him a watch, which he refused to accept. Last night Rachel tried to hang herself in her room.

Data from American Psychiatric Association. Diagnostic and Statistical Manual of Mental Disorders (DSM III-R), 3d ed., revised. Washington DC: American Psychiatric Association, 1987.

Table 17–3 • PERSONALITY DISORDERS DESCRIBED AS ANXIOUS AND FEARFUL

CHARACTERISTICS	EXAMPLES
Avoidant	
Exhibits hypersensitivity to potential rejection, humiliation, or shame. Socially withdrawn with low self-esteem but desires social relations if given guarantee of uncritical acceptance.	Sal has worked for a public relations firm for three years. He is successful and is liked by his coworkers. His nickname in the office is "Shy Sal." He has made several attempts to date female clients but finds himself unable to ask them out. He is active in a running club and bicycles 20 miles per week. He feels lonely and imprisoned in his body. He is aware of wanting to relate to others but is unable to take the necessary steps.
Dependent	
Passively allows others to take responsibility for her life or some major portion of it. Subordinates own needs to the needs of those whom she is dependent upon; lacks self-confidence.	Mona is a mother of three children. She enjoys caring for her family. She rarely does anything without approval or permission from her husband. She thought of going back to school, but her husband thought it was a stupid idea. She agreed with him after thinking it over. Once, she bought an expensive outfit to wear to a church affair and social. Her husband was outraged and struck her because she had spent $130. She later apologized and promised not to buy clothes without his permission.
Compulsive	
Restricted in ability to express warm and tender emotions. Preoccupied with conformity, such as rules, trivial details, and procedures. Exhibits superior attitudes when working with others; work and productivity are valued more than pleasure and relationships; tends toward perfectionism.	Jason worked in the accounting department of a community hospital. He was punctual, neat, and meticulous about his appearance and work. At home he was the same way with his family and hobbies. He was generally in the basement working on projects, and when interrupted, he became furious. His family complained that he was not a warm and emotionally feeling man, but he was able to provide the family with financial security.
Passive-Aggressive	
Habitually resents and resists demands and requests to perform adequately in both occupational and social functioning. This resistance is expressed indirectly, i.e., procrastination, stubbornness, intentional inefficiency, and forgetfulness.	Maurice has had four jobs in two years. He works as an artist for art galleries. He has much talent and has won a few awards for his paintings in the community. He was fired because he was unable to meet deadlines. Many times while working on the paintings he would procrastinate. His employer would give him extensions, but he still failed to meet the deadlines.

Data from American Psychiatric Association. Diagnostic and Statistical Manual of Mental Disorders (DSM III-R), 3d ed., revised. Washington DC: American Psychiatric Association, 1987.

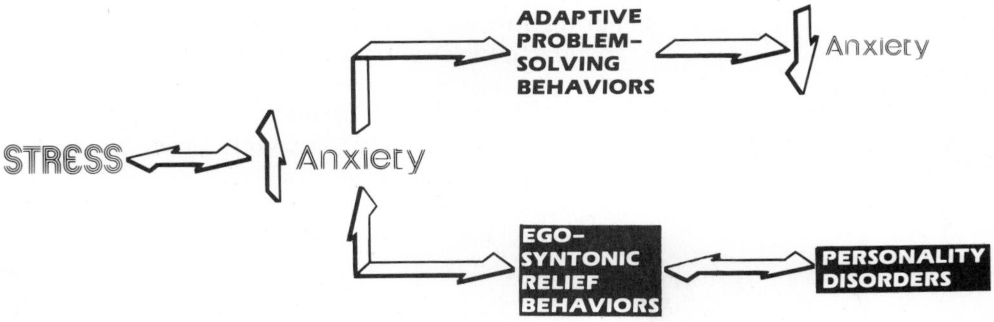

Figure 17-1. *Conceptualization of the process in the development of personality disorders.*

ing behaviors continue and are usually met with strong negative reactions from others.

4. *Capacity to "get under the skin" of others.* "Getting under the skin" of others refers to the uncanny ability of people with personality disorders to "merge personal boundaries" with others. This merging is manifested by the profound affect they have on others (Vaillant and Perry 1985). It is likened to the affect that lovers have on each other, except in the personality disorders the process is often unconscious and the results undesirable.

Recent research in the identification of biological markers and biogenetic predispositions for many of the personality disorders is yielding important findings. Many theorists, however, still believe that the origin of personality disorders is the failure to develop an identity compatible with society. The loss or absence of parents or parental substitutes and limited contact with adults and peers in the early stages of development deprive a child of establishing an ego identity through the process of identification. A defect in personality may also occur as a result of frustration when the child is unable to achieve satisfaction of fundamental needs such as love, security, recognition, respect, and success.

Personality disorders are characterized by their long term nature and repetitive, maladaptive, and often self-defeating behaviors. These behaviors are not experienced as uncomfortable or disorganized by the individual, as are the symptoms experienced by a client with a "neurotic disorder." It is important to note that, with personality disorders, other areas of personal functioning may be very adequate. The predominant maladaptive behaviors may affect only one aspect of the person's life. Therefore, many individuals with personality disorders do not seek treatment unless a severe crisis or trauma precipitates other symptoms.

The personality disorders seen most often in the health care system are the borderline personality and the antisocial personality. Since the behaviors central to these disorders often cause upheaval and disruption on psychiatric units, as well as on medical-surgical wards, clinics, and elsewhere, these two disorders will be examined.

ANTISOCIAL PERSONALITY DISORDERS

Kem B. Louie

OBJECTIVES

After studying this section on antisocial personality disorders, the student will be able to:

1. Discuss four characteristics common to all personality disorders.
2. Indicate where personality disorders fit on the mental health continuum.
3. Differentiate between the psychodynamic etiological theory and the family etiological theory for the antisocial personality disorder.
4. For the following areas of assessment, describe the characteristics commonly found in people with antisocial disorders: (a) affect, (b) relationship with others, and (c) behavioral patterns.
5. Identify three possible nursing diagnoses for the antisocial client.
6. Discuss three common reactions health care workers often experience when working with antisocial clients.
7. Outline nursing interventions for the following client behaviors: (a) manipulation, (b) impulsiveness, (c) aggression, and (d) detachment.
8. Contrast and compare five possible therapies for use with selected antisocial clients.

Prior to the DSM III, individuals diagnosed as having **antisocial personalities** were referred to as **psychopaths, sociopaths,** or impulsive characters (Millon 1981). These terms are often used interchangeably.

One of the earliest studies of antisocial personality disorders was conducted by McCord and McCord (1956). In their classic book, *The Psychopath*, the authors delineate six behavioral traits:

- Being antisocial or performing crimes against society.
- Driven by uncontrollable desires to seek excitement.
- Highly impulsive, with no stable goals.
- Aggressive and reacts to frustration with fury.
- Feels little guilt or remorse when committing an amoral act.
- Has a warped capacity for love in that he is cold and compassionless.

The authors emphasize that it is the total personality that makes up this syndrome rather than a single behavior. Modlin (1983) points out that antisocial behaviors solely (e.g., fighting, drinking, stealing, sexual assaults) do not constitute an antisocial personality disorder. Pathology in antisocial personalities is more interpersonal than internal. Diagnosis is made on the client's history rather than on the Mental Status Exam (Vaillant and Perry 1985).

In working with people with antisocial personality disorders, Cleckley (1964), a psychiatrist, describes the main features of this group (Box 17–1). Cleckley asserted that these traits are found not only in criminal personalities but also in society's most respected roles and settings, e.g., businessmen, scientists, physicians, and psychiatrists. Harrington (1972) quotes William Krasner:

> (These people) . . . do well in the more unscrupulous types of sales work, because they take such delight in 'putting it over on them,' getting away with it, and having so little conscience about defrauding their customers. They become private detectives, police, bodyguards, strikebreakers. Many go much higher to become politicians and industrialists where . . . their complete lack of scruples overcomes their more or equally able rivals.

There has been limited progress in understanding and treating antisocial syndromes. Reid (1985) cites four reasons for this:

1. It has been difficult to study syndromes that do not come to medical attention.
2. Because of the unpopularity of antisocial syndromes, mental health research funds go to support study in other needed areas (e.g., depression, cancer).
3. Since the success rate of treating these clients has been markedly poor, there is little motivation to inspire interest.
4. Because of the injuries, hurts, and loss of property and freedoms, there is limited compassion for these clients.

However, *some* progress has been made in understanding and treating antisocial syndromes.

Box 17–1. MAIN FEATURES OF ANTISOCIAL PERSONALITY DISORDERS

- Superficial charm and good intelligence.
- Absence of delusions and other signs of irrational thinking.
- Absence of nervousness or neurotic manifestations.
- Unreliability.
- Untruthfulness and insincerity.
- Lack of remorse and shame.
- Antisocial behavior without apparent compunction.
- Poor judgment and failure to learn from experience.
- Pathologic egocentricity and incapacity for love.
- General poverty in major affective reactions.
- Specific loss of insight.
- Unresponsiveness in general interpersonal relations.
- Fantastic and uninviting behavior with alcohol and sometimes without.
- Suicide rarely carried out.
- Sex life impersonal, trivial, and poorly integrated.
- Failure to follow any life plan.

Data from Cleckley H. The Mask of Sanity, 4th ed. St. Louis: C.V. Mosby Company, 1964, pp. 364–400.

Standard I: Theory

The DSM III-R has identified diagnostic criteria for the diagnosis of antisocial personality disorder (Box 17–2).

However, compared with other mental disorders, little research has been conducted on people with antisocial personalities, because they are not confined to one

Box 17–2. DSM III-R CRITERIA FOR ANTISOCIAL PERSONALITY DISORDER

A. Current age at least 18 years.
B. Evidence of conduct disorder with onset before age 15, as indicated by a history of **three** or more of the following:
   1. Was often truant
   2. Ran away from home overnight at least twice while living in parental or parental-surrogate home (or once without returning)
   3. Often initiated physical fights
   4. Used a weapon in more than one fight
   5. Forced someone into sexual activity with him or her
   6. Was physically cruel to animals
   7. Was physically cruel to other people
   8. Deliberately destroyed other's property (other than by fire setting)
   9. Deliberately engaged in fire setting
   10. Often lied (other than to avoid physical punishment)
   11. Has stolen with confrontation of a victim (e.g., mugging, purse-snatching, extortion, armed robbery)
   12. Has stolen without confrontation of a victim on more than one occasion (including forgery)
C. A pattern of irresponsibility and antisocial behavior since the age of 15, as indicated by at least **four** of the following:
   1. Is unable to sustain consistent work behavior, as indicated by any of the following (including similar behavior in academic settings if the person is a student):
      a. Significant unemployment for six months or more within five years when expected to work when work was available
      b. Repeated absences from work unexplained by illness in self or family
      c. Abandonment of several jobs without realistic plans for others
   2. Fails to conform to social norms with respect to lawful behavior, as indicated by repeatedly performing antisocial acts that are grounds for arrest (whether arrested or not), e.g., destroying property, harassing others, stealing, pursuing an illegal occupation
   3. Is irritable and aggressive, as indicated by repeated physical fights or assaults (not required by one's job or to defend oneself)
   4. Repeatedly fails to honor financial obligations, as indicated by defaulting on debts or failing to provide child support or support for other dependents on a regular basis
   5. Fails to plan ahead, or is impulsive, as indicated by **one or both** of the following:
      a. Traveling from place to place without a prearranged job or clear goal for the period of travel or clear idea about when the travel terminates
      b. Lack of a fixed address for a month or more
   6. Has no regard for the truth, as indicated by repeated lying, uses of aliases, or "conning" others for personal profit or pleasure
   7. Is reckless regarding his or her own or other's personal safety, as indicated by driving while intoxicated or recurrent speeding
   8. If a parent or guardian, lacks ability to function as a responsible parent, as indicated by **one or more** of the following:
      a. Malnutrition of child
      b. Child's illness resulting from lack of minimal hygiene
      c. Failure to obtain medical care for a seriously ill child
      d. Child's dependence on neighbors or nonresident relatives for food and shelter
      e. Failure to arrange for a caretaker for young child when parent is away from home
      f. Repeated squandering, on personal items, of money required for household necessities
   9. Has never sustained a totally monogamous relationship for more than one year.
   10. Lacks remorse (feels justified in having hurt, mistreated, or stolen from another)
D. Occurrence of antisocial behavior not exclusively during the course of schizophrenia or manic episodes

---

institution or setting. There is strong evidence, though, to support four theoretical hypotheses regarding the etiology for the antisocial individual: (1) psychodynamic issues, (2) family influences, (3) social and environmental influences, and (4) biological explanations.

PSYCHODYNAMIC ISSUES

The formal diagnosis of antisocial personality disorder requires specific overt behaviors that are characterized as illegal or immoral. However, antisocial personality is not just a term used for misbehavior. From a psychodynamic viewpoint, it is thought that psychopathology is caused by a fixed disturbance of developmental growth (MacKinnon and Michels 1971).

A child who has drifted through a series of foster homes, whose parents have abandoned him, or who has severe emotional deprivations may show antisocial traits early in life. Lack of validation, emotional warmth, and physical security interfere with normal ego development. Ego pathology in early life is further compounded during the stage of superego development (3–5 years). At this time, the child's ego lacks the maturity to identify with role models and social standards. Therefore, there are disturbances in superego formation. This is manifested in the individual's failure to develop control over the expression of his basic needs. Consequently, personality defenses are designed for gratification of impulses and to provide immediate relief of tension. Since mature ego functioning is impaired, the person is incapable of experiencing mature pleasure. The pleasures that are experienced have a primitive, oral quality and are more related to physiological responses, such as drinking, drugs, sex, or acquiring property (MacKinnon and Michels 1971). The capacity to experience pleasure in interpersonal relationships is lacking, as is the capacity for warm and sincere relationships. Missing is the ability to love, form friendships, and experience loyalty.

Since people with antisocial personalities fail to develop stabilizing egos and socialized superegos, primitive drives are not socially or morally modified by the ego or the superego. The individual pursues immediate gratification without regard to the welfare of others or the demands of external reality (MacKinnon and Michels 1971).

FAMILY INFLUENCES

The family histories of antisocial persons seem to play an important etiological role. Frequently, the antisocial individual was an unwanted child and/or illegitimate. Often parents of antisocial individuals are divorced or deserted their families. As children, many antisocial individuals were exposed to violent tempers, physical abuse, cruelty, and sexual abuse by their caretakers (Kolb and Brodie 1982). Societal goals are not usually clearly established in these families; therefore, the children are not able to introject the social values of the community through identification with the parents. The individual exhibits "primarily defensive modes of living related to some form of arrested behavior development, or to the development of a particular pattern or trait" (Kolb and Brodie 1982, 30).

SOCIAL AND ENVIRONMENTAL INFLUENCES

Society and environment influence the family's childrearing practices. In view of frequent family crises related to socioeconomic pressures, parents may develop negative attitudes toward their children (Zamora 1982). Inconsistent and ineffective discipline can teach the child to be deceitful, superficial, and narcissistic. The teaching of moral values and behaviors may also be lacking.

Antisocial personality disorder can be detected in early adolescence (APA 1987). Predominant characteristics include emotional immaturity and impulsive need for gratification. These preadolescents or adolescents may steal, run away, suffer from neurosis, act destructively, be quarrelsome, demonstrate guiltlessness, and act openly rebellious. This behavior is generally directed toward parents and teachers.

BIOLOGICAL THEORIES

Physical and biological studies concerning the antisocial individual yield interesting data. McCord (1982) summarizes the conclusions based upon studies of antisocial individuals with criminal records:

1. These individuals are physiologically insensitive and relatively incapable of learning from physically punishing treatments. This may be attributed to some form of neurological dysfunction or to some forms of training in early life that desensitize the person to certain emotional situations.
2. Slow wave and spike electroencephalographic (EEG) activity related to aggression is a common finding. Certain pieces of research indicate that this characteristic is inheritable.
3. Often these individuals are found to have a normal to superior range of intelligence.

4. Hormonal secretions, such as a lack of epinephrine, may have a partly hereditary link to antisocial behavior.
5. Defects in the hypothalamus have also been associated with this disorder. Such defects can be caused by genetics, prebirth injuries, early infant disease, or environmental influences.
6. Depletion of serotonin and its metabolic 5-hydroxyindoleacetic acid (5-HIAA).

It is important to note, however, that many people with antisocial personalities do not exhibit any of these characteristics. Caution should be used when interpreting and generalizing to all clients diagnosed with antisocial personality disorders. Further research is needed on noncriminal people with this disorder.

Standard II: Data Collection

The nurse will encounter individuals with antisocial personality patterns in a variety of settings. These include emergency rooms, prisons, general hospital settings, clinics, and psychiatric units. People brought into clinics and hospital settings are usually brought in against their will. The person with an antisocial personality may appear to health care professionals of the opposite sex as colorful, seductive, and engaging. Health care workers of the same sex often find them manipulative and demanding (Vaillant and Perry 1985).

Antisocial traits are found in everyone (depending on the time or situation when needs feel urgent, or if inner controls have not been developed). At times, behavior gives way to satisfying basic needs. *For the person with an antisocial personality, immediate gratification of needs overrides all social or moral dictates* (MacKinnon and Michels 1971).

Assessment of antisocial individuals should focus on (1) affect, (2) relationships with others, and (3) behavioral patterns.

AFFECT

ANXIETY. People with antisocial personalities can appear charming, self-confident, and verbally glib and can make social contacts easily. Such a person may appear free of anxiety or depression. It has been said that people with antisocial personality structures do not experience anxiety or depression. However, some clinicians believe that the antisocial behavior is a defense against a very low tolerance for anxiety (MacKinnon and Michels 1971). Indeed, antisocial behavior may be viewed as a defense against overwhelming anxiety and chronic depression (Vaillant and Perry 1985.) The antisocial person may project anxiety by picking on sensitive areas or habits in another, shifting the focus from himself to someone else in the environment.

GUILT. There does seem to be a total lack of guilt after participation in a lie, swindle, theft, or murder. If the person does experience remorse, the emotion is fleeting and soon forgotten and in no way alters the person's behavior (Stanton 1978). The individual explains his actions by denying doing something or denying finding anything wrong in what he or she does. Rationalizations include "everyone else does it" or "no one cares about that anyway . . . it's all built into the system."

SHALLOWNESS. There is a shallow quality to the antisocial person's affective responses. Although the person may be dramatic, engaging, and filled with apparent emotion, the emotions are superficial and aimed at influencing the listener. The listener is often left with feelings of detachment and a lack of connectedness, although the emotions displayed were intense (MacKinnon and Michels 1971).

RELATIONSHIPS WITH OTHERS

A person with antisocial character traits is unable to love, cherish, or even care about another person. All emotional energy is focused on the self, and other people exist only to fulfill personal needs. When people are no longer needed, they are discarded and easily replaced by others. People associated with such an individual, especially family and friends, suffer. Relationships with an antisocial individual are punctuated with brutal and irresponsible behavior (Harrington 1972). A sadomasochistic relationship typically exists between the client and his family (MacKinnon and Michels 1971).

A person with an antisocial personality structure is incapable of forming relationships and is often hurtful and deceitful to those close to him or her. However, such a person can often elicit loyalty and adoration. Charles Manson is such an example. Manson inspired blind devotion to his followers who, on command, would kill as a means of social protest, revenge, for pleasure, at random, and for no reason. Harrington (1972) quotes a speech of Albert Speer's regarding Adolph Hitler:

> . . . Hitler could fascinate, he wallowed in his own charisma, but he could not respond to friendship. Instinctively he repelled it. The normal sympathies men and women enjoyed were just not in him. At the core, in the place where the heart should be, Hitler was a hollow man. He was empty. . . . We who were really close to

> him, or thought we were, all came to sense this, however slowly. . . . We were all, all of us, simply projections of his own gigantic ego. . . . And yet, Hitler was my destiny. As long as he was alive, he dominated my spirit. . . . The man's drive, his iron will, his daemonism fascinated even while it repelled. . . . It was he who manipulated me. I was enthralled.

BEHAVIORAL PATTERNS

Lying, cheating, swindling, murdering, deceiving others, prostitution, rebelliousness, irresponsibility, and drug addiction are just a few behaviors associated with the antisocial personality. Lying is often pathological—lying for no apparent reason. Cheating and swindling family, friends, and business associates is done cleverly and without remorse. Murder may have no motive, give pleasure, or act as revenge for a minor slight. Sex is often used as a tool to manipulate or punish or as a lark. Sex is not within the context of sharing joy and love, as in an intimate relationship. Drug addiction is common among people with antisocial personality disorders, as is chronic alcoholism. Physical and verbal aggression is a frequent outlet for frustration. These individuals display a lack of responsibility that is manifested by an inability to hold a permanent job. Antisocial individuals often engage in illegal occupations, such as selling drugs and stolen goods and prostitution. Inability to function in the role of parent is often manifested in neglect, sadistic abuse, and desertion. Box 17–3 lists other areas the nurse may assess.

Surprisingly, many people with this disorder are extremely talented or have high IQs but never function to their potential. People with antisocial personality disorders do *not* have thought disorders. Even though they choose not to take responsibility for their actions, *they are held responsible in a court of law.*

Box 17–3. AREAS TO ASSESS WITH AN ANTISOCIAL CLIENT

1. What is the presenting problem according to the client? What is it according to others (e.g., family and police)?
2. Who has identified and defined the problem?
3. What functions does the problematic behavior serve for the client at this time?
4. What are the emotional state and reactions to the problems?
5. In what way and to what extent does the client perceive the antisocial behavior as a problem?
6. What particular circumstances or stress precipitated the behavior?
7. How is the client handling the problem? How has the client handled the problem in the past?
8. How would the client like to see the problem resolved?
9. What is the client's developmental history?
10. Is the client employed? What is the pattern of employment?
11. How does the behavior affect the job or role functioning?
12. What is the client's physical condition and status?
13. What substances (i.e., drugs and alcohol) are abused? How much is taken? When was the last time it was taken?
14. Has the client ever been arrested or convicted of a crime?

Standard III: Diagnosis

The data collected provides the nurse with information concerning the presenting problem or behaviors, emotional state, precipitating situations, and maladaptive coping behaviors. The antisocial client may exhibit any number of problematic behaviors. These behaviors are not in themselves pathological or maladaptive. Behaviors that are repetitive or rigid or present an obstacle to meaningful relationships or functioning are of concern to the management and care of the client.

Nursing diagnoses must be consistent with the treatment plan agreed upon by each member of the interdisciplinary team. *All involved in the care of the antisocial client must agree to the diagnoses, goals, and plan.*

Nursing diagnoses may be many. The person with a diagnosis of antisocial personality disorder often presents with gross behavioral problems. These behaviors usually cause a great deal of difficulty in interpersonal relationships. Therefore, *ineffective individual coping* may be diagnosed. *Ineffective coping* may be evidenced by overt hostility, manipulation of others, egocentricity, habitual disregard of social norms, or dependence on drugs or alcohol or both.

Many people with antisocial personality disorders end up in jail, juvenile courts, and houses of detention because of unlawful behavior and physical aggression toward others. Therefore, the nursing diagnosis of *potential for violence directed at others* is often applicable. Potential for violence directed at others may be evidenced by lack of impulse control, overt aggression and hostility, or emotional immaturity.

Often a person with an antisocial personality may have a parenting role. Since, by definition, a person with an antisocial personality disorder is unable to empathize, cherish, or support the needs of another human being, children suffer emotionally from such a parent. Therefore, the nursing diagnosis of *altered parenting* as evidenced by abuse, rejection, inadequate resources, or impaired judgment is possible.

It is important to remember when formulating nursing diagnoses that the diagnoses are modified to reflect the individuality of the client. Some clients will have areas of functioning that are quite adequate, whereas in others, the total functioning of the person may be disrupted.

Standard IV: Planning

Planning nursing interventions for a person with antisocial characteristics is done on the (1) content level—planning goals—and the (2) process level—nurses' reactions and feelings.

CONTENT LEVEL—PLANNING GOALS

The goals identified are dependent upon the analysis of the assessment data. Goals need to be prioritized based upon the dominant problem presented by the client. Many of the behaviors are related, and intervention aimed at one specific behavior may effect change in other behaviors.

Setting the goals for people with antisocial personality disorders is at best not easy. Too often, goals are set that are way beyond the capabilities of the client. Since antisocial behaviors reflect lifelong habits of coping with the world, change comes very slowly, if at all. When goals are too high, health care personnel become frustrated and angry with the client for not meeting the goals. Therefore, it is important that the goals be set with the client. The difficulty here is that the client often is not motivated to change, since he usually sees nothing wrong with his behavior.

The degree of psychopathology differs from person to person, and so must the goals. Building on a person's strengths and offering alternative behaviors can be useful. Telling the person "not to do" something often meets with resistance from the client, resulting in frustration on the part of the helping person and power struggles between the two.

For the nursing diagnosis, *potential for violence directed at others* the following goals may be appropriate:

Long Term Goals

- Client will avoid situations that stimulate potential aggressive acts by (state the date).
- Client will demonstrate alternate and acceptable behaviors to deal with aggressive thoughts or feelings by (state the date).
- Client will show an increase in ability to control unacceptable impulses.

Short Term Goals

- Client will name two situations that trigger aggressive acts (state the date).
- By (state the date) client will verbalize anger and frustration related to one incident that stimulated aggressive behavior.
- Client will develop one alternative behavior to relieve frustration and anger by (state the date).
- Client will demonstrate a decrease in aggressive behaviors by (state the date).

Ineffective individual coping is always present. Most evident are projection of blame onto others and manipulation. Often this manipulation is used in the service of getting immediate gratification of some wish or desire. Other times, manipulation is used to keep individuals or groups so confused and distracted that there is little to stop him from getting his way. The aim of intervention is to decrease the unacceptable behaviors. Possible goals follow:

Long Term Goals

- Client will adhere to rules and laws (state the date).
- Client will develop more healthy relationship with one other individual or group (state the date).

Short Term Goals

- Client will acknowledge manipulative behaviors pointed out by staff (state the date).
- Client will verbalize awareness of manipulative behaviors (state the date).
- Client will state one appropriate method of getting some of his needs met (state the date).

PROCESS LEVEL—NURSES' REACTIONS AND FEELINGS

Initially, nurses working with antisocial clients may find them charming and intelligent. After a while, nurses react with frustration and anger when these individuals resist or defy their assistance. As clients continue to test the limits of the treatment program or to manipulate others, including the staff, nurses experience increased anger, disappointment, helplessness, and despair. It is sometimes difficult to understand how a person who is reasonably intelligent repeatedly gets in trouble with family, friends, employer, and the law. Crimes include theft, embezzlement, forgery, robbery, rape, and other acts of violence. Often the nurse's response when hearing about these crimes is moralistic condemnation and contempt.

Beginning students and practitioners in psychiatric nursing are educated toward helping clients gain insight into their problems. The antisocial client does not experience subjective anxiety or guilt that ordinarily motivates people to change, nor do they perceive a need for change. This attitude on the part of the client can elicit feelings of frustration, hopelessness or anger in the nurse.

Nurses may unwittingly foster the problematic behaviors of their clients. For example, a nurse may admire and be envious of the manner in which a client is able to con or manipulate the system. At other times, a client's rebellious behavior may meet some unconscious need for vicarious enjoyment or punishment for the nurse. When this occurs, the nurse and client can support a pathological situation. Being aware of these feelings and responses to antisocial clients can assist nurses in working with them in a more therapeutic manner. Frequent staff meetings and peer supervision are crucial in maintaining objectivity when working with antisocial individuals.

The goal of treatment with these clients is movement toward behavioral change, particularly those behaviors that are judged by society to be inappropriate and that present an obstacle in developing and maintaining meaningful relationships.

Standard V: Intervention

V-A: PSYCHOTHERAPEUTIC INTERVENTIONS

Amid the many problematic behaviors presented by the antisocial personality, the following behaviors are more predominant and precipitate the most frustration among nurses and health care professionals. The behaviors are (1) manipulation, (2) impulsiveness, (3) aggression, and (4) detachment.

MANIPULATION. Manipulation of and by itself is not a maladaptive behavior. It can be understood as purposeful behavior directed at getting needs met. However, the term manipulative behavior, in the field of psychiatry, often has a negative connotation. **Maladaptive use of manipulation** is defined here as follows (Chitty and Maynard 1986):

Manipulation is maladaptive when

1. It is the primary method used to get needs met.
2. The needs, goals, and feelings of others are disregarded.
3. Others are dehumanized and treated as objects in order to fulfill the needs of the manipulator.

Clients can manipulate and attempt to control the staff by using a variety of scenarios (Chitty and Maynard 1986), which are discussed subsequently.

The Seducer. In the role of **seducer,** the manipulative client is initially extremely responsive to the nurse's therapeutic endeavors. He or she wants only to talk to "his" or "her" nurse. The client appears to share great "insights" with the nurse early on and always says just what the nurse wants to hear. The seduction may include bringing gifts and doing thoughtful "favors" for "his" or "her" nurse. Once the groundwork is set, this "special relationship" or "closeness" with the nurse is used to gain special favors. For example, staying out an hour later on pass, making bargains with the nurse (if I do . . . can I then have . . .), and asking for special privileges. If the nurse turns down these requests, the client instills guilt, "I thought you liked me" or "I thought we understood each other." The nurse now is in a no-win situation. If the requests are refused, the nurse loses the "therapeutic" relationship with the client. If the nurse gives in, the manipulative behaviors are reinforced, and the nurse feels controlled and put down by the client.

The Passive-Aggressor. Instead of wooing the nurse, as in the seducer, the **passive-aggressor** manipulates in ways that push the nurse away. People with antisocial personalities have an uncanny ability for detecting weak spots in others. The manipulator intuitively knows what will make others anxious and uses this knowledge for exploitation. For example, if the nurse is young and sexually inexperienced, one passive-aggressive approach would be to make sexual overtures or to try to touch the nurse. Or, if the nurse is highly obsessional—and many are—the client can get at the nurse by "exposing" how imperfect the nurse really is. This is done by pointing out the nurse's errors or commenting on the nurse's personal or professional problems in front of other clients and staff.

Keep the Ball in the Air. This is an often used and highly successful maneuver to get staff so crazy and befuddled that the manipulator can pretty much do as he or she chooses and get what he or she wants with little opposition. The technique **keep the ball in the air** is also used by a person in the manic phase of a bipolar depression (see Chapter 19). Eric Berne (1964) calls this "Let's You and Him Fight." This can be played out in a number of scenarios. One is to tell Nurse X, "You really are interested in the patients. I don't at all believe what Nurse Y said about you." The manipulator then goes to Nurse Y with false tales or part truths about Nurse X. Of course, this is carried out with nurses Z and Q as well. Pretty soon the staff is split and distrustful of one another. Staff energies are soon channeled into squabbling and trying to straighten out who said what to whom. While the staff are thus occupied, the manipulator goes about pretty much as he or she pleases. This same game can be played by telling Nurse Z that "Nurse X said I could stay out an hour later on pass" after Nurse Y told the manipulator that he could not stay out later. Again, staff becomes confused as to the guidelines for treatment.

Help Me If You Can. In **help me if you can,** the manipulator controls by evoking feelings of helplessness in others. All he has to do is act helpless, cry a lot, and refuse to talk. Pretty soon everyone is trying to find out what the crying is about, stop the crying, and get the client to talk. Staff members are now focused on getting at the "key" to helping this client and are feeling frustrated by their efforts.

An important step in decreasing manipulative behaviors is to set clear and realistic limits on specific behaviors. A manipulative client may overtly react to the limit setting with resentment and resistance; however, manipulative clients really want some limits placed on their behaviors. **Five steps in setting limits** follow (Chitty and Maynard 1986):

1. Set limits ONLY in those areas in which there is a clear need to protect the client or others.
2. Establish realistic and enforceable consequences of exceeding limits.
3. The client should be aware of the limits and the consequences when limits are not adhered to. The client should be told in a clear, polite, and firm manner what the limits and consequences are and should be given the opportunity to discuss any feelings or reactions to these limits and consequences.
4. All limits should be supported by *all the staff*. The limits should be *written in the care plan*.
5. When the limits are consistently adhered to, a decision to discontinue the limits may be made by the staff and noted on the nursing care plan. The decision should be made based upon consistent behavior, not on promises or sporadic efforts.

Table 17–4 outlines some goals and interventions aimed at decreasing manipulative behaviors.

IMPULSIVENESS. Antisocial behavior often in-

Table 17–4 • GOALS AND INTERVENTIONS FOR MANIPULATIVE BEHAVIOR

GOAL	INTERVENTION
1. Client will demonstrate a decrease in manipulative behavior by (state the date).	1a. Identify manipulative behaviors by client.
	1b. Set limits on manipulative behaviors by communicating expected behaviors.
	1c. Convey to the team consistency of approach in setting limits.
	1d. Be realistic as to which behaviors can be limited.
	1e. Assist client in developing means of setting limits on own behavior.
	1f. Assess degree of insight into manipulative behavior and motivation to change.
	1g. Avoid getting into power struggles by accusing and arguing with client.
2. Develop two alternative nonmanipulative behaviors by (state the date).	2a. Discuss client's behaviors in nonjudgmental and nonthreatening manner.
	2b. Assist client in identifying personal strengths and effective communication skills.
	2c. Assist client in testing out alternative behaviors for obtaining needs or fulfilling expectations.
	2d. Support client and provide feedback in trying new behaviors.

cludes impulsive actions. **Impulsiveness** is an action that is abrupt, unplanned, and directed toward immediate gratification. Thinking things over or considering the consequences of the action upon others does not occur. These clients have a history of unpredictable and hasty decisions. Frustration is poorly tolerated and often precipitates an impulsive response. A client's impulsive behavior has been described in terms of being erratic, self-serving, and thoughtless. In certain situations, the antisocial client's impulsive behavior is able to generate fear and aggression in others. The nurse can work with the client on modifying this impulsive behavior. Table 17–5 identifies a goal and possible interventions to aid in decreasing impulsive behavior.

AGGRESSION. Aggression is a frequently described behavior with antisocial clients. **Aggression** is "any verbal and/or nonverbal, actual or attempted, forceful abuse of the self upon another person or thing" (Clack 1963). Aggressive behaviors often lead to violence. Aggression is but one expression of anger and can occur in the steps outlined by Peplau (Clack 1963):

1. The person anticipates the fulfillment of needs for prestige and status, wants, wishes, or desires.
2. These needs or expectations are not met.
3. The person experiences anxiety and frustration.
4. Aggression results, providing temporary relief (relief behavior).
5. Rationalizations are offered for the aggression.

Table 17–6 identifies some goals and interventions to aid in decreasing aggressive behavior.

Refer to Chapter 19 for the therapeutic use of chemical restraints and the seclusion room when dealing with assaultive behaviors.

DETACHMENT. Detachment refers to interpersonal and intrapersonal disassociation from affective expression (Beck 1984). Therefore, individuals who manifest these behaviors have been labeled as cold, aloof, and distant. This behavior is thought to be learned and is defensive. The individual also dissociates him or herself from society and does not internalize social standards and values. Right and wrong have little personal meaning for this person. Table 17–7 identifies one goal and several interventions useful for working with a detached client.

V-F: PSYCHOTHERAPY

During counseling sessions, the antisocial person will challenge therapists and seek to outwit them. Antisocial clients are known to set up situations to test the therapist's skills, catch inconsistencies, arouse anger, and whenever possible, belittle or humiliate the therapist. The goals of the therapist are to see things from the client's point of view, convey a sense of trust, and create a feeling of sharing an alliance. A balance of professional firmness, authority, and tolerance for client's behaviors must be maintained (Millon 1981).

Unfortunately, psychotherapy has proved to be unsuccessful with this personality disorder (McCord 1982; Frosch 1983). Since people with this disorder neither experience subjective anxiety nor view their behavior as a problem, they have no motivation for change. Also, they are not able to form attachments to others. Without strong interpersonal relationships, a therapeutic alliance cannot evolve, since the therapeutic alliance or relationship is the cornerstone of psychotherapy. Other therapies have met with somewhat more success in selected clients. For example:

1. *Group therapy* has been successful with some antisocial clients. Often, however, aggressive behaviors have disrupted group functions. Generally these clients are unable to identify with their therapists or even keep appointments. Group therapy is not recommended on an outpatient basis.
2. *Self-help groups* in which clients share and discuss their feelings and behaviors may encourage development of group responsibility and loyalty. This is especially true if the group is composed of other individuals with antisocial personality disorders.
3. *Therapy based on modeling* also seems successful with the less aggressive antisocial individuals (McCord 1982). **Modeling** is demonstrating the desired behaviors. The client learns to imitate these behaviors in appropriate situations (Closurdo 1975).

Table 17–5 • GOALS AND INTERVENTIONS FOR IMPULSIVE BEHAVIOR

GOAL	INTERVENTION
1. Client will be able to identify impulsive acts and give examples of situations in which they occur.	1a. Identify the needs and feelings preceding impulsive acts. 1b. Discuss current and previous impulsive acts. 1c. Explore impact of such acts upon self and others. 1d. Recognize cues of impulsive behaviors that may injure others.

Table 17-6 • GOALS AND INTERVENTIONS FOR AGGRESSIVE BEHAVIOR

GOAL	INTERVENTION
1. Client will demonstrate control and responsibility in two situations in which he previously used aggressive action.	1a. Encourage client to spend time talking out instead of acting out intense feelings of frustration.
	1b. Communicate positive expectations to the client.
	1c. Assist client in developing concrete external controls.
	1d. Assist client in problem-solving techniques to cope with frustration or tension.
	1e. Provide feedback on results.
	1f. Limit choices to those that are safe and appropriate.
2. Client will cope with stress and aggression in a nonviolent manner most of the time by (state the date).	2a. Assist client in identifying feelings of anxiety, expectations, anger, frustration, disappointment, or perceived threats.
	2b. Assist client in verbalizing these feelings.
	2c. Assist client in describing precipitating events or situations leading to aggressive behavior.
	2d. Assist client in exploring present situation with situations in the past that have aroused similar feelings.
	2e. Assist client in identifying previous coping behaviors.
	2f. Assist client in exploring consequences of behavior upon self and others.
	2g. Assist client in developing more effective coping behaviors and interpersonal skills.

4. *Transactional therapists* have had some success with certain antisocial adolescents (McCord 1982). The emphasis of the treatment is on current and future situations in which the individual and therapist develop a contract outlining specific responsibilities and goals for both the therapist and the client. The individual learns eventually to incorporate responsibility when the person's "adult" monitors the "parent" and "child" messages (see Chapter 2).
5. *Behavior modification* has helped in extinguishing certain problematic behaviors. Positive reinforcement or conditioning using monetary rewards has shown to be more successful than using negative reinforcement such as punishment (McCord 1982). Positive

Table 17-7 • GOALS AND INTERVENTIONS FOR DETACHMENT BEHAVIOR

GOAL	INTERVENTION
1. Client will develop an increased sense of relatedness to others.	1a. Assist client in establishing rapport in interpersonal relationships.
	1b. Assist client in identifying patterns of past relationships with significant others.
	1c. Assist client in describing feelings related to detachment.
	1d. Assist client in exploring more effective interpersonal skills that increase sense of belonging.
	1e. Expect client to maintain the rules of the treatment and milieu.

reinforcements (e.g., tokens, privileges) are given when desired behaviors occur. For example, positive reinforcement can be used to decrease aggressive behaviors. When a client demonstrates a decrease in aggressive behavior, the client receives a token, which may be exchanged for privileges or other desired rewards.

6. *Family therapy* should begin immediately after the client is admitted to an inpatient unit, because the family or spouse may be consciously or unconsciously contributing to and supporting the problematic behaviors (Frosch 1983). Therapy is directed toward assisting each member of the family in understanding his or her own role and in dealing with the client's behaviors.

McCord (1982) reports that specific changes in social groups, such as families, schools, or entire communities, may beneficially affect the antisocial client. For example, instruction in effective family communication, the use of behavioral contracts, and immediate responses to individual or family crisis have decreased the rate of second time offenders among adolescents (Wade 1977). Academic training and job placement also have been responsible for lower rearrest rates (Quay and Love 1977).

Drugs have been used to control aggressive behaviors among antisocial individuals. Lithium has been successful with adolescents and adults (McCord 1982; Reid 1981).

Standard VI: Evaluation

Due to the nature of the dynamics of antisocial personality disorders, change in the client's behavior will occur very slowly. Therefore, many of the goals of treatment are long term. Short term goals and interventions need to be realistic. Revisions of the treatment plan may involve alternate approaches and reassessment of the goals. Equally important is the nurse's awareness of personal feelings and reactions to the client. This awareness can be gained by talking to other nurses and in the supervision process with another nurse.

If the goals are not met within a specific time period (while the client is hospitalized), further referrals need to be made to the family, community, or legal system.

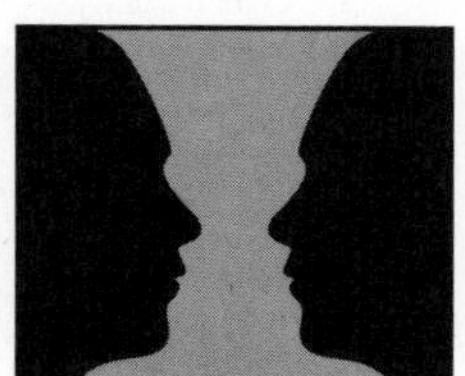

Case Study: Working With a Person Who Has an Antisocial Personality Disorder

Donald Mann, a 32-year-old divorced man, was hospitalized for uncontrollable aggressive impulses. Upon admission, there was no indication of thought disorders, hallucinations, or depressed affect. He was angry because he felt "forced" to voluntarily admit himself into the hospital. His boss had stated that if he didn't, he would be fired from his job. He was threatening a fellow history teacher and later assaulted him. The client stated, "I was only arguing a historical point, and I got carried away." He smiled and winked his eye as he was relating the course of events to the nurse, Ms. Burke. He stated he was unable to finish writing a book because his third wife divorced him. When asked about his childhood, he commented, "Fighting is synonymous with being a street kid." He has a history of wife abuse and frequent barroom fights. For the past year, he has been employed as a teacher of history in a private college. He has had numerous teaching positions in various states. Donald stated he enjoyed teaching and especially liked the students.

On the unit, Donald was generally cooperative. However, on two occasions he violated the rules of the unit. Once he was found with a bottle of alcohol ("I was celebrating one of our famous presidents"). The second incident involved threatening to harm another client on the unit. On both occasions, he responded glibly, "I'm sorry." The female staff usually had no difficulty in dealing with him, but the male staff generally complained about him.

It was the third day after admission when Donald threatened another client. The unit coordinator asked Ms. Burke to write a comprehensive care plan on Donald. His infractions of the rules and aggressiveness were disrupting the unit. Ms. Burke, who had admitted him to the unit had spent time with him over the past few days. She often felt flattered by his attention. He had told her that he found her "the best nurse on the unit." That afternoon, his case was to be presented at a staff conference.

During the meeting, each female member stated that Donald had stated that she was his favorite. He would also "tell tales" to each staff member about the other staff members. The female staff would often do special favors for Donald, e.g., getting him cigarettes, the paper, or

Continued on following page

Case Study: Working With a Person Who Has an Antisocial Personality Disorder *(Continued)*

candy. The male members found him argumentative, infuriating, and contemptuous. They tried to avoid him as much as possible. It was clear that almost everyone had strong positive or negative reactions to Donald. During the meeting, many of the females felt annoyed and angry at being manipulated. The staff together decided on goals and a plan of approach.

Assessment

Ms. Burke divided her data into subjective and objective components.

OBJECTIVE DATA

1. Two incidents of infractions of the rules
2. Past history of spouse abuse
3. Assaulted coworker prior to admission
4. Three marriages
5. Is argumentative with male staff
6. Rationalizes improper and aggressive behaviors—sees nothing wrong
7. Difficulty with interpersonal relationships at work
8. Physically threatened another client
9. Verbally aggressive with male staff
10. Sexual advances toward female staff
11. Manipulates "special favors" from female staff

SUBJECTIVE DATA

1. Sets one staff member against another, "Nurse Y said this about you . . ."
2. States he was "forced into coming to the hospital"
3. Tells each female nurse that she is his favorite

Nursing Diagnosis

Two nursing diagnoses were thought by staff to be the most important initially.

1. *Ineffective Individual Coping* related to inadequate psychological resources, as evidenced by verbal manipulation
   - Tells each female nurse that she is his favorite
   - Sets one staff member against another
   - Manipulates "special favors" from female nurses
   - Sexual advances toward female staff
   - Insincere and superficial
2. *Potential for Violence Directed at Others* related to antisocial character, as evidenced by history of overt, aggressive acts
   - Verbally aggressive with male staff
   - Threatened physical assault toward another client
   - History of spouse abuse
   - Rationalizes violent behavior; does not see behavior as undesirable
   - Two episodes of infraction of rules
   - Assaulted a coworker prior to admission

Planning

CONTENT LEVEL—PLANNING GOALS

Ms. Burke and the rest of the staff decided upon a number of strategies that would, it was hoped, cut down on Donald's manipulations and aggressiveness. Long term and short term goals were set. The aim of the goals was to alter Donald's behavior while on the unit and to elicit more appropriate behaviors for meeting needs and responding to frustration.

Nursing Diagnosis	Long Term Goals	Short Term Goals
1. *Ineffective Individual Coping* related to inadequate psychological resources, as evidenced by verbal manipulation	Client will ask directly for basic needs.	1a. Client will state awareness of manipulative behavior by (state the date). 1b. Client will state aware-

		ness of thoughts and expectations surrounding two situations of manipulation by (state the date).
2. *Potential for Violence Directed at Others* related to antisocial character, as evidenced by history of overt, aggressive acts	Client will demonstrate appropriate behaviors in response to frustration, without violence, most of the time.	2a. Client will talk about his anger and frustration rather than acting out by (state the date). 2b. By (state the date) client will develop two appropriate alternative behaviors to relieve frustration.

PROCESS LEVEL—NURSES' REACTIONS AND FEELINGS

During the planning it was decided that Ms. Burke would be the primary nurse during the day, and Ms. Hubb during the evening shift. Ms. Burke was to get supervision from the psychiatric clinical nurse specialist on the unit. The nursing coordinator suggested that communication regarding Donald be given in some detail during shift reports until modification of his aggressive and manipulative behavior was evident.

Intervention

The nursing care plan involved input from all staff members. It was anticipated that Donald would become easily frustrated and angry when limits were set on his manipulative and aggressive behavior. Ms. Burke on days and Ms. Hubb on evenings would be the two staff members primarily working with Donald. All requests, favors, and sharing of personal information would be channeled through these two nurses. Setting limits was an important aspect of the care plan. Both Ms. Burke and Ms. Hubb were to set the limits on flattery, gifts, and compliments. When such behavior occurred, interaction would be refocused back to Donald.

Very clear limits were set regarding aggressive behavior. He was told that angry and inappropriate verbal aggressiveness would result in losing a privilege on the unit for that day (e.g., no telephone calls, no television at night). Physical acting out had more severe consequences. For any physical assault, weekend passes would be withheld, and any other appropriate precautions would be taken, such as time in the quiet room or administration of medication.

Expected client behaviors were clearly explained, and when elicited, would meet with recognition and positive feedback. The following is an interview between the nurse and Donald following Donald's threat to strike another client:

Dialogue	Therapeutic Tool/Comment
N: I would like to talk with you about what happened this morning.	Be clear as to the purpose of the interview.
Mr. M: O.K., shoot.	
N: Tell me what started the incident.	Use open-ended statements. Maintain a nonjudgmental attitude.
Mr. M: Well, as I told you before, I always had to fight to get what I wanted in life. My father and mother abandoned me emotionally when I was a child.	
N: Yes, but tell me about this morning.	Redirect client to present problem/situation.
Mr. M.: O.K., I never liked Richard since I met him; he has it in for me. I just know it. He doesn't get along with anyone here. Just two days ago he almost had a fight.	

Continued on following page

Intervention *(Continued)*	N: Donald, what do you mean Richard has it in for you?	Explore situation.
	Mr. M.: When I'm talking to one of the nurses, he stares and makes comments under his breath.	
	N: What does he say?	Encourage description.
	Mr. M: How I'm "in" with the nurses. I'm just trying to do what is expected of me here.	
	N: You mean that Richard is envious of your relationship with the nurses?	Validate the client's meaning.
	Mr. M.: Right, he really doesn't want to be here. He doesn't care about all that therapeutic junk.	
	N: You seem to know a lot about how Richard thinks. I wonder how that is?	Assist client to make association to present situation.
	Mr. M.: He reminds me of someone I knew when I was young. His name was Joe Brown. We called him "Bones."	
	N: Tell me more about "Bones."	Explore situation further.
	Mr. M.: We called him "bones" because he was skinny as bones. He was into drugs and never ate. He was also called "Bones" because he was selfish. He never shared anything. He never even had a girl that I knew about.	
	N: So Richard reminds you of someone who is selfish and lonely?	Making interpretation of information. Note increasing anxiety.
	Mr. M.: That's right. I've had three marriages and girlfriends on the side. No one can take them away from me, just let them try (angrily).	
	N: What makes you so angry now?	Identify feelings and explore threat/anxiety.
	Mr. M.: Richard—I know he wants to be like me, but he can't. I'll hurt him if he makes any more comments about me.	
	N: Donald, you will not hurt anyone here on the unit.	Set limits on and expectations of client's behavior.
	Mr. M.: I'm sorry. I didn't mean that.	
	N: It's important that we examine your part in the incident this morning and how to cope without threats or violence.	Focus on client's responsibility and suggesting alternative methods of coping with situation.
	Mr. M.: Listen, I know I've gotten into trouble because I can't control my temper, but that's due to the fact that I won't get any respect until I can show them I don't fear them.	Exhibiting rationalization.
	N: Who are they?	Clarification of pronoun.
	Mr. M.: People like Richard.	
	N: You've told me that fighting was a way of survival as a child, but as an adult, there are	Show empathy and suggest other means of coping.

Dialogue	Thoughts/Techniques
other ways of handling situations that make you angry.	
Mr. M.: You're right. I've thought about this. Do you think it would help if you gave me some meds to control my anger?	Exhibiting superficial and concrete thinking—possible manipulation.
N: I wasn't thinking of medications but rather a plan of being aware of your anger and talking it out instead of fighting it out.	Clarify meaning toward behavioral change.
Mr. M.: I told you before, I have to fight.	
N: Have you thought about the consequences of your fighting?	Identify results of impulsive behavior.
Mr. M.: I feel bad afterwards. I sometimes wish it hadn't happened.	
N: Tell me about a time when you felt this way.	Explore previous situations of impulsiveness.
Mr. M.: I really loved my third wife, but she made me mad. I didn't want to hurt her, but I couldn't help myself.	
N: Couldn't help yourself?	Use reflection to get client to further describe situation.
Mr. M.: She wanted me to stay home and not go out with the guys, but I didn't want her to tell me what to do.	
N: And then what happened?	Continue to explore situation.

Refer to Donald's written care plan (Nursing Care Plan 17–1).

Evaluation

As expected, Donald became outraged when limits were set. He started to shout at the doctor and called him names. The staff calmly told him that because of his inappropriate shouting he was unable to use the phone for the rest of the day, as outlined in his plan. Over the next few days, he did some more testing, for example, yelling and throwing a can of soda at one of the evening staff. He was taken to the seclusion room for an hour. That weekend, he was refused pass. By the end of the third week, his behavior on the unit showed marked modification. His pitting of staff against staff was thwarted. By discharge, his verbal aggressiveness flared up once in a while, but much less often than on previous occasions.

Nursing Care Plan 17–1 • A PERSON WITH ANTISOCIAL PERSONALITY DISORDER: Mr. Mann

NURSING DIAGNOSIS

Ineffective individual coping related to inadequate psychological resources, as evidenced by verbal manipulation

Supporting Data

- Sexual advances toward female staff.
- Infraction of rules on unit.
- Attempts to set staff at odds with each other.
- Insincere and superficial.
- Manipulates "special favors" from nurses.

Continued on following page

Nursing Care Plan 17–1 • A PERSON WITH ANTISOCIAL PERSONALITY DISORDER: Mr. Mann *(Continued)*

Long Term Goal: Mr. Mann's manipulative behavior on the unit will be minimal by discharge.

Short Term Goal	*Intervention*	*Rationale*	*Evaluation*
1. Mr. Mann will state awareness of manipulative behavior by (state the date).	1a. Mr. Mann will relate to one nurse on both evening and day shifts. 1b. Mr. Mann will have one-to-one interaction with primary care staff on a day-to-day basis.	1a–b. Limits chance of mixed communication. Decreases ability to manipulate staff.	<u>Goal Partially Met</u> After two weeks client would acknowledge some manipulative behaviors and state he understood the consequences of continuing some of his manipulative behaviors.
	1c. Communicate clear limits on manipulative behavior. 1d. Communicate expected behavior. 1e. Spell out the consequences of manipulation. 1f. Share limits, expected behavior, and consequences of manipulation with all staff daily at report time and at team conferences.	1c–f. Clear expectations, expected behavior, and consequences provide sound framework for intervention.	
	1g. Avoid power struggles; do not be defensive.	1g. Arguments take focus away from client and issue.	
	1h. Offer positive reinforcement and feedback when expected behavior is evident.	1h. Can increase expected behavior.	
2. Mr. Mann will state awareness of thoughts and expectations surrounding two situations of manipulation by (state the date).	2a. Identify situations in which client is manipulative. 2b. Explore needs or expectations in each manipulative situation. 2c. Discuss impact of manipulative behavior on self and others.	2a–c. Change in behavior facilitated when client is aware of each manipulation.	<u>Goal Partially Met</u> Client was able to discuss one incidence with primary nurse in terms of expectation and thoughts.

NURSING DIAGNOSIS

Potential for violence directed at others related to antisocial character, as evidenced by history of overt aggressive acts

Supporting Data

- Past history of wife abuse.
- Past history of fighting.
- Assaulted a co-worker prior to admission.
- Threatened another client on the unit.
- Rationalizes behavior—does not see anything wrong.
- Two episodes of infraction of rules.
- Verbally aggressive with male staff.

Long Term Goal: Mr. Mann will demonstrate appropriate behaviors in response to frustration, without violence, most of the time.

Short Term Goal	*Intervention*	*Rationale*	*Evaluation*
1. Client will verbalize anger and frustration rather than act out by (state the date).	1a. Identify feelings of anxiety, anger, and frustration. 1b. Encourage appropriate verbalization of these feelings with the nurse. 1c. Discuss events that lead to aggressive behavior.	1a–b. Client will learn to talk it out instead of act it out. 1c. Client will learn to acknowledge and anticipate feelings of frustration that can lead to aggression.	Goal met Client continues to test staff by throwing things and name calling. By third week, the incidence of verbal and physical acting out had sharply declined.
2. By (state the date) client will develop two appropriate alternative behaviors to relieve frustration.	2a. Explore relief felt when aggression is utilized by client. 2b. Discuss impact or consequences of behavior upon self and others. 2c. Explore alternative behaviors in coping with anger and/or frustration. 2d. Assist client in developing effective communication skills. 2e. Provide feedback to client on behaviors. 2f. Reward client when not using aggressive behaviors.	2a–d. Learning to deal appropriately with aggression will allow client to take responsibility for his own behavior. 2e–f. Positive feedback and rewards help elicit desired behaviors.	Goal Partially Met Client initiated discussions twice with nurse when he "felt like wasting" another client. Physical acting out had decreased in incidence by end of third week.

Summary — Antisocial Personality Disorders

This section has described a group of personality disorders classified on Axis II of the DSM III-R. Individuals with personality disorders generally do not seek assistance or intervention because their defense mechanisms are ego-syntonic, that is, the defenses are not at odds with their sense of self. The three major groups of personality disorders are (1) paranoid, schizoid, and schizotypal; (2) histrionic, narcissistic, antisocial, and borderline; and (3) avoidant, dependent, compulsive, and passive-aggressive.

Antisocial personality disorders are characterized by acts against society, impulsiveness, aggressiveness, lack of remorse or guilt, shallow affect, and superficial interpersonal relationships. Various biological, cultural-environmental, and psychological theories have been presented to explain the dynamics of this personality disorder.

Clients with antisocial personality disorders, when hospitalized, evoke strong emotions in nurses. Frustration, anger, disappointment, and despair are usually experienced by health care professionals when caring for these clients. Being aware of these feelings and responses to antisocial clients can assist nurses in understanding and caring for them.

Areas to be assessed include (1) affect, (2) relationships with others, and (3) behavioral patterns. A number of nursing diagnoses may be identified. These include *ineffective individual coping, potential for violence directed at others*, and *altered parenting*. Goals and interventions are aimed at behavioral change. Most goals are long term in nature. Four specific problematic behaviors (manipulation, impulsiveness, aggression, and detachment) were presented, along with guidelines for intervention. Firm limits need to be set. This is done in a nonjudgmental and calm manner. Clear expectations for change in behavior need to be stated. A consistent approach among team members is vital. Other therapies that have been beneficial include the use of lithium to control aggression, behavior modification, group therapy, family therapy, and changes in the social environment.

Self-study exercises 1 through 12 at the end of this chapter will help you review antisocial personality disorders.

Borderline Personality Disorders

Suzanne Lego

OBJECTIVES

After studying this section on borderline personality disorders, the student will be able to:

1. Describe a textbook picture of a client with a borderline personality disorder.
2. Discuss three etiological theories of borderline personality disorder.
3. Act out five characteristics of the borderline personality.
4. Discuss five reactions health care workers could experience when working with a borderline client.
5. Identify three possible nursing diagnoses applicable to the borderline client.
6. For the following typical behaviors seen in borderline clients, discuss the nursing interventions and rationale for each: (a) hostility, (b) self-destruction, (c) demanding behavior.
7. Indicate three possible outcomes of successful interventions when working with a borderline client.

The diagnosis *borderline personality disorder* has received a great deal of attention in the past several years. Many papers, books, lectures, and professional presentations have focused on this problem. These clients are given much attention on inpatient units and in emergency rooms, where they are often branded "trouble makers" or "problem patients." The committee that devised the DSM III seriously contemplated substituting the term "unstable" for borderline, and others have called clients in this category "the personality disorder who decided not to specialize." (Vaillant and Perry 1985).

Reference was first made to the type of client on the borderline between psychosis and neurosis in 1938 (Vaillant and Perry 1985). Over the years, these clients were labeled "ambulatory schizophrenics," "pseudoneurotic schizophrenics," and "as if" personalities. The latter term arose because these clients identified so completely with the person on whom they were dependent and because their own emotional experiences were derived to such a great extent from those of others (Vaillant and Perry 1985).

Recently the borderline personality has been called "the most controversial topic in the mental health field today" (Sass 1982). The borderline personality as a diagnosis today has been compared with the hysterical neurotic of Freud's day. Just as in Freud's time we saw hysterics plagued with conflict over conscience versus desire, now we see people plagued with problems of identity and unstable interpersonal relationships. It has been postulated that the fragmentation of contemporary society has played a role in the increased numbers of borderline personalities (Sass 1982).

In an editorial for a special issue on borderline personality disorders in the Journal of Psychosocial Nursing, Shirley Smoyak points out that borderline patients separate the professionals from the amateurs in psychiatric nursing (Smoyak 1985). She observes that "nurses are in an excellent position to observe the rapid mood shifts, the unanticipated lashing out at other patients and staff, the clever and devious games of pitting one staff member against another, the emotional lability, and the covert and overt self-destructive behaviors. Such challenging behaviors require skilled intervention strategies."

Standard I: Theory

Three theoretical contributions to the study of the etiology and development of the borderline personality disorders are presented: (1) constitutional theory, (2) Kernberg's contribution, and (3) Masterson's contribution.

CONSTITUTIONAL THEORY

Some authors have hypothesized that borderline clients have inherited an incapacity to tolerate stress. Others believe they have a constitutional inability to regulate affect, predisposing them to psychic disorganization under certain early adverse environmental conditions (Vaillant and Perry 1985).

KERNBERG'S CONTRIBUTION

Otto Kernberg hypothesizes that in infancy these clients perceive their mothers as strongly nurturing, loving, and protective, as well as hateful, depriving, and punishing without warning. These mothers let needs go unmet for long periods of time and abandon the infants unpredictably. The infant perceives both contradictory views of the mother and becomes highly anxious. To reduce anxiety, the mother is "split" into a "good" and "bad" mother. **Splitting** is a primitive defense in which persons see themselves or others as all good or all bad, unable to integrate the positive and negative qualities of the self or others into an integrated whole. The person may alternately idealize and devalue the same person (APA 1987). This primitive defense is carried into adult life, and others are experienced either as strongly nurturing and objects of inordinate attachment or as hateful, mean, and sadistic. The "good" person is idealized, and the "bad" person is devalued. The client can feel good only by a flight into omnipotence. When the client experiences hate toward another person, along with feelings of extreme dependence, anxiety ensues. The client reduces the anxiety triggered by these conflicting feelings through the use of projective identification and denial. **Projective identification** is a "primitive form of projection used to externalize aggressive feelings. Once projection has occurred, fear of the person is coupled with a desire to control the person" (Smith and Lego 1984).

MASTERSON'S CONTRIBUTION

James Masterson has described the borderline client's problems as beginning during Mahler's rapprochement subphase of the separation-individuation process of development, between 18 and 36 months of age. At this time, the toddler begins to move away from the mother but returns from time to time for "emotional refueling," reassurance that the mother will not disappear. The developmental task is to learn that separation is acceptable and rewarding. However, mothers of these clients do not reward separation but rather discourage it by emotionally abandoning the child. That is, the child is punished for autonomous behavior and rewarded for crying, clinging, dependent behavior. This clinging behavior leads to an "emotional reunion" with the mother that comes to be longed for and repeated throughout life. By the same token, moves toward autonomy and independence lead the patient to experience what Masterson calls "abandonment depression" (Masterson 1976).

Box 17–4 identifies the DSM III-R diagnostic criteria for borderline personality disorder.

Standard II: Data Collection

The nurse assesses the client for behaviors that are consistent with the diagnosis of borderline personality disorders. On an inpatient unit, some of these behaviors include the following:

1. Hostile, demanding behavior.
2. Splitting—hating some nurses and loving others.
3. Devaluation—constant, biting criticism of staff.
4. Manipulation—playing staff against one another by lying or distortions.
5. Clinging, lonely behavior.
6. Self-mutilation.
7. Suicide threats or gestures.
8. Alcohol or drug abuse.
9. Sexual promiscuity.
10. Inappropriate overreactions to stress.
11. Projection of own hostility onto others on whom the client feels dependent.
12. Occasional psychotic behavior.

Standard III: Diagnosis

The behavior of a person with a borderline personality is punctuated with angry outbursts, impulsive acts, and manipulation. Often these clients carry out physically self-damaging acts such as suicidal or self-mutilating behaviors. Since these acts are usually impulsive, hospitalization may be necessary to ensure a safe environment. When this happens, an appropriate nursing diagnosis would be *potential for violence to self or others*. Violence to self or others may be evidenced by a number of

Box 17–4. DIAGNOSTIC CRITERIA FOR BORDERLINE PERSONALITY DISORDER

A pervasive pattern of instability of mood, interpersonal relationships, and self-image, beginning by early adulthood and present in a variety of contexts, as indicated by at least **five** of the following:

1. A pattern of unstable and intense interpersonal relationships characterized by alternating between extremes of overidealization and devaluation.
2. Impulsiveness in at least two areas that are potentially self-damaging, e.g., spending, sex, substance use, shoplifting, reckless driving, binge eating. (Do not include suicidal or self-mutilating behavior covered in 5.)
3. Affective instability: marked shifts from baseline mood to depression, irritability, or anxiety, usually lasting a few hours and only rarely more than a few days.
4. Inappropriate, intense anger or lack of control of anger, e.g., frequent displays of temper, constant anger, recurrent physical fights.
5. Recurrent suicidal threats, gestures, or behavior, or self-mutilating behavior.
6. Marked and persistent identity disturbance manifested by uncertainty about at least two of the following: self-image, sexual orientation, long-term goals or career choice, type of friends desired, preferred values.
7. Chronic feelings of emptiness or boredom.
8. Frantic efforts to avoid real or imagined abandonment. (Do not include suicidal or self-mutilating behavior covered in 5.)

behaviors such as anxiety, self-mutilation, frequent displays of temper, and poor impulse control.

These clients often complain of chronic boredom or emptiness. Uncertainty about such things as gender identity, self-image, and career choice may add to the client's already high anxiety state. Therefore, *severe or panic levels of anxiety* may be related to a number of internal or external factors or conditions.

Borderline persons are often very manipulative. They use manipulative tactics to get their needs met. Like the person with an antisocial personality, their manipulations may result in hurt or harm to others. At other times, they act out anxiety in the form of impulsive acts. Impulsive acts may include promiscuity, gambling, shoplifting, binge eating, excessive spending, drug use, and more. Therefore, their ability to cope with anxiety is maladaptive. *Ineffective individual coping* may be evidenced by manipulation of others, inability to solve problems, impulsive acts, or chronic use of maladaptive behaviors.

Standard IV: Planning

In planning intervention with borderline clients, the nurse keeps in mind the etiology of this condition. The key concepts are, first, the client's extreme, primitive dependency upon the nurse (mother) and, second, the client's extreme, primitive anger at the nurse. When each of the client's symptoms or problem behaviors is examined, these two issues will be seen to exist.

Considering this, the nurse provides a consistent, nurturing environment in which the appropriate expression of anger is tolerated. This is easier said than done. In order to achieve this, the nurse deals directly and openly with the client's manipulation, splitting, devaluation, and other aspects of the neediness and anger.

CONTENT LEVEL—PLANNING GOALS

Many goals formulated in the hospital setting are short term. Usually, when a client with a borderline personality is hospitalized, it is for short periods. Extended hospital stays can result in the client's becoming less functional in daily life.

For the nursing diagnosis *potential for self-directed violence*, the following goals could apply:

Long Term Goals

- Client denies any ideas of self-harm.
- Client will name two people to contact if suicidal thoughts occur in the future.

Short Term Goals

- Client will remain safe while in the hospital.
- By (state the date) client will discuss desire to hurt self rather than do it.
- Client will express feelings in a nondestructive manner (talking, physical activity, writing) by (state the date).

For the nursing diagnosis, *severe to panic levels of anxiety*, the following goals may be considered:

Long Term Goals

- Client will state how to lower anxiety using an appropriate outlet by (state the date).
- Client will state feeling more relaxed than anxious by (state the date).

Short Term Goals

- By (state the date) client will state he or she is relaxed in a situation that usually produces anxiety.
- Client will talk about feeling anxious and identify increases in anxiety by (state the date).
- Client will name activities that help to decrease anxiety (exercise, dancing, talking, singing, jogging) by (state the date).

Goals appropriate for the nursing diagnosis *ineffective individual coping* related to inadequate psychological resources could be the following:

Long Term Goals

- Client will solve most problems in a straightforward manner that injures neither self nor others by (state the date).
- Client will state ability to solve most life situations by problem-solving adaptive and acceptable solutions by (state the date).
- Client will name two people available to discuss problems and problem-solve solutions by (state the date).

Short Term Goals

- Client will discuss feelings of frustration and deal with them appropriately rather than acting them out.
- Client will name two acceptable alternatives to maladaptive coping skills by (state the date).
- By (state the date), client will solve one situation that was usually acted out maladaptively.

PROCESS LEVEL—NURSES' REACTIONS AND FEELINGS

Because these clients exhibit such strong anger and dependency, they evoke equally strong feelings in nurses. Their need to "split" others into "good" and "bad" people extends to the nurse and other staff. In addition, these clients are highly tuned into the vulnerable spots in others and, therefore, can make nurses feel highly anxious. Drawing from Burnham (1966), Epstein (1979), and Kernberg (1978), Smith and Lego (1984) in The American Handbook of Psychiatric Nursing devised the following lists of individual and group reactions of nurses to borderline clients:

INDIVIDUAL REACTIONS

1. Feelings of massive responsibility for the client's welfare.
2. Feelings of guilt because of failure to help the client.
3. Omnipotent urges to rescue the client from the mishandling of others.
4. Feelings of intense love and attachment to the client.
5. Promises to keep secrets for the client as a token of trust and esteem.
6. Feeling honored that the client "finally opened up."
7. Feeling highly confirmed in professional identity.
8. Feeling highly repudiated in professional identity.
9. Experiencing a need for excessively firm limits on the amount and quality of attention given to the client.
10. Guilt by association with some value or person viewed as hostile by the client.
11. Feelings of disappointment in one's work.
12. Feelings of being emotionally drained to the extent that one's personal relationships suffer.
13. Manifestations of the nurse's latent personality difficulties.
14. Hostile acting out toward the clients by discharging them or resigning them from the setting.
15. Contempt, jealousy, or envy of the seemingly "normal" client who manages to get considerable attention.
16. Feelings of general paranoia and fear of the client's "next projection."
17. Feeling emotionally exposed and vulnerable because of the client's "part-true" projections.
18. Defensiveness, counterattacking, rejection, and appeasement of the client.

GROUP REACTIONS

1. Diagnostic uncertainty, with contradictory evaluations of clients, occurs.

2. Groups of staff members may feel emotionally isolated from one another.
3. Two or more staff members may become suspicious of the motives and behaviors of other staff members toward the client.
4. Lunch hour and coffee break time may be dominated by discussion of specific clients.
5. The nucleus of an in-group may believe that they are the only ones who can help the client.
6. Loss of morale and confusion may be seen in the "out group."
7. Staff cleavage, with excessive clash of opinions, is seen by outside observers.
8. Blurring of staff-client role boundaries is seen in many forms (for example, client and staff discuss another staff member, or staff share personal information with the client).
9. Split in- and out-groups make the following accusations:
   a. "Ins" accuse "outs" of being cold and insensitive.
   b. "Outs" accuse "ins" of being too permissive and gullible and of spoiling the client.
10. Splits within departments in a hospital structure may be seen.
11. Administrative decisions to change client's therapist occur when the therapist is part of the "bad" split.

Consistent supervision and peer support are a must in order to maintain objectivity and avoid staff confusion. Conferences with all members of the health team can be extremely valuable.

Standard V: Intervention

Health care workers must deal with a variety of challenging behaviors when working with a borderline client. The client's hostility, self-destructive behaviors, and demanding behaviors are perhaps the most difficult. Table 17–8 shows examples, interventions, and theoretical rationales for borderline clients who display hostile, self-destructive, and demanding behavior. Borderline clients are nearly always treated with individual psychotherapy while in the hospital. The nurse supports the goals of psychotherapy. Team meetings are held often to counteract the effects of the clients' attempts to split staff.

Table 17–8 • EXAMPLES, INTERVENTIONS, AND THEORETICAL RATIONALES FOR TYPICAL BEHAVIORS OF CLIENTS WITH BORDERLINE PERSONALITY DISORDER

EXAMPLE OF BEHAVIOR	NURSING INTERVENTION	THEORETICAL RATIONALE
Hostility: "You are the worst nurse on this unit. I'm surprised they let you graduate from nursing school. You're a disgrace to your profession! I'm so mad, I could tear this unit apart. Maybe I will!"	In a calm way, the nurse asks the client to talk about what is causing all this anger, clarifies what has happened, sets limits, and provides safety for all the clients.	The client's rage has been touched off by anxiety about being cared for properly or about separation from caregivers. The nurse provides reassurance that anything can be discussed, that emotional security will not be withheld, and that the environment is safe. The client is helped to see that hostility can be faced and is manageable.
Self-destruction: The client gets angry during a therapeutic community meeting, runs to her room, breaks a lightbulb, and cuts her wrist superficially.	The nurse provides first aid but does not focus inordinate attention on the injury. Rather, attention is paid to the thoughts and feelings that led to the self-mutilation.	Self-destructive acts are unconsciously motivated by self-hatred, anger toward others, and a desire for "reunion" with the mother. The nurse helps the client explore these feelings without reinforcing the clinging, needy feelings.
Demanding Behavior: The client demands a pass even though she has been told she cannot leave for one week because she returned from her last pass drunk. "My doctor is hereby fired! I demand a new doctor and a transfer to another unit!"	The nurse calmly sets limits, pointing out they are a result of the client's inappropriate acting out. "Because you got drunk on pass, you cannot have another pass for a week. You knew the rule before you left on pass. You cannot change doctors or nurses, but must stay and deal with what you are thinking and feeling. That is the only way to change."	The client's acting out and demanding behavior cover her need for ego boundaries and control, her anger at earlier deprivation, and her fear of growth and separation. The nurse provides the missing ego, attempts to supply the previously missing emotional attachment, and provides reality testing about separation.

Standard VI: Evaluation

Nurses evaluate their interventions with borderline clients throughout the nursing process. When intervention is successful, the client

1. Communicates in a nondefensive way.
2. Displays less anger.
3. Displays less neediness.
4. Displays less acting out.

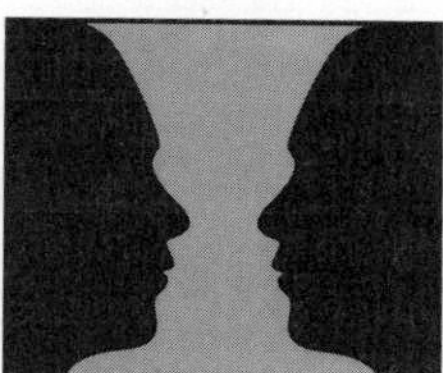

Case Study: Working With a Person Who Has a Borderline Personality Disorder

Mary Drake is a 24-year-old single secretary who lives alone. She has been seen in the emergency room several times for superficial suicide attempts. She was admitted because she has cut her wrists, ankles, and vagina with glass and has lost a lot of blood. This event was precipitated by her graduation from a community college.

Upon admission she is sweet, serene, and grateful to all the nurses, calling them "angels of mercy." Within one week she is angry at half the nurses, demanding a new primary nurse, saying that the one she has (whom she has grown attached to) hates her. She has managed to sneak alcohol onto the unit and was found in bed with a young male client. She continually breaks unit rules and then pleads to have this behavior forgiven and forgotten. When angry, she threatens to cut herself again. When asked why she cut herself, Mary states, "I was tired." She appears restless and tense and frequently asks for antianxiety medication. When asked what she is anxious about, she says "Uh . . . I don't know . . . I feel so empty inside." Mary frequently paces up and down the halls looking both angry and bored.

Assessment

Ms. McCarthy, a recent graduate and Mary's primary nurse, organizes the data into subjective and objective components.

OBJECTIVE DATA	SUBJECTIVE DATA
1. Makes frequent, superficial suicide attempts	1. Initially "loved" her primary nurse; now "hates" her and wants another nurse
2. Requests prn anti-anxiety medication frequently	2. States she is restless and tense
3. Paces up and down the hall much of the day	3. Complains of feeling empty inside
4. Threatens self-mutilation when anxious	4. Describes self as angry and bored much of the time
5. Brought alcohol onto the unit after pass	
6. Was found in bed with male client	

Nursing Diagnosis

Ms. McCarthy formulated three initial nursing diagnoses that had the highest priority during this time.

1. *Moderate to Severe Anxiety* related to threat to self-concept, as evidenced by inability to relax
   - States she feels "empty"
   - Is restless and tense
   - Requests prn antianxiety medication frequently
2. *Ineffective Individual Coping* related to inadequate psychological resources, as evidenced by inability to solve problems
   - After stating that she feels frustrated, client goes on pass and comes back with alcohol
   - After stating that she loves her therapist, client is found in bed with a male client
   - After stating that she hates her primary nurse, client demands a new primary nurse
3. *Potential for Self-Directed Violence* related to role changes, as evidenced by suicidal gestures and poor impulse control
   - Is admitted following self-mutilation
   - Threatens self-mutilation when anxious
   - Threatens self-mutilation on the unit

Continued on following page

Planning

CONTENT LEVEL—PLANNING GOALS

The nurse decided on the following goals:

Nursing Diagnosis	Long Term Goals	Short Term Goals
1. *Moderate to Severe Anxiety* related to threat to self-concept, as evidenced by inability to relax	Client will state that she feels relaxed more than she feels tense by discharge.	1. By (state the date) client will state she is relaxed in a situation that usually produces anxiety, e.g., after visiting hours.
2. *Ineffective Individual Coping* related to inadequate psychological resources, as evidenced by inability to problem-solve	Client will solve problems in a manner that injures neither self nor others by (state the date).	2. By (state the date) client will discuss feelings of frustration and deal with them appropriately rather than act them out.
3. *Potential for Self-Directed Violence* related to role changes, as evidenced by suicidal gestures and poor impulse control.	Client will state that she will use an alternate coping device when thoughts of self-mutilating occur.	3. By (state the date), client will discuss desire to mutilate self rather than do so.

PROCESS LEVEL—NURSES' REACTIONS AND FEELINGS

Ms. McCarthy talks to Mary's therapist twice a week in staff meetings. The therapist impressed upon Ms. McCarthy the difficulty health care workers have in working effectively with people with borderline personality disorders. These clients constantly act out their feelings in self-destructive and maladaptive ways. They usually are not aware of their feelings or what triggered their actions. The most difficult area for many health care workers is dealing with the intense feelings and reactions these clients can instill and provoke in others. Ms. McCarthy set a time twice a week for supervision with Mary's therapist. At the next meeting, common goals and intervention strategies were discussed.

Intervention

Working with Mary, the nurse found, was not easy. Many times the nurse felt angry and frustrated with Mary when acting-out behaviors occurred. With supervision, Ms. McCarthy was better able to deal with her feelings. The nurse became better able to focus on Mary's actions and work with Mary to figure out what feelings and events triggered the actions. See Mary's nursing care plan including interventions and rationales (Nursing Care Plan 17–2).

Evaluation

Mary appeared to come a long way in the three weeks she was on the unit. Her acting-out behaviors decreased. She had not threatened or attempted to mutilate herself in two weeks. Although Mary's sessions with her therapist were often stormy, there was more discussion of feelings. Her pacing the halls had decreased, and she appeared less tense most of the time. She still continued to ask for her antianxiety medication at frequent intervals but was willing to talk about what she thought the anxiety was about with both her primary nurse and the therapist. She agreed to continue therapy with her therapist on a bi-weekly basis after discharge.

Nursing Care Plan 17–2 • A PERSON WITH BORDERLINE PERSONALITY DISORDER: Mary

NURSING DIAGNOSIS

Moderate to severe anxiety related to threat to self-concept, as evidenced by inability to relax

Supporting Data

- States that she feels "empty."
- Is restless and tense.
- Requests prn antianxiety medication frequently.

Long Term Goal: Mary will state that she feels relaxed more than she feels tense by discharge.

Short Term Goal	*Intervention*	*Rationale*	*Evaluation*
1. By (state the date) Mary will state she is relaxed in a situation that usually produces anxiety (e.g., after visiting hours).	1a. Talk to client prior to event to help her observe and describe what she is expecting from the event.	1a. Understanding expectations that may or may not be met helps to identify source of anxiety and opens the way to more effective problem solving for unmet needs.	Goal met Client is able to discuss situation that was potentially anxiety provoking and appears relaxed after discussion.
	1b. Engage client in physical activity such as jogging or aerobic class.	1b. Exercise reduces physical tension and can increase endorphins, thereby increasing feelings of well-being.	Instead of pacing the halls today, she talked pleasantly with other clients after exercise class.

NURSING DIAGNOSIS

Ineffective individual coping related to inadequate psychological resources, as evidenced by inability to problem-solve.

Supporting Data

- After stating that she feels "frustrated," client goes on pass and returns with alcohol.
- After stating that she loves her therapist, client is found in bed with another client.
- After stating that she hates her primary nurse, client demands a new primary nurse.

Long Term Goal: Mary will solve problems in a manner that injures neither self nor others by (state the date).

Short Term Goal	*Intervention*	*Rationale*	*Evaluation*
1. By (state the date), Mary will discuss feelings of frustration and deal with them appropriately rather than act out.	1. Talk with client when she is frustrated regarding her goal, the block to the goal, and ways to either change the goal or reach it in an appropriate way.	1. Discussing and understanding the dynamics of frustration help to reduce the frustration by helping the client take positive action.	Goal met Mary is able to experience problems and deal with them appropriately. Acting out is minimal or absent. For example, client had an appointment for a job interview. She wanted to stay in bed and avoid the interview. Instead, she talked with the nurse about the fear of "growing up" and was able to get up and go to the interview.
2. By (state the date), Mary will discuss transference feelings and deal with them appropriately rather than act out.	2. Talk with client when she is experiencing strong positive or negative transference feelings, helping her to understand and experience all her feelings without acting them out.	2. Discussing and understanding the meaning of transference feelings and splitting help to reduce the potential for acting out.	

NURSING DIAGNOSIS

Potential for self-directed violence related to role changes, as evidenced by suicidal gestures and poor impulse control

Supporting Data

- Is admitted following self-mutilation.
- Threatens self-mutilation when anxious.
- Attempts self-mutilation on the unit.

Continued on following page

Nursing Care Plan 17–2 • A PERSON WITH BORDERLINE PERSONALITY DISORDER: Mary *(Continued)*

Long Term Goal: Mary will state that she no longer has the desire to mutilate herself.

Short Term Goal	*Intervention*	*Rationale*	*Evaluation*
1. By (state the date) Mary will discuss desire to mutilate self rather than do so.	1a. Nurse assists client in observing potential situations for self-mutilation.	1a–b. Observing, describing and analyzing thoughts and feelings reduces the potential for acting them out destructively.	Goal met Mary is able to experience troubling thoughts and feelings without self-mutilation. States, "I was mad at my therapist today and decided to cut my arms after the session. Instead, I told her I was angry, and together we figured out why."
	1b. Talk with client about these situations, eliciting thoughts and feelings.		
	1c. Encourage more appropriate ways to deal with these feelings.	1c. Offers alternative behaviors that can be more satisfying and growth promoting.	
	1d. Take care to safeguard environment at times when staff is busy and client's anxiety is acute.	1d. Times of increased anxiety/frustration/anger without external controls could increase probability of client self-mutilating behaviors.	

Summary — Borderline Personality Disorders

The borderline personality disorder has come to be known as the "neurosis of our time." These clients are recognizable by their highly unstable, angry, manipulative, and self-destructive behaviors, which are derived from primitive defenses. These defenses cover extreme neediness, anger, and fear of separation from nurturance. They present unique nursing challenges and stir up irrational, uncomfortable feelings in nurses. Intervention is directed toward providing emotional consistency, exploration of anger in appropriate ways, and gradual separation-individuation.

Self-study exercises 13 through 30 will help you review borderline personality disorders.

References

American Psychiatric Association. Diagnostic and Statistical Manual of Mental Disorders, 3d ed., revised. Washington DC: American Psychiatric Association, 1987.

Beck CM, Rawlins RP, Williams SR (eds). Mental Health-Psychiatric Nursing. St. Louis: C.V. Mosby Company, 1984.

Berne E. Games People Play: The Psychology of Human Relationships. New York: Grove Press, 1964.

Burnham DL. The special problem patient: Victim or agent of splitting? Psychiatry. Journal of the Study of Interpersonal Process, 29:2, 1966.

Carpenito AJ. Handbook of Nursing Diagnosis. Philadelphia: J.B. Lippincott Company, 1980.

Chapman AH. Textbook of Clinical Psychiatry: An Interpersonal Approach, 2nd ed. Philadelphia: J.B. Lippincott Company, 1976.

Chitty KK, Maynard CK. Managing manipulation. Journal of Psychosocial Nursing and Mental Health Services, 24(6):9, 1986.

Clack J. Nursing intervention into the aggressive behavior of patients. *In* Burd SF, Marshall MA (eds). Some Clinical Approaches to Psychiatric Nursing. London: Macmillan, 1963.

Cleckley H. The Mask of Sanity, 4th ed. St. Louis: C.V. Mosby Company, 1964.

Closurdo JS. Behavior modification and the nursing process. Perspectives in Psychiatric Care, 13:25, 1975.

Epstein L. Countertransference with borderline patients. *In* Epstein L, Feiner AH (eds). Countertransference. New York: Jason Aronson, 1979.

Frosch JP. The treatment of antisocial and borderline personality disorders. Hospital and Community Psychiatry, 34:243, 1983.

Harrington A. Psychopaths. New York: Simon & Schuster, 1972.

Kernberg OF. Borderline Conditions and Pathological Narcissism. New York: Jason Aronson, 1975.

Kernberg OF. Leadership and organizational functioning: Organization regression. International Journal of Group Psychotherapy, 28:1, 1978.

Kolb LC, Brodie HK. Modern Clinical Psychiatry, 10th ed. Philadelphia: W.B. Saunders Company, 1982.

Loomis ME. Nursing management of acting-out behavior. Perspectives in Psychiatric Care, 8:169, 1970.

MacKinnon RA, Michels R. The psychiatric interview in clinical practice. Philadelphia: W.B. Saunders Company, 1971.

Masterson JF. Psychotherapy of the Borderline Adult. New York: Brunner-Mazel, 1976.

McCord WM. The Psychopath and Milieu Therapy. New York: Academic Press, 1982.

McCord WM, McCord J. The Psychopath: An Essay on the Criminal Mind. Princeton: D. Van Nostrand Company, 1956.

Millon T. Disorders of Personality: DSM III: AXIS II. New York: John Wiley & Sons, 1981.

Modlin HC. The antisocial personality. Bulletin of the Menninger Clinic, 47:129, 1983.

Pasquali EA, Arnold HM, DeBasio N, Alesi EG. Mental Health Nursing, 2nd ed. St. Louis: C.V. Mosby Company, 1985.

Quay HC, Love CT. The effect of a juvenile diversion program on rearrests. Criminal Justice and Behavior, 5:410, 1977.

Reid WH (ed). The antisocial personality: A review. Hospital and Community Psychiatry, 36(8):831, 1985.

Reid WH (ed). The Treatment of Antisocial Syndromes. New York: Van Nostrand Reinhold Company, 1981.

Sass L. The borderline personality. The New York Times Magazine, August 22, 1982, p. 12.

Smith MC, Lego S. The client who has a borderline personality disorder. *In* Lego, S. (ed). The American Handbook of Psychiatric Nursing. Philadelphia: J.B. Lippincott, 1984.

Smoyak SA. Borderline personality disorder (editorial). Journal of Psychosocial Nursing, 23:5, 1985.

Stanton AH. Personality disorders. *In* Nicholi AM (ed). The Harvard Guide to Modern Psychiatry. Cambridge, MA: The Belknap Press of Harvard University, 1978.

Stringer AY, Josef NC. Methylphenidate in the treatment of aggression in two patients with antisocial personality disorder. American Journal of Psychiatry, 140:1365, 1983.

Toch H. An interdisciplinary approach to criminal violence. Journal of Criminal Law and Criminology, 71:216, 1980.

Vaillant GE, Perry JC. Personality disorders. *In* Kaplan HI, Sadock BJ (eds). Comprehensive Textbook of Psychiatry/IV, 4th ed. Baltimore, MD: Williams & Wilkins, 1985.

Wade TC. A family crisis intervention approach to diversion from the criminal justice system. Juvenile Justice Journal, 7:230, 1977.

Winshnie H. The Impulsive Personality. New York: Plenum Press, 1977.

Zamora LC. Anger. *In* Haber J, Leach AM, Schudy SM, Sideleau BF (eds). Comprehensive Psychiatric Nursing, 2nd ed. New York: McGraw Hill Book Company, 1982.

Self-Study Exercises

ANTISOCIAL PERSONALITY DISORDERS

Place T (true) or F (false) next to the possible backgrounds of those children who grow up to have an antisocial personality.

1. ________ They are born to parents who reject them.
2. ________ Parents of antisocial clients have had a fulfilling childhood.
3. ________ As children, antisocial clients were generally exposed to abuse, violent tempers, and cruelty.
4. ________ Authority, goals, and identification of role models were present for these children.

Write a few sentences in answer to the following:

5. Discuss the current thinking regarding the role of anxiety and guilt as they relate to the antisocial personality disorders.
6. Name four behaviors commonly observed in people with antisocial personality disorders.
7. Discuss five steps in setting limits in manipulation.

Multiple Choice

8. Choose the characteristic that is NOT *common to* ALL personality disorders.

   A. Ineffective and maladaptive responses to stress
   B. Difficulty in working and loving
   C. Evokes interpersonal conflict
   D. Always gets in trouble with the law; has no conscience

9. A nurse working with a person diagnosed as antisocial may experience all of the following EXCEPT:

   A. Anger
   B. Put-down
   C. Fear
   D. Adoration
   E. True intimacy

10. Choose the least effective therapeutic modality for an antisocial client.

    A. Behavior therapy
    B. Therapy based on modeling
    C. Psychotherapy
    D. Change in social setting

11. Nurse Gonzales said to another nurse that she admired the way Mr. Smith, an antisocial client, 'handled' the psychologist during the community meeting. Later in the day, Mr. Smith asked Nurse Gonzales if he acted inappropriately. Nurse Gonzales responded, "No. I wish I had thought of it. I don't get along with him." This is an example of

    A. Setting limits with the client
    B. Being honest with the nurse's feelings
    C. Supporting the pathological situation
    D. Confidential information

12. The treatment plan for Mr. Smith consisted of rewarding him with privileges when he acted appropriately. This is referred to as

    A. Modeling behavior
    B. Cognitive therapy
    C. Civil treatment
    D. Behavior modification

BORDERLINE PERSONALITY DISORDERS

Place T (true) or F (false) next to the characteristics of a borderline client according to the DSM III-R.

13. ________ Impulsive behavior that is self-damaging, e.g., promiscuity, gambling, overeating, overspending.
14. ________ Extreme paranoia, thinks people are poisoning him and out to hurt him.
15. ________ Relationships intense and very unstable, marked by devaluation and idealization.
16. ________ Great need to be perfect; very compulsive regarding hygiene and work habits.
17. ________ Inability to tolerate being alone; chronic feelings of boredom.
18. ________ Very withdrawn behavior; does not like to call attention to self.
19. ________ Inappropriate intense anger; problem with impulse control.
20. ________ Identity disturbances; questions self-image, gender identity, career goals, and more.
21. ________ Given to flights of mania when limits are set on impulsive behavior.
22. ________ Frequent impulsive suicidal gestures or self-mutilation.

Next to the theory of borderline etiology, place a C (constitution), K (Kernberg), or M (Masterson).

23. ________ As an infant, needed to split mother into all "good" or all "bad" to lower anxiety. Since needs went unmet and care was contradictory, this splitting is carried over into adult life.
24. ________ The inability to tolerate stress is an inherited personality trait.
25. ________ During the normal separation-individuation stage, the child's effort toward autonomy and independence was met with disapproval by the mothering one; clinging and dependent behaviors were rewarded.

Multiple Choice

26. Choose the defensive maneuver that is NOT readily used by the borderline client to reduce anxiety or get needs met.

    A. Splitting
    B. Manipulation
    C. Projection
    D. Sublimation

Short Answer

27. List behavioral outcomes of successful therapeutic intervention.

    A. ______
    B. ______
    C. ______

28. Name three nursing diagnoses which could be used with a borderline client.

    A. ______
    B. ______
    C. ______

29. Give the nursing intervention and the rationale for the following behaviors frequently seen in borderline clients:

    A. Hostility______
    ______
    B. Self-destructive______
    ______
    C. Demanding______
    ______

Circle the Correct Letters

30. Circle ONLY the personal reactions nurses and other health care workers may experience when working with a borderline client.

    A. Need to "rescue" client from others.
    B. Feelings of intense love or attachment toward client.
    C. Feeling comfortable after soon establishing a good working relationship.
    D. Contempt, jealousy, and envy of how client gets attention.
    E. Finding that the client quickly learns appropriate ways to solve problems.
    F. Emotionally exposed and vulnerable related to the client's "part-true" projections.

PEOPLE IN SEVERE TO PANIC LEVELS OF CHRONIC ANXIETY

UNIT V

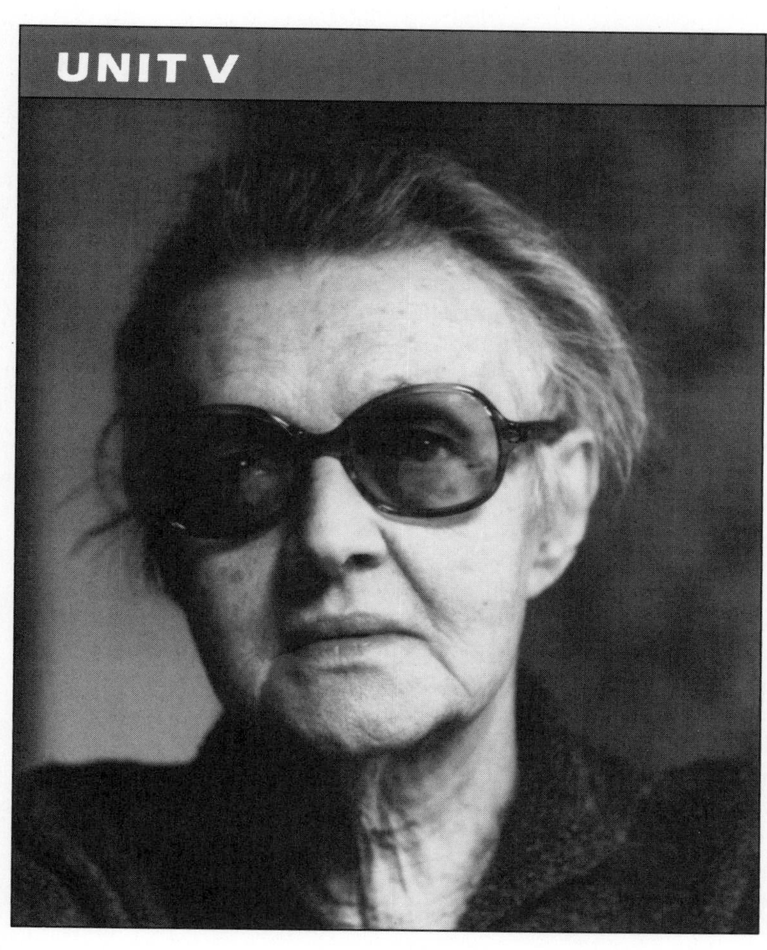

There is a language of the life more imminent than pain—'tis pain's successor—when the soul has suffered all it can.

EMILY DICKINSON

A Nurse Speaks

by Miriam Socias Perez

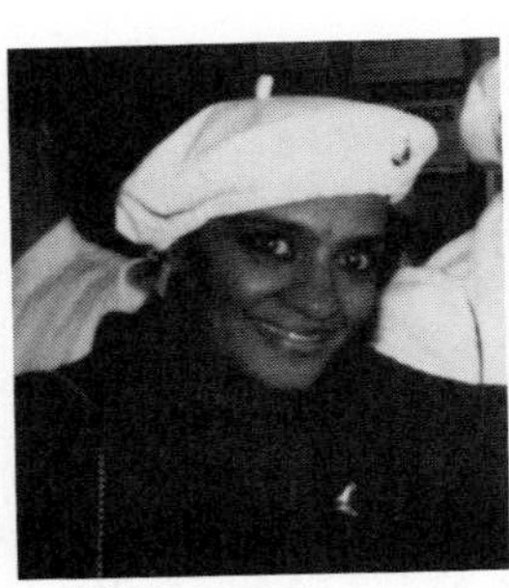

Two years after graduation from a two-year associate degree college, I chose to work in a hemodialysis unit. I found the work intense—at times stressful—and the possibility of death for many of our clients ever present.

Many of the conferences held for staff were geared toward coping with personal feelings should death of one of our clients occur. Death of a client was never easy to deal with. However, depending on the client's condition, death was more acceptable in some cases and more difficult to accept in others.

Ms. John was one of my clients in the hemodialysis unit. She was a great lady. She was 50 years old, separated, and unable to bear children. She had worked hard in a factory, had a great personality, and was loved by the staff. Ms. John had accepted her diagnosis, chronic end-stage renal failure, quite well. She respected her doctors wholeheartedly and *adored* her nurses. Ms. John had been maintained on a hemodialysis machine for ten years. She had an arteriovenous fistula in her left arm, which years later had to be replaced by a bovine graft in her right arm. Despite several complications, such as congestive heart failure and endocarditis, she always managed to spring back stronger after her recuperation. Ms. John was our unit's pride. She was quite knowledgeable about her disease and served as a valuable inservice resource person and support for our clients. She was great at comforting new clients and explaining all the routine procedures and the do's and don'ts in dialysis. She represented success and endurance, which can be rare in such a high-risk population.

Then, one day, Ms. John had a cardiac arrest while on the machine and died. I was working on the evening shift, but this had occurred during the day. When I arrived, the unit was so quiet, and the faces of the staff and clients were so sorrowful that I knew someone had died. When I found out who, I could not hold back the tears. The staff and I had been so good at dealing with and accepting death in the past. Why could we not control ourselves then? Ms. John had represented so much hope for our other clients that we now feared the thoughts going through the minds of the other clients concerning their own future on dialysis. For a moment, I wondered if perhaps I was the only one experiencing such feelings of grieving and sadness, but I noticed that even our unit director and supervisor were crying! It was such an empty, helpless, defeated type of feeling. At first I felt guilty for not being on the day shift. I wanted to know who had had the cardiac arrest code. My final question was, "Why did it have to be her?" That evening, when I returned home, I still felt that I must do something for her. She was so very special. I then wrote a poem.

The poem was read during her funeral service. Not only were Ms. John's friends and family at her funeral but also the members of the hemodialysis unit were there to say good bye. I shall never forget her.

CHAPTER 18

Alterations in Mood—Grief and Depression

Elizabeth M. Varcarolis

KEY TERMS AND CONCEPTS ◆ ◆ ◆ ◆ ◆ ◆ ◆ ◆ ◆ ◆

The key terms and concepts listed here also appear in bold where they are defined or discussed in this chapter.

MOOD
MOOD SYNDROME
DEPRESSIVE MOOD SYNDROME
MOOD EPISODE
PRIMARY AND SECONDARY DEPRESSIONS
ANHEDONIA
VEGETATIVE SIGNS OF DEPRESSION
SECONDARY GAINS
MAJOR DEPRESSION
DYSTHYMIA
TRICYCLICS (TCAs)
MONOAMINE OXIDASE INHIBITORS (MAOI)
ATYPICAL ANTIDEPRESSANTS
SEASONAL AFFECTIVE DISORDER (SAD)
PSYCHOMOTOR RETARDATION
PSYCHOMOTOR AGITATION
HYPERSOMNIA
GRIEF
MOURNING
PROLONGED GRIEF
DELAYED GRIEF
PHENOMENA EXPERIENCED DURING MOURNING
ANTICIPATORY GRIEF

Mood refers to a prolonged emotion that colors a person's whole psychic life (APA 1987). Joy, grief, elation, and sadness are all terms used to describe a particular mood.

Normal moods (sadness, grief, and elation) are universal experiences. Happiness and unhappiness are appropriate responses to life events. When sadness, grief, or elation is extremely intense and the mood is unduly prolonged, a disorder in mood results.

Mood disorders, also referred to as affective dis-

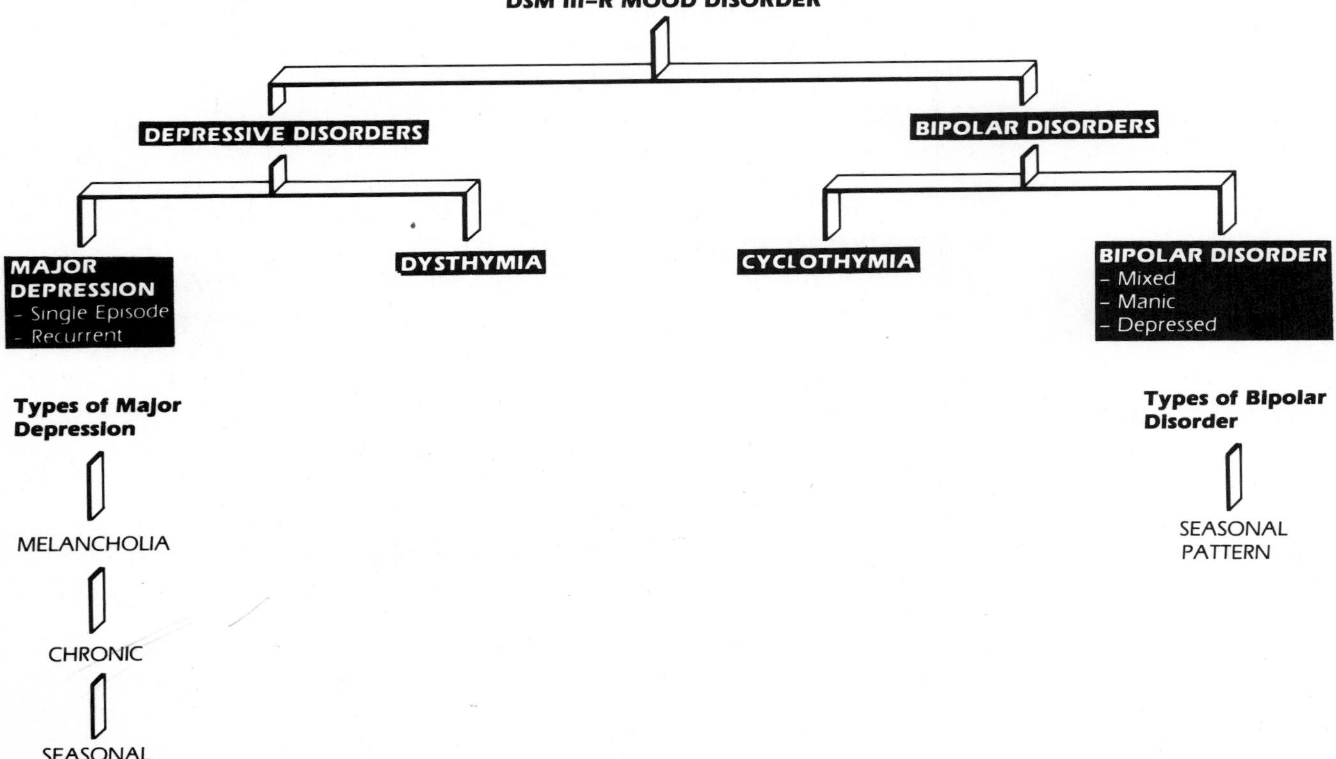

Figure 18–1. *Overview of mood disorder.*

orders, are divided into two general categories according to the DSM III-R classification: *bipolar disorders* and *depressive disorders* (Fig. 18–1).

Grief is not a mood disorder, although a depressive syndrome is often part of the grieving process. Grief is the normal response to a significant loss. Although grief is a normal phenomenon, it may be, at times, the focus of treatment.

This chapter will discuss grief and the depressive disorders. Chapter 19 will discuss the bipolar disorders.

Grief

OBJECTIVES

After studying this section on grief, the student will be able to:

1. Discuss the three phases of Engel's *acute stage* (four to eight weeks) of mourning.
2. Give examples of five phenomena people may experience during the *long term stage* (one to two years) of mourning.
3. Identify possible personal reactions a nurse might experience when working with a grieving client.
4. Describe two pathological grief reactions.
5. Name two nursing diagnoses appropriate for a client who is grieving.
6. Discuss five nursing interventions for a family who is grieving.
7. Identify when the work of mourning has been successful.
8. List six factors that can negatively affect the successful work of mourning.

Change is a part of life, and every change involves a loss and a gain. People come and go in our lives. As we gain experience, we lose our youth—dreams are realized or hopes abandoned. We are constantly faced with giving up one mode of life for another.

Loss is a part of the human experience, and grief is the normal response to a loss. The loss may be a relationship (divorce, separation, death, abortion), loss of health (body function or part, mental or physical capacity), loss of status or prestige, loss of security (occupational, financial, social, cultural), loss of self-confidence, loss of a dream, loss of self-concept, or a symbolic loss. Other losses include changes in circumstances, such as retirement, promotion, marriage, or aging. All losses affect a person's self-concept. People undergoing therapy may grieve as they give up old, familiar—although maladaptive—ways of viewing the world. A loss can be a real loss or a perceived loss.

In this chapter, **grief** refers to the subjective feelings and affect that are precipitated by a loss. The term **mourning** refers to the processes (grief work) by which grief is resolved (Carr 1985).

The depression experienced during the process of mourning is not a depressive disorder, although the bereaved may experience a clinical depressive syndrome. Mourning is a process of which depression is an important stage. A normal grief reaction is self-limiting and self-healing, in one to two years. Recovery occurs after the final stage of depression in the process of mourning (Parkes 1972). Depression may be *experienced* by the person as inertia, purposelessness, and helplessness. It may be *observed* by others as sad or disorganized behavior (Mendelson 1974).

Standard I: Theory

Mourning is a distinct psychological process. This process involves the disengagement of strong emotional ties from a significant relationship and reinvesting these ties in a new and productive direction. This reinvestment of emotional energy into new relationships or creative activities is necessary for a person's mental health and future in society. When the grieving process is successful, the griever is released from one interpersonal relationship and able to form new relationships. The complete process of mourning may take a year or more to complete.

A number of theorists have studied the grief process. Some of the most widely known are George Engel, Colin Parkes, Elizabeth Kubler-Ross, Erich Lindemann, John Bowlby, and Edgar Jackson. Although different terminology is used, the process outlined by these theorists is basically the same. Each describes commonly experienced psychological and behavioral characteristics. These characteristics follow a pattern of response:

1. Shock and disbelief.
2. Sensation of somatic distress.
3. Preoccupation with the image of the deceased.
4. Guilt.
5. Anger.
6. Change in the conduct behavior (e.g., depression, disorganization, restlessness).
7. Reorganization of behavior directed toward a new object or activity.

A person may demonstrate a different clinical picture at each of the varying stages of mourning. Each stage of grieving has its own characteristics, and individuals may vary considerably in regard to the duration and form of each stage. People react within their own value and personality structure, as well as their social environment and cultural patterns. Essentially, people are preprogrammed in their response to death. Distinct characteristics, however, can be identified throughout the grieving process.

The process of mourning is often divided into stages. The stages have been identified by Engel as (1) *acute* and (2) *long term*.

ACUTE STAGE (Four to Eight Weeks)

SHOCK AND DISBELIEF. The bereaved's first response is that of *denial*. The person is emotionally unable to accept his or her terrible loss. Denial functions as a buffer against intolerable pain and allows the person to acknowledge the reality of death slowly. The mourner may appear to be functioning in a robot-like fashion. Often, the bereaved person feels numb. A death may be "accepted" intellectually during this stage—"It's just as well; she was suffering"—although the emotional responses are still repressed. Denial is an important and needed defense and may last a few hours to a few days. *Denial that persists for longer than a few days could indicate difficulty in progressing through the process of mourning.*

DEVELOPING AWARENESS. As denial fades, painful feelings begin to surface. The finality of the loved one's death becomes more of a reality. Waves of anguish and pain are experienced and may be localized in the chest or epigastric area. *Anger* often surfaces at this time. It is not uncommon for doctors and nurses to be the subject of blame. Awareness by staff that anger is often displaced onto people in the hospital environment may decrease defensive staff behaviors. *Guilt* is often experienced, and the bereaved blames him- or herself for failing to do or not do specific tasks. Impulsive and self-destructive acts by the mourner may be evidenced by such behaviors as pushing one's hand through a window or beating one's head against the wall. *Crying* is a common phenomenon during this stage. "It is during this time that the greatest degree of anguish or despair, within the limits imposed by cultural patterns, is experienced or expressed" (Engel 1964). Crying can afford a welcome release from pent-up anguish and tension. Assessment of cultural patterns is important for making clinical judgments regarding the appropriateness of the behavior of the bereaved. Not crying can be the result of cultural programming or environmental restraints. The person may cry in private. *Inability to cry*, however, may be the result of a high degree of ambivalence toward the deceased. *A person who is unable to cry may have difficulty successfully completing the work of mourning.*

RESTITUTION. This stage is the formal ritualistic stage or the institutionalization of mourning during the acute stage. It brings friends and family together in the rites of the funeral service and serves to emphasize the finality of death. The viewing of the body, the lowering of the casket, and the various religious and cultural rituals all help shed any residual denial in the atmosphere of support. Every human society has its own moral and ethical standards according to which death can take place (Benton 1978). The gathering in ritualistic farewell for the deceased provides support and sustenance for the family.

LONG TERM STAGE (One to Two Years)

After the acute stage, the main work of mourning goes on intrapsychically and may take a year or two to complete. During this time, the bereaved may experience the various **phenomena experienced during mourning** described in Table 18–1.

Table 18-1 • PSYCHOLOGICAL AND BEHAVIORAL PHENOMENA EXPERIENCED DURING THE LONG TERM STAGE OF MOURNING

SYMPTOMS	EXAMPLES
Sensation of Somatic Distress	
Tightness in the throat, shortness of breath, sighing, "mental pain," exhaustion. Food tastes like sand; things feel unreal. Pain or discomfort may be identical to the symptoms experienced by the dead person. Normally symptoms are brief.	A woman whose husband died of a stroke complains of weakness and numbness on her left side.
Preoccupation with the Image of the Deceased	
The bereaved brings up and thinks and talks about numerous memories of the deceased. The memories are positive. This process goes on with great sadness. The idealization of the deceased lets the bereaved relive the gratifications associated with the deceased and helps resolve any guilt the bereaved has toward the deceased. The bereaved may also take on many of the mannerisms of the deceased through identification. Identification serves the purpose of holding onto the deceased. Preoccupation with the dead person takes many months before it lessens.	A man whose wife just died states, "I just can't stop thinking about my wife. Everything I see reminds me of her. We picked up this seashell on our honeymoon. I remember every wonderful moment we had together. The pain is so great, but the memories just keep coming." His friends noticed that when he talks his hand gestures and expressions are very like those of his recently deceased wife.
Guilt	
The bereaved reproaches him- or herself for real or fancied acts of negligence or omissions in the relationship with the deceased.	"I should have made him go to the doctor sooner." "I should have paid more attention to her, been more thoughtful."
Anger	
The anger the bereaved experiences may not be toward the object that gives rise to it. Often the anger is displaced on the medical or nursing staff. Often it is directed toward the deceased. The anger is at its height during the first month but often intermittent throughout the first year. The overflow of hostility disturbs the bereaved, resulting in the feeling that he or she is going "mad" or "insane."	"The doctor didn't operate in time. If he had, Mary would be alive today." "How could he leave me like this . . . how could he?"
Change in Conduct Behavior (Depression, Disorganization, Restlessness)	
A person may exhibit marked restlessness and an inability to organize his or her behavior. Routine activities take a long time to do. Depressive mood is common as the year passes and as the intensity of the grief declines. Absence of depression is more "abnormal" than its presence. Loneliness and aimlessness are most pronounced six to nine months after death.	Six months after her husband died, Mrs. Faye stated, "I just can't seem to function, I have a hard time doing the simplest tasks. I can't be bothered socializing." "I feel so down . . . so, so empty."
Reorganization of Behavior Directed Toward a New Object or Activity	
Gradually the person renews his or her interest in people and activities. The grieving thus releases the bereaved from one interpersonal relationship, and new ones are free to take its place.	Twenty months after her husband's death, Mrs. Faye tells a friend, "I'll be away this weekend. I am going fishing with my brother and his friend. This is the first time I've felt like doing anything since Harry died."

Standard II: Data Collection

Nurses are constantly confronted with clients and their families who are mourning significant losses. Assessing the mourner's level of anxiety and signs of unresolved grief reactions can alert the nurse to potential problems.

ASSESSING THE MOURNER'S LEVEL OF ANXIETY

Anxiety is always present when one is confronted with a change whose outcome is uncertain. Mild to moderate anxiety levels are useful and can motivate people in constructive directions. Severe to panic levels are temporarily disabling. When a client's anxiety levels are mild to moderate, he or she is able to solve problems and realistically appraise the situation. If a client is in severe or panic levels of anxiety, interventions are needed to reduce the client's anxiety.

ASSESSING UNRESOLVED GRIEF REACTION

Most bereaved persons resolve their loss over time and go on to resume their lives. However, unresolved grief reactions have been called the "hidden disease" and may account for many of the physical symptoms seen in doctors' offices and hospital units (Dempsey 1975). The "broken heart syndrome" is supported by statistics that show surviving spouses die within a year of their husband or wife at a much higher rate than control groups (Carr 1985). In some cases, the bereaved go to pieces, neglect themselves, do not eat, turn to alcohol or drugs, and become susceptible to physical disease. Often the disease is a direct reaction to an emotional loss (Dempsey 1975). Several studies show that the health of widows and close relatives decline within one year of bereavement, and medical and psychiatric problems increase (Bowlby and Parkes 1970; Carr 1985).

Two specific atypical reactions to grief have been identified: *prolonged grief* and *delayed grief* (Jackson 1957, Parkes 1972).

In **prolonged grief,** the bereaved remains intensely preoccupied with the memories of the deceased many years after the person has died.

Mrs. Green has lived by herself since her husband died five years ago. When her nephew came to visit, he found everything as it was five years ago. Mr. Green's coat was still on the hook in the front hall, and his slippers were by the day bed where he used to nap. Mrs. Green talked tearfully of how much she missed him and mentioned many incidents in their life together.

In **delayed grief** a person may not experience the pain of loss; however, that pain is modified by chronic depression, intense preoccupation with body functioning (hypochondriasis), phobic reactions, or acute insomnia. Suicidal thinking should always be assessed in a person experiencing a pathological grief response, especially if depression is the presenting symptom. Hallucinations, delusions, or obsessions may be seen. These symptoms may not surface for months or years after the death.

Sidney Bolla's wife died of cancer three years ago. Everyone remarked how well he handled himself and how well he did after the funeral was over. He was always a quiet man and kept to himself. Mr. Bolla started getting severe anxiety attacks one day while in the supermarket. As time progressed, he became fearful of going out and suffered from severe insomnia. A neighbor brought him to the hospital when he developed pneumonia and was too fearful to go outside of the house to seek medical attention.

Standard III: Diagnosis

Within the general hospital setting, patients often experience losses. Some of the losses may be loss of function (musculoskeletal, cardiovascular, sensory), or body part (mastectomy, limb, colostomy). Other patients may have losses associated with chronic pain or terminal illness or may have to make some change in lifestyle related to surgical or medical treatments. The nurse needs to be aware that withdrawn or apathetic behavior, crying, anger, denial, or guilt on the part of the client could signal a grief reaction or a potential pathological grief reaction. The nursing diagnoses of *grieving related to an actual or perceived loss* or *grieving related to an anticipated loss* could be used.

Anticipatory grief is grief that occurs before an actual loss. Anticipatory grief can allow for a gradual recognition of the loss. During this time, painful feelings may be partially resolved. *Dysfunctional grieving* would be appropriate for a person experiencing a *prolonged grief* or *delayed grief* reaction.

Standard IV: Planning

Planning effective care takes into consideration (1) content level—planning goals and (2) process level—nurses' reactions and feelings.

CONTENT LEVEL—PLANNING GOALS

Planning care for a client who is grieving should, whenever possible, include important family members. Possible goals for the nursing diagnosis *grieving related to an actual or perceived loss* could be

Long Term Goals

- In 12 to 18 months, client will state he remembers both the pleasures and the disappointments of the lost loved one.

Short Term Goals

- By (state the date) client will discuss with another person(s) painful thoughts and feelings resulting from the loss.
- Client will express feelings of anger, guilt, or loneliness to others by (state the date).
- By (state the date) client will name two people or organizations available when emotional support is needed.

PROCESS LEVEL—NURSES' REACTIONS AND FEELINGS

Culture plays an important part in the responses called forth in the face of death and dying. Our capacity to grieve stems from our view of death. In contemporary American society, there is a strong denial of death and growing old and becoming sick (Benton 1978). Rakoff (1973) stated:

> America conjured into its superficial stereotype, is a country of the eternal now, of the young, face lifting, good teeth into the seventies, old ladies in Bermuda shorts, hair colored at will, endless euphemisms for chronic disease, affliction and death.

Denial and fear of death are strong in the American culture. This denial and fear affect the behavioral responses of the bereaved, the family, and those who support the family in the face of death. Nurses are affected by cultural myths in the same way as the rest of society. When faced with a person who is dying, nurses remember their own losses. Difficult memories and feelings are often awakened. When staff members have not been able to resolve their own conflicts with death, the ability to help others is minimized. Psychological support needs to be available to help staff better understand the grieving process. When nurses examine their own feelings and their personal experience of loss, verbal and nonverbal clues to the needs of a grieving family member of a dying patient become more apparent (Marks 1976).

Sometimes, nurses grieve with family members at the death of a person they have cared for and became fond of. Sometimes an entire staff may mourn the death of a client. Just such a situation is described in A *Nurse Speaks* (p. 422).

Standard V: Intervention

Prolonged and serious alterations in social adjustment as well as potential medical diseases may develop in the absence of proper management during a grief reaction. The essential task is sharing the client's grief work (Lindemann 1944).

Most important in handling acute grief are talking and listening (Chapman 1976; Benton 1978). The nurse should keep her own talking to a minimum. Banal advice and philosophical statements are useless and can serve to increase the client's feelings of isolation. Unhelpful responses by others, such as, "He's no longer suffering" or "You can always have another child" or "It's better this way," can lead the bereaved to believe that others do not understand his or her acute pain and that the personal impact of the loss is being minimized. Such statements can compound feelings of isolation. More helpful responses are, "His death will be a terrible loss" or "No one can replace her" or "He will be missed for a long time." Statements such as these validate the bereaved's experience of loss and communicate the message that the bereaved is understood and supported.

Talking by the bereaved can serve the purpose of releasing negative emotions. When a person is faced with an unwanted loss, strong feelings of anger, guilt, and hate are normal reactions that need to be expressed in order to facilitate the process of mourning. It is important that the nurse plan time to be with the client to listen and encourage the expression of feelings surrounding the person's loss or anticipated loss.

If the bereaved is desperately lacking sleep, an antianxiety agent used sparingly may be appropriate (Chapman 1976). Some authorities think that the use of drugs to suppress the pain of grief could prolong the course of mourning (Parkes 1972; Jackson 1957).

The nurse's intervention is dependent upon the client's situation, as well as the environment. For example, within the hospital settings, many patients encounter pain. Facilitating the expression of feelings surrounding the loss of well-being and loss of control is vital. On maternity and pediatric units, parents may be anticipating the loss of a terminally ill child or experiencing the loss of a stillborn baby. Here the focus of intervention is facilitating the family's mourning. Specific guidelines the nurse can use in the general hospital setting with families of dying or deceased clients are described in Table 18–2.

Standard VI: Evaluation

The work of mourning is over when the bereaved can remember realistically both the pleasures and the disappointments of the lost loved one.

If after a normal period of time (12 to 24 months) a person has not completed the grieving process, reassessment and reevaluations are indicated.

Some of the factors that can affect the successful completion of the mourning process have been described by Engel (1964).

1. *The level of dependency in the relationship.* The more dependent the mourner was on the deceased, the more difficult the resolution of the loss.

Table 18–2 • NURSING INTERVENTIONS FOR GRIEVING FAMILIES

SITUATION	NURSING INTERVENTIONS	RATIONALE
1. The death or imminent death of family member.	1a. Communicate news to the family in area of privacy.	1a. Family can support each other in an atmosphere in which they can behave naturally.
	1b. If only one family member is available, stay with that member until clergy or family or friend arrives.	1b. Presence and comfort of nurse during initial stage of shock can help minimize feelings of acute isolation and anxiety.
	1c. If nurse feels unable to handle the situation, enlist the aid of another who can support the family.	1c. Individual or family will need support, questions answered, and guidance as to immediate tasks and information.
2. The family requests to see and take leave of the dying or dead person.	2. Request should always be granted.	2. Need to take leave can be of overwhelming importance for some—to kiss goodbye, ask for forgiveness, or take a lock of hair. Helps people face the reality of death.
3. Angry family members accuse the nurse or doctor of abusing or mismanaging the care of the deceased.	3. Continue to provide the best care for the dying or final care to the dead. Avoid becoming involved in angry and painful arguments and power struggles.	3. Complaints are not directed toward the nurse personally. The anger may be serving the purpose of keeping the grieving relatives from falling apart. Or, projected anger may be an attempt to deal with aggression and guilt toward the dying person.
4. Relatives may behave in a grossly disturbed manner (e.g., refuse to acknowledge the truth, collapse, lose control).	4a. Show patience and tact and offer sympathy and warmth.	4a. Shock and disbelief are the first responses to the news of death, and people need ways to protect themselves from the overwhelming reality of loss.
	4b. Encourage the person to cry.	4b. Helps to provide relief from feelings of acute pain and tension.
	4c. Provide a place of privacy for grieving.	4c. Facilitates natural expression of grief.
5. The family may request specific religious, cultural, and social customs strange or unknown to the nurse.	5. The nurse helps facilitate steps necessary for the family to carry out the desired arrangements.	5. Institutionalized mourning rituals of various cultures provide important external supports for the grief-stricken person.

Data from Engel GL. Grief and grieving. American Journal of Nursing, 64(9):93, 1964.

2. *The degree of ambivalence in the relationship*. Persistent, unresolved conflicts interfere with successful grief work.
3. *The age of the deceased*. The death of a child may have a more profound effect than that of an older person.
4. *The bereaved person's support system*. A person with few meaningful relationships will have more difficulty letting go of his ties with the deceased.
5. *The number of previous losses*. Present losses can trigger the pain of past losses. Unresolved feelings from past losses can complicate the present grief process.
6. *The physical and psychological health of the person grieving*. These factors greatly affect a person's capacity for grief work.

Summary — Grief

The process of mourning is a distinct psychological process and is the normal reaction to a loss. A loss can be real or perceived. It can include loss of a person, loss of security, loss of self-confidence, or loss of a dream. Essentially, the loss results in the loss of self-concept.

The stages of *acute grief* may take from four to eight weeks; the complete process of mourning (*long term stage*) may take a year or two. Characteristics of the acute stage as outlined by Engel include (1) shock and disbelief, (2) developing awareness, and (3) restitution. *Normal phenomena encountered during the process of mourning* over the next year or two include (1) *sensation of somatic distress*, (2) *preoccupation with the image of the deceased*, (3) *guilt*, (4) *anger*, (5) *depression*, and (6) *reinvestment of energy into new relationships and activities* and are reviewed in Table 18–1.

Culture greatly affects the patterns of mourning. Grief in another can reactivate distressing feelings of previous losses in health care workers. If the nurse has unresolved issues of grief and depression, ability to help others is greatly minimized. Staff members need psychological support when working with people who are grieving.

Unresolved grief reactions can lead to physical illness, disorganization in thinking and behavior, and personal neglect. Two specific atypical grief reactions are *prolonged grief* and *delayed grief*.

Specific nursing diagnoses can be used for a grieving client: (1) *grieving related to actual or perceived loss*, (2) *grieving related to anticipated loss*, and (3) *dysfunctional grieving*.

Grief work is successful when specific phenomena identified with the process have been experienced. Time should be given to a person in mourning for talking and reliving memories in the presence of a caring person who can share the pain. Guidelines for nurses have been outlined for interventions for a family who is grieving in Table 18–2.

The work of mourning is complete when the bereaved can remember realistically both the pleasures and the disappointments of the lost relationship. A number of factors affect the normal process of mourning: level of dependence in the relationship, degree of ambivalence in the relationship, the age of the deceased, the bereaved person's support system, the number of previous losses, and the physical and psychological health of the person grieving.

Self-study exercises 1 through 21 at the end of this chapter will help the student review material covered in this section.

Depressive Disorders

OBJECTIVES

After studying this section on depressive disorders, the student will be able to:

1. Compare and contrast major depression and dysthymia.
2. Discuss four theories of etiology for depression.
3. Identify possible behaviors for each of the following areas when assessing a depressed client: (a) affect, (b) thought processes, (c) feelings, (d) physical behavior, (e) communication, and (f) indications of masked depression.

4. Write five nursing diagnoses for a client who is depressed, including a long term goal and a short term goal for each.
5. Name three unrealistic expectations a nurse may have while working with a depressed person that can result in increased feelings of anxiety in the nurse.
6. Identify at least six principles of communication appropriate for a depressed client.
7. Name three interventions and rationales regarding the physical needs of depressed clients in each of the following categories: nutrition, elimination, rest and sleep, hygiene, and activities and recreation.
8. Discuss nursing considerations when administering the tricyclic antidepressants (TCAs), including (a) common side effects, (b) the serious side effects, and (c) the drugs that can trigger an adverse drug reaction.
9. Name (a) two common side effects of the monoamine oxidase inhibitors (MAOI) and (b) one serious adverse reaction and the appropriate medical intervention.
10. Identify five foods and four drugs contraindicated with the MAOIs.
11. Discuss the three atypical antidepressants, and name one indication for each.
12. Describe the procedure used in electroconvulsive therapy (ECT) and state the most important nursing action after an ECT treatment.

Depression, elation, anger, and anxiety are common examples of universally experienced alterations in mood. A **mood** is a "pervasive and sustained emotion that, in the extreme, markedly colors the person's perception of the world" (APA 1987).

A depressed mood is the most common presenting problem encountered by mental health professionals (Beck and Young 1985). A depressive illness is painful and can be debilitating. Many well-known and highly creative people have suffered from severe depressions, for example, Sigmund Freud, Winston Churchill, Ernest Hemingway, Marilyn Monroe, and Sylvia Plath.

A vivid and accurate example of the experience of depression is expressed by a client (Goldstein et al. 1980):

> When I get depressed, I feel like a drain and burden on my friends . . . the guilt and resentment are overwhelming. Everything I see, say or do seems extraordinarily flat and pointless; there is no color, there is no point of anything. Things drag on and on, intermittently. I am exhausted, dead inside. I want to sleep, to escape somehow, but if I really could sleep, I must again wake to the dullness and apathy of it all. I doubt completely my ability to do anything well; my mind has slowed down and burned out . . . it's virtually useless. The wretched thing works well enough to torment me with a dreary litany of my inaccuracies and to haunt me with the total desperate hopelessness of it all. What is the point of going on like this; it is crazy.

Most of us will experience a normal lowering of mood in response to various stressful life events. However, about 8–12% of males and 20–26% of females will experience a depressive episode during their lifetime (Cancro 1985). A depressive episode is one that usually warrants some kind of treatment.

When moods become severe or prolonged or affect a person's occupational or interpersonal functioning, the alteration in mood may constitute a mood disorder. The DSM III-R recognizes two categories of mood disorders: (1) depressive disorder and (2) bipolar disorder (see Fig. 18–1). This chapter covers the depressive disorder, and Chapter 19 covers the bipolar disorder.

A depressive illness can be precipitated by a variety of factors. For example, some environmental events are more likely than others to trigger the onset of depression. Death in the family is the first most common precipitator of depression. Second are separation and divorce. The third is physical illness followed by a sexual identity threat, work failures, and disappointment in a child (Goodwin 1982).

Depressive illnesses can occur in various *medical disorders*, such as hepatitis, mononucleosis, and multiple sclerosis.

A depressive syndrome may also accompany other *psychiatric disorders*, such as schizophrenia, psychoactive substance dependence disorder, or eating disorders.

The DSM III-R uses the terms *mood syndrome* and *mood episode* when discussing the mood disorders. A **mood syndrome** is an alteration of mood along with associated symptoms that occur for a minimal period of time. DSM III-R defines **depressive mood syndrome** as a "depressed mood or loss of interest, of at least two weeks' duration, accompanied by several associated symptoms, such as weight loss and difficulty concentrating" (APA 1987). A mood syndrome can occur as part of a physical illness, another psychiatric disorder, or as part of an organic mental disorder. When it does occur as part of an organic mental disorder or other nonmood psychiatric disorder, the depression is labeled **secondary depression.**

A **mood episode** (major depressive, manic, or hypomanic) is a mood syndrome that is *not due to* a known organic factor and is *not part of* another nonmood psychotic disorder, such as schizophrenia (APA 1987). Since these depressions are not secondary to any other process, mood episodes are labeled as **primary depressions.** Box 18–1 provides the DSM III-R diagnostic criteria for a major depressive episode.

There are two main primary depressive disorders: (1) major depression and (2) dysthymia (Fig. 18–2).

MAJOR DEPRESSION. In a major depression there is a history of one or more major depressive episodes (see Box 18–1), with no history of manic or hypomanic episodes. In a major depression, the symptoms often interfere with the person's social or occupational functioning and in some cases may include psychotic features. The emotional, cognitive, and behavioral symptoms an individual exhibits during a major depressive episode represent change in the person's usual functioning. When the symptoms of a major depressive episode have subsided, there is usually complete remission, and people return to their premorbid level of functioning (APA 1987).

DYSTHYMIA. Dysthymia (depressive neurosis) is mild to moderate in degree and characterized by a chronic depressive syndrome usually present for many years (Box 18–2). The depressive mood disturbance, because of its chronic nature, cannot be distinguished from the person's usual pattern of functioning (APA 1987). Since the individual has minimal social and occupational impairment, hospitalization is rarely necessary unless the person becomes suicidal. The age of onset varies from early and middle teens to late life. These clients are at risk for developing major depressive episodes as well as other psychiatric disorders (Hirschfeld and Goodwin 1988).

Identifying when a depression is a major depression or dysthymia can be difficult since both disorders share similar symptoms. The main difference is in duration and severity of the symptoms (APA 1987).

Another depressive pattern that has received recent attention is seasonal affective disorder (SAD).

SEASONAL AFFECTIVE DISORDER (SAD). It has been noted for centuries that depression and "hypomania or mania" appear to follow seasonal patterns. Today there is evidence to show that mania appears more frequently in the summer than at other times of the year (Hirschfeld and Goodwin 1988). Depression, on the other hand, seems to appear with a higher frequency in the winter (usually beginning in October and November) and is characterized by hypersomnia, fatigue, weight gain, irritability, and interpersonal difficulties (Hirschfeld and Goodwin 1988; Kaplan and Saddock 1988). The symptoms are atypical of depression

Box 18–1. DIAGNOSTIC CRITERIA FOR MAJOR DEPRESSIVE EPISODE

NOTE: A *Major Depressive Syndrome* is defined as criterion A below.

A. At least **five** of the following symptoms have been present during the same two-week period and represent a change from the previous functioning; at least one of the symptoms is either (1) depressed mood or (2) loss of interest or pleasure. (Do not include symptoms that are clearly due to a physical condition, mood-incongruent delusions or hallucinations, incoherence, or marked loosening of associations.)
   1. Depressed mood (or can be irritable mood in children and adolescents) most of the day, nearly every day, as indicated by either subjective account or observation by others
   2. Markedly diminished interest or pleasure in all, or almost all, activities most of the day, nearly every day (as indicated by either subjective account or observation by others of apathy most of the time)
   3. Significant weight loss or weight gain when not dieting (e.g., more than 5% of body weight in a month) or decrease or increase in appetite nearly every day (in children, consider failure to make expected weight gains)
   4. Insomnia or hypersomnia nearly every day
   5. Psychomotor agitation or retardation nearly every day (observable by others, not merely subjective feelings of restlessness or being slowed down)
   6. Fatigue or loss of energy nearly every day
   7. Feelings of worthlessness or excessive inappropriate guilt (which may be delusional) nearly every day (not merely self-reproach or guilt about being sick)

Continued

Box 18–1. DIAGNOSTIC CRITERIA FOR MAJOR DEPRESSIVE EPISODE *(Continued)*

8. Diminished ability to think or concentrate, or indecisiveness, nearly every day (by either subjective account or observation by others)
9. Recurrent thoughts of death (not just fear of dying), recurrent suicidal ideation without a specific plan, or a suicide attempt or a specific plan for suicide

B. 1. It cannot be established that an organic factor initiated and maintained the disturbance
2. The disturbance is not a normal reaction to the death of a loved one (uncomplicated bereavement)

NOTE: Morbid preoccupation with worthlessness, suicidal ideation, marked functional impairment or psychomotor retardation, or prolonged duration suggest bereavement complicated by major depression.

C. At no time during the disturbance have there been delusions or hallucinations for as long as two weeks in the absence of prominent mood symptoms (i.e., before the mood symptoms developed or after they have remitted)

D. Not superimposed on schizophrenia, schizophreniform disorder, delusional disorder, or psychotic disorder NOS (not otherwise specified)

Major Depressive Episode Codes: Fifth Digit Code Numbers and Criteria for Severity of Current State of Bipolar Disorder, Depressed, or Major Depression

1–Mild: Few, if any, symptoms in excess of those required to make the diagnosis, **and** symptoms result in only minor impairment in occupational functioning or in usual social activities or relationships with others

2–Moderate: Symptoms or functional impairment between "mild" and "severe."

3–Severe, Without Psychotic Features: Several symptoms in excess of those required to make the diagnosis, **and** symptoms markedly interfere with occupational functioning or with usual social activities or relationships with others

4–With Psychotic Features: Delusions or hallucinations. If possible, **specify** whether the psychotic features are *mood-congruent* or *mood-incongruent*

Mood-Congruent Psychotic Features: Delusions or hallucinations whose content is entirely consistent with the typical depressive themes of personal inadequacy, guilt, disease, death, nihilism, or deserved punishment

Mood-Incongruent Psychotic Features: Delusions or hallucinations whose content does *not* involve typical themes of personal inadequacy, guilt, disease, death, nihilism, or deserved punishment; included here are such symptoms as persecutory delusions (not directly related to depressive themes), thought insertion, thought broadcasting, and delusions of control

5–In Partial Remission: Intermediate between "in full remission" and "mild," **and** no previous dysthymia. (If major depressive episode was superimposed on dysthymia, the diagnosis of dysthymia alone is given once the full criteria for a major depressive episode are no longer met.)

6–In Full Remission: During the past six months no significant signs or symptoms of the disturbance

0–Unspecified

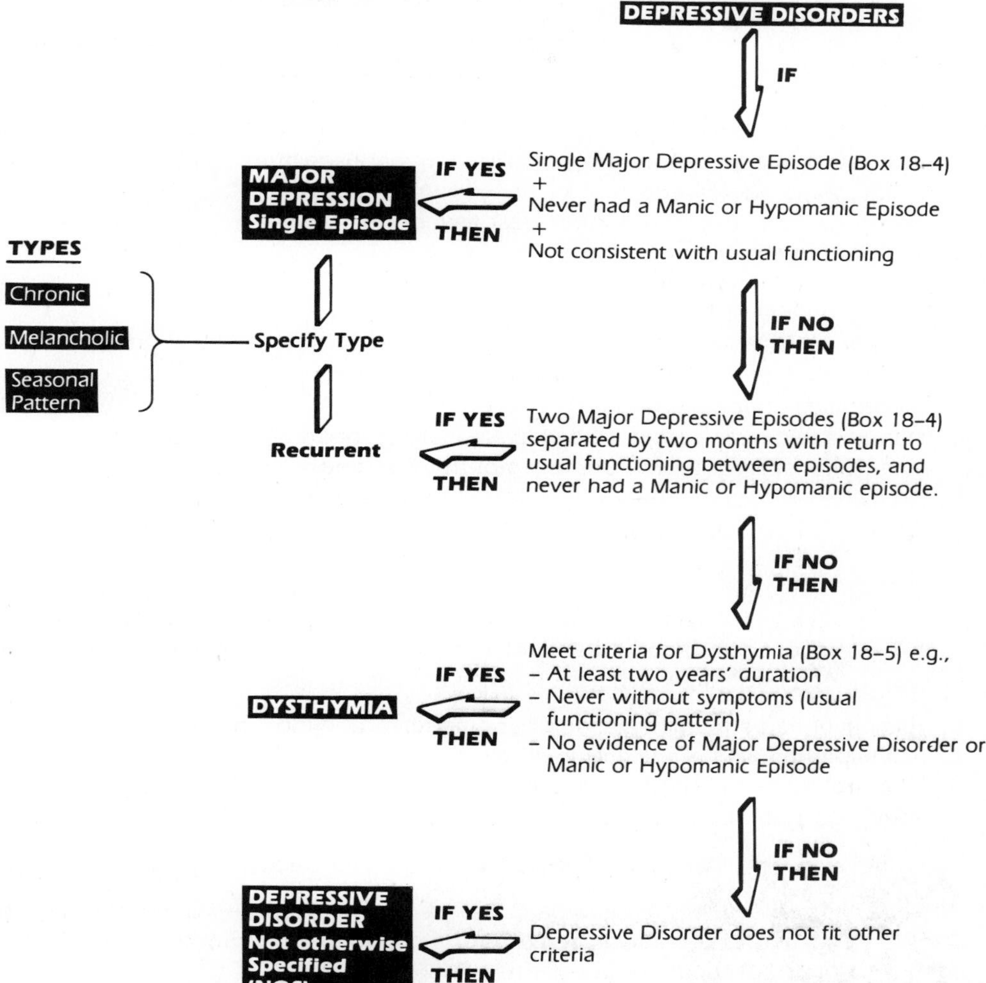

Figure 18–2. *Decision tree for depressive disorders.* (*Adapted from* Diagnostic and Statistical Manual of Mental Disorders (DSM III-R), *3d ed., revised.* Washington DC: American Psychiatric Association, 1987.)

and are more compatible with people who have a bipolar disorder. The syndrome of seasonal affective disorder (SAD) has only recently been studied. It appears to affect women mostly (80%) with a mean age of 40 (Kaplan and Saddock 1988). Interestingly, clients with SAD appear to respond to two to three hours of bright light a day (about 200 times brighter than usual indoor lighting). Clients report positive results after two to four days of treatment and also report a relapse two to four days after treatment is stopped.

Grief and the depressive line of disorders can be conceptualized as shown in Figure 18–3.

Standard I: Theory

Although there are many theories that attempt to explain the cause of depression, there are many psychological, biological, and cultural variables that make identification of any one cause difficult.

Four common theories of depression will be discussed: (1) *psychoanalytical*, (2) *cognitive*, (3) *learned helplessness*, and (4) *psychophysiological*.

PSYCHOANALYTICAL THEORY

Psychoanalytical theory emphasizes unconscious conflicts. Depression is thought to be the result of a harsh and punitive superego. Two themes central to the psychoanalytical theory of depression are *loss* and *aggression*. According to psychoanalytical theory, depression is triggered by a loss, and the depressive mood is the result of aggression turned inward toward the self.

LOSS. Freud identified both grief and depression as reactions to a loss, real or symbolic, in his classic *Mourning and Melancholia* (1917). When a person loses a crucial source of security, he or she may become depressed. The condition of depression is characterized by a sense

Box 18–2. DIAGNOSTIC CRITERIA FOR DYSTHYMIA

A. Depressed mood (or can be irritable mood in children and adolescents) for most of the day, more days than not, as indicated by either subjective account or observation by others, for **at least two years** (one year for children and adolescents)

B. Presence, while depressed, of at least **two** of the following:
   1. Poor appetite or overeating
   2. Insomnia or hypersomnia
   3. Low energy or fatigue
   4. Low self-esteem
   5. Poor concentration or difficulty making decisions
   6. Feelings of hopelessness

C. During a two-year period (one year for children and adolescents) of the disturbance, never without the symptoms of A for more than two months at a time

D. No evidence of an unequivocal major depressive episode during the first two years (one year for children and adolescents) of the disturbance

   NOTE: There have been many a previous major depressive episode, provided there was a full remission (no significant signs or symptoms for six months) before the development of dysthymia. In addition, after these two years (one year for children and adolescents) of dysthymia, there may be superimposed episodes of major depression, in which case both diagnoses are given.

E. Has never had a manic episode or an unequivocal hypomanic episode

F. Not superimposed on a chronic psychotic disorder, such as schizophrenia or delusional disorder

G. It cannot be established that an organic factor initiated and maintained the disturbance, e.g., prolonged administration of an antihypertensive medication

Specify Primary or Secondary Type

Primary Type: The mood disturbance is not related to a pre-existing, chronic, nonmood, Axis I, or Axis III disorder, e.g., anorexia nervosa, somatization disorder, a psychoactive substance dependence disorder, an anxiety disorder, or rheumatoid arthritis

Secondary Type: The mood disturbance is apparently related to a pre-existing, chronic, nonmood, Axis I, or Axis III disorder

Specify Early Onset or Late Onset

Early Onset: Onset of the disturbance before age 21

Late Onset: Onset of the disturbance at age 21 or later

of helplessness and hopelessness that is central to the experience of depression (White 1977).

When an infant between the ages of six months and 36 months experiences the physical or emotional loss of the mothering figure, the biological response is a depressive affect. The loss of mother's love can be a physical loss (death or divorce) or an emotional loss (withdrawal of affection because of depression, alcohol, or narcissism, for example) (Ripley 1977). The loss of the mother disrupts the normal development of the child. This early loss leaves the child extremely vulnerable to losses later in life. The young child interprets the withdrawal of affection (loss) as rejection of his or her self-worth and feels unworthy of love and approval. Numer-

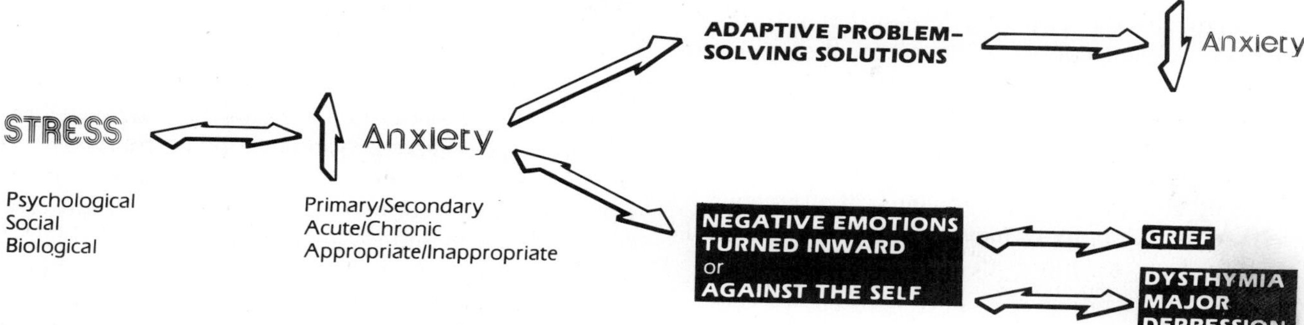

Figure 18–3. *Conceptualization of the process of grief and depression.*

ous studies support the relationship between early loss of a parent (death or divorce) and increased incidence and severity of depressive illness in an individual's later life (Ripley 1977; Bowlby 1961).

AGGRESSION. Psychoanalytical theory states depression is the result of anger turned inward against the self. The steps in the process of directing anger toward the self are outlined by Chapman (1976).

1. The child experiences emotional rejection and his needs for affection are not met.
2. The child feels hurt and unworthy of love; self-esteem is lowered.
3. Hostility is aroused toward those who have hurt and rejected him.
4. A state of ambivalence is experienced. The child needs and longs for love from the same people he rages against for not giving him love.
5. The need for acceptance and approval from the parents is so great that the child represses feelings of hostility.
6. Since these feelings of hostility could jeopardize receiving acceptance and approval from the parents, hostile feelings are pushed out of awareness and turned against the self to maintain acceptance and approval from the parents. Apathy and helplessness are experienced instead.
7. This pattern is set and continues throughout life. Hostility toward others is turned inward against the self in order to maintain acceptance and approval of others.

Measures aimed at promoting appropriate expressions of anger and activities planned to mobilize aggression are nursing interventions useful for many clients suffering from depression.

COGNITIVE THEORY

Albert Ellis, a well-known cognitive behavior therapist, views emotional disturbance as the product of irrational or illogical thinking. Ellis's rational emotive therapy (RET) has had success with people who are shy, nonassertive in social situations, experiencing marital problems, or have fears surrounding sexual situations. Expanding on Ellis's work, Aaron T. Beck applied the cognitive behavioral theory (CB) to depression. Beck proposed that illogical thinking and irrational beliefs are causative factors in the development of depression. Beck's cognitive triad of thinking believed to result in depression is as follows (1970):

1. Negative, self-depreciating view of self.
2. A pessimistic view of the world.
3. Belief that negative reinforcement or no validation for the self will continue in the future.

The goal of CB therapy is to change the way clients think and thus relieve the depressive syndrome. This is accomplished by assisting the client in the following (Gershon et al. 1983):

1. Identifying and testing negative cognitions.
2. Developing alternative thinking patterns.
3. Rehearsing new cognitive and new behavioral responses.

LEARNED HELPLESSNESS

One of the most popular theories in this category is Martin Seligman's theory of *learned helplessness*. Seligman (1973) states that although anxiety is the initial response to a stressful situation, anxiety is replaced by depression if the person feels that he or she has no control over the outcome of the situation. A person who believes that an undesired event is his or her fault and that nothing can be done to change it is prone to depression.

The theory of learned helplessness has been used to help explain the development of depression in certain social groups, such as the aged, the ghetto population, and women (Levitt 1983).

A study by Gulesserian and Warren (1987) found data that support this theory that "depression is linked with poor adaptational/coping abilities that may lead to learned helplessness, panic and depression." The lack of specific coping skills identified that appear to increase the likelihood of depression were the lack of social supports, tension-reduction skills, self-confidence, and effective problem-solving skills. The behavioral therapeutic approach includes teaching depressed individuals new and more effective coping skills.

PSYCHOPHYSIOLOGICAL THEORIES

Psychophysiological theories include (1) *genetic theories* and (2) *biochemical theories*.

GENETIC THEORIES. Twin studies provide evidence for the presence of genetic factors in the development of the depressive disorders. Studies of identical twins found that if one twin had a depressive disorder there was a 72% chance the other twin would also develop a depressive disorder. However, with fraternal twins, only 14% would be similarly affected (Allen 1976). There is also an increased incidence of mood disorders among relatives of people diagnosed with mood disorders (Goodwin and Guze 1984). Two studies support a possible "genetic marker" (human leukocyte antigen [HLA]) for transmission of mood disorders (Matthysse and Kidd 1981; Weitkamp et al. 1981). Although a genetic factor may not be exclusively responsible for the development of depression, studies bear out a genetic component in disorders of mood (Gershon et al. 1987).

BIOCHEMICAL RESEARCH. There is a great deal of research being done in the biochemical area. Specific neurotransmitters in the brain are believed to be related to altered mood states. The two main neurotransmitters are serotonin and norepinephrine, both catecholamines.

It is thought that low levels of serotonin and norepinephrine at the synaptic-receptor sites in the brain cause depression, and high levels trigger mania. Some drugs, like reserpine, can lower serotonin and norepinephrine levels in the brain. Such drugs are thought to be responsible for the depressive syndrome experienced by clients taking these drugs. The use of antidepressant drugs supports the biological theory of depression, since all antidepressant drugs inhibit the re-uptake of serotonin and norepinephrine, thereby increasing the amount of time these neurotransmitters are available to the postsynaptic receptor in the central nervous system.

Standard II: Data Collection

Although there is controversy regarding etiologies of depression, the symptoms of depression seem well accepted. Depressive reaction is generally characterized by dejection and sadness. Thinking is slow, and memory and concentration are usually affected. Depressed people dwell on and exaggerate their perceived faults and failures and are unable to focus on their strengths and successes. A person with major depression may experience delusions of being punished for "doing bad deeds" or "being a terrible person." Feelings of anxiety, worthlessness, guilt, anger, and helplessness are common. *Psychomotor agitation* may be evidenced by constant pacing and wringing of hands. The slowed movements of *psychomotor retardation*, however, are more common. Somatic complaints (headaches, malaise, backaches) are also common. *Vegetative signs* of depression (change in bowel movement and eating habits, sleep disturbances, and disinterest in sex) are usually present. An inability to find pleasure or meaning in any aspect of life **(anhedonia)** pervades the existence of a depressed person.

Although there are individual variations in depression, commonalities are revealed through the assessment of (1) affect, (2) thought processes, (3) feelings, (4) physical behavior, and (5) communication. Sometimes the symptoms of depression are not so obvious and are masked by other kinds of complaints. Therefore, (6) assessing symptoms that mask depression is useful in all hospital settings.

ASSESSING AFFECT

A person who is depressed sees the world through "gray-colored" glasses. Posture is poor; the client may look older than his or her stated age. Facial expressions reflect sadness and dejection, and the person may be given to frequent bouts of weeping. Feelings of hopelessness and despair are readily reflected in the person's affect.

ASSESSING THOUGHT PROCESSES

Identifying the presence of suicidal thoughts and suicide potential has the highest priority in the initial assessment. Asking a depressed person openly, "Have you thought about killing yourself?" can encourage the expression of painful pent-up feelings. (Refer to Chapter 22 for assessing risk factors and lethality of plan.) The risk of suicide is not necessarily correlated with the severity of the symptoms. Although depressed persons can attempt suicide at any time, the highest mortality occurs during the six- to nine-month period following improvement in depressive symptoms (Klerman 1978).

During the time a person is depressed, ability to solve problems and think clearly is negatively affected. Judgment is poor, and indecisiveness is common. People complain of their mind slowing down. Memory and concentration are poor. Evidence of delusional thinking may be seen in a major depression. Common examples of delusional thinking are, "I have committed unpardonable sins" or "God wants me dead" or "I am wicked and should die."

ASSESSING FEELINGS

Frequently reported feelings experienced by people when depressed include (1) anxiety, (2) worthlessness, (3) guilt, (4) helplessness and hopelessness, and (5) anger. Feelings of *anxiety* are present in 60–70% of people who are clinically depressed (Klerman 1978).

Feelings of *worthlessness* range from feeling inadequate to having an unrealistic evaluation of self-worth. These feelings reflect the low self-esteem that is a painful partner to depression. Such statements as, "I am no good; I'll never amount to anything," are frequently quoted sentiments. Themes of one's inadequacy and incompetence are repeated relentlessly.

Guilt is a common accompaniment to depression. Present or past failings are constantly belabored. Extreme guilt can take psychotic proportions, "I have committed such terrible sins, God is punishing me for my evil ways."

Helplessness is evidenced by the inability to carry out the simplest tasks. Everything is too difficult to accomplish (e.g., grooming, housework, job, caring for children). With feelings of helplessness come feelings of *hopelessness*. Even though most depressive states are usually time-limited, during a depressed period people believe things will never change. This feeling of utter hopelessness can lead people to look at suicide as a way out of constant mental pain. An analysis of the concept of hopelessness by Campbell (1987) cites findings in the literature that have identified hopelessness as one of the core characteristics of depression and suicide, as well as a characteristic of schizophrenia, alcoholism, sociopathy, and physical illness. Campbell (1987) identifies the common cognitive and emotional components of hopelessness defined in common usage as having the following attributes:

- Negative expectations for the future.
- Loss of control over future outcomes.
- Passive acceptance of the futility of planning to achieve goals.
- Emotional negativism as expressed in despair, despondency, or depression.

Anger and irritability are natural outcomes of profound feelings of helplessness (Drake 1975). Anger in depression is often expressed inappropriately. For example, anger may be expressed in destruction of property, hurtful verbal attacks, or physical aggression toward others. However, in people who are depressed, anger is directed most often toward the self, resulting in feelings of low self-esteem and worthlessness. An example of turning aggression against the self is suicide. Often the impulse to commit suicide is related to an impulse to murder someone else.

ASSESSING PHYSICAL BEHAVIOR

Complaints of lethargy and fatigue can result in **psychomotor retardation.** Movements are extremely slow, facial expressions are decreased, and gaze is fixed. The continuum in psychomotor retardation may range from slowed and difficult movements to complete inactivity and incontinence. At other times the nurse will note **psychomotor agitation.** For example, the clients may constantly pace, bite their nails, smoke, tap their fingers, or engage in some other tension-relieving activity. At these times, complaints of feeling "fidgety" and "unable to relax" are common.

Grooming, dress, and personal hygiene are markedly neglected. A person who usually takes pride in his or her appearance and dress may become sloppy, poorly groomed, and look shabby and unkempt.

Vegetative signs of depression are universal. Vegetative signs refer to alterations in those activities necessary to support the phenomenon of physical life and growth (eating, sleeping, elimination, and sex). For example, changes in *eating patterns* are common. Sixty to 70% of people who are depressed report anorexia. Overeating may occur in milder depressions. Changes in *sleep patterns* vary. Often people complain of insomnia, waking at 3:00 A.M. or 4:00 A.M. and staying awake or sleeping only for short periods. For some, sleep is increased **(hypersomnia)** and provides escape from painful feelings. In any event, sleep is rarely restful or refreshing. Changes in *bowel habits* are common. Constipation is seen most frequently in psychomotor retardation. Less frequently diarrhea may occur, often in conjunction with psychomotor agitation. *Interest in sex declines* (loss of libido) during depression. Some men may experience impotence, which can further complicate marital and social relationships.

ASSESSING COMMUNICATION

A person who is depressed speaks very slowly. Comprehension is slow. Often, it is not that a client does not hear or chooses not to reply when spoken to, he or she just needs more time to compose a reply. In extreme depression, however, a person may be mute.

ASSESSING INDICATIONS OF MASKED DEPRESSION

Masked depressions are depressions that are not recognized in the familiar form. The manner in which depression is masked is dependent upon (1) culture, (2) age and sex, (3) socioeconomic background, and (4) heredity (Lesse 1983).

In children, truancy, school phobias, underachievement, hyperactivity, learning disorders, and sociopathic behaviors may be the dominant characteristics of underlying depression. In adolescents, underachieving, dropping out of school, compulsive use of drugs and sex, delinquent behavior, and hostile outbursts may be masks for depression. Adults in the United States may mask depression behind hypochondriasis and psychosomatic disorders (Donlon 1982). The depressive mask may also take the form of compulsive gambling, compulsive work, or some behavior patterns. Behavior patterns associated with underlying depressions include accident proneness, eating disorders (anorexia, bulimia), or psychoactive substance dependence disorders (Lesse 1981).

Some adults who present with a masked depression have a characteristic personality profile (Lesse 1983). They are described as intelligent, capable, perfectionistic, hard working, and rigidly inflexible in everyday life. These personality characteristics are felt to be defenses against long-standing feelings of inferiority and inadequacy. Often parents of people who present with masked depressions are also very perfectionistic, obsessive compulsive, highly critical, and domineering (Lesse 1983).

The symptoms of depression are experienced by people on a continuum from mild-moderate to severe. Table 18–3 organizes the symptoms of depression on a continuum.

Standard III: Diagnosis

A high priority for the nurse during the initial assessment is to identify the presence of suicide potential. Therefore, the nursing diagnosis of *potential for self-directed violence* should always be considered. The diagnosis of potential for self-directed violence may be related to a pathophysiological condition (e.g., terminal illness) or treatment related (e.g., dialysis) or situational (e.g., divorce, child abuse) or related to a maturational issue (e.g., social isolation in the elderly). Suicide rates are high among adolescents, the elderly, and other specific populations. Potential for self-directed violence needs to be explored when data support this possibility. (See Chapter 22 for significant risk factors.)

Since concentration, judgment, and memory are usually poor, and psychotic behavior may be evidenced, *altered thought processes* is observed. Altered thought processes might be evidenced by such symptoms as inaccurate interpretation of stimuli, delusions, or memory deficits.

Feelings of worthlessness, guilt, helplessness, anger, and hopelessness all increase feelings of low self-esteem. Therefore, *disturbance in self-esteem, chronic low self-esteem*, or *powerlessness* is often present. For some, the feelings of hopelessness and despair may be viewed as *spiritual distress*, and spiritual distress may be the most appropriate diagnosis.

Many people experiencing a major depressive episode are withdrawn and demonstrate psychomotor retardation. In this case, the nurse may choose to focus care on *social interactions impaired* or *activity intolerance*.

Most depressed clients exhibit some of the vegetative signs of depression. When depression is severe, nursing and medical interventions are often warranted. For example, the nurse may identify *altered nutrition, constipation, diarrhea, and sleep disturbance*.

Since some clients may experience a disturbance in their ability to function in their usual occupational and interpersonal roles, *ineffective individual coping* related to poor self-esteem, helplessness, excessive negative beliefs about self, or lack of motivation to respond is possible. The nurse is often the first one to identify family problems through talking with family members, and *altered family processes* often surface. The nurse is in a key position to alert other members of the health team to support the family and mobilize additional supports (e.g., financial, psychological).

Standard IV: Planning

There are two levels of planning nursing care for a person who is depressed: the content level—planning long term and short term goals—and the process level—nurses' reactions and feelings.

Table 18-3 • DEPRESSION ON A CONTINUUM

MILD TO MODERATE	SEVERE
Communication	
Slow speech, long pauses before answering; monotone voice.	Slow in extreme—may be mute and not talk at all.
Affect	
Crying and weeping, slumped in chair, shoulders drooped, look of gloom and pessimism. Anxiety may or may not be manifested. **Anhedonia**—inability to experience pleasure.	May appear without affect—may be experiencing "nothingness"—can sit for hours staring into space.
Thinking	
No impairment in reality testing. Thinking slow, concentration and memory poor, interest narrows; loses perspective in situations, e.g., • "Everyone always lets me down." • "No one cares." Reflects doubts and indecisons. Thinking often repetitive in negative cycle, i.e., • "Why was I born; what's life all about" Mild feelings of guilt and worthlessness. **May have suicidal ideation.**	*Grasp of reality may be tenuous.* Thoughts may reflect *delusional thinking* reflecting feelings of • Low self-esteem • Worthlessness • Helplessness e.g., • "I'm no good." • "God is punishing me for my terrible sins." • "My insides are rotting." • "My heart has stopped beating." Concentration extremely poor. Severe feelings of guilt and low self-esteem. **May have suicidal ideation.**
Physical Behavior	
Fatigue and lethargy—hallmark symptoms. Does not prevent person from working, although often works below potential. Initiative and creativity are impaired.	Severe and extreme chronic fatigue and lethargy that markedly interfere with occupational functioning, social activities, or relationships with others.
Grooming and hygiene usually neglected.	Extreme neglect with personal grooming and hygiene.
Vegetative Signs	
Sleep—insomnia or hypersomnia nearly every day.	*Sleep*—usually insomnia; may have early morning waking at 3:00 or 4:00 A.M.
Energy often highest in A.M., *lowest in* P.M.	*Energy often lowest in* A.M., *highest* P.M.
Eating—may have anorexia or overeat.	*Eating*—usually has anorexia—weight loss of more than 5% in one month.
Bowels—Constipation if psychomotor retardation; may have diarrhea if psychomotor agitation.	*Bowels*—usually constipation.
Psychomotor Retardation (slow motor movements)—everything an effort or	*Psychomotor Retardation*—usually most common; may see
Psychomotor Agitation (agitated depression)—pacing up and down halls, wringing hands.	*Psychomotor Agitation*

Data from Chapman 1976; APA 1987; Swanson 1982.

CONTENT LEVEL—PLANNING GOALS

Long term and short term goals are formulated for each nursing diagnosis. Each client is different, and goals are devised according to each person's individual needs. Some, but not all, possible goals are presented.

When possible, the nurse and client discuss desired outcomes of hospital and health care interventions. The long range goals are identified, and concrete measurable steps are formulated as short term goals. For the following diagnoses, some long term goals and short term goals are presented.

For the nursing diagnosis *potential for self-directed violence*, as evidenced by suicidal ideation, the following are possible considerations:

Long Term Goals

- Client will remain safe while in hospital.
- By discharge, client will deny any suicidal thoughts or impulses.
- By (state the date) client will name three places/people he can turn to if suicidal thoughts or impulses arise in the future.

Short Term Goals

- Client will make suicide contract that he will talk to the nurse/therapist before harming self while in the hospital.
- Client will discuss with nurse feelings of anger and frustration by (state the date).
- By (state the date) client will explore with nurse thoughts, feelings, and circumstances that precede impulses to harm self.
- By (state the date) client will demonstrate two alternative actions he can take when experiencing impulses to harm self.
- Client will name two activities he is looking forward to participating in after discharge.

For the nursing diagnosis *altered thought processes*, the following goals might be considered:

Long Term Goals

- By discharge, client will state that her memory has improved.
- By discharge, client will demonstrate an increase in ability to make appropriate decisions regarding self.
- By discharge, client will accurately interpret events happening in the environment.
- By (state the date) client will state that she was able to participate in an activity that takes moderate concentration (reading, chess, Scrabble).

Short Term Goals

- Client will remember to keep appointments, attend activities, and attend to grooming with aid of medication and nursing interventions while in hospital.
- Client will make two decisions about future with aid of medications and nursing counseling by (state the date).
- Client will discuss with nurse irrational thoughts about self and others by (state the date).
- Client will demonstrate ability to concentrate on two five-minute activities (e.g., grooming, recreational) with the aid of medication and nursing interventions by (state the date).

Goals for a nursing diagnosis of *disturbance in self-esteem* should reflect an increase in the client's sense of self-worth. For example:

- By (state the date) client will name one/two/three things he likes about himself.
- Client will demonstrate an increased interest in personal appearance (grooming, hygiene, dress,) by (state the date).

Nursing diagnoses concerning *powerlessness* might include the following:

- By (state the date) client will discuss one new coping skill he has learned.
- By (state the date) client will name three alternative solutions to a particular problem.

Often when people feel hopeless and isolated, they are no longer able to find strength or sustenance from previous religious or spiritual beliefs. General goals for a person in *spiritual distress* are

- Client will state he once again finds strength and meaning in life through personal spiritual beliefs.
- Client will resume usual spiritual activities by (state the date).

Clients who are depressed are often withdrawn and unwilling or unable to participate in usual activities. General goals for *impaired social interaction* or *activity intolerance* may include the following:

Long Term Goals

- Client will interact freely with at least five other clients throughout the day by (state the date).
- Client will initiate attending two group activities a day by (state the date).

Short Term Goals

- By (state the date) client will discuss three alternative actions to take when he feels the need to withdraw.
- Client will participate in one activity with the nurse by the end of the day.
- Client will participate in two activities with other clients by the end of the week.
- By (state the date) client will identify two personal behaviors that might push others away.

Goals formulated for any of the vegetative signs of depression should be stated to show evidence of weight gain, return to normal bowel activity, sleeping six to eight hours per night, or increase in sexual desire.

For an individual whose work and interpersonal relationships had been negatively affected during the depressive episode, an ability to use previous adaptive coping skills would be a long range goal. For a family in which *altered family processes* have occurred, the long range goal would be resumption of previously satisfying and desired family coping styles.

PROCESS LEVEL—NURSES' REACTIONS AND FEELINGS

The depressed person has enormous needs for recognition and affection; however, he or she may be unable to acknowledge these needs. These intense needs for recognition and affection may be kept unconscious, since their recognition could bring up painful feelings of loneliness and rejection. One way a depressed person avoids recognition of painful feelings is by withdrawing. Withdrawal is a defense against perceived hurts and feelings of rejection. During this time, the client has a great need for communication and human company, even though there appears to be a lack of interest in either (Swanson 1978).

These clients often reject the overtures of the nurses, do not appear to respond to nursing interventions, and appear resistant to change. When this occurs, nurses can experience feelings of frustration, hopelessness, and annoyance. Nurses can alter these problematic responses by (1) recognizing any unrealistic expectations of self and client and (2) identifying feelings picked up by the nurse but originating in the client.

Unrealistic Expectations of Self

When they begin working in the hospital settings, many nurses have expectations of self and clients that may not be realistic. When these expectations of self and client are unrealistic, problems result when these expectations are not met. Unmet expectations usually result in anxiety, feeling hurt, angry, helpless, or incompetent. Many of the expectations the nurse has may not be conscious. However, when these expectations are made conscious and are worked through with peers and supervisors, more realistic expectations can be formed. Realistic expectations of one's self and one's client can decrease feelings of helplessness and increase the nurse's self esteem and therapeutic potential.

Unrealistic expectations are common, especially for nursing students and nurses new to the psychiatric setting. Common experiences and reactions are outlined in Table 18–4.

Identifying Feelings Picked up by the Nurse But Originating in the Client

Intense feelings of anxiety, frustration, annoyance, and helplessness may be experienced by the nurse but originate in the client. These feelings can be important diagnostic clues to the client's experience. Often the nurse senses what the client is feeling through empathy. Sometimes, the client has pushed these feelings out of awareness, and the feelings are manifested behaviorally in psychosomatic complaints, substance dependence, or destructive behaviors. Assisting clients to recognize these intense negative unconscious feelings is part of the therapeutic process moving toward healing the client.

When the nurse's feelings of annoyance, hopelessness, and anxiety are the result of empathetic communications with the client, the nurse can discuss these feelings with peers and supervisors in order to separate personal feelings from those originating in the client. If personal feelings are not separated out and examined, withdrawal by the nurse is likely to occur. People naturally stay away from situations and people that arouse feelings of frustration, annoyance, or intimidation. If the nurse is dealing with personal unresolved feelings of anger and depression, the complexity of the situation is bound to be compounded. There is no substitute for competent and supportive supervision to facilitate growth both professionally and personally. Supervision and sharing with peers helps minimize feelings of confusion, frustration, and isolation and can increase therapeutic potential and self-esteem in the nurse. The nurse is then free to intervene more directly with the client, and more direct communication can result in increased opportunities for the client to learn new coping skills.

Table 18–4 • POSSIBLE UNREALISTIC EXPECTATIONS

EXPECTATION	POSSIBLE RESULTS	POSSIBLE OUTCOMES
1. Nurse expects to feel needed and helpful to the client.	1a. Client does not respond, shows lack of interest.	1a. Nurse feels useless and ineffectual.
	1b. Client tells nurse to leave him alone and may show hostility.	1b. Nurse feels hurt. Avoids client to avoid arousing these feelings.
2. Nurse expects to form "therapeutic relationship" with the client.	2. Client acts aloof and cold.	2. Nurse feels rejected and may avoid feelings of rejection.
3. Nurse expects client to show signs of improvement after spending a lot of time with client.	3a. Client does not improve or slips back to being withdrawn and depressed.	3a. Nurse feels impatient and loses interest in such a "hopeless case."
	3b. Client shows contempt for nurse after nurse has worked with client.	3b. Nurse's self-esteem is lowered. Nurse interprets client's behavior as sign of personal incompetence.
	3c. Client's feelings of hopelessness and helplessness are picked up empathetically by the nurse.	3c. Nurse feels helpless and anxious around client. Withdraws from client to get away from feeling helpless. OR
		3d. Nurse becomes angry at client, "Why doesn't he shape up" or "Stop acting like a baby." Anger may also trigger withdrawal.

Data from Schwartz MS, Shockley EL. The Nurse and the Mental Patient: A Study in Interpersonal Relations. New York: John Wiley & Sons, 1956.

Standard V: Intervention

Shmagin and Pearlmutter (1977) alert nurses to the secondary gains a client may experience in depression. The **secondary gains** are those satisfactions the client derives from the depressive symptoms. As mentioned in Chapter 16, secondary gains may take the form of (1) escaping from responsibilities, (2) getting extra attention from others, or (3) exerting control through manipulation of others in the environment. Secondary gains can be extremely gratifying and provide rewards an individual was perhaps unable to obtain premorbidly. When the secondary rewards of depression meet previously unmet needs, they can serve to reinforce the symptoms of depression. Therefore, it is necessary for the nurse to minimize any secondary gains. The nurse assists clients in meeting unmet needs for attention and control in more appropriate and meaningful ways.

V-A: PSYCHOTHERAPEUTIC INTERVENTIONS

Nurses often have great difficulty communicating with a client without talking. However, some depressed clients are so withdrawn that they are unwilling or unable to speak. Just sitting with a client in silence may seem like a waste of time to the nurse. Often the nurse becomes uncomfortable not "doing something," and as anxiety increases, the nurse may start daydreaming, feel bored, remember something that "must be done now," and so forth. It is important to be aware that this time spent can be very meaningful to the depressed person, especially if the nurse has a genuine respect for people and interest in learning about the depressed individual.

Doris Chan, a senior nursing student, was working with a very depressed, withdrawn woman. The instructor noticed the second week that the student spent a lot of time talking with other students and their clients and little time with her own client. In supervision, Doris acknowledged feeling threatened and useless and said that she wanted a client who would interact with her. After reviewing the dynamics of depression, behavioral manifestations, and needs people have when they are depressed, Doris turned her attention back toward her client and spent time rethinking her plan of care. At the end of six weeks of sharing her feelings in post-conferences, working with her instructor, and trying a variety of approaches with her client, Doris was rewarded. On her last day, the client told Doris how important their time together was for the client. "I actually felt someone cared." The staff stated that up until this time, the client had not responded to anyone.

It is difficult to say when a withdrawn and depressed person is able and ready to respond. It is, however, known that certain techniques are useful in guiding effective nursing interventions. Some techniques of communication useful with a person who is depressed are listed in Table 18–5.

V-B: HEALTH TEACHING

It is important for both clients and their families to understand that depression is a legitimate medical illness over which the client has no voluntary control.

Depressed clients and families can greatly benefit from learning about the biological symptoms of depression, as well as the psychosocial and cognitive changes in depression (Jacob et al. 1987). Review of the medications, side effects, and toxic effects helps families evaluate clinical change and stay alert for reactions that might affect client compliance. Refer to V-D: *Somatic Therapies* for side effects of antidepressants.

When a client is leaving the hospital, predischarge counseling should be done with the client and his relatives. One purpose is to clarify the interpersonal stresses and steps that can alleviate tension for the family system. Predischarge counseling can be done by the psychiatrist, the psychiatric nurse clinician, or the psychiatric social worker.

Buckwalter and Abraham (1987) conducted a study involving predischarge nursing interventions with depressed clients and their families. Their findings suggest that including families in discharge planning can bring about the following results:

1. Increase family's satisfaction with the depressed family member during the after-care period.
2. Increase the client's use of after-care facilities in the community.
3. Contribute to a high overall adjustment score in the client three months after discharge.

Overall, the findings of the study indicated that the quality of social, family, and community readjustment was positively influenced.

V-C: ACTIVITIES OF DAILY LIVING

A depressed person presents many physical complaints. Since the depressed clients may view themselves as worthless, it is often up to the nurse to notice signs and symptoms of physical neglect. Nursing measures toward improving physical well-being and promoting adequate self-care are then initiated. Some effective interventions geared to physical needs are listed in Table 18–6.

V-D: SOMATIC THERAPIES

The nurse's main responsibility associated with somatic therapies involves (1) administering medications and (2) applying knowledge of electroconvulsive therapy when caring for a person who is depressed.

Psychopharmacology

Antidepressant drugs can *positively alter* poor self-concept, degree of withdrawal, the vegetative signs of depression, and activity level. However, one main drawback is that the client may have to take antidepressant agents from one to three weeks before noticing improvement. There are two major classifications of antidepressant drugs: (1) the tricyclics (TCAs) and (2) the monoamine oxidase inhibitors (MAOI). More recently, newer, non-traditional antidepressants have been made available, and these drugs are discussed under *Atypical Antidepressants*.

TRICYCLICS (TCAs). The tricyclic antidepressants (TCAs) inhibit the re-uptake of norepinephrine and serotonin by the presynaptic neurons in the central nervous system (Scherer 1985). Therefore, the amount of time that norepinephrine is available to the postsynaptic receptor is increased. This increase in norepinephrine in the brain is thought by many to be responsible for mood elevations when tricyclics are given to depressed persons.

About 70% of people diagnosed as having acute depressive disorder respond favorably to the tricyclic antidepressants (Donlon 1982). The tricyclics seem to be the most effective with severe agitated and retarded depressions with or without psychotic features (major depression). The tricyclics are less effective in depressions caused by traumatic life events or in a person whose depression is an inherent part of his or her personality, as in dysthymia (Beeber 1984).

Currently, a person who has had a positive response to tricyclic therapy will likely be maintained on that medication from six to 12 months in order to prevent an early relapse. some clients may continue to receive favorable results on lower doses after three to four months on the higher dose. If depressive symptoms do re-emerge, the higher dose of the TCA is reordered (Schatzberg and Cole 1986).

The most commonly used tricyclic antidepressants are amitriptyline hydrochloride (Elavil) and imipramine hydrochloride (Tofranil). These and other commonly

Table 18–5 • COMMUNICATION WITH A DEPRESSED CLIENT

INTERVENTION	RATIONALE
1. Spend short periods of time (5–10 minutes) frequently throughout the day.	1. Frequent short periods minimize anxiety for both nurse and client.
2. Let client know beforehand when, and for how long, the visits will be.	2. Clear expectations minimize anxiety. Scheduled times bring structure and purpose to empty periods of time.
3. Be on time and stay the full time contracted, even when the client does not acknowledge the nurse's presence.	3. Consistency and reliability lay the foundations for trust. The client experiences attention without "having to earn it." When the nurse does not come on time or stay the stated time, a depressed person may personalize the experience, "I'm not worthy of attention."
4. When the client is not speaking, sit with the person in silence for short periods.	4. Even if the client does not acknowledge you, he knows you are there. Your presence and interest over time can reinforce that you view him or her as worthwhile.
5. When a client is mute, make observations of happenings in the environment, "There are many new pictures on the wall" or "You are wearing your new shoes."	5. When a person is not ready to talk, direct questions can raise the client's anxiety and frustrate the nurse. Pointing to commonalities in the environment draws the client into and reinforces reality.
6. Use simple, concrete words.	6. Slowed thinking and difficulty concentrating impair comprehension.
7. Allow time for client to respond.	7. Slowed thinking necessitates time to formulate a response.
8. Listen and ask about suicidal plans.	8. People often experience relief and a decrease in feelings of isolation when sharing thoughts of suicide.
9. Spend time listening and sharing feelings.	9. Feeling understood can help diminish feelings of loneliness and isolation and facilitates sharing painful feelings necessary for healing.
10. *Avoid* laughing, joking, and "acting cheerful."	10. The nurse's cheerful attitude increases feelings of alienation and isolation in the client by contrasting the nurse's "up" feelings with the client's own feelings of low worth.
11. *Avoid* platitudes, such as "Things will look up" "Everyone gets down once in awhile."	11. This tends to minimize client's feelings and can increase feelings of guilt and worthlessness, since he cannot "look up" or "snap out of it."
12. Accept expressions of anger without becoming defensive. Work at not taking anger personally when expressed by the client.	12. Arguing or self-righteous responses serve to diminish both the client's and the nurse's self-esteem.
13. Encourage the client's verbalization of anger.	13. Sharing difficult feelings can minimize the need to act them out in inappropriate ways.
14. If client's anger is justified, admit an error was made.	14. Encourage appropriate expressions of anger and validate that it is all right to have angry feelings.
15. Avoid use of value judgments:	15. When depressed, a person sees the negative side of everything, for example:
"You look nice this morning."	Can be interpreted as "I didn't look nice yesterday morning."
"I like the way you did your hair."	Can be thought of as being done to please the nurse, "If I do my hair another way, maybe he/she will not like it."
Better to say, "You are wearing a new dress this morning" and "You've changed your hair style."	Neutral comments avoid negative interpretations.

Table 18–6 • PHYSICAL NEEDS OF THE DEPRESSED CLIENT

INTERVENTION	RATIONALE
Nutrition (When Anorexic)	
1. Offer small high-caloric and protein snacks frequently throughout the day and evening.	1. Low weight and poor nutrition render the client susceptible to illness. Small frequent snacks are more easily tolerated than large plates of food when one is anorexic.
2. Offer high-protein and high-caloric fluids frequently throughout the day and evening.	2. Prevents dehydration; can minimize constipation.
3. When possible, remain with the client during meals.	3. Reinforces the idea that someone cares, can raise self-esteem, and can serve as an incentive to eat.
4. Ask client which foods/drinks he or she likes. Offer choices. Involve dietitian.	4. Provide foods client is more likely to eat.
5. Weigh weekly and observe eating patterns.	5. Monitor status—signals needed for revising intervention.
Elimination	
1. Monitor intake and output; especially bowel movements.	1. Many depressed clients are constipated. If this condition is not checked, fecal impaction can occur.
2. Offer foods high in fiber and provide periods of exercise.	2. Roughage and exercise stimulate peristalsis and help evacuation of fecal material.
3. Encourage intake of fluids.	3. Helps prevent constipation.
4. Evaluate need for laxatives and enemas.	4. Prevent occurrence of fecal impaction.
Rest and Sleep	
1. Provide rest periods after activities.	1. Fatigue can intensify the feelings of depression.
2. Encourage client to get up and dress and stay out of bed during the day.	2. To minimize sleep during the day and increase likelihood of sleep at night.
3. Provide relaxation measures in the evening (e.g., backrub, tepid bath, warm milk).	3. To induce relaxation and sleep.
4. Reduce environmental and physical stimulants in the evening—provide decaffeinated coffee, soft lights, soft music, and quiet activities.	4. Decrease caffeine and epinephrine levels in order to increase the possibility of sleep.
5. Spend time with client before bedtime.	5. Help allay anxiety and increase feelings of security.
Hygiene	
1. Encourage the use of and provide toothbrush, washcloth, soap, make-up, shaving equipment, and so forth.	1. Being clean and well groomed can temporarily raise self-esteem.
2. Give step-by-step reminders, ie, "Wash the right side of your face, now the left . . . "	2. Slowed thinking and difficulty concentrating make organizing simple tasks difficult.
Physical Activities and Recreation	
1. While the client is most severely depressed, one-to-one activities are appropriate.	1. Since concentration is impaired, maximizes potential for interacting and may minimize anxiety levels.
2. Activities involving gross motor activity calling for minimal concentration are best, i.e., taking a walk, making beds with nurse, setting up chairs, and so forth.	2. Physical activities are thought to help temporarily mobilize aggression and relieve tension.
3. Provide activities that require very little concentration, (e.g., simple card games, looking through a magazine, drawing, playing with clay).	3. Concentration and memory are poor in depression. Activities that have no "right" or "wrong" minimize opportunities for client to put him- or herself down.
4. Eventually, bring client into contact with one other person and then into a group of three.	4. Distracts client from self preoccupations and provides opportunity for spending more time with people and activities that are based in reality.

Table continued on following page

Table 18–6 • PHYSICAL NEEDS OF THE DEPRESSED CLIENT *Continued*

INTERVENTION	RATIONALE
Physical Activities and Recreation *Continued*	
5. Eventually, involve client in group activities (e.g., dance therapy, art therapy, group discussions).	5. Socialization can decrease feelings of isolation. Genuine regard from others can increase feelings of self-worth.
6. In *psychomotor agitation*, providing activities that involve use of hands and gross motor movements is helpful (e.g., Ping-Pong, volley ball, finger painting, drawing, working with clay).	6. Gives client more appropriate discharge of motor tension than pacing and wringing hands.

administered tricyclic antidepressants (TCAs) are listed in Table 18–7.

Common Side Effects. The chemical structure of the tricyclics is similar to that of the antipsychotic medications. Therefore, the *anticholinergic* actions are similar (e.g., dry mouth, blurred vision, tachycardia, postural hypotension, constipation, urinary retention, and esophageal reflux). These side effects are both more common and more severe in clients taking antidepressants. Most of these side effects are not serious and are often transitory, but **urinary retention and severe constipation warrant immediate medical attention.**

The administration of the total daily doses of tricyclics at night is beneficial for two reasons. *First*, most tricyclics produce sedative effects, thereby aiding sleep. *Second*, the minor side effects occur during sleep, thereby increasing compliance with the drug therapy. Therefore, the client experiences fewer side effects during his or her waking hours (Hart et al. 1981).

Serious Side Effects. The most serious side effects of the tricyclics are cardiovascular. Arrhythmias, tachycardia, myocardial infarction, and heart block have been reported (Scherer 1985). Since the cardiac side effects are so serious, these agents are considered a risk in clients with cardiac disease and in the elderly. Clients to be started on the TCA antidepressants should have a thorough cardiac workup before beginning TCA therapy.

Adverse Drug Interactions. Individuals taking tricyclics can have adverse reactions to a number of other medications. For example, use of a MAOI along with a tricyclic is often contraindicated. A few of the more common medications usually *not* given while the tricyclics are being administered are listed in Table 18–8. Any client who is taking any of those medications along with the tricyclics should have medical clearance, since some of the reactions can be fatal (Donlon 1982).

MISUSE OF ANTIDEPRESSANT DRUGS. Antidepressants may cause a psychotic episode in a person with schizophrenia. Also, an antidepressant alone can cause a manic episode in a bipolar client. Depressed bipolar clients should receive lithium along with the antidepressant.

Careful suicide assessment should be made with all depressed clients (see Chapter 22). A fatal dose of antidepressant medications is 10 to 15 times the prescribed daily dose. It is suggested that only a week's supply of *any* antidepressant should be given to a severely depressed person (Lickey and Gordon 1983).

MONOAMINE OXIDASE INHIBITORS (MAOI). The

Table 18–7 • COMMONLY ADMINISTERED TRICYCLIC ANTIDEPRESSANT DRUGS

TRADE NAME	GENERIC NAME	USUAL THERAPEUTIC DOSAGE RANGE (mg/day)*
Elavil	amitriptyline hydrochloride	150–300
Tofranil	imipramine hydrochloride	150–300
Sinequan	doxepin hydrochloride	150–300
Norpramin	desipramine hydrochloride	150–300
Aventyl/Pamelor	nortriptyline hydrochloride	50–150
Vivactil	protriptyline hydrochloride	15–60
Asendin	amoxapine	150–450
Ludiomil	maprotiline	150–200

* These dosage ranges are approximate. Some clients need higher doses; others respond to lower doses. The physician usually starts with relatively low doses, which can be increased slowly.

Table 18–8 • DRUGS USED WITH CAUTION WHEN TAKING A TRICYCLIC DRUG (TCA)

DRUG	TYPE OF INTERACTION
Phenothiazines	↑ Plasma levels of TCA; may enhance cardiotoxic effects; ↑ anticholinergic effects or hypotensive effects
Alcohol	Addictive sedative effects
Barbiturates	↓ Plasma levels of TCA
Cigarette smoking	↓ Plasma levels of TCA
MAOIs	↑ Incidence of weight gain; hyperthermia; hyperreflexia, convulsions; or death (very rare)
Disulfiram	↑ Plasma levels of TCA
Oral contraceptives (or other estrogen preparations)	↓ Plasma levels of TCA
Anticoagulants	↑ Serum levels of TCA and prolongs prothrombin times
Some antihypertensives (clonidine, guanethidine, reserpine)	Reversal of hypotensive effects
Benzodiazepines	Reduced side effects in low dose combination; enhanced toxicity in overdose

Data from Blackwell B, Schmidt GL. Drug interactions in psychopharmacology. Psychiatric Clinics of North America, 7(3):625, 1984.
↑ = increased; ↓ = decreased

monoamine oxidase inhibitors (MAOI) are not as widely used as the tricyclics, since they have dangerous side effects. The most serious side effect of this drug is high blood pressure. For that reason, the MAO inhibitors are usually contraindicated for people who are debilitated, elderly, or hypertensive or who have cardiac or cerebrovascular disease or severe renal and hepatic disease (Donlon 1982; Hart et al. 1981; Lickey and Gordon 1983). The MAOIs are usually given when the tricyclics prove ineffective. Presently the MAOIs are also being tried with "atypical" depressions. Depressions that respond well to MAO inhibitors are characterized by pananxiety, phobias, panic attacks, hypochondriasis, and dysphoria (Beeber 1984). The most common MAOIs are isocarboxazid (Marplan), phenelzine sulfate (Nardil), and tranylcypromine sulfate (Parnate).

The MAOIs, like the tricyclics, block the re-uptake of norepinephrine and serotonin in the central nervous system. However, MAO is also responsible for the metabolism of tyramine. Therefore, a person taking a MAO inhibitor will be unable to metabolize tyramine. High levels of tyramine in the blood can cause high blood pressure, leading to hypertensive crisis, or stroke. Certain foods containing high tyramine levels are contraindicated for people taking MAO inhibitors. The MAO inhibitors also interact with a variety of drugs, as well as certain foods and beverages, to produce potentially dangerous increases in blood pressure. Table 18–9 lists foods and drugs not permitted or restricted with the monoamine oxidase inhibitors.

Even a clear-thinking person can have difficulty in restaurants and in the homes of friends keeping the list of "forbidden foods" constantly in mind. It is easy to understand why prescribing the MAOIs for someone who is having cognitive difficulty with memory and concentration could be risky.

Common Side Effects. Some common and troublesome side effects reported are orthostatic hypotension, weight gain, change in cardiac rate and rhythm, constipation, urinary hesitancy, vertigo, overactivity, muscle twitching, hypomanic and manic behavior, insomnia, weakness, and fatigue (Scherer 1985; Schatzberg and Cole 1986).

Adverse Reactions. The most serious reactions involve an increase in blood pressure, with the possible development of intracranial hemorrhage, hyperpexia, convulsions, coma, and death. Therefore, routine monitoring of blood pressure, especially during the first six weeks of treatment, is advised.

Since so many other drugs, foods, and beverages can have adverse reactions to the MAOIs, increase in blood pressure is a constant concern. The beginning of a hypertensive crisis occurs usually within a few hours after ingestion of the contraindicated substance. The crisis may begin with headaches, stiff or sore neck, palpitations, increase or decrease in heart rate often associated with chest pain, nausea and vomiting, and/or increase in temperature (pyrexia). When a hypertensive crisis is suspected, immediate medical attention is warranted. Antihypertensive medications, such as phen-

Table 18–9 • MONOAMINE OXIDASE INHIBITOR (MAOI) RESTRICTIONS

TYPE	EXAMPLE
Food Restrictions	
High Tyramine—Not Permitted	
Aged, matured cheeses	Cheddar, Camembert, Stilton, blue, Swiss
Smoked or pickled meats, fish, poultry	Herring, sausage, corned beef
Aged meats, fish, poultry	Chicken or beef liver paté
Yeast or meat extracts	Brewer's yeast, "Bouil," marmite (check labels in drinks, stews, soups)
Red wines	Chianti, burgundy, sherry, vermouth
Italian broad beans	Fava beans
Moderate Tyramine—Limited Amount Allowed	
Meat extracts	Bouillon, consommé
Pasteurized, light, pale beers	
Ripe avocado	
Low Tyramine—Permitted	
Distilled spirits *in moderation*	Vodka, gin, scotch, rye
Cheese	Cottage cheese, cream cheese
Beverages containing chocolate and caffeine	
Fruits	Bananas, figs, raisins, grapes, pineapple, oranges
Yogurt, sour cream	
Soy sauce	
Drug Incompatibilities	
Stimulants	Amphetamines, cocaine
Decongestants	Any product containing ephedrine, phenylephrine hydrochloride, or phenylpropanolamine hydrochloride
Tricyclics	TCAs
Narcotics	
Antihypertensives	Methyldopa, guanethidine, reserpine
Amine precursors	L-dopa, L-tryptophan
Sedatives	Alcohol, barbiturates, benzodiazepines
General anesthetics	

From Murphy DL, Sunderland T, Cohen RM. Monoamine oxidase inhibiting antidepressants. Psychiatric Clinics of North America, 7(3):555, 1984.

tolamine (Regitine), are administered slowly intravenously, and pyrexia is treated with hypothermia blankets or ice packs (Scherer 1985).

Some people do not respond to the MAOIs or the TCAs. For others side effects with either group prohibit use of either of these drugs. Therefore, the search for more effective drug therapy continues. Some newer atypical antidepressants are in current use and are proving effective in relieving depression.

ATYPICAL ANTIDEPRESSANTS. The atypical antidepressant drugs that will be introduced here are trazodone hydrochloride (Desyrel), bupropion hydrochloride (Wellbutrin), and fluoxetine hydrochloride (Prozac). These new antidepressant drugs are neither tricyclics nor monoamine oxidase inhibitors. The new antidepressant drugs have a lesser incidence of anticholinergic side effects, less cardiotoxicity, and a faster onset of action than the tricyclics (Karb et al. 1989).

Trazodone Hydrochloride (Desyrel). Trazodone hydrochloride has been found effective in outpatients with mild to moderate depression and anxiety, especially those depressed individuals who have difficulty falling asleep (Schatzberg and Cole 1986). The main side effects of this drug appear to be sedation, acute dizziness and fainting (particularly if taken on an empty stomach), and priapism. *Priapism* is persistent erection of the penis due to organic causes, not sexual desire. This condition is serious and may require surgical intervention. If not treated within a few hours, priapism can result in impotence (Schatzberg and Cole 1986). The dosage starts at 150 mg daily in divided doses and is increased by 50 mg daily until a therapeutic dose is reached. The maximum dose for outpatients is 400 mg. Usually the maintenance dose is approximately 150 to 300 mg per day.

Bupropion Hydrochloride (Wellbutrin). Bupropion hydrochloride appears to be effective in clients who are depressed, but *not* in those with panic-related disorders. Bupropion has a favorable side-effect profile, although nausea can occur in some clients. Rarely, seizures have occurred (Schatzberg and Cole 1986). The recommended daily dose is 75 to 600 mg (Karb et al. 1989).

Fluoxetine Hydrochloride (Prozac). Fluoxetine hydrochloride has been found effective in treating major depressions. Fluoxetine has a much more favorable side-effect profile than that of the tricyclic antidepressant drugs. Its major side effects include nausea, tremor, drowsiness, headache, and nervousness. This drug does seem to facilitate weight loss and does *not* potentiate seizures in humans. The drug is started at 20 mg per day and can be increased gradually to 40 mg or 60 mg per day. The maximum recommended daily dose is 80 mg per day, with many clients responding at dosages of 60 mg per day or less (Schatzberg and Cole 1986).

Electroconvulsive Therapy (ECT)

There are three main indications for electroconvulsive therapy (ECT). *First*, it is indicated when antidepressant drugs have no effect. Fifty percent of people who do not respond to antidepressant medication will respond to ECT (Major 1984). *Second*, it is indicated for acutely suicidal clients. The usual one- to three-week period before a person begins to experience a decrease in depressive symptoms from antidepressants is too long a period to risk for such a client. *Third*, it is indicated for depressed persons experiencing psychotic symptoms.

ECT is not particularly useful in those depressions associated with stress (Chapman 1976; Freedman and Kaplan 1976; Lickey and Gordon 1983). Chapman (1976) states ECT should never be employed in treating any conditions except some severely depressed clients and a small percentage of schizophrenic (catatonic) and manic clients.

The usual course of ECT is from six to 12 treatments; the average, eight to ten. ECT is often contraindicated for clients with cardiac problems, since a very small number of cardiac arrests have been reported. ECT is also contraindicated for clients with brain tumors.

The procedure is explained to the client, and an informed consent must be obtained when treating voluntary clients. For an involuntary client, when an informed consent cannot be obtained, it is possible to obtain permission from next of kin (Major 1984).

The client is NPO after midnight or at least four hours before treatment is to take place. Vital signs are taken, and the client is requested to void. Hairpins, contact lenses, and dentures are removed. Atropine is usually given to reduce tracheobronchial secretions.

The client is positioned on a padded table, and a short-acting sedative is given intravenously—usually methohexital sodium (Brevital) or thiopental (Pentothal)—to induce a short sleep. Succinylcholine chloride (Anectine), a muscle relaxant, is then administered intravenously to prevent tonic-clonic seizures when the electrical current is passed through the cortex. The reduction of tonic-clonic seizures reduces fractures to the cervical spine and long bones. Fractures used to be a serious side effect of ECT before the administration of Anectine became popular. However, Anectine also produces paralysis of the respiratory muscles, which necessitates the administration of 100% oxygen, usually by an anesthesiologist. The electrical shock passes through electrodes placed on either side of the client's skull bilaterally or on one side (unilaterally). The treatment lasts about two to three minutes, and the client may sleep from 20 to 30 minutes after the treatment is over.

The major side effect people complain of with bilateral treatments is confusion and memory loss following treatments. Upon awakening, the client will be confused and disoriented. The nurse needs to orient the client frequently, "Mr. Taylor, you are in Mercy Hospital. It's 9:00 A.M., and I will take you back to your room, where you will have breakfast." The client will have to be oriented frequently during the course of the treatments. Many people state that they have had memory deficits for the first few weeks before and after the course of treatment. Memory usually recovers completely. ECT is not a permanent cure for depression, and maintenance treatment with tricyclics or lithium decreases the relapse rate to about 20% (Lickey and Gordon 1983).

V-E: THERAPEUTIC ENVIRONMENT

When a person is severely depressed, hospitalization is usually indicated. The depressed person will need protection from suicidal acts, a supervised environment for regulating antidepressant medications, and when indicated, a course of ECT. Often being removed from a stressful interpersonal situation in itself has therapeutic value. Most hospitals have protocols regarding care and protection of the suicidal client. Chapter 22 covers the nurse's responsibilities in providing a safe therapeutic environment against self-inflicted harm.

V-F: PSYCHOTHERAPY

A number of treatment modalities have been applied in the treatment of depression. Studies demonstrate that traditional psychotherapies are only slightly more effective than placebos in reducing depressive symptoms (Hollon and Beck 1978; Beck and Young 1985).

Most recently there has been an increased emphasis on *short term therapies*. Those therapies that have received the most attention in outcome research include behavior therapy, interpersonal psychotherapy, brief psychodynamic therapy, and cognitive therapy (Beck and Young 1985; Bergin and Lambert 1978).

The *cognitive therapy* of Beck has been gaining momentum. The use of specific cognitive interventions meets with promising success in individual therapy with depressed persons. Covi and colleagues (1982) propose that group therapy utilizing Beck's cognitive therapy approach can be of great value in the treatment of depressed individuals.

The use of *behavior therapy* has also gained some recognition for success in the treatment of depression. Behavior therapists attempt to teach depressed people effective coping skills that will increase positive reinforcements from other people and the environment.

The cognitive-behavioral approaches to therapy are thought to be at least as effective as the tricyclic antidepressants, although pharmacology remains the standard against which all other treatments are compared (Beck and Young 1985). The National Institute for Mental Health (NIMH) has done research showing that drug therapy and psychotherapy in combination are more effective than either treatment alone (Lickey and Gordon 1983).

Group treatment can be an important modality for the treatment of depression. One study demonstrated how, through the use of group therapy, women diagnosed as depressed increased self-esteem, gained reassurance, and achieved a stronger sense of identity (van Servellan and Dull 1981). The treatment of people in groups provides for an increase in the number of people who can receive treatment at decreased individual cost.

Standard VI: Evaluation

Frequent evaluation of the short term and long term goals is made. For example, if the client comes into the unit with suicidal thoughts, the nurse evaluates whether suicidal thoughts are still present, whether the depressed person is able to state alternatives to suicidal impulses in the future, whether he or she is able to explore thoughts and feelings that precede suicidal impulses, and so forth. Goals relating to thought processes, self-esteem, and social interactions are frequently formulated, since these are areas often problematic in people who are depressed. Physical needs often warrant nursing or medical attention. If a person has lost weight because of anorexia, is appetite returning? If a person was constipated, are bowels now functioning normally? If the person was suffering from insomnia, is he or she now getting six to eight hours of sleep per night?

If goals have not been met, an analysis of the data, nursing diagnoses, goals, and planned nursing interventions is made. The care plan is reassessed and reformulated when necessary.

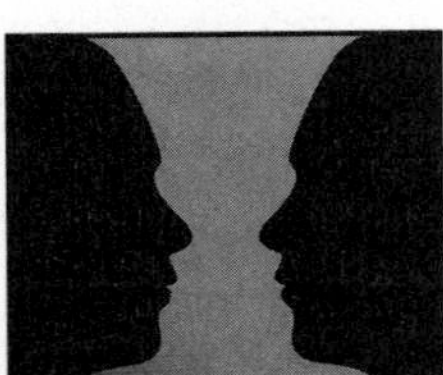

Case Study: Working With a Person Who Is Depressed

June Olston is a 35-year-old executive secretary. She has been divorced for three years and has two sons, 11 and 13 years old. She was brought into the emergency room (ER) by her neighbor. She had tried to kill herself by turning on the gas. The neighbor stated that both of June's sons were visiting their father for the summer. June had become more and more despondent after terminating a two-year relationship with a married man four weeks earlier. According to the neighbor, for three years after her divorce, June constantly talked about not being pretty or "good enough" and doubted that anyone could really love her. The neighbor stated that June had been withdrawn for at least three years. After the relationship with her boyfriend ended, June became even more withdrawn and sullen. June was about twenty pounds overweight, and her neighbors stated that June often stayed awake late into the night, drinking by herself and watching TV. She would sleep through most of the day. For the past four weeks, June's care of the children had become erratic, and often her sons would go to the neighbors for meals and to spend time.

After receiving treatment in the emergency room, June was seen by a psychiatrist. The initial diagnosis was dysthymia with suicidal ideation. A decision was made to hospitalize June for suicide observation and for evaluation for appropriate treatment.

The nurse, Ms. Weston, admitted June to the unit from the emergency room.

NURSE:	Hello Mrs. Olston, I'm Marcia Weston. I will be your primary nurse.
MRS. OLSTON:	Yeah . . . I don't need a nurse, a doctor, or anyone else. I just want to die.
NURSE:	You want to die?
MRS. OLSTON:	I just said that didn't I? Oh, what's the use. No one understands.
NURSE:	I would like to understand, Mrs. Olston.
MRS. OLSTON:	Look at me. I'm fat . . . ugly . . . and no good to anyone. No one wants me anyway.
NURSE:	Who doesn't want you?
MRS. OLSTON:	My husband didn't want me . . . and now Jerry left me to go back to his wife.
NURSE:	You think that because Jerry went back to his wife that no one else could care for you?
MRS. OLSTON:	Well . . . he doesn't anyway.
NURSE:	Because he doesn't care, you believe that no one else cares about you?
MRS. OLSTON:	Yes . . .
NURSE:	Who do you care about?
MRS. OLSTON:	No one . . . except my sons . . . I do love my sons even though I don't often show it.
NURSE:	Tell me more about your sons.

The nurse continues to speak with Mrs. Olston. Mrs. Olston talks about her sons with more affect and apparent affection; however, she continues to state that she does not think of herself as worthwhile and that she wants to die.

Assessment

The nurse divides the data into objective and subjective components.

OBJECTIVE DATA

1. Tried to kill herself by inhaling gas fumes
2. Recently broke off with boyfriend
3. Has thought poorly of herself three years since divorce
4. Has two sons she cares about
5. Twenty pounds overweight
7. Stays awake late at night drinking by herself
8. Sleeps into the day
9. Withdrawn since divorce

SUBJECTIVE DATA

1. "No one could ever love me."
2. "I'm not good enough."
3. "I just want to die."
4. "I'm fat and ugly . . . no good to anyone."
5. "I do love my sons, although I don't always show it."

Continued on following page

Nursing Diagnosis

The nurse evaluated Mrs. Olston's strengths and weaknesses. The nurse decided to concentrate on two initial nursing diagnoses that seemed to have the highest priority.

1. *Potential for Self-Directed Violence* related to separation from two-year relationship, as evidenced by actual suicide attempt
   - Tried to kill self by inhaling gas fumes
   - Recently broke off with boyfriend
   - Drinks at night by herself
   - Withdrawn for three years since divorce
2. *Disturbance in Self-Esteem* related to divorce and recent termination of love relationship, as evidenced by derogatory statements about self
   - "I'm not good enough."
   - "No one could ever love me."
   - "I'm fat and ugly . . . no good to anyone."
   - Works as an executive secretary
   - "I do love my sons, although I don't always show it."

Planning

CONTENT LEVEL—PLANNING GOALS

Because Mrs. Olston was acutely suicidal, she was put on suicide precautions (see Chapter 22 for suicide precaution protocol). The nurse discussed with Mrs. Olston possible goals related to issues of self-esteem. Although initially Mrs. Olston was very negative about herself, she was able to discuss with the nurse some of her strengths and identify some thoughts, feelings, and behaviors she would like to change about herself. The nurse devised the following long term and short term goals with some input from Mrs. Olston:

Nursing Diagnosis	Long Term Goals	Short Term Goals
1. *Potential for Self-Directed Violence* related to separation from two-year relationship, as evidenced by actual suicide attempt	Client will remain safe while in the hospital.	1a. Client will state she has a reason to live by (state the date). 1b. Client will state two alternative actions she can take when feeling suicidal in the future.
2. *Disturbance in Self-Esteem* related to divorce and recent termination of love relationship, as evidenced by derogatory statements about self	By discharge, client will name two things she likes about herself.	2. By (state the date) client will name two things she would like to change about herself.

PROCESS LEVEL—NURSES' REACTIONS AND FEELINGS

Ms. Weston is aware that when clients are depressed, they can be very negative, think life is hopeless, and at times be hostile toward those who want to help. At first, when Ms. Weston was new to the unit, she withdrew from depressed clients and sought out clients who appeared more hopeful and appreciative of her efforts. The unit coordinator had been very supportive of Ms. Weston when she was first on the unit. Ms. Weston, along with other staff, were sent to inservice education regarding working with depressed clients, and she was encouraged to speak up in staff meetings about the feelings many of these depressed clients evoked in her. As a primary nurse, she was now assigned a variety of clients. She found that as time went on, and with the support of her peers and speaking up at staff meetings, she was able to take less personally what the client said and not feel so responsible when clients did not respond as fast as she would like. After two years she had had the experience of seeing many clients who seemed hopeless and despondent upon admission respond well to nursing and medical interventions and go on to lead full and satisfying lives. This also made it easier for Ms. Weston to understand that, even though the client may think life is hopeless and believe there is nothing in his or her life to live for, change is always indeed possible.

Intervention

Mrs. Olston was put on 24-hour suicide precautions for the first three days. She appeared to respond positively to the attention from the nurses, as well as from some of the other clients on the unit. She told the nurse that since her divorce, she had become more withdrawn and had stopped socializing with others and participating in her usual outside activities. Her married boyfriend never took her out, and together they did not share any social activities. Just being around people who seemed interested in her made her feel better.

Her therapist on the unit used a variety of cognitive therapy approaches with Mrs. Olston. She was encouraged to look at her life and herself differently and evaluate her strengths and those things she valued. The therapist assisted Mrs. Olston in questioning and changing inaccurate thoughts and beliefs she held toward herself and her future. The therapist assisted Mrs. Olston in learning new behaviors to cope with her loneliness, lack of motivation, and negative thinking.

Ms. Weston, the nurse, worked closely with Mrs. Olston's therapist, and together they discussed ways to reinforce what Mrs. Olston was learning in therapy.

For example, the nurse together with Mrs. Olston scheduled activities throughout the day, including short rest periods. A record of these activities would be kept by the client and discussed with the therapist. The nurse also role played with Mrs. Olston some of the new behaviors being taught Mrs. Olston in her therapy sessions. Refer to Mrs. Olston's nursing care plan (Nursing Care Plan 18–1).

Evaluation

At the end of three days, Mrs. Olston was no longer thought to be suicidal. At the end of the week, she was much less withdrawn and sought out people on the unit and readily participated in activities. By discharge, she stated she was anxious to see her children and admitted to missing them terribly when they spent the whole summer away with their father. She was to continue her therapy session once discharged and had decided to go to some meetings of Parents Without Partners. She stated she was looking forward to getting back to work and felt much more hopeful about her life. She had also lost three pounds while in the hospital and was going to attend Weight Watchers once discharged, stating, "I need to get back into the world."

Although Mrs. Olston still had negative thoughts about herself, she admitted to feeling much better about herself. She was no longer suicidal and stated she was ready to resume previous activities and seeing old friends.

Nursing Care Plan 18–1 • A PERSON WITH DEPRESSION: Mrs. Olston

NURSING DIAGNOSIS

Potential for self-directed violence related to separation from two-year relationship, as evidenced by actual suicide attempt

Supporting Data

- Tried to kill self by inhaling gas fumes.
- Recently broke off with boyfriend.
- Withdrawn for three years since divorce.
- Drinks at night by herself.
- "I just want to die."

Continued on following page

Nursing Care Plan 18–1 • A PERSON WITH DEPRESSION: Mrs. Olston *(Continued)*

Long Term Goal: Client will remain safe while in hospital.

Short Term Goal	*Intervention*	*Rationale*	*Evaluation*
1. Client will state she has a reason to live by (state the date).	1a. Staff to observe client every 15 minutes while she is suicidal.	1a–b. Ensure client safety. Minimize impulsive self-harmful behavior.	1. *Goal met.* By end of second day, Mrs. Olston broke down in tears saying how much she loved and missed her children.
	1b. Remove all dangerous objects from client.		
	1c. Spend regularly scheduled periods of time with client throughout the day.	1c. Reinforces that she is worthwhile; builds up experience to begin to better relate to nurse on a one-to-one basis.	
	1d. Assist client in evaluating the positive as well as the negative aspects of her life.	1d. A depressed person is often unable to acknowledge any positive aspects of her life unless they are pointed out by others.	
	1e. Encourage expression of angry feelings in appropriate manner.	1e. Providing for expression of pent-up hostility in safe environment can reinforce more adaptive methods of releasing tension and may minimize need to act out self-directed anger.	
	1f. Accept client in her negativism.	1f. Acceptance enhances feelings of self-worth.	
2. Client will state two alternative actions she can take when feeling suicidal in the future.	2a. Explore usual coping behaviors.	2a. Identify those behaviors that need reinforcing and new coping skills that need to be introduced.	2. *Goal met.* By discharge, Mrs. Olston stated that she was definitely going to continue her cognitive-behavior therapy.
	2b. Assist client in identifying members of her support system.	2b. Evaluate strengths and weaknesses in support available.	She also discussed joining a women's support group that meets once a week in a neighboring town.
	2c. Suggest a number of community based support groups she might wish to discuss or visit (e.g., hotlines, support groups, women's groups, and so forth).	2c. Clients need to be aware of community supports in order to use them.	
	2d. Assist client in problem solving realistic alternatives that she is willing to use.	2d. Unless client is in agreement with any plan, she will be unable or unwilling to follow through in a crisis.	

NURSING DIAGNOSIS

Disturbance in self-esteem related to divorce and recent termination of love relationship, as evidenced by derogatory statements about self

Supporting Data

- "I'm not good enough.
- "No one could ever love me."
- "I'm fat and ugly . . . no good to anyone."
- "I do love my sons, although I don't always show it."

Long Term Goal: By discharge, client will name two things she likes about herself.

Short Term Goal	*Intervention*	*Rationale*	*Evaluation*
1. By (state the date) client will name two things she would like to change about herself.	1a. Assist client to identify two realistic things about herself that she would like to change.	1a. Help client to problem-solve two important areas of her life that are amenable change.	1. *Goal met.* By end of first week, client stated she (1) wanted to lose weight and (2) wanted to get back to being with some of her friends she had stopped seeing.
	1b. Work with the client to identify the various steps needed to help make these changes come about.	1b. Depressed clients often have difficulty problem solving owing to poor concentration and faulty judgment.	
	1c. Identify specific skills the client might need to attain goals, e.g., • assertiveness training • more effective communication skills • tension-reducing activities.	1c. Identifying and teaching more effective coping skills can increase perception of control and decrease feelings of hopelessness.	
	1d. Work with therapist to reinforce skills taught in therapy.	1d. Aids health team to monitor client progress and reinforce positive coping skills.	
	1e. Role play new coping skills with client.	1e. Aids in incorporating new skills into more automatic behavior.	
	1f. Encourage participation in group activities.	1f. Increase arena in which client can gain positive reinforcement.	
	1g. Assist client in planning a structured daily routine.	1g. Reduces time spent in negative rumination and helps client in thinking more in terms of goal directedness.	
2. Client will identify personal strengths by (state the date).	2a. Have client list those things she has been told are her strong points.	2a. A depressed person is often unable to see positive aspects in self but is able to identify others' perceptions.	2. By discharge, client was able to admit that (1) even when depressed, she was considered the best secretary in the office, and (2) with the exception of the past few weeks, she prides herself on being a good mother to her sons.
	2b. Discuss with client those positive qualities she most admires in herself.	2b. Helps client integrate positive aspects of self.	
	2c. Encourage client to give nurse examples of when client demonstrates these strengths.	2c. Helps to reinforce other more positive aspects of self and abilities.	

Summary — Depressive Disorders

Primary and secondary depression is probably the most common mental disorder seen in the health care system. The two *primary* depressive disorders are major depression and dysthymia. The symptoms in a *major depression* are usually severe enough to interfere with a person's social or occupational functioning. A person in a major depression may or may not have psychotic symptoms, and the symptoms a person usually exhibits during a major depression are very different from his or her normal premorbid personality.

In *dysthymia*, the symptoms are often chronic in nature (lasting two or more years) and are considered mild to moderate. Usually a person's social or occupational functioning is not greatly impaired. The symptoms in a dysthymic depression are often congruent with the person's usual pattern of functioning.

There are a number of theories regarding the etiology of depression. Four common theories include (1) psychoanalytical theory, (2) cognitive theory, (3) learned helplessness theory, and (4) psychophysiological theory.

Nursing assessment includes assessment of (1) affect, (2) thought processes. (3) feelings, (4) physical behavior, and (5) communication. The nurse also needs to be aware of (6) the symptoms that mask depression.

Nursing diagnoses can be numerous. Evaluation for *potential for self-directed violence* is always done with depressed individuals. Some other common nursing diagnoses are *altered thought processes, disturbance in self-esteem, altered nutrition, bowel elimination, sleep pattern disturbance, ineffective individual coping,* and *ineffective family coping.*

When planning care, the nurse sets measurable and individualized goals for each nursing diagnosis. Working with people who are depressed can evoke intense feelings of hopelessness and frustration in health care workers. Initially, nurses need support and guidance to clarify realistic expectations of self and client and sort out personal feelings from those communicated by the client via empathy. Peer supervision and individual supervision with an experienced nurse clinician/psychiatric social worker or psychologist is useful in increasing therapeutic potential.

Interventions with clients who are depressed involve a number of approaches. The nurse intervenes therapeutically, using specific principles of communications, planning activities of daily living, administering or participating in somatic therapies, and maintaining a therapeutic environment.

Evaluation is ongoing throughout the nursing process, and the client's outcomes are compared with the stated short term and long term goals. Revision of the care plan is done throughout the client's hospital stay by use of the evaluation process.

Self-study exercises 22 through 56 will help the student review the material covered in this section.

References

Allen MG. Twin studies of affective illness. Archives of General Psychiatry, 33:1476, 1976.

American Psychiatric Association. Diagnostic and Statistical Manual of Mental Disorders, 3rd ed., revised. Washington DC: American Psychiatric Association, 1987.

Arieti S. Affective disorders: Manic-depressive psychosis and psychotic depression. *In* Arieti S (ed). American Handbook of Psychiatry, 2nd ed. New York: Basic Books, 1974.

Beck A. The Diagnosis and Management of Depression. Philadelphia: University of Pennsylvania Press, 1967.

Beck AT. The core problem in depression: The cognitive triad. *In* Masseman J (ed). Depression: Theories and Therapies. New York: Grune & Stratton, 1970.

Beck AT, Young JE. Depression. *In* Barlow DH (ed). Clinical Handbook of Psychological Disorders. New York: The Guilford Press, 1985.

Beck MC, Rawlins RP, Williams SR. Mental Health Psychiatric Nursing: A Holistic Life Cycle Approach. St. Louis: C.V. Mosby Company, 1984.

Beeber LS. Antidepressant medications. *In* Lego S (ed). The American Handbook of Psychiatric Nursing. Philadelphia: J.B. Lippincott Company, 1984.

Benton RG. Death and Dying: Principles and Practices in Patient Care. New York: Van Nostrand Company, 1978.

Bergersen BS. Pharmacology in Nursing. St. Louis: C.V. Mosby Company, 1979.

Bergin AE, Lambert MJ. The evaluation of therapeutic outcomes. *In* Garfield SI, Bergin AE (eds). Handbook of Psychotherapy and Behavior Change: An Empirical Analysis, 2nd ed. New York: John Wiley & Sons, 1978.

Bowlby J. Separation anxiety: A critical review of the literature. Journal of Child Psychology and Psychiatry, 1:251, 1961.

Bowlby J, Parkes C. Separation and loss within the family. *In* Anthony E, Koupenik C (eds). New York: John Wiley & Sons, 1970.

Buckwalter KC, Abraham II. Alleviating the discharge crisis: The effects of cognitive-behavioral nursing intervention for depressed patients and their families. Archives of Psychiatric Nursing, 1(5):350, 1987.

Bunney WE, Murphy DL, Goodwin FK, Borge GF. The switch process from depression to mania: Relationship to drugs which alter brain amines. Lancet, 1:1022, 1970.

Campbell L. Hopelessness. Journal of Psychosocial Nursing, 25(2):18, 1987.

Cancro R. Overview of affective disorders. *In* Kaplan HI, Saddock BJ (eds). Comprehensive Textbook of Psychiatry, 2nd ed. Baltimore: Williams & Wilkins Company, 1985.

Carr AL. Grief, mourning, and bereavement. *In* Kaplan HI, Saddock BJ (eds). Comprehensive Textbook of Psychiatry, (4th ed). Baltimore: Williams & Wilkins, 1985.

Chapman AH. Textbook of Clinical Psychiatry, 2nd ed. Philadelphia: J.B. Lippincott Company, 1976.

Corfman E. Depression, manic depressive illness and biological rhythms. Rockville, MD: U.S. Department of Health and Human Services, National Institute of Mental Health, 1979.

Covi L, Roth D, Lipman RS. Cognitive group therapy of depression: The close-ended group. American Journal of Psychotherapy, 36:459, 1982.

Crary WG, Crary GC. Depression. American Journal of Nursing, 73:472, 1973.

Davison GC, Neale JM. Abnormal Psychology: An Experimental Clinical Approach, 3rd ed. New York: John Wiley & Sons, 1982.

DeGennaro MD, Hymen R, Crannell AM, Mansky PA. Antidepressant drug therapy. American Journal of Nursing, 83:1305, 1981.

Dempsey D. The way we die: An investigation of death and dying in America today. New York: MacMillan Company, 1975.

Donlon PT, Rockwell DA. Psychiatric Disorders, Diagnosis and Treatment. Bowie, MD: Robert J. Brady Company, 1982.

Drake RE, Price JL. Depression: Adaptation to disruption and loss. Perspectives in Psychiatric Care, 13:163, 1975.

Engel GL. Grief and grieving. American Journal of Nursing, 64:93, 1964.

Fitzgerald RG, Long I. Seclusion in the treatment and management of disturbed manic and depressed patients. Perspectives in Psychiatric Care, 11:59, 1973.

Freedman AM, Kaplan HI, Saddock BJ. Modern Synopsis of Comprehensive Textbook of Psychiatry, 2nd ed. Baltimore: Williams & Wilkins Company, 1976.

Gershon ES, Berretini WH, Nurnberger JI Jr, et al. The genetics of affective illness. *In* Meltzer HY (ed). Psychopharmacology: The Third Generation of Progress. New York: Raven Press, 1987.

Gershon ES, Nurnberger JI, Berretini WH, Goldin LR. Affective disorders: Genetics. *In* Kaplan HI, Saddock BJ (eds). Comprehensive Textbook of Psychiatry, 2nd ed. Baltimore: Williams & Wilkins Company, 1985.

Gitlin MJ, Jamison KR. Lithium clinics: Theory and practice. Hospital and Community Psychiatry, 35:363, 1984.

Goldstein MJ, Baker BL, Jamison KR. Abnormal Psychology: Experiences, Origins and Interventions. Boston: Little Brown & Company, 1980.

Goodwin DW, Guze SB. Psychiatric Diagnosis. New York: Oxford University Press, 1984.

Goodwin FK. Depression and manic-depressive illness. Bethesda, MD: U.S. Department of Health and Human Services, National Institute of Mental Health, 1982.
Gulesserian B, Warren CJ. Coping resources of depressed patients. Archives of Psychiatric Nursing, 1(6):392, 1987.
Guze SB, Robins E. Suicide and primary affective disorders. British Journal of Psychiatry 117:437, 1970.
Harris E. Lithium. American Journal of Nursing, 81:1310, 1981.
Hart CA, Turner MS, Orfitelli MK, Applebaum B. Introduction to Psychotropic Drugs. New York: Medical Examination Publishing Company, 1981.
Hinsie LE, Campbell RJ. Psychiatric Dictionary, 4th ed. New York: Oxford University Press, 1973.
Hirschfeld RMA, Goodwin FK. Mood disorders. *In* Talbott JA, Hales RE, Yudofsky SC (eds). Textbook of Psychiatry. Washington DC: American Psychiatric Press, 1988.
Hirschfeld RMA, Shea MT. Affective disorders: Psychosocial treatment. *In* Kaplan HI, Saddock BJ (eds). Comprehensive Textbook of Psychiatry, 2nd ed. Baltimore: Williams & Wilkins Company, 1985.
Hollon SD, Beck AT. Psychotherapy and drug therapy: Comparison and combination. *In* Garfield SI, Bergin AE (eds). Handbook of Psychotherapy and Behavior Change: An Empirical Analysis, 2nd ed. New York: John Wiley & Sons, 1978.
Jackson EN. Understanding Grief: Its Roots, Dynamics and Treatment. Nashville: Abingdon, 1957.
Jacob M, Frank E, Kupfer DJ, Cornes C, Carpenter L. A psychoeducational workshop for depressed patients, family and friends: Description and evaluation. Hospital and Community Psychiatry, 38(9):968, 1987.
Jacobs LI. Cognitive therapy of postmanic and post depressive dysphoria in bipolar illness. American Journal of Psychotherapy, 36:450, 1982.
Kaplan HI, Saddock BJ. Synopsis of Psychiatry: Behavioral Sciences and Clinical Psychiatry, 5th ed. Baltimore: Williams & Wilkins, 1988.
Karb VB, Queener SF, Freeman JB. Handbook of Drugs for Nursing Practice. St. Louis: C.V. Mosby Company, 1989.
Klerman GL. Affective disorders. *In* Nicholi AM Jr. (ed). The Harvard Guide to Modern Psychiatry. Cambridge, MA: Belknap Press of Harvard University Press, 1978.
Lesse S. The masked depression syndrome—Results of a seventeen year clinical study. American Journal of Psychotherapy, 37:456, 1983.
Lesse S. The relationship of anxiety to depression. American Journal of Psychotherapy, 36:332, 1982.
Lesse S. Unmasking the masks of depression. New Jersey: Carrier Foundation Letter, Number 74, 1981.
Levitt E, Lubin B, Brooks JM. Depression Concepts, Controversies and Some New Facts, 2nd ed. New York: Lawrence Erlbaum Associates, 1983.
Lickey ME, Gordon B. Drugs for Mental Illness: A Revolution in Psychiatry. New York: W.H. Freeman & Company, 1983.
Lindemann E. Symptomatology and management of acute grief. American Journal of Psychiatry, 101:141, 1944.
Major LF. Electroconvulsive therapy in the 1980's. Psychiatric Clinics of North America, 7(3):613, 1984.
Marks MJ. The grieving patient and family. American Journal of Nursing, 76:1488, 1976.
Matthysse S, Kidd KK. Evidence of HLA linkage in depressive disorders. New England Journal of Medicine, 305:1340, 1981.
McCoy SM, Garritson S. Seclusion, the process of intervening. Journal of Psychosocial Nursing and Mental Health Services, 21:8, 1983.
Mendelson M. Psychoanalytic Concepts of Depression, 2nd ed. New York: Books Division of Spectrum Publications, 1974.
Merck Manual, 14th ed. New Jersey: Merck & Company, 1982.
Parios R, Taylor CM. Electroconvulsive treatment. *In* Lego S (ed). The American Handbook of Psychiatric Nursing. Philadelphia: J.B. Lippincott Company, 1984.
Parkes CM. Bereavement: Studies of Grief in Adult Life. New York: International Universities Press, 1972.
Pilkonis PA, Frank E. Personality pathology in recurrent depression: Nature, prevalence, and relationship to response. American Journal of Psychiatry, 145(4):435, 1988.
Poznanski EO. The clinical phenomenology of childhood depression. American Journal of Orthopsychiatry, 52: 1982.
Rakoff VM. Psychiatric aspects of death in America. *In* Mack A (ed). Death in American Experience. New York: Schocken Books, 1973.
Rees WD, Lutkins S. Morality of bereavement. British Medical Journal, 23:31, 1967.
Ripley HS. Depression and the life span epidemiology. *In* Usdin D (ed). Depression Clinical, Biological and Psychological Perspectives. New York: Brunner/Mazel, 1977.
Schatzberg AF, Cole JO. Manual of Clinical Psychopharmacology. Washington DC: American Psychiatric Press, 1986.
Scherer JS. Lippincott's Nurses' Drug Manual. Philadelphia: J.B. Lippincott, 1985.
Schultz JM, Dark SL. Manual of Psychiatric Nursing Care Plans. Boston: Little, Brown & Company, 1982.
Schwartz MS, Shockley EL. The Nurse and the Mental Patient: A Study in Interpersonal Relationships. New York: John Wiley & Sons, 1956.
Seligman ME. Fall into hopelessness. Psychology Today, 7:43, 1973.
Seligman MEP, Abramson LV, Semmell A, Baeyer C. Depressive attributal style. Journal of Abnormal Psychology, 88:242, 1979.
Shmagin BG, Pearlmutter DR. The pursuit of unhappiness, the secondary gains of depression. Perspectives in Psychiatric Care, 15:63, 1977.
Swanson AR. Communicating with depressed persons. *In* Backer BA, Dubbert PM, Eisenman EJP (eds). Psychiatric/Mental Health Nursing: Contemporary Readings. New York: Van Nostrand Company, 1978.
Swanson AR. Depression. *In* Haber J, et al. (eds). Comprehensive Psychiatric Nursing, 2nd ed. New York: McGraw-Hill Book Company, 1982.
van Servellan GM, Dull LV. Group psychotherapy for depressed women: A model. Journal of Psychosocial Nursing and Mental Health Services, 19:25, 1981.
Warheit GJ. Life events, coping, stress, and depressive symptomatology. American Journal of Psychiatry, 136 (4B):502, 1979.
Weitkamp LR, Stancer HC, Persad E, Flood C, Guttormsen S. Depressive disorders and HLA: A gene on chromosome 6 that can affect behavior. New England Journal of Medicine, 305:1301, 1981.
White B, et al. Psychodynamics of depression: Implications for treatment. *In* Usdin D (ed). Depression: Clinical, Biological and Psychological Perspectives, New York: Brunner/Mazel, 1977.
Whitlock FA. Symptomatic Affective Disorders. New York: Academic Press, 1982.

Self-Study Exercises

GRIEF

Identify the phase of grief (shock, developing awareness, restitution) occurring in the acute stage of mourning.

1. ________ A person begins to feel intense feelings of anguish and despair. Anger, guilt and crying are common at this phase.
2. ________ A person gathers together with family and friends in rituals of saying good bye and ending the last remnants of denial.
3. ________ A person is not capable of emotionally accepting the intense feelings of pain and may have difficulty accepting the fact of death or intellectualizing feelings instead of feeling them.

True or False

4. ________ Completing the work of mourning takes four to eight weeks.
5. ________ Being with a person who is grieving can bring up one's own feelings of loss and sadness.
6. ________ Nurses have no difficulties dealing with people who are grieving and dying, since they are around death so often.

The following are examples of the normal phenomena experienced during the mourning process. Match the example from the left column with the expected phenomena from the right column.

7. ________ "If his brother had not been so hard on him, he would not have had the heart attack."
8. ________ "There were so many things I wanted to tell him . . . how much he meant to me . . . I should have said more kind things."
9. ________ "It sounds silly, but I am having difficulty swallowing, just the way John did before he died."
10. ________ "I just can't do anything . . . everything is so confusing. I don't even feel like eating or dressing."
11. ________ "Thoughts and memories just keep popping into my head . . . everything I see or do reminds me of the things we used to do together, everything."
12. ________ "I am thinking of resuming typing lessons . . . last night was the first night in a long time that I went to Bingo at church."

A. Sensations of somatic distress
B. Preoccupation with the deceased
C. Guilt
D. Anger
E. Disorganization and depression
F. Reorganization behavior

Put S (successful) or U (unsuccessful) for the evaluation of the work of mourning.

13. ________ "She was so strong. Why, I don't even think she cried the whole time—went through the whole process with a 'stiff upper lip.'"

14. ________ "She was a wreck when her sister died. Cried and carried on . . . why, it took her a year or more before she returned to church duties with any zest and started doing things again."
15. ________ "You know, Sid still talks about his mother as if she were alive today—weeps every time he talks about her. Well . . . she's been dead for four years."
16. ________ "I remember the good times we had together, but we had our rough times too before she died."

Multiple Choice

17. Regina, a 24-year-old woman whose mother has just died a painful death from cancer, tells the nurse tearfully she does not think she will ever get over her mother's death. *Which of the following would be the most appropriate response for the nurse to make:*

    A. "Time heals all wounds, and yours will heal in time also."
    B. "It was the best thing that could happen to her; she was in so much pain."
    C. "The loss must be very painful for you."
    D. "The hardest part will be the next couple of months. In a year you will feel fine again."

18. Three of the following are factors that could interfere with Regina's successful resolution of the grief process. Choose the one factor that would NOT negatively affect the mourning process.

    A. Regina said she loved her mother, but so often their relationship was stormy, and at other times she stated she hated her mother.
    B. Regina had lost her job two months before, and she and her husband had recently separated.
    C. Regina had always been a good problem solver, and she had many friends whom she counted on as a sounding board and for support.
    D. Regina was always complaining of physical illnesses, and two months ago she had been hospitalized with hepatitis.

List three nursing actions that can facilitate a family's grieving process (refer to Table 18–2).

19. ______________________________
20. ______________________________
21. ______________________________

DEPRESSIVE DISORDERS

Place an MD (major depression) or a D (dysthymic depression) next to the most likely depressive disorder.

22. ________ May have psychotic symptoms.
23. ________ Usually chronic course, two years or more.
24. ________ The symptoms are NOT congruent with the person's premorbid personality.
25. ________ Usually considered mild to moderate in nature. The symptoms do not greatly interfere with the person's occupational or interpersonal functioning.

Identify the corresponding theoretical approach: P (psychoanalytical), C (cognitive), B (biological), and L (learning theory).

26. ________ The success of the tricyclics (TCAs) and monoamine oxidase inhibitors (MAOIs) helps to support this theory.
27. ________ Thoughts can affect a person's mood.
28. ________ Loss and aggression turned against the self are two of the basic components of this theory.
29. ________ If a person believes he or she has no power to change a situation, and the situation is hopeless, the person becomes depressed.

Name two pieces of data one might find with a depressed person upon assessment for each of the following:

30. Affect 1. ________ 2. ________
31. Thinking 1. ________ 2. ________
32. Feelings 1. ________ 2. ________
33. Physical Behavior 1. ________ 2. ________
34. Communications 1. ________ 2. ________
35. Indications of Masked Depression 1. ________ 2. ________

For each of the following possible nursing diagnoses formulated for the depressed client, write one long term goal and one short term goal:

36. Potential for self-directed violence:
    LTG: ________
    STG: ________
37. Altered thought processes:
    LTG: ________
    STG: ________
38. Social isolation:
    LTG: ________
    STG: ________

Feelings of frustration, anger, and worthlessness may be feelings originating in the depressed client and experienced by the nurse. Which of the following actions by the nurse would be P (productive) or NP (non-productive):

39. ________ Say little and realize that these feelings will go away.
40. ________ Discuss these feelings in team meetings and validate feelings, perceptions, and ways to handle these feelings when with the client.
41. ________ Ask for supervision by an experienced nurse clinician/social worker/psychologist in order to increase self-awareness and therapeutic skills.

Label the following responses made by a nurse as H (helpful) or NH (not helpful) with a depressed client.

42. __________ "Don't worry, we all get down once in awhile."
43. __________ Don't talk of suicide, the person might get ideas.
44. __________ "Debra, I like your new dress."
45. __________ "I will stay with you for five minutes at 10:00 A.M., 1:00 P.M., and 3:30 P.M. today."
46. __________ Try to cheer the person up with a personal story or joke.
47. __________ If a client says an angry word, help him control his anger.

State a common physical problem a depressed person may have for each of the following areas, and offer two suggestions for intervention:

48. Nutrition:
    Problem: ____________________
    Intervention: 1. ____________________
    2. ____________________

49. Elimination:
    Problem: ____________________
    Intervention: 1. ____________________
    2. ____________________

50. Rest and Sleep:
    Problem: ____________________
    Intervention: 1. ____________________
    2. ____________________

51. Physical activity:
    Problem: ____________________
    Intervention: 1. ____________________
    2. ____________________

Multiple Choice

52. Mr. Smith has been put on Elavil. The intern asks the nurse how often and when the best time might be to give this drug. Which of the following would be the nurse's best response:

    A. Every morning, since it has a stimulant effect.
    B. With meals, since it is irritating to the gastric mucosa.
    C. At night—the full dose—to aid sleep and minimize side effects when awake.
    D. In four divided doses throughout the day.

53. Serious side effects can occur in people with heart conditions when they are given a tricyclic (TCA). Adverse drug reactions can also occur with all the following drugs EXCEPT:

    A. Insulin
    B. MAOI
    C. Alcohol
    D. Digitoxin

54. When Mr. Smith did not respond to the tricyclics (TCAs), Nardil (MAOI) was ordered. Which of the following would NOT be a nursing consideration for Mr. Smith:

    A. Wait ten days after the Elavil has been stopped.
    B. Monitor blood pressure closely after MAOI is started.
    C. Stop the medication if client complains of dizziness and constipation.
    D. Careful teaching of client and family regarding certain foods and drugs that may NOT be taken with MAOI.

55. Which of the following is an important nursing consideration with ECT:

    A. Permanent brain damage occurs with several treatments.
    B. ECT has had good results with paranoid schizophrenia and "neurotic" depressions.
    C. There are virtually no physical contraindications to ECT.
    D. During the course of treatment, a client will need frequent orientation to time, place, and person.

56. Which of the following types of therapy for depressed clients has shown a great deal of promise.

    A. Psychoanalytical
    B. Cognitive
    C. Drug therapy used alone
    D. Ego psychology

CHAPTER 19

Alterations in Mood— Elation

Elizabeth M. Varcarolis

OUTLINE

KEY TERMS AND CONCEPTS

The key terms and concepts listed here also appear in bold where they are defined or discussed in this chapter.

BIPOLAR DISORDER
CYCLOTHYMIA
MANIA
HYPOMANIA
SCHIZOAFFECTIVE DISORDER
FLIGHT OF IDEAS
PRESSURE OF SPEECH
CLANG ASSOCIATIONS
LITHIUM CARBONATE
ANTICONVULSANT DRUGS

OBJECTIVES

After studying this chapter, the student will be able to:

1. Describe characteristics observed during the assessment of a manic client's (a) mood, (b) behavior, and (c) thought processes.
2. Formulate three nursing diagnoses appropriate for a manic client, including supporting data.

3. Identify one long term and two short term goals for each of the three nursing diagnoses.
4. Give examples of unconscious tactics used by a person who is manic to maintain the manic defense.
5. Discuss the rationale for five principles of communication for use with a manic client.
6. For each of the following areas, identify two interventions a nurse may use when caring for the physical needs of the manic client: nutrition, rest and sleep, elimination, dress and hygiene, and physical activities.
7. Name four (a) expected side effects for a person on lithium therapy, (b) early signs of lithium toxicity, (c) advanced signs of lithium toxicity, and (d) indications of severe toxic effects of lithium.
8. Write a care plan specifying five areas of client teaching regarding lithium carbonate.
9. Describe indications for the use of seclusion with a manic client.

Mood disorders, also referred to as affective disorders, are divided into the bipolar and depressive disorders. The depressive disorders are covered in Chapter 18. This chapter discusses the bipolar disorders. Essentially the biopolar disorders include the occurrence of depressive episodes and one or more elated mood episodes (Fig. 19–1). Box 19–1 defines a variety of moods that will be discussed in this chapter.

An elated mood can range from normal elevated mood to hypomania to mania. The distinction between

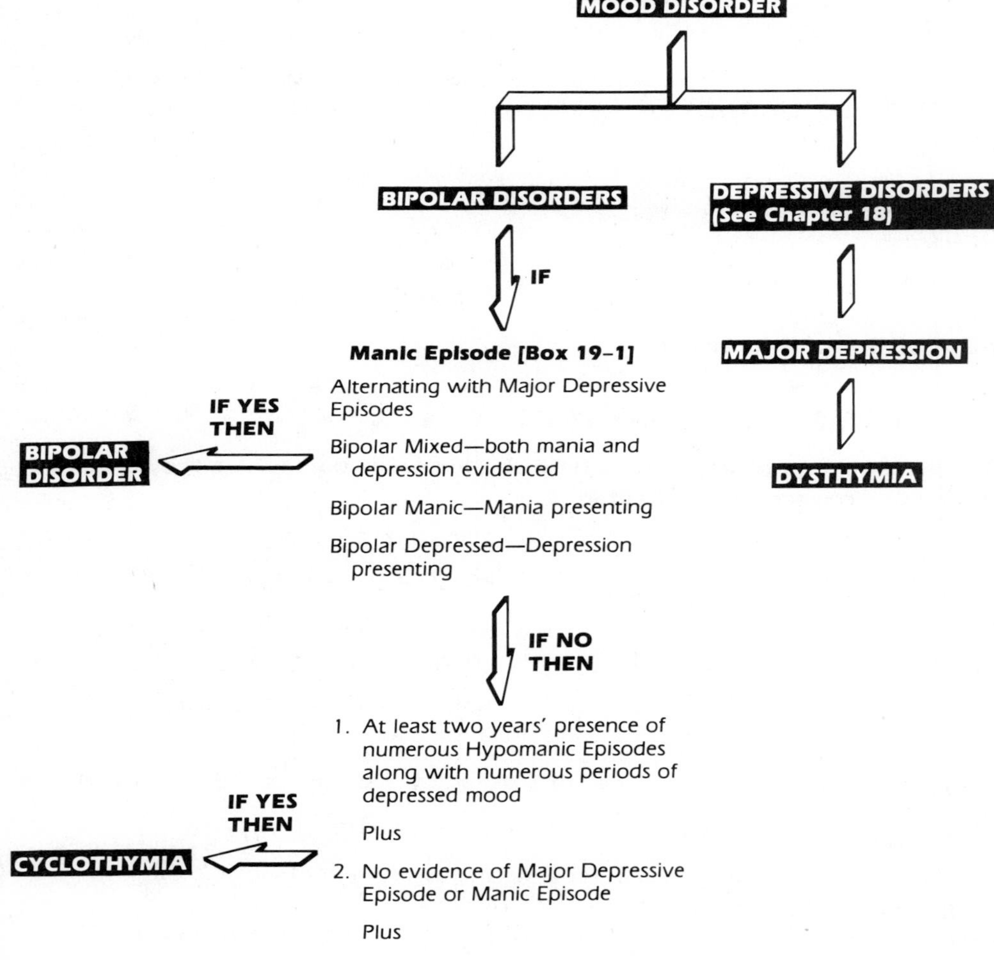

Figure 19–1. *Overview of mood disorder and decision tree for bipolar disorders.*

Box 19–1. EXAMPLES OF MOOD REFERRED TO IN PSYCHIATRIC NURSING

Dysphoric Mood An unpleasant mood, such as depression, anxiety, or irritability.

Elevated Mood A mood that is more cheerful than normal; it does not necessarily imply pathology.

Euphoric Mood An exaggerated feeling of well-being. As a technical term, euphoria implies a pathological mood. Whereas the person with a normally elevated mood may describe himself or herself as being in "good spirits," "very happy," or "cheerful," the euphoric person is likely to exclaim that he or she is "on top of the world" or "up in the clouds" or to say "I feel ecstatic," "I'm flying," or "I am high."

Euthymic Mood Mood in the "normal" range, which implies the absence of depressed or elevated mood.

Expansive Mood Lack of restraint in expressing one's feelings, frequently with an overevaluation of one's significance or importance. There may also be elevated or euphoric mood.

Irritable Mood Internalized feeling of tension associated with being easily annoyed and provoked to anger.

Data from Diagnostic and Statistical Manual of Mental Disorders, Third Edition, Revised. Washington DC: American Psychiatric Association, 1987.

hypomania and mania is based on loss of reality testing.

In **mania,** delusions, poor judgment, and other signs of impaired reality testing are often evident. During a manic episode, a person has marked impairment in his or her social, occupational, and interpersonal functioning.

The symptoms of **hypomania** are less severe than those of mania. A person in hypomania does *not* experience impairment in reality testing, nor do the symptoms markedly impair the person's social, occupational, or interpersonal functioning. Elevated mood along the continuum is shown in Figure 19–2.

Mania is thought by some theorists to be a reaction-formation to depression. A person in a manic state is said to be literally running from the psychogenic pain of underlying depression. The frenetic running behavior is evidenced in both the constant physical activity and the racing speech and thought patterns demonstrated by the manic client. Although outwardly the person may act elated, arrogant, and superior, there is almost always a strong depressive force behind the unstable and gay facade. The elation and hyperactivity serve as attempts to keep feelings of worthlessness and hopelessness at bay. Ths closer the feelings associated with the depression are to consciousness, the faster the manic must run. Mania can escalate to psychotic proportions. Therefore, hyomania and mania can be conceptualized as shown in Figure 19–3.

The two major bipolar disorders are (1) bipolar disorder and (2) cyclothymia. Schizoaffective disorder, which is briefly discussed here, is an atypical bipolar disorder.

BIPOLAR DISORDER. Bipolar disorder is a mood disorder that includes one or more manic episodes and usually one or more depressive episodes. Box 19–2 presents the DSM III-R criteria for manic episode. The symptoms observed in a bipolar disorder are more severe than those seen in cyclothymia.

The manic episode in bipolar disorder may begin suddenly and last a few days to months. Impairment in reality testing may take the form of grandiose or persecutory delusions. There is considerable impairment in social, occupational, and interpersonal functioning. Hospitalization is often warranted to protect the person from the consequences of poor judgment and hyperactivity.

A bipolar disorder is subclassified as follows:

- *Bipolar Mixed*: Presenting both major depressive and manic episodes intermixed or rapidly alternating every few days.
- *Bipolar Manic*: Currently in a manic episode.

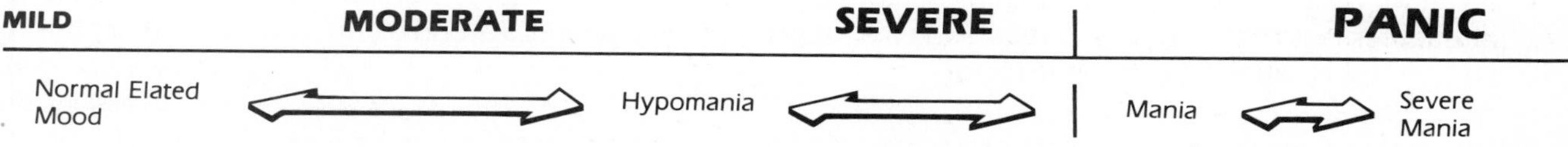

Figure 19–2. *Elated mood along the anxiety continuum.*

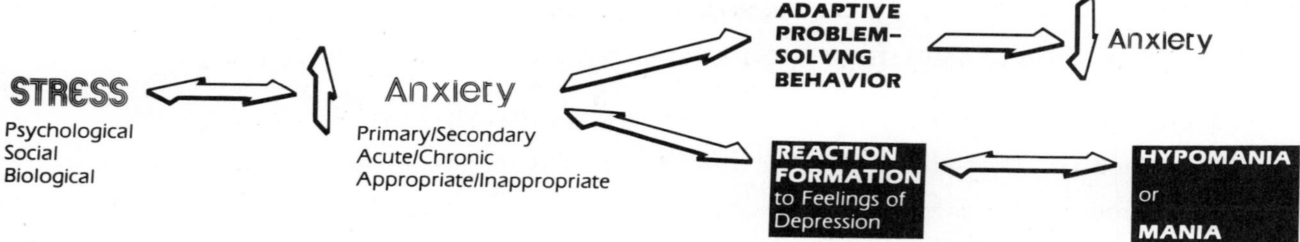

Figure 19–3. *Conceptualization of the process of mania and hypomania.*

- *Bipolar Depressed*: Has had one or more manic episodes currently in a major depressive episode.

CYCLOTHYMIA. Cyclothymia is a chronic mood disturbance (at least two years) involving both hypomanic and dysthymic mood swings. The episodes of hypomania or depression are not usually severe enough to warrant hospitalization. Delusions are *never* present, and the person's social, occupational, and interpersonal functioning are not grossly impaired. Box 19–3 presents the DSM III-R criteria for cyclothymia. Hospitlization is rarely warranted.

SCHIZOAFFECTIVE DISORDER. Kasanin identified this disorder and named it schizoaffective disorder in 1933. A schizoaffective disorder has the following features:

1. A mixture of schizophrenic and affective symptoms.

Box 19–2. DIAGNOSTIC CRITERIA FOR MANIC EPISODE

NOTE: A *Manic Syndrome* is defined as including criteria A, B, and C below. A *Hypomanic Syndrome* is defined as including criteria A and B but not C, i.e., no marked impairment.

A. A distinct period of abnormally and persistently elevated, expansive, or irritable mood

B. During the period of mood disturbance, at least **three** of the following symptoms have persisted (*four* if the mood is only irritable) and have been present to a significant degree:
   1. Inflated self-esteem or grandiosity
   2. Decreased need for sleep, e.g., feels rested after only three hours of sleep
   3. More talkative than usual or pressure to keep talking
   4. Flight of ideas or subjctive experience that thoughts are racing
   5. Distractibility, i.e., attention too easily drawn to unimportant or irrelevant external stimuli
   6. Increase in goal-directed activity (either socially, at work or school, or sexually) or psychomotor agitation
   7. Excessive involvement in pleasurable activities that have a high potential for painful consequences, e.g., the person engages in unrestrained buying sprees, sexual indiscretions, or foolish business investments

C. Mood disturbance sufficiently severe to cause marked impairment in occupational functioning or in usual social activities or relationships with others or to necessitate hospitalization to prevent harm to self or others

D. At no time during the disturbance have there been delusions or hallucinations for as long as two weeks in the absence of prominent mood symptoms (i.e., before the mood symptoms developed or after they have remitted)

E. Not superimposed on schizophrenia, schizophreniform disorder, delusional disorder, or psychotic disorder NOS (not otherwise specified)

F. It cannot be established that an organic factor initiated and maintained the disturbance. **NOTE:** Somatic antidepressant treatment (e.g., drugs, ECT) that apparently precipitates a mood disturbance should not be considered an etiological organic factor.

Continued

Box Box 19–2. DIAGNOSTIC CRITERIA FOR MANIC EPISODE *(Continued)*

Manic Episode Codes: Fifth Digit Code Numbers and Criteria for Severity of Current State of Bipolar Disorder, Manic, or Mixed

1–Mild: Meets minimum symptom criteria for a manic episode (or almost meets symptom criteria if there has been a previous manic episode)

2–Moderate: Extreme increase in activity or impairment in judgment

3–Severe, Without Psychotic Features: Almost continual supervision required in order to prevent physical harm to self or others

4–With Psychotic Features: Delusions, hallucinations, or catatonic symptoms; if possible, **specify** whether the psychotic features are *mood-congruent* or *mood-incongruent*

Mood–Congruent Psychotic Features: Delusions or hallucinations whose content is entirely consistent with the typical manic themes of inflated worth, power, knowledge, identity, or special relationship to a deity or famous person

Mood–incongruent psychotic featues: Either a or b:

a. Delusions or hallucinations whose content does *not* involve typical manic themes of inflated worth, power, knowledge, identity, or special relationship to a deity or famous person; included here are such symptoms as persecutory delusions (not directly related to grandiose ideas or themes), thought insertion, and delusions of being controlled

b. Catatonic symptoms, e.g., stupor, mutism, negativism, posturing

5–In Partial Remission: Full criteria were previously, but are not currently, met; some signs of symptoms of the disturbance have persisted

6–In Full Remission: Full criteria were previously met, but there have been no significant signs or symptoms of the disturbance for at least six months

0–Unspecified

Box 19–3. DIAGNOSTIC CRITERIA FOR CYCLOTHYMIA

A. For at least two years (one year for children and adolescents), presence of numerous hypomanic episodes (all of the criteria for a manic episode except criterion C, which indicates marked impairment) and numerous periods with depressed mood or loss of interest or pleasure that did not meet criterion A of major depressive episode

B. During a two-year period (one year for children and adolescents) of the disturbance, never without hypomanic or depressive symptoms for more than two months at a time

C. No clear evidence of a major depressive episode or manic episode during the first two years of the disturbance (one year for children and adolescents)

NOTE: After this minimum period of cyclothymia, there may be superimposed manic or major depressive episodes, in which case the additional diagnosis of bipolar disorder or bipolar disorder NOS (not otherwise specified) should be given

D. Not superimposed on a chronic psychotic disorder, such as schizophrenia or delusional disorder

E. It cannot be established that an organic factor initiated and maintained the disturbance, e.g., repeated intoxication from drugs or alcohol

2. Good premorbid adjustment.
3. Acute onset.
4. Family history of affective illness.

Schizoaffective disorder has been given many names, such as schizophreniform psychosis and reactive psychosis (Hirschfeld and Goodwin 1988). It is presently believed that schizoaffective disorder is a severe form of bipolar disorder.

Standard I: Theory

Many authorities believe that the bipolar disorders are a distinct diagnostic entity. Bipolar disorders (having one or more episodes of both elated and depressed moods) are thought to be distinctly different from the nonpolar depressive disorders, e.g., major depression or dysthymia (Weissman and Boyd 1985). A vast amount of research is being conducted to identify causal factors for the mood disorders. Most of this research is being done in the biological sphere. Some theoretical data pertaining specifically to the etiology of the bipolar disorders are (1) genetic, (2) interactive transmitters system (biogenic amines), (3) social, and (4) psychosocial.

GENETIC. Significant evidence exists to support the theory that bipolar disorders are a result of genetic transmission. For example, there is a higher rate of bipolar disorder and cyclothymia in relatives with a bipolar disorder than in those with a major depression or in those in the general population (Gershon et al. 1985; Weissman and Boyd 1985). Twin studies bear out a genetic marker for both the bipolar disorders and the depressive disorders; however, the incidence of illness is significantly higher in the bipolar disorders (Cancro 1985). Identical twins are 65–75% more concordant than fraternal twins (14–19%) (Hirschfeld and Goodwin 1988).

BIOGENIC AMINES. The neurotransmitters (norepinephrine, dopamine, and serotonin) have been studied since the 1960's as a causal factor in the mood disorders (mania and depression). Subsequent developments through research have found that the interrelationships among the neurotransmitter system are very complex. More complex hypotheses have developed since the amine hypotheses were originally proposed. One hypothesis is the "permissive" hypothesis by serotonin. This hypothesis proposes that serotoninergic dampenings of other neurotransmitter systems allow for the alteration between mania and depression in bipolar illness (Hirschfeld and Goodwin 1988).

SOCIAL STATUS. Some evidence suggests that the bipolar disorders may be more prevalent in the upper socioeconomic classes. The exact reason for this is unclear; however, people with bipolar disorders appear to achieve higher levels of education and occupational status, whereas there is no difference across various socioeconomic classes with the nonbipolar depressions. Also, there is evidence that a high proportion of bipolar clients has been found among creative writers and professional people (Weissman and Boyd 1985).

PSYCHOSOCIAL. Although there is increasing evidence for genetic and biological markers in the etiology of the mood disorders, psychosocial factors are still thought relevant (Carson et al. 1988). For example, manic and hypomanic episodes are viewed by some psychoanalytic theorists as extreme defenses against depression. The manic or hypomanic defense can be viewed as an attempt to avoid inner pain through exhausting activity and an exaggerated, elevated, or expansive mood. In short, the person unconsciously acts out the exact opposite of his or her underlying feelings. Thus, the manic defense can be conceptualized as a reaction-formation to an underlying depression.

Standard II: Data Collection

Three main characteristics of **mania** are (1) euphoria, (2) hyperactivity, and (3) flight of ideas. Not all people in the manic state experience euphoria; some people become extemely irritable, especially when limits are set on their behavior (Goodwin and Guze 1984). The nurse evaluates these characteristics when assessing a manic client's (1) mood, (2) behavior, and (3) thought processes.

ASSESSING MOOD

The euphoric mood associated with a bipolar illness is unstable and not constant. The mood may change to irritation and quick anger when the elated person does not get his or her way. The irritability and belligerence may be short-lived, or it may become the prominent feature of a person's manic illness. When elated, the person's overjoyous mood may seem out of proportion to what is going on around him, and a cheerful and gay mood may be inappropriate to his circumstances (Arieti 1974).

The person in a manic state may laugh, joke, and talk in a continuous stream, with uninhibited familiarity. People demonstrate boundless enthusiasm and treat everyone with confidential friendliness and incorporate everyone into their plans and activities. "They know no strangers." Energy and self-confidence seem boundless (Chapman 1976).

Elaborate schemes to get rich and famous and acquire unlimited power are frantically pursued despite objections and realistic constraints. Excessive phone calls are made and telegrams sent to famous and influential people all over the world. The manic is busy all hours of the day and night furthering his or her grandiose plans and wild schemes. To the manic person, there are no limits too high nor distances too far. There are no boundaries in reality to curtail the elaborate schemes.

In the manic state, a person often gives away money, prize possessions, and expensive gifts. The manic throws lavish parties, frequents expensive nightclubs and restaurants, and spends money freely on friends and strangers alike. This spending, charging, and high living continue even in the face of bankruptcy. Intervention is needed to prevent financial ruin.

As the clinical course progresses, sociability and euphoria are replaced by a stage of hostility, irritability, and paranoia. The high-spirited, jovial, confident, and enthusiastic mood eventually slips, and the forced gaiety and frantic running are revealed as a brittle defense against painful feelings (Chapman 1976; Klerman 1978). A client describes the painful transition from **hypomania** to mania (Goldstein el al. 1980):

Hypomania

> At first when I'm high, it's tremendous . . . ideas are fast . . . like shooting stars you follow 'til brighter ones appear . . . all shyness disappears, the right words and gestures are suddenly there . . . uninteresting people, things become intensely interesting. Sensuality is pervasive, the desire to seduce and be seduced is irresistible. Your marrow is infused with unbelievable feelings of ease, power, well being, omnipotence, euphoria . . . you can do anything . . . but somewhere this changes . . .

Mania

> The fast ideas become too fast and there are far too many . . . overwhelming confusion replaces clarity . . . you stop keeping up with it—memory goes. Infectious humor ceases to amuse—your friends become frightened . . . everything now is against the grain . . . you are irritable, angry, frightened, uncontrollable, and trapped in the blackest caves of the mind —caves you never knew were there. It will never end. Madness carves its own reality.

ASSESSING BEHAVIOR

When manic, a person constantly flits from one activity to another, one place to another, one project to another. Inactivity is impossible, even for the shortest period of time. Hyperactivity may range from mild, constant motion to frenetic, wild activity. Writing flowery and lengthy letters and making numerous and excessive long distance telephone calls are common. The spending of large sums of money on frivolous items and giving money away indiscriminately can leave a family in debt.

When a person is *hypomanic*, there exists a voracious appetite for food as well as indiscriminate sex. Although the constant activity of the hypomanic prevents proper sleep, short periods of sleep are possible. However, the *manic* person is too busy to eat, sleep, or engage in sexual activity. **This nonstop physical activity, and lack of sleep and food can lead to physical exhaustion and death.**

Mode of dress often reflects the person's grandiose yet tenuous grasp on reality. Dress may be described as outlandish, bizarre, colorful, and noticeably inappropriate. Make-up is garish or overdone. The manic client is highly distractible. Concentration is poor, and he or she flits from one activity to another without completing anything. Judgment is poor. Impulsive marriages and divorces take place. People often emerge from a manic state startled and confused by the shambles in which their life is left. The following description conveys one client's experience (Goldstein et al. 1980):

After Mania

> Now there are only other's recollections of your behavior—your bizarre, frenetic, aimless behavior—at last mania has the grace to dim memories of itself . . . now it's over, but is it? . . . Incredible feelings to sort through . . . Who is being too polite? Who knows what? What did I do? Why? and most hauntingly, will it, when will it, happen again? Medication to take, to resist, to resent, to forget . . . but always to take. Credit cards revoked . . . explanations at work . . . bad checks and apologies overdue . . . memory flashes of vague men (what did I do?) . . . friendships gone, a marriage ruined.

ASSESSING THOUGHT PROCESSES

Flight of ideas is a nearly continuous flow of speech. The person jumps rapidly from one topic to another. At times, the attentive listener can keep up with the changes, even though direction changes from moment to moment (Hinsie and Campbell, 1973). The talk as a whole is rapid, verbose, and circumstantial (including minute and unnecessary details). The goal is to maintain superficiality and escape from thoughts that would activate the underlying depression. The incessant talking often includes jokes, playing on words (puns), and teasing.

> How are you doing kid, no kidding around, I'm going home . . . home sweet home . . . home is where the heart is, the heart of the matter is I want out and that ain't hay, . . . hay, Doc . . . get me out of this place . . .

The content of speech is often sexually explicit and ranges from grossly inappropriate to vulgar. Themes in the communications of the manic may revolve around his or her extraordinary sexual prowess, brilliant business ability, unparalleled artistic talents (writing, painting, dancing) and so forth. The person may have average ability in these areas, at best.

Some of the manic's tension is drained off by what is termed **pressure of speech.** One can hear the force and energy behind the rapid words.

As mania escalates, flight of ideas may give way to clang associations. **Clang associations** is the stringing together of words because of their rhyming sounds, without regard to their meaning, for example: "Good luck, buck, chuck, duck" or "red, bed, said, ted, led . . . " Pressure of speech is easily detected in the staccato, rapid outpouring of clang associations.

In mania, grandiose persecutory delusions are common. For example, a manic client may think that God is speaking to him or that the F.B.I. is out to stop him from accomplishing some great feat such as "saving the world." Sensory perceptions may become altered as the mania escalates, and hallucinations may occur. In hypomania there is no evidence of delusions or hallucinations.

Table 19–1 illustrates mania along a continuum from hypomania to mania to severe levels of mania. Observations include communication, affect and thinking, and physical behavior.

Standard III: Diagnosis

Nursing diagnoses can be many and varied for the manic client. Some, but not all possible, nursing diagnoses are suggested here.

When a client comes into the hospital acutely manic, the primary consideration is the prevention of exhaustion and death from cardiac collapse. Because of the client's poor judgment, excessive and constant motor activity, probable dehydration, and difficulty evaluating reality, *potential for injury* is likely. Potential for injury is an appropriate diagnosis if the client's activity level is dangerous to his or her health. Immediate medical and nursing intervention is often vital to prevent physical exhaustion. Bruises or wounds resulting from falls and bumping into objects or secondary infections resulting from lack of nutrition, lack of sleep, and personal neglect indicate the client has potential for injury.

Potential for violence to self or others related to rage reaction, as evidenced by inability to control behavior, occurs frequently when excitation becomes so severe that the client may be destructive, hostile, and aggressive (Klerman 1978). More often, however, clients' intrusive and taunting behavior can induce others to strike out against them.

Grandiosity, poor judgment, and giving away possessions can result in bankruptcy, neglect of family, and impulsive major life changes (divorce, marriage, job changes, moving). These behaviors suggest *altered thought processes.* Getting involved in impossible schemes, shady legal deals, and questionable business ventures may be a result of *ineffective individual coping* related to altered affect caused by changes in body chemistry or inadequate psychological resources.

The client in the acutely manic state may have numerous unmet physical needs. The manic client is too busy to eat and sleep, is often constipated and poorly groomed, and dress may be flamboyant and bizarre. *Fluid volume deficit, altered nutrition (less than body requirements), constipation, sleep pattern disturbance,* or *self-care deficit* are considerations.

Because of the manic's rapid speech (flight of ideas), poor attention span,and difficulty concentrating, *altered family process* related to an ill family member should always be part of the assessment. The family, as well as the client, will need questions answered, understanding, and support.

Standard IV: Planning

Planning interventions for a person who is manic is planned on two levels: (1) the content level—planning goals—and (2) the process level—nurses' reactions and feelings.

CONTENT LEVEL—PLANNING GOALS

After the assessment has been made and the nursing diagnoses placed in order of priority, short term and long term goals are formulated. Goals are made for each nursing diagnosis according to the client's unmet needs. Listed subsequently are some—by no means

Table 19–1 • MANIA ON THE ANXIETY CONTINUUM

MODERATE TO SEVERE	PANIC	
Hypomanic	**Acute Manic**	**Severe Manic**
	Communication	
1. Talks and jokes incessantly, is the "Life of the Party," gets irritated when not center of attention.	1. May go suddenly from laughing to anger or depession. *Mood labile.*	1. Totally out of touch with reality.
2. Treats everyone with familiarity and confidentiality; often borders on crude.	2. Becomes inappropriately demanding of people's attention, and intrusive nature repels others.	—
3. Talk often very sexual in nature—can reach obscene, inappropriate propositions to total strangers.	3. Speech may be marked by profanities and crude sexual remarks to everyone (nursing staff in particular).	—
4. Talk is fresh; flits from one topic to the next. Marked by *pressure of speech*.	4. Speech marked by *flight of ideas*, where thoughts racing and flying from topic to topic. May hear *clang association*.	4. Most likely *clang associations*.
	Affect and Thinking	
1. Full of pep and good humor, feelings of good humor, feelings of euphoria and sociability; may show inappropriate intimacy with strangers.	1. Good humor gives way to increased irritability and hostility, short-lived period of rage, especially when not getting one's way or controls are set on behavior. May have quick shifts of mood from hostility to being very docile.	1. May become destructive or aggressive—totally out of control.
2. He feels boundless self-confidence and enthusiasm. Has elaborate schemes for becoming rich and famous. Initially schemes may seem plausible.	2. Grandiose plans are totally out of contact with reality. Plans and thinking musician, prominent businessman, great politician, or religious figure, without any basis in fact.	2. May experience undefined hallucinations and delirium.
3. Judgment often poor. Gets involved with schemes in which his job, marriage, or financial status may be destroyed.	3. Judgment extremely poor.	—
4. May get involved with writing large quantities of letters to rich and famous people regarding his schemes or make numerous world-wide telephone calls.	—	—
	Physical Behavior	
1. Overactive, distractible, buoyant, and busily occupied with grandiose plans (not delusions); goes from one action to the next.	1. Extremely restless, disorganized, and chaotic. Physical behavior may be difficult to control. May have outbursts, e.g., throwing things, or become briefly assaultive when crossed.	1. *Dangerous State*. Incoherent, extremely restless, disoriented, and agitated. Hyperactive. Motor activity is totally aimless (must have physical or chemical restraints to prevent exhaustion and death).
2. Increased sexual appetite; sexually unresponsible and indiscreet. Illegitimate pregnancies in hypomanic female and venereal disease in both male and female are common. Sex used for escape, not for relating to another human being.	2. Too busy—no time for sex. Poor concentration, distractibility, and restlessness too severe.	2. In the extreme.
3. May have voracious appetite, eat on the run, or gobble food during brief periods.	3. No time to eat—too distracted and disorganized.	3. Same as acute manic but in the extreme.
4. May go without sleeping; unaware of fatigue. However, may be able to grab short naps.	4. No time for sleep—psychomotor activity too high; if unchecked can lead to exhaustion and death.	
5. Financially extravagant, goes on buying sprees, gives money and gifts away freely, can easily go into debt.	5. In the extreme.	5. Too disorganized to do anything.

Data from Arieti 1974; Chapman 1976; Klerman 1978.

all—possible goals for the following diagnoses:

1. Potential for injury.
   - The client's cardiac status will remain stable during hospitalization.
   - While in acutely manic state, the client will drink eight ounces of high-caloric, high-protein drink every hour throughout the day.
   - The client will spend time with the nurse in a quiet environment each hour between 7 A.M. and 11 P.M.
   - The client's skin will be free from abrasions and scrapes every day while in the hospital.
2. Potential for violence directed at others.
   - By (state the date) the client will display nonviolent behavior toward others while in the hospital, with the aid of medication and nursing interventions.
   - With the aid of seclusion or nursing interventions, the client will refrain from provoking others to physically harm themselves.
   - The client will respond to external controls (medication, seclusion, nursing interventions) when potential or actual loss of control occurs.
3. Ineffective coping or altered thought process.
   - Client will retain valuables or other possessions while in the hospital.
   - Client will make only one five-minute telephone call per hour.
   - Client will have competent medical assistance and legal protection when signing any legal documents regarding personal or financial matters.
4. Fluid volume deficit, altered nutrition (less than body requirements), constipation, sleep pattern disturbance, and self-care deficit.
   - Client will have good skin turgor by 8:00 P.M.
   - Client will have normal bowel movements within two days with the aid of high-fiber foods and fluids.
   - Client will take a ten-minute rest period every two hours during the day (8:00 A.M. to 10:00 P.M.) with the aid of the nurse.
   - Client will sleep six hours in 24 hours with the aid of medication and nursing measures, within three days.
   - Client will wear appropriate make-up/shave each day while in the hospital.
   - Client will wear appropriate attire for age and sex each day while in the hospital.
5. Altered family process. Usually, when an episode of mania ceases (a few days to a few months), people return to normal functioning. Often, however, during a manic flight an individual may unknowingly violently overthrow what was once a "normal" life. People may come out of their manic sprees startled to find themselves broke, without a job, without friends, and without a spouse. Families need to understand what is happening and need support and counseling for themselves. The goals a nurse will set will depend on the complexity of the situation. Often many members of the health team become involved with supporting the families. For example, social workers, psychologists/psychiatrists, psychiatric nurse clinicians, and staff nurses give important information and realistic reassurances and can make appropriate referrals. Goals may include
   - Family/spouse will meet with the nurse to assess family needs by the end of the week.
   - Family/spouse will understand prognosis, use of medications, and how to recognize prodromal signs of mania before discharge.

PROCESS LEVEL—NURSES' REACTIONS AND FEELINGS

A nurse working with a manic client for the first time needs guidance and support and needs to become aware of possible client behaviors resulting from the manic defense. The manic client poses problems and requires interventions very different from the withdrawn and depressed individual.

First, the manic client, unlike most all other clients on the psychiatric unit, needs to be directed *away* from active environmental stimuli (upbeat music, activity groups, games, large meetings) in order to minimize the escalation of the mania.

A quiet, dimly lit, and calm atmosphere is ideal for the manic. Getting a client to stay in such an environment is a task. The manic needs to be up, to be high, to keep depressive feelings from surfacing. Therefore, the individual rarely stays put for very long. Firmness and a neutral approach usually work best. *Because the manic client is so distractible, the nurse can use this distractibility to move him or her from potentially problematic situations to more productive activities.* Often activities that involve some motor activity, using large muscle groups (ping-pong, punching bag, writing), provide constructive outlets for energy. A few hours of keeping up with a person who is manic can deplete the nurse's energy. Often nurses take turns monitoring a manic's behavior while the client is still extremely hyperactive.

Second, the manic client can elicit a number of intense emotions from the nurse. A manic client is out of control and fights being controlled. Fear of underlying painful feelings is great. Therefore, the client may use humor, manipulation, power struggles, or demanding behavior to prevent or minimize the staff's ability to set limits on and control dangerous behavior.

When the manic is joking, punning, and being the life of the party, the mood can be infectious. A manic client can be genuinely funny and entertaining. The nurse needs to remain uninvolved or neutral and take measures to prevent further escalation of the mania. To joke with or encourage the manic's humor is meeting the nurse's needs at the client's expense. The client is running from pain, not to a good time.

Since one motivation of the manic's behavior is to keep painful feelings out of awareness, the behavior of a manic client is often aimed at decreasing the effectiveness of staff control. He or she might accomplish this by getting involved with power plays. For example, the client might taunt the staff by pointing out "faults" or "oversights," drawing negative attention to one or more staff. Usually this is done in a loud and disruptive manner. This serves to get staff defensive, thereby escalating the environmental tension and the client's degree of mania.

Another unconscious tactic is to divide staff in order to keep the environment unsettled. The manic is very sensitive to the vulnerabilities and conflicts within a group. Often, a manic client will manipulate staff by turning one group of staff against another in an unconscious attempt to discourage outside controls. For example, a client might tell the day shift, "You are the only nurse(s) that listen(s). On evenings they hardly look at you. You could drop dead, and the nurses wouldn't even know it." To the evening shift the client might say, "Thank God you're here. At last someone who cares. All the day people do is push pills and drink coffee."

In the attempt to ward off painful feelings by maintaining mania, the client can become aggressively demanding, another manic defense. This behavior often triggers frustration and exasperation from the staff. Again, the manic distracts the staff into a defensive position and sets up an environment that allows the manic defense to go unchecked.

When the staff start to feel angry at each other and confused, it is often an indication that a client is splitting the staff. Frequent staff meetings dealing with the behaviors of the client and the nurses' responses to these behaviors can help minimize splitting and feelings of anger and isolation by the staff. The consistent setting of limits is the main theme with a person in mania. *Consistency among staff is imperative* if the limits set are to be carried out effectively.

Standard V: Intervention

V-A: PSYCHOTHERAPEUTIC INTERVENTIONS

Table 19–2 suggests some basic principles of communication for use with the client who is manic.

V-C: ACTIVITIES OF DAILY LIVING

A person in mania has great difficulty meeting personal physical needs. Thus, the nurse finds that much attention is directed toward interventions associated with activities of daily living. Table 19–3 suggests interventions appropriate for safeguarding the physical health of the manic client.

V-D: SOMATIC THERAPIES

Lithium Carbonate

Lithium Carbonate ($LiCO_3$) is considered the drug of choice for treating the manic phase of a bipolar disorder. Lithium is a mood stabilizer and is often referred to as an *antimanic* drug. When effective, it can calm manic clients, prevent or modify future manic episodes, and protect against future depressive episodes (Lickey and Gordon 1983).

Initially when a client comes into the hospital in severe mania, a neuroleptic (antipsychotic) drug, often Thorazine, is given. Neuroleptics act promptly to slow speech, inhibit aggression, and decrease psychomotor activity. The immediate action of the neuroleptic medication is to prevent exhaustion, coronary collapse, and death. See Chapter 20 for a discussion of the neuroleptic (antipsychotic) drugs. Electroconvulsive therapy (ECT) may also be used to subdue severe manic behavior (Kaib et al. 1989).

In order for lithium to work, it must reach therapeutic levels in the client's blood. This usually takes from seven to 14 days, or longer. As lithium levels become effective in reducing manic behavior, the neuroleptics are usually discontinued. Lithium is 70% to 80% effective in treating the manic phase in a bipolar disorder (Harris 1989); however, it is not a cure. Many clients are on indefinite lithium maintenance and will suffer manic and depressive episodes if the drug is discontinued.

Trade names for lithium carbonate include Lithane, Eskalith, and Lithonate. *Initially*, 300–600 mg by mouth is given three times a day to reach a therapeutic lithium level of 1.0–1.5 mEq/l when a person is in severe mania. Then, a maintenance dose of 300–600 mg by mouth is given three times a day to maintain lithium blood levels of 08–1.2 mEq/l (Hart et al. 1981). However, each client has individual reactions to lithium. So, although 0.8–1.2 mEq/l is presumed to be appropriate maintenance blood level, 0.8 mEq/l may be too high for some people. Others can avoid a manic or depressive episode on 0.4–0.6 m Eq/l (Schatzberg and Cole 1986).

There is a small range between the therapeutic dose and the toxic dose. Initially, blood levels are drawn weekly or biweekly until the therapeutic level has been

Table 19–2 • PRINCIPLES OF COMMUNICATION WITH THE MANIC CLIENT

NURSING INTERVENTION	RATIONALE
1. Use a firm and calm approach, "John, come with me, Eat this sandwich."	1. Provides structure and control for a client who is out of control. Can result in feelings of security: "Someone is in control."
2. Use short and concise explanations or statements.	2. Short attention span limits comprehension to small bits of information.
3. Work at remaining neutral—avoid power struggles and value judgments.	3. Client can use inconsistencies and value judgments as justification for arguing and escalating mania.
4. Be consistent in approach and expectations.	4. Consistent limits and expectations minimize potential for client manipulating staff.
5. Avoid getting caught up in joking and repartee. Maintain a calm and neutral manner.	5. Minimizes the manic spiral. Joking and laughing with the manic client is disrespectful of client needs.
6. Have frequent staff meetings to plan consistent approaches and to set agreed-upon limits.	6. Consistency of all staff is needed to maintain controls and minimize manipulation by client.
7. When limits are decided upon by staff, they need to be told to the client in simple, concrete terms, including the consequences, e.g., "John, do not yell/hit Peter. If you cannot control yourself, we will help you." or "The seclusion room will help you feel less out of control and prevent harm to yourself and others."	7. Clear expectations help client experience outside controls, as well as understand reasons for medication, seclusion, restraints, if he or she is not able to control behaviors.
8. Legitimate complaints should be heard and acted upon.	8. Reduces underlying feelings of helplessness and can raise self-esteem.
9. Accept acting-out behavior calmly (obscene remarks, crude jokes, and gestures).	9. Acceptance thwarts the unconscious attempt to trigger anger and get the nurse to act irrational (out of control) thus maintaining the manic defense.
10. Firmly redirect energy into more appropriate and constructive channels.	10. Distractibility is the nurse's most effective tool with the manic client.

reached. After therapeutic levels have been reached, blood levels are drawn every month. Blood should be drawn eight to 12 hours after the last dose of lithium.

Many hospital policies state that if during maintenance therapy, blood lithium levels go over 1.5 mEq/l, the drug should be withheld for 24 hours and restarted at a lower dose. Toxic effects are usually associated with levels of 2.0 mEq/l or more, although they can occur at much lower levels (Bergersen 1979; Goodwin and Guze 1984).

INDICATIONS FOR USE OF LITHIUM. Lithium use can be divided into four general clinical situations (Schatzberg and Cole 1986):

1. To control rapidly acute, overt psychopathology, as in mania or psychotic agitation.
2. To attempt to modify milder ongoing or frequent but episodic clincal symptoms, such as chronic depression or episodic irritability.
3. To establish a prophylactic maintenance regimen to avert future affective or psychotic episodes.
4. To enhance the effect of antidepressants in clients with a major depressive disorder.

Lithium has been used with success in some clients who have a schizoaffective disorder. Schizoaffective disorder is considered an atypical bipolar disorder. Also, in some cases, chronically impaired schizophrenics have improved when placed on lithium, especially those who had proved resistant to other treatments.

It has been noted that some people with depressions improve on lithium alone. Recent studies suggest that adding lithium to tricyclic or MAOI antidepressant therapy in a client who has not responded favorably to the antidepressant may increase the chance of a favorable response (Schatzberg and Cole 1986).

CONTRAINDICATIONS FOR USE OF LITHIUM. Prior to administration of lithium, a medical evaluation is given to assess a client's ability to tolerate the drug. In particular, baseline physical and laboratory examinations should include the following (DePaulo 1984):

1. Renal function.
2. Thyroid status, including thyroxine (T_4) and thyroid-stimulating hormone (TSH).

Table 19–3 • PHYSICAL NEEDS OF MANIC CLIENTS

NURSING INTERVENTION	RATIONALE
Nutrition	
1. Monitor intake, output, and vital signs.	1. Ensure adequate fluid and caloric intake; minimize dehydration and cardiac collapse.
2. Offer frequent high-caloric protein drinks and finger foods (sandwiches, fruit, milk shakes).	2. Constant fluid and caloric replacement needed. Too active to sit at meals. Finger foods allow "eating on the run."
3. Frequently remind client to eat. "Tom, finish your milk shake." "Sally, eat this banana."	3. The manic client is unaware of bodily needs and is easily distracted. Needs supervision to eat.
Rest and Sleep	
1. Encourage frequent rest periods during the day.	1. Lack of sleep can lead to exhaustion and death.
2. Keep client in areas of low stimulation.	2. Promote relaxation and minimize manic behavior.
3. At night, provide warm baths, soothing music, and medication when indicated. Avoid caffeine.	3. Promote relaxation, rest, and sleep.
Elimination	
1. Monitor bowel habits; offer fluids and food high in fiber. Evaluate need for laxative. Encourage to go to bathroom.	1. Prevent fecal impaction resulting from dehydration and decreased peristalsis.
Dress and Hygiene	
1. Supervise choice of clothes, minimize flamboyant and bizarre dress, i.e., garish stripes, plaids, loud unmatching colors.	1. Lessens the potential for ridicule, which lowers self-esteem thus increasing the need for manic defense. Assist client in maintaining dignity.
2. Give simple step-by-step reminders for hygiene and dress. "Here is your razor. Shave the left side . . . now shave the right side. Here is your toothbrush. Put the toothpaste on the brush . . . "	2. Distractibility and poor concentration are countered by simple, concrete instructions.
Activities and Recreation	
1. When possible, provide an environment with minimal stimuli (quiet, soft music, dimly lit).	1. Reduced stimuli lessen distractibility.
2. Solitary activities requiring short attention span with mild physical exertion are best initially: writing, painting, ping-pong, woodwork, walks with staff.	2. Solitary activities minimize stimuli; mild physical activities release tension constructively.
3. When less manic, client may join one or two other clients in quiet, nonstimulating activities (board games, drawing, cards). AVOID GAMES OF COMPETITION.	3. As mania subsides, involvement in activities that provide a focus and social contact becomes more appropriate Games of competition can stimulate aggression and increase psychomotor activity.
4. Protect client from giving away money and possessions. Hold valuables in hospital safe until rational judgment returns.	4. Client's "generosity" is a manic defense consistent with irrational, grandiose thinking.
Physical Safety	
1. Acute mania may warrant use of phenothiazines and seclusion to minimize physical harm.	1. Exhaustion and death can result from dehydration, lack of sleep, and constant physical activity.
2. Observe for signs of lithium toxicity.	2. There is a small margin of safety between therapeutic dose and toxic dose.

3. Evaluation for dementia or neurological disorders, as these signal a poor response to lithium.

Other clinical and laboratory assessments (including a cardiogram) are done as needed, depending on the individual's physical condition (DePaulo 1984).

Lithium is not given to people who are pregnant, have brain damage, or have cardiovascular, renal, or thyroid disease. Lithium is also contraindicated in mothers who are breast-feeding or have myasthenia gravis and in children under 12 years of age.

EXPECTED SIDE EFFECTS. Fine mild hand tremors, polyuria, and mild thirst often occur and may persist throughout therapy. Mild nausea and general discomfort may occur initially, and the client can be reassured that these side effects usually subside with treatment. Weight gain is sometimes an undesirable side effect of long term use (Hart et al. 1981; Scherer. 1985). Table 19–4 identifies early, advanced, and severe signs of toxic poisoning with lithium. "The major long-term risks of lithum therapy are hypothyroidism and impairment of the kidney's ability to concentrate urine" (Harris 1989).

CLIENT TEACHING. The client and the client's family should be instructed regarding the following points (Hart et al. 1981; Bergersen 1979; Scherer 1985; Harris 1989).

1. Maintain a normal diet and normal salt and fluid intake (2500–3000 ml/day). Lithium decreases sodium reabsorption by the renal tubules, which could cause sodium depletion. A low sodium intake causes a relative increase in lithium retention, which could lead to toxicity.
2. Withhold drug if excessive diarrhea, vomiting, or diaphoresis occurs. Dehydration can raise lithium levels in the blood to toxic levels.
3. Diuretics are contraindicated with lithium.
4. Lithium is irritating to the gastric mucosa; take lithium with meals.

Table 19–4 • SIGNS OF LITHIUM TOXICITY

LEVEL	SIGNS*	INTERVENTIONS
	Early Signs	
Less than 1.5 mEq/l	Nausea, vomiting, diarrhea, thirst, polyuria, slurred speech, muscle weakness.	Medication should be withheld, blood lithium levels drawn, and the dose re-evaluated.
	Advanced Signs	
1.5 mEq/l to 2 mEq/l	Course hand tremor persistent gastrointestinal upset, mental confusion, muscle hyperirritability, electroencephalographic changes, incoordination.	Use interventions outlined above or below, depending on severity of circumstances.
	Severe Toxic Effects	
2.0 m Eq/l to 2.5 mEq/l	Ataxia, serious electroencephalographic changes, blurred vision, clonic movements, large output of dilute urine, seizures, stupor, severe hypotension, coma. Fatalities are usually secondary to pulmonary complications.	There is no known antidote for lithium poisoning. The drug is stopped and excretion is hastened. Gastric lavage and treatment with urea, mannitol, and aminopylline all hasten lithium excretion.
Greater than 2.5 mEq/l	Confusion, incontinence of urine or feces, coma, cardiac arrhythmia, peripheral circulatory collapse, abdominal pain, proteinuria, oliguria, hypothyroidism.	Hemodialysis may also be used in severe cases.

* Careful monitoring is needed because the toxic levels of lithium are close to the therapeutic levels.
Data from Scherer JC. Nurses' Drug Manual. Philadelphia: J.B. Lippinott Company, 1985. p. 631–632.

5. Periodic monitoring of renal functioning and thyroid function is indicated with long term use.
6. Avoid taking over-the-counter medications without checking first with a physician.
7. If weight gain is significant, the client may need to see a physician for a low-calorie diet.
8. NSAIDs (nonsteroidal antiinflammatory drugs), alcohol, and tetracycline can *raise* lithium levels.
9. Carbamazepine (Tegretol), sodium bicarbonate, and theophylline/aminophylline can *lower* lithium levels.

Other Antimanic Drugs

Recently, several **anticonvulsant drugs** have been useful in treating mania and appear to have mood-stabilizing effects. For example, carbamazepine (Tegretol), valproic acid (Depakene), and clonazepam (Klonopin) are used in current practice. *Carbamazepine* has antimanic effects equal to those of the neuroleptics but does not have the side effects of these drugs. In particular, carbamazepine does not add the risk of tardive dyskinesia. Carbamazepine is especially useful in clients who have not responded to lithium in the past and who are rapid cyclers, that is, they go from a euphoric mood to a dysphoric mood in rapid succession (Hirschfeld and Goodwin 1988). Carbamazepine (Tegretol) is also being evaluated for use in the treatment of dysphoria, episodic violence or wrist cutting, borderline personality disorder, chronic pain, and diabetes insipidus. It also may be useful as an adjunct to antipsychotic treatment in clients with schizophrenia (Schatzberg and Cole 1986). *Clonazepam* is especially useful when rapid sedation is required. All of these drugs are particularly indicated for clients who fail to respond to more standard treatment (lithium or tricyclic antidepressants). These drugs can be used either along with other mood stabilizers or as alternatives to more traditional mood stabilizers.

V-E: THERAPEUTIC ENVIRONMENT

Hospitalization is indicated for people in the acutely manic state. Hospitalization helps the client gain control over extreme hyperactive behavior and allows for medication stabilization. Control of hyperactive behavior most always includes immediate treatment with a neuroleptic such as Thorazine. However, when a client is dangerously out of control, use of the seclusion room may be indicated as well.

Seclusion serves the following purposes (Fitzgerald and Long 1973):

1. Reduces overwhelming environmental stimuli.
2. Protects a client from injuring self, others, or staff.
3. Prevents destruction of personal property or property of others.

Seclusion is warranted when *documented data* by the nursing and medical staff reflect the following points (Roper et al. 1985):

1. Other measures have failed.
2. Behavior has been sustained.
3. Substantial risk or harm to others is clear.
4. Client is unable to control his or her actions.

The use of seclusion or restraints involves complex therapeutic, ethical, and legal issues. Therefore, most hospitals have well-defined protocols for treatment with seclusion. Protocols include a proper reporting procedure through the chain of command when a client is to be secluded. When and what to document and specific nursing responsibilities aimed at safeguarding the client are outlined. For example, a protocol usually spells out who can make the decision for seclusion when a physician is not available, how long a client can be in seclusion without a doctor's written order (e.g., 15–30 minutes) whom to call if a doctor is not available to write an order (within 15–30 minutes).

Seclusion protocols also identify specific nursing responsibilities. For example, how often the client's behavior is to be observed and documented (e.g., every 15 minutes), how often the client is to be offered food and fluids (e.g., every 30–60 minutes), and how often the client is to be toileted (e.g., every one to two hours).

Since phenothiazines are often used with clients in seclusion, vital signs should be taken frequently (every 15 minutes), especially when a client is undergoing frequent neuroleptization (Baradell 1985).

When a client does require seclusion to prevent harm to self, it is ideal to have one nurse on each shift work with the client on a continuous basis. Communications with a client in seclusion should be concrete and direct but kind and limited to brief instructions (Baradell 1985). Clients should be reassured that the seclusion is only a *temporary measure*, and that they will be returned to the unit when they gain control of their behavior (Baradell 1985).

Frequent staff meetings regarding personal feelings about seclusion are necessary to prevent possible dangers. Dangers include the use of seclusion as a form of punishment and leaving a client in seclusion for long periods of time without proper supervision (Fitzgerald and Long 1973). Refer to Chapter 3 for legal and ethical issues when employing restraints or seclusion.

V-F: PSYCHOTHERAPY

Psychotherapy is often useful, especially in conjunction with drug therapy. A survey of lithium clinics revealed that psychotherapy and group psychotherapy were offered in about 94% of the clinics (Gitlin and Jamison 1984).

A client describes her feelings about drug therapy and psychotherapy (Jamison and Goodwin 1983):

> I cannot imagine leading a normal life without lithium. From startings and stoppings of it, I now know it is an essential part of my sanity. Lithium prevents my seductive but disastrous highs, diminishes my depressions, clears out the weaving of my disordered thinking, slows me, gentles me out, keeps me in my relationships, in my career, out of a hospital, and in psychotherapy. It keeps me alive, too. But psychotherapy heals, it makes some sense of the confusion, it reins in the terrifying thoughts and feelings, it brings back hope, and the possibility of learning from it all. Pills cannot, do not, ease one back into reality. They bring you back headlong, careening, and faster than can be endured at times. Psychotherapy is a sanctuary, it is a battleground, it is where I have come to believe that someday I may be able to contend with all of this. No pill can help me deal with the problems of not wanting to take pills, but no amount of therapy alone can prevent my manias and depressions. I need both.

Standard VI: Evaluation

Depending on the goals the nurse has set, evaluation of goals is done periodically. If goals are not met, the factors that prevented the attainment of the goals are analyzed. Were there incorrect or insufficient data? Inappropriate nursing diagnoses? Unrealistic goals? Was the intervention poorly planned? After analysis of the goals and reassessment of the care plan, the plan is reworked if indicated.

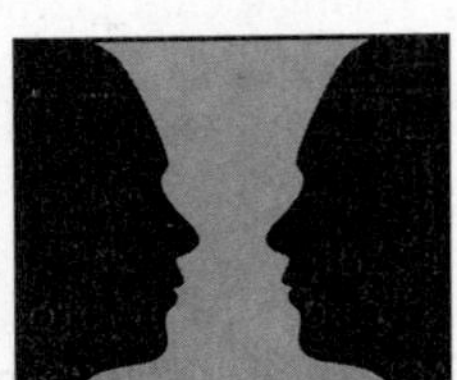

Case Study: Working With a Person Who is Manic

Mary Horowitz was brought into the emergency room after being found on the highway shortly after her car had broken down. When the police came to her aid, she told them that she was "driving herself to fame and fortune." She appeared overly cheerful, constantly talking and laughing and making jokes. At the same time, she walked up and down beside the car, sometimes tweaking the cheek of one of the policemen. She was coy and flirtatious with the police, saying at one point, "Boys in blue are fun to do."

She was dressed in a long red dress with a blue and orange scarf around her neck, many long chains of various colors, and a yellow and green turban on her head. It was when she reached into the car and started drinking from an open bottle of bourbon that the police decided that her behavior and general condition might result in harm to herself or others. When the police explained to Mary that they wanted to take her to the hospital for a general check-up, her jovial mood turned to short-lived anger and rage. Two minutes after getting into the polic car, she was singing "Carry Me Back to Ole Virginia."

Upon admission to the emergency room, she was seen by a psychiatrist, and her sister was called. The sister stated that Mary had stopped taking her lithium two weeks ago and was becoming more and more agitated and out of control. She stated that Mary had not eaten in two days, had stayed up all night calling friends and strangers all over the country, and had finally fled the house when the sister called the ambulance to take her to the hospital. The psychiatrist got in touch with Mary's physician, and it was decided to hospitalize Mary in order to restart her on lithium. It was hoped that medications and a controlled environment would prevent further escalation of the manic state and prevent possible exhaustion and cardiac collapse.

Assessment

Upon admission to the unit, Mr. Atkins was assigned as Mary's primary nurse. Mary was unable to sit down. She strode ceaselessly up and down the halls, talking loudly and pointing to other clients and making loud sexual or hostile comments. Some of the other clients laughed at her actions and her dress.

Mr. Atkins suggested that they go to a quieter part of the unit. Mary turned to him angrily and said, "Let me be . . . set me free, lover . . . I am untouchable . . . I'll get the F.B.I. to set me free."

Mr. Atkins divided the data into subjective and objective components:

OBJECTIVE DATA

1. Little if anything to eat for days
2. Little if any sleep for days
3. A history of mania
4. A history of lithium maintenance
5. Constant physical activity—unable to sit
6. Very loud and distracting to others
7. Becomes angry when wishes are curtailed
8. Flight of ideas
9. Dress is loud and inappropriate
10. Remarks suggested sexual themes
11. Some clients found her behavior amusng
12. Remarks suggested grandiose thinking
13. Poor judgment

SUBJECTIVE DATA

1. "Driving myself to fame and fortune."
2. "I'm untouchable . . . I'll get the F.B.I. to set me free."
3. "Let me be . . . set me free."

Nursing Diagnosis

Mr. Atkins discussed with the admitting psychiatrist Mary's immediate needs. Mary was immediately given 400 mg of Thorazine intramuscularly and was to have 300 mg every three hours as needed. Mary was to be observed for behaviors that might indicate harm to herself or others. The medical staff stated that if medication and nursing interventions did not reduce her activity level, the nurses should allow for possible periods of rest and ingestion of fluids and minimize her provocative behavior toward others. Failing that, the use of seclusion would have to be considered. It was agreed that her physical safety was greatly jeopardized.

Mr. Atkins's initial diagnoses reflected the nursing and medical staff's main concern: Mary's physical condition. Although Mary presented many possible nursing diagnoses and needs at the time, the following two nursing diagnoses were formulated because they focus on her physical safety:

1. *Potential for injury* related to dehydration and faulty judgment, as evidenced by lack of awareness of safety precautions
   - Has not slept for days
   - Has not taken in food or fluids for days
   - Constant physical activity—unable to sit
2. *Ineffective Individual Coping* related to inadequate psychological resources, as evidenced by change in usual communication patterns
   - Very loud and distracting to others
   - Remarks suggested sexual themes
   - Some clients found her behavior amusing
   - Remarks suggested grandiose thinking
   - Flight of ideas
   - Loud, hostile, and sexual remarks to other clients

Planning

CONTENT LEVEL—PLANNING GOALS

Mr. Atkins formulated the following goals:

Nursing Diagnosis	Long Term Goals	Short Term Goals
1. *Potential for Injury* related to dehydration and faulty judgment, as evidenced by lack of awareness of safety precautions	Client's cardiac status will remain stable during manic phase.	1a. Client will be well hydrated, as evidenced by good skin turgor and normal urinary output and specific gravity within 24 hours.
		1b. Client will sleep/rest three hours during the first night in hospital, with the aid of medica-

Continued on following page

Planning (Continued)

		tion and nursing intervention. 1c. Client's blood pressure and pulse will be within the normal limits within 24 hours with the aid of medication and nursing measures.
2. *Ineffective Individual Coping* related to inadequate psychological resources, as evidenced by change in usual communication patterns.	Within three days, client will respond to external controls when aggression escalates.	2a. Client will engage in safe activities aimed at reducing aggressive energy within 24–48 hours.

PROCESS LEVEL—NURSES' REACTIONS AND FEELINGS

Mr. Atkins had worked on the psychiatric unit for two years. He had learned to deal with many of the challenging behaviors associated with the manic defense. For example, he no longer took most of the verbal insults personally, although many of the remarks could be very cutting and "close to home." He was also better able to recognize and set limits on some of the tactics used by the manic to split the staff. The staff on this unit worked very closely with each other, which made the atmosphere more positive and supportive, therefore communication was good among staff. Frequent and effective communication is needed when working with clients who try to split staff. Clear staff communication is vital in order to maximize external controls and maintain consistency in nursing care.

The only aspect of Mary's behavior that Mr. Atkins thought he might have some difficulty with was the sexual assaults and loud sexual comments she might make toward him. He knew that this could make him anxious, and his concern was that his anxiety might be picked up by the client.

When discussing this with the unit coordinator, they both decided that two nurses should provide care for Mary. A female nurse would spend time with Mary in her room, and Mr. Atkins would spend time with Mary in quiet areas on the unit. It was decided that neither Mr. Atkins nor any male staff member would be alone with Mary in her room at any time. Mr. Atkins should ask for relief if Mary's sexual remarks and acting-out behaviors were making him anxious.

Intervention

Since the most immediate concerns for Mary upon admission were those of physical safety, 400 mg of Thorazine intramuscularly was given immediately. Other clients were moved to provide Mary with a single room. Mary would not allow vital signs to be taken at first; however, eventually vital signs were taken and recorded at regular intervals. After two hours of pacing with Mary and coaxing Mary into less stimulating areas of the unit, she started taking some fluids. Within five hours she was drinking 8 ounces of high-caloric fluids per hour, after much reminding and encouragement.

By the next day, Mary's behaviors were much less hyperactive, and although her verbal sexual and aggressive assaults were less intense, she continued to provoke other clients. At this time, Mr. Atkins began to channel some of Mary's phsycial energy into less disruptive activities. He and Mary did some slow exercises to relaxing music in a quiet part of the unit; he provided writing paper for Mary, and she spent five to ten minutes writing furiously. She continued to pace and yell out to other clients, but with continued medication and nursing intervention, Mr. Atkins saw that this behavior was decreasing.

When Mary's sister came to visit, she brought clothes for Mary, and Mr. Atkins spent some time with the sister finding out more about Mary. He learned that Mary was a school teacher, had been depressed for three months prior to her first manic attack two years ago, and was recently coming out of her second depressive episode. Although the second depressive episode was less severe than the first, the sister was concerned that Mary would "do something foolish," meaning suicide. Mary was separated from her husband and was having a difficult time adjusting to being back at work.

Mr. Atkins and the female nurse encouraged Mary to dress and groom herself more appropriately, since some of the other clients were beginning to laugh at Mary because of her appearance. Mr Atkins was aware that ridicule could further lower Mary's self-esteem, thus increasing her anxiety and need for the manic defense.

Mary's behavior was beginning to be controlled by the lithium about 12 days later, and she was being weaned off Thorazine. At this time, Mary was able to talk to Mr. Atkins about how upset and depressed she was about her life (job and separation) and the fact that she had to take medication for the "rest of my life." See Nursing Care Plan 19–1.

Mr. Atkins reviewed the side effects and toxic effects of lithium and reviewed dietary and other precautions. At the end of her hospital stay, Mary stated that she was resigned to continuing her lithium. After talking to Mr. Atkins, she decided to re-enter therapy to "help me get back into life."

Evaluation

After two days, the medical staff thought Mary's cardiac status was stable. Her vital signs were within normal limits, she was taking in sufficient fluids, and her urinary output and specific gravity were normal. Although her hyperactivity persisted, it did so to a lesser degree, and she was able to get periods of rest during the day and was sleeping three to four hours during the night.

Mary's hyperactivity continued to be a challenge to the nurses; however, Mary was able to attend to some activities with the nurse that required gross motor movement and channeled some of her aggressive energy. Shortly after arrival to the unit, Mary had started a fight with another client, but seclusion was avoided since Mary was able to refrain from further violent episodes as a result of medication and nursing interventions. She could be directed toward solitary activities, which drained off some of her energies, at least for short periods of time.

As the effectiveness of the drugs progressed, Mary's activity level decreased, and by discharge she was able to discuss real issues of concern with the nurse and make some useful decisions about her future.

Nursing Care Plan 19–1 • A PERSON WITH MANIA: Mary

NURSING DIAGNOSIS

Potential for injury related to dehydration and faulty judgment, as evidenced by lack of awareness of safety precautions

Supporting Data

- Has not slept for days.
- Has not taken in food or fluids for days.
- Constant physical activity—is unable to sit.

Long Term Goal: Client's cardiac status will remain stable during manic phase.

Short Term Goal	*Intervention*	*Rationale*	*Evaluation*
1. Client will be well hydrated, as evidenced by good skin turgor and normal urinary output and specific gravity within 24 hours.	1a. Give Thorazine immediately and as needed.	1a. Continuous physical activity and lack of fluids can eventually lead to cardiac collapse and death.	Goal met After three hours Mary would take small amounts of fluids (2–4 ounces per hour).
	1b. Check vital signs frequently (every 15 minutes).	1b. Monitor cardiac status—Thorazine can lower blood pressure.	
	1c. Place client in private or quiet room (whenever possible).	1c. Reduce environmental stimuli—minimize escalation of mania and distractibility.	

Continued on following page

Nursing Care Plan 19-1 • A PERSON WITH MANIA: Mary *(Continued)*

Short Term Goal	*Intervention*	*Rationale*	*Evaluation*
	1d. Stay with client and divert away from stimulating situations.	1d. Provide support with nurse's presence. Ability to interact with others is temporarily impaired.	
	1e. Offer high-caloric high-protein drink (8 ounces) every hour in quiet area.	1e. Proper hydration is mandatory for maintaining cardiac status.	After five hours, Mary started taking 8 ounces per hour with a lot of reminding and encouragement.
	1f. Frequently remind client to drink: "Mary take two more sips."	1f. Client's concentration is poor; she is easily distracted.	
	1g. Offer finger food frequently in quiet area.	1g. Client is unable to sit; snacks she can eat while pacing are more likely to be consumed.	
	1h. Maintain record of intake and output.	1h. Enables staff to make accurate nutritional assessment for client's safety.	
	1i. Weigh client daily; take specific gravity at end of each shift as ordered.	1i. Monitor nutritional status.	Goal met After 24 hours, specific gravity as within normal limits.
2. Client will sleep/rest three hours during the first night in hospital with aid of medication and nursing intervention.	2a. Continue to direct client to areas of minimal activity.	2a. Lower levels of stimulation can decrease excitability.	Client awake most of first night. Slept for two hours from 4 A.M. to 6 A.M.
	2b. When possible, try to direct energy into productive and calming activities (pacing to slow, soft music; slow exercise; drawing alone; writing in quiet area, so forth).	2b. Directing client to paced, nonstimulating activities can help minimize excitability.	Was able to rest on second day for short periods and engage in quiet activities for short periods of time (5–10 minutes).
	2c. Encourage short rest periods throughout the day (e.g., 3–5 minutes every hour) when possible.	2c. Client may be unaware of feelings of fatigue. Can collapse from exhaustion if hyperactivity continues without periods of rest.	
	2d. Client should drink decaffeinated drinks only—decaffeinated coffee, teas, or colas.	2d. Caffeine is a CNS stimulant. Inhibits needed rest or sleep.	
	2e. Provide nursing measures at bedtime that promote sleep—warm milk, soft music, backrubs, and so forth.	2e. Promotes nonstimulating and relaxing mood.	
3. Client's blood pressure (BP) and pulse (P) will be within normal limits within 24 hours with the aid of medication and nursing interventions.	3a. Continue to monitor blood pressure and pulse frequently throughout the day (every 30 minutes).	3a. Physical condition is presently a great strain on client's heart. Thorazine can lower blood pressure. Since client will be getting frequent intramuscular doses of Thorazine for next 24 hours, close monitoring is needed to maintain client safety.	Baseline on unit not obtained owing to hyperactive behavior. Information from family physician stated BP 130/90 and P 88 baseline.
	3b. Keep staff informed by verbal and written reports of baseline vital signs and client progress.	3b. Alerting all staff regarding client status can increase medical intervention if a change in status occurs.	BP at end of 24 hours 130/70; P 80.

NURSING DIAGNOSIS

Ineffective individual coping related to inadequate psychological resources, as evidenced by change in usual communication patterns

Supporting Data

- Remarks suggested sexual themes.
- Some clients found her behavior amusing.
- Remarks suggested grandiose thinking.
- Flight of ideas.
- Loud hostile and sexual remarks to other clients.

Long Term Goal: Within three days, client will respond to external controls when aggression escalates.

Short Term Goal	*Intervention*	*Rationale*	*Evaluation*
1. Client will engage in safe activities to drain off hostile and aggressive energy within 24–48 hours with aid of medication and nursing interventions.	1a. Maintain a calm and matter-of-fact (neutral) attitude.	1a. Anxiety can be transmitted from staff to client.	Goal partially met Six hours after admission, client started fight with another client. Staff explained that seclusion might be needed to help her gain control over her behavior.
	1b. Avoid power struggles and defensive postures when client is verbally abusive.	1b. Client does not mean abuse personally; it is part of manic defense. Power struggles and defensive remarks by staff can escalate mania and potentiate acting out violently.	
	1c. Set limits and provide controls when necessary, e.g., "Mary, you are not to hit George. Come with me now." or "If you have trouble controlling yourself, we will help you."	1c. When client is out of control, external controls are needed to prevent client from acting out violently.	
	1d. Engage client in solitary activities that use large muscle groups (punching bag, ping-pong, pacing with nurse, exercise).	1d. Activities client can do alone or with nurse that require large muscle groups can help drain physical tension.	2nd day, client able to participate with nurse in solitary activities using large muscle groups for short periods of time (5–10 minutes).

Summary

Genetic factors appear to play a role in the etiology of the bipolar disorder. However, the outward gaiety and expansive self-confident facade of a manic client is seen as an attempt to keep feelings of depression out of awareness. Mania can be observed on a continuum from hypomania to actute mania.

The three main features of mania are (1) euphoria, (2) hyperactivity, and (3) flight of ideas. The nurse assesses the client's mood, behavior, and thought processes in order to plan the appropriate nursing interventions.

The analysis of the data helps the nurse choose appropriate nursing diagnoses. Some of the nursing diagnoses appropriate for a client who is manic are *potential for violence, ineffective individual coping, altered thought processes*, and *self-esteem disturbance*. Physical needs often take priority and demand nursing interventions. Therefore, *fluid volume deficit, altered nutrition*, or *elimination*, as well as *sleep pattern disturbance*, are usually part of the nursing plan. *Altered family process* is a very important consideration. Support, information, and guidance for the family can greatly affect the client's eventual recovery from his or her manic episode.

Planning nursing care involves setting realistic and measurable short term and long term goals for each of the nursing diagnoses. It is helpful for the nurse to understand that the manic symptoms help keep painful feelings out of awareness. Therefore, the client will go to great lengths to prevent outside controls from limiting manic flight. The manic client has a number of unconscious tactics to keep the nursing staff defensive, divided, and confused. When these tactics are successful, staff are less able to set consistent limits and monitor erratic behaviors. Unconscious tactics include splitting members of the staff against each other through manipulation, loudly and persistently pointing to faults and shortcomings in staff, constantly demanding attention and favors of the staff, and provoking clients as well as staff with profane and lewd remarks. The manic client is constantly distracting activities and groups with his or her continuous physical motion and incessant joking and talking. The feelings aroused in such situations are usually ones of anger and frustration toward the client. When these feelings are not examined and shared, the therapeutic potential of the staff is reduced, and feelings of confusion and helplessness remain.

Working with a manic client can be challenging. Interventions involve using specific principles of therapeutic communications, assisting with activities of daily living and somatic therapies, maintaining a therapeutic environment, and when certified, intervening as a nurse therapist.

Evaluation includes examining the effectiveness of the nursing interventions, changing the goals as needed, and reassessing the nursing diagnoses. Evaluation is an ongoing process and is part of each of the other steps in the nursing process.

References

American Psychiatric Association. Diagnostic and Statistical Manual of Mental Disorders, 3rd ed., revised. Washington DC: American Psychiatric Association, 1987.

Arieti S. Affective disorders: Manic-depressive psychosis and psychotic depression. *In* Arieti S (ed). American Handook of Psychiatry, 2nd ed. New York: Basic Books, 1974.

Baradell JC. Humanistic care of the patient in seclusion. Journal of Psychosocial Nursing, 23(2):9, 1985.

Bergersen BS. Pharmacology in Nursing. St. Louis: C.V. Mosby Company, 1979.

Campbell L. Hopelessness. Journal of Psychosocial Nursing, 25(2):18, 1987.

Cancro R. Overview of affective disorders. *In* Kaplan HI, Sadock BJ (eds). Comprehensive Textbook of Psychiatry, 4th ed. Baltimore, MD: Williams & Wilkins, 1985.

Carson R, Butcher JN, Coleman JC. Abnormal psychology and modern life. Glenview, IL: Scott, Foresman & Company, 1988.

Chapman AH. Textbook of Clinical Psychiatry, 2nd ed. Philadelphia: J.B. Lippincott Company, 1976.

DePaulo JR. Lithium. Psychiatric Clinics of North America, 7(3):587, 1984.

Fitzgerald RG, Long I. Seclusion in the treatment and management of disturbed manic and depressed patients. Perspectives in Psychiatric Care, 11:59, 1973.

Gershon ES, Nuenberger JI, Berretitini WH, Goldin LR. Affective disorder genetics. *In* Kaplan HI, Sadock BJ (eds). Comprehensive Textbook of Psychiatry, 4th ed. Baltimore, MD: Williams & Wilkins, 1985.

Gitlin MJ, Jamison KR. Lithium clinics: Theory and practice. Hospital and Community Psychiatry, 35:363, 1984.

Goldstein MJ, Baker BL, Jamison KR. Abnormal psychology: Experiences, origins and interventions. Boston: Little Brown & Company, 1980.

Goodwin DW, Guze SB. Psychiatric Diagnosis. New York: Oxford University Press, 1984.

Harris E. Lithium: in a class by itself. American Journal of Nursing, 89:190, 1989.

Hart CA, Turner MS, Orfitelli MK, Applebaum B. Introduction to psychotropic drugs. New York: Medical Examination Publishing Company, 1981.

Hinsie LE, Campbell RJ. Psychiatric Dictionary, 4th ed. New York: Oxford University Press, 1973.

Hirschfeld RMA, Goodwin FK. Mood disorders. *In* Talbott JA, Hales RE, Yudofsky SC (eds). Textbook of Psychiatry. Washington, DC: The American Psychiatric Press, 1988.

Jamison KR, Goodwin FK. Psychotherapeutic treatment of manic-depressive patients on lithium. *In* Greenhill M, Gralnick A (eds). New York: Macmillan Company, 1983.

Karb VB, Queener SF, Freeman JB. Handbook of Drugs for Nursing Practice. St. Louis: C.V. Mosby Company, 1989.

Klerman GL. Affective disorders. *In* Nicholi AM Jr. (ed). The Harvard Guide to Modern Psychiatry. Cambridge, MA: Belknap Press of Harvard University Press, 1978.

Lickey ME, Gordon B. Drugs for mental illness, a revolution in psychiatry. New York: W.H. Freeman & Company, 1983.

Roper JM, et al. Restraint and seclusion. Journal of Psychosocial Nursing, 23(6):18, 1985.

Schatzberg AF, Cole JO, Manual of Clinical Psychopharmacology. Washington DC: American Psychiatric Press, 1986.

Scherer JC. Nurses' drug manual. Philadelphia: J.B. Lippincott Company, 1985.

Weissman MM, Boyd JH. Affective disorders; epidemiology. *In* Kaplan HI, Sadock BJ (eds). Comprehensive Textbook of Psychiatry, 4th ed. Baltimore, MD: Williams & Wilkins, 1985.

Self-Study Exercises

Choose the most appropriate answer.

1. All of the following may be observed in a person who is manic except:

   A. "Hey baby, don't baby me . . . me and you can have some fun, fun and games and sugar and spice . . . "
   B. Quick short periods of anger, quickly changing to another euphoria or depression.
   C. Splitting staff members against each other in order to prevent controls upon his or her manic defense.
   D. Although thoughts may be fast, thoughts are never illogical or irrational.

2. Mrs. Jack has been on lithium for months. Her most recent blood level was 2.2 mEq/l. What reactions might the nurse expect to see?

A. Fine hand tremors, mild thirst, and polyuria. S/E
B. Diarrhea, vomiting, and slurred speech.
C. Electroencephalographic changes, ataxia, and seizures.
D. No untoward effects, since her blood level is within normal limits.

Complete the nursing diagnosis by filling in the related factor(s). For the nursing diagnosis presented, give two pieces of data that would support the diagnosis for a manic client.

3. Potential for injury related to ______________ as evidenced by:
   Data 1 ______________
   Data 2 ______________
4. Impaired verbal communication related to ______________ as evidenced by:
   Data 1 ______________
   Data 2 ______________
5. Altered family process related to ______________ as evidenced by:
   Data 1 ______________
   Data 2 ______________

For each of the preceding nursing diagnoses, state one long term and two short term goals.

6. Potential for injury:
   LTG: ______________
   STG: ______________
   STG: ______________
7. Impaired verbal communication:
   LTG: ______________
   STG: ______________
   STG: ______________
8. Altered family process:
   LTG: ______________
   STG: ______________
   STG: ______________

Identify four unconscious tactics used by a manic client in order that he or she may disrupt the environment and maximize the manic defense.

9. ______________
10. ______________
11. ______________
12. ______________

Name two interventions for each of the following areas, giving the rationale for the action.

13. Nutrition:
    1. ______
    2. ______
    Rationales: ______
14. Rest and sleep:
    1. ______
    2. ______
    Rationales: ______
15. Dress and hygiene:
    1. ______
    2. ______
    Rationales: ______
16. Activities and recreation:
    1. ______
    2. ______
    Rationales: ______

List at least three cautions a person on lithium should know.

17. ______
18. ______
19. ______

Name three indications for seclusion.

20. ______
21. ______
22. ______

Place an H (Helpful) or NH (Not Helpful) for each of the statements made by the nurse to a manic client.

23. ______ "Tom come with me to the quiet room."
24. ______ "Comb the left side of your head . . . now the right side."
25. ______ "That's a funny joke, Tom . . . have you heard this one?"
26. ______ "I know the other nurses don't want you to join this group, but I'll let you."
27. ______ "I don't like those remarks. They aren't true, and that kind of behavior is disgusting."
28. ______ "Come away from this group. Let's write instead."

CHAPTER 20

Schizophrenic Disorders

Elizabeth M. Varcarolis

OUTLINE

KEY TERMS AND CONCEPTS

The key terms and concepts listed here also appear in bold where they are defined or discussed in this chapter.

DOUBLE BIND MESSAGE
SCAPEGOATING
AFFECT
ASSOCIATIVE LOOSENESS
DECODE
AMBIVALENCE
AUTISM
IDEAS OF REFERENCE
HALLUCINATIONS
DELUSIONS
NEOLOGISMS
FANTASY
STUPOR
WAXY FLEXIBILITY
EXTREME MOTOR AGITATION
ECHOPRAXIA
STEREOTYPED BEHAVIORS
ILLUSIONS
AUTOMATIC OBEDIENCE
NEGATIVISM
CONCRETE THINKING
DEPERSONALIZATION
DEREALIZATION
ECHOLALIA
CLANG ASSOCIATION
WORD SALAD
EXTRAPYRAMIDAL SIDE EFFECTS
ACUTE DYSTONIA
AKATHISIA
PSEUDOPARKINSONISM
TARDIVE DYSKINESIA
NEUROLEPTIC MALIGNANT SYNDROME
NEUROLEPTIC (ANTIPSYCHOTIC) MEDICATIONS
PARANOIA
BLOCKING
CONSENSUAL VALIDATION

OBJECTIVES

After studying this chapter, the student will be able to:

1. Discuss the progression of the disorders known as schizophrenia.
2. Compare four theories that explain the etiology of schizophrenia.
3. Give examples of affect, associative looseness, autism, and ambivalence.
4. Give two examples of (a) withdrawal, (b) disturbance in behavior, (c) disturbance in thinking, and (d) disturbance in speech patterns as they relate to the schizophrenic disorders.
5. Formulate three possible nursing diagnoses appropriate for a person with schizophrenia.
6. Describe three countertransference reactions a nurse may experience with a schizophrenic client.
7. Act out interventions for a client who is (a) hallucinating, (b) delusional, and (c) demonstrating looseness of associations.
8. Explain three areas of health teaching appropriate for a family with a schizophrenic member.
9. Discuss four desired effects of the antipsychotic drugs.
10. Assess six side effects of antipsychotic medication and the nursing intervention for each.
11. Identify six positive outcomes of group work that nurses can do in the hospital setting.

12. Identify the kind of individual, group, and family therapies most useful for schizophrenic clients and their families.
13. Discuss how frequent evaluation of a schizophrenic client's nursing care plan can improve nursing skills and client progress.
14. Give the rationale for five specific interventions useful for each of the following: (a) paranoid schizophrenia, (b) catatonic schizophrenia, and (c) disorganized schizophrenia.

"Then the world became embryonic in Africa—and there was no need for communication . . . I have been living in vaporous places peopled with one-dimensional figures and tremulous buildings until I can no longer tell an optical illusion from a reality . . . that head and ears incessantly throb and roads disappear" (Vidal 1982; written by Zelda Fitzgerald to her husband, the writer Scott Fitzgerald, in an account of going "mad").

Schizophrenia is a psychotic disorder. It is marked by a profound withdrawal from interpersonal relationships and a retreat into a world of fantasy. This flight into fantasy results in a loss of contact from reality that can vary from mild to severe (Chapman 1976).

There is no one acceptable definition for psychosis. The psychoses differ from other groups of psychiatric disorders in their degree of (1) severity, (2) withdrawal, (3) alteration in affect, (4) impairment of intellect, and (5) regression (Hinsie and Cambell 1981).

SEVERITY. The psychoses are considered major disorders and involve disruptions in all segments of a person's life. Psychosis is seen in the major mood disorders, a wide range of organic disorders, and schizophrenia. These disorders are severe, intense, and disruptive. The person with a psychotic disorder suffers greatly, as do those in his immediate environment.

WITHDRAWAL. Withdrawal is so severe in psychosis that psychotic individuals are said to be autistic. That is, the person withdraws from reality into a private world. The psychotic individual is more withdrawn than a person with a neurotic disorder, personality disorder, psychophysiological disorder, or any other mental disorder.

AFFECT. The affect, mood, or emotional tone in a person with a psychotic disorder is vastly different from that of "normal" affect. In the mood disorders (see Chapters 18 and 19), one observes the exaggeration of sadness and lightheartedness in the form of depression and mania, respectively. In the schizophrenic disorders, affect may be exaggerated, flat, or inappropriate.

INTELLECT. In psychotic disorders, the intellect is involved in the actual psychotic process, resulting in disturbances of language, thought, and judgment. Schizophrenia is called a formal thought disorder. Thinking and perceptions of reality are usually severely impaired.

REGRESSION. The most severe and prolonged regressions are seen in the psychoses. There is a falling back to earlier behavioral levels. In schizophrenia this may include returning to primitive forms of behavior, such as curling up in a fetal position, eating with one's hands, and so forth.

In 1886 Emil Kraepelin first recognized that a number of clinical syndromes could be seen as one specific disease, which Kraepelin called dementia praecox. Today we call these disorders schizophrenia. Freud viewed schizophrenia as untreatable by psychotherapeutic methods. Sullivan and Fromm-Reichmann, however, engaged in extensive psychoanalytical work with schizophrenic persons. Sullivan believed schizophrenia to be the result of destructive experience with significant others during the formative years of life. Today increased research is being conducted in the biological, genetic, and neuropathological realms in order to find a singular explanation for schizophrenia.

Recent data from the National Institute of Mental Health show that 1 in 100 people (that is, 1% of the general population) have or will suffer from the symptoms of schizophrenia (Roy 1986). People with schizophrenia occupy about 50% of the hospital beds for the mentally ill and about 25% of all available hospital beds (Merck Manual 1987).

The symptoms of schizophrenia usually become manifest during adolescence or early adulthood, except for paranoid schizophrenia, which usually has a later onset. The process of schizophrenia is often slow, with the exception of catatonia, which may have an abrupt onset.

As an adolescent, a person who later develops schizophrenia is often withdrawn from others, lonely, and perhaps depressed. Plans for the future may appear to others as vague or unrealistic (Kolb and Brodie 1982).

There may be a transitional "preschizophrenic" phase a year or two before the disorder is diagnosed. This phase may include neurotic symptoms such as acute or chronic anxiety, phobias, obsessions, and compulsions or may reveal dissociative features (Chapman 1976). As anxiety mounts, indications of a thought disorder may be present. An adolescent may complain of difficulty with concentration and with the ability to complete school work or job-related work. Eventually there is severe deterioration of work along with the deterioration of the ability to cope with the environment. Such complains as mind wandering and needing to devote more time to maintaining one's thoughts are heard. Finally, the ability to keep out unwanted intrusions into one's thoughts becomes impossible. Eventually, the person finds that his mind becomes so confused and thoughts so distracted, that the ability to have ordinary conversations with others is lost (Kolb and Brodie 1982).

The person may initially feel that something strange or wrong is going on. He misinterprets things going on in his environment and may give mystical or symbolic meanings to ordinary events. For example, he may think that certain colors hold special powers, or that a thunderstorm is a message from God. The person often mistakes other people's actions or words as signs of hostility or evidence of harmful intent.

As the disease develops, the person suffers from strong feelings of rejection, lack of self-respect, loneliness, and feelings of hopelessness. Emotional and physical withdrawal increase feelings of isolation, as does an inability to trust or relate to others. The withdrawal may become severe, and withdrawal from reality may become evident in hallucinations, delusions, and odd mannerisms. Some persons think their thoughts are being controlled by others or that their thoughts are being broadcast to the world. Others may think that people are out to harm them or are spreading rumors about them. Voices are most often heard in the form of commands or derogatory statements about their character. The voices may seem to appear from outside the room, from electrical appliances, or from other sources.

Early in the disease, there may be preoccupation with religion, matters of mysticism, or metaphysical causes of creation. Speech may be characterized by obscure symbolisms. Later, words and phrases may become indecipherable, and these can be understood only as part of the person's private fantasy world. Sometimes the person makes up words. People who have been ill with schizophrenia for a long time often have speech patterns that are incoherent and rambling and devoid of meaning to the casual observer.

Sexual activity is frequently altered in mental disorders. Homosexual concerns may be associated with all psychoses but are most prominent with paranoia. Doubts regarding sexual identity, exaggerated sexual needs, altered sexual performance and fears of intimacy are prominent in schizophrenia. The process of regression in schizophrenia is accompanied by increased self-preoccupation, isolation, and masturbatory behavior (Donlon 1976).

The schizophrenic person finds himself in a painful dilemma. He retreats from personal intimacy or closeness because of his intense fear that closeness will be followed by subsequent rejection or harm. However, this retreat from others leaves him lonely and isolated.

This dilemma often becomes the nurse's dilemma. The nurse wishes to establish a constructive emotional bond but at the same time seeks to diminish the client's anxiety. For the schizophrenic person, moves toward emotional closeness will inevitably increase anxiety.

Prior to the 1950's, prior to the advent of antipsychotic drugs, the prognosis for schizophrenia was poor. Today, the outlook is much brighter. With good follow-up therapy and well-controlled maintenance drug treatment, only 10 to 15% of clients in remission relapse within a year, compared with 65 to 70% of relapses without such treatment (Lehmann and Cancro 1985). The less adherence there is to following a medical maintenance program, the greater the possibility of relapse.

Usually, an abrupt onset is a favorable prognostic sign. A slow insidious onset over a period of two or three years is more ominous. Those whose prepsychotic personalities show good social, sexual, and occupational functioning have greater chances for a good remission or a complete recovery. Childhood histories of withdrawn, seclusive, eccentric, and tense behavior is

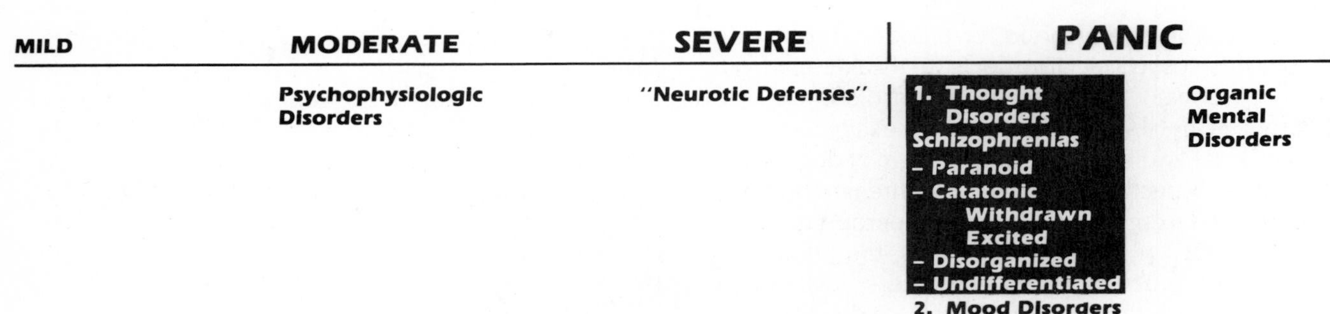

Figure 20–1. *Schizophrenic disorders on the Anxiety Continuum.*

an unfavorable diagnostic sign. The younger the client is at the onset of schizophrenia, the more discouraging the prognosis. Interestingly, the presence of depression often signifies a better prognosis (Lehmann and Cancro 1985).

Since schizophrenia is a psychotic disorder, it is placed on the high end of the anxiety continuum (Fig. 20–1). Using anxiety as a framework, we can conceptualize the schizophrenic disorders as shown in Figure 20–2.

Early psychiatric and medical treatment helps secure a more favorable eventual outcome. A delay in terms of months or years allows the psychotic process to become more entrenched (Chapman 1976). No single symptom is always present in all cases of schizophrenia or occurs only in schizophrenia alone (Harvard Medical School 1986). The different DSM III-R syndromes of schizophrenia with symptoms are outlined in Figure 20–3. The first section of this chapter deals with the basic symptoms of schizophrenia. The remaining sections discuss paranoia, catatonia, and disorganized schizophrenia.

Standard I: Theory

Many diverse theories of schizophrenia have been hypothesized by scholars from a variety of disciplines. As mentioned, the DSM III-R (APA 1987) presents schizophrenia as a group of disorders of differing etiologies. Furthermore, there is no consensus in the literature as to what is meant by the classification "schizophrenia" (Weiner 1985). Schizophrenia is most reliably classified by a cluster of symptoms and signs, no one of which is specific only to schizophrenia (Weiner 1985). The process of schizophrenia appears complex, and the etiology is perhaps dependent upon a variety of factors. Most cases are thought to be a complex interaction between inherited and environmental factors.

There are numerous hypotheses relating to the etiology of schizophrenia. Basically, these hypotheses can be divided into two general categories: (1) The biological models are those that regard schizophrenia as primarily biological in origin, and (2) the environmental models believe that the origin of schizophrenia is rooted in environmental factors (Merck Manual 1987).

BIOLOGICAL MODELS

The most commonly accepted biological models are the (1) dopamine hypothesis, (2) genetic hypotheses, and (3) neuroanatomical studies.

Dopamine Hypothesis

Bioamines (brain enzymes) are neurotransmitters to those areas of the brain that mediate emotions, feelings of pleasure and pain, awareness, levels of consciousness, and more. These bioamines are broken down into the following categories (Rickelman 1979):

Catecholamines	Indolamine
Epinephrine	Serotonin
Dopamine	
Norepinephrine	

The presence of high levels of metabolites (products of metabolism) of the brain bioamines has been found in the urine of clients who are frankly psychotic. When the symptoms worsen, the level of metabolites of catecholamines and indolamine increases in the client's urine.

The dopamine theory of schizophrenia is based on the action of the neuroleptic drugs (antipsychotic drugs). Neuroleptics are the drugs of choice for treating the symptoms of schizophrenia. The neuroleptics are believed to block the dopamine receptors in the brain, thereby limiting the activity of dopamine and reducing

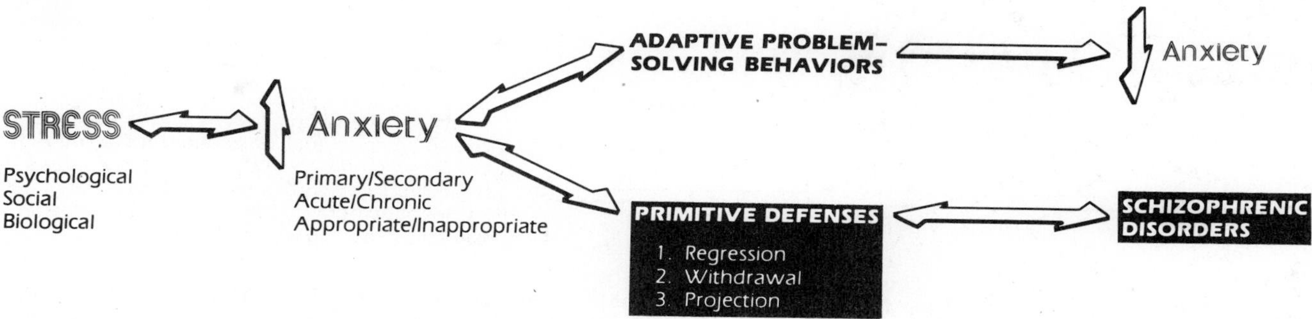

Figure 20–2. *Conceptualization of the Process of Schizophrenia.*

DSM III–R CHART OF SCHIZOPHRENIC DISORDERS

Key diagnostic criteria include the following:

A. Presence of psychotic symptoms in Active Stage 1, 2, or 3 for at least one week.

1. Two of the following:
- **a.** Delusions
- **b.** Hallucinations—prominent—lasting several days or occurring several times a week
- **c.** Incoherence, loosening of association, poverty of content of speech, markedly illogical thinking
- **d.** Catatonic behavior
- **e.** Flat or inappropriate affect

2. Bizarre delusions (e.g., thought broadcasting, being controlled by a dead person)

3. Prominent hallucinations (e.g., auditory—voice of running commentary on things that are happening, two voices talking to each other)

B. Funtioning in work, social relations, and self-care markedly below highest level achieved before onset of the disturbance; not due to any organic mental disorder, mental retardation, or other mental disorders

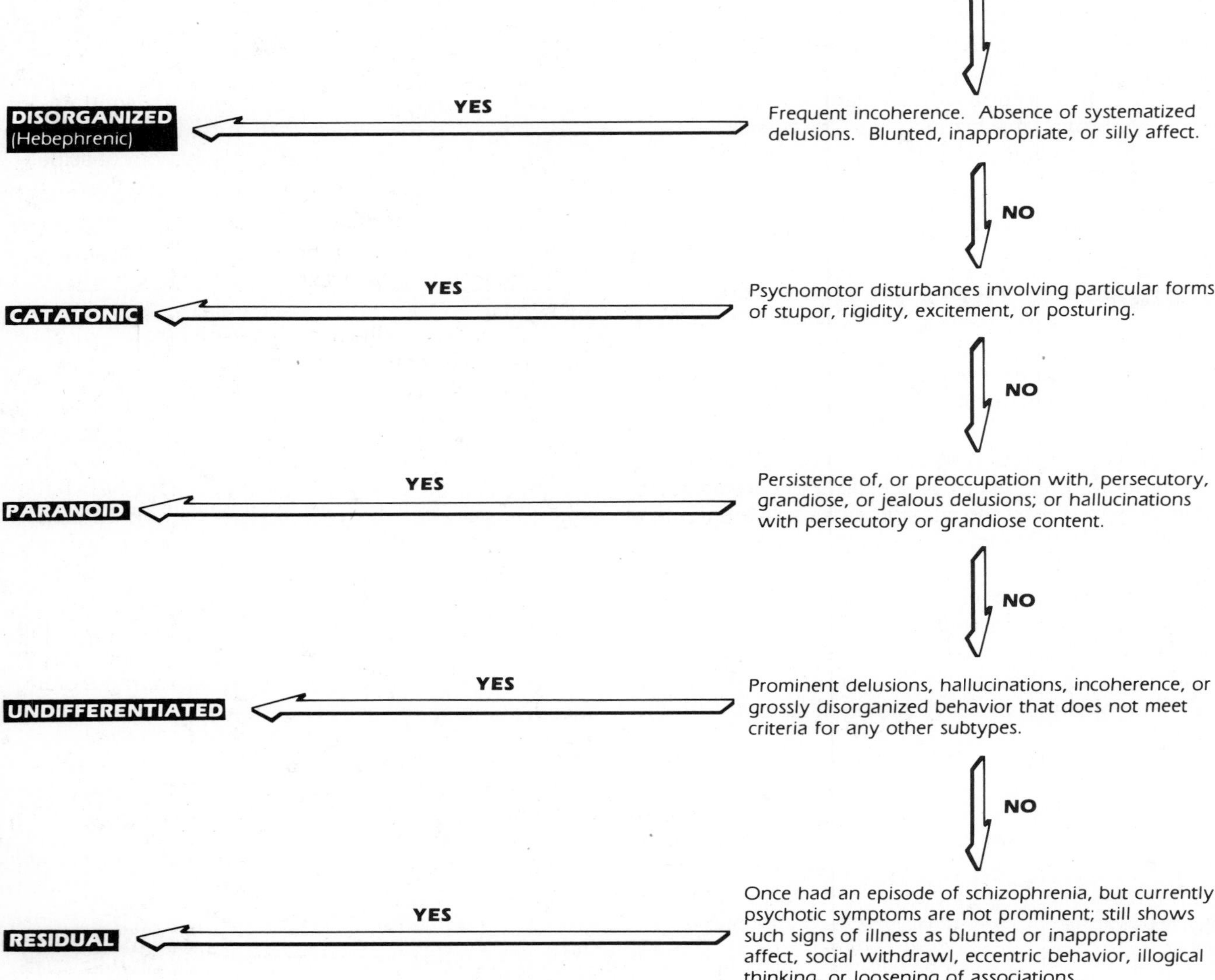

Figure 20–3. *Decision tree for the schizophrenic disorders.* (*Adapted from* Janicak PG, Andriukaitis SN. DSM III: *Seeing the Forest Through the Trees. Psychiatric Annals,* 10(8):17, 1980, *and* Diagnostic and Statistical Manual of Mental Disorders [DSM III-R], *3d ed., revised.* Washington DC: American Psychiatric Association, 1987.)

the symptoms of schizophrenia (Black et al 1988). Amphetamines, on the other hand, enhance dopamine transmission. Amphetamines produce an excess of dopamine in the brain and can exacerbate the symptoms of schizophrenia in a schizophrenic client. In large doses, amphetamines can simulate symptoms of paranoid schizophrenia in a nonschizophrenic person. Crow (1980) suggests that some of the symptoms of schizophrenia (e.g., delusions, hallucinations, and thought disorders) are due primarily to hyperdopaminergic activity. Other symptoms, such as apathy and poverty of thought, are related to neuronal loss.

Genetic Hypotheses

Gottesman and Shield (1982) summarized the contribution of genetic studies in the literature to support the genetic hypotheses of schizophrenia. For example:

1. Identical twins. Concordance rate (co-twin similarly affected) for schizophrenia is 35 to 60% greater than that of the general population.
2. Identical twin concordance is three times that of fraternal twins.
3. Children of schizophrenics placed early for nonfamilial adoption develop schizophrenia as adults at higher rates than the general population.
4. Children of "normal" parents placed in foster homes in which a foster parent later developed schizophrenia do not show an increased rate of schizophrenia.

No individual schizophrenic gene has been identified. Genes may be necessary as a predisposing factor to schizophrenia (Gottesman and Shield, 1982; Black et al 1988).

Neuroanatomical Studies

New technology has been able to support the hypothesis that the symptoms in schizophrenia may be linked to some type of functional or structural brain abnormality. The new brain imaging techniques, including computed tomography (CT), magnetic resonance imaging (MRI), and positron emission tomography (PET), identify substantial evidence that some schizophrenics have structural brain abnormalities (Black et al. 1988).

The most common finding is ventricular enlargement. Cerebellar atrophy is also a frequent finding. Some evidence associates ventricular enlargement with poor premorbid functioning, poor response to treatment, and cognitive impairment (Black et al 1988).

ENVIRONMENTAL MODELS

The most prominent theoretical models in this group are the developmental model and the family theory model.

Developmental Model

Harry Stack Sullivan (1953) developed the interpersonal theory for the development of schizophrenia. Sullivan proposed that when an infant grows up in an environment of tenderness, consistent care, warmth, and respect in an atmosphere of minimal anxiety, the child incorporates these values into his sense of self, or ego. Peplau states that when these conditions are met, the child grows to see himself as someone worthy of respect and love. The world is perceived as positive. The child can trust that his needs will be met and the environment is safe and secure. This sense of trust stimulates growth (Field 1979).

When hostility, inconsistency of care, ridicule, and rejection are communicated toward the infant, trust in the environment is never achieved. The world is perceived as a frightening, hostile, and dangerous place. The child's innate trust toward growth becomes thwarted.

According to Sullivan, each person maintains contact with reality by consistently checking feelings, thoughts, and actions through interpersonal relationships. Initially, the infant validates reality with the mothering one. As the child grows, validating one's perceptions involves more people. This reality checking of thoughts, feelings, and actions with others Sullivan calls **consensual validation** (Chapman 1976).

If a child grows up in an environment of fear and anxiety, the chances to validate feelings, thoughts, and behaviors are decreased. The child's ability to perceive reality will be greatly impaired. Therefore, a personality deficit or schizophrenia might result.

Family Theory Model

Family factors originally proposed have not been supported by systematic clinical investigation, and parental influences are no longer considered to be a cause of schizophrenia. However, the family influence on the course of the illness is now an interactive study (Black et al 1988). For example, schizophrenic clients who come from families who are highly critical, hostile, or overinvolved tend to relapse more than those who come from families that are supportive (Falloon 1986).

Two phenomena observed in excess among some schizophrenic families will be presented briefly: these are double bind communication and scapegoating.

DOUBLE BIND COMMUNICATION. The double bind is a form of disturbed communication that takes place within schizophrenic families. Although the double bind form of communication may take place in all families, it is thought to be excessive among schizophrenic families.

A **double bind message** contains two contradictory messages given by the same person at the same time, to which the receiver is expected to respond. Most often the receiver is a child. Constant double bind situations result in feelings of helplessness, fear, and anxiety in the receiver of the double bind messages.

Message	Example
1. An overt message is given, indicating a command or threat to reply.	"Come, give your mother a kiss."
2. A covert message (posture, gesture, tone of voice) implies the opposite.	Mother stiffens and turns head in disgust as child approaches.
3. The person is left in a no-win situation. If he responds to the verbal message, he gets rejected. If he responds to the covert message, he gets reprimanded.	After a period of constant double bind messages, the child feels paralyzed to act.

SCAPEGOATING. Murray Bowen's work with schizophrenic families (1978) revealed profound emotional distance between parents of schizophrenic children. He found that often the parents experienced loneliness, feelings of isolation, and emptiness. Feelings of helplessness, inadequacy, and poor self-esteem can trigger painful levels of anxiety. Many of these parents project personal feelings of pain and anxiety onto an event, situation, or person outside the self. For example, instead of acknowledging the anxiety-provoking feelings of emptiness and poor self-esteem, the couple projects inner problems onto outward events (e.g., the wife projects the cause of her feelings of isolation and loneliness on the "fact" that the husband pays more attention to television sports that he does to her). The husband defends against his feelings of emptiness and despair by projecting the root of these feelings on the "fact" that his wife appears to care more for her job than for her family.

Scapegoating comes in when the child is the focus of the pain and anxiety within the family. For example, the mother denies her own feelings of inadequacy and helplessness and projects these feelings onto the child. The child then becomes the target of the mother's painful feelings. The *child* is now perceived as inadequate and helpless by the whole family. The mother's projections are then perceived as a reality. The feelings that began in the mother become a reality in the child (Bowen 1978). Therefore the child becomes the "identified client" or scapegoat for the problems of the parents. The focus of attention onto the child's "problems" relieves the tension between the parents and helps to repress the painful feelings within the parents.

Family studies do suggest that the family life of schizophrenic persons is disturbed. However, a clear etiological relationship between family pathology and schizophrenia has not been established (Weiner 1985; Black et al 1988).

Standard II: Data Collection

A group of symptoms identifies the schizophrenia syndrome (Lehmann and Cancro 1985). Many of the signs and symptoms of schizophrenia are presented below and will become evident when working with people diagnosed as schizophrenic.

Bleuler's fundamental signs of schizophrenia, referred to as the four A's, will be presented here as the primary symptoms in schizophrenia. Other characteristic clinical features of schizophrenia will be presented as the secondary symptoms of schizophrenia.

ASSESSING PRIMARY SYMPTOMS OF SCHIZOPHRENIA

At the end of the nineteenth century, Eugene Bleuler described four fundamental signs of schizophrenia that are still used by clinicians today. The four A's include (1) affect, (2) associative looseness, (3) ambivalence, and (4) autism.

Affect

Affect is the feeling tone a person experiences during a specific period of time. It is sometimes referred to as mood or emotion. The affect of a schizophrenic person usually falls into one of three categories: flat or blunted, inappropriate, or bizarre.

In a *flat or blunted affect* there is no show of emotions. The tone of voice may be a monotone, and the response appears mechanical. Feelings and emotions are deeply repressed. The person with schizophrenia is very much out of touch with his painful feelings.

Inappropriate affect is also commonly seen in schizophrenia. Inappropriate affect refers to an emotional response to a situation which is not congruent with the tone of the situation. For example, a young man, told that his father is ill, breaks out laughing. Ambivalence may play a role in neutralizing feelings.

Bizarre affect is especially prominent in the disorganized form of schizophrenia. Grimacing, giggling, and mumbling to oneself come under this heading. Bizarre affect is marked when there is inability to relate logically to the environment.

Associative Looseness

Associations are the threads that tie one thought to another and one concept to another. In schizophrenia, these threads are missing, and the connections become interrupted. In **associative looseness,** thinking becomes haphazard, illogical, and confused (Hinsie and Cambell 1981). An example follows:

NURSE: Are you going to the picnic today?
CLIENT: Only five dollars at the top.

Initially, this client's response is not in keeping with the question asked by the nurse. However, to the client, his response has meaning. This young man always referred to his emotional security in dollars and cents. When he was feeling secure and confident, he spoke of himself as having plenty of money: "I have $500.00 at the top." At times, the nurse may be able to decipher or **decode** the client's messages and begin to understand the client's feelings and needs. Any exchange in which a person feels understood is useful. Therefore the nurse might respond to the client in this way:

NURSE: Are you saying, Tony, that you don't feel secure enough to go out with the others today?
CLIENT: Yeah . . . not much at the top today.

If the nurse does not understand what the client is saying, it is important to let the client know this. Clear messages and complete honesty are an important part of the work with schizophrenic persons. Letting the person know *you don't understand* but *would like to understand*, or you *will try to understand*, is honest. If the nurse is confused by the client's message but indicates understanding, the nurse contributes to increasing this type of message. The client then sees no reason to change his communication (Cook 1971).

Ambivalence

Ambivalence is defined as holding, at the same time, two opposing emotions, attitudes, ideas, or wishes toward the same person, situation, or object (Hinsie and Cambell 1981). Ambivalence occurs normally in all relationships throughout life. In the adult, only part of the ambivalent feeling is conscious; the other part of the feeling often remains unconscious. Pathological ambivalence is paralyzing and incongruous. Normal ambivalence is part of the mixed emotions of everyday life (Arieti 1974). Two examples of ambivalence follow:

Joan, a schizophrenic girl, waits by the door of the unit every Thursday, the day "her student nurse" comes. When the student nurse comes into the unit, Joan hides in her room or bathroom. Joan is acting out her ambivalence between her need for human relationships and her fear of relating.

Sam, a 25-year-old man soon to be discharged from the hospital, constantly tells the social worker he wants his own apartment. When Sam was told that an apartment had been found for him, he stated "But who will take care of me?" Sam is acting out his ambivalence between his desire to be independent and his desire to be taken care of.

Autism

Bleuler described **autism** as a type of thinking that is not bound to reality, but follows the inner fantasy world of the individual (Hinsie and Cambell 1981). Autistic thinking is not only found in schizophrenics but also is used by healthy adults as well as by children when at play. A healthy person is aware, however, that his thoughts are private, may be illogical, and are not based upon reality. He can relate his fantasies or daydreams to others. Pathological examples of autistic thinking follow:

1. **Ideas of reference** are false impressions that outside events have special meanings for oneself.

   James hears on the radio that it is going to snow. He takes that as a sign that the FBI is going to kill him.

2. **Delusions** are fixed ideas. See Table 20–1 for types of delusions with examples.

   James *thinks* the FBI is going to kill him.

3. **Hallucinations** are false sensory perceptions. See Table 20–2 for types of hallucinations and examples.

Table 20–1 • DELUSION*

DEFINITION	EXAMPLE
Jealousy	
The false belief that one's mate is unfaithful. May have pieces of so-called "proof."	Harry kept accusing his girlfriend of going out with other men, even though this was not the case. His "proof" was that she came home from work late twice that week. He persisted in his belief even when the girlfriend's boss explained that everyone had worked late.
Persecution	
The false belief that one is being singled out for harm by others. This belief often takes the form of a plot by people in power against the person.	Sam believed that the secret service was planning to kill him. He became very wary of what food he ate, since he believed that the secret service was poisoning his food.
Grandeur	
The false belief that one is a very powerful and important person.	Sally believed that she was Mary Magdalene and that Jesus controlled her thoughts and was telling her how to save the world.
Ideas of Reference	
Misconstruing trivial events and remarks and giving them personal significance.	When Maria saw the doctor and nurse talking together, she believed they were talking against her. When she heard on the radio that a hurricane was coming, she believed this to be a message that "bad weather" or harm was going to befall her.
Delusions of Control	
The false belief that one's actions or thoughts are controlled by an external person or force.	Sam stated that his thoughts were being controlled by electrical currents operated by bad people.
Somatic Delusions	
The false belief that the body is changing in an unusual way—e.g., rotting inside.	David kept telling the doctor that his brain was rotting away.

*A false belief held and maintained as true even with evidence to the contrary. This is not a belief that is maintained by one's culture or subculture.

James *hears* the voice of God telling him that the FBI is going to kill him.

4. **Neologisms** are words a person makes up which have special meaning for the person.

James told the nurse that the M*ase-do-dues* told the FBI where he could be found and killed.

Normal children at times make up their own words. This creation of neologisms by children is creative, constructive, and adaptive. Neologisms in the schizophrenic reaction represent regression and disruption in reality functioning (Weich 1978).

ASSESSING SECONDARY SYMPTOMS OF SCHIZOPHRENIA

A number of clinical characteristics are associated with the schizophrenia syndrome. (1) Withdrawal, (2) disturbances in behavior, (3) disturbances in thinking and perceiving, (4) disturbances in feeling, and (5) disturbances in speech patterns are presented here as secondary symptoms.

Withdrawal

Withdrawal can be seen as a defense against uncomfortable levels of anxiety. Withdrawal on a continuum may stretch from moderate shyness to stupor. Behaviors become maladaptive in terms of their *frequency*, *intensity*, and *duration* of use. Most normal persons have personal patterns of withdrawal during stress. For example, a person might sleep late after going to bed early the night before, watch TV for long periods and hardly remember what he is watching, or read detective stories and other escapist materials. Or, a person can withdraw physically. A man who has had a fight with his wife may

Table 20–2 • HALLUCINATION*

DEFINITION	EXAMPLE
Visual	
Seeing a person, object, or animal that does not exist in the environment.	Charles, who is experiencing alcohol withdrawal delirium, "sees" hungry rats coming toward him.
Auditory	
Hearing voices or sounds that do not exist in the environment but are projections of inner thoughts or feelings.	Anna "hears" the voice of her dead mother call her a whore and a tramp.
Tactile	
Feeling strange sensations where there are not external objects to stimulate such feelings. Common in delirium tremens (DT's).	A paranoid schizophrenic "feels" electrical impulses controlling his mind. A person experiencing alcohol withdrawal delirium "feels" snakes crawling on his body.
Gustatory	
Tasting sensations which have no stimulus in reality.	Sal will not eat the hospital food because he "tastes" the poison the FBI is putting in his food.
Olfactory	
Smelling odors that are not present in the environment.	Theresa "smells" her insides rotting.

**False sensory perception* for which there is no external stimuli.

Hallucinations are different from **illusions** in that illusions are misperceptions or misinterpretations of a real experience. For example, a man *saw* his coat hanging on a coat rack and believed it to be a bear about to attack him. He *did* see something real but *misinterpreted* what it was.

go out for a walk with the dog. A student who has been studying for an exam to the point of frustration goes out to a movie. As long as withdrawal activities do not interfere with interpersonal relationships or become a substitute for activities in the real world, they may be viewed as adaptive.

Fantasy represents a retreat from reality and an attempt to solve problems in a private world. The difference between a normal person and a person with schizophrenia, however, is that the schizophrenic person is not sure where his fantasy ends and reality begins.

A person with schizophrenia withdraws not just from the activities of life, but from his own feelings as well. This often gives the clinical picture of the blunting or flat affect. Where there is no evidence of actual physical withdrawal, there is more often a delusional paranoid structure, which defends against anxiety.

Catatonic stupor is perhaps the most severe form of physical withdrawal. A schizophrenic who responds to his own autistic world (fantasy world), and who is unable to interact with the real world, is severely withdrawn from reality.

Disturbances in Behavior

Because the person's extreme withdrawal from reality, a number of alterations in behavior may become evident. These alterations in behavior are described subsequently.

STUPOR. The person who is in a stupor may sit motionless for long periods of time and may be motionless to the point of apparent coma.

WAXY FLEXIBILITY. Waxy flexibility consists of excessive maintenance of posture evidenced when a person's arms or legs can be placed in any position and the position is held for long periods of time.

EXTREME MOTOR AGITATION. Extreme motor agitation is agitated physical behavior, such as running about, in response to inner and outer stimuli. The person may become dangerous to others or suffer exhaustion or collapse or die if not stopped.

ECHOPRAXIA. Echopraxia is a stance in which the person will mimic the movements of others around him.

STEREOTYPED BEHAVIORS. Stereotyped behaviors are motor patterns that originally had meaning to the person (e.g., sweeping the floor, washing windows), but that have become mechanical and lack purpose.

AUTOMATIC OBEDIENCE. A catatonic client may perform, without hesitation, all simple commands in a robot-like fashion. This behavior is termed automatic obedience.

NEGATIVISM. Negativism is equivalent to resistance. In *active negativism* the person does the opposite of what he or she is told to do. When the person does not do things he or she is expected to do (e.g., does not get out of bed, does not dress, does not eat), such behavior is termed *passive negativism*.

DETERIORATION IN APPEARANCE AND MANNERS. This is evidenced in poor grooming and deterioration in self-care.

Regressive patterns of behavior may be present and are especially evident in disorganized schizophrenia. The first seven behavior disturbances described above are most often seen in catatonic schizophrenia.

Disturbances in Thinking and Perceiving

Schizophrenia is said to be a disorder of thought. Looseness of associations, previously discussed, demonstrates to the listener the person's difficulty in responding to reality. Other disturbances in thought and perception that frequently present themselves in the schizophrenia syndrome are (1) delusions, (2) hallucinations, and (3) concrete thinking.

DELUSIONS

A popular definition of **delusion** is a false, fixed belief not amenable to change by reason or experience. The three components of a delusion are as follows (Hinsie and Cambell 1981):

1. A false belief
2. Manufactured without appropriate or sufficient evidence in reality to support it
3. Held by one despite proof that the belief is in error

Most common delusional thinking includes the following:

1. Ideas of reference
2. Delusions of persecution
3. Delusions of grandeur
4. Somatic delusions
5. Delusions of jealousy
6. Delusions of control

Refer to Table 20–1 for definitions and examples of delusions.

About 75% of schizophrenic persons experience delusions at some time during their illness. In schizophrenia, persecutory and grandiose delusions are the most common (Chapman 1976).

Peplau described the commonalities of delusions and hallucinations as pathologies both stemming from anxiety. Anxiety greatly influences a person's ability to perceive reality accurately. Disorganizing levels of anxiety make it difficult or impossible for a person to describe or interpret what is going on around him. If a person is emotionally or physically isolated from others and suffers an inability to trust others, the opportunity to validate personal experiences and clarify confusion is greatly diminished. Recall the steps in developing relief behavior for anxiety (see Chapter 9):

1. An expectation is held.
2. The expectation is not met.
3. Extreme discomfort occurs (anxiety).
4. Relief behaviors are called into play.
5. The behavior(s) are rationalized.

In the acute phase of schizophrenia, the person is overwhelmed by panic levels of anxiety and is not able to distinguish what is inside of him (thoughts) from what is outside of him (reality). Therefore, a delusion may become the inadequate behavior to relieve the excruciating pain of panic levels of anxiety, whether the anxiety is biologically or psychologically induced.

By the time most people come to the hospital, step 5, rationalization, is fixed. When delusions become fixed, they are difficult to alter, and the person has arrived at the chronic phase of his illness. When the delusions become stable, the feeling of intense anxiety subsides. Delusions can provide a person with feelings of safety.

HALLUCINATIONS

Hallucinations can be defined as sensory perceptions to which there is *no external stimulus*. The most common types of hallucinations are listed subsequently.

1. Auditory—hearing voices
2. Visual—seeing persons or things
3. Olfactory—smelling odors
4. Gustatory—experiencing tastes
5. Tactile—feeling body sensations

Refer to Table 20–2 for examples of common hallucinations.

Peplau states that hallucinations, like delusions, have three fundamental characteristics (Field 1979):

1. The perceptions are created within (e.g., voices).
2. The perceptions are then projected onto the real world.
3. The projected perceptions (voices) are then interacted with as if they were real.

It is estimated that 90% of people with schizophrenia experience hallucinations at some time during their illness (Chapman 1976). Although manifestations of hallucinations are varied, auditory hallucinations are most common in schizophrenia. These voices may seem to come from outside or inside the person's head. The voices may be familiar, single, or multiple. Voices speaking directly to the person or commenting on the person's behavior are most common in schizophrenia. *Command hallucinations* must be assessed for, since the "voices" may command the person to hurt himself or others (APA 1987). As mentioned previously, Crow (1980) believes hallucinations and delusions are a response to excessive dopamine activity in the brain.

Evidence of possible hallucinatory behavior may be the turning or tilting of the head "as if" talking to someone or frequent blinking of the eyes and grimacing by the client. Sometimes even audible responses are heard.

Hallucinations may be understood as a process that a person has adopted to relieve panic levels of anxiety. Peplau has described the process of hallucinations, which usually begins in an anxious and lonely person. Box 20–1 operationally defines this process described by Peplau (Field 1979; Field and Ruelke 1973).

CONCRETE THINKING

In psychiatry, the term **concrete thinking** usually implies overemphasis on specific details as opposed to general and abstract thinking. For example, during an assessment the nurse might ask what brought the client to the hospital. The client might answer, "A cab." When asked to give the meaning of the proverb "people in glass houses shouldn't throw stones," the person might answer concretely, "Don't throw stones or the windows will break." The answer is literal; the ability to use abstract reasoning is absent.

Disturbances in Feeling

As it has been mentioned, a person with schizophrenia is usually not in touch with his feelings, and his affect is often flat or bizarre. Feelings such as (1) depression, (2) depersonalization, and (3) derealization are often present.

DEPRESSION. Depression is often seen in people with schizophrenia. The incidence of suicide may be 5 to 7% higher in schizophrenia than in the general population (see Chapter 22).

DEPERSONALIZATION. Depersonalization is a nonspecific feeling that a person has lost his identity—that he is different or unreal. The person may be concerned that parts of his body do not belong to him. Or, the person may have an acute sensation that his or her

Box 20–1. THE HALLUCINATION PROCESS (PEPLAU)

PHASE ONE	A person who is lonely, anxious, and under stress calls to mind a helping person. The person then interacts with the perception of the helping person as if the person were real. For the first time in a long time, the painful level of anxiety is lowered, and loneliness is temporarily relieved.
PHASE TWO	The "helping person" is called back again and again to relieve the recurring anxiety and loneliness. A ritual of controlling anxiety begins.
PHASE THREE	The person experiences great relief of anxiety by calling up the projected helping person, and the need for this kind of interaction grows. More time is set aside for interactions with the "created projection" than with people in the real world.
PHASE FOUR	The person loses the ability to focus on the outside world and spends more time with hallucinations. Control over the appearance of the hallucination is lost. When this happens, others notice the person's interaction with the "voices." The person may feel embarrassed, and anxiety and withdrawal increase.
PHASE FIVE	With the loss of control, the persons's own loss of self-esteem and low self-worth become projected onto the voices. The voices now become derogatory, accusatory, and threatening.
PHASE SIX	This negative experience of threatening voices increases the person's anxiety and withdrawal and decreases the person's ability to focus onto the real world.
PHASE SEVEN	The voices continue to threaten and terrorize. The individual promises not to reveal the presence of the voices if the voices will only once more treat him or her kindly.

Data from Field WE, Ruelke W. Hallucinations and how to deal with them. American Journal of Nursing, 73(4):638, 1973.

body has drastically changed. For example, people may see their fingers as snakes or their arms as rotting wood.

DEREALIZATION. Derealization is the false perception by a person that his environment has changed. For example, everything seems bigger or smaller, or familiar surroundings have become somehow strange and unfamiliar.

Disturbances in Speech Patterns

The most common disturbance in speech pattern is looseness of associations, which has been previously addressed. Other patterns of speech that may be evidenced in schizophrenia include (1) echolalia, (2) clang association, (3) neologisms, and (4) word salad.

ECHOLALIA. Echolalia is the pathological repeating of words of another by imitation and is often seen in people with catatonia.

NURSE: Mary, come for your medication.
MARY: Mary, come for your medication.

CLANG ASSOCIATION. Clang association is the meaningless rhyming of words, often in a forceful manner (e.g., red, bed, ted, ned, said, fed). This form of speech pattern may be seen in schizophrenia; however, it also may be seen in the manic phase of a bipolar disorder or in an organic condition.

NEOLOGISMS. Neologisms are words a person makes up that make no sense to the listener, although they have special meaning for the schizophrenic person. For example, a young man told the nurse that the *Niplaps* are near and the *Ruses* are coming.

WORD SALAD. Word Salad is a term used to identify a mixture of phrases meaningless to the listener, and perhaps to the speaker as well. It may include a string of neologisms, as in the following example: "Birds and fishes, . . . HiHo's, . . . trees . . . mud and stars, . . . thump, bump, . . . no more time."

CATEGORIZING SYMPTOMS

There has been renewed interest in categorizing the symptoms of schizophrenia into *positive* and *negative* symptoms. This classification was originally proposed by Fish and Jackson in the nineteenth century. Crow (1980) states that the positive symptoms (hallucinations, delusions, and thought disorder) have a different etiology than the negative symptoms (affective flattening, apathy, and poverty of thought). Some psychiatric nurses find classifying symptoms into positive and negative useful in deciding appropriate treatment approaches. Refer to Table 20–3 for an overview of positive and negative symptoms and suggested interventions summarized by Maxine Loomis (1986).

Standard III: Diagnosis

As indicated by the assessment, a person with schizophrenia may have a variety of symptoms. Although there may be many clients on a unit with schizophrenia, each may present with different personal needs and defensive behaviors. Each client requires a nursing care plan that reflects individual needs and strategies appropriate to the client's behaviors and level of functioning. Some nursing diagnoses that are appropriate to nurses' work with schizophrenic clients are discussed.

During the course of schizophrenia, a client is likely to experience hallucinations or delusions. During this time impairment in thought processes may be evident in the client's ability to reason, problem-solve, make decisions, and concentrate. These distortions alter the client's ability to perceive reality accurately (hallucinations or delusions) and usually impair the client's judgment. A nursing diagnosis of *altered thought process* is appropriate. *Altered thought process* may be related to alteration in biochemical compounds, panic anxiety, emotional trauma, and so forth.

With alteration in thought process come changes in language and speech. Therefore, *impaired verbal communication* may be problematic to varying degrees. When looseness of associations is severe, the person is unable to communicate needs or feelings. The nurse interacts in a variety of ways to try to understand and help reduce the client's anxiety. Use of neologisms, echolalia, clang associations, and word salad contribute to the client's *impaired verbal communication*.

When a person is unable to interpret the world around him accurately, his ability to cope with his environment is also impaired. Therefore, *ineffective individual coping* is most always present. A person's *ineffective individual coping* may be evidenced by inappropriate use of defense mechanisms and inability to meet role expectations. Behaviors may include withdrawal or excitability, disorganized or regressive behaviors, paranoia, and inability to meet basic needs.

A person who is extremely paranoid may have special problems. For example, if the person is refusing to eat anything because he thinks his food is being poisoned, then *altered nutrition: less than body weight* is used.

"Voices" that tell the person to harm others or himself can result in bodily harm or even death to the client or others. *Potential for violence directed at others or self-directed* would take priority (refer to section on paranoia).

Table 20–3 • POSITIVE AND NEGATIVE SYMPTOMS IN SCHIZOPHRENIA

POSITIVE SYMPTOMS (+)	NEGATIVE SYMPTOMS (−)
Characteristics	
1. Appears quickly in first phase of illness.	1. Develops over long periods of time.
2. Least important prognostically.	2. Interferes with person's ability to survive.
3. Person has some control over the negative impact of these symptoms.	3. Part of chronic psychiatric disability.
Examples	
1. Hallucinations	1. Apathy
2. Delusions	2. Inability to initiate and maintain relationships.
3. Paranoia	3. Inability to initiate and maintain conversations
4. Depersonalization	4. Difficulty making decisions
5. Concrete thinking	5. Inability to hold jobs
6. Word salad, clang associations	6. Poor personal hygiene
7. Posturing	
Most Useful Interventions	
1. Neuroleptic (antipsychotic) medication.	1. Skill training interventions: A. Identify areas of skill deficit person is willing to work on. B. Prioritize skills important to the person.
2. Medical assessment to rule out physiological process that may be contributing to symptoms.	2. Working with person to identify stressors: A. Identify which stressors contribute to maladaptive behaviors. B. Work with person on increasing appropriate coping skills.

Data from a paper presented by Maxine Loomis. Psychiatric Nursing Update Convention, 1986, Philadelphia, PA.

During the acute phase of catatonia, a client may be highly agitated and can exhaust him- or herself to a dangerous degree if rest and high caloric fluid replacement are not immediately provided. Extreme hyperactivity can lead to cardiac or respiratory collapse and indicates an *activity intolerance*.

During extreme withdrawal, attention to physical care is vital. Some useful nursing diagnoses might be (1) *constipation/incontinence*, (2) *impaired physical mobility*, or (3) *self-care deficit: feeding, bathing, dressing/grooming and toileting*.

When the disease has been long term, it is not uncommon to note multiple admissions to a unit. Problems with compliance with medications is thought to be a major factor. Families with schizophrenic members may have their own confused patterns of communication and insufficient knowledge of the client's problems or may feel powerless in coping with the client at home. *Ineffective family coping: compromised or disabling* may be an important area for intervention by members of the health team, especially in relation to discharge planning.

Most all people with schizophrenia suffer from a low self-concept. There is often confusion of sexual identity, as well as unrealistic and distorted perception of self. Depersonalization further confuses the person's perception of body image. *Disturbance in self-esteem* is usually present.

Refer to Figure 20–3 for an overview of DSM III-R criteria for the individual schizophrenic disorders.

Standard IV: Planning

Planning involves more than the identification of measurable and attainable goals. Identification of personal reactions and feelings regarding the client is necessary if the interventions in the nursing care plan are to be carried out effectively. Therefore, planning involves (1) content level—planning goals— and (2) process level—nurses' reactions and feelings.

CONTENT LEVEL—PLANNING GOALS

It is important that goals be both meaningful and attainable by nursing action. The goals are usually directed toward the "related to" component of the nursing diagnosis. Therefore, *altered thought process related to isolation* and *altered thought process related to unclear communications* would have different short term and long term goals. The goals listed subsequently are offered as examples and guidelines for nursing actions.

1. *Altered thought process* related to panic levels of anxiety, as evidenced by hallucinations or delusions.
   - By (state the date) client will go from panic to severe level of anxiety with the aid of medication and nursing intervention.
   - Client will meet with nurse once a day for 15 minutes in an activity in which client feels safe.
   - By (state the date) client will state that "the voices" or "the thoughts" are less frequent, with the aid of medication and nursing intervention.
   - By (state the date) client will engage in one unit activity per day that provides reality testing.
   - By (state the date) client will be able to talk about concrete happenings without talking about delusions or hallucinations for short periods.
   - By (state the date) client will be able to make needs and wants clearer with the aid of medication and nursing interventions.
2. *Ineffective individual coping* related to lack of motivation to respond, as evidenced by alteration in social participation.
   - By (state the state) client will meet with nurse for ten minutes per day in an activity in which the client feels safe.
   - By (state the date) client will meet with the nurse and one other client in simple activity.
   - Client will state that he feels more comfortable with nurse by (state the date).
   - Client will state that he feels more comfortable with one other client or staff member by (state the date).
   - Client will attend one simple group activity each day by (state the date).
3. *Potential for violence directed at others* related to misperceived messages from others, as evidenced by persecutory delusions and hallucinations.
   - By (state the date) client will state that the voices are less angry, with the aid of medication.
   - By (state the date) client will state he thinks that the nurse(s)/staff want to help him.
   - Client will join the nurse for one activity per day in which he states that he feels safe.
   - By (state the date) client will state that he feels safe on the unit with the staff.
4. *Activity intolerance* related to extreme stress, as evidenced by constant physical agitation and increased respiration and pulse.
   - Client will cease dangerous levels of activity within 20 minutes after intramuscular medication.
   - Client will take 8 ounces of a high-caloric fluid every 30 minutes.
   - Client will have 5-minute rest periods every 30 minutes.

PROCESS LEVEL—NURSES' REACTIONS AND FEELINGS

Working with individuals diagnosed as schizophrenic is bound to bring up strong emotional reactions from health care workers. The psychotic client is intensely anxious, lonely, dependent, and distrustful. The intensity of these emotions can stir up intense, uncomfortable, and frightening emotions in all health care workers. The identification of transference and countertransference phenomena is an important part of the work of the therapeutic process. (See Chapter 6 to review the transference and countertransference phenomena).

If personal countertransferential reactions are ignored by the nurse, feelings of helplessness follow. Increased feelings of helplessness escalate anxiety. Without the support, opportunity, and willingness to explore these reactions with more experienced nursing staff, defensive behaviors emerge. Defensive behaviors in the nurse, such as denial, withdrawal, and avoidance, thwart the client's progress and undermine the nurse's self-esteem. These behaviors are associated with staff burnout. Statements such as "These clients are hopeless," "You can't understand these people," "You waste your time with them" are examples of unexamined or unrecognized emotional reactions to client's behaviors or feelings.

For new nurses introduced into the psychiatric setting, especially for student nurses, the availability of supportive supervision is a *must* if learning is to take place. The student's part in the supervisory process is a willingness to discuss and identify personal feelings, as well as to identify problematic behaviors. This can be and often is done in group supervision. Experienced psychiatric nurses call this process *peer group supervision.*

Individual supervision provides the greatest opportunity for a better understanding of the interpersonal issues involved in establishing a working relationship with the client. Individual supervision can increase the learner's understanding of the client and his situation, competence with therapeutic skills, and self-confidence. Unfortunately, many schools of nursing do not have the time or faculty to provide this learning opportunity for students. Some psychiatric settings encourage the practice of supervision and provide time and personnel for psychiatric nurses and other staff.

Kahn (1984) identifies three strong transferences on the part of schizophrenic clients that can trigger equally strong countertransference reactions among mental health workers. These three transferences are (1) the dependent transference, (2) the angry transference and (3) the eroticized transference. These issues are best dealt with during supervision. During this time the transference phenomena are identified, personal reactions of the nurse are explored, and appropriate intervention strategies are suggested and evaluated.

For example, when dealing with *dependency issues*, decisions need to be made about when to gratify modest dependency needs without hindering the development of the client's autonomy. What feelings does the nurse experience in relationship to the client's exhaustive dependency needs? Which responses are rational and which irrational? Do the irrational feelings toward the client block effective therapeutic work?

During supervision of the *angry transference* feelings, the nurse learns to inhibit the urge to act on angry personal responses, to provide a corrective experience with anger for the client, and to understand the function the anger serves for the client (e.g., maintaining distance).

Eroticized transference is difficult and may be threatening to both the client and the nurse. Supervision may involve exploring ways to set clear limits while maintaining effective contact with the client (Kahn 1984).

Menninger (1984) discusses the extreme frustration that staff have with the slow progress of schizophrenic clients. This sense of frustration and feelings of helplessness can lead to burnout. Periodic reassessment of treatment goals and scaling down of expectations can benefit both staff and clients.

These are some, but by no means all, of the kinds of issues that may come up when dealing with a schizophrenic client. Clinical practice with adequate supervision increases the nurse's skills, lowers personal anxiety, increases confidence, and can improve the quality of interpersonal relationships with clients as well as relationships with others.

Standard V: Intervention

The detrimental effect of stress on a schizophrenic person's environment has been long observed by clinicians. Environmental stress can result in a remission of schizophrenic symptoms. Much of the work with schizophrenic clients involves decreasing taxing levels of environmental stress, thereby lowering the client's level of anxiety. Lowered anxiety levels can decrease the intensity of schizophrenic symptoms and make the client more amenable to engaging in activities and relationships that are reality-based. Lowering anxiety levels is accomplished with the aid of medications, therapeutic relationships with health professionals, improved family interactions, and involvement in nonthreatening activities. Lowered anxiety levels make it possible for all people, including people with schizophrenia, to define problems and focus on issues.

When planning interventions, it is important not to overlook the adaptive skills of a psychotic client. *Attention should be given to the client's assets and healthy functioning as well as to areas of deficiencies* (MacKinnon and Michels 1971).

V-A: PSYCHOTHERAPEUTIC INTERVENTIONS

Therapeutic strategies for working with schizophrenic clients often involve interventions that address specific behaviors. Psychotherapeutic interventions are aimed at lowering the client's anxiety, decreasing defensive patterns, encouraging participation in the environment and raising the client's level of self-esteem. Refer to the appropriate sections for useful intervention strategies for paranoid, withdrawn, excitable, and regressed behaviors.

All nurses should be familiar with the principles of dealing with certain phenomena that are certain to arise with most all schizophrenic clients. These are the phenomena of (1) hallucinations, (2) delusions, and (3) looseness of associations.

Hallucinations

Understanding the process of hallucinations offers useful guidelines for working with clients who are actively hallucinating. The hallucinatory process starts out in a painfully lonely and isolated person under stress. Hallucinations are a means to allay terrorizing feelings of alienation and the resulting panic levels of anxiety.

As mentioned, voices are the most common hallucinatory experience reported by schizophrenic clients. Initially, it is important to understand what the voices are saying or telling the person to do. The presence of suicidal or homicidal messages indicates priority measures for all members of the health team.

When working with a client who is hearing voices, one does not argue that the voices are or are not real but indicates that the nurse does not hear the voices the client hears. Emphasizing reality can also be done by casting doubt on the client's own misinterpretation of reality. Peplau suggests discrediting the voices by referring to the voices as "the so-called voices" or "the voices that you hear" (Field and Ruelke 1973).

Since hallucinations can defend against anxiety, they serve a purpose. When the client is asked to give up something important to him, no matter how maladaptive, something more adaptive and useful should be available to take its place—namely, receptive and interested people in the client's environment. Establishing a relationship that minimizes anxiety and is built on honesty, consistency of care, and genuine concern for the client is an important first step. See Peplau's interventions with hallucinating clients in Box 20–2 (Field 1976).

Delusions

Delusions can also defend against anxiety and can provide a feeling of safety. The decrease in anxiety is important to the client's ability to focus on and accurately perceive reality. It is useful if the nurse attempts to see the world as it appears through the eyes of the client (MacKinnon and Michels 1971). In that way, the nurse can better understand the client's delusional experience. For example:

CLIENT You people are all alike . . . all in on the CIA plot to destroy me.

NURSE I do not want to hurt you, Tom. Thinking that people are out to destroy you must be very frightening.

First, the nurse clarifies the reality of his or her intent. Second, the nurse empathizes with the client's apparent experience, the feelings of fear. The nurse does not get drawn into the conversation regarding the content of the delusion (CIA and plot to destroy) but looks for the feelings the person may be experiencing. Talking

Box 20–2. SUGGESTED STEPS WHEN INTERVENING WITH HALLUCINATION (PEPLAU)

These steps are carried out by the nurse within the context of an established relationship with the client:

1. The client learns to name his anxiety. The nurse helps the client connect his feelings of anxiety with the occurrence or increase in intensity of his "voices." This first step is necessary for the client to gain a sense of control over the hallucinatory process.
2. A relationship with the client is established. Time spent with the client includes focus on various aspects of the client's life and interests, not just the hallucinatory process.
3. The nurse discredits the reality of the voices with such terms as "so-called voices" or "the voices you hear." The nurse does *not* deny that the client hears the voices, but emphasizes that the nurse does not hear the voices.
4. Since hallucinations were originally manufactured to reduce anxiety, the nurse anticipates that the client could experience panic levels of anxiety and feelings of terror when asked to give them up. The client himself must dismiss the voices.
5. The nurse alerts other members of the health team, when the appropriate time nears for the client to dismiss the voices. Interest and support from other members of staff temporarily provide replacement for the invented voices.

Data from Field WE, Ruelke W. Hallucinations and how to deal with them. American Journal of Nursing, 73(4):638, 1973.

about the client's feeling experience can be useful for the client; talking about delusional material is not.

It is *not* useful to argue with the client regarding the content of the delusion. Doing so can intensify the client's retention of irrational beliefs. Although the nurse does not argue with the client's delusions, clarifying misinterpretations of the environment is useful. For example:

CLIENT I see the doctor is here, and he is out to get me and destroy me.

NURSE: It is true the doctor wants to see you, but he wants to talk to you about your treatment. Would you feel more comfortable talking to him in the day room?

Interacting with the client on concrete realities in the environment can be useful in minimizing the client's time spent with delusional ruminations. Often, specific manual tasks within the scope of the client's abilities can be useful as distractions from delusional thinking. The more time the client spends with reality-based activities or people, the more opportunity the client has to learn to be comfortable with reality.

Looseness of Associations

As mentioned earlier, the speech patterns of a schizophrenic client often reflect looseness of associations. This speech pattern mirrors the client's autistic thoughts. The client's autistic and disorganized ramblings may leave the nurse confused and frustrated. MacKinnon and Michels (1971) state that the most common defense encountered in an interview with the schizophrenic is the client's unconscious use of disorganization. Therefore, the client's autism can be seen as a symptom of his inability to handle anxiety (Cook 1971). Increase in the client's autistic speech patterns can indicate increased anxiety on the part of the client.

"Decoding" is a term used for interpreting the meaning of autistic communications. Cook (1971) stated that "decoding is not always possible, but when possible can help in understanding the client's experience and needs."

The following guidelines may be useful when spending time with a client whose speech is confused and disorganized (MacKinnon and Michels 1971; Cook 1971):

1. Do not pretend understanding of the client's communications when you are confused by the client's words or meanings.
2. Tell the client you are having difficulty understanding his communications.
3. Place the difficulty in understanding on yourself, *not* the client—e.g., say, "I am having trouble following what you are saying," *not* "You are not making any sense."
4. Look for recurring topics and themes in the client's communications—for example, "You've mentioned trouble with your brother several times. I guess your relationship with your brother is on your mind."
5. When understanding the client's autistic communications is not possible, just listening to and being accepting of the client can be meaningful.

V-B: HEALTH TEACHING

Teaching methods of health management to clients, families, and other care-givers can be important in stabilization of the schizophrenic person's future adjustment. Falloon (1986) suggests that it is not just the level or source of stress in the client's environment that is crucial; also important is the manner in which people involved deal with the stress, and how effectively stressful issues are resolved.

Psychological strategies aimed at reducing exacerbation of the psychotic symptoms follow (Falloon et al. 1982):

1. Educate the client and his family about the illness. Emphasize how stress and medication affect the illness. Such knowledge may increase medication compliance and motivate involvement in psychosocial activities.
2. Assist the client to increase his ability to solve problems related to environmental stress.
3. Teach the client coping strategies to deal with the source of symptoms of schizophrenia and the stresses in his or her social environment.

Studies indicate the importance of the family environment for a schizophrenic client. When a schizophrenic client is returned to a family environment consisting of warmth, concern, and supportive behavior, he is less likely to suffer a relapse. An environment highly critical of the client's behavior, or consisting of intrusive involvement into his life, is more likely to correlate with recurrent episodes of schizophrenia (Falloon 1986).

Some of the critical attitudes toward people with schizophrenia results in a lack of understanding of the symptoms of schizophrenia. For example, the client's apathy, lack of drive, and motivation may be wrongly interpreted as laziness. This erroneous assumption can encourage hostility on the part of family members, care-givers, or people in the community in general. Therefore, further teaching of the disease process of schizophrenia can reduce tensions within families and communities. Educating the client, families, and others is most effective when carried out over a period of time.

Both the client and his or her family should be informed of the long term need for antipsychotic medication and the positive effects possible. Effective teaching in this area can help to increase medical compliance. Side effects and toxic effects should be carefully explained, and medical contact should be made readily available when questions or problems arise (see section V-D: *Somatic Therapies*).

The client and his family should be cautioned regarding the use of marijuana and amphetamines. These drugs can potentiate the symptoms of schizophrenia.

Hertz (1984) cites recent studies demonstrating that schizophrenic clients experience exacerbations and remissions throughout their illness. Results of a study by Hertz showed that during the prodromal period, families and clients noticed certain symptoms that can indicate a potential relapse.

The symptoms identified in this study were the same symptoms that a nonpsychotic person experiences under stress. Symptoms include dysphoria, feeling tense, nervousness, eating less, difficulty concentrating, having trouble sleeping, and seeing friends less. Early warning signs of possible relapse recognized by both family and client may ward off a possible psychotic relapse if medical attention is immediately obtained. The client and his family should be aware of the prodromal signs and symptoms indicating a potential exacerbation of the disease.

V-C: ACTIVITIES OF DAILY LIVING

Those clients who have the most difficulty with the rudiments of self-care usually include the disorganized and catatonic schizophrenic in the acute phase of the illness. The paranoid client usually manages basic activities of daily living more competently. Specific interventions regarding basic activities of daily living for paranoid, catatonic, and disorganized clients will be discussed in separate sections of this chapter.

Providing for the basic needs for schizophrenics once discharged from the hospital is a larger and even more complex problem. The deinstitutionalization of thousands of schizophrenic persons in the 1970's resulted in their release into communities unable to cope with the needs of these clients. Basic needs for housing, food, medical care, safety, employment, and social support went unmet for many. Under the guise of "least restrictive alternatives," thousands of people with chronic thought disorders ended up living in vermin-infested boarding houses, single-room occupancy hotels, cardboard housing on the fringes of town, or on park benches. Because of their confusion and inability to articulate needs, most of these people were unable to attain aid such as food stamps, simple and suitable occupation, and social supports. Too many ended up lonely, alienated, and misunderstood — the victims of muggers, rapists, and homelessness (Torrey 1986).

V-D: SOMATIC THERAPIES

Medication

Appropriate drugs for the psychotic disorders are called **neuroleptic** or **antipsychotic medications.** These drugs used to be popularly referred to as the major tranquilizers. Drugs once termed the minor tranquilizers are now called anxiolytic or antianxiety agents. A comparison of the properties of the neuroleptics (e.g., phenothiazines) and the anxiolytic or antianxiety agents (e.g., benzodiazepines) is outlined in Table 20–4.

Desired therapeutic responses to neuroleptic/antipsychotic medications are summarized subsequently (Hart et al. 1981; Lickey and Gordon 1983; Harvard Medical School 1986):

1. Reduction in disruptive and violent behavior
2. Increase in activity, speech, and sociability in withdrawn or mute clients
3. Improvement in self care
4. Improvement in sleep patterns
5. Reduction in the disturbing quality of hallucinations and delusions
6. Improvement in thought processes
7. Decreased resistance to psychotherapy/supportive psychotherapy
8. Reduced rate of relapse (about 2.5 times)
9. Decrease in the intensity of paranoid reactions

Other uses for these neuroleptic/antipsychotic agents are as *antiemetics* (postoperatively, in radiation and chemotherapy for intractable vomiting) and to *potentiate narcotic analgesics* (treatment of pain) in terminal cancer (Karb et al. 1989).

Schizophrenia is the most common indication for neuroleptic/antipsychotic medication. People in acute mania or psychotic depression may respond to a short course of neuroleptics. These agents frequently are effective in the treatment of the behavioral disorders associated with organic brain disease.

The five chemical classes of neuroleptic/antipsychotic medications are the phenothiazines, thioxanthenes, butyrophenones, dibenzoxazepines and dihydroindolones (Karb et al. 1989). The properties and side

Table 20–4 • COMPARISON OF PROPERTIES OF ANTIPSYCHOTIC AND ANTIANXIETY MEDICATIONS

NEUROLEPTICS (Antipsychotic Medications)	ANXIOLYTICS (Antianxiety Medications)
1. Are not central nervous system (CNS) depressants: A. Produce lassitude and drowsiness* but do *not* induce general anesthesia. B. Always possible to elicit some response, even when a patient is "snowed under."	1. Are central nervous system (CNS) depressants. Stages of CNS depression include: A. Drowsiness* B. Sleep C. General anesthesia D. Coma An overdose can lead to respiratory and circulatory failure and death.
2. Can precipitate convulsive seizures in those with epilepsy or abnormal EEGs.	2. Are effective anticonvulsants. Often used in withdrawal syndromes to control and prevent seizures—e.g., Librium or Valium used in alcohol withdrawal delirium.
3. Can alter thought processes—e.g., lessen looseness of associations and diminish hallucinations and delusions, which are symptoms of psychosis.	3. Have *no* effect on the mental process in psychotic disorders.
4. Are *not* habit forming and do *not* produce physiological dependence.	4. Can be habit-forming, can produce physiological dependence, and can cause withdrawal symptoms if drug is stopped suddenly.

***NOTE:** *The sedative properties of both categories of medications are potentiated by alcohol.* This is more dangerous in the antianxiety medications since CNS depression can lead to respiratory failure, circulatory failure, and death.

effects of all are similar. The phenothiazines usually are considered the prototype when assessing the action and side effects of these medications. Table 20–5 identifies the commonly used drugs in some of these categories and specific properties of each.

Often, specific drugs chosen are made on the basis of side effects. For example, Thorazine (chlorpromazine) is the most sedating and has fewer extrapyramidal side effects (EPS) than other antipsychotic agents but causes hypotension in large doses. Haldol (haloperidol) is least sedating and is often used in high doses to reduce assaultive behavior but has a high incidence of EPS. The value of Haldol for treating violent behaviors is its effectiveness in controlling hallucinatory phenomena with a low incidence of hypotension (Hart 1981; Kolb and Brodie 1982). People who are functioning at work or at home may prefer less sedating drugs; clients who are agitated and excitable do better on a more sedating medication.

Neuroleptic/antipsychotic agents are usually effective within three to six weeks. When a client fails to improve after six months of drug therapy, he probably is not going to improve at all with that particular medication. The continuation of drug treatment beyond this point increases the client's risk of side effects (e.g., tardive dyskinesia). Only about 10% of schizophrenic clients do not respond to antipsychotic drugs. These clients should not continue to take medication that, for them, holds only risks and no benefits (Lickey and Gordon 1983).

Neuroleptic medications are fairly safe for most clients. It is difficult to take a lethal overdose. Tolerance does not develop, nor does a potential for abuse (Harvard Medical School 1986). Most of the side effects are minor or temporary. Common side effects include drowsiness, postural hypotension, constipation, blurred vision, and dry mouth. These drugs are used with caution in people with seizure disorders, since neuroleptics can lower the seizure threshold.

More disturbing side effects include the **extrapyramidal side effects.** Three of the more common extrapyramidal side effects are (1) **acute dystonia** (muscle cramps of the head and neck), (2) **akathisia** (restless pacing or fidgeting), and (3) **pseudo parkinsonism** (stiffening of muscular activity in the face, body, arms, and legs). These side effects are reversible and not considered medically serious. Treatment usually consists of lowering the dosage or prescribing an antiparkinsonism medication. Commonly used antiparkinsonism drugs include Artane (trihexyphenidyl), Cogentin (benztropine), Akineton (biperiden), and Benadryl (diaphenhydramine). See Table 20–6 for common side effects,

Table 20–5 • COMMONLY PRESCRIBED NEUROLEPTIC/ ANTIPSYCHOTIC MEDICATIONS

DRUG	GENERIC NAME AND MAINTENANCE DOSE	SPECIAL CONSIDERATIONS
Phenothiazines		
Thorazine	Chlorpromazine 30–75 mg/day, oral	1. Most frequently prescribed. 2. Time-release capsule. 3. Increased sensitivity to sun (seen with other phenothiazines as well). 4. Highest sedation and hypotensive effects. Least potent. 5. Low incidence of extrapyramidal side effects (EPS).
Prolixin Prolixin-E	Fluphenazine 1.0–5.0 mg/day, oral 25–50 mg IM	1. Injection form can be effective for 1 to 2 weeks.
Prolixin-D	25–50 mg IM	2. Injection form can be effective for 3 to 4 weeks.
Mellaril	Thioridazine 100–300 mg/day, oral	1. Known to cause retinitis pigmentosa in high doses. Any diminished vision or brown discoloration should be investigated. 2. Low incidence of EPS. 3. High incidence of low blood pressure and cardiac effects.
Stelazine	Trifluoperazine 5–15 mg/day, oral	1. Low sedation—good for withdrawn or paranoid symptoms. 2. High incidence of EPS.
Butyrophenones		
Haldol	Haloperidol 1–15 mg/day, oral	1. Has low sedative properties; is used in high doses for assaultive patients, thus avoiding the severe side effect of hypotension. 2. Appropriate for the elderly for the same reason as above. Lessens the chance of falls from dizziness or hypotension. 3. Available in long-acting injection form. 4. High incidence of EPS.
Thioxanthenes		
Taractan	Chlorprothixine 75 mg/day, oral	1. This drug group is very similar to phenothiazines.
Navane	Thiothixene 6–60 mg/day, oral	

Table 20–6 • NURSING MEASURES FOR SIDE EFFECTS OF NEUROLEPTIC/ANTIPSYCHOTIC MEDICATIONS

SIDE EFFECTS	NURSING MEASURES
Automatic Nervous System Effects	
1. **Dry mouth**	1. Frequent sips of water and sugarless candy/gum.
2. **Urinary retention**	2. Check patient's voiding; possible catheterization.
3. **Constipation**	3. Encourage diet high in fiber; evaluate need for mild laxative.
4. **Blurred vision**	4. Usually abates in 1 to 2 weeks. If patient is on Mellaril, hold and check with physician.
5. **Nasal congestion**	5. Nasal decongestants; body will adjust in a few weeks.
6. **Tachycardia**	6. Patients with existing cardiac problems should *always* be worked up before administering the antipsychotic drugs. Haldol is usually the preferred drug, due to its low anticholinergic effects.
7. **Inhibition of ejaculation or impotence in men**	7. Alert physician; may require alternative medication.
Extrapyramidal Side Effects	
1. **Pseudoparkinsonism:** Mask-like faces, drooling, shuffling gait, tremors, pill-rolling hand movements, muscular rigidity (cogwheel rigidity).	1. Alert medical staff. Physician may lower dosage, switch to another phenothiazine, or administer an antiparkinsonian drug (e.g., Artane or Cogentin). Artane and Cogentin are used with caution, since a "high" may result; Cogentin is becoming a popular abused drug.
2. **Akathisia:** Occurs in 20% of patients. Regular rhythmic motor movements usually of lower limbs; jiggling an arm while sitting or pacing up and down.	2. Physician may change antipsychotic or give antiparkinsonian agent or muscle relaxant such as diazepam. Tolerance does not develop to akathisia, but akathisia disappears when neuroleptic is discontinued.
3. **Acute dystonic reactions:** Very painful spasms of voluntary muscles. Muscles of the neck, back, jaws, limbs, and eyes may be involved; extremely distressful for persons experiencing such a reaction. Usually seen in first 5 days of neuroleptic therapy.	3. Rapid relief can be obtained with intramuscular injection of Benadryl or Cogentin. Nursing measures include taking patient to quiet spot and staying with him or her while orders and medication are being made available.
4. **Tardive dyskinesia (TD):** Extremely severe and irreversible side effect. Usually appears with long term use. Effects may be grotesque, i.e.: protruding tongue, puffing of the checks, chewing motions. People who develop TD may become socially disabled.	4. No known treatment. Discontinuing the drug does not always relieve symptoms. It has been reported by the APA that 10 to 20% of patients taking drug for over 1 year may develop TD. Nurses and doctors should encourage patients to be screened for TD at least every 3 months.
Other Side Effects	
1. **Postural hypotension**	1. Check blood pressure before giving; advise patient to dangle feet before getting out of bed to prevent dizziness and subsequent falls. A systolic pressure of 80 when standing is indication to hold the current dose. This usually subsides when drug is stabilized in 1 to 2 weeks.
2. **Dermatologic changes:** Hives, contact dermatitis, photosensitivity; these can reflect hypersensitivity to the drug.	2. Notify physician; withdrawal of the drug may be indicated. Teach client to stay out of sun and to use sunscreen, hat, and sunglasses.

Table continued on following page

Table 20-6 • NURSING MEASURES FOR SIDE EFFECTS OF NEUROLEPTIC/ANTIPSYCHOTIC MEDICATIONS *Continued*

SIDE EFFECTS	NURSING MEASURES
Other Side Effects	
3. **Phototoxicity:** Extreme sensitivity in sun; patient is easily sunburned.	3. Advise patient to wear protective clothing and sunscreen when in the sun.
4. **Increased weight:** Distressing side effect for many; increase in appetite is attributed to metabolic changes caused by the drug.	4. Nurse can work with patient to monitor weight gain and to work with diets; if severe, alternate drugs may be used.
5. **Endocrine changes:** Lactation, moderate breast enlargement, and galactorrhea in women; in both men and women, changes in sexual drive—usually loss of libido. Amenorrhea seen occasionally in women.	5. Alert physician; may change neuroleptic.
Rare Side Effects	
1. **Agranulocytosis:** Usually becomes evident after 4 to 10 weeks; symptoms include sore throat, fever, and malaise. It is a rare occurrence, but one the nurse should be aware of. Any flulike symptoms should be carefully evaluated.	1. Nurse notifies medical staff STAT. Hold medication. Physician may order blood work done to determine leukopenia or agranulocytosis. If test results are positive, the drug is discontinued, and reverse isolation may be initiated. CBC every 3 to 6 months should be routine.
2. **Cholestatic jaundice:** Rare, reversible, and usually benign if caught in time. Prodromal symptoms are fever, malaise, nausea, and abdominal pain; jaundice appears one week later.	2. Drug is discontinued; bed rest and high-protein, high-carbohydrate diet given. Liver function tests every 6 months should be routine.
3. **Neuroleptic Malignant Syndrome:** Occasionally fatal and always serious, this disease is manifested by *hyperpyrexia* (up to 107°F), *severe parkinsonian muscle rigidity* with *elevated creatinine phosphokinase* blood levels and elevated white count. *Liver enzymes* are *usually elevated*, and *renal shutdown is possible*.	3. Medical treatment is symptomatic (e.g., cooling body to decrease fever and administering antispasmodics such as dantrolene to reduce muscle spasms).

Data from Hart et al. 1981; Lickey and Gordon 1983; Scherer 1985; Karb et al. 1989; Schatzberg and Cole 1986.

toxic effects, and nursing/medical interventions for the neuroleptic/antipsychotic drugs. Most clients develop a tolerance to these extrapyramidal symptoms after a few months. Effective nursing and medical management is important during this time to encourage compliance with the medications until the disturbing and frightening side effects have been properly managed. *Tardive dyskinesia*, another extrapyramidal side effect, is more serious and not always reversible.

Torrey (1986) states that the most troubling side effects in outpatient management are weight gain, impotence, and tardive dyskinesia. Weight gain is most frequently a problem with women and can result in a 100-lb gain with some clients. Discontinuation of the antipsychotic medication may be necessary with the use of an alternative drug. Impotence is occasionally reported by males and may necessitate the switching to alternative drugs as well.

As mentioned, **tardive dyskinesia** (TD) can be irreversible. Tardive dyskinesia consists of involuntary tonic muscular spasms typically involving the tongue, fingers, toes, neck, trunk, or pelvis. This potentially serious extrapyramidal side effect most frequently affects women, older clients, and up to 50% of people on long-term high-dose therapy. TD varies from mild to moderate and can be disfiguring or incapacitating. Early symptoms of TD are fasciculations of the tongue or constant smacking of the lips. These early oral movements can develop into uncontrollable biting, chewing, sucking motions, open mouth, and lateral movements of the jaw (Harvard Medical School 1986; Scrak and Greenstein 1986). In most cases the early symptoms of TD will disappear when the antipsychotic medication is discontinued. In a few cases, however, early symptoms are not reversible and may progress (Torry 1986). There is yet no proven cure for advanced TD.

The National Institute of Mental Health (NIMH) has developed a brief test for the detection of TD. The test is referred to as AIMES.* The three areas of examination are facial and oral movements, extremity movements, and trunk movement.

Neuroleptic malignant syndrome is serious and sometimes fatal. It can occur in clients who are maintained on stable doses of antipsychotics for months, or it may occur suddenly when medication is being started. Symptoms and signs include hyperpyrexia up to 107°F, severe rigidity, elevated white blood cell count, and elevated liver enzyme levels. Unstable BP and P and altered states of consciousness are common (Schatzberg and Cole 1986). Immediate treatment is necessary. Table 20-6 outlines the common side effects of neuroleptic/antipsychotic agents and suggests nursing measures when working with a client taking these medications.†

Other Somatic Therapies

Besides the use of the antipsychotic medications, the only recognized somatic treatment for schizophrenia is electroconvulsive therapy. It is indicated when antipsychotic drug therapy fails or is not advised for treatment with the client. Mostly it is employed for violent, suicidal, and severely catatonic clients (Harvard Medical School 1986).

V-E: THERAPEUTIC ENVIRONMENT

Activities

Effective hospital care involves more than protection of the client from a threatening family, social, or vocational environment. It should also provide for healthy substitutes for erecting new identifications, resources for resolving conflicts, and opportunities for learning social and vocational skills (Kolb and Brodie 1982).

Beard and coworkers (1978) cite numerous studies that support the use of structured group activities with schizophrenic clients. Participation in activity groups, determined by the client's level of functioning, has been found to decrease withdrawal, promote motivation, modify unacceptable aggression, and increase social competence.

Lancaster (1976) conducted a study that resulted in an increase in self-concept scores of those clients who participated in activity group therapy, as opposed to no increase in the control group. Activities such as drawing pictures, reading poetry, and listening to music were used as a focus of conversation to reduce anxiety and promote socialization. Group functions such as picnics at different points in time reflected growth in social concern for others and the ability to set limits on self and others. Nurses can utilize activity group therapy in a variety of settings. Lancaster states that "success at tasks and increased involvement with objects and individuals will lead to greater self-esteem in a multiplicity of settings."

In the hospital and in outpatient settings the nurse may participate with other members of the health team to provide appropriate, structured and useful activities for the clients. Recreational, occupational, art, and dance therapists are available on many psychiatric units (see Chapter 5).

Safety

A client may become physically violent, often in response to hallucinations or delusions. During this time, measures need to be taken to ensure client safety as well as the safety of others. Measures such as restraints and isolation may be indicated. See Chapter 19 for indications and general guidelines for management of a client in seclusion.

V-F: PSYCHOTHERAPY

Medication maintenance has been shown to be the single most important factor in the prevention of relapse in a schizophrenic person. Drugs reduce most of the disturbing, disorganizing, and destructive aspects of the schizophrenic person's behavior (*primary symptoms*). Drugs, however, do not improve or affect the underlying apathy, unresponsiveness, lack of initiative, and symbolic defects (*secondary symptoms*) (Bruch 1980; Harvard Medical School 1986). Torrey (1986) cites a study which demonstrates that "supportive psychotherapy," in addition to drug therapy, results in an even lower rate of relapse than drug therapy alone.

A number of disciplines provide training in individual and group therapy for professionals working with schizophrenic clients. For example, psychiatrists, psychologists, psychiatric nurse specialists, and social workers are all active in providing therapy for schizophrenic

---

*Copy of the AIMES test is free. Write NIMH, Schizophrenic Disorders Section, Somatic Treatments Branch, Rockville, Maryland 20857.

†For a detailed account of the nursing care and psychotrophic medications, see Beeber LS. Antipsychotic medications. *In* Lego S (ed). The American Handbook of Psychiatric Nursing. Philadelphia: J.B. Lippincott Company, 1984, pp. 556-559.

clients. Hilde Bruch (1980) cites a study which identified the elements that made for successful therapeutic outcomes with schizophrenics, even though the therapists' disciplines were diverse. "*The highest improvement rate was associated with 'active participation' with the therapist showing initiative in a sympathetic inquiry, challenging the client's self-deprecatory attitude, and identifying realistic limits as to what is acceptable in the client's behavior.*"

Individual Therapy

Intensive insight-oriented psychotherapy is of questionable value with schizophrenic clients. Supportive psychotherapy, however, over long periods of time has great value and results in helping the person make adjustments to a more useful and satisfactory life. Individual therapy, ideally combined with group therapy, should be made available to the client on an outpatient basis as well as being part of inpatient treatment.

Group Therapy

Group therapy is particularly useful for clients who have had one or more psychotic breaks. It has been shown that groups can benefit the client in the development of *interpersonal skills, resolution of family problems*, and the *effective use of community supports*. Groups provide opportunities for socialization in safe settings, the expression of tensions, and sharing problems (Spitz 1984).

The most useful types of groups for schizophrenics are groups that help the client develop abilities to deal with such issues as day-to-day problems, sharing relevant experiences, learning to listen, asking questions, and keeping topics in focus (Mosher 1982). Groups available on an outpatient basis over a long period of time allow for individual growth in these areas.

Family Therapy

It is unfortunate that more families are not more involved with the therapy of their schizophrenic members, since families play such an important role in the course of the illness (Hertz 1984). Family education and family therapy are known to diminish the negative effects of family life on schizophrenic clients.

In family therapy sessions, the family can identify family fears, faulty communications, and distortions. Improved problem-solving skills can be taught, and healthier alternatives to situations of conflict can be explored. Family guilt and anxiety can be lessened, facilitating change. In some studies, family treatment was even more effective than individual treatment in reducing the severity of symptoms and preventing rehospitalization (Falloon et al. 1982).

The family self-help movement has been an important development in the mental health field. Families of schizophrenics have formed local and national self-help and advocacy organizations. Families with schizophrenic members do have needs. They need to be part of the decision-making process, to have adequate and appropriate help in crises, and to have periodic respite from the hard work of coping with a schizophrenic member (Lamb et al 1986). Families need help in understanding the disease and the role of medications, setting realistic goals, and developing problem-solving ways to handle the tensions and misunderstandings within the family environment. Whether this is in the form of formal family therapy or educational counseling, the family unit needs inclusion and counsel if the schizophrenic member is to become stabilized.

Discharge planning is a vital part of managing schizophrenic clients. Nurses, doctors, and social workers should all be aware of the community resources for clients who are to be discharged. Some clients may feel more comfortable with self-help community groups such as *Recovery Inc.* and *Schizophrenics Anonymous*. Information on available community resources should be made available to clients and families alike. (See appendix for address of self-help group clearing houses in the United States.)

Standard VI: Evaluation

Evaluation is always an important step in planning care. Evaluation is especially important when working with people who have chronic psychotic disorders. Modifications may have to be made in the goals set for specific clients. All goals need to be realistic and obtainable. It is not uncommon for the goals set for people with chronic disorders to be too ambitious. Often a former short term goal becomes a long term goal. Change is a process that occurs over time. With a person diagnosed as schizophrenic, the time period may be pronounced. Therefore, to prevent both client frustration and staff burnout, short term goals should be realistic and obtainable.

Another advantage to regularly scheduled evaluation with chronically ill clients is that it allows the staff to bring in new data and to reassess the client's problems. Is the client not progressing because a more important need is not being met? Is the staff using the client's strengths and interest to reach identified goals? Are there more appropriate interventions available for this client to facilitate his or her progress?

The active involvement of staff with the client's progress can help sustain interest and prevent feelings of helplessness and burnout. Input from the client can offer valuable data on why a certain desired behavior or situation has not occurred.

Paranoia

Any intense and strongly defended irrational suspicion can be regarded as **paranoia.** Paranoid ideas cannot be corrected by experiences and cannot be modified by facts or reality. Projection is the most common defense mechanism used by people who are paranoid. For example, when paranoid individuals feel self-critical, they experience others as being harshly critical toward them. When they feel anger, they experience others as being unjustly angry at them.

Paranoid states may occur in a variety of mental or organic disorders. For example, a person experiencing a psychotic depression or manic episode may display paranoid thinking. Paranoid symptoms can be *secondary* to physical illness, organic brain disease, or drug intoxications.

Primary paranoid disorders (that is, those in which the primary symptom is paranoid thinking) are (1) paranoid delusional disorder, (2) paranoid personality disorder, and (3) paranoid schizophrenia. One theory is that these three disorders represent different degrees along a schizophrenic continuum (Harvard Medical School 1986).

Essentially, the person with a paranoid schizophrenic disorder has more prominent hallucinations and more disorganized and bizarre delusions than individuals with either of the other primary paranoid disorders. For example, the person might believe that forces from outer space are controlling his or her life through invisible space rays. A person with paranoid schizophrenia is more confused and hesitant and less arrogant and self-assertive than people in either of the other two conditions. Features associated with paranoid schizophrenia include unfocused anxiety, anger, argumentativeness, and violence, as well as a stilted, formal quality and extreme intensity in interpersonal relationships (APA 1987). The person with a paranoid disorder is usually terrified. Although not always consciously aware of them, the paranoid person has deep feelings of loneliness, despair, helplessness, and fear of abandonment. The paranoid facade is a defense against painful feelings.

COMMUNICATIONS. Since a person who is paranoid is unable to trust the actions of those around him, he is usually guarded, tense, and reserved. Although he may keep himself aloof from interpersonal contacts, his impairment in functioning may be minimal. In order to ensure interpersonal distance, he may adapt a superior, hostile, and sarcastic attitude. A common defense to maintain self-esteem used by paranoid individuals is to disparage others and dwell on their short-comings. Frequently the client will misinterpret the messages of others or give private meaning to the communications of others. Minor oversights are often interpreted as personal rejection.

During hospitalization, a paranoid client may make offensive yet accurate criticisms of staff and ward policies. It is important that staff not react to these criticisms with anxiety or rejection of the client. Staff conferences, peer group supervision, and working with one's clinical supervisor are effective ways to look behind the behaviors to the motivations of the client. This provides the opportunity to reduce the client's anxiety and increase staff effectiveness.

PHYSICAL NEEDS. A person with a paranoid schizophrenic disorder usually has stronger ego resources than individuals with the other schizophrenic disorders, particularly with regard to occupational functioning and capacity for independent living (APA 1987). Grooming, dress, and self-care, therefore, may not be a problem. In fact, in some cases grooming may be meticulous. Nutrition, however, may pose a problem. A common distortion or delusion is that the food is poisoned. In this case, special foods should be provided in self-contained containers in order to minimize the suspicion of tampering. If the client thinks that others will harm him when he is sleeping, he may be fearful of going to sleep. Therefore, proper rest may become a problem that warrants nursing interventions.

PHYSICAL BEHAVIORS. A paranoid person may become physically aggressive in response to hallucinations or delusions. Hostile drives are projected onto the environment and then acted upon. Homosexual urges may be projected to the environment as well, and fear of sexual advances from others may stimulate aggression.

Therefore, an environment that provides the client with a sense of security and safety should minimize anxiety and environmental distortions. Activities that distract the client from rumination of his hallucinations and delusions can also help to decrease anxiety. Table 20–7 suggests some basic nursing interventions for clients who are experiencing paranoia.

Table 20-7 • NURSING CONSIDERATIONS FOR PEOPLE WHO ARE PARANOID

NURSING INTERVENTION	RATIONALE
Communications	
1. Honesty and consistency are imperative. If you say, "I'll be back at 11 A.M." or "I'll call your social worker this morning," *always* follow through with what you say you will do.	1. A person who is paranoid will be quick to pick up dishonesty. Honesty and consistency provide an atmosphere in which trust can grow.
2. Avoid a warm and gushing approach. A nonjudgmental, respectful, and consistent approach is most effective.	2. Warmth and gushing can be frightening to a person who needs emotional distance. Matter-of-fact consistency is not threatening.
3. Eliminate physical contact; do *not* touch the client.	3. Touch may be interpreted as a physical or sexual assault.
4. Evaluate themes in hallucinations and delusions. Do not argue with the content.	4. The themes are important to know (e.g., kill self or others), since protective action may have to be taken. Arguing with hallucinations and delusions makes the person defend his beliefs more vigorously.
5. When speaking of the client's "voices," do use terms such as "so-called voices" or "the voices you say you hear."	5. Helps cast doubt on reality of hallucinations.
6. Resist getting caught up in content; rather, look for the feelings behind the delusions and hallucinations.	6. One cannot logically discuss illogical material, but one *can* discuss feelings—e.g., "I don't know about the FBI trying to harm you, but thinking that must be frightening."
7. Clarify and restate your role. Repeat with patience and understanding.	7. Prevents misinterpretation and minimizes misconstruing the relationship.
8. Use simple and clear language when speaking to client. Explain everything you are going to do before you do it.	8. Prevents misinterpretations and clarifies nurse's intent and actions.
9. Diffuse angry and hostile verbal attacks with a nondefensive stand. Explore with client origin of angry feelings.	9. The anger a client expresses is often displaced. When staff become defensive, anger of both client and staff escalates. A nondefensive and nonjudgmental attitude provide an atmosphere in which feelings can be explored more easily.
Physical Needs	
1. Grooming and dress are rarely a problem.	1. Provide necessary toilet articles and facilities for client to care for clothes.
2. When client thinks food is poisoned, nurse can taste food, eat food with client, or provide foods in their own containers—e.g., milk cartons, hard boiled eggs, apples.	2. Delusions that food is poisoned are common with paranoid clients. Usually these measures promote adequate nutrition. Tube feeding is instituted as a *last* resort.
3. When the client is unable to sleep, staying with the client for specific time periods can be helpful.	3. Client may feel too vulnerable to sleep. The nurse's presence often helps the client feel more secure—e.g., "I will stay with you 15 minutes," or "until you fall asleep."
Physical Behaviors	
1. Provide verbal and physical limits to client's hostility—e.g., "We won't allow you to hit or hurt anyone here; if you can't control yourself, we will help you."	1. When anxiety is high, client may feel out of control. Often, firm verbal limits are effective in calming client; if not, a quiet room or medication may be necessary.
2. Assign solitary, noncompetitive activities that take some concentration (e.g., crossword puzzles, picture puzzles, photography, typing); when client feels less threatened, bridge and chess may be more appropriate, requiring increased concentration.	2. When client is extremely distrustful of others, solitary activities are best. Activities that demand concentration keep attention of client on reality and minimize hallucinatory and delusional preoccupation.

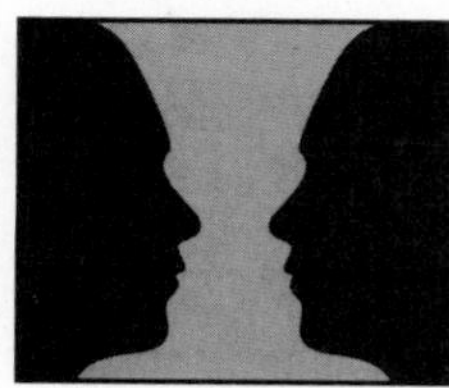

Case Study: Working With a Person Who Is Paranoid

Tom is a 37-year-old man who is currently an inpatient at the Veterans Administration (VA) Hospital. He has been separated from his wife and four children for six years. His medical records state that he has been in and out of hospitals frequently for 17 years for his illness, which Tom describes as "hearing voices alot." Tom is an ex-marine who first "heard voices" at the age of 19 while he was stationed in Okinawa; he subsequently received a medical discharge.

This hospitalization was precipitated by an exacerbation of auditory hallucinations. "I thought people were following me. I hear voices, usually a woman's voice, and she's tormenting me. People say that it happens because I don't take my medications. The medications make me tired and I can't have sex." Tom also admits to using cocaine and marijuana. He is aware that marijuana and cocaine increase his paranoia and that taking drugs usually precedes hospitalization, but says that "they make me feel good." Tom finished 11 years of school but did not graduate from high school. He denies having any close friends. He was in prison for five years for manslaughter and told the nurse, "I was in prison because I did something bad." He was abusing alcohol and drugs at the time, and drug abuse has been related to each subsequent hospitalization.

Ms. Lally is Tom's primary nurse. When Tom meets the nurse, he is dressed in pajamas and bathrobe. His hygiene is intact, and he is well nourished. He tells the nurse that he does not sleep much because "the voices get worse at night." Ms. Lally notes in Tom's medical record that he has had two episodes of suicidal ideation. During those times the voices were telling him to jump "off rooftops" and "in front of trains."

During the first interview, Tom only occasionally makes eye contact and speaks in a low monotone. At times he glances about the room as if distracted, mumbles to himself, and appears visibly upset.

NURSE: Tom, my name is Ms. Lally. I will be your nurse while you're in the hospital. We will meet every day for 30 minutes at 10:00 A.M. During that time we can discuss areas of concern for you.

TOM: Well . . . don't believe what they say about me. I want to start new . . . are you married?

NURSE: This time is for you to talk about *your* concerns.

TOM: Oh . . . (*Looks furtively around the room then lowers his eyes.*)
Someone is trying to kill me . . . I think . . .

NURSE: You appear to be focusing on something other than our conversation. Is something making you uncomfortable?

TOM: The voices tell me things . . . I can't say . . .

NURSE: I don't hear any voices except yours and mine. I am going to stay with you. Tell me what is happening and I will try to help you.

TOM: The voices tell me bad things . . .

Ms. Lally stayed with Tom and encouraged him to communicate with her. As Tom focused more on the nurse, his anxiety appeared to lessen. His thoughts became more connected; he was able to concentrate more on what the nurse was saying, and he mumbled less to himself.

Assessment

After the initial interview, Ms. Lally divides the data into objective and subjective components:

OBJECTIVE DATA

1. Speaks in low monotone voice
2. Poor eye contact
3. Well-nourished and hygiene intact
4. Admits to auditory hallucinations
5. Has history of drug abuse—cocaine and marijuana
6. Has no close friends
7. Has been hospitalized since age 19 and has not worked since that time.
8. Has had suicidal impulses twice
9. Imprisoned five years for violent acting out
10. Thoughts scattered when anxious

Continued on following page

Assessment *(Continued)*

SUBJECTIVE DATA

1. "Someone is trying to kill me . . . I think . . . "
2. "I don't take my medicine. It makes me tired and I can't have sex."
3. "The voices get worse at night and I can't sleep."
4. Voices have told him to "jump off rooftops" and "in front of trains."

Nursing Diagnosis

Ms. Lally formulates two nursing diagnoses based on her assessment data.

1. *Altered Thought Processes* related to unclear communication and alteration in biochemical compounds, as evidenced by persecutory hallucinations and intense suspiciousness
   - Voices have told him to "jump off rooftops" and "in front of trains."
   - "Someone is trying to kill me . . . I think . . . "
   - Abuses cocaine and marijuana, although paranoia increases, because "it makes me feel good."
2. *Noncompliance with medications* related to side effects of therapy, as evidenced by verbalization of noncompliance and persistence of symptoms
   - Does not take prescribed medication because "it makes me tired and I can't have sex."
   - Chronic history of relapse of symptoms when out of hospital

Planning

CONTENT LEVEL—PLANNING GOALS

Ms. Lally decides that initial concentration should be placed on establishing a relationship in which Tom can feel safe with the nurse and comfortable enough to discuss his voices and events that precipitate them. Over time, the nurse aims to provide a temporary replacement for the hallucinatory experience. The nurse is also aware that if Tom's anxiety level can be lowered and his suspicions diminished, he will be able to participate more comfortably in reality-based activities and have an increased ability to problem-solve. Since noncompliance with his medications appears to be a major factor in the persistence of Tom's disturbing symptoms, this becomes an important focus for discussion. Ms. Lally plans to evaluate the medication and side effects with the physician and to work with Tom on alternatives to increase his medical compliance.

The following goals are outlined:

Nursing Diagnosis	Long Term Goals	Short Term Goals
1. *Altered Thought Processes* related to unclear communication and alteration in biochemical compounds, as evidenced by persecutory hallucinations and intense suspiciousness	Tom will state he is able to function without interference from "his voices" or thoughts by discharge.	1a. By (state the date) Tom will state that he feels comfortable with the nurse. 1b. By (state the date) Tom will name two actions that precipitate the voices and paranoia. 1c. By (state the date) Tom will name two actions he can take if the voices start to become upsetting to him.
2. *Noncompliance with medications* related to side effects of therapy, as evidenced by verbalization of noncompliance and persistence of symptoms	Tom will adhere to medication regime by (state the date).	1. By (state the date) Tom will name actions he can take to offset the side effects of medication. 2. Tom will attend weekly support group for people with schizophrenia.

PROCESS LEVEL — NURSES' REACTIONS AND FEELINGS

On the first day of admission, Tom assaulted another male client, stating that the other client accused him of being a homosexual and touched him on the buttocks. After assessing the incident, the staff agreed that Tom's provocation came more from his own projections (Tom's sexual attraction to the other client) than from anything the other client had done or said.

Tom's difficulty with impulse control frightened Ms. Lally. She had some real concerns regarding Tom's impulse control and the possibility of Tom's striking out at her, especially when Tom was hallucinating and highly delusional. Ms. Lally mentioned her concerns to the nursing coordinator, and it was suggested that Ms. Lally meet with Tom in the day room until he demonstrated more control and less suspicion of others. After five days Tom was less excitable, and the sessions were held in a room set aside for client interviews. Ms. Lally also spoke with a senior staff nurse regarding her fear. By talking to the senior nurse and understanding more clearly her own fear, Ms. Lally was able to identify interventions to help Tom regain a better sense of control.

Intervention

Ms. Lally made out an initial nursing care plan (Nursing Care Plan 20–1). An important part of her plan was conferring with the physician about the legitimate concerns Tom had regarding his medication. The physician decided to try giving Tom a larger dose of medication at bedtime to minimize his insomnia, and a lighter dose during the day to minimize the sedative side effects. The concerns Tom had regarding not being able to sustain an erection were legitimate, and the physician stated that he would try another medication if Tom's complaint of impotence continued. Ms. Lally worked with Tom on continuing his participation in the support group. During team conference, the social worker suggested that if Tom was able to maintain contact with a support group, he might be a good candidate for a group home in the future.

Medications appeared to greatly lower Tom's suspiciousness and his hallucinatory symptoms. This enabled Tom to discuss with the nurse more reality-based concerns and to be more amenable to attending the weekly support group. After the fourth meeting, Tom seemed to view the group more favorably and even spoke of making a friend in the group.

Evaluation

By discharge, Tom said he had a better understanding of his medications and what to do. He knew that marijuana and cocaine would increase his symptoms, but he said sometimes he got lonely and needed to "feel good." He did say he planned to continue with the support group and with outpatient counseling. The reason he gave for deciding to attend outpatient therapy was that he felt Ms. Lally had really cared about him, and that made him feel good. By the time of discharge he was sleeping much better and said he had more energy during the day.

Nursing Care Plan 20–1 • A PERSON WITH PARANOIA: Tom

NURSING DIAGNOSIS

Altered thought processes related to unclear communication and alteration in biochemical compounds, as evidenced by persecutory hallucinations and intense suspiciousness.

Supporting Data

- Voices have told him to "jump off rooftops" and "in front of trains."
- "Someone is trying to kill me . . . I think . . . "
- Abuses cocaine and marijuana although paranoia increases: "It makes me feel good."

Continued on following page

Nursing Care Plan 20–1 • A PERSON WITH PARANOIA: Tom *(Continued)*

Long Term Goal: Tom will state that he is able to function without interference from "his voices" by discharge.

Short Term Goal	*Intervention*	*Rationale*	*Evaluation*
1. By (state the date) Tom will state that he feels comfortable with the nurse.	1a. Meet with Tom each day for 30 minutes. 1b. Use clear, unambiguous statements. 1c. Provide activities that need concentration and are noncompetitive.	1a. Short, consistent meetings help establish contact and decrease anxiety. 1b. Minimize potential for misconstruing messages. 1c. Increase time spent in reality-based activities and decrease preoccupation with delusional and hallucinatory experiences.	*Goal met* By end of first week Tom said he looked forward to meeting with "my nurse."
2. Tom will name two events that precede the hallucinations and delusions, by (state the date).	2a. Investigate content of hallucinations with Tom. 2b. Explore those times that voices are most threatening and disturbing.	2a. Identify suicidal or aggressive themes. 2b. Identify events that increase anxiety.	*Goal met* Tom was able to identify that the voices were worse at nighttime. He also stated that after smoking marijuana and taking cocaine, he always thought people were trying to kill him.
3. Tom will name two actions that he can take if the voices start to become upsetting to him by (state the date).	3. Explore with Tom possible actions that can minimize anxiety.	3. Offer him alternatives while anxiety level relatively low.	*Goal met* Tom has the number of a doctor he can call when hallucinations start to escalate.

NURSING DIAGNOSIS

Noncompliance with medications related to side effects of therapy, as evidenced by verbalization of noncompliance and persistence of symptoms

Supporting Data

- Does not take prescribed medication: "It makes me tired and I can't have sex."
- Chronic history of relapse of symptoms when out of hospital.

Long Term Goal: Tom will adhere to medication regimen by (state the date).

Short Term Goal	*Intervention*	*Rationale*	*Evaluation*
1. By (state the date) Tom will name actions he can take to offset side effects of medication.	1a. Evaluate medication response with physician in hospital. 1b. Educate Tom regarding side effects—how long they last and actions to take.	1a. Identify drugs and dosage that have increased therapeutic value and decreased side effects. 1b. Can give increased sense of control over symptoms.	*Goal partially met* Physician readjusted dose—highest dose at bedtime to increase sleep; low dose during the day to decrease fatigue. Tom stated he slept better at night, still tired during the day.
2. Tom will attend weekly support group for people with schizophrenia.	2. Encourage Tom to join support group for people with schizophrenia.	2. Mutual concerns and problems discussed in an atmosphere of acceptance—concerns such as housing, expenses, loneliness, and jobs. Group also provides peer support for drug therapy maintenance.	*Goal met* Week 1—Tom attended meeting. Week 2—Tom stated that he made a friend. Spoke in group about "not feeling good" at times. Week 3—Tom said that he might go to group, once discharged from hospital.

Catatonia

The essential feature of catatonia is abnormal motor behavior. A major defense mechanism used by a person in a catatonic state is repression. One theory regarding the symptoms of catatonia is that they are an attempt to deal with feelings of intense rage. The extreme muscular immobility (repression of rage) often gives way to uncontrollable outbursts of physically destructive behavior when repression lifts. Therefore, the two extreme motor behaviors seen in a client with catatonia are extreme motor agitation and extreme psychomotor retardation. Other behaviors identified with catatonia include mutism, waxy flexibility, stereotyped behavior, negativism, echolalia, and echopraxia. The onset of catatonia is usually abrupt and the prognosis favorable.

THE WITHDRAWN PHASE

COMMUNICATIONS. Clients in the withdrawn phase of catatonia can be so withdrawn that they appear comatose. They can be mute and may remain so for hours, days, weeks, or months. Although such a client may not appear to pay attention to events going on around him or her, the client is acutely aware of things that go on in his or her environment and may remember them accurately at a later date (Chapman 1976).

PHYSICAL NEEDS. When a client is extremely withdrawn, physical needs take priority. A client may need to be hand fed or tube fed to maintain adequate nutritional status. Normal control over bladder and bowel functions can be interrupted. Assessment of urinary or bowel retention must be made and acted upon when found. Incontinence of urine and feces poses the problem of skin breakdown and potential infection. Since physical movements may be minimal or absent, range-of-motion exercises need to be carried out to prevent muscular atrophy, calcium depletion, and contractures. Dressing and grooming will most likely need direct nursing interventions.

The negativistic client may trigger resistance in the staff to nursing interventions, since the client refuses to participate in activities or cooperate voluntarily.

PHYSICAL BEHAVIORS. During the withdrawn state, the catatonic person may be on a continuum from complete stupor to pronounced decrease in spontaneous movements. *Waxy flexibility* is often seen. As mentioned, this is the ability to hold distorted postures for extensive periods of time. The term "waxy" refers to the holding of any posture that the staff may place the person in. For example, if the nurse raises the client's arms over his head, the client can maintain that position for hours, days, or longer. This phenomenon is often used as a diagnostic sign. When less withdrawn, a client may demonstrate *stereotyped behavior, echopraxia, echolalia,* or *automatic obedience*.

Caution is advised, because even after holding a single posture for long periods of time, the client may suddenly and without provocation have brief outbursts of destructive violence, in response to inner hallucinations or delusions. Table 20–8 suggests specific nursing interventions for a catatonic client when withdrawn or in a catatonic stupor.

EXCITED PHASE

COMMUNICATIONS. During the excited, or hyperactive, stage the person talks or shouts continuously and the verbalizations may be incoherent.

PHYSICAL NEEDS. A person who is constantly and intensely hyperactive can become completely exhausted and die if medical attention is not available. Most often a phenothiazine (Thorazine) is administered intramuscularly. The client may continue to be agitated, but within limits this should not be physically harmful. During this time of heightened physical activity, the client's body has an increased need for fluids, calories, and rest. During the hyperactive state a client can be destructive and violent to others in response to inner hallucinations or delusions. Table 20–9 suggests nursing interventions during the excited phase of catatonia. Table 20–8 highlights some basic nursing care. Many of these concerns and interventions are the same as for a bipolar client in a manic phase.

Table 20–8 • NURSING CONSIDERATIONS FOR PEOPLE WHO ARE WITHDRAWN

NURSING INTERVENTION	RATIONALE
Communications	
1. Stay with the person and sit in silence for short intervals. This is often the first step.	1. Do not demand that the client reply; meet the person at his or her own level. The client may be too anxious or confused to speak.

Table continued on following page

Table 20–8 • NURSING CONSIDERATIONS FOR PEOPLE WHO ARE WITHDRAWN *Continued*

NURSING INTERVENTION	RATIONALE
Communications	
2. Initiate frequent, short, regular contacts with the withdrawn person.	2. Initially, short intervals are more tolerable for both client and nurse.
3. Before you leave, be very specific as to when you will be back—e.g., "I will be back at 1 P.M. for ten minutes." Always be on time and always keep your word.	3. Visit the patient regularly and be back when you say you will. Disappointments caused by you could interfere with forming a relationship. If a delay is unavoidable, explain this to the client.
4. When speaking to the client, use simple, short sentences.	4. The client's thoughts may be confused, and attention span short.
5. Make observations about happenings in the environment—e.g., "I see you brought your Bible with you this morning."	5. Focuses attention on common realities in the environment.
6. When the client begins to speak, keep topics neutral and simple.	6. Helps to minimize anxiety and frustration.
7. Clarify the client's use of the generalized "they."	7. Clients with weak ego boundaries have difficulty with differentiating others from self. Ask, "Who are *they*?"
8. Meet hostility and rejection with a nonjudgmental and neutral response—e.g., "If you don't want to visit now, I'll be back at 1 P.M. to spend time with you."	8. Often clients are verbally abusive to or rejecting of the nurse; this is rarely personal. When the client can experience acceptance and caring for how he or she is at that moment, feelings of self-worth may increase.
9. Always tell the client you do not understand when you do not.	9. Clients may erroneously think the nurse can "read their mind" or "know" what they are thinking. By correcting this false belief, the nurse clarifies communications and delineates ego boundaries.
Physical Needs	
1. Talk to the client who appears comatose while giving physical care, and explain everything that you are doing. Talk as if the client fully understands. Address the client respectfully—e.g., "Mr. Jones, I am going to shave the other side of your face. The water may feel cold."	1. Even though clients may appear comatose, they may be *aware of everything that is going on*. Often, clients can remember verbatim conversations of others around them during the time they were comatose.
2. Monitor intake.	2. Client may be too disorganized to eat or drink.
3. Monitor output—urine and bowel.	3. Client may retain urine and feces or be incontinent of urine and feces.
4. Encourage involvement with hygiene and dressing at the client's own level. *Do not do for a client what he or she is able to do.*	4. Sometimes giving short, simple reminders is sufficient for a disorganized client. At other times the nurse may have to assist the client with grooming and dressing.
Physical Behaviors (Recreation)	
1. Increase participation with others at client's level of tolerance.	
A. Stuporous to very withdrawn: one-to-one simple activities with the nurse—e.g., talking, looking through a magazine, painting, working with clay.	A. Those activities that require no verbal response and have no time limit or "right or wrong" are the least threatening.
B. Less withdrawn: simple, concrete activity with nurse and perhaps with one other client—e.g., card games, drawing, ping pong.	B. Brings the client slowly into contact with others. This provides a greater opportunity for reality orientation and consensual validation.
C. Eventually, offer client group activities—e.g., ward meetings, occupational therapy, dance therapy, bingo games.	C. Increased participation with others can increase client's ability to validate reality and to experience satisfaction in reality-based activities.

Table 20–9 • NURSING CONSIDERATIONS FOR PEOPLE WHO ARE HYPERACTIVE

NURSING INTERVENTION	RATIONALE
Communications	
1. Use firm, clear statements.	1. Client may be disorganized; needs clear statements. Firmness provides a sense of outside control.
2. Keep patient in a quiet area.	2. Helps to decrease environmental stimuli and anxiety.
Physical Needs	
1. Monitor weight and dietary intake.	1. Client may lose calories, fluids, and essential nutrients.
2. Offer frequent high-caloric fluids and "finger goods"—e.g., milk, bananas, sandwiches, candy bars, hard-boiled eggs.	2. Foods that a client can carry with him or her when too active to sit during meals help to replace and maintain adequate nutrition.
3. Provide rest periods.	3. Minimizes exhaustion and fatigue.
4. Supervise grooming and physical appearance.	4. Client may be too agitated to care for physical appearance.
Physical Behaviors (Recreation)	
1. Watch closely for signs of increased agitation.	1. Client may become increasingly agitated and need a decrease in environmental stimuli or medication. Intervention should be made before anxiety escalates to panic levels, when intervention becomes traumatic for both client and staff.
2. Simple physical activity using large muscles groups may help discharge some physical tension—e.g., pace with the client, ping-pong, volleyball.	2. Gross motor activity that requires minimal concentration can reduce anxiety and tension.

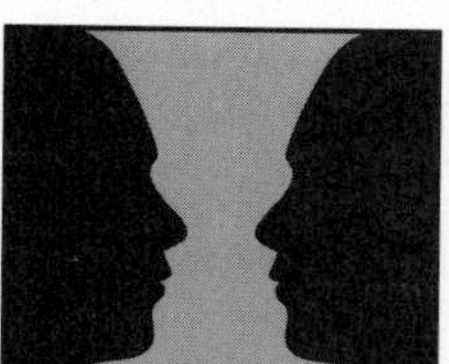

Case Study: Working With a Person Who Is In Withdrawn Catatonia

Mrs. Ling Chou is a 25-year-old pregnant woman. She left China for the United States six months ago to join her husband. Before she came to the United States she lived with her parents and worked in a button factory. In China Mrs. Chou had been educated to speak and understand English. She has always been shy and looked to her parents and now to her husband for guidance and support. Shortly after she arrived in the United States, her mother developed pneumonia and died, and Mrs. Chou was not able to go back to China for the funeral. Mr. Chou states that his wife thought that if she had stayed in China her mother would not have become ill. Recently, she told him that evil would come to the newborn baby because she was unable to take proper care of her mother. Three days before admission, Mrs. Chou became lethargic and spent most of the day staring into space and mumbling to herself. When Mr. Chou asked whom she was talking to she would answer, "My mother." She had not eaten for two days, and at the time of admission, Mrs. Chou sits motionless and mute and appears stuporous.

The physician noticed that when he took Mrs. Chou's pulse, her arm remained in mid-air until he replaced it by her side. Mr. Chou said that once his wife became extremely agitated and started to scream and cry while tearing the curtains and knocking over objects. Shortly afterward she returned to a withdrawn, mute state. Mr. Chou is extremely distraught and confused, and he fears for the safety of their baby. George Nolan is assigned to Mrs. Chou as her primary nurse.

Mrs. Chou is sloppily dressed, her hair and nails are dirty, and she appears greatly unkempt. She is very pale, and her skin turgor is poor. She sits motionless and appears unaware of anything going on around her. Mr. Nolan introduces himself and explains what he will be doing

Case Study: Working With a Person Who Is In Withdrawn Catatonia *(Continued)*

beforehand—for example, that he will be taking her blood pressure and pulse and offering her fluids.

While taking her vital signs, he tells Mrs. Chou the date, time, and where she is. When he is finished taking her vital signs, he offers Mrs. Chou some fluids. She is able to take sips from a straw when the straw is placed in her mouth. Mrs. Chou is put on intake and output. She is placed in a four-bed room next to the nurses' station.

Assessment

Mr. Nolan assesses his data:

OBJECTIVE DATA

1. Motionless and mute for two days
2. Has not taken nourishment for two days
3. Is pregnant
4. Has had one episode of violent and destructive activity
5. Appears to be comatose, eyes not focused, body limp
6. Has had recent shock with mother's death
7. Skin turgor poor
8. Poorly groomed
9. Waxy flexibility

SUBJECTIVE DATA

1. Told husband "evil" would come to the baby because she did not take proper care of her mother.

Nursing Diagnosis

Mr. Nolan notes that Mrs. Chou is unable to take care of any basic needs (e.g., nutrition, hygiene, or proper toileting). He identifies *self-care deficit* as the primary initial priority.

Planning

CONTENT LEVEL—PLANNING GOALS

Mr. Nolan formulated the following long term and short term goals:

Nursing Diagnosis	Long Term Goals	Short Term Goals
1. *Self-Care Deficit* related to immobility, as evidenced by inability to feed, bathe, dress or toilet herself.	1. Mrs. Chou will maintain nutritional intake and body weight while in the hospital.	1a. Mrs. Chou will take in 2000 cc of fluid each day. 1b. Mrs. Chou will eat three meals per day.
	2. Mrs. Chou will maintain normal bladder and bowel function while in the hospital.	2a. Mrs. Chou will void 1000–1500 cc per day. 2b. Mrs. Chou will have one BM per day.
	3. Mrs. Chou will maintain present muscle tone and flexibility while in the hospital.	3a. Mrs. Chou will participate in passive ROM exercises three times per day for 15 minutes.

PROCESS LEVEL—NURSES' REACTIONS AND FEELINGS

Mr. Nolan found that initially he became impatient with Mrs. Chou. He was used to carrying out nursing procedures quickly and efficiently. Mrs. Chou's morning care demanded a great deal of time. For example, he found himself being impatient with the long periods it took to feed Mrs.

Chou. He discussed his impatience with a colleague. During the discussion it became apparent that it was more Mrs. Chou's total dependency on him that made him anxious. Mr. Nolan sees himself as highly organized and in control, often suppressing many of his own needs and desires to be taken care of. "I guess her total dependency triggers off some of my own unmet dependency needs." Once he was able to separate some of his own personal concerns that triggered his reaction, he was able to focus on Mrs. Chou's needs with more patience. He found that the more he talked to Mrs. Chou as if she were able to understand everything he said, the easier it was for him to maintain a certain level of relatedness and interest.

Intervention

Mr. Nolan assigned the psychiatric aide to bathe and dress Mrs. Chou in the mornings. He spent time with Mrs. Chou each morning and afternoon doing range-of-motion exercises, offering her frequent sips of juice or milk, and talking to her—that is, making observations about neutral happenings in the environment. Mr. Chou visited every day, and Mr. Nolan encouraged Mr. Chou to talk to his wife about everyday occurrences in his life and about their future. He also cautioned Mr. Chou that there was a possibility that Mrs. Chou could suddenly become agitated and aggressive, and that this was part of the disease.

With the aid of medication therapy and nursing management, Mrs. Chou began to show signs of comprehension. By the end of the seventh day, Mrs. Chou was talking, feeding herself, and able to bathe herself. She appeared to have developed a strong attachment to Mr. Nolan, and told her husband how kind he was to her while she was "away." She even remembered that Mr. Nolan brought in a Chinese music tape during the period when she was stuporous. The psychiatrists thought that Mrs. Chou's catatonic reaction was triggered by her mother's death, and strongly suggested counseling after discharge to facilitate the work of mourning.

Evaluation

Generally, catatonic episodes are acute and related to identifiable stressors, and the disorder has a favorable prognosis. Mrs. Chou responded rapidly to medication and Mr. Nolan's nursing intervention. Although much of Mrs. Chou's passivity was culturally determined, the psychiatrists suggested that Mrs. Chou develop more outlets for release of emotional tensions. Mrs. Chou agreed to counseling after discharge.

Disorganized Schizophrenia

The most regressed and socially impaired of all the schizophrenic disorders is the disorganized form. A person diagnosed with disorganized schizophrenia (formally hebephrenia) may have marked loosening of associations, grossly inappropriate affect, bizarre mannerisms, and incoherence of speech and may display extreme social withdrawal (APA 1987). Although delusions and hallucinations are common, they are fragmentary and not well organized. Behavior may be considered "odd," and giggling or grimacing in response to internal stimuli (hallucinations or delusions) is common. The onset is usually early, the course insidious, and the prognosis poor.

COMMUNICATIONS. People with disorganized schizophrenia live almost entirely in a private fantasy. Verbal responses are marked by looseness of associations or incoherence. Clang associations or word salad may be present. **Blocking,** which is a sudden cessation in the train of thought, is frequently observed.

PHYSICAL NEEDS. Grooming is neglected. Hair may be dirty and matted, and clothes inappropriate and stained. There is no awareness of social expectations. A client may be too disorganized to carry out simple activities of daily living (ADL).

Basic goals for nursing intervention include encouraging optimal level of functioning, preventing further regression, and offering substitutes for inappropriate behaviors whenever possible. Refer to Table 20–10 for basic nursing considerations.

PHYSICAL BEHAVIORS. Behavior is often described as bizarre. A client may twirl around the room or make strange gestures with his or her hands and face. Social behavior is often primitive or regressed. For example, a client may eat with his or her hands, pick his or her nose, or masturbate in public. Typical behaviors include posturing, grimacing or giggling, and mirror gazing.

Table 20–10 • NURSING CONSIDERATIONS FOR PEOPLE WHO ARE DISORGANIZED

NURSING INTERVENTION	RATIONALE
Communications	
1. Speak in short, simple sentences.	1. Thought patterns are disorganized. Simple phrases are best understood.
2. Constantly reinforce reality—e.g., call client by name, state the date, state your name, and so forth.	2. Thinking is often autistic and confused. Stressing common environmental realities provides a tie with reality.
3. Initiate short, frequent contacts.	3. Helps to establish rapport and personal contact in a manner less threatening to client.
4. Allow client time to respond.	4. Since thought process of client is disorganized, time is needed for client to take messages in and compose a response.
Physical Needs	
1. Observe for signs and symptoms of physical illness—e.g., cold, thirst, pain.	1. Clients are often disorganized, out of touch with feelings, and unable to assess personal needs or ask for what they need.
2. Check for incontinence and provide fresh clothes when necessary. Use nonpunitive, matter-of-fact approach.	2. Client may be too disorganized to use toilet. Encourage appropriate dress and hygiene.
3. Help clients with hygiene prn, e.g., set up shaving, give step-by-step instructions; if unable to shave, help with shaving; help with putting on make-up, brushing hair, teeth, and so forth.	3. Can minimize anxiety and help client maintain self-esteem. Meets client at own level. When client is able to do partial care, even though slowly, this type of assistance encourages independent functioning.
4. Lay out clothes that are clean and appropriate. Give simple step-by-step instructions for dress—e.g., "Put in left arm . . . now right arm . . . pull sweater over your head."	4. Maintains optimal level of functioning and self-esteem.
5. Encourage appropriate social behaviors—e.g., have clients eat with utensils and cover front with napkin.	5. Increases social interactions. When taking something away—e.g., eating with hands—offer alternatives such as large spoon with which to eat food, protecting front from fallen food particles with napkin.
Physical Behavior (Recreation)	
1. Plan and initiate simple, daily routine.	1. Consistent daily routine helps client maintain contact with reality with minimal anxiety.
2. Plan simple, concrete tasks that require minimal concentration and skill—e.g., drawing, walking with nurse, dancing, ward meetings, folding linen.	2. Tasks that match client's concentration and interest can promote socialization, increase contact with reality, provide exercise, and increase self-esteem.

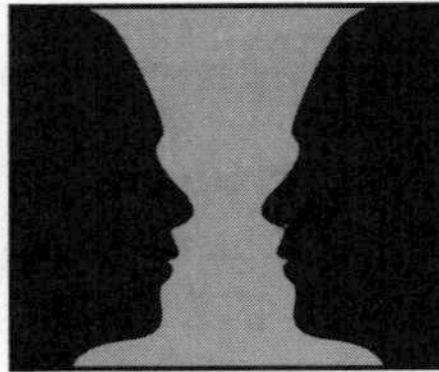

Case Study: Working With a Person Who Is Disorganized

Martin Taylor, a 36-year-old white unemployed man, has been transferred to an inpatient psychiatric unit for further evaluation. He is accompanied to the unit by his mother and sister. He has been previously hospitalized for three years with the diagnosis of chronic schizophrenia. His only employment was for five months as a janitor, after high school graduation. Other significant family history includes a twin brother who died of a cerebral aneurysm in his teens. Martin tells the nurse he has used every street drug available, including LSD and IV heroin. His mother states that as a teenager, prior to his substance abuse, he was an excellent athlete who received average grades. At the age of seventeen he had his first psychotic break in the setting of polysubstance abuse. His behavior became markedly bizarre (e.g., eating cat food and swallowing a rubber-soled shoe that required an emergency laporotomy).

Ms. Lamb is Martin's primary nurse. Ms. Lamb meets with Martin after speaking with his mother and sister. Martin is unshaven and his appearance is disheveled. He is wearing a red headband in which he has placed popsicle sticks and scraps of paper. He chain-smokes during the interview and frequently gets up and paces back and forth. He tells the nurse that he is Alice from the book *Alice in The Underground*, and that people from space hurt him with needles. His speech pattern is marked by associative looseness and occasional blocking. For example, he often stops in the middle of a phrase and giggles to himself. At one point when he started to giggle, Ms. Lamb asked him what he was thinking about. He stated, "You interrupted me." At that point he began to shake his head while repeating in a sing-song voice, "Shake them tigers . . . shake them tigers . . . shake them tigers . . . " He denies suicidal or homicidal ideation. Ms. Lamb notes that Martin has a great deal of difficulty accurately perceiving what is going on around him. He has markedly regressed social behaviors. For example, he eats with his hands and picks his nose in public. He has no apparent insight into his problems; he tells Ms. Lamb that his biggest problem is the people in space.

Assessment

OBJECTIVE DATA

1. Associative looseness
2. Giggles and mumbles to self
3. Poorly and bizarrely dressed
4. Low level of functioning
5. History of bizarre behavior
6. Restless, pacing, and chain-smoking
7. Regressed social behaviors
8. Occasional blocking

SUBJECTIVE DATA

1. "I am Alice in the Underground."
2. "People from space hurt me with needles."
3. "You interrupted me." In response to being asked what he was thinking.
4. Denies suicidal or homicidal impulses.
5. "My biggest problems are the people from space."

Nursing Diagnosis

Ms. Lamb identifies Martin's deterioration of functioning as one priority for intervention. Ms. Lamb's first diagnosis follows:

1. *Ineffective Individual Coping* related to confused thought processes and lack of motivation to respond, as evidenced by inability to meet basic needs.
   - Regressed social behaviors
   - Poorly and bizarrely dressed
   - Low level of functioning
   - Frequent looseness of association

Planning

CONTENT LEVEL — PLANNING GOALS

Nursing Diagnosis	Long Term Goals	Short Term Goals
1. *Ineffective Individual Coping* related to confused thought processes and lack of motivation, as evidenced by inability to meet basic needs	Martin will be able to perform three skills in daily living within one month.	1a. Martin will be able to bathe independently in one week. 1b. Martin will make his bed in two weeks. 1c. Martin will be able to make a sandwich with the aid of the nurse in three weeks.

PROCESS LEVEL — NURSES' REACTIONS AND FEELINGS

Working with a client who has limited potential for relating, poorly defined ego boundaries, and limited social skills and who demonstrates regressed bizarre behaviors requires a great deal of

Continued on following page

Planning *(Continued)*

skill, patience, and peer support. In the presence of delusions, bizarre behaviors, and regressed social skills, health care workers can experience helplessness, feel overwhelmed, and become anxious. Some anxiety may be caused by empathizing or acknowledging the client's deeply repressed feelings of inferiority, fear, and anger. At times, nurses may have similar repressed feelings that they are unable to deal with. This may motivate withdrawal from the client in an attempt to minimize the nurse's awareness of personal uncomfortable feelings. Often, the more withdrawn and regressed the client is, the more health care workers tend to withdraw. The process of increasing independence in a regressed client can be taxing. Team involvement is necessary to promote success and continued interest in the client. For example, frequent team meetings among the recreational therapist, occupational therapist, nurses, social worker, and psychiatrist can sustain interest in a client's progress, provide mutual support for members of the health care team, and provide new data for reformulating goals and interventions.

Intervention

Ms. Lamb discussed Martin at the weekly health team conference. Since Martin has a chronic history of deterioration, all members of the health team agreed to work together on a few concrete goals. A trial daily checklist for activities in daily living was devised for use during the first week and to be reviewed at the next meeting. It included such items as the following:

- Makes bed
- Brushes teeth
- Combs hair
- Shaves
- Showers
- Makes two meals a week
- Wears clean clothing

The psychiatrist stated that when Martin takes his neuroleptic medication regularly, he is less withdrawn, his behavior is less bizarre, and he is better able to concentrate.

Evaluation

After one month, Martin is able to carry out basic ADLs when constant reminders are given. He is able to bathe, shave, comb his hair, and dress more appropriately when given simple instructions and encouragement. The goal of making a sandwich or fixing a simple lunch has not yet been met, since Martin starts to eat the food before the task of finishing the sandwich is completed. The social worker is trying to place Martin in a group home where his socialization skills can be increased, his isolation decreased, and his level of functioning maintained.

Summary

Psychotic symptoms are more pronounced and disruptive than those symptoms found in other disorders. The basic differences are in the degree of severity, withdrawal, alteration in affect, impairment of intellect, and regression.

Four theoretical hypotheses for explaining the symptoms of schizophrenia were discussed: biological (catecholamines and serotonin), genetic, family, and interpersonal theories. However, no one theory at present can account for all phenomena found in the schizophrenic process.

During the nurse's work with schizophrenic clients, specific symptoms are evident. No one symptom is found in all cases of schizophrenia. Named here as primary were Bleuler's four A's: affect, associative looseness, ambivalence, and autism. Secondary symptoms discussed were withdrawal, disturbances in thinking, disturbances in behavior, disturbances in feeling, and disturbances in speech patterns.

Some nursing diagnoses were discussed, including, *altered thought process, impaired communications, ineffective individual coping*, and others.

Planning on the content level was discussed, and a variety of short term and long term goals were proposed for each of the nursing diagnoses. Planning on the process level involves awareness of personal feelings and reactions to clients' feelings and behaviors. The schizophrenic's strong dependent, angry, and eroticized transferences, among other feelings and reactions, warrant supervision and peer support.

Interventions for people with schizophrenia include therapeutic interventions, health teaching, activities of daily living, somatic therapies, therapeutic environment, and psychotherapy. Each area was discussed and examples were given.

A brief overview of paranoid, catatonic (withdrawn

and excited), and disorganized schizophrenia was given. Specific nursing interventions were outlined, and a case study for each was presented.

References*

Aaronson LS. Paranoia as a behavior alienation. Perspectives in Psychiatric Care, 15(1): 1977.

American Psychiatric Association. Diagnostic and Statistical Manual of Mental Disorders, 3d ed., revised. Washington DC: American Psychiatric Association, 1987.

Arieti S. American Handbook of Psychiatry, Vol 3. New York: Basic Books, 1974.

Beard MT, et al. Activity therapy as a reconstructive plan in the social competence of chronic hospitalized patients. Journal of Psychosocial Nursing and Mental Health Services, 16(2):33, 1978.

Black DW, Yates WR, Andreasen NC. Schizophrenia, schizophreniform disorders and delusional paranoid disorders. *In* Talbott JA, Hales, RE, Yudofsky, SC (eds). Textbook of Psychiatry. Washington DC: American Psychiatric Press, 1988.

Bowen M. Family Therapy in Clinical Practice. New York: Jason Aronson, 1978.

Bruch H. Psychotherapy in schizophrenia: historical considerations. *In* Strauss J (ed). The Psychotherapy of Schizophrenia. New York: Plenum Book Company, 1980.

Cancro R. Individual psychotherapy in the treatment of chronic schizophrenic patients. American Journal of Psychotherapy, 37(4):493, 1983.

Chapman AH. Textbook of Clinical Psychiatry: An Interpersonal Approach. Philadelphia: J.B. Lippincott Company, 1976.

Cook JC. Interpreting and decoding autistic communication. Perspectives in Psychiatric Care, 9(1): 1971.

Crow TJ. Positive and negative schizophrenic symptoms and the role of dopamine. British Journal of Psychiatry, 137:383, 1980.

Donlon PT. Sexual symptoms of incipient schizophrenic psychoses. Medical Aspects of Human Sexuality, 10:69, 1976.

Falloon IRH. Family stress and schizophrenia: theory and practice. Psychiatric Clinics of North America, 9(1):165, 1986.

Falloon IRH, et al. Family management in the prevention of exacerbations of schizophrenia. New England Journal of Medicine, 306:1437, 1982.

Field WE Jr. The Psychotherapy of Hildegard E. Peplau. New Braunfels, TX: Atwood Printing, 1979.

Field WE, Ruelke W. Hallucinations and how to deal with them. American Journal of Nursing, 73(4):638, 1973.

Gottesman II, Shield S. Schizophrenia—the Epigenetic Puzzle. New York: Cambridge University Press, 1982.

Hart CA, et al. Introduction to Psychotropic Drugs. Rochester, NY: Medical Examination Publishing Company and Excerpta Company, 1981.

Harvard Medical School Mental Health Letter. Care of schizophrenia, 2(12):1, 1986.

Hertz MI. Recognizing and preventing relapse in patients with schizophrenia. Hospital and Community Psychiatry, 35 (4):344, 1984.

Hinsie L, Cambell RJ. Psychiatric Dictionary, 5th ed. New York: Oxford University Press, 1981.

*Many older references are those of primary sources and are considered classics by some practitioners.

Irving S. Basic Psychiatric Nursing, 3rd ed. Philadelphia: W.B. Saunders Company, 1983.

Johnson-Soderberg S. Theory and practice of scapegoating. Perspectives in Psychiatric Care, 15(4):1977.

Kahn ME. Psychotherapy with chronic schizophrenics: alliance, transference and countertransference. Journal of Psychosocial Nursing, 22(7):20, 1984.

Karb VB, Queener SF, Freeman JB. Handbook of Drugs for Nursing Practice. St. Louis, MO: C.V. Mosby, 1989.

Kolb LC, Brodie HKH. Modern Clinical Psychiatry, 10th ed. Philadelphia: W.B. Saunders Company, 1982.

Lamb RH, et al. Families of schizophrenics: a movement in jeopardy. Hospital and Community Psychiatry, 37(4):353, 1986.

Lancaster J. Schizophrenic patient activity groups as therapy. American Journal of Nursing, 76(6):949, 1976.

Lehmann HE, Cancro R. Schizophrenia: clinical features. *In* Kaplan HI, Sadock BJ (ed). Comprehensive Textbook of Psychiatry/IV, 4th ed. Baltimore, MD: Williams & Wilkins, 1985.

Lickey ME, Gordon B. Drugs for Mental Illness: A Revolution in Psychiatry. New York: W.H. Freeman Company, 1983.

MacKinnon RA, Michels R. The Psychiatric Interview in Clinical Practice. Philadelphia: W.B. Saunders, 1971.

Menninger WW. Dealing with staff reactions to perceived lack of progress by chronic mental patients. Hospital and Community Psychiatry, 35(8):805, 1984.

Merck Manual (15th ed). Berkow R, et al (eds). Rahway, NJ: Merck Sharp & Dohme Research Laboratories, 1987.

Mosher LR. A psychosocial approach to returning schizophrenia. The Schizophrenic Outpatient, 1:1, 1982.

Rickelman B. Brain bio-amines and schizophrenia: a summary of research findings and implications for nursing. Journal of Psychosocial Nursing and Mental Health Services, 17(9):28, 1979.

Roy A. Foreword. The Psychiatric Clinics of North America, 9(1):1, 1986.

Schatzberg AF, Cole JO. Manual of Clinical Psychopharmacology. Washington, DC: American Psychiatric Press, Inc., 1986.

Scherer JC. Nurses' Drug Manual. Philadelphia: J.B. Lippincott Company, 1985.

Schwartz LH, Schwartz JL. The psychodynamics of patient care. Englewood Cliffs, NJ: Prentice-Hall, 1972.

Schwartz MS, Schockley EL. The nurse and the mental patient. New York: John Wiley & Sons, 1956.

Scrak BM, Greenstein RA. Tardive dyskinesia evaluation in a nurse managed prolixin program. Journal of Psychosocial Nursing, 24(5):10, 1986.

Spitz HI. Contemporary trends in group psychotherapy: a literature survey. Hospital and Community Psychiatry, 35(2):132, 1984.

Sullivan HS. The interpersonal theory of psychiatry. New York: W.W. Norton & Company, 1953.

Torry ER. Management of chronic schizophrenic outpatients. Psychiatric Clinics of North America, 9(1):143, 1986.

Vidal G. The second American revolution and other essays (1976–1982). New York: Random House, 1982.

Weich MJ. Transitional language. *In* Grolnick SA, Barkin L (eds). Between Reality and Fantasy. New York: Jason Aronson, 1978.

Weiner H. Schizophrenia: etiology. *In* Kaplan HI, Sadock BJ (eds). Comprehensive Textbook of Psychiatry/IV, 4th ed. Baltimore, MD: Williams & Wilkins, 1985.

White EM, Kahn ME. Use of modification in group psychotherapy with chronic schizophrenic outpatients. Journal of Psychosocial Nursing and Mental Health Services, 20(2):1982.

Self-Study Exercises

Match the theory of schizophrenia (right column) next to the concepts central to that theory (left column).

1. ________ Catecholamines
2. ________ Identical twin 35–60% concordant schizophrenia
3. ________ Double bind
4. ________ Hostile environment and lack of consensual validation for the infant
5. ________ Scapegoating
6. ________ Children of normal parents placed for adoption in homes in which schizophrenia later develops do not show increase in rate of schizophrenia
7. ________ Ventricular enlargement

A. Neuroanatomical
B. Developmental
C. Genetic
D. Dopamine hypothesis
E. Family

Place T (True) or F (False) next to each statement.

8. ________ It is impossible to understand a person when his speech is characterized by looseness of association.

9. ________ Hallucinations, delusions, and neologisms are examples of autistic thinking.

10. ________ Ambivalence in relationships is found only in the mentally ill.

11. ________ A man hears that the stock market is down and takes that as a sign that God will destroy the world. This is an example of an idea of reference.

Write brief responses in answer to the following:

12. Discuss the difference between a hallucination and a delusion and give examples.

13. Depression, depersonalization, and derealization were presented here under *disturbance in* ________________.

14. Give an example of (A) clang association, (B) neologism, and (C) word salad.

15. Name two possible short term goals for *alteration in thought processes*.
    A. ________________________________
    B. ________________________________

Circle all correct answers.

16. Circle possible outcomes of unresolved countertransferential reactions by a nurse.

    A. Denial
    B. Withdrawal from client
    C. Increase in nurse's self-esteem
    D. Burnout

17. Circle the possible outcomes of effective health teaching with client and family. Cross out those that are not possible outcomes.

    A. Increase compliance with medication
    B. Increase problem-solving skills

C. Minimize misunderstanding of the schizophrenic member within the family or community group
D. Reduce the occurrence of schizophrenic symptoms from the ingestion of certain drugs (e.g., marijuana, amphetamines)
E. Help the family identify those symptoms which may signal a possible relapse

18. Circle the desired effects of neuroleptics/antipsychotic medication.
    A. Reduction in intensity of hallucinations and delusions
    B. Improvement in thought process
    C. Increase in affect and motivation
    D. Decrease in the intensity of paranoid reactions

Place H (Hallucinations, D (Delusions), or HD (Hallucinations and Delusions) next to the appropriate intervention.

19. ________ Look for themes in the client's speech patterns.
20. ________ Tell the client you do not hear the voices he hears.
21. ________ Point out reality and attempt to empathize with the client's experience.
22. ________ Discredit the validity of perceptions—e.g., "those so-called voices."
23. ________ Do not argue with the client over the validity of this thinking.
24. ________ Always validate reality.
25. ________ Clarify misinterpretations of the environment.
26. ________ Do not pretend to understand the client when you do not.
27. ________ Place the focus of difficulty in understanding on yourself—e.g., "I am having a difficult time understanding you."

Place T (True) or F (False) next to each statement.

28. ________ *All* the extrapyramidal side effects (EPS) are reversible.
29. ________ Specific antipsychotics are often ordered because of their specific side effects.
30. ________ The only problem with antipsychotics is that a tolerance develops.
31. ________ Tardive dyskinesia, weight gain, and impotence are the most troubling side effects in outpatient management.
32. ________ Fatal side effects from the neuroleptics (antipsychotics) are rare.
33. ________ A person in a catatonic stupor is totally unaware of anything going on around him or her.
34. ________ Physical needs may take the highest priority when a person is in either extreme catatonic excitement or stupor.

True (T) *or False* (F). *The following can result from frequent team evaluation of the treatment plan for a chronic schizophrenic client:*

35. ________ Reassess problems; may have missed important needs.
36. ________ Reevaluate client's strengths and identify alternative interventions.
37. ________ Reassess goals and renew interest in client.

True (T) *or False* (F). A *person with paranoid schizophrenia*

38. ________ often has better ego functions than a person with any other schizophrenic disorder.
39. ________ uses sarcasm and hostility to maintain emotional distance.
40. ________ needs help with grooming and dress.
41. ________ uses projection as a main defense mechanism.

Mutiple Choice

42. Jerry P., a 17-year-old youth, had a paranoid psychotic break following the death of his twin brother. He was sure everyone wanted him dead and that his food was poisoned. He heard the voice of God demanding that he join his brother. He would not bathe or change his clothes because he believed that the WARLOCKS could then take over his body. Of the following possible nursing diagnoses, which has the highest priority?

    A. Alteration in nutrition: less than body weight
    B. Alteration in health maintenance
    C. Potential for self-harm
    D. Alteration in thought processes

43. If Tom thought his food was poisoned, the nurse should first

    A. Discuss nutrition with Tom.
    B. Get an order for tube feedings.
    C. Offer Tom food in its own containers (e.g., milk, oranges).
    D. Show him how irrational his thinking is.

44. When Tom says, "You are wearing a red sweater. That means you are against me today," he is experiencing a/an

    A. Delusion
    B. Hallucination
    C. Idea of reference
    D. Fantasy

45. When speaking to a person who is paranoid, you would consider all of the following EXCEPT:

    A. Use simple, clear language.
    B. Refrain from touching the client.
    C. Be warm and enthusiastic.
    D. Clarify and restate your role in a patient manner.

46. Which activity would you choose INITIALLY for a person who was paranoid?

    A. Listening to music alone.
    B. Poker with two other people.
    C. Team volley ball.
    D. Model airplanes, concentrating by self.

47. Medication appropriate for a person in extreme psychomotor agitation is

    A. Lithium
    B. Thorazine
    C. Librium
    D. Artane

Write a short paragraph in answer to each of the following questions:

48. Discuss two issues for each of the following transferences that the nurse would work on during supervision: (A) angry transference, (B) dependent transference, (C) eroticized transference.

49. Recount a situation of a disorganized client and identify at least five interventions.

CHAPTER 21

Organic Mental Syndromes and Disorders

Brenda Lewis Cleary
Elizabeth M. Varcarolis

OUTLINE

KEY TERMS AND CONCEPTS

The key terms and concepts listed here also appear in bold where they are defined or discussed in this chapter.

ORGANIC MENTAL SYNDROME
ORGANIC MENTAL DISORDER
HYPERVIGILANT
DELIRIUM
DEMENTIA
DYSTONIA
DYSGRAPHIA
ILLUSIONS
HALLUCINATIONS (TACTILE, VISUAL)
UNCOMPLICATED ALCOHOL WITHDRAWAL
ALCOHOL WITHDRAWAL DELIRIUM
PRIMARY DEMENTIA
SECONDARY DEMENTIA
PSEUDODEMENTIAS
CONFABULATION
PERSEVERATION
APHASIA
APRAXIA
AGNOSIA
MNEMONIC DISTURBANCE
AGRAPHIA
HYPERORALITY
HYPERMETAMORPHOSIS
ALZHEIMER'S DISEASE

OBJECTIVES

After studying this chapter, the student will be able to:

1. Differentiate between the terms *organic mental syndrome* and *organic mental disorder.*
2. Describe the clinical picture of delirium and contrast it with the clinical picture of dementia.
3. Identify three nursing diagnoses useful for a client with delirium, including supportive data.
4. Formulate three realistic and measurable goals for a client with delirium.
5. Summarize the essential somatic and psychotherapeutic interventions for a client in alcohol withdrawal delirium.
6. Discuss three essential features for each of the four stages of Alzheimer's disease presented in this text.
7. Give an example of the following phenomena assessed during the progression of Alzheimer's disease:
   A. Apraxia
   B. Agnosia
   C. Aphasia
   D. Confabulation
   E. Hyperorality
8. Choose two nursing diagnoses suitable for a client with Alzheimer's disease, and formulate two goals for each.
9. Identify at least three specific nursing interventions for a client with Alzheimer's disease for each of the following areas:
   A. Communication
   B. Activities of daily living
   C. Health teaching with the families
   D. Therapeutic environment

Organic mental syndromes and organic mental disorders occur when temporary or permanent neuron damage results in psychological or behavioral dysfunction.

Organic mental syndrome is a general term used to refer to disturbances in orientation, memory, intellect, judgment, and affect due to physiological changes in the brain, without reference to the etiology. For example, delirium and dementia are organic mental syndromes.

Organic mental disorders are specific brain syndromes in which an etiology is known. For example, alcohol withdrawal delirium and Alzheimer's disease are specific organic mental disorders (APA 1987). The term disorder is used most correctly when the etiology is known.

The DSM III-R (APA 1987) identifies six categories of organic mental syndromes. These six categories follow:

1. Delirium and dementia

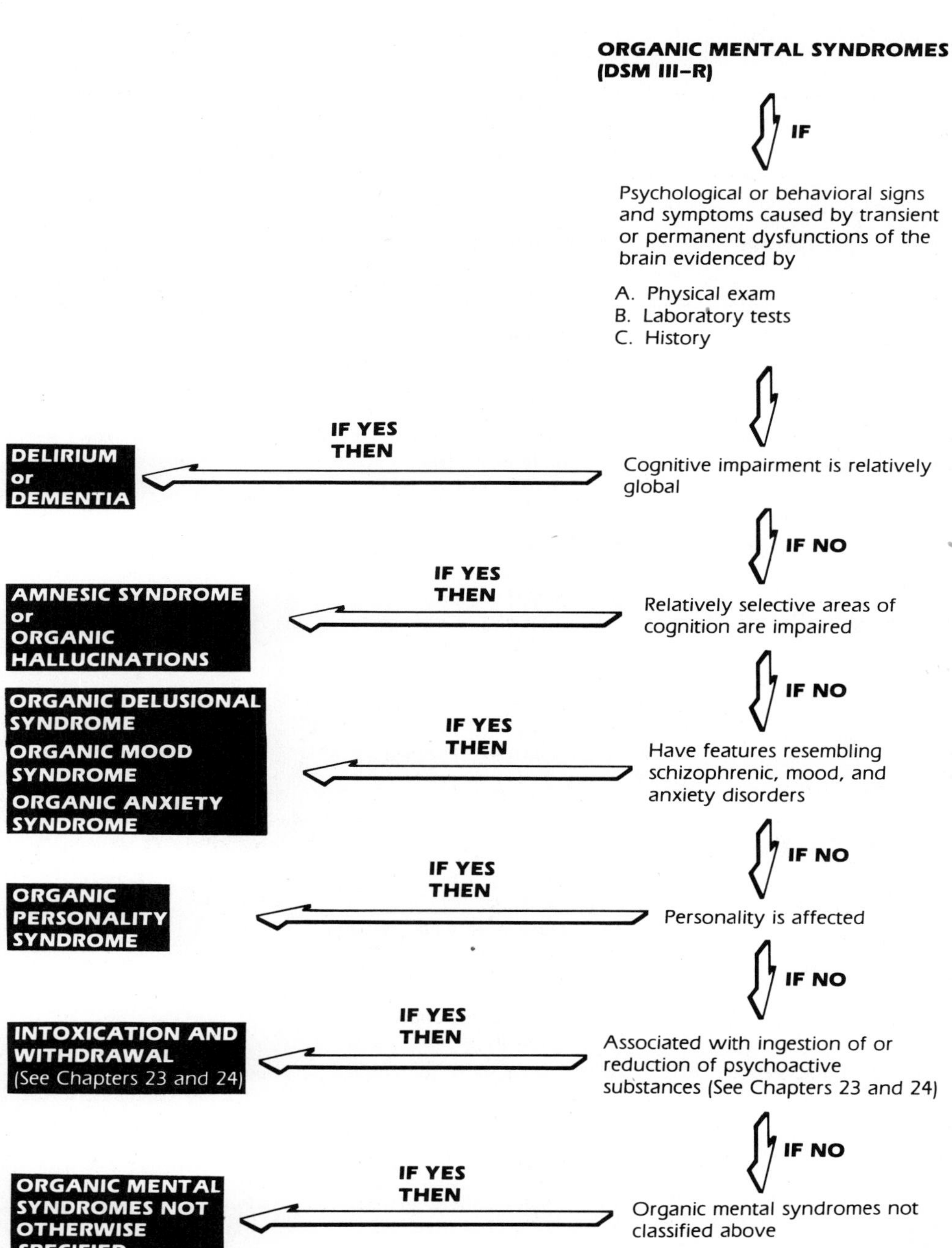

Figure 21-1. *Decision tree for the organic mental syndromes.* (Adapted from Diagnostic and Statistical Manual of Mental Disorders [DSM III-R], 3rd ed., revised. Washington DC: American Psychiatric Association, 1987.)

2. Amnesic syndrome and organic hallucination
3. Organic delusional syndrome, organic mood syndrome, and organic anxiety syndrome
4. Organic personality syndrome
5. Intoxication and withdrawal
6. Organic mental syndromes not otherwise specified

Figure 21 – 1 gives an overview of the organic mental syndromes. Table 21 – 1 gives a brief description of each of the organic mental syndromes identified in the DSM III-R (APA 1987).

This chapter addresses the broad categories of delirium and dementia, since these are by far the most common conditions that nurses encounter.

Delirium usually has a sudden onset and is generally reversible with proper treatment of the underlying cause(s). **Delirium** can be defined as an acute, reversible brain syndrome with multiple etiologies (APA 1987).

Dementia most often has a slow and insidious onset and in many cases has an irreversible course. **Dementia** is referred to as an insidious, chronic, often irreversible brain syndrome (APA 1987). However, the prognosis depends on the underlying cause. Dementias such as

Table 21 – 1 • BRIEF DESCRIPTION OF ORGANIC MENTAL SYNDROMES

SYNDROME	CHARACTERISTICS	IMPAIRMENT IN SOCIAL AND OCCUPATIONAL FUNCTIONING	POSSIBLE CAUSES
Group 1: Cognitive Impairment Is Relatively Global			
Delirium	• *Fluctuating levels of awareness* • *Clouding of consciousness* (confused and disoriented) • Perceptual disturbances (illusions and hallucinations) • *Memory*, especially *recent* memory, is *disturbed* • Alteration in sleep-wake cycle • EEG *changes* • *Abrupt onset* may last about one week • *Reversible* when underlying cause has been treated.	Severe	Metabolic, Nutritional or Toxic Disorders — e.g.: • Hypoxia • Hepatic/renal disorders • Postoperative states • Psychoactive substances • Intoxication or withdrawal
Dementia	• *Slow, insidious onset* • Impaired long and short term memory • *Deterioration of cognitive abilities* — judgment, abstract thinking • *Often irreversible* if untreatable • Personality change • No or slow EEG changes	Severe	• May be primary (Alzheimer's disease, Pick's disease, Multi-infarct dementia) • May be secondary (Parkinson's disease, multiple sclerosis, AIDS, hypothyroidism, Huntington's chorea) • Prolonged or untreatable delirium
Group 2: Selective Areas of Cognition Are Impaired			
Amnestic Syndrome (Relatively uncommon)	• Impairment in short and long term memory • Inability to learn new material • Remote memory better than that of recent events • *Confabulation* • Apathy, lack of initiative • Emotionally bland	Moderate to severe	• Head trauma • Hypoxia • Herpes simplex encephalitis • Thiamine deficiency • Chronic use of alcohol (ETOH)
Organic Hallucinations	• Prominent, persistent, or recurring hallucinations • Hallucinations range from pleasant to terrifying, depending on etiology • The person may be aware that hallucinations are not real or be convinced of their reality.	Depends on degree of impairment and if person acts on the hallucinations.	Most Common: • Long-term use of alcohol • Hallucinogens Sensory deprivation: • Auditory (for some, deafness) • Visual (for some, blindness) Seizure foci (especially in temporal and occipital lobes)

Table 21-1 • BRIEF DESCRIPTION OF ORGANIC MENTAL SYNDROMES *Continued*

SYNDROME	CHARACTERISTICS	IMPAIRMENT IN SOCIAL AND OCCUPATIONAL FUNCTIONING	POSSIBLE CAUSES
Group 3: Have Features Resembling Schizophrenia and Mood and Anxiety Disorders			
Organic Mood Syndrome	• Persistently depressed, elevated, or expansive mood • Mild cognitive impairment • Associated features may include panic attacks, suspiciousness, somatic concerns, labile mood, hallucinations/delusions • Specifies manic, depressed, mixed	Mild to severe	• Toxic or metabolic factors, drugs—e.g., methyldopa, reserpine, hallucinogens • Endocrine disorders • Viral infections
Organic Anxiety Syndrome (Note: To diagnose, need prominent anxiety symptoms and an organic factor)	• Prominent recurrent panic attacks or • Generalized anxiety • Mild cognitive impairment	Mild to severe	• Endocrine disorder—e.g., hyper/hypothyroidism, hypoglycemia • Psychoactive substances—e.g., caffeine, cocaine, amphetamines • Withdrawal, central nervous system (CNS) depressants, alcohol, sedatives • Pulmonary embolus • Chronic obstructive pulmonary disease (COPD)
Organic Delusional Syndrome	• Delusions (e.g., persecutory) • Hallucinations may be present • Mild cognitive impairment • Speech may ramble or be incoherent • Hyperactivity (pacing or rocking) or apathetic immobility may occur • Ritualistic or stereotypical behavior	Severe. May harm self or others when reacting to delusion.	Diverse Causes: • Psychoactive substances—e.g., amphetamines, cannabis, hallucinogens • Temporal lobe epilepsy • Cerebral lesions • Huntington's chorea
Group 4: Personality Is Affected			
Organic Personality Syndrome	Persistent Personality Disturbance—e.g.: • Affective instability • Recurrent outbursts, rage • Socially inappropriate actions (e.g., sexual indiscretion) • Marked apathy, indifference • Mild cognitive impairment	Behavior may lead to legal difficulties; may be dangerous to others	• Neoplasms • Temporal lobe epilepsy • Multiple sclerosis
Group 5: Ingestion or Reduction of Psychoactive Substances			
Intoxication and Withdrawal	Substance-specific syndrome after ingesting specific psychoactive substance Substance-specific syndrome following reduction of specific psychoactive substance	Mild to moderate to severe, depending on frequency, intensity, and duration of use	• Alcohol (see Chapter 23) • CNS Stimulants—e.g., cocaine, crack • CNS Depressants—e.g., sedatives, hypnotics, anxiolytics • Narcotics • Designer drugs • Hallucinogens (See Chapter 24)
Group 6: Organic Syndromes Not Classifiable As Above-Mentioned Syndromes			
Organic Mental Syndromes Not Otherwise Specified	Variable	Variable	Variable

Data from American Psychiatric Association. Diagnostic and Statistical Manual of Mental Disorders (DSM III-R) 3rd ed., revised. Washington DC: American Psychiatric Association, 1987.

those of the Alzheimer type, which involve *primary* encephalopathy, have no precisely known cause or cure; thus, at the present time, they are considered irreversible. On the other hand, dementias that are *secondary* to other pathological processes (e.g., neoplasms, trauma, infections, or toxic disturbances) may be improved when the underlying cause is eliminated.

In the section *Delirium — An Organic Mental Syndrome*, alcohol withdrawal delirium will be discussed as an example of an *organic mental disorder*. In the section *Dementia — An Organic Mental Syndrome*, Alzheimer's Disease will also be discussed as an example of an *organic mental disorder*.

Using anxiety as a framework, the organic mental disorders and syndromes can be conceptualized as shown in Figure 21-2.

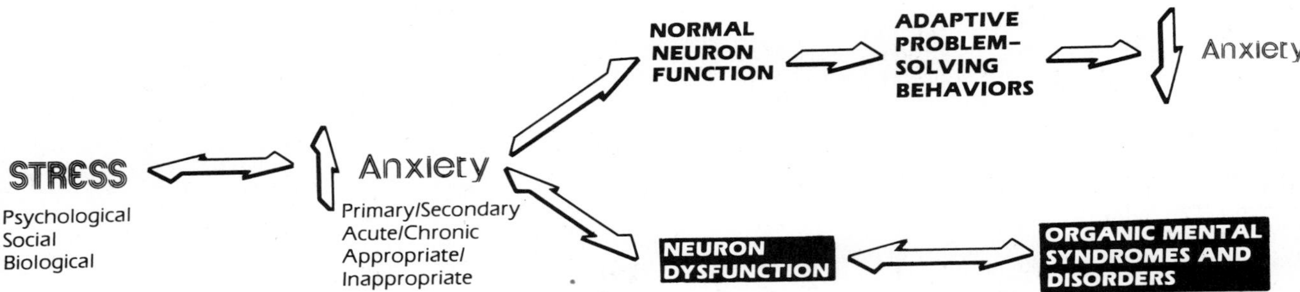

Figure 21-2. *Conceptualization of the process of the organic mental syndromes and disorders.*

Delirium — An Organic Mental Syndrome

Nurses frequently encounter delirium on medical and surgical units in the general hospital setting. During specific phases of a hospital stay, *confusion* may be noted — for example, after surgery or after the introduction of a new drug. The second or third hospital day may herald the onset of confusion for older people with difficulty adjusting to an unfamiliar environment.

Delirium is a syndrome caused by transient malfunctioning, but with no destruction of brain cells. Delirium is *always* secondary to an underlying medical condition or toxic agent. Delirium may be followed by complete recovery; however, if left untreated or if it is untreatable, delirium may progress to a chronic mental syndrome (dementia) or to irreversible coma and death. Delirium is most often seen in children and those over 60 years of age, although it does occur in all age groups.

The DSM III-R (APA 1987) states that the essential feature of delirium is a *clouded state of consciousness* and that delirium in general is marked by cognitive difficulties. Thinking, memory, attention, and perception are generally disturbed. The clinical manifestations of delirium develop over a short period of time (hours to days) and appear on a continuum from mild to severe.

Delirious states usually *fluctuate in intensity*; consequently, nurses may note varying levels of consciousness and orientation during a short period of time. The condition is often more intensified at night. Delirium is characterized by progressive disorientation to time and place. Since delirium increases psychological stress, interventions that lower anxiety and reduce manifestations of the delirium can minimize or in some instances even alleviate the confusional state (Trockman 1978).

Standard I: Theory

Delirium can be caused by any number of pathophysiological conditions. Some of the most common causes of delirium include infections, postoperative states, metabolic abnormalities, hypoxic conditions, drug withdrawal states, and drug intoxications. Multiple drug use, or polypharmacy, is frequently implicated in acute organic mental syndromes (Gomez and Gomez 1987). Some drugs commonly responsible for delirium states are digitalis preparations and antihistamines, as well as medications used for treatment of hypertension, depression, and Parkinson's syndrome (Dwyer, 1987; Ellison 1984; Lipowski, 1983). See Box 21–1 for common causes of delirium.

Standard II: Data Collection

Problems in accurate assessment of delirium or an acute confusional state often arise. *First*, the degree of reversibility can only be determined retrospectively. *Second*, the relative acuity of the onset depends on how noxious the stimuli are. *Third*, a reversible confusional state (delirium) can occur simultaneously with an irreversible mental syndrome (dementia), further complicating accurate identification (Foreman 1986).

Generally, the nurse therapist suspects the presence of delirium when a client rather *abruptly develops a clouded state of consciousness. Confusion is a hallmark of delirium*. The person may have difficulty with orientation first to time, then to place, and last to person. For example, a client with delirium may think the year is 1972 instead of 1990, that the hospital is home, and that the nurse is his wife. Orientation to person is usually intact; that is, the person is aware of his or her own identity (Kaplan and Sadock 1988).

Fluctuating levels of consciousness tend to be unpredictable. Disorientation and confusion are usually markedly worse at night and during the early morning. In fact, some clients may only be confused or delirious at night and remain lucid during the day.

Data collection should include assessment of (1) cognitive and perceptual disturbances, (2) physical needs, and (3) moods and physical behaviors.

Box 21–1. DELIRIUM: ETIOLOGICAL FACTORS

Some major categories that can cause alteration in neural function are outlined below.

A. Drug intoxications/withdrawals
  1. Alcohol, anxiolytics, opioids, central nervous system (CNS) stimulants (cocaine, crack) and others
B. Infections
  1. Systemic: pneumonia, typhoid fever, malaria, urinary tract infection, septicemia
  2. Intracranial: meningitis, encephalitis
C. Metabolic disorders
  1. Hypoxia (pulmonary disease, heart disease, anemia)
  2. Hypoglycemia
  3. Sodium, potassium, calcium, magnesium and acid-base imbalances
  4. Hepatic encephalopathy, uremic encephalopathy
  5. Thiamine (Vitamin B_1) deficiency (Wernicke's encephalopathy)
  6. Endocrine disorders (e.g., thyroidism, parathyroidism)
  7. Hypo- or hyperthermia
  8. Diabetic acidosis
D. Neurological diseases
  1. Seizures
  2. Head trauma
  3. Hypertensive encephalopathy
E. Drugs
  1. Digitalis, steroids, lithium, levodopa, anticholinergics
F. Postoperative states
G. Psychosocial stressors
  1. Relocation or other sudden changes
  2. Sensory deprivation or overload
  3. Sleep deprivation
  4. Immobilization

Data from Dwyer 1987; Foreman 1986; Perry and Markowitz 1988; Seltzer and Frazier 1980.

ASSESSING COGNITIVE AND PERCEPTUAL DISTURBANCES

It may be difficult to engage delirious persons in conversation, since they are easily distracted and their attention wanders. *Memory* is often impaired. In mild delirium, memory deficits are noted upon careful questioning. In more severe delirium, memory difficulties usually take the form of obvious difficulty in processing and remembering recent events. For example, the person might ask when a son is coming to visit when the son has left only an hour before.

Perceptual disturbances are common. Perception is the processing of information about one's internal and external environment (Dwyer 1987). Various misinterpretations of reality may take the form of illusions or hallucinations.

An **illusion** is an error in perception of a sensory stimulus. For example, a person may mistake folds in the bedclothes for white rats, or the cord of a window blind for a snake. The stimulus is a real object in the environment; however, it is misinterpreted and often becomes the object of the client's projected fear. Illusions, unlike delusions or hallucinations, can be explained to and clarified for the individual.

Hallucinations are false sensory stimuli (see Chapter 20). **Visual hallucinations** are a diagnostic symptom of organic mental syndrome. **Tactile hallucinations** may also be present. For example, people in alcohol withdrawal delirium might become terrified when they "see" giant spiders crawling over the bedclothes or "feel" bugs crawling on their bodies. Auditory hallucinations occur more often in other psychiatric disorders, such as schizophrenia or depression (Clunn and Payne 1986).

The delirious individual generally possesses an awareness that something is very wrong (Ronsman 1988). For example, the delirious person may state, "My thoughts are all jumbled." When perceptual disturbances are present, the emotional response is one of fear and anxiety. Verbal and psychomotor signs of agitation should be noted.

Two abilities requiring high cortical functioning may be impaired in delirium: the ability to name an object and the ability to write. **Dystonia** refers to the inability to name objects. **Dysgraphia** refers to the inability to write (APA 1987).

ASSESSING PHYSICAL NEEDS

PHYSICAL SAFETY. A person in delirium becomes disoriented and may try to "go home." Or, a person may think he or she is home and jump out of a window trying to get away from "invaders." Wandering, pulling out tubes such as intravenous (IV) lines and Foley catheters, and falling out of bed are common dangers that require nursing intervention and supervision.

An individual experiencing delirium has difficulty processing stimuli in the environment. Confusion magnifies the inability to recognize reality. The physical environment should be made as concrete and clear as possible. Elevating the head of the bed slightly can maximize orientation to place. Objects such as clocks and calendars can maximize orientation to time. Eye glasses, hearing aids, and a well-lit environment can maximize the person's ability to interpret more accurately what is going on in the environment. Nagley (1986) recommends nurse-client interaction for periods of at least 5 to 10 minutes, when no other nursing actions are being carried out, to help decrease anxiety and increase awareness of reality.

BACTERIOLOGICAL SAFETY. Self-care deficits may lead to skin breakdown and leave a person prone to infection. Often this condition is compounded by poor nutrition, forced bedrest, and possible incontinence. These are areas requiring nursing assessment and intervention.

MEDICAL SAFETY. Autonomic signs such as tachycardia, sweating, flushed face, dilated pupils, and elevated blood pressure often occur. In some acute mental syndromes such as alcohol withdrawal, these changes have to be monitored and documented carefully and may require immediate medical attention.

There are usually changes in the sleep-wakefulness cycle, and the level of consciousness may range from lethargy to stupor or from semi-coma to hypervigilance. The **hypervigilant** person is extraordinarily alert and may have difficulty getting to sleep or may be actively disoriented and agitated throughout the night.

ASSESSING MOODS AND PHYSICAL BEHAVIORS

Physical behavior and mood may change dramatically within a short period of time. Moods may swing back and forth from fear, anger, and anxiety to euphoria, depression, and apathy. These moods are often accompanied by physical behaviors associated with feeling states. A person may strike out from fear or anger or may cry, call for help, curse, moan, and tear off clothing one minute and become apathetic the next. In short, behavior and emotions are characterized by an erratic and fluctuating nature. Lack of concentration and disorientation complicate interventions (Davison and Neale 1982). The following vignette illustrates delirium (Goodwin and Guze 1979):

Mrs. Yates, 70, lived with her daughter, Pam, and son-in-law, Bob. Mrs. Yates took care of the house, did the cooking and cleaning and was active in church activities. She had a number of lady friends and once a week would go to the movies or play cards "with the girls." One day after work, her daughter Pam came home to find her mother huddled in a darkened room, terrified. When asked what was wrong, Mrs. Yates stated that the house was under siege and she had to hide in the dark, "Can't you hear them?" Outside, the sound of drilling and pounding by construction workers was what Pam heard. Mrs. Yates was experiencing illusions. That night when Pam went in to check on her mother, she discovered that her mother was gone. Pam found her wandering in her night clothes three blocks from the house.

Pam became terribly alarmed, even though her husband insisted that "it's normal for old people to become confused" and that they had just been fortunate up to now. Mrs. Yates was taken to the emergency room. Upon admission she was oriented to person, but not to time and place. She thought it was 1942 and that she was back in London during World War II. She kept shouting, "Get those men out of my house!" She would "pick" at things in the air and was so restless, agitated, and incoherent that a mental examination was postponed.

Physical examination of Mrs. Yates revealed bilateral rales in the lower lobes of the lungs, a high white blood cell count, temperature of 101.3° F, and mild dehydration. Diagnosis of bilateral lower lobe pneumonia was made, and within 24 hours of treatment with IV fluid, antibiotics, and diligent nursing care, Mrs. Yates became oriented to time, place, and person, and her "clouded state of consciousness" disappeared.

The doctor explained to the family that Mrs. Yates's temporary delirium was secondary to the infectious process and that the symptoms of delirium often may appear hours before the signs or symptoms of the underlying disorder.

Standard III: Diagnosis

The nurse analyzes the data and considers those areas that warrant the highest priority. Delirium is always secondary to some physical illness or drug toxicity. The priority in medical care is to identify the cause and take appropriate medical or surgical intervention. If the underlying disorder is corrected and reversed, complete recovery is possible. If, however, the underlying disorder is not corrected and persists, sustained neuron damage can lead to irreversible changes such as dementia and even death.

Therefore, nursing concerns center on (1) assisting with proper medical management to eradicate the underlying cause, (2) prevention of physical harm due to confusion, aggression, or electrolyte and fluid balance, and (3) supportive measures to relieve distress.

Safety needs play a substantial role in nursing care. Clients often perceive the environment as distorted. Objects in the environment are often misperceived (illusions), and people and objects may be misinterpreted as threatening or harmful. These misinterpretations are often acted upon. For example, feeling threatened or thinking that common medical equipment is harmful, the client may pull off an oxygen mask, pull out an IV or nasogastric tube, or try to flee. In such a case a person demonstrates *potential for injury* related to altered cerebral function as evidenced by sensory deficits or perceptual deficits.

Fever and dehydration may be present; thus, fluid and electrolyte balance must be managed. If the underlying cause of the client's delirium results in fever, decreased skin turgor, decreased urinary output, decreased fluid intake, dry skin or dry mucous membranes, then the nursing diagnosis *fluid volume deficit* must be made. Fluid volume deficit may be related to fever, electrolyte imbalance, reduced intake, or infection.

Since there may be disruption in the sleep-wake cycle, the client may be less responsive during the day and become disruptively wakeful during the night. At no time, either day or night, does the client experience a restful sleep; instead, the person suffers from a fragmented and fluctuating state of consciousness (McHugh and Folstein 1987). Therefore, *sleep pattern disturbance* related to impaired cerebral oxygenation or disruption in consciousness is possible.

Since the delirious person is usually dazed or drowsy, he or she can rarely sustain attention on any mental task. The client may be roused for a moment and coaxed to respond before slipping back to unresponsiveness. Memory is often impaired. Since it is difficult to sustain communication with a delirious client, *impaired verbal communication* related to cerebral hypoxia or decreased cerebral blood flow as evidenced by confusion may be evident.

Perceptions are disturbed during delirium. Hallucinations, distractibility, illusions, and disorientation are often part of the clinical picture. If any of these are evident, then *altered thought processes* related to alteration in biochemical compounds, cerebral anoxia, or such must be considered.

Standard IV: Planning

Planning involves planning on the (1) content level—planning goals and (2) process level—nurses' reactions and feelings.

CONTENT LEVEL—PLANNING GOALS

The client may present various needs; however, *potential for injury* is usually present. Appropriate goals might include the following:

- Client will remain safe while in the hospital.

- During lucid periods, client will be oriented to time, place, and person with the aid of nursing interventions such as clocks, calendars, and other orienting information.
- Client will refrain from removing tubes (e.g., IV, nasogastric, catheter, oxygen) while confused, with the aid of frequent orientation by nurse and medications as necessary.
- Client will remain free from falls while confused, with the aid of nursing safety measures.
- Client will respond to external controls if he or she becomes physically aggressive toward self, other clients or staff.

Maintaining fluid and electrolyte balance is crucial if the underlying disorder increases the person's metabolic rate and results in increased temperature and decrease in circulating fluid volume. Goals for *fluid volume deficit* could include the following:

- Client will be well hydrated within 24 hours.
- Client will take 8 ounces of protein fluid orally once every hour.
- Client's skin turgor will be normal within 24 hours.
- Client's specific gravity (urine) will be within normal limits by (state the time).
- Client's vital signs will become/remain stable by (state the time).

Sleep pattern disturbance can cause a problem not only for the client in terms of sleep deprivation and increased anxiety, but also for the other clients. Creative nursing measures are often necessary. Possible goals follow:

- Client will sleep four to six hours per night within three days.
- Client will state that he or she is comfortable at night with aid of nursing measures (e.g., back rub, light, frequent orientation, nurse's presence) within (state the time).
- Client will state accurately that he knows where he is and what is happening to him when awake at night within (state the date).
- Client's anxiety level will decrease from panic levels to severe or moderate, with aid of medication and nursing interventions.

Since *impaired verbal communication* and *altered thought processes* are usually evident, goals that enhance the client's ability to interpret reality are useful. For example:

- Client will demonstrate accurate perception of the environment by discharge.
- Client will be able to tell nurse where he or she is by (state the date).
- Client will state that he or she understands nurse will support him or her when "hearing" or "seeing" frightening things.
- Client will name correct environmental object(s) or sound(s) after experiencing an illusion, with aid of nursing interventions.

PROCESS LEVEL—NURSES' REACTIONS AND FEELINGS

In many cases, delirium is more easily associated with a medical disease than with a mental disorder by many nurses. *First*, delirium is usually treated on a medical or surgical unit, and *second*, delirium usually responds to specific medical or surgical interventions, depending on the underlying cause. Frequently this syndrome reverses within a few days or less when the underlying cause is identified and treated. Since the behaviors exhibited by the client can be directly attributed to temporary medical conditions, intense countertransferential reactions are less likely to occur. At any rate, intense conflicting emotions are less likely to occur when working with a client in delirium than when working with a client with dementia, which will be discussed later in this chapter.

There are a few behaviors associated with delirium, however, that the nurse may find especially "challenging." Since delirium is predictably more severe and incapacitating during the night and early morning hours, night staff often find that a loud, frightened, agitated, and perhaps aggressive client can take up much of their time. Experienced nurses are aware that even though people in delirium may appear "out of it," they often respond to a calm and caring approach. Maximizing the person's contact with reality during the night can be helpful in reducing the anxiety and terror these patients often experience.

However, there are certain instances which may cause staff to experience strong negative feelings toward a client in delirium. Such incidents might include delirium resulting from psychoactive substance withdrawal. For example, nurses working with clients in alcohol withdrawal delirium might think a person "did it to herself" or is "getting what he deserves." Often, nurses exhibit judgmental attitudes toward persons in withdrawal. Unfortunately, negative attitudes by staff serve only to increase the client's anxiety, intensifying feelings of terror, confusion, and defensive behavior.

One explanation is that the nurse might be projecting onto the client intense feelings of anger and condemnation originally experienced in response to an alcoholic parent, spouse, or other individual. If a nurse has lived with an alcoholic parent or caregiver, these feelings and reactions may have been painful. Children of alcoholics often suffer from related problems in later life, such as difficulty experiencing satisfying relationships, resulting in depression. Support groups found all over the country for *adult children of alcoholics* (AC of A) assist people to live more satisfying lives by helping the person work through the burdensome and negative emotions that continue to affect one's life negatively unless dealt with.

Also, many health care workers are not well informed regarding the disease of alcoholism. Sometimes education about the disease can increase understanding and change attitudes (see Chapter 23).

Standard V: Interventions

Delirium is seen in all areas of hospital nursing, but most commonly in postoperative, intensive care, and medical units. Whatever the setting, *delirium requires medical intervention*. As mentioned, if the underlying cause of delirium is not treated, permanent brain damage may ensue. The nurse is usually involved with meeting many of the physical needs of the delirious person. In addition, lowering the client's anxiety and fear and increasing the client's orientation to reality can help promote comfort, reduce secondary injury, and minimize behaviors stimulated by fear and misinterpretation of the environment (e.g., climbing out of bed, fighting staff, pulling out IV tubes). Continuous reality orientation is a major emphasis in working with a delirious client, although the same information may have to be repeated many times an hour. Table 21–2 suggests some basic nursing interventions for use with a delirious client. Suggested interventions cover communication and physical needs.

Standard VI: Evaluation

The long term goals of (1) the client will remain safe while in the hospital and (2) the client will be oriented to time, place, and person by discharge. However, it is the short term goals that need constant assessment.

For example, are the client's pulse and blood pressure within normal limits? Are all IV and nasogastric (NG) tubes, Foley catheters, hyperalimentation lines, and so forth intact? Is the client's urine specific gravity within normal limits? Is the client oriented to time and place? Has the client's anxiety level decreased from panic levels to severe or moderate? Constant and frequent checking of short term goals helps monitor successful treatment of the client's underlying medical condition as well as responses to nursing interventions and helps prevent possible progression to more profound levels or irreversible neuron changes.

The Clinical Picture of an Organic Mental Disorder

Although alcohol and alcohol-related problems are covered in Chapter 23, alcohol withdrawal delirium is presented here as an example of an organic mental disorder.

Table 21–2 • DELIRIUM: INTERVENTIONS

NURSING INTERVENTION	RATIONALE
Communication	
1. Introduce self and call client by name at the beginning of each contact.	1. Short term memory impairment; person often confused and needs orienting to time, place and person.
2. Maintain face-to-face contact.	2. Easily distracted; needs help to focus on one stimulus at a time.
3. Use short, simple, concrete phrases.	3. Cannot process complex information.
4. Briefly explain everything you are going to do before doing it.	4. Prevent misinterpretation of action.
5. Encourage the presence of family and friends (one at a time) to take quiet, supportive role.	5. To lower anxiety and increase orientation.
6. Keep room well lit.	6. Provide accurate environmental stimuli to maintain/increase orientation.

Table continued on following page

Table 21-2 • DELIRIUM: INTERVENTIONS *Continued*

NURSING INTERVENTION	RATIONALE
Communication	
7. Keep head of bed elevated.	7. Provide important environmental clues.
8. Provide clocks and calendars.	8. Help orient to time.
9. Encourage meaningful articles from home (pictures, figurines).	9. Provide comfort and support.
10. Encourage client to wear personal eyeglasses and/or hearing aid.	10. Increase accuracy of incoming stimuli.
11. Make an effort to assign the same personnel on each shift to care for client.	11. Minimize confusion, which allows for relationships to take place.
12. When *hallucinations* are present, acknowledge the person's feelings and point out reality. For example: "I know you are frightened, but I do not see spiders on your sheets."	12. Person feels understood. Can be reassuring.
13. When *illusions* are present, clarify reality. For example: "This is a coat rack, not a man with a knife . . . see. You seem frightened. I'll stay with you for a while."	13. Misinterpreted objects or sounds can be clarified, once pointed out.
14. Inform client of progress during lucid intervals.	14. Consciousness fluctuates; will lower anxiety for client to know where he or she is and who you are during lucid periods.
15. Ignore insults and name calling, and acknowledge how upset the person may be feeling. For example: CLIENT: You incompetent jerk, get me a real nurse, someone who knows what they are doing. NURSE: You are very upset. What you are going through is very difficult. I'll stay with you.	15. Terror and fear often projected onto environment. Arguing or becoming defensive only increases client's aggressive behaviors and defenses.
16. If client behavior becomes physically abusive, *First,* set limits on behavior—for example: "Mr. Jones, you are not to hit him. Tell me how you feel." OR "Mr. Jones, if you have difficulty controlling your actions, we will help you until you gain control." *Second,* check orders for use of chemical or physical restraints (e.g., posey)	16. Clear limits need to be set to protect client, staff, or others. Often client can respond to verbal controls. Use physical restraints as a last resort *if at all.*
Physical Needs	
1. Check pulse periodically—e.g., every hour or every four hours, depending on underlying conditions.	1. Pulse is a good indicator of course of delirium.
2. Check temperature regularly.	2. Hyperthermia possible.
3. Schedule medications and treatments so as not to interfere with client's sleep/rest.	3. Fluctuating levels of consciousness prevent adequate needed rest.
4. Check for skin breakdown and apply appropriate interventions—e.g., turn every two hours; lotion for bony prominences; proper positioning.	4. Breakdown can develop rapidly when client is on bedrest, combined with dehydration.
5. Monitor fluid intake and output.	5. Monitor electrolyte balance.
6a. Check skin turgor and urine specific gravity. If client appears dehydrated, then forcing fluids may be appropriate.	6a. Replace fluid volume.
6b. If skin turgor and urine specific gravity are within limits, or if client is overhydrated, then fluids would *not* be forced.	6b. Prevent fluid volume overload.

Alcohol withdrawal syndromes occur after the intake of ethyl alcohol (ETOH) has been reduced or has ceased in a person who has had chronic exposure to large amounts of alcohol over a period of time. For example, the classic withdrawal state occurs when a person reduces intake of alcohol after having ingested one pint of hard liquor (or the equivalent in beer or wine) for at least ten consecutive days (Butz 1982). The phenomena of tolerance and dependence are discussed in Chapter 23.

Alcohol withdrawal reactions range from mild to severe. The severity of the withdrawal reaction is dependent on the length of the drinking period and the amount of alcohol consumed.

The DSM-III-R (APA 1987) identifies two alcohol withdrawal syndromes: (1) *uncomplicated alcohol withdrawal* and (2) the more severe *alcohol withdrawal delirium* (often referred to as delirium tremens or DTs).

ASSESSMENT

Nursing and medical assessments include (1) assessing the severity of withdrawal (2) assessing for possible traumatic injuries, and (3) assessing for withdrawal from other drugs.

Assessing the Severity of Withdrawal

Uncomplicated Alcohol Withdrawal. (6 to 8 hours following cessation or reduction of ETOH). The early signs of withdrawal develop within a few hours after cessation or reduction of ETOH intake; they peak after 24 to 36 hours and then rapidly and dramatically disappear, unless the withdrawal progresses to alcohol withdrawal delirium.

Early signs of withdrawal include anxiety, anorexia, insomnia, and tremor. The person may appear hyperalert, manifest jerky movements and irritability, startle easily, and experience subjective distress often described as "shaking inside" (Butz 1982). The person may also report transient, poorly formed hallucinations, illusions, or vivid nightmares. Nausea and vomiting may also occur (Kaplan and Sadock 1988).

Pulse and blood pressure are usually elevated. Grand mal seizures may also develop, usually during the first 36 to 48 hours after cessation of ETOH intake; however, they may occur later. It is rare for seizures to occur during alcohol withdrawal delirium (Butz 1982).

A client in uncomplicated alcohol withdrawal should be monitored to prevent progression into alcohol withdrawal delirium. Careful assessment followed by appropriate medical and nursing interventions can prevent the more serious withdrawal reactions of delirium. Sedatives are useful on a temporary basis (3 to 5 days) to reduce the symptoms of withdrawal (e.g., chlordiazepoxide [Librium] or diazepam [Valium]). The pulse and blood pressure should be checked hourly for the first 8 to 12 hours after admission, at least every 4 hours during the first 48 hours, and then 4 times a day thereafter (Smith-DeJulio 1982). *The pulse is a good indication of progress through withdrawal.* Elevation may indicate impending alcohol withdrawal delirium, signaling the need for more rigorous sedation.

ALCOHOL WITHDRAWAL DELIRIUM. (40 to 48 hours after cessation or reduction of ETOH). Alcohol withdrawal delirium is considered a medical emergency and has a 20% mortality rate if left unattended (Kaplan and Sadock 1988). Usually death is due to myocardial infarction, peripheral vascular collapse, hyperthermia, or aspiration pneumonia. The state of delirium usually peaks after three days (72 hours) of abstinence (can occur later) and lasts from two to three days.

Along with anxiety, insomnia, anorexia, and delirium, additional features include (Kaplan and Sadock 1988):

1. Autonomic hyperactivity (e.g., tachycardia, diaphoresis, elevated blood pressure),
2. Severe disturbance in sensorium (e.g., disorientation, clouding of consciousness),
3. Perceptual disturbances (e.g., visual or tactile hallucinations),
4. Fluctuating levels of consciousness (e.g., ranging from hyperexcitability to lethargy).

Delusions (paranoid), agitated behaviors, and fever (100°F to 103°F) are usually present.

Whenever possible, an accurate history of *what* the person has been taking (ETOH and other drugs), *when*, and *how much* is vital for effective treatment. Such information is a crucial part of the nurse's assessment to be passed on to the medical team. Sometimes family or friends who come in with the individual in withdrawal can supply such information.

Assessing for Possible Traumatic Injuries

In the emergency room, a person may come in after a fight or accident, with head injuries as well as the noticeable odor of alcohol on his or her breath. Many of these clients have high serum alcohol levels when injuries occur. These high levels of alcohol can greatly interfere with an accurate physical and neurological assessment. Intracranial hematomas, subdural hematomas, and other conditions can go unnoticed if symptoms of acute alcohol intoxication and withdrawal are not distinguished from the symptoms of a brain injury. Therefore, neurological signs (pupil size, equality, and reaction to light) should be assessed, especially with comatose clients suspected of trauma injuries (Smith-DeJulio 1982).

Assessing for Multiple Withdrawal

One danger frequently encountered today is that of multiple drug abuse, or polypharmacy. Multiple drug and alcohol dependencies are common, and simultaneous withdrawal syndromes are becoming a common phenomenon. The presence of two or more simultaneous withdrawal syndromes can present a bizarre clinical picture and pose problems for safe withdrawal. Again, family and friends may be helpful in gaining important information that can enhance safe withdrawal. Answers to *how much* of *what* was taken and *when* can save people's lives.

INTERVENTIONS FOR ALCOHOL WITHDRAWAL DELIRIUM

Somatic Therapy

A variety of drugs may be used to prevent or treat alcohol withdrawal delirium. The best treatment of alcohol withdrawal delirium is prevention, and adequate sedation is the most important aspect of medical prevention. Sedation also can prevent progression to a deeper and more dangerous level of delirium.

Sedation, in effect, allows for safe withdrawal from the drug ETOH; therefore, a *long-acting central nervous system* (CNS) *depressant* is substituted for the shorter-acting drug of dependence (ETOH). Although various detoxification procedures may be practiced in different regions of the country, *benzodiazepines* are the drugs of choice (especially Librium and Valium) in many areas because of their high therapeutic safety index and anticonvulsant properties. Barbiturates, meprobamate, and other CNS depressants are also safely used in some areas. For example, in uncomplicated withdrawal 25 to 50 mg of Librium may be given every two to four hours. However, once alcohol withdrawal delirium appears, doses of 50 to 100 mg are given (Kaplan and Sadock 1988). Ten to 20 times the normal doses of these drugs may be needed, since cross-tolerance from the drug of dependence often develops. *Danger of an inadvertent overdose is always possible, and close nursing and medical observation is needed, especially during the first* 24 *hours* (Butz 1982).

Thiamine (*vitamin* B_1) *deficiency* is often present owing to poor dietary intake and malabsorption. Thiamine replacement is given to prevent Wernicke's syndrome (encephalopathy). Wernicke's syndrome is characterized by nystagmus, ptosis, ataxia, confusion, coma, and possible death (Frances and Franklin 1988).

Hypomagnesemia is another condition found in people with long term drinking problems. *Magnesium sulfate* is often given (1) to increase the body's response to thiamine and (2) to raise the seizure threshold.

Anticonvulsants may or may not be used. Diazepam (Valium) or phenobarbital may be used on a short term basis to control a client's seizures and prevent status epilepticus. Phenytoin (Dilantin) is less frequently used because seizures usually occur within the first 48 hours of withdrawal and Dilantin takes days to reach an effective blood level (Smith-DeJulio 1982). See Table 21–3 for a summary of drugs used in treatment.

Fluid and electrolyte replacements may be necessary, especially if the client is vomiting, has diarrhea, and is diaphoresing. In these cases, the client may be dehydrated and may need proper fluids and electrolyte replacement (e.g., potassium). However, caution should be taken. Diuresis occurs when blood alcohol levels *rise*, but fluid retention may occur as blood ETOH levels fall; therefore, a person in withdrawal may be *overhydrated*. Rigorous fluid therapy could cause serious complications, such as congestive heart failure.

Psychotherapeutic Measures

People experiencing withdrawal are often terrified, confused, and anxious. When the nurse has a kind, warm, and supportive manner, this often can allay anxiety and provide a sense of security. Consistent and frequent orientation to time and place may be necessary. Encouraging the family (one at a time) or close friends to stay with the client in quiet surroundings can also help increase orientation and minimize confusion and anxiety. Pulse and blood pressure need to be monitored frequently. Illusions are usually terrifying for the client. *Illusions* can be clarified, which reduces the client's terror. Interventions are often needed for a client who is hallucinating. Kaplan and Sadock (1988) warn against the use of physical restraints because a client may struggle against the restraints to the point of exhaustion. General guidelines for psychotherapeutic interventions appropriate for the client in withdrawal delirium are given in Table 21–2.

Clinical Vignette: A Client With Alcohol Withdrawal Delirium

After her divorce, Mary started having a few drinks after coming home from work. Initially, she found that these drinks helped her relax and "put me in a good mood."

Table 21–3 • MEDICATION FOR TREATMENT OF ALCOHOL WITHDRAWAL DELIRIUM

DRUG	DOSE	PURPOSE
Sedatives		
Benzodiazepines		
Librium (chloriazepoxide) (drug of choice)	25–100 mg p.o. q 4 h (for 5–7 days) tapering doses	Librium and Valium provide *safe* withdrawal and have *anticonvulsant* effects
Valium (diazepam)	5–10 mg p.o. q 2–4 h in tapering doses	
Phenobarbital/Pentobarbital	100 mg p.o. in tapering doses	Control withdrawal; caution: can depress respiration
Thiamine (Vitamin B_1) Given intramuscularly (IM) or intravenously (IV) prior to glucose loading	100 mg p.o. qid	Prevent Wernicke's encephalopathy
Magnesium Sulfate (Especially if history of seizures)	1 g IM q 6 h for 2 days	Increases effectiveness of Vitamin B_1 Helps reduce status postwithdrawal seizures
Anticonvulsant		
Phenobarbital		For seizure control
Benzodiazepams		Most effective in short time
Dilantin (phenytoin)		Takes days to reach therapeutic level
Folic Acid	1 mg p.o. qid	Nutritional deficiencies and malabsorbtion due to heavy long term alcohol abuse
Multivitamins	1 daily	causes deficiencies in many vitamins

Data from American Psychiatric Association 1987; Frances and Franklin 1988; Smith-DeJulio 1982.

Over time, Mary found that two drinks no longer did the trick, and that she required three and then four drinks to achieve the relaxed feeling and mild euphoria she sought. Mary's body was building up a tolerance for the drug, and it took higher and higher doses to get the desired effect. The body is able to adjust to gradually increased doses of certain drugs over a period of time and begins to require a certain level of the drug to function "normally" (see Chapter 23). After ten years, Mary was drinking a couple of drinks at lunch, before dinner, and during the evening. However, on first glance the effects of alcohol did not show. Mary was able to "appear normal" with a high blood alcohol level (BAL). Eventually, Mary developed the habit of taking a drink every morning to settle the "shakes" and prevent tremulousness. She drank in the morning not so much to feel good but to prevent feeling bad.

In the fall of 1989, after suffering an acute attack of pancreatitis, Mary was hospitalized, given IV fluids, and had an NG tube in place. After three days, suddenly Mary became extremely agitated. She screamed that she was being held hostage by Iranian spies. She mistook her water carafe for a time bomb *(illusion)*. She became terrified at night, believing she saw giant ants on the walls.

Mary's blood pressure increased from 120/70 on admission to 150/100. Her pulse increased from 88 to 140. She thought it was the winter of 1978, about the time of her divorce.

Once alcohol withdrawal delirium was diagnosed, Mary was given 100 mg of Librium intramuscularly (IM), and then orally every four hours. Her pulse and blood pressure were monitored every hour. She was given 100 mg of thiamine IM prophylactically against encephalopathy, as well as magnesium sulfate. Mary had normal skin turgor, and her urine specific gravity was within normal limits; therefore, fluids were not forced.

Her terror at "seeing large ants" was reduced by the nurse's presence and assurances that the nurse did not see the ants. Once the nurse showed her the carafe and poured some of the water into a glass, Mary understood that it was not a bomb.

Mary's agitation and aggressiveness became worse at night, and a friend stayed with her, talking in a calm manner and orienting her to her surroundings. When the nurses came to give medication and check vital signs and urinary output, they carefully explained everything they were going to do beforehand, to allay misinterpretation of their actions by Mary.

Mary was placed in a private, well-lit room. A minimal amount of environmental stimuli was allowed (e.g., no radios or TV, one visitor at a time). A clock was placed in clear view. The head of her bed was kept elevated to increase environmental orientation, and her bed faced the window to provide further orientation to time of day.

Three days later, Mary was fully oriented, although still taking Librium. The episode had frightened her. She agreed to go to an Alcoholics Anonymous (AA) meeting and learn about other available avenues to sobriety (see Chapter 23).

Dementia—An Organic Mental Syndrome

Severe memory loss is *not* a normal part of growing older. Slight forgetfulness is a common phenomenon of the aging process, but not to the extent that it interferes with one's activities of daily living. A decided majority of people who live to very old age never experience a significant memory loss or any other symptoms of dementia. Most of us know people in their 80's and 90's who lead active lives, with their intellect intact. Margaret Mead, Pablo Picasso, Duke Ellington, Count Basie and Ansel Adams are all examples of people who were still active in their careers when they died; all were past 75 years of age (Picasso was 91) (Mace and Rabins 1981). The slow, mild cognitive changes associated with aging should not impede social or occupational functioning.

Dementia, on the other hand, is marked by progressive deterioration in intellectual functioning, memory, and ability to problem-solve and learn new skills. Judgment and moral and ethical behaviors decline.

Teusink and Mahler (1984) stress the progressive decline of the demented person in activities of everyday life, the failure of memory and intellect, and the disorganization of the personality. A person's declining intellect often leads to emotional changes, lack of self-care (ADL), and finally to hallucinations and delusions—that is, psychotic symptoms brought on by organic changes.

A person may have progressive dementia from a variety of etiologies; Alzheimer's disease, Pick's disease, Huntington's chorea, multi-infarct dementias, advanced alcoholism (such as in Korsakoff's syndrome), and Creutzfeldt-Jakob's disease are a few examples.

Dementias can be classified as primary or secondary in nature. **Primary dementias** are not reversible, are progressive in their course, and are not secondary to any other disorder. For example, Alzheimer's disease accounts for about 65% of all dementias, and multi-infarct dementia accounts for about 10% of all dementias (Kaplan and Sadock 1988). Both Alzheimer's and multi-infarct dementias are *primary*, progressive, and irreversible.

Secondary dementias occur as a result of some other pathological process (e.g., metabolic, nutritional, or neurological). AIDS-related dementia is an example of a secondary dementia increasingly seen in health care settings. The exact prevalence of AIDS-related dementia is not known, but it may occur in up to 70% of hospitalized AIDS clients. Some clinicians refer to this phenomena as HIV *encephalopathy* (McArthur 1987). Refer to Chapter 26. Other secondary dementias result from

Box 21–2. DEMENTIA: ETIOLOGICAL FACTORS

A. Primary dementias
   1. Alzheimer's disease (senile and presenile dementia)
   2. Multi-infarct dementia
   3. Pick's disease
B. Secondary dementias
   1. Infections
      a. Tuberculosis
      b. Tertiary neurosyphilis
      c. Fungal, bacterial, and viral infections of the brain (Creutzfeldt-Jacob disease)
   2. Trauma; subdural hematoma, hypoxia
   3. Toxic and metabolic disturbances
      a. Korsakoff's syndrome; Wernicke's encephalopathy (thiamine deficiency)
      b. Pernicious anemia (vitamin B_{12} deficiency)
      c. Folic acid deficiency
      d. Thyroid, parathyroid, or adrenal gland dysfunction
      e. Liver or kidney dysfunction
      f. Metal poisoning
      g. Carbon dioxide (CO_2) and some drugs
   4. Neoplasms
   5. Other neurological diseases
      a. Huntington's chorea
      b. Parkinson's disease
      c. Multiple sclerosis
      d. Cerebellar degenerations
   6. Normal pressure hydrocephalus
   7. AIDS related dementia (HIV encephalopathy)

Data from Mac and Rabins 1981; Seltzer and Frazier 1980.

viral encephalitis, pernicious anemia, folic acid deficiency, and hypothyroidism.

Korsakoff's syndrome is an example of secondary dementia due to thiamine deficiency that may be associated with prolonged, heavy alcohol ingestion. Along with progressive mental deterioration, Korsakoff's syndrome is marked by peripheral neuropathy, cerebellar ataxia, confabulation, and myopathy (APA 1987).

Some secondary dementias are treatable. In about 15% of dementia cases, when the underlying cause is eliminated the symptoms of dementia can be reversed (Cohen 1984; Kaplan and Sadock 1988; Pajik 1984). Refer to Box 21 – 2 for illnesses which can cause dementia. At times it is necessary to distinguish delirium from dementia. Some major differences are outlined in Table 21 – 4.

Since dementia of the Alzheimer type accounts for 65% of all dementias and is the fourth most prevalent cause of death after heart disease, cancer, and stroke in the adult population, Alzheimer's disease will be discussed in detail as an example of dementia (Powell and Courtice 1983).

Table 21 – 4 • DIFFERENTIATION BETWEEN DELIRIUM AND DEMENTIA

DELIRIUM	DEMENTIA
Onset	
Acute development of impairment in orientation and memory, intellectual function, judgment and affect	Slow, insidious deterioration in cognitive functioning
Essential Feature	
Clouded state of consciousness, fluctuating levels of consciousness, and cognitive impairment	Progressive deterioration in memory, orientation, calculation, and judgment; symptoms do not fluctuate
Etiology	
The syndrome is *secondary* to any number of underlying disorders that cause temporary, diffuse disturbances of brain function	The syndrome is either *primary* in etiology or *secondary* to other disease states or conditions
Course	
The clinical course is usually brief (hour to days); prolonged delirium may lead to dementia	Progresses over months or years; often irreversible
Speech	
May be slurred; reflects disorganized thinking	Generally normal in early stages; progressive aphasia; confabulation
Memory	
Short term memory impaired	Short term, then long term memory destroyed
Perception	
Visual or tactile hallucinations; illusions	Hallucinations not prominent
Mood	
Fear, anxiety, and irritability most prominent	Mood labile; previous personality traits become accentuated, e.g., paranoid, depressed, withdrawn, obsessive-compulsive
EEG	
Pronounced diffuse slowing or fast cycles	*Normal* or mildly slow

Data from Foreman 1986; Kaplan and Sadock 1988.

Alzheimer's Disease—An Organic Mental Disorder

Alzheimer's disease attacks indiscriminately. Its victims are male and female, black and white, rich and poor, and are people with varying degrees of intelligence. Although the disease can strike at a younger age, most victims are 65 years of age or older. Alzheimer's is "a thief of minds, a destroyer of personalities, wrecker of family finances and filler of nursing homes" (AARP 1986).

Yasmin Aga Khan (the daughter of the famous actress, Rita Hayworth, who was stricken with Alzheimer's disease) once stated that to watch a once proud, beautiful, independent, dignified human being transformed into a dependent, mentally disabled person is terrifying. An estimated 4 million Americans are afflicted with the disease; it affects up to 11% of the population over 65 years of age and 25% of the population over 85 years (McHugh and Folstein 1987).

A wide range of problems may masquerade as dementia and be mistaken for Alzheimer's disease. For example, depression in the elderly is often misdiagnosed as dementia. Disorders that can often mimic dementia include drug toxicity, metabolic disorders, infections, and nutritional deficiencies. Disorders that mimic dementia are sometimes referred to as **pseudodementias.** That is, although the symptoms may suggest dementia, a careful examination may reveal another diagnosis altogether. When an organic mental syndrome is suspected, clinical evaluation includes the following (Perry and Markowitz 1988):

1. Confirm the diagnosis.
2. Search for underlying causes.
3. Identify psychosocial stressors that may exacerbate related emotional and behavioral problems.

Assessment and diagnosis of Alzheimer's disease include initially ruling out other pathophysiological conditions through the history and physical and laboratory tests. Burnside (1988) suggests the following laboratory tests:

- Chest and skull x-rays
- Electroencephalography
- Electrocardiography
- Urinalysis
- SMA 12/60 (sequential multiple analyzer—12 test serum profile)
- T_3, T_4 (serum triiodothyronine and thyroxine) tests
- CBC (complete blood count)
- VDRL (Venereal Disease Research Laboratory) test
- Serum creatinine assay
- Electrolytes
- Serum vitamin B_{12} assay
- Serum folate assay
- Evaluation of vision and hearing

Computed tomography (CT) and positron emission tomography (PET) scans possess diagnostic capabilities by revealing brain atrophy and ruling out other conditions such as neoplasms. Mental status questionnaires and a variety of other tests to determine mental status deterioration and brain damage are an important part of the assessment.

Since depression in the elderly is most often confused with dementia, Table 21–5 identifies features that aid in distinguishing depression from dementia. Medical and nursing personnel should be cautioned, however, because dementia and depression *can* coexist in the same person (Burnside 1988).

Table 21–5 • DEPRESSION VERSUS DEMENTIA IN THE ELDERLY

DEMENTIA	DEPRESSION
1. Recent memory is impaired. In early stages, patient attempts to hide cognitive losses; is skillful in covering up.	1. Patient readily admits to memory loss; other cognitive disturbances may or may not be present.
2. Symptoms progress slowly and insidiously; difficult to pinpoint onset.	2. Symptoms are of relatively rapid onset.
3. Approximate or "near-miss" answers are typical; tries to answer.	3. "Don't know" answers are common; patient does not try to recall or answer.
4. Patient struggles to perform well but is frustrated.	4. Little effort to perform; is apathetic; seems helpless and pessimistic.
5. Affect is shallow or labile.	5. Depressive mood is pervasive.
6. Attention and concentration may be impaired.	6. Attention and concentration are usually intact.
7. Changes in "personality"—e.g., from cheerful and easy-going to angry and suspicious.	7. Personality remains stable.

Distributed by Dr. Beverly Richards at Indiana State Nurses Association Clinical Sessions, November 1982. Reprinted with permission.

Standard I: Theory

Although the cause of Alzheimer's disease is not known, there are a number of hypotheses regarding etiology. These include the (1) genetic model, (2) acetylcholine model, (3) toxin model, and (4) abnormal protein model.

GENETIC MODEL. It has been found that 40% of people with Alzheimer's disease have first-degree relatives with the disease. Also, family members have a risk of acquiring the disease that is higher than that of the general population. Most people with Down's syndrome who survive into the second or third decade of life eventually develop Alzheimer's disease. Recently, a defect on chromosome 21 was found in people with Alzheimer's disease; this is the same chromosome that is damaged in Down's syndrome (St. George-Hyslop et al. 1987; Kaplan and Sadock, 1988).

ACETYLCHOLINE MODEL. Some studies have indicated that people with Alzheimer's dementia have drastically reduced levels of the enzyme acetyltransferase. This is the enzyme needed to synthesize the neurotransmitter acetylcholine. Some theorists propose that the cognitive defects that occur in Alzheimer's disease, especially memory loss, are a direct result of the reduction in acetylcholine available to the brain.

TOXIN MODEL. High levels of aluminum have been found in some people who have died from Alzheimer's disease. It is known that aluminum toxicity can cause dementia in animals (Wells 1982). Research continues in this area.

ABNORMAL PROTEIN MODEL. Alzheimer's disease results in neuritic plaques and neurofibrillary tangles that are microscopic abnormalities in brain tissue as well as cerebral atrophy. These pathological changes involve an accumulation of proteins not normally found in the brain (Wurtman 1985). A more detailed description follows.

1. **Neurofibrillary tangles** form mostly in the hippocampus, the part of the brain responsible for recent (short term) memory as well as the emotions. Therefore, memory and emotions are negatively affected. Neurofibrillary tangles are actually pairs of filaments wrapped around each other within a neuron.
2. **Senile plaques** are cores of degenerated neuron material lying free of the cell bodies on the ground substances of the brain. The quantity of plaques has been correlated with the degree of mental deterioration.
3. **Granulovascular degeneration** is the filling of brain cells with fluid and granular material. Increased degeneration accounts for increased loss of mental function. Brain atrophy is observable with the use of CAT scanning (Gershon and Herman 1982; Heston and White 1983; Reisberg 1984).

Other etiologies under investigation include a slow viral infection, an autoimmune process, and decreased blood flow to the brain (Burnside 1988); Perry and Markowitz 1988).

Standard II: Data Collection

Alzheimer's disease is characterized by progressive deterioration of cognitive functioning. Initially, deterioration may be so subtle and insidious that others may not notice. In early stages of the disease, the affected person may be able to compensate for loss of memory. Some people may have superior social graces and charm that give them the ability to "hide" severe deficits in memory, even from experienced health care professionals (Burnside 1988). This "hiding" is actually a form of *denial* which is an unconscious protective defense against the terrifying reality of losing one's place in the world. Family members may also unconsciously deny that anything is wrong as a defense against the painful awareness of deterioration in a loved one. As time goes on, other defensive maneuvers become evident. **Confabulation** (making up stories or answers to maintain self-esteem when the person does not remember) is noticed. For example, the nurse addresses a client who has remained in a hospital bed all weekend:

NURSE: Good morning Ms. Jones. How was your weekend?

CLIENT: Wonderful. I discussed politics with Jesse Jackson, and he took me out to dinner.

Confabulation is not the same as lying. When lying, a person is aware that he or she is making up an answer; confabulation is an *unconscious* attempt to maintain self-esteem.

Perseveration (the repetition of phrases or behavior) is eventually seen and often is intensified under stress. The *avoidance of answering questions* also is a mechanism by which the client is able to maintain self-esteem unconsciously in the face of severe memory deficits.

Therefore, (1) denial, (2) confabulation, (3) perseveration, and (4) avoidance of questions are four defensive behaviors the nurse might notice during the assessment.

The following four signs of Alzheimer's disease have been described (Wolanin and Fraelich-Philips 1981):

1. **Aphasia** (loss of language ability), which progresses with the disease. Initially, the person has difficulty finding the correct word and then is reduced to a few words, finally reduced to babbling or becoming mute.
2. **Apraxia** (a loss of purposeful movement in the absence of motor or sensory impairment). The person is unable to perform once familiar and purposeful tasks. For example, in apraxia of gait, the person loses the ability to walk. In apraxia of dressing, the person is unable to put his clothes on properly (may put his arms in his trousers or put his jacket on upside down).
3. **Agnosia** (loss of sensory ability to recognize objects). For example, the person may lose the ability to recognize familiar sounds (auditory agnosia), such as the ring of the telephone, a car horn, the door bell, and so forth. Loss of this ability extends to the inability to recognize familiar objects (visual or tactile agnosia), such as a glass, magazine, pencil, or toothbrush. Eventually the person is unable to recognize those people whom he or she loves or even part of his or her own body.
4. **Mnemonic disturbance** (memory loss). Initially the person has difficulty remembering recent events. Gradually deterioration progresses to include both recent and remote memory.

The degeneration of neurons in the brain is the wasting of working components in the brain. These cells contain memories, receive sights and sounds, cause hormones to secrete, produce emotions, and command muscles into motion.

Essentially, with Alzheimer's disease one loses a personal history, place in the world, ability to recognize the environment, and eventually loved ones. Alzheimer's disease robs family and friends, husbands and wives, sons and daughters of valuable human relatedness and companionship, resulting in a profound grieving process. Alzheimer's disease robs society of productive and active participants. Because of these devastating effects, it challenges mental health professionals and social agencies, the medical and nursing professions, and researchers looking for possible solutions.

Alzheimer's disease has been classified according to the stages of the degenerative process. The number of stages ranges from three to seven depending on the source. However, four stages, discussed subsequently, are commonly used to categorize the progressive deterioration seen in victims of Alzheimer's disease (Reisberg 1984).

PHASE 1—MILD ALZHEIMER'S DISEASE

The loss of intellectual ability is insidious. The person with mild Alzheimer's disease loses energy, drive, and initiative and has difficulty learning new things. Personality and social behavior remain intact, which often influences others to minimize and underestimate the loss of the individual's abilities. The individual may still continue to work, with the extent of the dementia becoming evident in a new or demanding situation. Depression may occur early in the disease but usually lessens as the disease progresses. Activities such as doing the marketing or managing finances are noticeably impaired during this phase.

Sam Collins, 56, was a lineman for a telephone company. He felt that he was getting old. He kept forgetting things and would write notes to himself on scraps of paper. One day on the job, he forgot momentarily which wires were to connect and connected all the wrong ones, causing mass confusion for a few hours. At home, Sam flew off the handle when his wife, Jean, suggested they invite the new neighbors for dinner. It was hard for him to admit that anything new confused him, and he often forgot names *(aphasia)* and sometimes lost the thread of conversations. Once he even forgot his address when his car broke down on the highway. He was moody and depressed and became indignant when Jean found three months of unpaid bills stashed in his sock drawer. Jean was bewildered, upset, and fearful that something terrible was wrong.

According to studies quoted by Reisberg (1984), one third of individuals with Alzheimer's disease at this stage decline quickly and may be dead within three years. Another third, although their condition worsens, may still function within the community with support. The final third usually remain at this level for three years or more.

PHASE 2—MODERATE ALZHEIMER'S DISEASE

Deterioration becomes evident during the moderate phase. Often the person with moderate Alzheimer's disease cannot remember his or her address or the date. There are memory gaps in the person's history that may fluctuate from one moment to another. Hygiene suffers, and ability to dress appropriately is markedly affected. The person may put on clothes backward, button the buttons incorrectly, or not zip zippers (this inability to carry out simple activities is *apraxia*). Often the person has to be coaxed to bathe.

Mood becomes labile, and the individual may have bursts of paranoia, anger, jealousy, and apathy. Activities such as driving become hazardous; the person may suddenly speed up or slow down for no apparent reason or go through stop signs. Care and supervision become a full-time job for family members. Denial mercifully takes over and protects the person from the realization that he is losing control not only of his mind but also of his life. Along with denial, the person begins to withdraw from activities and people, since he often feels overwhelmed and frustrated doing things that were once easy. He may also have moments of becoming tearful and sad.

For a short period, Sam was transferred to a less complicated work position after his inability to function was recognized. Jean drove him to work and picked him up. Sam would often forget what he was doing and stare blankly. He would accuse the supervisor of spying on him. Sometimes he would disappear at lunch and be unable to find his way back to work. The transfer lasted only a few months, and Sam was forced to take an early retirement. At home, Sam slept in his clothes. He lost interest in reading and watching sports on TV and often broke into angry outbursts over seemingly nothing. Often he would become extremely restless and irritable and wander around the house aimlessly.

PHASE 3—MODERATE TO SEVERE ALZHEIMER'S DISEASE

At this stage, the person is often not able to identify familiar objects or people, even a spouse (*severe agnosia*). The person needs repeated instructions and directions for the simplest tasks (*advanced apraxia*): "Here is the facecloth, pick up the soap . . . now, put water on the facecloth and rub the facecloth with soap . . . " Often the individual cannot remember where the toilet is and becomes incontinent. Total care is necessary at this point, and the burden on the families can be emotionally, financially, and physically devastating. The world becomes very frightening to the person with Alzheimer's disease, since nothing makes sense any longer. Agitation, violence, paranoia, and delusions are more commonly seen once the mechanisms of denial and withdrawal are no longer effective. Institutionalization may be the most appropriate recourse at this time, since the level of care is so demanding, and violent outbursts and incontinence may be crises that the family can no longer handle. Some criteria for placement in a nursing home follow:

1. The person wanders.
2. The person is a danger to himself or others.
3. The person is incontinent.
4. The person's behavior affects the sleep of others.

Sam was terrified. Memories would come and then slip away. People came and went, but they were strangers. Someone was masquerading as his wife, and it was hard to tell what was present reality and what was memory. Things never stayed in the same place. Sometimes they hid the bathroom where he couldn't find it. He in turn had to hide things to keep them safe, but he would forget where he hid them. Buttons and belts were confusing, and he didn't know what they were doing there, anyway. Sometimes he would try to walk away from the terrifying feelings and the strangers. He would try to find something he had lost long ago . . . if he could only remember what it was.

PHASE 4—LATE ALZHEIMER'S DISEASE

Williams (1986) described what is called a Klüver-Bucy–like syndrome in late Alzheimer's disease. **Agraphia** (inability to read or write), **hyperorality** (the need to taste, chew, and put everything in one's mouth), blunting of emotions, **visual agnosia** (loss of ability to recognize familiar objects), and **hypermetamorphosis** (touching everything in sight) are all associated with this syndrome.

At this stage, the ability to talk, and then eventually the ability to walk, is lost. If death due to secondary causes (e.g., infection, choking) has not come, the end stage of Alzheimer's disease is characterized by stupor and coma.

Jean and the children kept Sam at home until his outbursts became frightening. After he was lost for two days when he had somehow unlocked the front door, Jean had Sam placed in a Veterans Administration (VA) Hospital. When Jean came to visit, Sam would sometimes cry. Sam never talked and was always tied into his chair when she came to visit. The staff explained to her that although Sam could still walk, he kept getting into other people's beds and scaring them. They explained to Jean that perhaps Sam wanted comfort and missed human touch. They encouraged her visits, even though Sam did not seem to recognize her. Sam did respond to music, and Jean brought a radio, and when she played the country and western music he always loved, Sam would nod and clap his hands.

Jean was torn between guilt and love, anger and despair. Jean was confused and depressed. She was going through the painful process of mourning the loss of the man she loved and had shared a life with for 34 years.

Three months after admission to the VA Hospital, and eight years after the incident of the crossed wires at the telephone company, Sam choked on some food, developed pneumonia, and died.

Standard III: Diagnosis

Care for a client with dementia, especially Alzheimer's disease, requires a great deal of patience, creativity, and maturity. The needs of such a client can be enormous for nursing staff and for families who care for their loved one in the home. As the disease progresses, so do the needs of the client and the demands on the caregivers, staff, and family.

One of the most important areas of concern identified by both staff and families is the client's safety. Many people with Alzheimer's disease wander and may be lost for hours or days. Seizures are not uncommon in the later stages of this disease. Injuries from falls and accidents can occur during any stage, as confusion and disorientation progress. There is potential for burns if the client is a smoker or is unattended at the stove. Prescription drugs can be taken incorrectly, or bottles of noxious fluids can be mistakenly drunk, resulting in a medical crisis. Therefore, *potential for injury* is always present.

Throughout the course of the disease, the nursing diagnosis may not change (e.g., potential for injury); however, the "related to" and "as evidenced by" components may, and these are the parameters from which meaningful and effective goals are formed. Potential for injury can be related to confusion, unsteady gait, faulty judgment, poisons, household hazards, loss of short term memory, and more. Potential for injury can be evidenced by impaired mobility, sensory deficits, history of accidents, and lack of knowledge of safety precautions. Depending on the etiology or evidence, goals are formulated.

Communicating with the client with Alzheimer's disease becomes progressively more difficult. Comprehension diminishes, and the person finds it difficult and then is unable to name objects (*aphasia*). Eventually the inability to recognize objects (*agnosia*) appears. As the person becomes more disoriented, memory diminishes and attention span decreases, and the person is unable to maintain continuity in relationships, events, and environment. Lowering the person's level of fear and anxiety, providing a sense of safety, and emphasizing visual and verbal clues are helpful when *impaired verbal communication* is assessed. Impaired verbal communication may be related to aphasia, cerebral impairment, and more. Supporting data include (1) difficulty in finding the correct word and (2) inappropriate speech or response.

As time goes on, the person loses the ability to perform tasks that were once familiar and routine (*apraxia*). For example, the person's ability to dress diminishes. At first, supervision or simple directions may be enough; eventually total assistance will be needed. This progression applies to bathing, hygiene, grooming, feeding, and toileting — in fact, to all areas of daily living. Therefore, *self-care deficit* occurs, to varying degrees. Depending on the affected person's disability, goals and interventions are planned. The most effective and respectful goals are those that allow the client to carry out as much of his or her own care as possible.

It may be difficult to view the person with Alzheimer's disease as a once-competent, humorous, caring person whose life included family and friends. Memory impairment robs people of their continuity and place in life, along with cherished relationships and the joy of living. Unfortunately, the affected person often *is* aware of what is happening to him or her. The losing of one's sense of self is experienced as terrifying, despairing, and isolating. Therefore, *disturbance in self-esteem*, *role performance*, and *disturbance in personal identity* need to be addressed in some fashion when planning care. *Powerlessness*, *hopelessness*, and *grieving* are important considerations.

Evidence of hallucinations, delusions (usually paranoid), illusions, and memory impairment signal *altered thought processes* related to dementia. The nursing diagnosis, *altered thought processes*, is usually part of any care plan for a person with Alzheimer's disease.

Ineffective individual coping is evident. Besides not being able to function in one's occupational and personal life, as previously discussed, long-standing personality traits may become intensified and manifested in inappropriate behaviors. Common behaviors include hording, regression, and being overly demanding. Therefore, nurses and family members often intervene in behaviors that signal ineffective individual coping.

Perhaps some of the most crucial aspects of the client's care are support, education, and referrals for the family. The family loses an integral part of its unit. Family members lose the love, the function, the support, the companionship, and the warmth that this person provided. There are always *altered family processes*. *Grieving* is an important process for the family to go through; it can make the task ahead somewhat clearer and, at times, less painful.

A recent study (Mass and Buckwalter, 1988) identified four of the most frequently used nursing diagnoses for clients with Alzheimer's disease on a special Alzheimer's unit as

1. Altered thought processes (52%)
2. Self-care deficit (48%)
3. Altered patterns of urinary elimination: incontinence (12%)
4. Altered nutrition: less than body requirements (10%)

Standard IV: Planning

Planning includes (1) on the content level—goals—and (2) on the process level—nurses' reactions and feelings.

CONTENT LEVEL—PLANNING GOALS

For the nursing diagnosis *potential for injury* a number of goals may be appropriate. Some, by no means all, follow:

- Client will remain safe in the (hospital/home).
- With the aid of ID bracelet and neighborhood/hospital alert, client will be returned within three hours of wandering.
- Client will remain free of danger during seizures.
- With the aid of nursing interventions client will not burn self.
- With the aid of nursing guidance and environmental manipulation, client will fall without hurting him- or herself.
- Client will ingest only correct doses of prescribed medications and food/fluids stuffs.

For the nursing diagnosis *impaired communication*, the following goals might be useful:

- Client will communicate needs.
- Client will answer yes or no to questions.
- Client will state needs in alternate modes when aphasic.
- Client will signal correct word upon hearing it.
- Client will refer to picture or label when aphasic.
- Client will wear prescribed glasses or hearing aid each day.

For a client with *self-care deficit*, possible goals follow:

- Client will participate in self-care at optimal level.
- Client can follow step-by-step instructions for dressing, bathing, grooming.
- Client will put on own clothes appropriately, with aid of Velcro tapes and nursing supervision.
- Client's skin will remain intact despite incontinence or prolonged pressure.

Disturbance in self-esteem needs to be addressed. Often nurses tend to treat older people or people with cognitive impairments as if they were children. Being treated like a child could very well foster childlike behaviors. Self-esteem is damaged, anxiety increases, and regressive behaviors are fostered. Some goals that might apply follow:

- Client will state both positive and negative comments about his or her personal level of functioning.
- Client will function at his or her highest level within the family.
- Client will state that he or she is aware that people care about him or her.
- Each day, client will participate in simple activities that bring enjoyment (singing with others, group exercises, recounting past successes to others).

Altered thought processes evidenced by hallucinations, delusions, illusions, and severe memory impairment may play a large role in the care provided by the nurse or families. Some nursing goals that might be appropriate follow:

- Client will acknowledge the reality, after it is pointed out, of an object or sound that was misinterpreted (illusion).
- Client will state that he or she feels safe after experiencing hallucinations.
- Client will remain nonaggressive when experiencing paranoid ideation.
- Client will discuss some aspects of his or her life which hold pleasant memories.

Ineffective individual coping evidenced by hoarding, regressive, or demanding behaviors can also be a challenge for nurses and families alike. Goals include the following:

- Client will retain only hoarded items that do not include potentially dangerous materials such as glass, metal, or food.
- Client will respond to suggestions by nurse to go to his or her room to masturbate when masturbating in a public area.
- Number and intensity of client's demands on staff/family will decrease with aid of nursing interventions.

Families with a demented member are under tremendous stresses. The stress of caring for an ill family member, who in many ways has become a stranger, can trigger intense feelings of anger, guilt, hopelessness, despair, and grief within the family. If the family is caring for the ill member in the home, the combination of intense emotional conflicts and overwhelming demands to meet the ill family member's multiple physical needs can be tremendous. There are almost always *altered family processes*. Divorces, separations, and other evidences of severe stress may be the result. Financial drains may leave the family bankrupt. A variety of supports are needed. Goals that need consideration follow:

- Family members will have the opportunity to express "unacceptable" feelings in a supportive environment.
- Family members will have access to professional counseling.
- Family members will name two organizations within their geographical area that can offer support.
- Family members will participate in ill member's plan of care, with encouragement from staff.
- Family members will state that they have outside help which allows family members to take personal time for themselves (1–7 days) each week or month.
- Family members will have the name of three resources that can help with financial burdens and legal considerations.

PROCESS LEVEL—NURSES' REACTIONS AND FEELINGS

Nurses working in any setting with cognitively impaired clients are aware of the tremendous responsibility placed on the caregivers. Severe confusion, psychotic states, and violent and aggressive behaviors can take their toll on staff/family (Burnside 1988). Taking care of clients who are unable to communicate and have lost the ability to relate and respond to others is extremely difficult, especially for student nurses and nurses who do not understand dementia or Alzheimer's disease (Burnside 1988).

Nurses working in areas that care for clients who are cognitively impaired (e.g., nursing homes, extended care facilities) need special training. Training needs to include education about the process of the disease and knowledge of psychiatric nursing needs and effective interventions, as well as knowledge regarding the neuroleptic (antipsychotic) drugs. Supportive and educational opportunities should be readily available, not just to nurses but to nurse's aides who are also often directly responsible for administering basic care.

Burnout of staff can be a problem. Burnside (1988) identifies three possible antidotes to burnout:

1. *Revise goals* so that they are realistic. Nurses sometimes set goals that are too high and not realistic. Frustration and discouragement ensue when the goals cannot be met.
2. *Refrain from being swept into a hopeless stance.* Concentrate on finding satisfaction in small accomplishments, (e.g., the client is comfortable, is participating in an activity, is less delusional than previously). Indeed, for this person, such a situation may mark quite an accomplishment.
3. *Research* is a prime factor for eliminating staff burnout (Lipkowitz 1982). Involving nurses in research helps involve staff in an important activity that can increase nurses' knowledge for caring for the demented client and add a feeling of purpose to what is a very demanding job, involving great patience and maturity.

Standard V: Intervention

Dementia is a progressive global deterioration of mental functioning, with impairment of recent memory and abstract reasoning and ultimate disorientation. Whether impairments are reversible or irreversible, several nursing interventions can be employed with the cognitively impaired. *The basic principle underlying all care for the cognitively impaired is to facilitate the highest level of functioning a person is capable of in all areas (self-care, social and family relationships). Prevention of further regression* is a long term goal.

Treatment of dementia is, at present, palliative and supportive in nature. Medical or surgical interventions that attempt to diminish the pathophysiology remain experimental.

Low-dose major tranquilizers may be administered to clients with severe agitation, aggression, or paranoid behavior. Nutrition, hygiene, safety, and elimination needs are all management concerns. There is a real and present need for further development of day-care programs, respite programs, and special long term Alzheimer's care units.

According to Ninos and Makohon (1985), assisting patients to cope within their environment is the basis for treatment or therapy, particularly nursing therapy. Thus, nurses must identify and modify, where possible, specific functional disturbances and assist clients and families in compensating for such disturbances.

Intervention with family members is also critical. The effects of losing a family member to dementia—that is, watching a person who has an important role within the family unit and who is loved and a vital part of his or her family's history deteriorate—can be devastating. The interventions discussed subsequently have been found useful.

V-A: PSYCHOTHERAPEUTIC INTERVENTIONS

Burnside (1988) suggests the following guidelines for use when implementing interventions or teaching a severely cognitively impaired person:

1. Do not provide more than one visual clue (object) at one time.
2. Know that the client may lack understanding of the task assigned.
3. Remember that relevant information is remembered longer than irrelevant information.
4. Break learning tasks into very small steps.
5. Give only *one* instruction at a time.
6. Report, record, and chart all data.

Table 21-6 gives special guidelines for nurses and family members to use when communicating with a cognitively impaired person.

Table 21-6 • USEFUL COMMUNICATION STRATEGIES FOR USE BY CAREGIVERS (NURSES OR FAMILY)

NURSING INTERVENTION	RATIONALE
1. Always identify yourself and call the person by name at each meeting.	1. Client's short term memory impaired—requires frequent orientation to time and environment.
2. Speak slowly.	2. Gives client time to process information
3. Use short, simple words and phrases.	3. Client's cognitive impairment too great to make sense of complex statements or abstract ideas.
4. Maintain face-to-face contact.	4. Maximizes verbal and nonverbal clues.
5. Be near client when talking, one or two arm lengths away. Focus on one piece of information at a time.	5. Attention span of client is poor and easily distracted; helps client focus. Too much data can be overwhelming and can increase anxiety.
6. Talk with client about familiar and meaningful things.	6. Allows self-expression and reinforces reality.
7. Encourage reminiscing about happy times in life.	7. Remembering accomplishments and shared joys helps to distract client from deficit and gives meaning to existence.
8. When client is delusional, acknowledge client's feelings and reinforce reality. Do not argue or refute delusions.	8. Acknowledging feelings helps client feel understood. Pointing out realities may help client focus on realities. Arguing can enhance adherence to false beliefs.
9. If a client gets into an argument with another client, stop the argument and get them out of each other's way. After a short while (5 minutes), explain to each client matter-of-factly why you had to intervene.	9. Prevents escalation to physical acting out. Shows respect for client's right to know. Explaining to person in adult manner helps maintain self-esteem.
10. Confusion and disorientation easily increase anxiety. When client becomes verbally aggressive, acknowledge client's feelings and shift topic to more familiar ground—e.g.: "I know this is upsetting for you, since you always cared for others. . . . Tell me about your children."	10. Acknowledging feelings makes the client feel more understood and less alone. Topics the client has mastery in can remind him or her of areas of competent functioning and increase self-esteem.
11. Have client wear prescribed eye glasses and/or hearing aid.	11. Increase environmental awareness; orientation, and comprehension, which in turn increases awareness of personal needs and the presence of others.
12. Keep client's room well lit.	12. Allows for maximum environmental clues.
13. Have clocks, calendars, personal items (e.g., family pictures, personal Bible, or other personally meaningful objects) in clear view of client while in bed.	13. Assists in maintaining personal identity.
14. Reinforce client's pictures, nonverbal gestures, X's on calendars, and so forth.	14. When aphasia starts to hinder communication, alternate methods of communication need to be instituted.

Table 21-7 • STRATEGIES FOR ACTIVITIES OF DAILY LIVING

NURSING INTERVENTION	RATIONALE
Dressing and Bathing	
1. Always have client perform all tasks that he or she is capable of.	1. Maintains client's self-esteem and uses muscle groups; impedes staff burnout; minimizes further regression.
2. Always have client wear own clothes, even in the hospital.	2. Helps maintain client's identity and dignity.
3. Use clothing with elastic, and substitute Velcro tape for buttons and zippers.	3. Minimizes client's confusion and eases independence of functioning.
4. Label clothing items with *client's name* and *name of item.*	4. Helps identify client if he or she wanders *and* gives client additional clues when *aphasia* or *agnosia* are operative.
5. Give step-by-step instructions whenever necessary—e.g.,: "Take this blouse . . . put in one arm . . . now the next arm . . . pull it together in the front . . . now . . ."	5. Client can focus on small pieces of information more easily; allows client to perform at optimal level.
6. Make sure that water in faucets is not too hot.	6. Judgment lacking in client; unaware of many safety hazards.
7. If client is resistant to doing self-care, come back later and ask again.	7. Moods may be labile and client may forget but often will comply after short interval.
Nutrition	
1. Monitor food and fluid intake.	1. Client may have anorexia or be too confused to eat.
2. Offer finger food that client can walk around with.	2. Increases input throughout the day; client may eat only a small amount at meals.
3. Weigh client regularly (once a week).	3. Monitors fluid/nutritional status.
4. During period of *hyperorality*, watch that client does not eat nonfood items (e.g., ceramic fruit, food-shaped soaps).	4. Client will put everything thought to be food into mouth; may be unable to differentiate nonedible objects made in the shape and color of food.
Bowel and Bladder Functions	
1. Begin bowel and bladder program early; start with bladder control.	1. Same time of day for bowel movements and toileting—in early A.M., after meals and snacks, and before bedtime—can help prevent incontinence.
2. Evaluate use of disposable diapers.	2. Prevents embarrassment.
3. *Label* bathroom door (as well as other rooms).	3. Additional environmental clues can maximize independent toileting.
Sleep	
Client may become awake, be frightened, and cry out at night. 1. Keep area well lit.	1. Reinforces orientation, minimizes possible illusions.
2. Give frequent reassurances.	2. Human contact can lower anxiety.
3. If possible, allow client to sit by desk (in hospital).	3. Increases orientation and feelings of safety and decreases sense of isolation.
4. Non-barbiturates may be ordered (e.g., chloral hydrate).	4. Barbiturates can have paradoxical reaction, causing agitation.
5. If medications are indicated, neuroleptics with sedative properties may be the most helpful (e.g., Haldol).	5. Helps clear thinking as well as offering sedation.
6. Avoid the use of restraints.	6. Client can become more terrified and fight against the restraints until exhausted to a dangerous degree.

V-B: HEALTH TEACHING

Educating families with a cognitively impaired member is one of the most important areas of teaching for nurses. Families who are caring for a member in the home need to know about communication strategies (Table 21–6), strategies for activities of daily living (Table 21–7), how to structure the environment (Table 21–8), and most important, where to get help. Help includes professional counseling and education regarding the process and progression of the disease. Families especially need to know about and be referred to com-

Table 21–8 • THERAPEUTIC ENVIRONMENT FOR THE COGNITIVELY IMPAIRED

NURSING INTERVENTION	RATIONALE
Safe Environment	
If living with family:	
1. Gradually restrict the use of car.	1. Judgment becomes impaired; client dangerous to self and others.
2. If wanders during night, put mattress on the floor.	2. Prevents falls when client is confused.
3. Remove throw rugs and other objects in person's path.	3. Minimizes tripping and falling.
In hospital or with family:	
4. Minimize sensory stimulation.	4. Decreases sensory overload, which could increase anxiety and confusion.
5. If client becomes verbally upset, listen briefly, give support, then change the topic.	5. Goal is to prevent escalation of anger. When attention span is short, client can be distracted to more productive topics/activities.
6. Label all rooms and drawers. Label often used objects (hairbrushes, toothbrushes).	6. May keep client from wandering into other clients' rooms. Increases environmental clues to familiar objects.
7. Install safety bars in bathroom.	7. Prevents falls.
8 Supervise client when smoking.	8 Danger of burns always present.
9. If client has history of seizures, keep padded tongue blades at bedside. Educate family and observe.	9. Seizure activity is common in advanced Alzheimer's disease.
For clients who wander:	
10. Have client wear Medi-Alert bracelet, which cannot be removed (with name, address, telephone number). Provide Police Department with recent pictures.	10. Client can be easily identified by police, neighbors, or hospital personnel.
11. Alert local police—hospital—neighborhood about wanderer.	11. May reduce time for returning client to home/hospital.
12. If in hospital, have wandering client wear brightly colored vest with name, unit, and phone number printed on back.	12. Client easily identifiable.
13. Have complex locks put on door when wandering is a problem.	13. Reduces opportunity to wander.
14. Encourage physical activity during the day.	14. Physical activity may decrease wandering at night.
15. Explore sensor devices.	15. Provides warning if client wanders.
Activities	
1. Provide picture magazines and children's books when client's reading ability diminishes.	1. Allows continuation of usual activities that the client can still enjoy; provides focus.
2. Provide simple activities that allow for exercise of large muscles.	2. Exercise groups, dance groups, walking, and so forth provide socialization, as well as increasing circulation and helping to maintain muscle tone.
3. Encourage group activities that are familiar and simple to perform.	3. Such activities as group singing, dancing, reminiscing, and working with clay and paint all help to increase socialization and minimize feelings of alienation.

munity-based groups that can help shoulder this tremendous burden, (e.g., day-care centers, senior citizen groups, Alzheimer's associations, organizations providing home visits and respite care, family support groups). Available information regarding housekeeping, home health aides, and companions should also be available. Such outside resources can help prevent total emotional and physical fatigue of family members.

Teusink and Mahler (1984) have labeled the processes that the family goes through as (1) denial, (2) overinvolvement, (3) anger, (4) guilt, and (5) resolution. They compare these steps to those of the mourning process, using the model of Kubler-Ross (see Chapter 18). Scott, Roberto, and Hutton (1986) confirmed in their research that family support was positively associated with the caregiver's coping effectiveness. According to the research findings of Chenoweth and Spencer (1986), each stage of Alzheimer's disease involves new and different stresses, which can at least be diminished by professional assistance.

Family members often feel guilty that they did not do or are not doing enough. They may feel frustrated and angry. It is not an uncommon reaction to blame staff, nurses, and doctors. The use of projection helps protect family members from their own feelings of helplessness and hopelessness. It is *vital* that the health care providers understand this phenomenon in order to minimize defensive responses. Consultation with family members and education about the disease are of enormous benefit.

Finally, family members need to know where and how to place the ill member when this becomes necessary. Eventually the ill family member's labile and aggressive behavior, incontinence, wandering, unsafe habits, or disruptive nocturnal activity can no longer be appropriately dealt with in the home. Families need information, support, and financial guidance at this time. When the nurse is unable to provide the relevant information, proper referrals by the social worker are needed.

V-C: ACTIVITIES OF DAILY LIVING

Nurses and family members are constantly involved with maintaining adequate self-care, rest, hygiene, and nutrition. Many useful interventions have been devised by health care workers over the years. Table 21-7 provides some suggestions.

V-E: THERAPEUTIC ENVIRONMENT

Providing a therapeutic environment is another area of great concern for care-givers of a cognitively impaired person. A therapeutic environment can be divided into (1) safety considerations and (2) activities that increase socialization and minimize loneliness. Table 21-8 gives some guidelines for providing a therapeutic environment.

Standard VI: Evaluation

It is very important that the goals set for clients with cognitive impairment be measurable, within their capabilities, and evaluated frequently. As the person's condition continues to deteriorate, goals will need to be altered to reflect the person's diminished functioning. Frequent evaluation and reformulation of goals will also help to diminish staff frustration as well as minimize the client's anxiety by assuring that tasks are not more complicated than the person can accomplish. The overall goals in treatment and nursing care are to promote the client's optimal level of functioning and retard further regression, whenever possible. Full staff involvement in the evaluation process may increase the likelihood that the goals will be realistic.

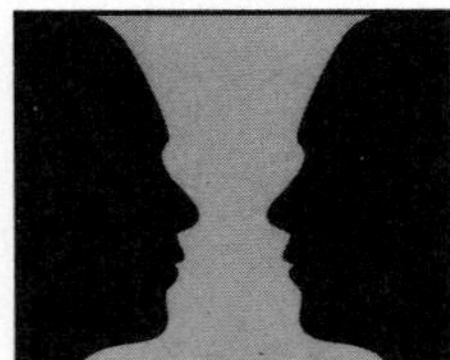

Case Study: Working With a Person Who Is Cognitively Impaired

During the past four years, Mr. Ludwik has demonstrated rapidly progressive memory impairment, disorientation, and deterioration in his ability to function, related to Alzheimer's disease. He is a 67-year-old man, who had retired at age 62 to spend some of his remaining "youth" with his wife, Helen, in order to travel, garden, visit family, and finally experience the plans they had made over the past forty years. He was diagnosed with Alzheimer's disease at age 63.

Mr. Ludwik has been taken care of at home by his wife and daughter, Daisy. Daisy was divorced and had come home to live with her two young daughters.

Progressively the family members found themselves close to physical and mental exhaustion. Mr. Ludwik has become increasingly incontinent when he cannot find the bathroom. He wanders constantly away from home despite close supervision. The police and neighbors bring him back home on the average of four times a week. Once he was lost for five days, after he somehow boarded a bus for Pittsburgh, 100 miles from home. He was robbed and beaten before being found by the police and returned home.

He frequently wanders into his granddaughters' rooms at night while they are sleeping, and tries to get into bed with them. Too young to understand that their grandfather is lonely and confused, they fear he is going to hurt them. Four times in the past two weeks he has fallen while getting out of bed at night, thinking he was in a sleeping bag camping out in the mountains.

After a conflicting and painful two months, the family placed him in a nearby nursing home.

Helen Ludwik told the admitting nurse, Mr. Jackson, that her husband wanders almost all of the time. He has difficulty finding the right words for things (*aphasia*) and becomes frustrated and angry when that happens. Sometimes, he does not seem to recognize the family (*agnosia*). Once he thought Daisy was a thief breaking into the house and attacked her with a broom handle. This caused Daisy to break down into heavy sobs—"What's happened to my father? He was so kind and gentle. O God . . . I have lost my father."

Helen Ludwik tells Mr. Jackson that sometimes Mr. Ludwik can participate in dressing himself; at other times, when he appears confused over what goes where, he needs to be completely dressed. At this point Mrs. Ludwik begins to cry uncontrollably, saying, "I can't bear to part with him . . . but I can't do it any more. I feel like I've betrayed him."

Mr. Jackson then focused his attention on Mrs. Ludwik and her experience. He stated that he knew what a difficult decision this was for her. He said that he believed the nursing home was a proper place for Mr. Ludwik at this time, but that he was also aware that families usually had conflicting and intense emotional reactions of guilt, depression, loss, anger, and other painful feelings. Mr. Jackson suggested that Mrs. Ludwik talk to other families with a cognitively impaired member. "It might help you to know that you are not alone, and having contact with others to share your grief can be healing." One of the groups he suggested was the Alzheimer's Disease and Related Disorders Association (ADRDA), a well known self-help group.

Assessment

Since, indeed, the family was just as much the client as the family member with Alzheimer's disease, Mr. Jackson tried to take the most pressing immediate needs into consideration. He identified the following data obtained on initial assessment:

OBJECTIVE DATA

1. Wanders away from home about four times a week
2. Was lost for five days, robbed, and beaten
3. Often incontinent when cannot find the bathroom
4. Has difficulty finding words
5. Has difficulty at times identifying members of the family
6. Has difficulty at times dressing himself
7. Falls out of bed at night
8. Has memory impairment
9. Disoriented much of the time
10. Gets into bed with granddaughters at night when wandering
11. Family undergoing intense feelings of loss and guilt

SUBJECTIVE DATA

1. "I can't bear to part with him."
2. "I feel I've betrayed him."
3. "I've lost my father."

Nursing Diagnosis

Mr. Jackson evaluated the data. Indeed, there were many potential nursing diagnoses that would be appropriate and several client needs that required intervention by the nursing staff. Mr. Jackson chose four initially; the first one deals with client safety, the following two address maintaining an optimal level of functioning and preventing further regression, and the fourth deals with the very real and immediate needs of a family in crisis. Therefore, Mr. Jackson made the following diagnoses:

1. *Potential for Injury* related to altered cerebral functioning, as evidenced by wandering
   - Wanders away from home about four times a week
   - Wanders despite supervision
   - Falls out of bed at night
   - Gets into other people's beds
   - Wanders at night

Continued on following page

2. *Altered Pattern of Urinary Elimination: Incontinence*, related to cerebral impairment or disturbed cognition, as evidenced by inability to find the toilet
   - Increasingly incontinent when cannot find the bathroom
3. *Self Care Deficit* (self-dressing deficits) related to impaired cognitive functioning, as evidenced by impaired ability to put on and take off clothing.
   - Sometimes is able to dress with help of wife
   - At other times, too confused to dress self at all
4. *Family Grieving* related to loss and deterioration of family member
   - "I can't bear to part with him."
   - "I feel I've betrayed him."
   - "I've lost my father."
   - Family undergoing intense feelings of loss and guilt

Planning

Mr. Jackson's plan took into account both content level — planning goals — and process level — his own emotional reactions to cognitively impaired individuals.

CONTENT LEVEL — PLANNING GOALS

Although Mr. Ludwik had many unmet needs that required nursing interventions, Mr. Jackson decided to focus on the four initial nursing diagnoses previously cited. As other problems arose, they would be addressed.

Nursing Diagnosis	Long Term Goals	Short Term Goals
1. *Potential for injury* related to altered cerebral functioning, as evidenced by wandering	Client will remain safe in nursing home.	1a. Client will not fall out of bed at any time. 1b. Client will wander only in protected area. 1c. Client will be returned within two hours if he leaves unit.
2. *Altered Pattern of Urinary Elimination: Incontinence*, related to disturbed cognition, as evidenced by inability to find the toilet	Client will be less incontinent (# of episodes) by the fourth week of hospitalization.	2a. Client will participate in toilet training. 2b. Client will find the toilet most of the time.
3. *Self-Care Deficit* (self-dressing) related to impaired cognitive functioning, as evidenced by impaired ability to put on and take off clothes	Client will participate in dressing himself most of the time.	3a. Client will follow step-by-step instructions for dressing most of the time. 3b. Client will don own clothes with aid of Velcro tape.
4. *Family Grieving* related to loss and deterioration of family member	All family members will state, in three months' time, that they feel more supported and able to talk about their grieving.	4a. Family members will state that they have opportunity to express "unacceptable" feelings in supportive environment. 4b. Family will state that they have found support from others who have a family member with Alzheimer's disease.

CONTENT LEVEL — NURSES' REACTIONS AND FEELINGS

Mr. Jackson had worked in this particular unit for a long time. It was a unit especially designed for cognitively impaired individuals, which made nursing care easier than on a regular unit. However, Mr. Jackson would be the first to admit that he had come a long way in the four years he had worked on the unit.

Four years ago, he found himself getting constantly frustrated and angry. He had entered this special unit very enthusiastically and had worked very hard setting goals and trying to implement them. However, he thought no one, especially the clients, cared about what he was doing for them. When the nursing coordinator asked him what made him come to that conclusion, he burst out, "Nothing I do seems to make any difference . . . no one listens to me."

Mr. Jackson had a lot to learn about Alzheimer's disease, and he found that the more he learned, the more he understood why change took so long or, in some cases, could not take place. He, like everyone before him, learned to become more realistic in formulating goals, which lessened his frustration.

He also learned from the other caregivers on the unit many nursing care strategies that increased competent care and decreased frustration. For example, he learned that he could distract certain clients away from inappropriate behaviors (e.g., arguing with others, taking things out of other people's rooms) by engaging them in another, enjoyable activity, such as talking about something they were interested in. This reduced Mr. Jackson's initial response of "scolding" the client, which usually resulted in escalating the client's anxiety, confusion, and sometimes aggression, and left Mr. Jackson annoyed and upset.

As time progressed, Mr. Jackson found that he was well suited to this kind of nursing. He had an enthusiastic manner, and his patience, wit, and genuine liking for his clients made him an ideal role model for staff new to the unit. He did a lot of teaching on the unit, both formal and informal. Presently he is working on a workbook for caregivers of the cognitively impaired, to be published in the near future.

Intervention

Mr. Jackson gave Mrs. Ludwik the names of two organizations in her community that worked with families with a cognitively impaired member. He emphasized the Alzheimer's Association support group composed of other family members who were going through similar circumstances. He gave Mrs. Ludwik the name of the social worker as well as the nurse clinician assigned to the unit, who could give the family information on the disease, answer questions, and provide support and further referrals. Mr. Jackson asked Mrs. Ludwik to let him know after one week how things were going, and he said that further plans could be made at that time.

Wandering is not an uncommon phenomenon, especially among male clients with Alzheimer's disease. However, since wandering at night may be indicative of cardiac decompensation, Mr. Jackson alerted the medical staff. Mr. Ludwik's mattress was placed on the floor in order to prevent falls, and there was a large area on the unit where he could wander safely. A bright orange vest was made for Mr. Ludwik with his name, unit, and phone number taped on the back, in case he did wander off the unit. A Medi-Alert bracelet was also made up for him, containing the same information. He was encouraged to participate in activities that encouraged the exercise of large muscle groups (e.g., exercise groups, dance groups). He seemed to wander less at night if he had been involved in physical exercise the day before. On those nights that he did wander out of his room, the staff would allow him to wander in the safe area. He was offered snacks, and the room was kept well lit. Sometimes Mr. Ludwik would curl up on the couch and fall asleep.

On the unit, Mr. Jackson and the staff began toilet training Mr. Ludwik; i.e., they took him to the toilet early in the morning, after each meal and snack, and in the evening. On this unit, all the rooms, including the bathrooms, were clearly labeled in large, colorful letters; clocks were placed in every room in clear view, and each room had a large calendar with X's marking off the days.

Mr. Jackson found that, most mornings, Mr. Ludwik was able to follow simple step-by-step instructions for dressing, but that he was much better at this after breakfast than in the early morning hours. Therefore, a schedule was set up including toileting, breakfast, toileting, and then dressing. When Mr. Ludwik became irritable and refused to dress, Mr. Jackson would involve Mr. Ludwik in another activity and, after 15 or 20 minutes, suggest dressing. This seemed to work most of the time. Mr. Ludwik always wore his own clothes, unchanged except for the

Continued on following page

Velcro tape that replaced the original buttons and zippers. This seemed to lessen Mr. Ludwik's frustration during dressing.

Mr. Ludwik's love for gardening was sublimated into activities such as finger painting and modeling clay. The activity therapist found that Mr. Ludwik was most content during these times. Refer to Nursing Care Plan 21–1.

Evaluation

By the end of four weeks, Mr. Ludwik was still free from injuries. Placing his mattress on the floor had solved one potential problem. Mr. Ludwik continued to wander at night but more often, in the past week or so, he would nap on the couch after having a snack. He did wander off the unit once, when visitors were coming in, but was returned to the unit by the security guard as he prepared to leave the hospital. The familiar orange vest had been spotted immediately.

Initially, when Mr. Ludwik came to the unit he was very disoriented. However, getting used to certain staff members and set routines helped to overcome his disorientation. With the aid of the Velcro tape fasteners and constant, short reminders, Mr. Ludwik dressed himself with minimal assistance.

Urinary incontinence showed great improvement over the four-week period. Although Mr. Ludwik was still incontinent, episodes were down to four times a week. He was amenable to the toileting schedule and usually complied without problems.

The family began short term counseling together. Counseling sessions not only gave Helen Ludwik and Daisy an opportunity to express pent-up feelings and receive guidance but also gave Mr. Ludwik's granddaughters time to express their own fears and confusion.

Mrs. Ludwik had been to two meetings of an Alzheimer's support group, at which she found great relief. She said she had felt isolated for so long. Her daughter Daisy was planning to go with her to the next meeting.

Nursing Care Plan 21–1 • A PERSON WITH COGNITIVE IMPAIRMENT: Mr. Ludwik

NURSING DIAGNOSIS

Potential for injury related to altered cerebral functioning, as evidenced by wandering

Supporting Data

- Wanders despite supervision.
- Falls out of bed.
- Gets into other people's beds.

Long Term Goal: Client will remain safe in nursing home.

Short Term Goal	*Intervention*	*Rationale*	*Evaluation*
1. Client will not fall out of bed at any time.	1a. Spend time with client upon admission.	1a. Lowers anxiety, provides orientation to time and place. Client's confusion will be increased by change.	*Goal met*
	1b. Label client's room in big, colorful letters.	1b. Offers alternate clues in new surroundings.	
	1c. Remove mattress from bed and place on floor.	1c. Prevents falling out of bed.	Mattress on floor prevented falls out of bed.
	1d. Keep room well lit at all times.	1d. Provides important environmental clues; helps lower possibility of delusions.	
	1e. Show client clock and calendar in room.	1e. Fosters orientation to time.	
	1f. Keep window shade up.	1f. Allows day-night variations.	

Short Term Goal	Intervention	Rationale	Evaluation
2. Client will wander only in protected area.	2a. At night take client to large, protected, well-lit room.	2a. Client able to wander safely in protected environment.	*Goal met* Client continued to wander at night; with aid of supervision kept out of other clients' rooms most of the time. By fourth week, client started to nap on couch in large room after snacks during the night.
	2b. Alert physician to check client for cardiac decompensation.	2b. Possible underlying cause of nocturnal wakefulness/wandering.	
	2c. Offer snacks when client is up—milk, decaffeinated tea, sandwich.	2c. Helps replace fluid and caloric expenditure.	
	2d. Allow soft music on radio.	2d. Helps induce relaxation.	
	2e. Spend short, frequent intervals with client.	2e. Decreases client's feelings of isolation and increases orientation.	
	2f. Take client to bathroom after snacks.	2f. Helps prevent incontinence.	
	2g. During day, offer activities that include use of large muscle groups.	2g. For some clients, helps decrease wandering.	
3. Client will be returned within two hours if he leaves the unit.	3a. Order Medi-Alert bracelet for client (with name, unit/hospital, phone number).	3a. If client gets out of hospital, he can be identified.	*Goal met* By fourth week, client wandered off unit only once; was found in lobby and returned by security guard within 45 minutes.
	3b. Place brightly colored vest on client with name, unit, and phone number taped on back.	3b. If client wanders in hospital, he can be identified and returned.	
	3c. Check client's whereabouts periodically during the day and especially at night.	3c. Helps monitor client's activities.	

NURSING DIAGNOSIS

Altered pattern of urinary elimination: incontinence, related to a cerebral impairment, as evidenced by incontinence when he cannot find the toilet

Supporting Data

- Increasingly incontinent when cannot find the bathroom

Long Term Goal: Client will be less incontinent by the fourth week of hospitalization.

Short Term Goal	*Intervention*	*Rationale*	*Evaluation*
1. Client will participate in toilet training.	1. Start toilet training (toilet client early A.M. after meals, before bed, and after snacks).	1. Reduces potential for incontinence.	*Goal met* For first two weeks, client was very confused in new environment. Gradually began to adjust to "toileting."
2. Client will find toilet and be less incontinent by the fourth week.	2a. Frequently identify large sign on bathroom.	2a. Frequent orientation to place.	By fourth week, incontinent episodes decreased from three times a day (first wk) to four times a week.
	2b. Evaluate use of incontinence pads.	2b. Can provide dignity and help maintain self-esteem.	Client not using incontinence pads at present.

Continued on following page

Nursing Care Plan 21-1 • A PERSON WITH COGNITIVE IMPAIRMENT: Mr. Ludwik *(Continued)*

NURSING DIAGNOSIS

Self-care deficit (self-dressing deficit) related to diminished cognitive functioning, as evidenced by impaired ability to put on and take off clothing

Supporting Data

- Sometimes is able to dress with help of wife.
- At other times too confused to dress self at all.

Long Term Goal: Client will participate in dressing himself most of the time.

Short Term Goal	*Intervention*	*Rationale*	*Evaluation*
1. Client will follow step-by-step instructions for dressing.	1a. Refrain from rotating staff.	1a. Minimizes confusion and disorientation.	*Goal met* By fourth week, client was able to follow instructions for dressing most of the time.
	1b. Always provide client's own clothes.	1b. Maintains client's identity and sense of dignity.	
	1c. Divide tasks into very small steps.	1c. Client can understand one simple comment at a time.	
	1d. Do not hurry client.	1d. Hurrying client can cause increased anxiety, agitation, and disorientation.	
	1e. Calmly give instructions: "Put one leg in trousers . . . now the next leg . . . "	1e. Support and encouragement help lower anxiety and maximize ability to follow instructions.	
2. Client will don own clothes with aid of Velcro tape.	2a. Have family replace buttons and zippers with Velcro tape.	2a. Easy to fasten shirts and pants.	*Goal met* Client was able to use Velcro much of the time to dress self, with the aid of close supervision.
	2b. Have client wear pants with elastic in waist.	2b. Lessens need for fastening.	
	2c. Work with client to use Velcro tape.	2c. Client responds to frequent orientation and step-by-step instruction.	
	2d. When client refuses or is too agitated to follow instructions, come back later.	2d. Client's moods often labile; forgets easily. Can be redirected later (15 to 20 minutes).	

NURSING DIAGNOSIS

Family grieving related to loss and deterioration of family member.

Supporting Data

- "I've lost my father."
- "I can't bear to part with him."
- "I feel like I've betrayed him."

Long Term Goal: All family members will state in three months' time that they feel more supported and able to talk about their grieving.

Short Term Goal	*Intervention*	*Rationale*	*Evaluation*
1. Family members will state that they have opportunity to express "unacceptable" feelings in supportive environment.	1a. Make arrangements for family to meet with counselor (e.g., nurse clinician, social worker, psychologist).	1a. Family in crisis: family needs to identify feelings and define some plan to regain sense of control and facilitate grief work.	*Goal met* By the third week, family started attending short term family counseling sessions.
	1b. Encourage spouse's input.	1b. Helps maintain spouse's involvement and may help reduce feelings of guilt.	

	1c. Encourage family members to stay with client and arrange outings (e.g., home visits for holidays, picnics, weekends, etc.).	1c. Increases client's personal identity and can aid family members in gradually "letting go."	
	1d. Encourage family members to express feelings; encourage ongoing sessions with counselor.	1d. Family members need to have a place where they can get support and understanding.	
2. Family will state that they have found support from others who have a family member with Alzheimer's disease.	2a. Offer family written names and phone numbers of available support groups in their vicinity.*	2a. The more supports a family has, the better they are able to cope with a complex and painful situation.	*Goal met* Mrs. Ludwik had attended two meetings of an Alzheimer's support group and found it enormously supportive. The daughter planned to attend the next meeting.
	2b. Follow up periodically.	2b. Continue to assess needs and encourage family members to obtain support.	

*A family caring for a client in the home would benefit from, along with the above, (1) companions, (2) other volunteers, (3) home health aids, (4) visiting nurse, (5) day care centers, (6) senior citizen groups, (7) respite care (8) financial and legal counseling. Caring for a cognitively impaired family member can quickly lead to physical and emotional exhaustion and throw the family into crisis.

Summary

Organic mental syndrome is the general term that refers to disturbances in orientation, memory, intellect, judgment, and affect due to changes in the brain, without regard to etiology. Of the six organic mental syndromes identified in the DSM III-R (APA 1987), delirium and dementia were discussed in this chapter, since they are most widely seen by health care workers.

Organic mental disorders are specific organic brain syndromes with specific etiology. Alcohol withdrawal delirium and Alzheimer's disease are two organic mental disorders that have been discussed in this chapter.

Delirium is marked by acute onset, a clouded state of consciousness, and symptoms of disorientation and confusion which fluctuate by the minute, hour, or time of day. Delirium is always secondary to an underlying condition; therefore, it is temporary, is transient, and may last from hours up to three to five days once the underlying cause is treated. If not treated, permanent damage to the neurons could result in dementia or death.

Nursing diagnoses for delirium were suggested. Nursing diagnoses included *potential for injury, fluid volume deficit, sleep pattern disturbance,* and *impaired verbal communication.* Goals for each of these nursing diagnoses were identified.

The clinical picture of *uncomplicated alcohol withdrawal* and *alcohol withdrawal delirium* was described, as well as specific medical and nursing interventions. The use of sedation (e.g., Librium, Valium, phenobarbital), thiamine (vitamin B_1), magnesium sulfate, and anticonvulsants was outlined.

Dementia usually has a more insidious onset. Global deterioration of cognitive functioning (e.g., memory, judgment, ability to think abstractly, orientation) is often progressive and irreversible, depending on the underlying cause. If dementia is primary (Alzheimer's disease, multi-infarct dementia, or Pick's disease), the course is irreversible. However, if the underlying cause is treatable, then the progression of the dementia at times may be halted or reversed.

Alzheimer's disease accounts for 65% of all dementias, and multi-infarct disease for about 10%; however, these percentages may change with the rising incidence of AIDS-related dementia (HIV encephalopathy).

There are various theories about the etiology of Alzheimer's disease, none of which is conclusive, although the genetic theory identifies familial tendencies. Signs and symptoms were noted during the progression of the disease through four phases: phase 1 (mild), phase 2 (moderate), phase 3 (moderate to severe), and phase 4 (late). The phenomena of confabulation, perseveration, aphasia, apraxia, agnosia, and hyperorality were explained.

People with Alzheimer's disease have many unmet needs and present many nursing problems. There is often a *potential for injury, impaired verbal communication, self-care deficit, disturbance in self-esteem, altered thought processes, ineffective individual coping,* and always *altered family processes.*

Goals for each of these nursing diagnoses were identified, and interventions for the client with Alzheimer's disease were presented, especially in the areas of (1) communication, (2) activities of daily living, (3) health teaching of families, and (4) therapeutic environment.

A case study of a cognitively impaired client was presented, and a nursing care plan was included. Self-study exercises at the end of this chapter will help you review the material presented throughout this chapter.

References

AARP. Coping & caring: Living with Alzheimer's disease. Washington DC: American Association of Retired Persons, 1986.

Adams M, Hanson R, Norkoal D, Beaulieu A, Bellville E, Morss K. Psychological responses in critical care units. American Journal of Nursing, 78:1504, 1978.

American Psychiatric Association. Diagnostic and statistical Manual of Mental Disorders, (DSM III-R), 3rd ed. revised. Washington DC: American Psychiatric Association, 1987.

Ansbaugh P. Emergency management of intoxicated patients with head injuries. Journal of Emergency Nursing, 3(3):9, 1977.

Burkhalter PK. Nursing care of the alcoholic and drug abuser. New York: McGraw-Hill Book Company, 1975.

Burnside IA. Alzheimer's disease: An overview. Journal of Gerontological Nursing, 5(4):14, 1979.

Burnside IM. Nursing and the Aged, 3rd ed. New York: McGraw-Hill Book Company, 1988.

Butz RH. Intoxication and withdrawal. *In* Estes NJ, Heinemann ME (eds). Alcoholism, 2nd ed. St. Louis, MO: C.V. Mosby Company, 1982.

Charles R, Truesdell M, Wood E. Alzheimer's disease: Pathology, progression and nursing process. Journal of Gerontological Nursing, 8(2):69, 1982.

Chenoweth B, Spencer B. Dementia: The experience of family caregivers. The Gerontologist, 26(3):267, 1986.

Clunn PA, Payne DB. Psychiatric Mental Health Nursing, 4th ed. New York: Medical Examination Publishing Company, 1986.

Cohen GD. The mental health professional and the Alzheimer patient. Hospital and Community Psychiatry, 35:115, 1984.

Cummings JL, Benson DF. Dementia: A Clinical Approach. Boston: Butterworths, 1983.

Davidhizar R, Gunden E, Wehlage D. Recognizing and caring for the delirious patient. Journal of Psychiatric Nursing, 16(5):38, 1978.

Davison GC, Neale JM. Abnormal psychology and experimental clinical approach, 3rd ed. New York: John Wiley & Sons, 1982.

Dwyer BJ. Cognitive impairment in the elderly: Delirium, depression or dementia? Focus on Geriatric Care and Rehabilitation, 1(4):1, 1987.

Ellison JM. DSM-III and the diagnosis of organic mental disorders. Annals of Emergency Medicine, 13(7):521, 1984.

Fisk A. Alzheimer's disease: A five article symposium (Introduction). Postgraduate Medicine, 73:204, 1983.

Foreman MD. Acute confusional states in hospitalized elderly: A research dilemma. Nursing Research, 35(1):34, 1986.

Frances RJ, Franklin JE. Alcohol and other psychoactive substance use disorders. *In* Talbott JA, Hales RE, Yudofsky SC (eds). Textbook of Psychiatry. Washington DC: American Psychiatric Press, 1988.

Gershon S, Herman S. The differential diagnosis of dementia. Journal of the American Geriatrics Society, 30(11):S58, 1982.

Gilmore GM. Behavioral management of the acutely intoxicated patient in the emergency department. Journal of Emergency Nursing, 12(1):13, 1986.

Gomez GE, Gomez EA. Delirium. Geriatric Nursing, 8(6):330, 1987.

Goodwin DW, Guze SB. Psychiatric diagnosis. New York: Oxford University Press, 1984.

Haber J, Hoskins P, Leach A, Sideleau B. Comprehensive Psychiatric Nursing, 3rd ed. New York: McGraw-Hill Book Company, 1983.

Heston L, White JA. Dementia: A practical guide to Alzheimer's disease and related illnesses. New York: W.H. Freeman & Company, 1983.

Kaplan HI, Sadock BJ. Synopsis of Psychiatry, 5th ed. Baltimore, MD: Williams & Wilkins, 1988.

Kelly FM. Caring for the patient in acute alcohol withdrawal. Critical Care Quarterly, 8(4):11, 1986.

Lipkowitz R. Research builds esteem: A model patient/family group program. Generations, 7(1):42, 1982.

Lipowski ZJ. Transient cognitive disorders (delirium, acute confusional states) in the elderly. American Journal of Psychiatry, 140:1426, 1983.

Lucas MJ, Steele C, Bognanni A. Recognition of psychiatric symptoms in dementia. Journal of Gerontological Nursing, 12(1):11, 1986.

Mace NL, Rabins PB. The 36 Hour Day. Baltimore, MD: Johns Hopkins University Press, 1981.

Mackey A. OBS and nursing care. Journal of Gerontological Nursing, 9(2):75, 1983.

Mass ML, Buckwalter KC. A special Alzheimer's unit: Phase I of baseline data. Applied Nursing Research, 1(1):41, 1988.

McArthur JC. Neurological manifestations of AIDS. Medicine, 66(6):407, 1987.

McHugh PR, Folstein MF. Organic mental disorders. *In* Michels R, Cavenar JO (eds). Psychiatry, Vol. 1. Philadelphia: J.B. Lippincott Company, 1987.

Nagley SJ. Predicting and preventing confusion in your patients. Journal of Gerontological Nursing, 12(3):27, 1986.

Ninos M, Makohon R. Functional assessment of the patient. Geriatric Nursing, 6:139, 1985.

Pajk M. Alzheimer's disease: Inpatient care. American Journal of Nursing, 84:215, 1984.

Perry SW, Markowitz J. Organic mental disorders. *In* Talbott JA, Hales RE, Yudofsky SC (eds). Textbook of Psychiatry. Washington DC: American Psychiatric Press, 1988.

Powell LS, Courtice K. Alzheimer's Disease: A Guide for Families. Reading, MA: Addison-Wesley Company, 1983.

Reisberg B. Stages of cognitive decline. American Journal of Nursing, 84:225, 1984.

Ricci M. All-out care for an Alzheimer patient. Geriatric Nursing, 4:369, 1983.

Schneider E, Emr M. Alzheimer's disease: Research highlights. Geriatric Nursing, 6:136, 1985.

Scott JP, Roberto KA, Hutton JT. Families of Alzheimer's victims: family support to the caregivers. Journal of American Geriatrics Society, 34:348, 1986.

Seltzer B, Frazier SH. Organic mental disorders. *In* Nicholi AA (ed). The Harvard Guide to Modern Psychiatry. Cambridge, MA: The Belknap Press of Harvard University, 1980.

Smith-DeJulio K. Care of the alcoholic patient during acute episodes. *In* Estes NJ, Heinemann ME (eds). Alcoholism, 2nd ed. St. Louis, MO: C.V. Mosby Company, 1982.

St. George-Hyslop PH, Tanzi RE, Polansky RJ, et al. The genetic defect causing familial Alzheimer's disease on chromosome 21. Science, 235:885, 1987.

Teusink JP, Mahler S. Helping families cope with Alzheimer's disease. Hospital and Community Psychiatry, 35:152, 1984.

Trockman G. Caring for the confused or delirious patient. American Journal of Nursing, 78:1495, 1978.

Tyler KL, Tyler HR. Differentiating organic dementia. Geriatrics, 39(3):38, 1984.

U.S. Department of Health and Human Services. Q & A: Alzheimer's Disease. Washington, DC, U.S. Department of Health and Human Services, 1985.

Wells CE. Chronic brain disease: An update on alcoholism, Parkinson's disease and dementia. Hospital and Community Psychiatry, 33:111, 1982.

Williams L. Alzheimer's: The need for caring. Journal of Gerontological Nursing, 12(2):21, 1986.

Wolanin MO, Halloway J. Relocation confusion: Intervention for prevention. Psychosocial Nursing Care of the Aged, 2nd ed. *In* Burnside IM (ed). Nursing and the Aged. New York: McGraw-Hill Book Company, 1980.

Wolanin MO, Fraelich-Philips LR. Confusion: Prevention and Cure. St. Louis, MO: CV Mosby Company, 1981.

Wurtman R. Alzheimer's disease. Scientific American, 252:62, 1985.

Zabourek RP. Identification of the alcoholic in the acute care setting. Critical Care Quarterly, 8(4): 1986.

Self-Study Exercises

Which of the following are organic mental syndromes (S) and which are organic mental disorders (D)?

1. ________ Dementia
2. ________ Intoxication
3. ________ Alcohol withdrawal delirium
4. ________ Withdrawal
5. ________ Pick's disease

Place DEL (delirium) or DEM (dementia), as appropriate, next to each of the following symptoms:

6. ________ Has acute onset.
7. ________ Eventually both short term and long term memory are affected.
8. ________ No or slow changes in EEG.
9. ________ Fluctuating levels of consciousness.
10. ________ Aphasia and Agnosia are commonly observed.
11. ________ Disorientation most severe at night; may be oriented during the day.
12. ________ Confabulation or perseveration commonly observed.
13. ________ Visual tactile hallucinations most common in this syndrome.

Match the following for use in treatment of alcohol withdrawal delirium:

14. ________ Can prevent Wernicke's encephalopathy	A. Magnesium sulfate
15. ________ Drug of choice for safe withdrawal from alcohol	
16. ________ Recommended if client has had seizures in the past and to speed the absorption of thiamine	B. Librium
	C. Haldol
17. ________ If a client is having seizures during withdrawal, this drug is effective and fast-acting	D. Paraldehyde
	E. Thiamine (vitamin B_1)
	F. Valium
	g. Dilantin

Match the terms in the right column with the definitions in the left column.

18. ________ The inability to name objects	A. Hypermetamorphosis
19. ________ Difficulty finding the right word—can deteriorate to become mute	
20. ________ Unable to perform once familiar and simple tasks	B. Perseveration
21. ________ The need to taste, chew, and put everything in one's mouth	C. Hyperorality

22. ________ Repeating the same word or behavior over and over again.

D. Apraxia

E. Mnemonic disturbance

F. Agnosia

G. Aphasia

H. Confabulation

Short Answer

Mark Peters, a Vietnam Veteran, has just been admitted and diagnosed with acute bacterial endocarditis. His temperature is 103°F, his skin turgor is poor, and his urine output is dark amber and scanty. He is agitated and screams in terror when he hears the bleeps from the ECG monitor. He thinks that he has been captured in Vietnam and that the bleeps are coming from a time bomb, and he is desperate to flee. He thinks it is 1971 and that you are the enemy.

23. Formulate two nursing diagnoses (ND) and identify at least one short term goal (STG) for each diagnosis.
    ND: ________
    related to ________
    as evidenced by ________
    STG: ________

    ND: ________
    related to ________
    as evidenced by ________
    STG: ________

24. Describe the deterioration of a client who is going through the four stages of Alzheimer's disease and identify essential features during each stage.

    A. Phase 1 (mild) ________

    B. Phase 2 (moderate) ________

    C. Phase 3 (moderate to severe) ________

    D. Phase 4 (late) ________

Mrs. Kendel is a 52-year-old woman who has progressive Alzheimer's disease. She lives with her husband, who has been trying to care for her in the home. Mrs. Kendel often wears evening gowns in the morning, puts her blouse on backward, and sometimes puts her bra on backward outside her blouse.

She often forgets where things are. She makes an effort to cook but often confuses frying pans and pots and sometimes has trouble turning on the stove.

Once in a while she can't find the bathroom in time, often mistaking it for a broom closet. She becomes very frightened of noises and is terrified when the telephone or doorbell rings.

At other times she cries because she is aware that she is losing her sense of her place in the world. She and her husband have always been close, loving companions, and he wants to keep her at home as long as possible.

25. Identify two nursing diagnoses (ND) for Mrs. Kendel as they relate to her being maintained at home.
    ND: ______________________________
    related to ______________________________
    as evidenced by ______________________________

    ND: ______________________________
    related to ______________________________
    as evidenced by ______________________________

26. Help Mr. Kendel by writing out a list of suggestions which he can try at home that might help facilitate (a) communication, (b) activities of daily living, (c) therapeutic environment.

27. Identify at least seven interventions appropriate to this situation for each of the areas.

28. Identify possible types of resources available for maintaining Mrs. Kendel in the home for as long as possible. Identify the name of one self-help group that you would urge Mr. Kendel to join.

PEOPLE WHO USE SELF-DESTRUCTIVE DEFENSES AGAINST ANXIETY

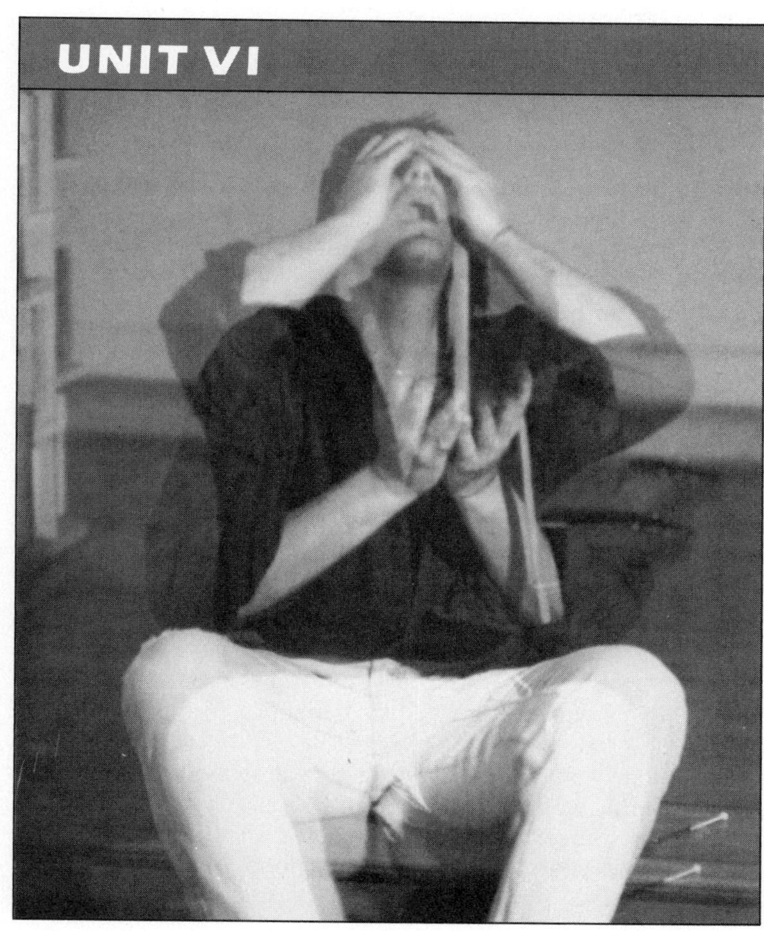

There is another way to go through life besides pulled through it kicking and screaming.

HUGH PRATHER

A Nurse Speaks

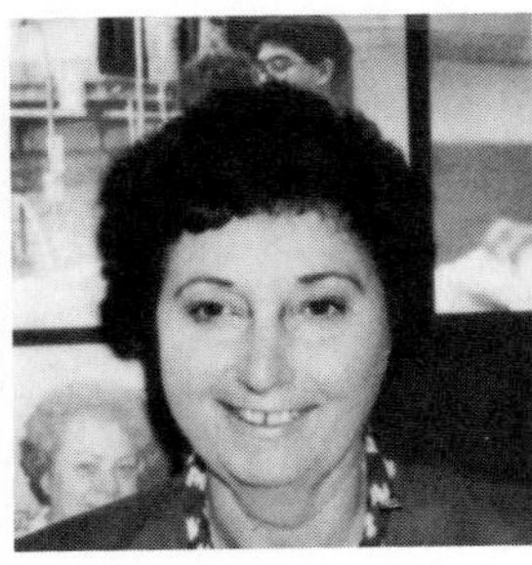

by Sara H. Withgott

I became involved in working with the chemically dependent as a graduate student. I needed some experience in group facilitating. One of my professors told me there was a new program starting in a local hospital that I should investigate, as there would be some groups that needed facilitators. I thought about whether or not I wanted to work with alcoholics and drug addicts. Ambivalence prevailed. I finally decided I could handle this experience one day a week for two semesters.

I was off and running very quickly. The next day I was in a planning meeting for aftercare with the agency staff. They were doubtful I could survive since I wasn't recovering. Ambivalence quickly faded into motivation. I *can do* this without being in recovery. I *will do* this without being in recovery.

The first two months were rough. I facilitated with a recovering person. That was a true educational experience. The program grew faster than was expected. By the fourth month I was facilitating a group of recovering clients alone.

The initial experiences are a blur but very soon I knew these clients were very special. I was only a facilitator; their recovery was their responsibility. This was the lesson that I had to learn. I could only facilitate their recovery. I must not ever think that I was the reason for their recovery.

As I look back I recall many people who came through my aftercare group. There was Willie. At times I still cry for Willie. After his wife died he was unable to gain access to their investments. Without money Willie was forced to give up his last two loves: Willie had to give up his beloved dogs. He could only afford to feed himself. After these losses Willie simply could not hold on to sobriety. He returned to the bars. His fate was death some six months later. I miss Willie's monthly phone calls very much.

Then there was Martha. Martha put her life back together after many suicide gestures. Martha was sure life did not hold much for her. Then she went through treatment and her tough-love husband went to Al-Anon. Martha has completed a BA in psychology with a 4.00 GPA since she began recovery. She has written and published three children's books. Last summer Martha produced a political play she wrote about her home town. It was a smashing success. It's not unusual to pick up the phone early on a Sunday morning and hear Martha saying, "Happy Sunday, isn't it great to be alive!"

Bryan came into aftercare hanging on to a thread of sobriety. After two rather severe slips/relapses he committed himself to sobriety. I knew Bryan would probably maintain his sobriety when he was able to grieve the death of his beloved father without drinking. I look forward to a Christmas card from Bryan every year. The card always has the family newsletter depicting Bryan's success at work and his celebration on his Alcoholics Anonymous sobriety birthdays.

It has been 15 years since I started facilitating the aftercare groups. I truly forgot to stop volunteering after I completed my master's degree. I am still volunteering for the same hospital. I have overcome the problem of not being a recovering person. Last year I joined the Behavioral Assistance Group

Board of Directors as secretary. I help other volunteers facilitate their groups now. Oh yes, and when one of the volunteers can't facilitate the group I jump at the opportunity to substitute. Participating in the recovery of another human being is most gratifying. I intend to volunteer for another 15 years if there is a need. Chemically dependent people are very special people!

CHAPTER 22

People Who Contemplate Suicide

Elizabeth M. Varcarolis

OUTLINE

KEY TERMS AND CONCEPTS

The key terms and concepts listed here also appear in bold where they are defined or discussed in this chapter.

SUICIDE
SUBINTENTIONED SUICIDE
SUICIDE ATTEMPT
COMPLETED SUICIDE
SUICIDAL IDEATION
SAD PERSONS SCALE
PRIMARY INTERVENTION
SECONDARY INTERVENTION
TERTIARY INTERVENTION
NO-SUICIDE CONTRACT

OBJECTIVES

After studying this chapter the student will be able to:

1. Describe the profile of suicide in the United States, including clues, professions at risk, most common psychopathology, population at risk, and when people may commit suicide.
2. Identify common precipitating events.
3. Act out two verbal and two nonverbal clues that might signal suicidal ideation.
4. Discuss three areas of assessment in determining lethality of plan according to Farberow.
5. Using the SAD PERSONS scale, list the ten risk factors to consider when assessing for suicide.
6. Describe three expected reactions a nurse may have when beginning work with suicidal clients.
7. Give examples of intervention: primary, secondary, and tertiary (postvention) intervention.
8. Give examples of psychotherapeutic interventions that a nurse may carry out (a) in the clinic, (b) in the hospital, and (c) on a telephone hotline.
9. Write two "no-suicide contracts."
10. Make up a care plan including two nursing diagnoses and four goals for a suicidal client.

Humans are the only creatures aware of their own mortality. They are able to contemplate the past as well as the future, to consider their personal end, and to be cognizant of their own death (Mowshowitz 1984).

Whether to live or die is a universal question that has been debated for centuries. Whether or not a person has the right to suicide is an intensely complex moral, ethical, religious, and legal issue.

People are granted the right to "life, liberty, and the pursuit of happiness." Health care professionals, however, are in frequent contact with people who are following more self-destructive pursuits. Schneidman (1963) has identified self-destructive behaviors as **subintentioned suicide.** Compulsive use of drugs and alcohol, hyperobesity, gambling, self-harmful sexual behaviors, and medical noncompliance are examples of covert, self-destructive behaviors, or subintentioned suicidal acts. By definition, in **subintentioned death,** a person takes part in hastening his or her own death. This participation with one's own death may be on a covert or unconscious level (Frederick 1980). These covert acts of self-destruction, however, are often easier for health care providers to deal with than the overt act of suicide.

Suicide is the ultimate act of self-destruction. In most cases of suicide, crisis precedes the attempt (Clayton 1985). Suicidal risk should always be assessed in any crisis situation. Suicidal thoughts, threats, or attempts are signals of a person or family in high anxiety. Sustained severe to panic levels of anxiety are seen in all crises.

The act of purposeful self-destruction by taking one's own life arouses intense and complex emotions in others. Suicide, which is the act of opting for nonexistence, is an option that some members of our society are adopting at increasing and alarming rates. Suicide is the tenth leading cause of death in the United States (Kaplan and Sadock 1988). This figure does not take into account the many suicides disguised as accidents. Suicide is the third leading cause of death after accidents and homicides among the 15 to 24-year-old group and is steadily increasing among our elderly population (Kaplan and Sadock 1988).

Not all suicides are committed by insane or severely disturbed individuals. Kavenaugh (1972) states that suicide can be a "tortuous ethical decision made by a moral and sane individual." Perhaps a third of those who have attempted suicide unsuccessfully are persons without known psychopathology (Kolb and Brodie 1982), although many of these deaths may have been precipitated by severe stressors including financial loss and illness. When psychopathology does exist, depression and alcoholism are most commonly seen. The 9- to 15-month period following recovery from a depressive episode is a high-risk period (Donlon and Rockwell 1982).

The "right to die" issue is presently controversial. The right to die dilemma is most debated in cases of terminal illness. Does someone with a terminal disease and who is in pain have a moral and ethical right to take his or her own life? Should life be sustained beyond a certain point? Is rational suicide in such cases legally and ethically sanctioned?

What about the right to suicide? The answer, if indeed there is an answer, lies between two extremes. Karl Menninger (1938), founder of the Menninger Clinic, states: "A man impelled to kill somebody must be prevented from doing so, if necessary by physical restraint. A man who is impelled to kill himself must similarly be restrained." However, Thomas Szaz (1963), an existential psychiatrist, thinks that adults have the right to suicide if they are not suffering from a major psychiatric illness. If this belief were adopted, questions would remain. At what age is someone considered an adult? What distinguishes a major from a minor psychiatric illness? A person's right to choose how and when he or she is to die remains in debate.

Transient thoughts of death and dying are a universal phenomenon. There is a time when most everyone will experience momentary self-destructive thoughts. Obsessive preoccupation with thoughts of suicide, however, is pathological (Kolb and Brodie 1982).

The Center for Study of Suicide Prevention of the United States Public Health Service has classified suicidal behavior into three categories, according to intent. The first category of suicidal behaviors is *completed suicide*, the second is *suicide attempt*, and the third is *suicidal ideation* (Beck, et al. 1973).

1. **Completed Suicide** includes all willful, self-inflicted, life-threatening acts leading to death.
2. **Suicide Attempt** includes all willful, self-inflicted life-threatening attempts which have not led to death. Attempted suicide is most often associated with hysteria, antisocial personality, thought disorders, and various paraphilias (Kaplan and Sadock 1985).
3. **Suicidal Ideation** means that the person is thinking about harming himself or herself.

The following summary of statistical findings provides a profile of suicide in America:

1. Most people who go on to commit suicide give out clues and warnings and often seek help. It has been estimated that about 75% of all suicide victims seek help within the four months before they take their lives.
2. Of those who commit suicide, 65 to 70% have made previous attempts. A person who has attempted suicide in the past is at great risk for successful suicide. The risk is highest in the first two years after a suicide attempt, *especially in the first three months*.
3. The incidence of suicide is higher in urban areas than in rural areas. It is also higher for those who are socially mobile or who are migrants. The suicide rate for white Americans is higher than for non-whites (except young black males). Surprisingly, suicide is more common among the affluent rather than among the poor.
4. There seems to be some correlation between certain groups of people and the suicide rate. For example, the suicide rate seems to be higher in students, young black males, gifted individuals, immigrants, and Indian-Eskimos.
5. The incidence of suicide also seems to be higher in some occupations. Doctors, dentists, lawyers, police, and air-traffic controllers have higher suicide rates than does the general population. People who are physically ill are also at higher risk than the general population. The suicide rate is higher for single people than for married persons and is higher for divorced males than for divorced females. See Table 22–1 for myths and facts related to suicide.
6. A significantly greater number of suicidal attempters than nonsuicidal attempters stated they were inactive in religious activities, according to one study.

Monday is the most frequent day for suicide, morning the most frequent time, and April the most frequent month.

People who have problems with impulse control (drugs/alcohol, violence), are depressed, are psychotic, or have a family member who committed suicide are at greater risk than the general public. Up to 75% of clinically depressed people have suicidal ideation or intent (Donlon and Rockwell 1982; Harvard Medical School 1986; Kolb and Brodie 1982; Mullis and Byers 1988; Simmons 1981).

Figure 22–1 conceptualizes the process of suicide as a self-destructive problem-solving behavior.

Standard I: Theory

Since the subject of suicide arouses strong feelings and reactions in all persons, it is wise to examine personal thoughts and ethical beliefs regarding another person's attempt at suicide.

Theoretical considerations and research findings can clarify or modify one's understanding of the phenomena surrounding overt self-destructive behavior. Three areas provide a framework for nurses' work with suicidal persons. They are (1) precipitating events, (2) motivating forces, and (3) theories.

Table 22-1 • MYTHS AND FACTS REGARDING SUICIDE

MYTH	FACT
1. Only people who are mentally ill commit suicide.	1. Suicide can be a decision made by a moral and sane individual.
2. Suicidal persons are fully intent on dying.	2. Most persons who contemplate suicide are highly ambivalent about dying.
3. If a nurse suspects that a person is thinking about suicide, the nurse should not bring up the subject lest the person kill himself.	3. Open dialogue is most often a relief for the suicidal person. Talking can decrease the risk of suicide.
4. Suicide is an impulsive act.	4. The act may be impulsive, but most often suicide has been carefully thought out.
5. The chance of suicide lessens as depression lessens.	5. When depression is lifting, there is more energy to carry out a previously pondered suicide plan.
6. Suicide can be an inherited trait.	6. Alcoholism and depression most likely are genetic, and having a relative who has committed suicide is a risk factor; however, there are no genetic markers for suicide.
7. Most suicidal persons give no warning.	7. About 75% of people who attempt or commit suicide give definite clues to intent.
8. All non-whites have a lower suicide rate than whites.	8. This is true with the exception of young black males.
9. Professionals such as lawyers, doctors, dentists, police, and air-traffic controllers have a low suicide rate.	9. All have higher suicide rates than people in the general population.
10. People who are psychotic have the greatest chance of killing themselves among those with definite psychopathology.	10. People with depression and alcoholism are at greatest risks for suicide among people with psychopathology.
11. Only people with grave problems, mental illness, or physical illness think about suicide.	11. At one time or another, almost everyone contemplates suicide.
12. People who just want attention use suicidal threats as manipulation.	12. Even if a suicide threat is manipulative, the person may actually go on to commit suicide. ALL *threats should be taken seriously*.
13. People who are sociopathic, hysterical, or who commit various paraphilias never attempt suicide.	13. Persons suffering from depression or alcoholism are at highest risk for contemplating suicide; however, sociopaths, hysterics, and paraphiliacs most often actually *attempt* suicide.
14. People who go from "rags to riches" are better protected against suicide than those who go from fortune to poverty.	14. Persons with sudden change in fortune (success, riches, acclaim) are also at risk for suicide.

Data from Donlon and Rockwell 1982; Harvard 1986; Kaplan and Sadock 1985; Simmons 1981.

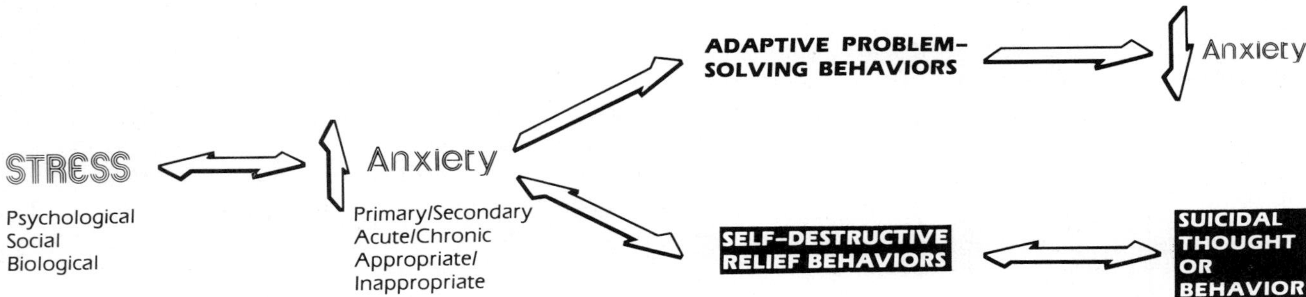

Figure 22-1. *Conceptualization of the process of suicidal thoughts or behaviors.*

PRECIPITATING EVENTS

The act of suicide may be precipitated by a variety of internal and external events. Adam (1985) summarized various events from studies in the literature and found that social isolation, severe life events, and sensitivity to loss often precede a suicide attempt.

SOCIAL ISOLATION. Suicidal individuals frequently have difficulty forming and maintaining relationships. Usually there is a high rate of divorce, separation, or single marital status. Norman Cousins maintains that all human history is an endeavor to shatter loneliness. He tells the story of a woman who had recently committed suicide. She had written in her diary every day during the week before her death, "Nobody called today, nobody called today, nobody called today" (Mowshowitz 1984).

SEVERE LIFE EVENTS. Severe life events often precede a suicide attempt. Paykel (1975) found that people who attempted suicide were four times as likely to suffer severe life events (e.g., divorce, death, sickness) in the six months prior to their attempts than were people in the general population. Serious arguments with a spouse, a new person in the home, and having to appear in court were more frequent occurrences in the lives of persons who attempted suicide than of nonsuicidal persons. A recent study by Parker (1988) found that among adolescents attempting suicide (1) they experienced more life changes than other adolescents, and (2) a history of emotional illness in the family was the most significant variable.

Stress results not only from tragic or disturbing life events, but also from desired events (refer to Chapter 8). A dramatic change in fortune or status can precipitate suicidal depression. Freddie Prinze, a brilliant young actor, committed suicide at the height of his career. He had recently signed a million dollar a year contract and was the toast of the entire TV industry (Mowshowitz 1984). Ross Lockridge, author of *Raintree County*, and Thomas Heggen, creator of *Mister Roberts*, were both catapulted into sudden fame and wealth. Both committed suicide, unable to live with the contradictions of success and fortune (Leggett 1974).

SENSITIVITY TO LOSS. People who are sensitive to losses may react tragically to separation or loss of a loved one. People who commit suicide after such a loss usually have had insecure or unreliable childhood experiences. Repeated studies demonstrate a significantly higher incidence of broken homes in the childhood of people who commit suicide than in the general population. People from broken homes may be more susceptible to loss of a significant relationship than someone whose background includes more stable or loving relationships.

MOTIVATING FORCES

The suicidal person may be stimulated by a variety of motivating forces. The suicide attempt may reflect a desire for reincarnation, a wish-fulfilling fantasy of reunion, or efforts to force love from others. Or, a suicide attempt may be an effort to get away from psychological pain, an effort to atone for past sins, or an attempt to escape from severe physical pain or deformity. Another motive could be the wish to instill guilt in a significant person who is perceived as abandoning or rejecting the suicidal person. In this case suicide can be seen as a means of control and revenge (Kolb and Brodie 1982). *All suicidal thoughts and ideas, no matter what the motivation or intent, should be taken seriously.*

THEORIES

A great deal of information has been gathered on suicide from clinical observations, studies, and research. However, no single theory can account for all the data available. Two theoretical models that have influenced suicidologists most are the (1) psychodynamic theories and (2) sociological theories. A more recent area of study is (3) biochemical genetic theories.

PSYCHODYNAMIC THEORIES. Psychodynamic explanations of suicide focus on the role of aggression and the internalizing of hostile or disappointing relationships. Freud described suicide as a murderous attack on an ambivalently loved, internalized significant person. In other words, there would not be a suicide without the repressed desire to kill someone else. This is sometimes referred to as "murder in the 180th degree." Others describe suicide as a wish to be at peace with the internalized significant person.

Other themes besides punishment of inner "objects" and the wish to be reunited with a deceased loved object are the wish for revenge and the wish to get rid of a hated part of the self. Suicide is either a phenomenon of disturbed internalizations of hostile or ambivalent significant persons or an effort to cope with the absence of comforting and deeply loved significant others (Malzberger and Buie 1980). Whatever the introjected or internalized object signifies, *suicide is an attempt to escape from an intolerable situation or intolerable state of mind* (Adam 1985).

SOCIOLOGICAL THEORIES. Suicidal crisis involves the unique characteristic of rejecting society, as well as rejection of the self (Farberow 1967). The threat of death carries enormous impact for all concerned. No other kind of death leaves family and friends with such long-lasting feelings of shame, guilt, puzzlement, and distress (Davison and Neale 1982; Van Dongen 1988).

Sociological theory refers to the social and cultural context in which a person lives. "Suicide or dying behaviors do not exist in a vacuum, but are an integral part of the life style of the individual" (Schneidman 1963). Circumstances in a person's cultural and social environment may correlate with a person's opting for death over life. Durkheim is the pioneer of sociological research in the study of suicide. The principal types of suicide found in his studies are the (1) egotistic suicide, (2) anomic suicide, and (3) altruistic suicide (Davison and Neale 1982).

1. *Egotistic suicide* occurs when a person is insufficiently integrated into society.
2. *Anomic suicide* occurs when a person is isolated from others through abrupt changes in social status or social norms.
3. *Altruistic suicide* occurs as a response to societal demands. The deaths of buddhist monks and of nuns who set themselves on fire to protest the Vietnam War are examples of altruistic suicide.

One extension of Durkheim's theory proposes that the more integrated individuals are in a given society, the lower the risk of suicide. For example, the more meaningful the occupational roles and the higher the status of integration, the lower the risk of suicide (Adam, 1985; Gibbs and Martin 1964). Others have established that suicide can be related to sudden change in status more than just to social status alone (Breed 1963; Mowshowitz 1984).

BIOCHEMICAL/GENETIC THEORIES. It is difficult to distinguish biochemical or genetic predispositions to suicide from predispositions to depression or alcoholism. Both of these disorders do run in families and most likely have a genetic component (Harvard Medical School 1986). However, it is thought that low levels of the neurotransmitter serotonin may play a part in whether someone commits suicide. Low serotonin levels are related to depressed moods. In a study of people hospitalized for suicide attempts, those with low serotonin levels were more likely to commit suicide than those with normal serotonin levels (Harvard Medical School 1986).

Also, low blood platelet levels of monoamine oxidase (MAO) have been found in persons with a higher familial incidence of suicide than in people with normal levels (Kaplan and Sadock 1988). Monoamine oxidase inhibitors (MAOI) are commonly given for the treatment of depression (see Chapter 18).

No theory completely explains why a person will choose to end his or her life. However, a framework for nursing assessment and intervention can borrow from all three theoretical models.

Standard II: Data Collection

Nurses in all areas of work are in contact with people who have a high potential for suicidal behaviors. Patients on the general medical-surgical units are often suffering losses in health or losses of function. Many people are hospitalized for alcohol-related medical problems or have alcoholism as a secondary diagnosis. Both depressed people and those with alcohol problems have a much higher rate of suicide than the general population. These two groups comprise about 50% of all completed suicides (Kaplan and Sadock 1985).

On maternity wards, women are often undergoing situational crises. These crises may be related to an unwanted newborn or loss of a newborn. On obstetrical units, removal of a breast or uterus can be experienced as traumatic mutilation, resulting in alteration in self-concept and personal identity. In specialized units, such as burn units and intensive care units, nurses are continually dealing with people in physical and emotional crises. Appropriate interventions through referral for a psychiatric consultation or for counseling can prevent a suicide attempt or the actual act of suicide (Kolb and Brodie 1982).

Three areas of assessment will be discussed: (1) assessing the verbal and nonverbal suicidal clues, (2) assessing the lethality of the suicide plan, and (3) assessing high-risk factors.

ASSESSING VERBAL AND NONVERBAL CLUES

Almost all people considering suicide will send out clues, especially to people they think of as supportive. Nurses often fit this category. Clues may be verbal, behavioral, somatic, or psychodynamic (Reubin 1979).

Verbal Clues	Examples
Overt Statements	"I can't take it anymore."
	"Life isn't worth living anymore."
	"I wish I were dead."
	"Everyone would be better off if I died."
Covert Statements	"It's OK now, soon everything will be fine."
	"Things will never work out."
	"I won't be a problem much longer."
	"Nothing feels good to me anymore, and probably never will."
	"How can I give my body to medical science?"

The nurse should always make overt what is covert. Most often it is a relief for a person contemplating suicide to finally talk to someone about his or her despair and loneliness. Asking someone if he or she is thinking of suicide does **not** "give a person ideas." Self-destructive ideas are a personal decision. Making covert indications of suicide overt **does** make possible a decrease in isolation and can increase problem-solving alternatives for living. Pallikkathayil and McBride (1986) found that suicide attempters were extremely receptive to talking about their suicide crisis, even those that regretted the failure of their attempt. Often these people expressed gratitude for the opportunity to talk to someone. Specific questions to ask include the following (Stevenson et al. 1988):

Are you experiencing thoughts of suicide?
Have you ever had thoughts of suicide in the past?
Have you ever attempted suicide?
Do you have a plan for committing suicide?
If so, what is your plan for suicide?

The following dialogue illustrates how the nurse can make covert messages overt.

NURSE:	You haven't eaten or slept well for the past few days, Mary.
MARY:	No . . . I feel pretty low lately.
NURSE:	How low are you feeling?
MARY:	Oh . . . I don't know . . . nothing seems to matter to me anymore . . . it's all so meaningless . . .
NURSE:	What is meaningless, Mary?
MARY:	Life . . . the whole thing . . . nothingness . . . life is a bad joke.
NURSE:	Are you saying that you don't think life is worth living?
MARY:	Well . . . yes . . . it's all so hopeless anyway . . .
NURSE:	Are you thinking of killing yourself, Mary?
MARY:	Yes . . . sometimes I think about it . . . I probably would never go through with it.
NURSE:	I am concerned about these thoughts. I need to share them with other members of the staff. For now, let's talk more about what you are thinking and feeling.

Be alert for behavioral clues, somatic clues, and emotional clues.

1. **Behavioral Clues** Sudden behavioral changes, especially when depression is lifting and when the person has more energy available to carry out a plan.	1. **Examples** • Giving away prized personal possessions. • Writing farewell notes. • Making out a will. • Putting personal affairs in order.
2. **Somatic Clues** Physiological complaints can mask psychological pain and internalized stress.	2. **Examples** Symptoms associated with chronic stress include headaches, muscle aches, trouble sleeping, irregular bowel habits, unusual appetite, or weight loss.
3. **Emotional Clues** Various emotions can signal possible suicidal ideation.	3. **Examples** Social withdrawal, feelings of hopelessness and helplessness, confusion, irritability, and complaints of exhaustion are some examples.

ASSESSING LETHALITY OF SUICIDE PLAN

The evaluation of a suicide plan is extremely important in determining the degree of suicidal risk. There are three main elements to be considered when evaluating the lethality of a suicide plan: (1) specificity of details, (2) lethality of proposed method, and (3) availability of means (Farberow 1967). If a person has definite plans as to the time, place, and the means, he or she is at high risk. Someone who is thinking of suicide but has not thought about how, where, or when is at a lower risk.

The lethality of method also indicates the level of risk—e.g., how quickly the person would die by that method, lessening the probability of intervention. *High-risk* methods include using a gun, jumping, hanging, carbon monoxide poisoning, and staging a car crash. Examples of *lower-risk* methods are slashing wrists, inhaling house gas, and ingesting pills. When the *means* are available, the situation is more serious. For example a person who states he will jump from, and has access to, a high building, or that he will shoot himself and has a gun, is a serious risk. When people are psychotic, they are at high risk regardless of the specificity of details, lethality of method, and availability of means, since impulse control, judgment, and thinking are all grossly impaired.

ASSESSING HIGH-RISK FACTORS

A variety of tools can be used to aid a health care worker in assessing suicidal potential. Patterson and coworkers (1983) have devised an assessment aid using a brief acronym (SAD PERSONS) to evaluate ten major risk factors in suicide potential (Box 22–1). The SAD PERSONS assessment is a simple, clear-cut, and practical guide to gauging suicide potential. Ten categories are

Box 22-1. SAD PERSONS ASSESSMENT

S Sex	Men kill themselves three times more than women, although women make attempts three times more than men.
A Age	High-risk group: 19 years or younger 45 years or older
D Depression	Studies report that 35 to 79% of those who attempt suicide manifested a depressive syndrome.
P Previous Attempts	Of those who commit suicide, 65 to 70% have made previous attempts.
E ETOH (Ethanol)	ETOH (alcohol) is associated with up to 65% of successful suicides. Estimates are that 15% of alcoholics commit suicide. Heavy drug use is considered in this group and given the same weight as alcohol.
R Rational Thinking Loss	People with psychoses (functional or organic) are more apt to commit suicide than those in the general population.
S Social Supports Lacking	A suicidal person often lacks significant others (friends, relatives), meaningful employment, and religious supports. All three of these areas need to be part of the assessment.
O Organized Plan	The presence of a specific plan (date, place, means) signifies a person at high risk.
N No Spouse	Repeated studies indicate that those persons who are widowed, separated, divorced, or single are at greater risk than those who are married.
S Sickness	Chronic, debilitating, and severe illness is thought to be a factor when assessing for suicide potential.

Patterson W. et al. Sad Persons Scale, Psychosomatics, 24:343, 1983.

Other data from Adam 1985; Hart and Keidel 1979; Patterson et al. 1983; Reubin 1979; Simmons 1981; Stevenson 1988.

described in the assessment tool. The person being evaluated is assigned one point for each applicable category. The person's total points are compared with a scale, which assists health care workers in determining whether hospital admission is necessary. The decision to admit someone to a hospital unit depends upon a number of variables, such as whether the person lives alone, whether the person has access to a high-risk weapon, and whether the person has attempted suicide previously. The following scale serves as a general guideline:

Points	Guidelines for Intervention
0-2	Home with follow-up care
3-4	Close follow-up and possible hospitalization
5-6	Strongly consider hospitalization
7-10	Hospitalize

Standard III: Diagnosis

The nursing diagnoses for a person who is suicidal may address a number of areas. However, the nursing diagnosis with the highest priority is *potential for self-directed violence.*

Potential for self-directed violence may be evidenced by a variety of emotional states. Feelings of hopelessness, anger, poor impulse control, frustration, abandonment, and rejection are common among people who are suicidal. Suicide is often related to a loss. The loss of a significant person can leave a person feeling isolated, panicky, and confused. Loss of job, status, money, and sickness can be overwhelming. Potential for self-directed violence can also be related to crises in adolescents, adults, and the elderly. Identity crisis in the adolescent and isolation and loss of spouse in the elderly are situations signaling individuals in trouble.

Ineffective individual coping is also usually present. For example, a person who is clinically depressed, relies heavily on drugs and alcohol, is facing a variety of situational or maturational crises, or has chronic mental or physical problems may have impaired problem-solving and coping skills. Therefore, ineffective individual coping may be evidenced by inability to meet role expectations or to meet basic needs related to heavy use of alcohol/drugs, inadequate psychological resources, or unsatisfactory support systems.

Ineffective family coping is often present. A child or teenager may be unable to get the guidance, support, and love he needs from home. Withdrawal of support from other family members can leave a child feeling abandoned, overwhelmed, and confused. This withdrawal of love and support may be related to the parent's own problems with alcohol/drugs, mental disorders, or perceived desertion through divorce or separation. When there are intense feelings of hostility and intolerance between parents, children often get left out or are manipulated and pitted against either or both parents. Therefore, examples of ineffective family coping may be evidenced by behavior problems in children, break-up of the family unit, chaotic family communication, or highly ambivalent family relationships.

Suicide is an attempt to alter an intolerable life situation or state of mind which people feel helpless or powerless to change. Therefore, feelings of *hopelessness* and *powerlessness* are feelings often described by people who contemplate suicide.

Hopelessness, the belief that nothing can help change an intolerable situation or experience plays a major role in most suicides. Hopelessness can be related to a multitude of physical conditions (e.g., AIDS, cancer) and situations (e.g., financial, alterations in significant relationships). Hopelessness is evidenced by verbal statements, cognitive difficulties (decreased judgment, decreased problem solving), and more.

Powerlessness (thinking one has no control over events) may be related to a lifestyle of helplessness or a current situation that the person perceives as untenable and unalterable. An interpersonal interaction may also be perceived to be unalterably painful or psychologically traumatic. The person may be left feeling powerless or isolated.

People who think of ending their lives often do not feel very good about themselves. Feelings of worthlessness and expressions of shame or guilt are common among some. Therefore *disturbance in self-esteem* or *chronic low self-esteem* need serious consideration.

Standard IV: Planning

Planning nursing care for a person who is suicidal involves planning on the (1) content level—planning goals—and (2) process level—awareness of personal reactions to suicide and the person who is suicidal.

CONTENT LEVEL—PLANNING GOALS

Long term and short term goals are set for each nursing diagnosis identified. The nurse works with the client to set goals that are consistent with the suicidal person's perceptions and ability to carry out the goals. If a person is thought to be actively suicidal, hospitalization may be appropriate. For the nursing diagnosis *potential for self-directed violence*, the following goals may apply:

Long Term Goals

- Client will state by (state the date) that he wants to live.
- By (state the date) client will name two people he can call if he starts to think of suicide.
- Client will name one acceptable alternative to his situation by (state the date).

Short Term Goals

- Client will remain safe while in the hospital.
- Client will talk about painful feelings (guilt, anger, loneliness) by (state the date).
- Client will make a *no-suicide contract* with the nurse covering the next 24 hours.

When people are depressed or suicidal, they are often unable to see choices or make decisions that could change their situation. This is referred to as "tunnel vision." Clarifying hazards for the client and facilitating the expression of negative feelings are basic interventions. When the client is able to explore alternatives to his or her situation, change in thinking and behavior is possible. When alternatives to suicide are acceptable, feelings of hopelessness diminish. Therefore, goals for *ineffective individual coping* evidenced by faulty problem solving could include the following:

Long Term Goals

- By (state the date) client will name signs and symptoms which indicate that he is starting to feel overwhelmed.
- By (state the date) client will name two persons that

he can talk to if he has suicidal thoughts in the future.
- By (state the date) client will state that he has used two new coping mechanisms successfully in a stressful situation.
- By (state the date) client will state one decision he has made that will improve his situation.

Short Term Goals

- Client will discuss with nurse situations that trigger suicidal thoughts and two feelings surrounding these situations by (state the date).
- Client will identify three past coping mechanisms and state which were useful and which were not useful by (state the date).
- Client will name two effective ways to handle difficult situations in the future by (state the date).
- Client will state that he feels comfortable with one new technique after three sessions of role-playing.

Often a suicidal person is living within a family unit—that is, spouse, children, parent(s), or other significant others. The hopelessness, and desperation, irritability, and withdrawal of the suicidal person profoundly affects other members of the family. Feelings of anxiety, denial, guilt, anger, frustration, and hopelessness arise in those close to a suicidal person. In many cases, the suicidal behavior is a reaction to dysfunctional family behavior. If the motive is to instill guilt in a significant person(s) as a means to control and extract revenge, the whole family unit would be in crisis. Therefore, the whole family needs support and counseling. For a diagnosis of *ineffective family coping* related to ineffective patterns of communication, the following goals could be included:

Long Term Goals

- Each family member will state that he or she feels less guilty, angry, or manipulated now, (using a scale from 1 to 10) than before working with the nurse.
- Each family member will state that he or she feels better able to communicate with the suicidal member by (state the date).
- Each family member will state that he or she feels supported (by nurse, counselor, therapist) and less confused and angry.
- By (state the date) each family member will state that the communication among all members of the family has improved.

Short Term Goals

- Each family member will state two feelings toward the suicidal member by (state the date).
- Each family member will state what he or she thinks the problem is by (state the date).
- Each family member will state three referral sources available for individual or family counseling, support, and guidance during the crises.

Although the motives for suicide may vary and the number of precipitating events may be infinite, all persons with suicidal ideation suffer similar feelings. Intense feelings of deprivation of affection, lack of hope for the future, and profound feelings of worthlessness and low self-esteem are common. The diagnosis of *disturbance in self-esteem* or *chronic low self-esteem* related to feelings of worthlessness may have the following associated goals:

Long Term Goals

- Client will name three things that he likes about himself by (state the date).
- Client will participate in two activities that he enjoys and does well by (state the date).
- Client will state that he feels more comfortable around people by (state the date).
- Client will name one project he has completed and feels proud of by (state the date).
- Client will state that he feels better about himself by (state the date).

Short Term Goals

- Client will state that he will continue meeting with the nurse on a regular basis.
- Client will make eye contact with the nurse 50% of the time that they are together.
- Client will talk about painful feelings with the nurse by (state the date).
- Client will begin to look at personal strengths as well as weaknesses by (state the date).
- Client will participate in his treatment plan by (state the date).

PROCESS LEVEL—NURSES' REACTIONS AND FEELINGS

People who are suicidal present affects and behavior that are difficult for nurses to deal with effectively. All health care professionals who work with people who are suicidal need supervision and guidance by a more experienced health care professional. Most people who are suicidal experience extreme hopelessness and helplessness; are withdrawn, keenly sensitive to rejection, and ambivalent; and may be hostile and angry. Affects such as these can stir up strong negative reactions in others. Birtchnell (1983) has identified in the literature a number of reactions that often arise in health care workers when working with a client who is suicidal. If these and other intense emotional responses are not made known and discussed in supervision, effective intervention will be limited, especially if these feelings are picked up by the suicidal client.

When these feelings are *not* identified, discussed, and worked out, the least that will happen is that the nurse will feel incompetent, experience low self-esteem, and become angry at the client for arousing these feelings. The worst that could happen is escalation or perpetuation of the client's painful feelings. The client may interpret the nurse's anxiety, irritation, and avoidance as validation for his own feelings of poor self-regard and self-hate. When feelings of hopelessness and poor self-esteem escalate, so does the potential for suicide.

The universal reactions of (1) anxiety, (2) irritation, (3) avoidance, and (4) denial by any health care worker caring for a suicidal person are discussed subsequently.

ANXIETY. Anxiety may have a number of sources. However, it is important to recognize that two common sources of anxiety are activated when working with a suicidal client. *First*, Birtchnell (1983) states that there are suicidal inclinations in all of us. A suicidal patient has the capacity to arouse these latent emotions and perhaps bring them out more strongly. *Second*, suicidal behavior or ideations on the part of the client may be interpreted by concerned health care personnel as personal rejection. Both sources of anxiety are usually working at an unconscious level. It is crucial that nurses become aware of their anxiety and attempt to identify the source, or unmet need or expectation. Personal anxiety can then be reduced and not transferred to the client.

IRRITATION. Often people who make repeated suicide attempts are accused by family as well as health care workers of just "trying to get attention" or "looking for sympathy." It is not uncommon to hear of friends of family members saying to a suicidal person out of frustration to "go ahead and get it over with." Such remarks by family and health providers strip the suicidal person of all hope and act as an encouragement for the suicidal person to kill himself or herself (Andriola 1973). No matter how trivial the suicidal attempt may appear; it is a genuine communication that the person is despairing and is unable to find a way out of a desperate situation or state of mind.

AVOIDANCE. People who are suicidal and people who are psychotic are frequently kept at a distance and "handled with kid gloves" by both medical and nursing personnel (Birtchnell 1983). Nurses and physicians may get caught up into taking responsibility for the actions of the suicidal person (rescue fantasy). Then, when things do not go the way the nurse or physician would like them to go, helplessness sets in. Staff then avoid situations or people that stimulate feelings of helplessness and incompetence. When the need to feel in control and responsible for other people's decisions is lessened through experience and supervision, the nurse is better able to refocus energies back to the client.

DENIAL. Denial of or minimizing suicidal ideation or gestures is a defense against experiencing the feelings aroused by a suicidal person. Denial can be seen in statements such as, "I can't understand why anyone would want to take his own life." Often family members and health care professionals are unable to acknowledge suicidal tendencies in someone close to them. Denial also operates in us when identification with a suicidal person is strong such as when a colleague commits suicide or a respected figurehead gives off covert suicidal messages.

PERSONAL STAGES HEALTH CARE WORKERS PASS THROUGH. Hammel-Bissell (1985) documents the "rites of passage" that psychiatric nurses must go through in order to work effectively with a suicidal person. Four stages are presented. Each stage progresses to the next as the nurse works through expected feelings and reactions.

- The first stage is *naiveté*, in which feelings of shock and denial are prominent.
- The second stage is termed *recognition*. This stage involves feelings of anxiety, fear, helplessness, and confusion.
- The third stage, *stage of responsibility*, brings with it a cycle of feeling responsible, guilty, and then angry. This is a very conflictual time for people working with suicidal persons. It is crucial that during this time the nurse is helped through supervision and peer support. The nurse needs to vent these feelings and benefit from the experience of others who have gone beyond this stage. Otherwise, nurses may suffer burnout, may distance themselves from colleagues and clients, or may leave the work situation altogether.
- The fourth and final stage, the *stage of individual choice*, comes through awareness gained through supervision, continuing education, and/or personal therapy. This is the stage when the nurse comes to the realization that the client is the only one in charge of his life. This frees the nurse to do whatever is humanly possible to help the client, while realizing that one person cannot ultimately control the decisions of another.

Standard V: Intervention

Suicide intervention can be divided into three distinct areas. Primary intervention, secondary intervention, and tertiary intervention.

Primary intervention includes those activities that provide support, information, and education in situations which could otherwise become more serious and even lethal. Primary intervention can be practiced in schools, home, hospitals, and industrial settings.

Secondary intervention is treatment of the actual suicidal crisis. Secondary intervention is practiced in clinics, hospitals, and on telephone hotlines. Most people who are suicidal do *not* necessarily want to die; they just *don't know how to go on living in an intolerable situation* or state of mind. Ambivalence is one of the most important tools a nurse has when working with a suicidal person.

Tertiary intervention (postvention) can refer to (1) interventions with family and friends of a person who has committed suicide or (2) interventions with a person who has recently attempted suicide. Tertiary intervention for the latter is geared toward minimizing the traumatic aftereffects of the suicide attempt.

V-A: PSYCHOTHERAPEUTIC INTERVENTIONS

Psychotherapeutic skills used by the nurse working with a client who is suicidal are practiced primarily (1) in clinics, (2) in hospitals, and (3) on telephone hotlines. The key element is the establishment of a workable relationship. There is general agreement by workers in this field on the importance of warmth, sensitivity, interest, concern, and consistency on the part of the helping person. Studies indicate that any treatment modality can be effective as long as it (1) includes the establishment of a personal relationship with the suicidal person, (2) encourages more realistic problem-solving behavior, and (3) reaffirms hope (Evans 1983).

There is no place for hostility, sarcasm, or power struggles in the work with a suicidal person. These responses will only enhance poor self-esteem and feelings of hopelessness. Efforts should be geared toward maintaining or raising the suicidal person's self-esteem and self-respect. Cassem (1980) states that "self-esteem or self-respect is the most basic psychic condition to be guarded if life is to continue."

In the Clinic

Usually, people in suicidal crisis are seen in emergency rooms and referred to an outpatient clinic. Indeed, if after initial assessment, the person is felt to be at low risk and not in need of hospitalization, referral to a clinic for crisis counseling is always indicated. Hoff (1984) names six techniques which are useful in an outpatient setting:

Technique	Action
1. **Relieve Isolation**	1. Arrange for person to stay with family or friends. If no one is available and the person is highly suicidal, hospitalization must be considered.
2. **Remove All Weapons**	2. Weapons and pills are removed by friends, relatives, or nurse.
3. **Encourage Alternative Expression of Anger**	3. Have person talk freely about feelings, unmet expectations, and disappointments. Plan with person alternative ways of handling frustration and anger.
4. **Avoid Final Decision of Suicide During Crisis**	4. Assure the person that the suicidal crisis is a temporary state. Encourage the person to avoid a decision until alternatives can be considered during a noncrisis state (see subsequent discussion of *No-Suicide Contract*).
5. **Re-establish Social Ties**	5. Contact family members. Arrange for family crisis counseling. Activate links to self-help groups—e.g., Widow-To-Widow, Parents Without Partners, Al-a-Teen, and others. (see Appendix for referral to self-help groups)
6. **Relieve Extreme Anxiety**	6. After thorough assessment, a tranquilizer may be prescribed to induce sleep and lower anxiety. *Note: only a one-to-three day supply should be given, and only with a return appointment for crisis counseling.*

All persons receiving crisis counseling for suicidal ideations or actual suicide attempts should be given the opportunity for follow-up counseling or psychotherapy after the immediate crisis is over. **No-suicide contracts** between a counselor and a suicidal client have been used successfully in a variety of settings, such as individual therapy, family therapy, group work, and behavior therapy (Hipple and Cimolic 1979a). The contract is outlined in clear and simple language. The purpose of the no-suicide contract is to give the counselor time to explore alternatives with the client. When the time of the contract is up, the contract is renegotiated. Examples of a no-suicide contract include

- "I won't kill myself without talking to my counselor first."
- "I won't kill myself until next week."
- "I will go to the hospital emergency room if I start to have suicidal impulses."
- "I won't kill myself, either on purpose or accidentally, for any reason."

Crisis counseling is imperative for a person who is suicidal. A suicidal person can be in an acute crisis situation or chronically suicidal. A person who is chronically suicidal usually has the following clinical history (Hatton et al. 1977b):

1. Has eliminated all resources — is isolated and withdrawn from significant others.
2. Abuses alcohol/drugs.
3. Has recurrent depression.
4. Has made several prior suicide threats or attempts over several years' time.
5. Has made numerous bids for help, with little or no relief.
6. Presents with instability in job performance and/or interpersonal relationships.

Crisis counseling can be effective for the chronically suicidal person; however, it cannot alter personality patterns. More research and clinical study are needed in the area of formulating a treatment plan and intervening successfully with the chronically suicidal person.

In the Hospital

How and when to use hospitalization is somewhat controversial. "*Danger to self or others*" is a general guideline. Legalities are often an important consideration. Either too much or too little restraint may be grounds for liability. Too much restraint may be grounds for abridgment of civil rights, and too little restraint may be grounds for malpractice (Schutz 1982). Generally, if the primary counselor (nurse, social worker, psychologist) determines that the person is highly suicidal, has no immediate supports, and is exhausted and unable to carry out an alternative to suicide, hospitalization is indicated (Hatton et al. 1977b). However, it is true that some people are more responsive to treatment when they are not under constant observation. Long term hospitalization may undermine a person's ability to function effectively "on the outside" (Harvard Medical School 1986).

Even when the decision for hospitalization is made, there are no hospitals that are 100% "suicide-proof." Every hospital should have a suicide protocol that attempts to ensure the suicidal client's safety. **Students are advised to become familiar with the suicide protocol in the hospital(s) they are affiliated with.** Box 22 – 2 lists guidelines for minimizing suicidal behavior on a psychiatric unit (Schultz 1982).

Suicidal precautions are meant to provide the client with a sense of security. If the client loses control and makes a suicidal attempt, the staff will step in and assume control. Built into the suicide protocol are frequent interactions between staff and the suicidal client, for example, once every 30 minutes or three times a day for 15 minutes. (See V-E: *Therapeutic Environment* for structuring a therapeutic environment while the suicidal person is in the hospital.)

When suicidal adolescents are admitted to a psychiatric unit, further restrictions may be imposed. Phone calls and visitation rights are often limited to just the family. Friends, schoolmates, and girlfriends and boyfriends are restricted. This is done to reduce the incidence of *secondary gains* and maintain personal dignity. (Secondary gains are discussed and defined in Chapters 15 and 16.) Positive reinforcement of suicide as a means of receiving attention and sympathy and temporarily relieving feelings of isolation should be minimized. Better problem-solving techniques and more satisfying ways of achieving attention, affection, and a sense of belonging are explored with the adolescent client (Kenny and Krajewski 1980).

On the Telephone Hotlines

A counselor on a telephone hotline is often a lay person or volunteer who has had special training. At other times, friends, neighbors, relatives, police, nurses, and the clergy find themselves at the other end of a telephone cry for help. Guidelines for what to do on the other end of a suicidal phone call are provided here (Hatton et al. 1977; Neville and Barnes 1985; Frederick 1980). Almost all persons who are suicidal are ambivalent. *Ambivalence is one of the best tools a nurse has when working with a suicidal individual.* Talking with a helping person can help increase the suicidal person's ambivalence toward staying alive and can allow time to evaluate alternative actions. Essentially, the helping person attempts to establish rapport, assess the lethality of the situation, identify the problem, determine appropriate resources, and establish a plan with the caller (Hipple and Cimolic 1979a).

ESTABLISH RAPPORT. The most important thing is to keep the person on the line as long as possible. As

Box 22–2. GUIDELINES FOR MINIMIZING SUICIDAL BEHAVIOR ON A PSYCHIATRIC UNIT

The Client*

1. *Suicide Precaution*, include 1 : 1 monitoring, having client in view *at all times* (one arm's length distance between staff member and client).
   a. *Includes* during toileting.
   b. *Includes* during the night.
2. *Suicide Observation* includes a 15-minute visual check of suicidal client.
3. For each of the above, behavior, mood, and verbatim statements are recorded in the chart every 15 minutes.

The Environment

1. Count silverware and all other sharp objects before and after use by clients.
2. Do not allow clients to spend too much time alone in their rooms, and abolish private rooms altogether.
3. Jump-proof and hang-proof the bathrooms by installing break-away shower rods and recessed shower nozzles.
4. Keep electrical cords to minimum length.
5. Install windows of unbreakable glass. Install tamper-proof screens or partitions too small to pass through. Keep all windows locked.
6. Lock all utility rooms, kitchens, adjacent stairwells, offices. All nonclinical staff (housekeepers, maintenance, and others) should receive instructions.
7. Take all potentially harmful gifts (flowers in glass vases, etc.) from visitors before allowing them to see clients.
8. Go through client's belongings with client and remove all potentially harmful objects (e.g., belts, shoelaces, metal nail files, tweezers, matches, razors).
9. Assure that visitors do not leave potentially harmful objects in client's room (e.g., matches, nail files).
10. Search clients on return from pass (for drugs, sharp objects, cords, and so forth).

* See Table 22–2 for suicide precautions for different behaviors.

long as the person keeps talking, he is not acting out suicidal threats. It is often helpful to acknowledge the person's distress. Although you do not know how the person feels, you can tell the person that you understand that he is in distress and is extremely unhappy. This lets the person know that (1) you take his concerns and him seriously, (2) there is no need to complete the suicidal act to make it clear that he is in distress, and (3) other alternatives are available. For example (Neville and Barnes 1985): "The fact that you are considering suicide makes it clear that you are feeling overwhelmed and need some assistance. Now that I know this, there is no need for you to hurt yourself without first talking about what can be done to help you."

Establishing rapport may also be contingent on allowing ventilation of the caller's feelings. The helping person often has to accept angry or manipulative communication. The goal is to keep the caller talking and provide a psychological life-line.

Reinforcing the caller's positive responses is also useful. Any positive responses, thoughts, and actions that the person tells you about need to be met with a validation that these were positive and in the person's best interests. For example, if the caller tells you that he was thinking about suicide but decided to wait to call you first, you want to reinforce that this was a positive move (Neville and Barnes 1985): "Your calling me at this time was a very positive move; I am glad you decided to call now."

IDENTIFY THE PROBLEM. The problem needs to be clearly identified. As with all crisis situations, the problem-solving approach is used. The use of reflection and restating are *not* useful in crisis situations (see Chapter 10 for interventions in crisis). The use of problem-solving approaches is helpful. Problem-solving statements help define the problem and explore avenues of action. For example:

Whom have you talked to about your parent's divorce?
How do you think the divorce will change your relationship with your parents?
Have you told them/him/her?
Do you think that they no longer love you?

ASSESS THE LETHALITY OF THE SITUATION

1. If the caller is threatening suicide, evaluate the lethality of the plan (see page 583).
2. If the caller has already taken pills, determine what kind and how many, whether the caller has been drinking, and so forth.
3. Determine if there is someone nearby—neighbor, bystander, housekeeper, manager. If the answer is yes, tell the caller that you want to speak to that "someone" right now.
4. If not, try to get the caller's address and explain that you want to get help for him or her.
5. If the caller does not want to give you the address, then instruct the caller on first aid:
   - Taking pills—induce vomiting
   - Stop bleeding—apply pressure with bandage
   - For inhalation poisoning—fresh air, loosen tight clothing

EVALUATE POSITIVE COPING AND ENCOURAGE ALTERNATIVES. Has the caller felt this way in the past? What did he or she do then? What works best? What could the caller do differently in this situation? What does the caller think would help change his or her situation? *Give referrals to appropriate places in the community* that may help alter the situation.

NEGOTIATE A NO-SUICIDE PLAN. As mentioned, a clearly worded contract with the caller may give the helping person time to work with the caller on more alternatives. Ideally, the aim is to get the caller into crisis counseling. If that is not possible, you can try to arrange a relationship over the phone. The wording in the contract should be clear and not conditional. Words such as "try" and "unless" are *not* used.

Not Useful		More Useful
"I will *try* not to kill myself."	→	"I *will not* kill myself."
"I will not kill myself *unless* my wife leaves me."	→	"I will not kill myself *at any time*."
"I will not kill myself until I *call* you."	→	"I will not kill myself before I *talk* to you."

It is necessary that the person manning the telephone hotline have a variety of community resources available for referral. Besides the names and addresses of the resource, telephone numbers and names of contact persons should also be given whenever possible. Dependence is placed on the caller to contact resources for more, long-term assistance (Hipple and Cimolic 1979b).

It is important that the caller is made aware that he does have control over his own decisions and believes that someone cares about his situation and is available to spend time with him.

Research on the ability of telephone counseling to reduce suicide rates and effect behavioral change is sparse. It is thought that severely suicidal people do not make use of life-sustaining avenues such as hotlines. One case study pointed out that only 2% of all suicide victims in Los Angeles County had called the prevention center (Harvard Medical School 1986). However, recent studies do indicate that telephone counseling may have considerable therapeutic potential (Glatt et al. 1986; Hornblow 1986).

V-B: HEALTH TEACHING

Primary intervention in the form of health teaching is an important method of lessening suicidal attempts. The goal is to reach people before they become so overwhelmed that suicide appears to be a rational alternative. *Primary intervention* relates to the principles of good mental health. The following programs provide support, information, and education (Hart and Keidel, 1979):

- Programs on emotional health in the junior and senior high schools.
- Drug and alcohol courses, allowing for "rap sessions," in grade schools, junior, and senior high schools.
- Special programs in industry for the drug/alcohol abuser.
- Seminars for all health care providers on assessment and intervention in suicide, especially for those working in schools, industry, and well-baby clinics.
- Seminars and group activities for the elderly that focus on (1) physical concerns such as reactions to medications and physical changes and (2) emotional concerns such as: how to handle loneliness, separations from family, and loss of friends through death.

V-C: ACTIVITIES OF DAILY LIVING

Since social isolation and withdrawal are often present, active encouragement and advice are given regarding contacting significant persons and loved ones. Renewing friendships and important relationships can help foster self-esteem. When the crisis pertains to a significant other (spouse, parent, child), therapies such as family, couple, or group counseling may be indicated.

Community agencies may be useful in helping a person renew or initiate activities related to work, special interests, hobbies, sports, and other activities that can help enhance self-esteem.

V-D: SOMATIC THERAPIES

In cases in which extreme anxiety and lack of sleep occur for several days, the risk of suicide can increase. A tranquilizer will usually take care of both the anxiety and the sleeping problem. If medication is given, the supply should be for one to three days only, with a return appointment scheduled for re-evaluation. Tranquilizers, however, should never be given to a highly suicidal individual. Generally, a lethal dose for tranquilizers is ten times the normal dose. When a drug is combined with alcohol, only half that amount can cause death (Hoff 1984).

When a coexisting psychiatric condition is present in a person who is suicidal, somatic intervention is dictated according to the psychopathology. For example, a person who is suicidal and also holds the diagnosis of schizophrenia may need increased medication. Similar considerations are made for people who are clinically depressed as well as suicidal. Electroconvulsive therapy (ECT) can save the life of a seriously depressed and highly suicidal person (Harvard Medical School 1986). It takes from one to three weeks of antidepressant therapy before the person experiences an elevation of mood. ECT can have more immediate effects.

V-E: THERAPEUTIC ENVIRONMENT

There are times when hospitalization is thought to be the most therapeutic. Placing a highly suicidal person in a controlled hospital environment can provide structure and control as well as give the person time to evaluate his or her situation with professional staff. During hospitalization, the client is continually assessed as to suicidal risk and level of suicidal precaution needed. (Refer to Table 22–2 for guidelines for suicide precautions.) Repeated monitoring of a suicidal person's suicide intent and extent of hopelessness is ongoing in suicide prevention. The decision to discontinue suicide precautions is ideally based on clinical observations of nursing staff, physicians, and social workers as well as on input from the client. Therefore, the decision to continue or discontinue suicide precautions should be based on subjective data and objective clinical observations (Busteen and Johnson 1983).

V-F: PSYCHOTHERAPY

Initial intervention for a suicidal person is crisis intervention. However, all persons should be offered the opportunity for further therapy after the crisis is over. A nurse educated at the master's level may work with suicidal clients in a variety of modalities. Suitable therapies have been mentioned. Couple, individual, family, and group counseling are all useful. This is especially true if a person is chronically suicidal or has coexisting psychopathology such as depression, borderline symptoms, schizophrenic disorders, and others.

Tertiary intervention for family and friends ("survivors") of a person who has committed suicide should be initiated as soon after the death as possible (e.g., within 72 hours) and continued at least through the first anniversary of the death. Mourning the death of a loved one who has committed suicide is painful at all times. A family of a person who has committed suicide is often faced with the process of mourning without the normal, informal social supports usually provided. Survivors often feel that they are "going crazy" or "losing their minds." They need to know that these feelings are normal (Van Dongen 1988). Survivors need to find outlets for the undercurrent of anger against the deceased, who is responsible for trauma, confusion, and pain inflicted on them. Unfortunately, few survivors of suicide seek out counseling (Van Dongen 1988). Pronounced feelings of anger and guilt are common reactions.

Self-help groups have been found to be extremely beneficial for survivors of a suicidal family member or friend. Many people join self-help groups even if the suicide took place 25 to 30 years ago (Roche Report 1982).

Self-help groups for the survivors of a family member or friend who committed suicide are similar to all other self-help groups. Essentially, self-help groups for family survivors are run by people who have lost someone through suicide. When a professional is involved, it is in the role of facilitator, consultant, or educator—not that of leader. Ideally, lay leaders should have some professional training in group processes and awareness of the limitations of the group experience. Professional therapists (nurses, social workers, psychiatrists, psychologists) should be used as a source of referral and should be available for consulting. Referral for individual and family therapy is advised once individual and

Table 22–2 • GUIDELINES FOR SUICIDE PRECAUTIONS

PSYCHIATRIC ASSESSMENT TOOL	EXAMPLES OF CLIENT SYMPTOMS	NURSING CARE
	Level I	
Those clients who are not verbalizing or suggesting suicidal ideation.	Level I includes all clients admitted to the unit who do not meet the criteria for Levels II through IV.	1. Check client's whereabouts at least every hour. 2. Frequent verbal contact while awake.
	Level II	
Those clients who have suicidal ideations and who, after assessment by staff, are assessed to be in minimal danger of activity attempting suicide.	1. The client with vague suicidal ideation but without plan. 2. The client who is willing to make a no-suicide contract. 3. The client with insight into existing problems.	1. Check client's whereabouts every 15 to 30 minutes. 2. Frequent verbal contact while awake. 3. Chart client's whereabouts, mood, verbatim statements, behavior every 15 to 30 minutes.
	Level III	
Those clients with suicidal ideations and who, after assessment by unit staff, present clinical symptoms that indicate a higher suicide potential than Level II.	1. The client with a concrete suicide plan. 2. The client who is ambivalent about making a no-suicide contract. 3. The client with minimal insight into existing problems. 4. The client with limited impulse control.	1. Close observation*—i.e., within visual range of staff while awake. Accompany to bathroom. Client placed in multiple client room. While asleep, client is to be checked every 15 to 30 minutes. 2. Chart client's whereabouts, mood, verbatim statements, behavior every 15 to 30 minutes. 3. Meal trays contain no glass or metal silverware.
	Level IV	
Those clients with suicidal ideations or delusions of self-mutilation who, according to assessment by unit staff, present clinical symptoms that suggest a clear intent to follow through with the plan or delusion.	1. The client who is currently verbalizing a clear intent to harm self. 2. The client who is unwilling to make a no-suicide contract. 3. The client who presents with no insight into existing problems. 4. The client with poor impulse control. 5. The client who has already attempted suicide in the recent past by a particularly lethal method—e.g., hanging, gun, or carbon monoxide.	1. One-to-one nursing observation and interaction 24 hours a day (never out of staff's sight). 2. Arm's length at all times. 3. Chart client's whereabouts, mood, verbatim statements, behavior every 15 to 30 minutes. 4. Meal trays contain no glass or metal silverware.

* Nurse and physician explain to the client what the nurse will be doing and why. Both nurse and physician document this in chart.

Adapted from Busteen EL, Johnstone C. The development of suicide precautions for an inpatient psychiatric unit. Journal of Psychosocial Nursing and Mental Health Services, 21(5):18, 1983.

family problems have been identified (Roche Report 1982).

Likewise, staff and therapists who have been working with a client who successfully commits suicide need support. The opportunity should be available for staff to make adequate emotional expression of feelings of self-blame, guilt, and anger. If one of the staff has been closely involved over a long period of time with the client who has committed suicide, the staff member will also pass through a period of grief (Birtchnell 1983). Suicide can be an occupational hazard for a therapist involved in direct client care. Feelings of anger and guilt, experiencing loss of self-esteem, and having intrusive thoughts about the suicide are common. Symptoms similar to those of post-trauma were experienced by a significant percentage of psychiatrists who had a client who committed suicide (Chemtob et al. 1988). Peer support and supervision help work through the loss.

A full-scale psychological postmortem assessment should be carried out among staff. The purpose is to reveal errors in judgment or overlooked clues that could be useful when evaluating future clients. Discussion should center on piecing together the pressures which led up to the client's taking his or her life, (Birtchnell 1983).

Tertiary intervention might also be viewed by some as

referring to a person who has survived a suicide attempt. In such a case, efforts to prevent a future attempt (primary intervention) and working with the individual on immediate problems and concerns (secondary intervention) are indicated.

Standard VI: Evaluation

Evaluation of a suicidal client is an ongoing part of the assessment. The nurse must be constantly alert to changes in the suicidal person's mood, thinking, and behavior. As has been mentioned, sudden behavioral changes can signal suicide intent, especially when the client's depression is lifting and more energy is available to carry out a preconceived plan. A person with a diagnosis of schizophrenia is also at risk when recovering from a psychotic episode. Anniversaries of losses and holiday seasons are particularly difficult times for some people.

Evaluation includes identifying the presence or absence of any clues or thoughts of suicide. The nurse also looks for indications suggesting that the person is communicating thoughts and feelings more readily and that his or her social network is widening. For example, if the person is able to talk about his or her feelings and engage in problem-solving with the nurse, this would be a positive sign. Is the client increasing his or her social activities and expanding his or her interests? Does the client state that he or she thinks more or less suicidal thoughts? Essentially, the nurse evaluates the goals and establishes new ones as different situations arise. Goals for a client who is in a crisis situation may differ from those for a client who is chronically suicidal.

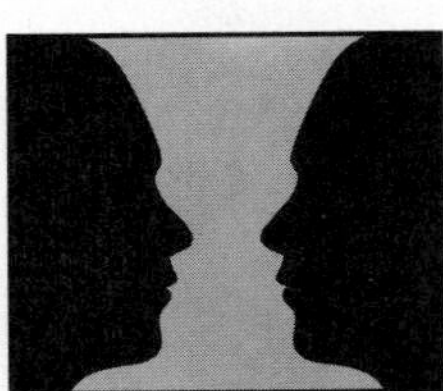

Case Study: Working With a Person Who is Suicidal

Thomas Martin, a 46-year-old social worker, was brought to the hospital for evaluation after an attempted suicide. When he did not show up for work, his coworker called to check on him. His landlady stated that his car was still in the driveway and that she would check his room. She found Mr. Martin lying on the bed, beside an empty bottle of sleeping pills. A strong smell of liquor filled the room and a nearly empty bottle of Scotch was on a table by the bed. An ambulance took Mr. Martin to the emergency room (ER), where his stomach was pumped. He stayed in the ER for 16 hours, until he was no longer groggy. He was then seen by a psychiatric nurse, Mrs. Ruiz, for evaluation.

He told Mrs. Ruiz that he has been separated from his wife for two years but has seen his eight-year-old son every week for the past 24 months. Three days prior to his suicide attempt, his wife sent him a letter stating that she wanted to remarry and move to Oklahoma with her son and new husband.

Assessment

Mr. Martin's manner was hostile and sarcastic. He told the nurse that it did not matter what anyone did, he would "do it again," and that next time he would succeed. He sat sneering at the nurse saying, "I never liked nurses anyway."

NURSE: What is it about nurses that you don't like?

MR. MARTIN: *Mimicking the nurse's tone.* What is it about nurses that you don't like—what dribble. Don't try that therapeutic garbage on me. I don't need help from you or anyone else.
Silence.
You're all castrating bitches . . . all women are. I hate all women.

NURSE: Tell me about one woman who has hurt you.

MR. MARTIN: *Angrily* . . . Stop prying into my business with your little therapeutic diddies.
Silence.
Well . . . my wife . . . she . . . she . . . oh God . . . *At this point Mr. Martin starts sighing deeply, then bursts into tears.*

NURSE: *Waits a few minutes.* This situation with your wife and son moving away has upset you deeply.

MR. MARTIN: I don't want to live if I can't see my son. He is all I have left. He is the only thing that ever mattered to me.

NURSE: You have no friends or family?

MR. MARTIN:	All my family died when I was a kid. As for friends . . . I don't need other people. Anyway, people don't seem to like me much. Look, don't spend time worrying about me. I've got a few more tricks up my sleeve.
NURSE:	Do you mean that you will try to kill yourself again?
MR. MARTIN:	What could it possibly mean to you?
NURSE:	I *am* concerned about you, Mr. Martin.
MR. MARTIN:	Well . . . isn't that the nursie thing to say. . . . Such great understanding.
NURSE:	I do understand that you are very troubled right now and have no one to go to.

Mrs. Ruiz organized her data into objective and subjective components.

OBJECTIVE DATA

1. Male, age 46, no support systems
2. Impending loss of significant relationship with son
3. Possible drinking problem, need more data
4. Suicide attempt
5. Holds responsible job
6. Estranged wife and son moving away from area
7. Appears articulate and bright

SUBJECTIVE DATA

1. "I don't want to live if I can't see my son."
2. "I've got a few more tricks up my sleeve."
3. "He (son) is the only thing that ever mattered to me."
4. "All my family died when I was just a kid."
5. "I don't need other people."
6. "People don't seem to like me much."

Nursing Diagnosis

Mrs. Ruiz analyzed her data and set up her nursing diagnoses in order of priority.

1. Potential for Self-Directed Violence related to suicidal behavior and believing he has no reason to live
   - Suicide attempt
   - "I don't want to live if I can't see my son."
   - "He is the only thing that ever mattered to me."
   - "I've got a few more tricks up my sleeve."
   - Is holding a responsible job
2. Social Interaction Impaired related to inability to engage in satisfying relationships
   - "He (son) is all I have left."
   - "All my family died when I was a kid."
   - "I don't need other people."
   - "People don't seem to like me much."

Mrs. Ruiz discussed the case with the admitting resident. Since Mr. Martin stated that he wanted to kill himself, had no family or friends that could stay with him, and had access to drugs, the decision was made to hospitalize him for further evaluation. Ordinarily, Mrs. Ruiz would follow him in clinic after discharge. In this case, Mrs. Ruiz told the physician that she thought it best for a male psychiatric nurse to work with Mr. Martin after discharge. Mrs. Ruiz explained she thought that Mr. Martin would have a strong negative transference with a female nurse and, at this time, working with him on alternatives in his life was the main goal. After the immediate crisis was over, working on his interpersonal relationships would take priority.

Planning

Mr. Martin was kept in the hospital for three days. During that time he was placed on suicide precautions as outlined in Table 22–2. He was discharged to the clinic after the staff thought that he was no longer a suicidal risk. When asked if he wanted a male nurse instead of a female nurse, he stated, "No . . . I'll talk to little nursie—nursie . . . she's got a thing for me."

CONTENT LEVEL—PLANNING GOALS

The nurse met with Mr. Martin, and both worked out the following goals:

Planning *(Continued)*

Nursing Diagnosis	Long Term Goals	Short Term Goals
1. *Potential for Self-Directed Violence* related to loss of a son	Mr. Martin will state that he wants to live.	1a. Mr. Martin will make a *no-suicide contract* with the nurse by the end of the first session. 1b. Mr. Martin will talk about painful feelings by (state the date). 1c. Mr. Martin will look at alternative ways he can keep in touch with his son by (state the date).
2. *Social Interaction Impaired* related to social isolation.	Mr. Martin will state that he feels less isolated and is participating in at least one activity involving other people.	2a. Mr. Martin will discuss feelings of isolation and loneliness by (state the date). 2b. Mr. Martin will identify three positive aspects of self and job by (state the date). 2c. Mr. Martin will state that he enjoys one new weekly activity by (state the date).

PROCESS LEVEL—NURSES' REACTIONS AND FEELINGS

Mrs. Ruiz knew that working with Mr. Martin was going to evoke high anxiety. When talking to her clinical supervisor, it became apparent that the "idea" of sending Mr. Martin to a male nurse therapist, while logical on the surface, was motivated by Mrs. Ruiz's own anxiety. She was trying to avoid Mr. Martin. "I guess I did try to shove him off. His sarcasm and belittling made me feel put down and angry."

Reviewing that first session with the supervisor clarified a number of important dynamics. *First,* it became evident that Mr. Martin was experiencing low self-esteem as a result of the impending loss of his son's companionship. The resulting anxiety was turned inward. Mr. Martin's rage at the loss and the inability to change the situation resulted in intense feelings of helplessness. *Second,* it appeared from the data that Mr. Martin was extremely isolated. It also appeared that most of this isolation was self-imposed. His sarcasm and belittling remarks appeared to be devices to (1) push people away, (2) temporarily lift sagging self-esteem through "one-upmanship," and (3) divert attention from his own fears. The supervisor and Mrs. Ruiz saw the need to relieve Mr. Martin's isolation without increasing his anxiety to severe levels.

It was important for Mr. Martin to talk about some of his feelings. Identifying and expressing feelings could have a number of benefits. *First,* talking about pent-up feelings could minimize feelings of isolation. *Second,* talking about feelings could reduce the need to act them out through self-destructive channels. *Third,* once identified, these feelings could be more positively discharged and worked through.

Intervention

At first, Mr. Martin was sarcastic, belittling, flirtatious, and hostile. Mrs. Ruiz kept her responses neutral and continued to focus her concern on Mr. Martin's situations and on working with alternatives. She gave him frequent opportunities to talk about his feelings. Initially, Mr. Martin would ridicule the nurse and belittle the idea: "Oh . . . you want to know about my precious painful feelings." Gradually, the testing-out behavior began to diminish. Slowly, and with some reluctance, Mr. Martin began talking about his feelings of loneliness and despair and sense of being a failure as a husband and father. He talked about the pain of his separation from his wife and his feelings of being a failure to his son.

The nurse continued to be neutral, not getting involved with power struggles or becoming defensive. Mrs. Ruiz began to see more clearly how these sarcastic and belittling behaviors helped Mr. Martin to defend against painful feelings of failure and low self-esteem. Refer to Nursing Care Plan 22–1 for specific interventions used with Mr. Martin.

Evaluation

After two months, Mr. Martin stated that although he missed his son desperately, he no longer thought of suicide. He did not want to leave his son that legacy. He was planning his next vacation in Oklahoma, camping with his son for two weeks. His interpersonal relationships were still strained. He was beginning to look at situations which gave rise to his sarcasm and belittling and to relate his actions to feelings that had been unconscious. His sarcasm and belittling toward Mrs. Ruiz had diminished a great deal, although he resorted to it when he felt threatened. He spent more time on examining his life, feelings, and where he wanted to go, and less on defensive behaviors. Although by this time the crisis was over, Mr. Martin continued counseling with Mrs. Ruiz. He was able to say that at times he felt more comfortable with his coworkers, although he still did not feel at home with others. He had resumed weekly bowling. He stated that he was surprised that he enjoyed it. He had even started talking to a "fellow there who is also divorced and got a rough deal. He's not a bad guy."

Nursing Care Plan 22–1 • A SUICIDAL CLIENT AFTER DISCHARGE: MR. MARTIN

NURSING DIAGNOSIS

Potential for self-directed violence related to loss of son

Supporting Data

- Suicide attempt.
- "I don't want to live if I can't see my son."
- "I've got a few more tricks up my sleeve."
- Impending loss of son.

Long Term Goal: Mr. Martin will state that he wants to live.

Short Term Goal	*Intervention*	*Rationale*	*Evaluation*
1. Mr. Martin will make a *no-suicide contract* with nurse by end of first session.	1a. Assess suicide status.	1a. Periodic check of suicidal status ongoing. Higher rate of suicide for those who have attempted suicide.	*Goal met.* Mr. Martin signed contract: "I will not kill myself until I talk to the nurse" (first session).
	1b. Even if Mr. Martin denies suicide, make a *no-suicide contract.*	1b. Demonstrates concern and offers alternatives if suicidal thoughts return.	
2. Mr. Martin will talk about painful feelings by (state the date).	2a. Remain neutral in face of hostility and put-downs.	2a. Diminishes power struggles and discourages continuing acting-out behaviors.	First to third week, hostile and sarcastic communication is constant.
	2b. Refocus attention back to Mr. Martin.	2b. Arguments and power struggles keep attention focused away from important issues.	By fourth week, Mr. Martin stated, "You really want to know."
	2c. Give frequent opportunities for discussion of feelings through verbal invitation and stated concern.	2c. Aggressive, hostile communications are cover for painful feelings. When client can express feelings in words, there is less need to act them out.	Mr. Martin talked of feeling like a failure as a husband and father.

Nursing Care Plan 22–1 • A SUICIDAL CLIENT AFTER DISCHARGE: MR. MARTIN *(Continued)*

Short Term Goal	Intervention	Rationale	Evaluation
3. Mr. Martin will look at alternative ways he can keep in touch with his son by (state the date).	3. Alternative solutions can be problem-solved once feelings and problems are identified.	3. Acceptable alternatives increase a future orientation and decrease hopelessness. Client can experience feelings of control over the situation.	By fifth week, Mr. Martin talked about taking son on a camping trip during summer recess.

NURSING DIAGNOSIS

Social interaction impaired related to social isolation

Supporting Data

- "He (son) is all I have left."
- "All my family died when I was a kid."
- "I don't need other people."
- People don't seem to like me much."

Long Term Goal: Mr. Martin will state that he feels less isolated and less frightened of people by (state the date).

Short Term Goal	Intervention	Rationale	Evaluation
1. Mr. Martin will discuss feelings of isolation and loneliness by (state the date).	1. Provide opportunities for Mr. Martin to express feelings and thoughts regarding his self-imposed isolation.	1. Before change can take place, clarification of personal feelings and thoughts is necessary.	*Goal met:* By fourth week Mr. Martin spoke of feeling alone—son is only contact to life.
2. Mr. Martin will identify three " positive aspects of self and job by (state the date).	2a. Validate Mr. Martin's strengths.	2a. Positive as well as negative feedback aid in more realistic perception of self.	By fifth week, Mr. Martin stated that he thinks he is a good worker and is respected (if not liked) by his peers.
	2b. Encourage self-evaluation of positive as well as negative aspects of Mr. Martin's life.	2b. Client can begin to see himself more clearly, with increase in self-esteem.	
3. Mr. Martin will state that he enjoys one new weekly activity with at least one other person by (state the date).	3a. Review previous activities that Mr. Martin enjoyed before his marriage broke up.	3a. Change focus from negative present to positive aspects of his past. Can help increase hope and self-esteem.	By seventh week, Mr. Martin stated that he started bowling again and was surprised that he had a good time.
	3b. Have Mr. Martin choose an activity that he is willing to participate in.	3b. Participating in own problem-solving and decision-making offers a sense of control and an increase in self-esteem.	

Summary

Suicide is the willful act of ending one's life. A person can also hasten one's death by covert self-destructive behaviors such as alcoholism, medical noncompliance, hyperobesity, anorexia nervosa, and gambling. Death from such causes is called subintentioned death.

Suicidal behavior can be classified into three categories: (1) completed, (2) attempted, and (3) ideation. Statistics surrounding suicide provide a profile that can be useful when assessing a person's suicidal intention. Many complex factors contribute to a person's decision to commit suicide. These factors include psychodynamic, sociological, and biochemical theories.

It is critical for the nurse to assess the client's suicidal intent. The nurse assesses verbal and nonverbal clues, lethality of suicide plan, and high-risk factors. Nursing diagnoses may include a number of problem areas; however, *potential for self-directed violence* is most crucial initially. When planning care, the nurse plans specific goals. Personal reactions to suicide and the suicidal client need to be dealt with. Common and expected reactions were discussed, and supervision with a more experienced health care professional has been emphasized.

Intervention in suicide can be on a *primary, secondary,* or *tertiary* level. Various interventions were spelled out using the Standards of Nursing Practice as a guide. Evaluation is ongoing, especially with a person who has a potential for suicide, since the incidence is often higher when depression is lifting or a person is recovering from a psychotic episode. Goals are evaluated and reset, according to change in the assessment and progress by the client toward mutually agreed upon goals. A case study was provided to highlight nurses' work with a suicidal client.

References

Adam KS. Attempted suicide. Psychiatric Clinics of North America, 8(2):183, 1985.

Andriola J. A note on the possible iatrogenesis of suicide. Psychiatry, 36:213, 1973.

Beck AT, et al. Classification and nomenclature. *In* Resnick H, Hawthorne B (eds). Suicide Prevention in the Seventies. Washington DC: U.S. Government Printing Office, 1973.

Benton RG. Death and Dying: Principles and Practices in Patient Care. New York: D. Van Nostrand Company, 1978.

Birtchnell J. Psychotherapeutic considerations in the management of the suicidal patient. American Journal of Psychotherapy, 37(1):24, 1983.

Breed W. Occupational mortality and suicide among males. American Sociological Review, 28:179, 1963.

Busteen EL, Johnstone C. The development of suicide precautions for an inpatient psychiatric unit. Journal of Psychosocial Nursing and Mental Health Services, 21(5):15, 1983.

Cassem NH. Treating the person confronting death. *In* Nicholi AM (eds). The Harvard Guide to Modern Psychiatry. Cambridge, MA: The Belknap Press of Harvard University Press, 1980.

Chemtob CM, Hamada RS, Baver G, Kinney B, Turiqoe RY. Patient's suicide: Frequency and impact on psychiatrists. American Journal of Psychiatry, 145(2):224, 1988.

Clayton PJ. Suicide. Psychiatric Clinics of North America, 8(2):203, 1985.

Davison GC, Neale JM. Abnormal Psychology. New York: John Wiley & Sons, 1982.

Donlon PT, Rockwell DA. Psychiatric Disorders: Diagnoses and Treatment. Bowie, MD: Robert J. Brady Company, 1982.

Evans DL. Explaining suicide among the young: An analytic review of the literature. Journal of Psychosocial Nursing and Mental Health Services, 21(5):9, 1983.

Farberow NL. Crisis, disaster and suicide: theory and therapy. *In* Schneidman ES (ed). Essays in Self-Destruction. New York: Jason Aronson, 1967.

Fitzpatrick JJ. Suicidology and suicide prevention: historical perspectives from the nursing literature. Journal of Psychosocial Nursing and Mental Health Services, 21(5):9, 1982.

Frederick CJ. Drug abuse: An indirect self-destructive behavior. *In* Farberow NL (ed). The Many Faces of Suicide: Indirect Self-Destructive Behaviors. New York: McGraw-Hill Book Company, 1980.

Gibbs J, Martin W. Status integration and suicide: a study in sociology. Eugene, OR: University of Oregon Press, 1964.

Glatt KM, Sherwood DW, Amisson TJ. Telephone hotlines at a suicide site. Hospital and Community Psychiatry, 37(2):178, 1986.

Hamlin WT. Adolescent suicide. Journal of the National Medical Association, 74(1):25, 1982.

Hammel-Bissell BP. Suicidal casework: assessing nurses' reactions. Journal of Psychosocial Nursing and Mental Health Services, 23(10):20, 1985.

Hart NA, Keidel GC. The suicidal adolescent. Americal Journal of Nursing, 79(1):80, 1979.

Harvard Medical School Mental Health Letter. Suicide—Part II, 2:1, 1986.

Hatton CL, et al. Intervention. *In* Hatton CL (ed). Suicide: Assessment and Intervention. New York: Appleton-Century-Crofts, 1977a.

Hatton CL, et al. Theoretical framework. *In* Hatton CL (ed). Suicide: Assessment and Intervention. New York: Appleton-Century Crofts, 1977b.

Hipple J, Cimolic P. The counselor and the suicidal crisis: diagnosis and prevention. Springfield, MA: Charles C Thomas, Publisher, 1979a.

Hipple J, Cimolic, P. The use of the telephone in treatment. Springfield, MA; Charles C Thomas, Publisher, 1979b.

Hoff LA. People in Crisis: Understanding and Helping, 2nd ed. Menlo Park, CA: Addison-Wesley Publishing Company, 1984.

Hopkins BW. Running away from it all: suicide among troubled youth. Family Life Developmental Center—Department of Human Developmental Studies: Cornell University, Ithaca, NY, July–August, 1983.

Hornblow AR. The evolution and effectiveness of telephone counseling services. Hospital and Community Psychiatry, 37(7):731, 1986.

Kaplan HI, Sadock BJ. Comprehensive textbook of psychiatry, 4th ed. Baltimore, MD: Williams & Wilkins, 1985.

Kaplan HI, Sadock BJ. Synopsis of Psychiatry, 5th ed. Baltimore, MD: Williams & Wilkins, 1988.

Kavenaugh RE. Facing Death. Baltimore, MD: Penguin Books, 1972.

Kenney EM, Krajewski KJ. Hospital treatment of the adolescent suicidal patient. *In* McIntyre MS, Angle CR (eds). Suicide Attempts in Children and Youth. New York: Harper & Row, Publishers, 1980.

Kliman AS. Psychological first aid for recovery. *In* (ed). The Will to Live vs. the Will to Die. New York: Human Sciences Press, 1984.

Kolb LC, Brodie HKM. Modern Clinical Psychiatry, 10th ed. Philadelphia: W.B. Saunders Company, 1982.

Leggett J, Ross and Tom: Two American Tragedies. New York: Simon & Schuster, 1974.

Malzberger JT, Buie D. The devices of suicide. International Review of Psychoanalysis 7:61, 1980.

Menninger K. Man Against Himself. New York: Harcourt, Brace & World, 1938.

Mowshowitz I. The special role of the pastoral counselor. *In* (ed). The Will to Live vs. the Will to Die. New York: Human Sciences Press, 1984.

Mullis MR, Byers PH. Social support. Journal of Psychosocial Nursing, 25(4):16, 1988.

Neville D, Barnes S. The suicidal phone call. Journal of Psychosocial Nursing, 23(8):14, 1985.

Pallikkathayil L, McBride AB. Suicide attempts. Journal of Psychosocial Nursing, 24(8):13, 1986.

Parker SD. Accidents or suicide: Do life changed events lead to adolescent suicide? Journal of Psychosocial Nursing, 26(6):15, 1988.

Patterson W, et al. Evaluation of suicidal patients: The SAD PERSONS Scale. Psychosomatics, 24(4):343, 1983.

Paykel ES, et al. Suicide attempts and recent life events. Archives of General Psychiatry, 33:327, 1975.

Peck ML. Adolescent suicide. *In* Harron CL, et al. (eds). Suicide: Assessment and Intervention. New York: Appleton-Century-Crofts, 1977.

Reubin R. Spotting and stopping the suicide patient. Nursing 79, 9(4):83, 1979.

Roche Report: Frontiers of Psychiatry. Suicide support groups: self-help for those left behind. December, 1982.

Schneidman ES. Orientation towards death: a vital aspect of the study of lives. *In* White RW (ed). The study of lives. New York: Atherton Press, 1963.

Schutz BM. Legal Liability in Psychotherapy. San Francisco, CA: Jossey-Bass, Publishers, 1982.

Simmons S. Suicide potentiality. U.S. Department of Health and Human Services (NIH Publication No. 82-2308). Washington DC: U.S. Government Printing Office, 1981.

Stevenson JM. Suicide. *In* Talbott JA, Hale RE, Yudofsky SC. Textbook of Psychiatry. Washington DC: American Psychiatric Press, 1988.

Szasz T. Law, Liberty and Psychiatry. New York: Macmillan & Company, 1963.

Van Dongen CJ. The legacy of suicide. Journal of Psychosocial Nursing, 26(1):9, 1988.

Self-Study Exercises

Place T (True) or F (False) next to each statement.

1. ________ Attempted suicide is associated with depression and alcoholism.
2. ________ People with antisocial disorders and people with hysterical disorders have a high suicide rate.
3. ________ Once a person is over the suicide crisis, he or she most likely will not attempt suicide in the future.
4. ________ Non-whites in a low socioeconomic status have the highest rates for suicide.
5. ________ If the nurse thinks that a client may be thinking of suicide, the nurse should not bring up the subject, lest the person get ideas.
6. ________ The suicide rate is higher among gifted individuals, immigrants, police, and doctors than in the general population.
7. ________ A person who has had a family member commit suicide, is divorced, and is a heavy drinker is a risk for possible suicide.

Choose the most appropriate response in each case.

8. Choose the event that would *least likely* precipitate suicide.

   A. Person is extremely socially isolated.
   B. Person has just won a million dollars with his picture on TV.
   C. Person who has grown up in an orphanage has just lost a spouse.
   D. Person who is a wealthy man who has gradually worked his way up the ladder of success.

9. Choose the type of suicide that is included in *Durkheim's* theory.

   A. Murder in 180th degree
   B. Low serotonin levels
   C. Anomic
   D. Alcohol abuse or depressed

10. The statement by a suicidal person, "How can I go about giving my body to medical science?" is an example of a (an)

    A. Overt statement
    B. Behavioral clue
    C. Emotional clue
    D. Covert statement

11. The best response to a client who states, "Things will never work out, but I have an answer now," is

    A. Things have a way of working out in time.
    B. I feel the same sometimes.
    C. I knew you would find a better solution.
    D. What things . . . What kind of answer have you found?

12. Charles Brown, age 52, just lost his wife in a car accident four months ago. Since that time he has been severely depressed and has taken to drinking to "numb the pain." Using the SAD PERSONS assessment scale, how many points does Mr. Brown have?

    A. Three points
    B. Four points

C. Five points
D. Six points

13. Which of the following is the BEST way to phrase a **no-suicide contract**?

A. "I will not kill myself until I call my therapist."
B. "I will not kill myself unless my husband leaves me."
C. "I will not kill myself, either by accident or on purpose, no matter what happens."
D. "I will not try to kill myself until next week."

Next to the intervention, put a P for primary intervention, an S for secondary intervention, or a T for tertiary intervention.

14. ________ Work with the family of a recent suicide victim.
15. ________ Relieve isolation, remove all weapons, and encourage alternative expressions of anger.
16. ________ Place the suicidal person on suicide precautions when first admitted to the hospital.
17. ________ Work with a teenager who has recently attempted suicide.
18. ________ Provide seminars for the elderly that focus on physical and emotional concerns.
19. ________ Keep the person on the telephone, find out if the person has taken anything, assess the lethality of plan, and work on alternatives.

Name two short term goals for the following nursing diagnoses:

20. *Potential for Self-Directed Violence* related to loss of a loved one
    1. ________________________________
    2. ________________________________

21. *Ineffective Family Coping* related to lack of sleep and inability to concentrate
    1. ________________________________
    2. ________________________________

For discussion

22. Name and briefly discuss three common and expected emotional reactions that a nurse might have when initially working with people who are suicidal.

CHAPTER 23

People Who Depend Upon Alcohol

Kathleen Smith-DiJulio

OUTLINE

KEY TERMS AND CONCEPTS

The key terms and concepts listed here also appear in bold where they are defined or discussed in this chapter.

ALCOHOLISM
ADDICTION
DEPENDENCE
DENIAL
CODEPENDENCY
INTERVENTION
DISULFIRAM (ANTABUSE)
AVERSIVE CONDITIONING
ALCOHOLICS ANONYMOUS (AA)
BLACKOUTS
TOLERANCE
WITHDRAWAL
MAST (MICHIGAN ALCOHOL SCREENING TEST)
PREFERRED DEFENSIVE STRUCTURE (PDS)

BLOOD ALCOHOL LEVEL (BAL)

AL-ANON

AL-A-TEEN

ADULT CHILDREN OF ALCOHOLICS (ACoA)

ENABLING

DUAL DIAGNOSIS

OBJECTIVES

After studying this chapter, the student will be able to:

1. Compare and contrast what is meant by alcohol addiction and alcohol withdrawal.
2. Define alcoholism.
3. Discuss three theories of etiology of alcoholism.
4. Identify significant data found in an alcoholic client, using the five areas of assessment covered in this chapter.
5. Describe the difference in the relationship of blood alcohol levels (BALs) and behavior between an alcoholic person and a nondrinker.
6. Formulate six nursing diagnoses that might apply to alcoholic clients, including related etiologies.
7. Identify two short term goals that might be useful steps in achieving long term sobriety.
8. Write at least four principles of psychotherapeutic intervention that a nurse would use with an alcoholic client.
9. Discuss two issues that a therapist should address when treating alcoholics.
10. Explain three issues that affect the alcoholic during phases of treatment.
11. Discuss five therapeutic modalities used with alcoholic people.
12. Identify four indications that a person is successfully recovering from alcoholism.

Alcohol is the most widely used — and misused — drug in America. It has only been in recent decades that alcoholism has begun to be thought of as a disease rather than a moral weakness. Attitudes change slowly and moral notions about this disease still prevail, resulting in missed diagnoses and lack of treatment for affected individuals. The impact of excessive alcohol use on human health and well-being is substantial, and no one is immune from the gamut of medical-social-emotional-familial-legal-economic problems that uncontrolled alcohol use creates. It is a problem that cannot be ignored.

Two thirds of the nation's adults consume alcohol regularly. One in ten of these develops problems associated with his or her alcohol use. It has been estimated that one third of hospital admissions are alcohol-related. Alcohol-related traffic accidents continue to be a major problem in our society. Alcohol contributes significantly to the incidence and severity of accidents in the home and workplace. In families with at least one alcoholic spouse, the rate of separation and divorce is seven times that of the general population (USDHHS 1984). Support groups for adult children of alcoholics (ACoA) are meeting all over the country, attempting to address childhood needs that were unmet in the chaotic emotional atmosphere of an alcoholic family.

Alcohol use occurs throughout the life span. Alcohol misuse during pregnancy can result in fetal alcohol syndrome (FAS). A baby born with FAS can show signs of mental retardation, abnormal behavior, abnormal features of the face and head, and growth retardation (Frances and Franklin 1988).

More than one third of adolescents have tried alcohol by age 13. By their senior year in high school 93% have done so. Six percent of seniors drink on a daily or near daily basis. One third of seniors approved of drinking one or two drinks daily, although two thirds felt that as many as four or five drinks per day would be harmful (USDHHS 1984). Adolescents tend to drink small amounts frequently, which is a pattern different from that for adults. They also tend to have problems with alcohol, not alcoholism. Alcoholism is normally a progressive illness. Most adolescents change their drinking practices as they mature and accept adult responsibilities. Those who are at a particularly high risk for ongoing problems and alcoholism are children of alcoholics. The nature of this risk should be explained, and abstinence encouraged.

Alcohol problems among the elderly are also difficult to ascertain because of the social isolation of many elderly people and because there is an attitude of letting the elderly do what they want—after all, "they deserve it." No one deserves an alcohol problem! Those elderly who had alcohol problems as adults will carry them into old age—if they survive. Some elderly people develop alcohol problems in old age in response to the myriad of life crises that may occur, including retirement, failing health, and the deaths of family members and friends (see Chapter 29).

Because of the broad social impact of alcohol use, it is critical that nurses learn to recognize the indicators of a developing alcohol problem. Because alcohol problems in most persons are progressive in nature, early detection is critical to ensure a positive prognosis. There is no arena of nursing practice that can ignore problems caused by excessive alcohol consumption. People with alcohol problems are seen in clinics, inpatient hospital units, and even in schools. Nurses need to know about alcohol-related problems in order to care for their clients effectively, wherever they may practice. In addition, the nursing profession is becoming more involved in the treatment of alcoholism, and many nurses are becoming actively involved in all aspects of treatment. This chapter will provide fundamental knowledge about alcoholism and focus on the role of the nurse in both assessment and treatment processes.

Figure 23-1 conceptualizes alcohol abuse as a self-destructive behavior in response to stress.

Standard I: Theory

Alcohol, a psychoactive substance, is used by the majority of the adult population in the United States. Most people that use this central nervous system depressant do so without problems. However, a certain percentage of people develop problems associated with their alcohol use. Alcohol use does occur on a continuum (Fig. 23-2). Movement along this continuum in either direction is a progressive process and takes time.

Alcoholism is the term applied to the end stage of the disease continuum that includes addiction and dependence. **Addiction** incorporates the concepts of loss of control of alcohol ingestion, drinking despite alcohol related problems, and a tendency to relapse. **Dependence** can be physical or psychological. Evidence of **tolerance** (increasing amounts of alcohol are required to achieve the desired effect) and **withdrawal** (stopping alcohol use results in specific signs and symptoms) indicates *physical* dependence. *Psychological* dependence involves craving for, and compulsive use of, alcohol. The alcoholic thinks he needs a drink to survive.

The reason one person becomes addicted and another does not seems to depend on a number of factors, including psychosocial and environmental factors as well as genetic predisposition. The difficulty in determining cause and effect is that the diagnosis of alcoholism generally occurs many years after the onset of drinking. Many different factors are involved over the course of those years and probably have an influence on the eventual development of alcoholism in any particular individual. Theories to be briefly examined here include biological, psychological, and sociocultural theories.

BIOLOGICAL THEORIES

Interest in biological theories was spurred by the observation that alcoholism seemed to run in families. If your ancestors had problems with alcohol, the likelihood seemed to be increased that you would too. The first studies that seemed to indicate a genetic component in the development of alcoholism were by Goodwin and coworkers (1973, 1974). They studied identical twins of alcoholic and nonalcoholic fathers. All twins studied were adopted at birth; half were placed in alcoholic homes, half in nonalcoholic homes. The children of al-

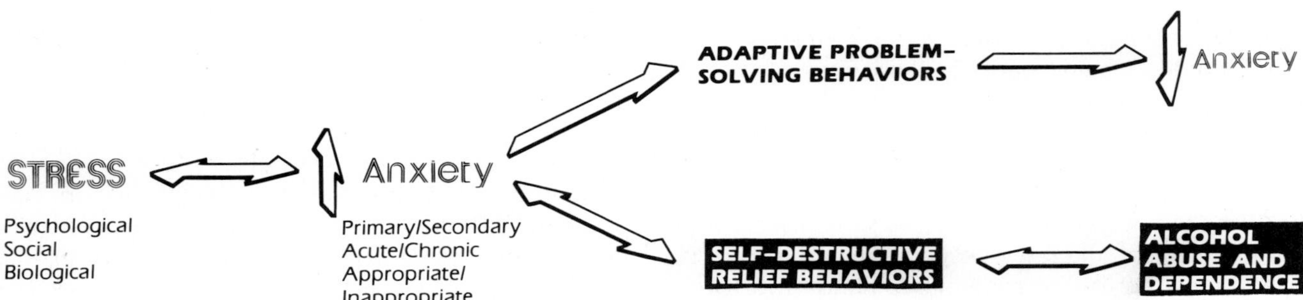

Figure 23-1. *Conceptualization of the process of alcohol addiction and dependence.*

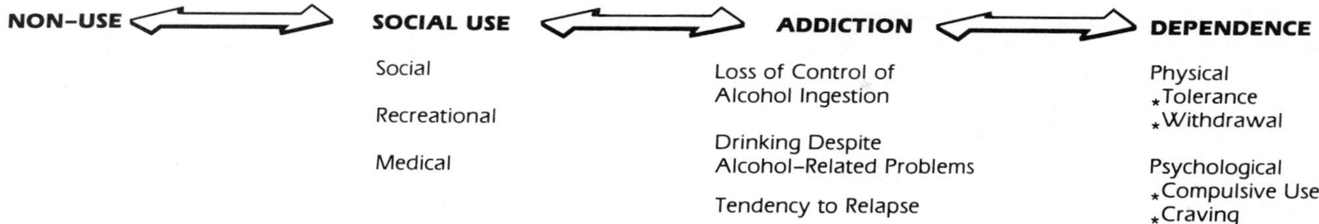

Figure 23-2. A *continuum of alcohol use.*

coholic fathers developed alcoholism at a rate significantly higher than did children of nonalcoholic fathers, even when the children of alcoholic fathers were raised in nonalcoholic homes. Twins raised in alcoholic homes whose biological fathers were not alcoholic did *not* develop alcoholism greater than that of the general population.

Current research has largely shifted from looking for an actual gene that causes alcoholism to looking at inherited abnormalities of biochemical factors that predispose to the development of alcoholism. The most promising research in this regard focuses on neuropeptides (also known as endogenous opiates), specifically enkephalins and endorphins. The theory is that a deficiency of these leads to dysphoria. In an attempt to feel better, the affected individual resorts to alcohol use, finds relief, and is thus reinforced for alcohol ingestion. When not drinking, the person again becomes dysphoric, knows that alcohol will improve mood, and so drinks again. Current research involves testing this hypothesis by restoring deficient neuropeptides in those at high risk for developing alcoholism (children of alcoholics) to see if alcoholism can be prevented. Much change in this area of research will likely be seen in the next five to ten years.

PSYCHOLOGICAL THEORIES

When addiction is conceptualized as a behavioral disorder, one looks to psychological theories for insight into the phenomenon. Knott (1987) described alcoholism as a behavioral impairment due to compulsive alcohol use. The affected individual is overwhelmingly preoccupied with procuring alcohol.

Although there is no addictive personality type, there are psychodynamic factors associated with alcoholism. These include the following (Knott 1987):

1. A *basic depressive personality organization*. Alcoholic persons are frequently described as having a depressed mood; yet they do not meet the DSM III-R criteria for either major depression or dysthymic disorder.
2. An *intolerance for frustration and pain*. This intolerance exhibits itself in response to both psychological and physical pain. Much research has centered on the ability of alcohol to reduce tensions. The tension-reduction hypothesis is a viable theory for explaining reasons for both alcohol intake and progression into alcoholism (Schuckit 1984).
3. *Lack of success in life*.
4. *Lack of affectionate and meaningful relationships*. Because of unmet needs, alcoholics require nurturance, which they usually cannot find as adults. Defense mechanisms protect them from associated anxiety.
5. *Low self-esteem; lack of self-regard*. Alcoholic people often feel worthless, hopeless, and helpless about themselves and the possibility of their lives ever being any different.
6. *Risk-taking propensity*.

According to psychological theories, a person drinks to feel better. The habit of drinking in response to psychological needs then becomes reinforced, and over time the drinking behavior develops into an addiction.

SOCIOCULTURAL THEORIES

Sociocultural theories attempt to explain differences seen in the incidence of alcoholism in various groups. Attitudes about alcohol use, which are derived from the society and culture, influence when and how a person drinks. For example, Italians and Jews are thought to have lower alcoholism rates because they have rules about when and how much to drink. In these two cultures, drinking occurs in the context of meals and serves specific social and religious purposes. Drunkenness is frowned upon. The French, in contrast, are said to have high alcoholism rates because it is socially acceptable to drink anywhere and any time, and drunkenness is tolerated.

Another theory correlates alcoholism rates with the degree of cultural stress. This theory is said to explain the higher incidence of alcoholism among black males. Black females are said to be protected because of their more active involvement in religious groups that promote abstinence (Harper 1976).

Women in general are said to have had lower alcoholism rates because of the cultural mores that have prohibited women from public drinking and heavy alcohol intake. Some speculate that as more opportunities for drinking alcohol become available to women, the rate of alcoholism among women will rise. The current ratio of male to female alcoholics is 3 : 1.

Theories centering on drinking practices in general place much emphasis on the learning experiences of adolescents. Social practices that encourage drinking as an adult mode of behavior may result in strong pressures to drink. Education about the role of alcohol in one's life and some exposure to it at home (e.g., sampling with meals), may mitigate some of the social pressures toward excessive, frequent alcohol consumption. The higher rates of alcoholism in alcoholic and teetotaling families are thought to derive from this lack of exposure to and thinking about the social role of alcohol.

In summary, *there is no single cause of alcoholism. Multiple factors come to bear to produce this disease in any specific individual.* For example, a child of an alcoholic may have a biochemical deficiency predisposing the child to alcoholism and may grow up with low self-esteem in a society that has no rituals governing alcohol use. Because of complex biological, psychological, and sociocultural factors, this person is at risk for developing alcoholism.

DEFINITIONS

The lack of consensus on the etiology has made precise definition of alcoholism difficult. The *World Health Organization* (WHO) (1952) defined alcoholics as those excessive drinkers whose dependence on alcohol has attained such a degree that there is an interference with the person's mental, physical, social, and economic well-being or those who show prodromal signs of such development. Put simply, if you have or are developing significant problems in any area of life functioning owing to your alcohol intake, then you have an alcohol problem.

In 1977, the Committee on Alcohol Related Disabilities of WHO endorsed the term *alcohol dependence syndrome* to emphasize the existence of a *recognizable pattern of clinical phenomena* (Edwards et al. 1977). The essential features of this syndrome follow (Mandell 1983):

- Regularity of drinking behavior
- Emphasis on drink-seeking behavior
- Increased tolerance for alcohol
- Repeated withdrawal symptoms that are alleviated by further drinking
- Subjective awareness of a compulsion to drink
- A tendency to relapse

The diagnostic scheme in the DSM III-R (APA 1987) focuses on the behavioral aspects and the pathological pattern of use, emphasizing the physical symptoms of tolerance and withdrawal. The term alcoholism is replaced by the label alcohol dependence. Also, a distinction is made between alcohol abuse and dependence (alcoholism).

The DSM III-R criteria for psychoactive substance dependence is presented in Box 23–1. In this scheme, the duration of symptoms is taken into account. In the case of abuse, the symptoms must last no less than one month; in the case of dependence symptoms, they last longer.

Diagnostic criteria for alcohol intoxication, alcohol hallucinosis, alcohol amnestic disorder, and dementia associated with alcoholism are shown in Box 23–2. Uncomplicated alcohol withdrawal and alcohol withdrawal delirium (D.T.'s) are organic mental disorders discussed in Chapter 21.

As can be seen, terms describing various patterns of alcohol use have been as confusing as definitions. Definitions of use shown in Figure 23–2 will be used throughout this chapter. The terms *addiction* and *alcoholism* will be used interchangeably. The term *abuse* will be avoided because it is value-laden. The most useful definition for assessment purposes is the WHO definition, which associates addiction with resultant problems.

Standard II: Data Collection

An objective assessment strategy allows nurses to obtain concrete data useful in diagnosis, planning, referral, and treatment. Most of the information needed for a complete and accurate health assessment is obtained by means of the nursing history. Nurses do basic screening histories on all of their clients. This is the time to begin asking about alcohol use. Since it is relatively recently that alcoholism has been considered a disease, many nurses are not sure of how to ask questions about what was formerly perceived as a "personal matter." The following pointers are helpful in the alcohol history–taking process:

1. Begin by asking the client about the use of *prescribed drugs*. The client is usually generally honest about these, since they are ordered by a physician and thus perceived to be needed. From the answer to this question an impression can be gained about the person's drug orientation. Some people will express their practice of using medications only when absolutely required (e.g., antibiotics for specific infections). Others will begin grumbling that they cannot get the correct prescriptions from any of the doctors

Box 23–1. DSM III-R CRITERIA FOR PSYCHOACTIVE SUBSTANCE DEPENDENCE

A. At least three of the following:
   1. Substance often taken in larger amounts or over a longer period than the person intended
   2. Persistent desire or one or more unsuccessful efforts to cut down or control substance use
   3. A great deal of time spent in activities necessary to get the substance (e.g., theft), taking the substance (e.g., chain-smoking), or recovering from its effects
   4. Frequent intoxication or withdrawal symptoms when expected to fulfill major role obligations at work, school, or home (e.g., does not go to work because is hung-over, goes to school or work "high," intoxicated while taking care of his or her children), or substance use when it is physically hazardous (e.g., drives when intoxicated)
   5. Important social, occupational, or recreational activities given up or reduced because of substance use
   6. Continued substance use despite knowledge of having a persistent or recurrent social, psychological, or physical problem that is caused or exacerbated by the use of the substance (e.g., keeps using heroin despite family arguments about it, cocaine-induced depression, or having an ulcer made worse by drinking)
   7. Marked tolerance: need for markedly increased amounts of the substance (i.e., at least 50% increase) in order to achieve intoxication or desired effect; or markedly diminished effect with continued use of the same amount

   NOTE: The following items may not apply to cannabis, hallucinogens, or phencyclidine (PCP):

   8. Characteristic withdrawal symptoms (see specific withdrawal syndromes under *Psychoactive Substance–Induced Organic Mental Disorders*)
   9. Substance often taken to relieve or avoid withdrawal symptoms

B. Some symptoms of the disturbance have persisted for at least one month or have occurred repeatedly over a longer period of time

Criteria for Severity of Psychoactive Substance Dependence

Mild: Few, if any, symptoms in excess of those required to make the diagnosis, and the symptoms result in no more than mild impairment in occupational functioning or in usual social activities or relationships with others

Moderate: Symptoms or functional impairment between "mild" and "severe"

Severe: Many symptoms in excess of those required to make the diagnosis, and the symptoms markedly interfere with occupational functioning or with usual social activities or relationships with others.*

In Partial Remission: During the past six months, some use of the substance and some symptoms of dependence

In Full Remission: During the past six months, either no use of the substance or some use of the substance with no symptoms of dependence

*Because of the availability of cigarettes and other nicotine-containing substances and the absence of a clinically significant nicotine intoxication syndrome, impairment in occupational or social functioning is not necessary for a rating of severe nicotine dependence.

they see. "Doctor shopping" and repeated client requests for medications, especially psychotropic medications, are indicators of a possible drug problem. Keep these responses in mind when asking other questions.

2. Next, question the person about *over-the-counter-drugs*. Many do not consider these substances drugs because they are so readily available and advertised. This questioning provides an opportunity for client education about drug effects.

Box 23–2. DSM III-R CRITERIA FOR ALCOHOL INTOXICATION, HALLUCINOSIS, AMNESTIC DISORDERS, AND ALCOHOLISM-ASSOCIATED DEMENTIA*

Alcohol Intoxication

A. Recent ingestion of alcohol (with no evidence suggesting that the amount was insufficient to cause intoxication in most people)
B. Maladaptive behavioral effects—e.g., fighting, impaired judgment, interference with social or occupational functioning
C. At least one of the following physiological signs:
   1. Slurred speech
   2. Incoordination
   3. Unsteady gait
   4. Nystagmus
   5. Flushed face
D. Not due to any other physical or mental disorder

Alcohol Idiosyncratic Intoxication

A. Maladaptive behavioral change—e.g., aggressive or assaultive behavior occurring within minutes of ingesting an amount of alcohol insufficient to induce intoxication in most people
B. The behavior is atypical of the person when not drinking
C. Not due to any other physical or mental disorder

Alcohol Hallucinosis

A. Organic hallucinosis with vivid and persistent auditory or visual hallucinations developing shortly (usually within 48 hours) after cessation of or reduction in heavy ingestion of alcohol in an individual who apparently has alcohol dependence
B. No clouding of consciousness, as in alcohol withdrawal delirium
C. Not due to any other physical or mental disorder

Alcohol Amnestic Disorder

A. Amnestic syndrome following prolonged heavy ingestion of alcohol
B. Not due to any other physical or mental disorder

Dementia Associated With Alcoholism

A. Dementia following prolonged, heavy ingestion of alcohol and persisting for at least three weeks after cessation of alcohol
B. Exclusion of all other causes of dementia, other than prolonged, heavy use of alcohol, by the history, the physical examination, and laboratory tests

---

*For uncomplicated alcohol withdrawal and alcohol withdrawal delirium, see Chapter 21.

3. Finally, ask the person about *self-prescribed drugs*. The client may be puzzled or bewildered about this category of drugs. An explanation that caffeine and nicotine are drugs, followed by an assessment of their use by the client, sets the stage for the drinking history. Emphasize the fact that alcohol is a commonly used drug. Elicit the role that alcohol plays in the everyday functioning of the client. For example, How much do you drink each day? Is alcohol used throughout the day? Under what circumstances is it used? Not used? How much is drunk on a given occasion? Is it beer, wine, or hard liquor? (See Figure 23–3 for alcohol equivalents.) What happens when drinking is curtailed? Questioning should not stop

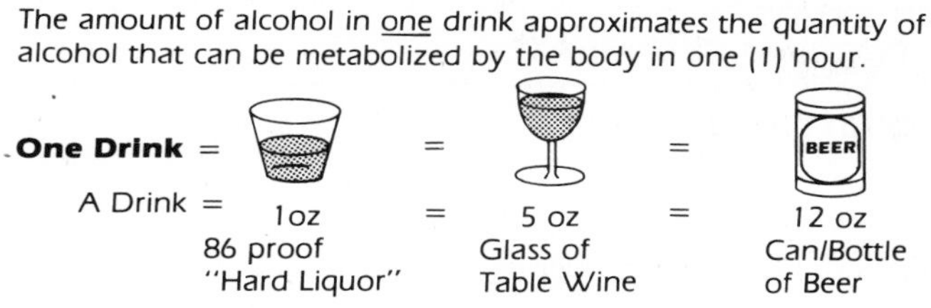

The amount of alcohol in one drink approximates the quantity of alcohol that can be metabolized by the body in one (1) hour.

Figure 23-3. *Alcohol equivalents.*

until you have asked the client about a whole array of prescribed and nonprescribed drugs. Multidrug use is the norm, and nurses must be on the lookout for it, since drugs determine the client's presenting symptoms.

How a person responds to interview questions is a significant factor for assessment purposes. The majority of people give thoughtful, matter-of-fact responses that suggest no alcohol problem. Some will express concern and ask for information and referral. It may have been the first time anyone has asked about their alcohol use! Others will say that they abstain from alcohol. The reasons for abstinence are important. Do they abstain for religious or health reasons? Are they acknowledged alcoholics in recovery? Are they trying to prove to someone else that they can be abstinent? For example: "My husband thinks I drink too much so I'm going to show him. I'm not going to have a drop for two weeks. I can take it or leave it." Such a response indicates possible problems, and further assessment is required. Other responses that serve as "red flag" indicators for the need for further assessment are rationalizations—"You'd drink, too, if . . . "; automatic responses, as if predicted; or very slow, prolonged responses, as if the person is being very careful about what to say. Last are the practicing alcoholics who admit they have a problem but project an air of hopelessness about ever achieving sobriety (Estes and Heinemann 1986).

ASSESSING SEVERITY OF ILLNESS

It is useful at this point to incorporate the CAGE questionnaire as part of the assessment protocol. This questionnaire consists of four questions that focus on the main idea of **C**utting down alcohol consumption. **A**nnoyance by criticism of drinking, **G**uilty feelings associated with alcohol use, and **E**ye-openers, or early morning drinking. The title of the questionnaire was derived by extracting the first letter of the four main ideas, formulating the acronym **CAGE.** The specific questions follow (Mayfield et al. 1974):

1. Have you ever felt you should **C***ut down on your drinking*?
2. Have people **A***nnoyed you by criticizing your drinking*?
3. Have you ever felt bad or **G***uilty about your drinking*?
4. Have you ever had a drink first thing in the morning to steady your nerves or get rid of a hangover (**E***ye-opener*)?

Two or three "yes" answers to these questions strongly suggest dependence on alcohol, especially physical dependence in terms of the inability to cut down and the need for an eye-opener (refer to Figure 23–2).

The **MAST (Michigan Alcohol Screening Test)** questionnaire is useful for determining the extent of life problems associated with alcohol use and is shown in Figure 23–4. The MAST questions can be asked verbally in interview form. When used in this manner, questions can be clarified. The more areas of life functioning that are affected by alcohol use, the more severe is the person's alcohol problem.

Note Question No. 3 in the MAST questionnaire regarding periods of amnesia, alcohol-induced amnesia, or blackouts. **Blackouts** are periods in which a person has no recollection of events and behaviors while intoxicated, although the person's state of consciousness may not be abnormal when observed by others. Blackouts can occur at any time during the progression of the disease; however, severity and duration of alcoholism usually correlate with the occurrence of blackouts (Frances and Franklin 1988).

ASSESSING LEVELS OF ANXIETY AND COPING STYLES

Alcoholic people are threatened on a number of different levels in their interactions with nurses. *First*, they are concerned about being rejected. Alcoholic clients are acutely aware of the fact that not all nurses are equally willing to care for people with alcoholism and, in fact, many clients may have experienced instances of rejection in past encounters with nursing personnel. Therefore, vulnerability is increased each time that they must interact with the health care system!

Second, alcoholic clients may be anxious about recovering because in order to do so they must give up the substance they think they need to survive—alcohol. *Third*, alcoholics are concerned about failing, not being able to succeed at recovering. Alcoholism is a chronic relapsing condition. In fact, relapse is one of the criteria for diagnosing addiction to alcohol (refer to Figure 23–2). Most alcoholics have tried recovery at least once before and have relapsed. As a result, many become discouraged about their chances of ever succeeding.

The above-mentioned concerns can threaten the alcoholic person's sense of security and sense of self, thus

• MICHIGAN ALCOHOL SCREENING TEST (MAST)

POINTS		QUESTIONS
(0)	1.	Do you enjoy a drink now and then?
(2)	2.	Do you feel you are a normal drinker?*
(2)	3.	Have you ever awakened the morning after some drinking the night before and found that you could not remember a part of the evening before?
(1)	4.	Does your spouse (or parents) ever worry or complain about your drinking?
(2)	5.	Can you stop drinking without a struggle after one or two drinks?*
(1)	6.	Do you ever feel bad about your drinking?
(2)	7.	Do friends and relatives think you are a normal drinker?*
(0)	8.	Do you ever try to limit your drinking to certain times of the day or to certain places?
(2)	9.	Are you always able to stop drinking when you want to?*
(4)x	10.	Have you ever attended a meeting of Alcoholics Anonymous (AA)?
(1)	11.	Have you ever gotten into fights when drinking?
(2)	12.	Has drinking ever created problems with you and your spouse?
(2)	13.	Has your spouse (or other family member) ever gone to anyone for help about your drinking?
(2)	14.	Have you ever lost friends or girl- or boyfriends because of drinking?
(2)	15.	Have you ever gotten into trouble at work because of drinking?
(2)	16.	Have you ever lost a job because of drinking?
(2)	17.	Have you ever neglected your obligations, your family, or your work for two or more days because you were drinking?
(1)	18.	Do you ever drink before noon?
(2)	19.	Have you ever been told you have liver trouble? Cirrhosis?
(2)	20.	After heavy drinking, have you ever had delirium tremens (D.T.'s), severe shaking, heard voices, or seen things that were not there?
(4)	21.	Have you ever gone to anyone for help about your drinking?
(4)	22.	Have you ever been in a hospital because of drinking?
(0)	23.	(a) Have you ever been a patient in a psychiatric hospital or on a psychiatric ward of a general hospital?
(2)x		(b) Was drinking part of the problem that resulted in hospitalization?
(0)	24.	(a) Have you ever been seen at a psychiatric or mental health clinic or gone to any doctor, social worker, or clergyman for help with an emotional problem?
(2)x		(b) Was drinking part of the problem?
(2)	25.	Have you ever been arrested, even for a few hours, because of drunk behavior?
(2)	26.	Have you ever been arrested for drunk driving after drinking?

*Positive responses are "alcoholic" responses.
A total of four or more points is presumptive evidence of alcoholism, and a 5-point total would make it extremely unlikely that the individual was not alcoholic.
A positive response to 10, 23, or 24 would be diagnostic; a positive response indicates alcoholism.
Reprinted with permission from Journal of Studies on Alcohol, vol. 36, pp. 117–126, 1975. Copyright by Journal of Studies on Alcohol, Inc., Rutgers Center of Alcohol Studies, New Brunswick, NJ 08903.

Figure 23-4. *Michigan Alcohol Screening Test* (MAST).

increasing anxiety levels. In order to protect against overwhelming anxiety, the alcoholic establishes a **preferred defensive structure (PDS)** (Wallace 1986). The elements of the PDS follow:

1. *Denial.* Deliberate denial of certain life difficulties is a useful method of coping.
2. *Projection.* The tendency to assume that others are very much like oneself and to perceive them as such, as in "*It takes one to know one.*"
3. *All-or-none thinking.* Allows for structured, restricted choices and highly certain communication.
4. *Conflict minimization and avoidance.* The alcoholic will go to great lengths to reduce conflict. Conflict, after all, increases anxiety.
5. *Rationalization.* "The alcohol made me do it." "You'd drink, too, if . . . "
6. *Self-centered selective attention.* Only attending to what can be coped with is an effective way to minimize anxiety.
7. *Preference for nonanalytical modes of thinking and perceiving.* For example, being influenced more by emotion and what "feels good."
8. *Passivity versus assertion.*
9. *Obsessional focusing.* When the alcoholic spends a lot of energy procuring and ingesting alcohol, there is

little left with which to focus on problems that the alcohol may be causing.

The PDS is a collection of skills and abilities for achieving one's ends. It should be challenged only when more functional tactics and strategies are in place for diminishing anxiety. This will be discussed further in V-F: *Psychotherapy*.

Manipulation is another behavior that the alcoholic uses in order to minimize anxiety. The alcoholic engages in manipulation merely to get needs met. Having had numerous experiences in which needs were not met, the alcoholic person may no longer trust nurses, or most people, to respond to their concerns. The alcoholic also is not able to communicate needs assertively (characteristic No. 8 in the PDS list). Manipulation occurs when there is a conflict of goals between the manipulator and the nurse. It involves intentional, deceptive behavior that, when successful, results in exhilaration at having put "something over" on the other party (Bursten 1972).

Manipulation need not be a frustrating experience for the nurse if it is recognized and thwarted. The following behaviors may indicate that manipulation is occurring (Burgess and Lazare 1976; Estes et al. 1980):

1. *Making many demands*. "I haven't eaten in a week. I'm hungry." "Can you please tell the doctor I'm very uncomfortable? I need more help with withdrawal." "When do I get to leave?"
2. *Pressuring a person or forcing an issue*. "Did you say anything to the doctor?"
3. *Violating rules, routines, procedures*. Examples are the people who sneak alcohol into the hospital rooms so that they will not be deprived of their drug.
4. *Requesting special privileges*. "I'm uncomfortable having people see me in this hospital gown. May I smoke in my room—just this once?"
5. *Playing staff and clients off; playing staff against each other*. An example of the former is one client saying to another: "What do you do to irritate the nurses so?" An example of the latter is: "The evening nurse said I could smoke in my room. Why won't *you* let me?"
6. *Threatening*. "Wait until my doctor hears about this!"
7. *Betraying confidences*. "He told me not to tell but . . . "

Acknowledging the manipulative behavior is useful in order to resolve the immediate issue effectively.

ASSESSING LEVEL OF ALCOHOL IN BODY SYSTEM AND PHYSIOLOGICAL CHANGES

In order to more thoroughly assess the client addicted to alcohol, it is important to know the person's **blood alcohol level (BAL).** Knowing the BAL assists in determining the level of intoxication, level of tolerance, and whether the person accurately reported recent drinking during the nursing history. These factors are also assessed by means of behavioral cues. The relationship between blood alcohol level and behavior in a *nontolerant* individual is shown in Table 23-1.

When tolerance is built up, there is a discrepancy between the blood alcohol level and expected behavior. A person who has developed a tolerance to alcohol may have high blood alcohol levels (BAL) with minimal signs of impairment. For example, a person presented in the emergency room with a BAL of 0.51. He was stuporous, ataxic, and had slurred speech. The fact that he was still alive indicated a high tolerance for alcohol. A nursing history conducted when the client sobered up revealed an extensive drinking history. When this is the case, assessing for withdrawal symptoms is important (see V-D: *Somatic Therapies*).

Table 23-1 • RELATIONSHIP BETWEEN BLOOD ALCOHOL LEVELS AND BEHAVIOR IN A NONTOLERANT DRINKER

BAL	BLOOD ALCOHOL ACCUMULATION (BAC)	BEHAVIOR
0.05 mg%	1-2 Drinks	Changes in mood and behavior; judgment is impaired
0.10 mg%	5-6 Drinks	Voluntary motor action becomes clumsy; legal level of intoxication in most states
0.20 mg%	10-12 Drinks	Function of entire motor area of the brain is depressed, causing staggering and ataxia; emotional lability is present
0.30 mg%	15-18 Drinks	Confusion; stupor
0.40 mg%	20-24 Drinks	Coma
0.50 mg%	25-30 Drinks	Death due to respiratory depression

BAL = Blood alcohol level.
BAC = Blood alcohol accumulation *in excess of* alcohol metabolized.

The presence of alcohol in the body results in associated physiological problems. A listing of physical problems associated with alcohol use is presented in Box 23–3. A nursing history, physical examination, and laboratory tests are methods used to gather data about alcohol-related physical problems. The extent of impairment depends on individual susceptibility as well as on the amount of heavy drinking.

A thorough nursing history is designed to elicit information about the various physical and psychosocial problems that can occur in people dependent on alcohol. A detailed guide entitled "Guide For Nursing History of Persons With Alcohol Problems" has been developed by Estes and Heinemann (1986). Questions are asked about the alcoholic person's view of current status, family, and psychosocial and drinking histories. Also, questions are designed, in a detailed health history, to elicit information about alcohol's effect on each body system. The client is also asked about the use of other drugs.

The drinking history component of this nursing history guide deserves special mention because it is useful for estimating the degree of addiction as well as the likelihood of withdrawal. Questions are asked to determine how long the client has been drinking, including asking about how long problems with alcohol have been present. Information about the quantity and frequency of drinking is important, and relevant questions

Box 23–3. PHYSIOLOGICAL EFFECTS OF ALCOHOL USE*

Metabolic

Hypoglycemia
Hyperlipidemia
Hyperuricemia

Gastrointestinal System

Increased incidence of cancer of the oral mucosa
Increased acid production
Nausea and vomiting; diarrhea
Esophagitis and varices
Malabsorption of nutrients, especially folic acid, vitamin B_1 (thiamine), and vitamin B_{12}
Ulcers—gastric and duodenal
Gastritis, enteritis, colitis, hemorrhoids
Fatty liver, alcoholic hepatitis, cirrhosis
Pancreatitis

Neurological System

Sleep disturbance
Peripheral neuropathies
Brain syndromes
Wernicke-Korsakoff's syndrome
Cerebellar degeneration

Cardiovascular System

Hypertension, tachycardia due to withdrawal
Decreased mechanical performance of the heart
Cardiomyopathy, after ten or more years

Respiratory System

Impaired diffusion
Increased incidence of lung infections—e.g., bronchitis, pneumonias
Smoking effects—e.g., chronic obstructive pulmonary disease (COPD)

Genitourinary System

Increased urinary excretion of potassium and magnesium leads to hypomagnesemia and hypokalemia
Hypogonadism, hypoandrogenization, hyperestrogenization in men
Diminished sexual performance
Impotency in males
Decreased menstruation, leading to infertility

Musculoskeletal System

Myopathies

Skin

Infections
Lesions, burns, scars

Hematological System

Anemias
Impaired phagocytosis, which reduces body's response to invasion by bacteria
Leukopenia, which can affect the body's immune system
Hematomas

*For discussion of uncomplicated alcohol withdrawal and alcohol withdrawal delirium, refer to Chapter 21.

Used with permission from Smith-DiJulio K. Nursing people experiencing dependence on alcohol and other drugs. *In* Luckmann J, Sorensen K.C. Medical-Surgical Nursing: A Psychophysiologic Approach, 3rd ed. Philadelphia: W.B. Saunders Company, 1987, pp. 1836–1866.

include the following:

- *What do you drink?*
- *How much do you drink? Do you ever drink more? How often?*
- *When did you start this drinking bout?*
- *When did you have your last drink?*
- *What have you been drinking? How much per day?* (*Be certain to ask about beer, wine, and liquor individually. The more you ask, the more information you are likely to obtain.*)
- *What kind of problems has alcohol caused for you? With your family? Friends? Job? Health? Finances? The law?*

With the preceding information, you can make more accurate plans for intervention.

ASSESSING PSYCHOLOGICAL CHANGES

It is self-evident that alcohol use affects a person's behavior. Certain psychological characteristics are associated frequently with alcohol use, including denial, depression, dependency, hopelessness, low self-esteem, and various psychiatric disorders. Often it is difficult to determine which came first, psychological changes or drinking behavior. Some people self-medicate in order to cope with psychiatric symptoms. For these people, symptoms of psychological difficulty remain even after months of sobriety. While obtaining a nursing history, questions that attempt to determine whether drinking occurred as an attempt to cope with either a dysphoric or an elated mood can be helpful. Psychological changes that occurred as a result of drinking clear rather quickly with sobriety.

Psychiatric disorders that may be seen concurrently in alcoholics include acute and chronic organic mental syndromes, attention deficit disorder, schizophrenia, borderline personality disorder, antisocial personality disorder, anxiety disorders, and disorders of mood (McKelvey et al. 1987; Schuckit 1984).

Mood disorders and schizophrenia are the two most commonly reported forms of mental illness seen in persons with alcoholism. Close attention to mental status will often provide clues to these disorders. If clear-cut alcohol dependency is present along with a well-defined psychiatric disorder, conservative treatment consists of viewing both disorders as primary **(dual diagnosis)** and treating each separately. Since most alcohol dependencies are great "mimickers," a long, well-monitored detoxification period, in order to observe for the appearance or disappearance of mental symptoms, is appropriate. This often requires skilled psychiatric nursing care to deal with the transition created when a detoxifying client begins to develop major psychiatric problems that must be treated also. Since the majority of psychotropic medications interact adversely with alcohol, trying to treat psychiatric illness in an active alcoholic is discouraged. Alcohol also interferes with medication compliance. Many clinicians are familiar with the well-stabilized bipolar or schizophrenic client who begins to use alcohol, subsequently disrupts or stops taking psychiatric medication, and ends up being rehospitalized for stabilization of his or her disorder.

Denial has become the hallmark psychological characteristic of alcoholism, with the alcoholic person bearing the brunt of the blame for not admitting to having a disease, seeking treatment, and getting cured. **Denial** is a defense mechanism used to avoid the anxiety associated with having to admit something painful or difficult. It is true that the alcoholic person tends to deny having a problem with alcohol, but family and friends often deny the same problem. Also, society denies the problem of alcoholism by failing to allocate funds for alcoholism research, prevention, treatment, and rehabilitation. Nurses and other health care professionals deny the problem by ignoring its existence in their clients. This can result from feelings of hopelessness and helplessness in treating alcoholism, owing to gaps in current knowledge of how to do so.

ASSESSING SOCIAL CHANGES AND AVAILABLE SUPPORT SYSTEMS

Deterioration in a person's social status and social relationships often occurs as a result of alcoholism. Job demotion or loss of job, with resultant reduced or nonexistent income may occur. Meeting basic needs for food, shelter, and clothing is thereby hampered. Marriages and other close relationships deteriorate and fail, and the person often finds him- or herself alone and isolated. This lack of interpersonal and social supports is an important factor in treatment planning for the alcoholic person.

Standard III: Diagnosis

Appropriate nursing diagnoses depend on an accurate assessment. While the DSM III-R criteria emphasize patterns of use and physical symptoms, nursing diagnoses identify how dependence on alcohol interferes with a person's ability to meet the activities and demands of daily living.

According to the physical, emotional, and social circumstances of the alcoholic person, nursing diagnoses can be many and varied. Table 23–2 identifies a variety of nursing diagnoses appropriate for use in all hospital settings.

Alcohol impairs health status. When intoxicated, the person is not concerned with being healthy, and often does not, or cannot, take responsibility for basic care. Therefore, *altered health maintenance* may be evident.

Alcohol impairs judgment and increases risk-taking behaviors. *Injury* often results. With long term dependence, changes in blood profiles occur. For example, liver function test results are elevated and hemoglobin (Hb) and hematocrit (Hct) are decreased. A multitude of changes occur after long term heavy alcohol use that affect the body's immune system and cardiovascular, gastrointestinal (GI), and genitourinary (GU) functioning. Potential for seizures, falls, and accidents is increased; therefore, the *potential for injury* is present.

Disturbance in self-esteem or *chronic low self-esteem* is evidenced by projection of blame/responsibility for problems, denial of problems obvious to others, rationalizations, and expressions of shame/guilt. Low self-esteem is also reflected in the person's self-destructive behaviors and in nonparticipation in health-seeking behaviors.

As with any other disease, alcoholism represents a dysfunction or maladaption to the requirements of everyday life (Gitlow 1988) affecting the person's family, social, and occupational functioning. The use of alcohol becomes the main coping device. The disease can progress to the point at which the individual is unable to meet basic needs. Also, related illnesses become prominent and perhaps life-threatening, accidents increase as a result of intoxication, and denial becomes a major barrier to change. Sometimes coping becomes impossible, and suicide is attempted. Therefore, *ineffective individual coping* is prominent.

The family goes through many changes as the disease progresses. Family members begin to assume responsibilities for the alcoholic member, communications become dysfunctional, and often the family's activities

Table 23–2 • NURSING DIAGNOSES COMMONLY ASSOCIATED WITH THE ABUSE OF ALCOHOL

NURSING DIAGNOSIS	COMMENTS
Activity intolerance	Malnutrition
Activity intolerance, potential	Peripheral neuropathies Bacterial endocarditis
Airway clearance, ineffective	Pneumonias
Anxiety	Actual or potential alcohol/drug withdrawal Abstinence
Diarrhea	Inflammation, irritation of the bowel due to alcohol ingestion Black, tarry stools from gastrointestinal bleeding
Breathing pattern, ineffective	Alcohol or drug overdose
Cardiac output, decreased	Alcoholic cardiomyopathy
Coping, ineffective family: disabling	Social patterns often become dysfunctional
Coping, ineffective individual	A drug-dependent person has come to see alcohol (drugs) as the solution to every problem; excessive drug-taking is maladaptive, and problem-solving abilities are impaired ● Loses most or all significant others ● Not able to perform on the job ● Usually does not meet basic needs ● Risk of suicide increases ● Denial becomes a major barrier to overcome in effecting change ● Illness rates increase owing to effects of lifestyle as well as drugs ● Accident rate increases owing to intoxication
Fluid volume deficit, potential	Secondary to protracted vomiting or diarrhea
Health maintenance, altered	Choosing to take alcohol and other drugs impairs health status; when intoxicated, the person is not concerned with being healthy and often does not take responsibility for basic care
Injury, potential for	Alcohol/drugs impair judgment and increase risk-taking behavior; injury often results; with alcohol dependence, the blood profile becomes abnormal—liver function test results are elevated and hemoglobin (Hb) and hematocrit (Hct) are decreased
Trauma, potential for	Driving accidents

Table 23–2 • NURSING DIAGNOSES COMMONLY ASSOCIATED WITH THE ABUSE OF ALCOHOL *Continued*

NURSING DIAGNOSIS	COMMENTS
Knowledge deficit	Ignorance of alcohol/drug effects Ignorance of withdrawal process
Noncompliance	Resumption of alcohol/drug taking behavior after treatment
Nutrition, altered: less than body requirements	Nutritional deficits are frequent because an intoxicated person is not interested in food; money is spent on alcohol
Oral mucous membrane, altered	Combined with the effects of smoking, leads to an increased incidence of carcinoma of the oropharynx
Parenting, altered: actual or potential	Adults focused exclusively on their own needs to manage drug dependence do not pay attention to the needs of their children Ineffective role modeling Emotional neglect Increased incidence of physical, sexual abuse
Powerlessness	Central feelings in alcohol- and drug-dependent people
Disturbance in self-esteem **Chronic low self-esteem**	Evidenced by the self-destructive nature of alcohol/drug dependence and by nonparticipation in treatment. Not taking responsibility for self
Sensory-perceptual altered: auditory-visual	Audiovisual hallucinations due to withdrawal
Sexual dysfunction	Alcohol/drug abuse and dependence interfere with sexual arousal and performance: • Impotence in men • Decreased vaginal lubrication in women
Sleep pattern disturbance	CNS depressants interfere with REM (rapid eye movement) and Stage IV (deep) sleep
Thought processes, altered	Judgment impaired; memory deficits with Wernicke-Korsakoff's syndrome; when intoxicated, the alcohol/drug dependent person is less able to grasp ideas, reason, solve problems, calculate, attend to task
Violence, self-harm, or potential for	Increased risk of suicide; increased incidence of child abuse, domestic violence, including battered woman syndrome

Used with permission from Smith-DiJulio K. Nursing people experiencing dependence on alcohol and other drugs. *In* Luckmann J, Sorensen KC. Medical-Surgical Nursing: A Psychophysiologic approach, 3rd ed. Philadelphia: W.B. Saunders Company, 1987, pp. 1861–1862.

and energies are organized around the disease and the affected member. Families may go from crisis to crisis, and maladaptions to crises may be evident in the form of spouse abuse or child abuse, and thus, *ineffective family coping* may be present.

Standard IV: Planning

On completion of the assessment process, identified problems are assigned priorities and a plan of care is developed. A plan of care is a guide to action toward improvement or recovery from alcoholism (Estes and Heinemann 1986). Planning care is guided by the (1) content level—goals—and (2) process level—nurses' reactions and feelings.

CONTENT LEVEL—PLANNING GOALS

Planning care that may be effective in treating alcoholism requires attention to social status, income, ethnic background, sex, and age, since all these contribute to an individual's personality, behavior, and growth. The goals guide nursing interventions; thus the goals need to be compatible with the person's personality, desired behaviors, and potential for growth. Therefore, goals for treatment need to be developed *with* the alcoholic person and reflect his or her desires and expectations for the future. Both short term and long term goals must be established.

Long term goals are usually more global and tend to be viewed as the end product of a hard struggle—for example, sobriety. Gitlow (1988) stated that sobriety or abstinence is not actually the aim of treatment but is a means to an end. The end, or real purpose of treatment, is to improve function and the person's quality of life.

However, improvement in life cannot take place without sobriety or abstinence for an alcoholic person. Improvement in life is not compatible with the ingestion of alcohol. According to Gitlow (1988), improvement can occur only when there is

1. Diminishment in psychomotor activity associated with alcohol ingestion. Use of alcohol results in prolonged and intermittent agitation, enormously uncomfortable for the alcoholic.
2. Control of organic pathology. Almost every complication of alcoholism requires abstinence for a maximal rate of improvement. Medical therapy in the presence of active drinking fails to achieve a satisfactory recovery.
3. Potential for change and insight. It is impossible to develop insight when cognitive functioning is impaired and the brain is sedated. "It's hard to learn to navigate from the deck of a sinking ship."

Therefore, for *ineffective individual coping* related to biochemical changes caused by alcohol ingestion, the goals would be as follows:

Long Term Goals

- Client will maintain sobriety.

Short Term Goals

- Client will attend Alcoholics Anonymous (AA) every night for one month.
- Client will be actively involved with his or her sponsor.
- Client will participate in treatment center after-care group and individual and/or family counseling.
- Client will name two people to call when experiencing an urge to drink.
- Client will participate in relapse prevention training (identifying the individual's high-risk situations for drinking).
- Client will name two "problem areas" that he or she wants to work on.

Another important area for initial intervention is in the area of self-esteem. Therefore, for the nursing diagnosis *disturbance in self-esteem* or *chronic low self-esteem* the goals might be as follows:

Long Term Goals

- Client will state that he or she feels good about himself or herself and about the potential for the future.
- Client will demonstrate responsibility in implementing personal treatment goals.
- Client will demonstrate responsibility in implementing personal life goals.

Short Term Goals

- Client will state that AA is assisting him or her to "live one day at a time."
- Client will participate in social skills training.
- Client will role-play assertive communication skills to get needs met and maintain self-esteem.
- Client will demonstrate one new skill learned each week.
- Client will discuss negative aspects of his or her life while keeping the focus on ways to effect positive change.
- Client will state that he or she is more comfortable accepting positive feedback from others regarding personal strengths and positive qualities.

PROCESS LEVEL—NURSES' REACTIONS AND FEELINGS

It is not only within the nursing community but also in the whole medical community that ambivalence, frustration, and confusion operate in the treatment of alcoholism. Gitlow (1988) states, "The special reticence with which the medical community has approached alcoholism demands a greater endeavor for its understanding. Does alcoholism, because of its societal and moral implications, awaken discomfort and fear within the physician? . . . and in the nurse?"

A nurse might want to help but may perceive the alcoholic to be willful, uncooperative, and unworkable. The nurse may doubt whether alcoholism is indeed a disease.

Alcoholism is a disease of complex etiology involving many factors—mental, physical, genetic, and environmental. Nurses and physicians must be convinced that alcoholism is a disorder, an illness, a disease, and not a weakness, a nastiness, or someone's "fault" (Block 1988). What do we think alcoholism is?

Are we affected by societal stereotypes—for example, middle aged, shabby, hedonistic, irresponsible, unemployed, or in some low status job? If alcoholics are viewed as somehow different from ourselves, it will be doubly difficult to recognize the disease in our clients, in our colleagues, or in ourselves until it is far advanced (Bissell 1988).

To really come to a personal understanding means that one must examine one's own attitudes, feelings, and beliefs about alcoholism and "alcoholics." It often means that one must examine one's own drinking and that of others, and this is not always pleasant work (Bissell 1988).

The presence of alcohol in a nurse's own family can overshadow the nurse's interactions with alcoholics.

The negative or positive experiences a nurse has had with alcoholics will color all interpersonal interactions with present or future alcoholic clients.

Therefore, it is important to attend to personal feelings that arise when working with alcoholic people. All health care professionals require supervision if they are not experienced in this area. Nurses who do not attend to and work through expected negative feelings that arise during treatment end up in power struggles with the clients, and the therapeutic process becomes generally ineffective.

Adult children of alcoholics (ACoA) may have problems of **codependency.** A codependent is a family member who alternately rescues and blames the alcoholic. The rescuing component is often referred to as **enabling.** Enabling is helping the alcoholic avoid experiencing the consequences of his or her drinking. Enabling behaviors include making social and job excuses, taking over the alcoholic's chores, and bailing him or her out of difficult situations resulting from the alcoholic's drinking behaviors. Children of alcoholics may end up "taking care of" the alcoholic parent in order to maintain stability within the family. The rescuing, or enabling, aspect of family members can help intensify the alcoholic's denial. There are nationwide self-help groups for family members and friends who are living with, or are closely involved with, an alcoholic. These will be briefly introduced here, since they will be mentioned throughout the chapter.

Self-help groups formed to help family members of alcoholics deal with many common issues are independent of Alcoholics Anonymous (AA) but share many elements of a common belief system structured by the use of AA's "twelve steps" as their philosophical and operational guide (Ablon 1986).

The twelve steps of AA are presented in Box 23–4. **Al-Anon** is a support group for spouses and friends of alcoholics. Al-Anon, like AA, Al-a-Teen, and ACoA (discussed below), works through a combination of educational and operational principles. For example, alcoholism is a disease of the body and the mind, not a moral or perverse whim of the alcoholic (Ablon 1986). This acceptance of the disease concept of alcoholism can remove burdens of guilt, hostility, and shame from family members (Ablon 1986). Al-Anon also offers pragmatic methods for avoiding "enabling."

Al-a-Teen is a nationwide network for children over ten years old who have alcoholic parents. It is structured under the guidance of members of Al-Anon. It offers the teenager the chance to exchange feelings and problems with other teenagers going through similar experiences, which can be tremendously therapeutic.

Groups of **Adult Children of Alcoholics (ACoA)** offer support for those who often experience similar difficulties and problems in their adult life as a result of having an alcoholic parent or parents. Adult children of alcoholics were often deprived of a nurturing parent in their formative years.

Box 23–4. THE TWELVE STEPS OF ALCOHOLICS ANONYMOUS

1. *We admitted we were powerless over alcohol—that our lives had become unmanageable.*
2. *Came to believe that a power greater than ourselves could restore us to sanity.*
3. *Made a decision to turn our will and our lives over to the care of* God ***as we understood* Him.**
4. *Made a searching and fearless moral inventory of ourselves.*
5. *Admitted to* God, *to ourselves, and to another human being the exact nature of our wrongs.*
6. *Were entirely ready to have* God *remove all these defects of character.*
7. *Humbly asked* Him *to remove our shortcomings.*
8. *Made a list of all persons we had harmed, and became willing to make amends to them all.*
9. *Made direct amends to such people whenever possible, except when to do so would injure them or others.*
10. *Continued to take personal inventory, and when we were wrong, we promptly admitted it.*
11. *Sought through prayer and meditation to improve our conscious contact with* God ***as we understood* Him,** *praying only for knowledge of* His *will and the power to carry that out.*
12. *Having had a spiritual awakening as the result of these steps, we tried to carry* His *message to alcoholics, and to practice these principles in all our affairs.*

The Twelve Steps reprinted with permission of Alcoholics Anonymous World Services, Inc.

Standard V: Intervention

Nurses interact with alcoholics in all areas of nursing practice. General approaches to intervention that apply to all contexts of care are described here.

The aim, in alcoholism treatment, is toward self-responsibility, not compliance. A major challenge is predicting treatment outcome and improving treatment effectiveness by matching subtypes of clients to specific types of treatment. Although alcoholics share some characteristics and dynamics as a group, there are significant differences within the alcoholic population in regard to physiological, psychological, and sociocultural processes. These differences argue against the idea of a single alcoholic personality, and they support the classifying of subtypes of alcoholics. These differences also influence the recovery process, either positively or negatively. Until we get better at defining subtypes, treatment outcomes across types of treatment approaches and programs will remain essentially the same. The choice of inpatient or outpatient care often depends on cost and whether or not insurance coverage is available. Outpatient programs work best for employed alcoholics with involved social support systems. Those people without support and structure to their day often do better in inpatient programs.

In addition, neuropsychological deficits have been associated with long term drinking. Impairment has been found in abstract reasoning ability, ability to use feedback in learning new concepts, attention and concentration spans, cognitive flexibility, and subtle memory functions. These deficits undoubtedly impact on the process of alcoholism treatment (Walker et al. 1986).

General interventions with supporting rationales are presented in Table 23–3. Specific interventions will be discussed throughout the rest of the chapter.

V-A: PSYCHOTHERAPEUTIC INTERVENTIONS

Principles for psychotherapeutic interventions include the following (Zimberg 1978):

1. Expect sobriety. The distortions, memory loss, and confusion that occur as a result of intoxication make communication and intervention ineffective when the person is intoxicated.
2. Individualize goals and interventions.
3. Set limits on behavior and on conditions under which treatment will continue.
4. Support and redirect defenses rather than attempting to remove them.
5. Recognize that the process of recovery is carried out in stages.
6. Look for therapeutic leverage. Make sobriety worthwhile for the alcoholic (e.g., for keeping one's job, family, friends).

A popular tool for helping the resistant alcoholic person develop a willingness to engage in treatment is **the intervention** process developed by Johnson (1986). This technique can be useful as a response to the first stage of treatment when the alcoholic person has more need for external control. The concept behind *the intervention* is that alcoholism is a progressive illness and very rarely goes into remission without outside help. The strategies for *the intervention* are outlined in Box 23–5.

Table 23–3 • GENERAL INTERVENTIONS, WITH RATIONALE, FOR PEOPLE AFFECTED BY ALCOHOLISM

NURSING INTERVENTION	RATIONALE
1. Support/kindness.	1. Promotes ability to engage in treatment; minimizes anxiety.
2. Reinforce disease concept of addiction.	2. Decreases guilt associated with alcoholic behavior.
3. Effective communication.	3. Establishes trust; role-modeling.
4. Limit setting.	4. Promotes ability to engage in treatment.
5. Maintain consistency.	5. Fosters an objective and nonjudgmental milieu.
6. Education.	6. Client has learning needs related to • alcoholism as a chronic disease; • the development of alternative coping skills to deal with stressful or problematic feelings or situations; • nutrition, hygiene, infection control.
7. Family therapy.	7. Promotes sharing of feelings and identification of destructive patterns that exist within the family system.

Box 23–5. STEPS IN THE INTERVENTION

1. All the people concerned about and affected by the person's drinking are gathered together to present their case. The intervention must be rehearsed before it is actually carried out, usually with the support and guidance of a counselor.
2. Specific evidence related to the drinking is presented by each person, and it is written down so that each person does not have to rely on memory in a tense situation.
3. Timing must be right:
   - There must be current evidence available.
   - It must take place after a crisis is precipitated by alcohol use and *not* when the person is intoxicated or in severe withdrawal.
4. The intervention requires privacy. Hold it in a place where no interruptions can occur.
5. Anticipate the use of defenses. Do not react to them.
6. Demonstrate genuine, but firm, concern.
7. Understand alcoholism as a disease.
8. Present treatment alternatives.
9. Prepare responses to possible outcomes. The goal is to get the affected person treatment. If the alcoholic says yes to treatment, then he or she is taken immediately to a detoxification unit where arrangements have been previously made. If the alcoholic refuses, then family members state his or her decision must force them to make decisions of their own, since they are no longer willing to live with the alcoholic's behavior.

From Johnson VE. Intervention: How to Help Someone Who Doesn't Want Help. Minneapolis, MN; Johnson Books, 1986.

V-B: HEALTH TEACHING

Nurses must be very clear, when communicating with people in all walks of life, in stating that alcohol is a drug and, as such, can have negative consequences. Primary prevention programs aimed at youth must emphasize a "decision about drinking" theme and educate youngsters about the effect of alcohol on mental processes, physical processes, and mood. Teaching about alcohol's effects on unborn babies (NIAAA 1987) should occur in the preteen and teenage years as well as in gynecologists' offices and obstetrics clinics. Nurses can and must play an active role in counteracting the all too prevalent social message that alcohol is a harmless beverage and, in fact, is required for inclusion in many social groups. Groups such as Mothers Against Drunk Drivers (MADD) and Students Against Drunk Drivers (SADD) are natural allies in this effort.

V-D: SOMATIC THERAPIES

The predominant somatic therapies used in alcoholism treatment are those used for detoxification (management of withdrawal from alcohol) and disulfiram (Antabuse).

Not all people who stop drinking require inpatient hospitalization and drug management. This decision depends on the length of time and the amount the client has been drinking, prior history of withdrawal complications, and overall health status. In some instances, withdrawal can be life-threatening and needs to occur slowly in a supervised setting. The key to effective detoxification is adequate sedation. Medication should not be given until the symptoms of withdrawal are seen. Early withdrawal symptoms are tremors, diaphoresis, rapid pulse (greater than 100), elevated blood pressure (greater than 150/90), and occasional hallucinosis. Grand mal seizures can occur and are self-limited. The withdrawal process, not the seizure, needs to be treated.

Alcohol withdrawal delirium (D.T.'s) need not occur if withdrawal is managed well. Central nervous system (CNS) depressants, especially benzodiazepines (e.g., Librium, Valium) are the drugs of choice for withdrawal management. The goal is to reduce withdrawal symptoms to prevent alcohol withdrawal delirium (see Chapter 21 for treatment of alcohol withdrawal delirium).

Oversedation must be avoided. Alcoholics usually require high doses of medications because they are tolerant of the effects of CNS depressants as a result of their alcohol use. After symptom control is achieved, the drug dosage is gradually reduced, frequency of administration is lengthened, and the drug is gradually eliminated from the body.

Disulfiram (Antabuse) has been used in the treatment of alcoholism for over 30 years. It works on the classical conditioning principle. Disulfiram inhibits *impulsive* drinking because the client tries to avoid the unpleasant physical reaction involved in the alcohol-disulfiram reaction. This reaction consists of facial flushing, tachycardia, respiratory distress, a potentially serious drop in blood pressure, and nausea and vomiting. The adverse reaction usually begins within minutes to half an hour after drinking and may last 30 to 60 minutes. Consequently, disulfiram should not be prescribed for individuals with a history of serious heart disease, stroke, serious hypertension, or diabetes (Schuckit 1984).

Disulfiram must be taken daily. The action of the drug can last about five days after the last dose (Zuska and Pursch 1988), and rarely up to two weeks. It is most effectively used early in the recovery process while the individual is making the major life changes associated with long term recovery from alcoholism. Disulfiram should always be prescribed with the full knowledge and consent of the client. The client needs to be told about the side effects and be well aware that any substances that contain alcohol can trigger an adverse reaction. Substances such as

- mouthwashes
- after-shave lotions
- cough medicines (any elixir)
- food sauces (if made with wine)
- flavor extracts

contain alcohol and should be avoided. Disulfiram should not be viewed as a cure for alcoholism.

Of course, the effectiveness of disulfiram as a deterrent to drinking depends entirely on the client's willingness to take the drug. As a result, its utility has been limited by the fact that more than half of alcoholic clients refuse it. In addition to the problem of initial rejection, voluntary compliance with the disulfiram regimen has often been quite poor. In order to take advantage of the deterrence potential of disulfiram, it seems necessary to increase acceptance of this drug (Brubaker et al. 1987).

The most commonly heard reason for not taking disulfiram is that it is a "crutch." If a client has such an objection, it can be discussed individually or in group therapy. It should be pointed out that an equally valid argument could be made for antidepressants and insulin. This kind of reasoning can be extended to alcohol rehabilitation programs, religion, AA, or even the acquisition of knowledge itself. If one wants to be strong and do it alone, why bother with any of these?

V-E: THERAPEUTIC ENVIRONMENT

It was formerly thought that you could not help alcoholics until they were ready for help. This is only partially true. It is true that most alcoholics do not present themselves readily for treatment. The motivation of an alcoholic, like that of anyone else who is facing changes in lifestyle, is mixed. Whatever motivation is there can be encouraged. It is part of the nurse's job to help clients become receptive to the possibility of change. *Johnson's intervention*, described earlier (see Box 23–5), is useful in this regard.

At all levels of practice, the nurse can play an important role in **the intervention** process by recognizing the signs of alcohol problems in both client and family and

Table 23–4 • SPECIFIC INTERVENTIONS FOR ALCOHOLICS

NURSING INTERVENTION	RATIONALE
1. Communicate empathy, focus on feelings. Avoid comments that seem judgmental.	1. Establish a therapeutic alliance based on understanding in an atmosphere of openness and support.
2. Evaluate extent of alcohol use (using a nursing history and standardized test), levels of anxiety, and coping styles as well as support systems.	2. Ascertain strengths/weaknesses, coping skills, available resources, and potential withdrawal reactions.
3. Continually assess • presence of PDS (preferred defensive structure); • psychophysiological responses.	3. Data collected in initial interview is not complete; assessment is ongoing.
4. Assess for relapse.	4. Alcoholism is a chronic condition; relapse should be addressed.
5. Assess the need for disulfiram (Antabuse).	5. May be an effective adjunct early in treatment.
6. Refer to local resources—always include AA.	6. Behavior change is long term; support, encouragement, and suggestions are needed throughout.
7. Refer to other community agencies as needed.	7. Assistance may be needed in other areas of life functioning—e.g., vocational rehabilitation, socialization, treatment of associated psychiatric disorders.

knowing available resources to help with the problem. Table 23–4 identifies important interventions for nurses working with people recovering from alcohol.

The nurse's ability to develop a warm, accepting relationship with the alcoholic can assist the client in feeling safe enough to start looking at problems with some degree of openness and honesty. If the nurse lacks acceptance and empathy, knowledge and skill will not be useful. If the nurse has not worked through strong negative feelings related to alcohol/alcoholism, he or she should refer the client to another nurse or alcoholism counselor who has dealt with these issues and can begin promoting recovery. The client-counselor relationship is often considered to be more important than the type of treatment pursued (Valle 1981).

Alcoholics often seem indifferent to the destruction they bring on themselves and their families. They also show marked dependency, and they may lean on others, most often loved ones, to solve their problems. This characteristic can give the family and friends an effective means of motivating the alcoholic toward treatment. When family and friends refuse to solve the alcoholic's problems, the alcoholic will be forced to face the consequences of his or her own drinking behavior. Al-Anon teaches family members the three Cs concept. Family members did not *cause* the disease, they cannot *control* it, nor can they *cure* it. They learn that they are not responsible for the disease or for the person affected by it.

A sex difference in willingness to acknowledge alcoholism as a problem has been observed (Thom 1986). There are many more barriers for women than for men in acknowledging the need for help with an alcohol problem. Sometimes it is more difficult for women to identify themselves as having alcoholism. This may be due in part to the social stigma against alcoholic behavior in women. Also, many women begin drinking heavily along with an alcoholic partner or spouse. Yet many women do not see their behavior as problematic enough to warrant help-seeking. Those who attempt to get help may find themselves thwarted by actively drinking spouses (Thom 1986). Practical problems, such as child care, may also be a barrier to seeking treatment. Given these issues, dealing with alcohol problems in women may be best accomplished at the primary care level.

In terms of treatment goals, it is safest to propose abstinence as a treatment goal for all alcoholics. Abstinence is strongly related to good work adjustments, positive health status, comfortable interpersonal relationships, and general social stability. Treatment must also address the client's major psychological and social problems as well as the drinking behavior. Involvement of appropriate family members is now considered essential by most treatment providers. As previously mentioned, Al-Anon and Al-a-Teen are useful support groups for families.

A significant relationship has been noted between a client's feelings of "belongingness" and treatment outcome (Machell 1987). The more a client feels socially involved with peers, the better the chance for successful treatment outcome, longer length of stay, and lower relapse rates. Nurses should evaluate the feelings of belongingness periodically by questioning clients as to how they perceive themselves within their peer group. A client may be immersed in social events but perceive him- or herself as isolated. Clients with an isolated perception stand a much greater chance of shorter lengths of stay in treatment programs and a higher rate of relapse.

Children of alcoholics (COA) deserve special consideration. One of every eight Americans comes from an alcoholic home, and 7 million of these are youngsters facing the daily fear, uncertainty, and problems that result from their parent's alcoholism. In the United States, there are 21 million *adult children of alcoholics* (ACoA) who may continue to suffer the long-lasting mental, emotional, and physical consequences caused by life with an alcoholic parent. In addition, they are at greatly increased risk for developing alcoholism themselves (Woodside 1986). National support groups for ACoA are helping many work through common life problems. Involvement in Al-a-Teen or Al-a-Tot (support groups for teenagers and children of alcoholics based on the Al-Anon style) can help alleviate the guilt and responsibility in those children currently living with an alcoholic parent or parents. Children learn that they did not *cause*, and cannot *control* or *cure*, their parent's disease.

School nurses and nurses in pediatric and family practice clinics should assess for alcoholism in the family whenever a child presents for behavioral, mental, or repeated physical complaints that seem to have no basis in fact. A willingness to talk about alcoholism, to respond in a nonjudgmental fashion, and to be a supportive listener allows children relief in knowing that they are not alone and that there is help available. Nurses need to take advantage of their key positions by identifying and providing assistance to children and youth suffering negative consequences of family drinking problems.

V-F: PSYCHOTHERAPY

Nurses with advanced training may be involved in psychotherapy with alcoholic clients. Psychotherapy assists clients in identifying and using alternate coping mechanisms in order to reduce reliance on alcohol.

Eventually, psychotherapy can assist recovering alcoholics in becoming comfortable with sobriety.

Psychotherapy with alcoholics takes many forms. It can be individual, group, or family therapy; directive or nondirective therapy; goal-centered or insight-oriented therapy. Whatever type is used, clients need to be informed of what they can expect and cannot expect from the therapy and, likewise, what is expected from them. *No psychotherapy should take place while the client is actively drinking.*

The therapist must be prepared to respond to a number of issues that arise when treating alcoholics. Drinking is one. It must be talked about and dealt with. The therapist should be prepared to do some active outreach to a client who may miss a session and may be drinking. What if a client comes to a session intoxicated? In this instance, it is usually best to remind the client that sobriety is a prerequisite for ongoing psychotherapy, to make another appointment as soon as possible, and to ask the client to stop drinking now in order to keep that appointment. Support for the person can be elicited by calling an AA sponsor or some other supportive person.

Nurses as therapists may also be asked about their own drinking habits. It is best to deal with this issue by exploring the client's underlying concerns about whether the alcoholic client thinks the nurse can understand and help him or her.

Confidentiality must be maintained throughout therapy except when this conflicts with events requiring mandatory reporting (e.g., child abuse).

A number of issues occur frequently during the first six months of sobriety that require addressing. These include the following:

1. Physical changes take place as the body adapts to functioning without alcohol.
2. Numerous signals occur in the client's internal and external world that previously have been cues to drink. Different responses to these cues need to be learned.
3. Emotional responses (feelings that were formerly diluted with alcohol) are now experienced full-strength. Because they are so unfamiliar, they can be anxiety-producing.
4. Responses of family and coworkers to the client's new behavior must be addressed. Sobriety disrupts a system, and everyone in that system needs to adjust to the change.
5. New coping skills must be developed in order to prevent relapse and to ensure prolonged sobriety. AA makes use of the acronym HALT: "Don't get too **H**ungry, **A**ngry, **L**onely, or **T**ired." When alcoholics experience these feelings, they are to HALT and implement alternative coping strategies.

Counseling during this early stage of treatment needs to be directive, open and honest, and friendly and caring. Slogans from AA can be helpful in providing initial as well as ongoing motivation for adjusting to life without alcohol. Some examples are: "One day at a time," "Easy does it," and "Utilize, don't analyze." These phrases can provide a focus for clients new to recovery. The therapeutic process involves teaching the client to identify the physical and emotional changes that are occurring in the "here and now." The nurse therapist can then assist in the problem-solving process.

In psychotherapy generally, anxiety is the price paid for increments in self-awareness and disclosure to others. Unfortunately, in alcoholics, anxiety is also one of the more important inner cues or "triggers" for drinking. Therefore, the most difficult task in alcoholism therapy is to encourage increased self-awareness and disclosure while simultaneously keeping anxiety at minimal levels. This means that the therapist must be content with a gradual deepening of self-awareness in the client, rather than demanding sudden, dramatic "breakthroughs." Moreover, the therapist must ensure a therapeutic context in which high levels of support are available as the client uncovers aspects of self and discloses these to others.

Therapy with alcoholics, as it is currently practiced, too often attempts to remove the alcoholic's PDS (preferred defensive structure) instead of using it effectively to help achieve abstinence. The elements of the PDS, which help the alcoholic cope with anxiety, can be directed at all other stressful situations that the alcoholic faces while achieving sobriety (e.g., family, job, financial problems). Therapeutic efforts that confront the alcoholic's PDS prematurely and too strongly will increase, rather than reduce, the probability of further drinking.

Recovery programs successful in producing abstinence, such as AA, partially owe their success to the intuitive recognition of the fact that an alcoholic's PDS is to be protected and capitalized on, rather than confronted and radically altered. In the early stages of recovery, the alcoholic protects self-esteem by attempting to minimize the anxiety associated with change and growth. After two to five years of sobriety, the need for PDS is reduced and it can be recognized for what it is. This is often the best time for a recovering alcoholic to engage in insight psychotherapy — once defenses have been loosened.

Alcoholism therapy must be viewed as a time-dependent process. A particular therapeutic intervention for a recently drinking alcoholic may be entirely inappropriate for one who has managed to achieve several years of sobriety, or vice versa. Besides individual therapy, other specific psychotherapeutic techniques used with alcoholics include behavior therapy and group, family, and marital therapy.

BEHAVIORAL THERAPY. Behavioral therapy is a highly individualized form of treatment. The alcoholic's behavior is carefully assessed before beginning specific intervention strategies. **Aversive conditioning** was the first behavioral technique applied to treatment of alcoholism. In this mode, an aversive event (e.g., electric shock, emetine-induced nausea and vomiting) is paired with the sight, smell, and taste of alcohol. This aversion needs to be reinforced periodically or it will disappear over time.

A variety of different behavioral techniques are employed for situations the client may face during recovery. Included are skills training (for situations requiring refusal of drinks), assertiveness training, relaxation training, and relapse prevention training, which focuses on interrupting signals to drink (Marlatt 1985). The latter approach realistically recognizes that alcoholism is a chronic condition marked by relapses. Therefore, the possibility of relapse should be discussed, and options for preventing escalation into a serious drinking episode should be explored. The goal is to help the person learn from those situations so that periods of sobriety can be lengthened over time and so that relapse is not viewed as total failure.

ALCOHOLICS ANONYMOUS. Alcoholics Anonymous (AA) is a self-help group of recovering alcoholics that provides support and encouragement to those involved in continuing recovery. The regular meetings provide role models for recovery as well as guidance from others who have experienced many of the same problems and temptations that the client is facing. One-to-one sponsorship allows a person to receive assistance from another AA member on a 24-hour basis as required. The twelve-step program (see Box 23–4) allows the alcoholic person to "let go" and to take the risks associated with growth and change. There are a variety of groups available in most communities so that a person, by "shopping around," can usually find a compatible group. Meetings may be open (for anybody) or closed (AA members only).

GROUP THERAPY. Group therapy has been helpful for many people recovering from alcoholism. The *advantages of group therapy are*

- social isolation is decreased;
- newly recovering alcoholics have models in those with longer histories of sobriety;
- alcoholics are encouraged to seek support and encouragement from a variety of people;
- the therapist can observe the interpersonal behavior of the clients, without always being directly involved.

Groups can be closed or open, homogeneous or mixed, education- or therapy-oriented. Clients should be screened for admission to the group, and the therapist should maintain good record-keeping throughout. *Ground rules* that include commitments to the following points must be developed (Vanicelli 1986):

- minimal tenure in the group;
- expectations of regular attendance or advance notice of absences;
- advance notice to the group if one is considering leaving;
- abstinence and willingness to talk about fears of drinking or actual slips should they occur;
- talk about other difficult issues in the client's life;
- talk about group dynamics;
- confidentiality.

Goals for therapy include

- sobriety;
- motivation to continue to grow and change;
- recognizing and identifying behavior patterns that led to drinking;
- learning new ways to handle old problems;
- developing an emergency plan for high-risk situations that might lead to relapse;
- recognizing and identifying feelings (especially guilt, anger, depression, fear);
- learning to enjoy life without alcohol.

FAMILY THERAPY. Family therapy in alcoholism recognizes that the disease is a "family illness"—that is, all members are affected. Alcoholic family members lack trust in each other, lack nurturing closeness, and solve problems in a piecemeal fashion. Children of alcoholics (COA) become used to extra and inappropriate responsibilities. Parental role models are distorted. In fact, family equilibrium is established around the alcoholism. Therefore, removal of the drinking behavior becomes a threat!

As with any form of therapy, abstinence from alcohol must be a goal. The family has to begin to learn healthy ways to solve problems. Children of alcoholics are at high risk for developing their own alcoholism. This should be discussed openly at family therapy sessions. The basic purpose of intervention is to assist the family to motivate a change in their ineffective communication and response patterns. Instilling hope in the family's future is one of the nurse's greatest responsibilities.

When the alcoholic is in inpatient treatment, the family frequently has the opportunity to learn about the disease of alcoholism, family dynamics, communication, and recovery. Structured family therapy may begin at this time. Past behavior, anger, and alcohol use—and the family's role in these—are brought up and dealt with. Plans are made to change behavior as sobriety becomes a part of daily life. The carrying out of these plans must be rehearsed and practiced.

Following inpatient treatment of the alcoholic, family

members are usually concerned about the alcoholic's returning to drinking. They frequently "walk on eggshells," not thinking or talking about drinking or other problems, in an attempt to prevent a relapse from happening. Ongoing therapy helps them change roles as the need for control is lessened. Spouses frequently are reluctant to give up the position of power they had when the alcoholic drank. Responsibility needs to be renegotiated. Children's roles and changes in behaviors need to be examined as well.

MARITAL THERAPY. For the married couple, issues about time spent at home and about sex are prominent. The alcoholic may not have much libido as he or she begins to recover. Sex is not a paramount urge. The spouse may secretly hope for more of everything. Having felt deprived in many areas when the alcoholic was actively drinking, the spouse wants gratification of those unmet needs soon after the alcoholic stops drinking. Couples need further education in the recovery process as they deal with major changes in how they function. Understanding these needs for the spouse may need to be pursued in Al-Anon or in groups designed to help families understand and cope with sobriety. For example, the wife may not understand the anger of the newly sober husband. She may balk at his attendance at AA meetings or his kindness to people in AA. She may feel rejected and not needed. These issues predominate in the early months of recovery.

In a study of types of marital therapy with alcoholic couples, it was found that alcohol-focused spouse involvement, as well as behavioral marital therapy, helped alcoholics stay in treatment, and that the couples maintained their marital satisfaction better after treatment (McCrady et al. 1986).

Standard VI: Evaluation

Treatment outcome is judged by maintenance of abstinence, decreasing symptomatic denial, acceptable occupational functioning, improving family relationships, and, ultimately, the client's ability to relate normally and comfortably with other human beings.

The ability to utilize existing supports and skills learned in treatment bodes well for ongoing recovery. For example, recovery is launched if, in response to cues to drink, the client calls his or her sponsor or other recovering alcoholics; increases attendance at AA, after-care, or other group meetings; or writes feelings in a log and considers alternative action.

In general, the nature and determinants of the alcoholic person's post-treatment functioning are unexplored. In a study of treated alcoholics and their families, it was found that extra-treatment factors such as environmental stressors, coping responses, and social resources had as much influence on the recovery process as did the client's treatment experiences and initial symptomatology (Billings and Moos 1983; Estes and Heinemann 1986).

Vaillant and coworkers (1983) concur, stating that alcoholic persons recover not so much because we treat them as because they treat themselves. These authors list four factors closely associated with remission from alcoholism:

1. Finding a substitute dependency, such as a compulsive hobby, to replace alcohol.
2. Experiencing a consistent aversive event related to drinking, such as use of disulfiram or an obvious adverse health effect.
3. Discovering a fresh source of hope and self-esteem.
4. Obtaining new social supports, such as new friends or a new job.

Awareness and clinical assessment of extra-treatment factors make the evaluation process more meaningful in that the nurse can more adequately understand post-treatment functioning and the process of recovery and relapse. Continuous monitoring and evaluation lead to a better chance for prolonged recovery.

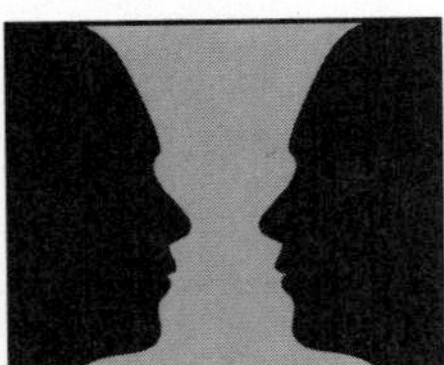

Case Study: Working With a Person Who Has Alcoholism

Mr. Young, age 49, and his wife arrived in the Emergency Department (ED) one evening, fearful that Mr. Young had had a stroke. His right hand was limp, and he was unable to hyperextend his right wrist. Sensation to fingertips in his right hand was impaired.

Mr. Young looked much *older than his stated age*. He looked to be about 65! His *complexion* was *ruddy* and *flushed*. *History taking was difficult*. Mr. Young answered only what was asked of him, volunteering no additional information. He stated that he had taken a nap that afternoon, and that when he awakened his right arm was as described.

Mr. Young revealed that he had been unemployed for four years because the company he had worked for had gone bankrupt. He had been unable to find a new job but had an appointment for an interview in ten days. His wife was now working full time, so the family finances were okay. They had two grown children who no longer lived at home.

He denied any significant medical illness except for *high blood pressure*, just diagnosed last year. His *family history* was negative for illness, with the exception of *alcoholism*. His mother was a recovering alcoholic who had been treated at an inpatient facility and was maintaining her sobriety. Ms. Dee, the admitting nurse, asked Mr. Young questions about his use of alcohol, including quantity, frequency, and withdrawal experiences. In general, he *denied* any significant alcohol involvement. Ms. Dee shared with him the fact that the disease of alcoholism runs in families. Ms. Dee asked Mr. Young whether (1) he knew that, and (2) if it concerned him with regard to his own drinking. Mr. Young said he knew and that he did not want to think about it.

Ms. Dee then spoke with Mrs. Young about the events of the day. Ms. Dee stated that she spoke with Mr. Young and that she was concerned that he might have an alcohol problem. Ms. Dee shared the impressions that had led her to that tentative conclusion and asked Mrs. Young to describe her husband's involvement with alcohol. Mrs. Young's shoulders slumped; she sighed and said, "I have spent the entire day talking to a counselor at the local treatment center to see if I can get him in. He won't admit that he has a problem." Mrs. Young then recounted a six-year history of steadily increasing alcohol use. She said that for a while she could not admit to herself that her husband was an excessive drinker. "He tried to hide it, but gradually I knew. I could tell from little changes that he was intoxicated. I couldn't believe it was happening because he had been through the same thing with his mother. And we'd always had such a good relationship. I thought I knew him. Actually, I guess I did, as a working man. Being unemployed and unable to find a job has really floored him. And now he's even going to job interviews intoxicated!"

Mrs. Young recounted how her husband's drinking worsened dramatically with unemployment and how she tried ridding their home of liquor, only to find bottles hidden in their mobile home one day when she went to clean it. She described her feelings, which were like an emotional roller coaster—elated, hopeful when he seemed to be doing okay; dejected, desperate on other occasions such as the time that she found the alcohol in their mobile home. Mrs. Young hated going to work for fear of what he would do while she was gone. She stated that she was terrified that one day her husband would crack up the car and kill himself, since he often drives when he is intoxicated. Ms. Dee discussed with Mrs. Young her own involvement as part of the family system. Options for Mrs. Young and her husband were discussed.

Meanwhile, the ED physician had examined Mr. Young. The diagnosis was radial nerve palsy. Mr. Young had most likely passed out and lay on his arm. Since Mr. Young was intoxicated, he had not felt the signals that his nerves sent out to warn him to move (i.e., numbness, tingling). Mr. Young had continued to lie in his position for so long that the resulting cutting off of circulation was sufficient to cause some temporary nerve damage.

Mr. Young's blood alcohol level (BAL) was .311 mg%! This is three times the legal limit of intoxication (.100 mg%). Even though he had a BAL of .311, Mr. Young was alert and oriented and not slurring his speech or giving any other outward signs of intoxication. The difference between Mr. Young's BAL and behavior indicated the development of tolerance, a symptom of physical dependence (refer to Table 23–1).

Assessment

Ms. Dee organized her data into objective and subjective components.

OBJECTIVE DATA

1. Drives when intoxicated
2. Nerve damage due to passing out while lying on arm
3. Alcohol use has increased during stress of unemployment
4. Alcohol use has impaired his capacity to obtain employment
5. Alcohol use is causing disruption in marital relationship
6. Client unable to see effect of his drinking
7. Family history of alcoholism
8. BAL three times legal limit of intoxication; has developed a tolerance

SUBJECTIVE DATA

1. Denies he has an alcohol problem

Nursing Diagnosis

From the data, the nurse formulates the following nursing diagnosis:

1. *Ineffective Individual Coping* related to alcohol use
   - Alcohol use has increased during stressful period of unemployment
   - Alcohol use has impaired client's capacity to obtain employment
   - Alcohol use is causing disruption in marital relationship
   - Client unable to see effect of his drinking on his life functioning

Planning

CONTENT LEVEL—PLANNING GOALS

It was decided to allow Mr. Young to sober up in the ED, since it is difficult to discuss goals when the client is intoxicated. When the client is sober, the nurse establishes goals with the client that are realistic, appropriate, and measurable.

Nursing Diagnosis	Long Term Goals	Short Term Goals
1. *Ineffective Individual Coping* related to alcohol use	1. Client will abstain from alcohol.	1a. Client will identify the role of alcohol in his life and his risk for alcoholism, given his family history. 1b. Client will agree to remain sober from now to job interview ten days hence. To assist in this effort, he agrees to • obtain an appointment at a community alcohol center; • attend at least one AA meeting/day; • seek out other support; • call the ED nurse to report on the job interviews and referral appointments. 1c. Client will state two alternative behaviors to engage in when experiencing the urge to drink. 1d. Client will name two ways to begin to rebuild trust in his relationship with his wife.

PROCESS LEVEL—NURSES' REACTIONS AND FEELINGS

The denial the alcoholic exhibits often results in rejection by nurses, who feel that the alcoholic causes his own problems. Nurses generally feel sympathetic toward spouses and other family members but have a sense of helplessness about being able to effect change.

Feelings of rejection, sympathy, and helplessness impair the nurse's ability to facilitate change. True, some alcoholic persons do maintain their denial and effectively resist intervention. But many others welcome the opportunity to begin to learn different ways to cope with life problems. Before dismissing alcoholics as "not wanting help" or being "the only ones that can change things,'' nurses need to ask themselves if they have done all that they can in an attempt to engage the client in the change process.

Ms. Dee had seen many clients with the disease of alcoholism make radical changes in their lives, and she had learned to view alcoholism as a treatable disease. She was aware also that it was the client who made the changes, and she no longer felt responsible when a client was not ready to make that change.

Intervention

Ms. Dee suggested that Mrs. Young attend Al-Anon meetings and gave her information on where she could find groups in her area. She also urged Mrs. Young to discuss what is going on with her grown children and told her about the problems that adult children of alcoholics (ACoA) often experience. She encouraged Mrs. Young to let her children know of support groups they could go to if they felt the need.

Ms. Dee also urged Mrs. Young *not* to drive in the car with her husband if he was driving while intoxicated. Ms. Dee stated that she should not protect him from the results of his drinking (e.g., bail him out of jail if DWI, make excuses for him). Ms. Dee added that Al-Anon could offer crucial support for her and assist her in minimizing her enabling behaviors, which family members often exhibit.

Ms. Dee outlined an initial care plan for Mr. Young (Nursing Care Plan 23–1). Attending AA was a central part of the treatment program, along with a variety of other interventions, e.g., skills training, education, medical intervention, family counseling, and evaluation for antabuse (disulfiram).

Evaluation

Mr. Young's willingness to become actively involved in planning short term goals is evidence that they were realistic and appropriate. In this case, the main opportunity to evaluate the short term goals is when and if Mr. Young calls back to report on steps he has taken to meet those goals. At that time, he should be supported and applauded for the progress he has made and encouraged to ''keep up the good work.'' Other referrals may be given if indicated.

Mr. Young did continue with AA. His denial persists, but he was highly motivated to keep his marriage. He gradually accepted a variety of referrals and, as time progressed, he found that the positive feedback and support from others increased his self-esteem, decreased his feelings of isolation, and reinforced his long term goal of sobriety.

Nursing Care Plan 23–1 • A PERSON WITH ALCOHOLISM: Mr. Young

NURSING DIAGNOSIS

Ineffective individual coping related to alcohol use

Supporting Data

- Alcohol use increases in response to the stress of job loss, lowered role status.
- Alcohol use has impaired client's capacity to obtain employment.
- Alcohol use is causing disruptions in relationship with wife.
- Family history of alcoholism.

Long Term Goal: Client will abstain from alcohol.

Short Term Goal	*Intervention*	*Rationale*	*Evaluation*
1. Client will identify role of alcohol in his life and his risk for alcoholism, given his family history.	1a. Point out relationship between no job and increased alcohol use.	1a. Use assessment data to clarify behavior patterns.	Goal met. Client listens to nurse—admitted that going to job interviews intoxicated would lower the chance of getting a job. Stated that he felt so down that he needed alcohol to feel OK.
	1b. Provide information on the disease of alcoholism.	1b. Stressing alcoholism as a disease can lower guilt and help increase self-esteem.	
	1c. Point out the factors placing person at risk for alcoholism.	1c. Children with alcoholic parents are at a greater risk for developing alcoholism themselves.	

Continued on following page

Nursing Care Plan 23–1 • A PERSON WITH ALCOHOLISM: Mr. Young *(Continued)*

Short Term Goal	*Intervention*	*Rationale*	*Evaluation*
	1d. Communicate concern, empathy, nonjudgmental acceptance, warmth.	1d. Helps establish a therapeutic relationship based on understanding and provides an atmosphere of openness and support. Helps client maintain self-esteem.	
2. Client will remain sober from now until job interview (ten days).	2a. Refer to AA. 2b. Refer to local resources for an appointment with alcohol counselor. 2c. List other available supports (e.g., friends, family).	2a–c. Much support and encouragement are needed when making major life changes, such as stopping drinking. A variety of support systems help decrease feelings of alienation and isolation.	Goal met. Client calls the ED to report on carrying out the plan; states that potential employer wants him back for second interview.
3. Client will state two alternative behaviors that he can exercise when experiencing the urge to drink.	3a. Evaluate client's situation by using a crisis intervention model—that is, assessing precipitating events, support systems, and coping skills.	3a. Identifies high-risk situations and opportunities for change.	Goal met. After three weeks, client stated that he attended AA every day. He was learning to identify situations that trigger the urge to drink and was learning new coping behaviors. After five weeks, client had a slip and drank for two days; he decided to try Antabuse.
	3b. Explore alternate coping skills. Skills training may be needed (e.g., assertion, socialization, problem-solving).	3b. Behavior change is a learning process. Relapse prevention can be practiced.	
	3c. Encourage participation in AA, group therapy, or other appropriate modalities.	3c. Provide support and minimize feelings of isolation while learning new skills.	
	3d. Referral to a physician for: • complete physical examination; • possible disulfiram (Antabuse) therapy.	3d. Antabuse may help provide the external control needed during early months of sobriety; because it can cause physiological crises when taken with alcohol, a physical examination is needed.	
4. Client will name two ways to begin to rebuild trust in his relationship with his wife.	4. Referral to a marital counselor.	4. Alcoholism is a "family illness" adversely affecting those close to the alcoholic.	Goal met. Wife has been attending Al-Anon for six weeks, three times per week, after finding a group that she felt comfortable with. Client and wife decided to start couples therapy in two weeks.

Summary

In this chapter it was shown that alcohol use occurs on a continuum and that the development of addiction and dependence is a time-related phenomenon. Various etiological theories attempt to explain why some drinkers develop alcoholism and others do not. Since there is no clear consensus about the nature of alcoholism, notions about treatment are also inconsistent. The more closely clinics are matched to a range of treatment alternatives, the greater the likelihood that sobriety will be achieved and overall life functioning improved.

Nurses encounter alcoholic people in all areas of practice and thus must be prepared for assessing, planning, implementing, and evaluating nursing care of alcoholics. Assessment strategies have been outlined for determining the severity of the illness, levels of anxiety, and coping styles, as well as physiological and psychosocial changes. Some of the nursing diagnoses applicable to alcoholic clients were outlined. Planning nursing care on both process and content levels was discussed. Principles and specific examples of psychotherapeutic intervention were listed. Specific approaches include behavior therapy; individual, group, family, and marital therapy; and Alcoholics Anonymous (AA). Whatever techniques are employed, the nurse must make clear to the client what expectations are reasonable. Issues common in early sobriety were discussed, as were some general approaches to relapse prevention. Factors to be considered in evaluation were described. A case study demonstrated the steps of the nursing process as applied to an alcoholic client.

References

Ablon J. Perspectives on Al-Anon family groups. *In* Estes NJ, Heinemann ME (eds). Alcoholism: Development, Consequences and Interventions. St. Louis, MO: C.V. Mosby Company, 1986.

American Psychiatric Association. Diagnostic and Statistical Manual of Mental Disorders, 3rd ed., revised. Washington DC: American Psychiatric Association, 1987.

Billings AG, Moos RH. Psychosocial processes of recovery among alcoholics and their families: Implications for clinicians and program evaluators. Addictive Behaviors, 8:205, 1983.

Bissell L. Diagnosis and recognition. *In* Gitlow SE, Peyser HS (eds). Alcoholism: A Practical Treatment Guide, 2nd ed. Philadelphia: Grune & Stratton, 1988.

Block MA. Motivating the alcoholic patient. *In* Gitlow SE, Peyser HS (eds). Alcoholism: A Practical Treatment Guide, 2nd ed. Philadelphia: Grune & Stratton, 1988.

Brubaker RG, Prue DM, Rychtarik RG. Determinants of disulfiram acceptance among alcohol patients: A test of the theory of reasoned action. Addictive Behaviors, 12:43, 1987.

Burgess AW, Lazare A. Psychiatric Nursing in the Hospital and the Community, 2nd ed. Englewood Cliffs, NJ: Prentice-Hall, 1976.

Bursten B. The manipulative personality. Archives of General Psychiatry, 26:318, 1972.

Edwards G, Gross MM, Keller M. Alcohol related disabilities. WHO Offset Publication No. 32. Geneva: World Health Organization, 1977.

Estes NJ, Heinemann ME. Alcoholism: Development, Consequences and Interventions. St. Louis, MO: C.V. Mosby Company, 1986.

Estes NJ, Smith-DiJulio K, Heinemann ME. Nursing Diagnosis of the Alcoholic Person. St. Louis, MO: C.V. Mosby Company, 1980.

Frances RJ, Franklin JE. Alcohol and other psychoactive substance use disorders. *In* Talbott JA, Hales RE, Yudofsky SC (eds). Textbook of Psychiatry. Washington DC: American Psychiatric Press, 1988.

Gitlow SE. An overview. *In* Gitlow SE, Peyser HS (eds). Alcoholism: A Practical Treatment Guide, 2nd ed. Philadelphia: Grune & Stratton, 1988.

Goodwin DW, Schulsinger F, Hermansen L, Guze SB, Winoker G. Alcohol problems in adoptees raised apart from alcoholic biological parents. Archives of General Psychiatry, 28:228, 1973.

Goodwin DW, et al. Drinking problems in adopted and nonadopted sons of alcoholics. Archives of General Psychiatry, 31:164, 1974.

Harper FD (ed). Alcohol Abuse and Black America. Alexandria, VA: Douglass Publishers, 1976.

Johnson VE. Intervention: How to Help Someone Who Doesn't Want Help. Minneapolis, MN: Johnson Books, 1986.

Knott DH. The addictive process. Lecture presented at the University of Utah Summer School on Alcoholism and Other Drug Dependencies, Salt Lake City, June, 1987.

Machell DF. Fellowship as an important factor in alcoholism residential treatment. Journal of Alcohol and Drug Education, 32(2):56, 1987.

Mandell W. Types and phases of alcohol dependence illness. *In* Galanter M (ed). Recent Developments in Alcoholism, Vol. 1. New York: Plenum Press, 1983, pp. 415–447.

Marlatt GA. Relapse Prevention: Maintenance Strategies in the Treatment of Addictive Behaviors. New York: Guilford Press, 1985.

Mayfield D, McLeod G, Hall P. The CAGE questionnaire: Validation of a new alcoholism screening instrument. American Journal of Psychiatry, 131:1121, 1974.

McCrady BS, Noel NE, Abrams DB. Comparative effectiveness of three types of spouse involvement in outpatient behavioral alcoholism treatment. Journal of Studies on Alcohol, 47:459, 1986.

McKelvey MJ, Kane JS, Kellison K. Substance abuse and mental illness: Double trouble. Journal of Psychosocial Nursing, 25(1):20, 1987.

NIAAA. Program strategies for Preventing Fetal Alcohol Syndrome and Alcohol Related Birth Defects. DHHS Publication No. (ADM)87-1482, Washington DC: U.S. Government Printing Office, 1987.

Schaef AW. Co-Dependence: Misunderstood — Mistreated. San Francisco: Harper & Row, 1986.

Schuckit MA. Drug and Alcohol Abuse, 2nd ed. New York: Plenum Press, 1984.

Smith-DiJulio K. Nursing people experiencing dependence on alcohol and other drugs. *In* Luckman J, Sorensen K (eds). Medical-Surgical Nursing. Philadelphia: W.B. Saunders Company, 1987, pp. 1836–1866.

Thom B. Sex differences in help-seeking for alcohol problems. 1. Barriers to help-seeking. British Journal of Addiction, 81:777, 1986.

U.S. Department of Health and Human Services. Fifth Special Report to the U.S. Congress on Alcohol and Health from the Secretary of Health and Human Services. DHHS Publication No. (ADM) 84-1291, Washington DC: U.S. Government Printing Office, 1984.

Vaillant GE, Clark W, Cyrus C, Milofsky ES, Kopp J, Wulsin VW, Moglienlnicki NP. Prospective study of alcoholism treatment: Eight-year follow up. American Journal of Medicine, 75:455, 1983.

Valle SK. Interpersonal functioning of alcoholism counselors and treatment outcomes. Journal of Studies on Alcohol, 42:783, 1981.

Vanicelli M. Group psychotherapy with alcoholics: Special techniques. *In* Estes NJ, Heinemann ME (eds). Alcoholism: Development, Consequences and Interventions. St. Louis, MO: C.V. Mosby Company, 1986, pp. 374–387.

Walker DR, Donovan DM, Kivlahan DR, Roszell DK. Prediction of alcoholism treatment outcome: Multiple assessment domains. *In* Grant I (ed). Neuropsychiatric Correlates of Alcoholism. Washington DC: American Psychiatric Press, 1986, pp. 109–125.

Wallace J. Alcoholism from the inside out: A phenomenologic analysis. *In* Estes NJ, Heinemann ME (eds). Alcoholism: Development, Consequences and Interventions. St. Louis, MO: C.V. Mosby Company, 1986, pp. 3–14.

Woodside M. Children of alcoholics: Breaking the cycle. Journal of School Health, 56:448, December, 1986.

World Health Organization, Expert Committee on Mental Health. Report on the First Session of the Alcoholism Subcommittee. WHO Organizational and Technical Report Series, No. 48, August, 1952.

Zimberg S. Principles of alcoholism psychotherapy. *In* Zimberg S, Wallace J, Blume SB (eds). Practical Approaches to Alcoholism Psychotherapy. New York: Plenum Press, 1978.

Zuska JJ, Pursch JA. Long term management. *In* Gitlow SE, Peyser HS (eds). Alcoholism: A Practical Treatment Guide, 2nd ed. Philadelphia: Grune & Stratton, 1988.

Bibliography

Annis HM. Is inpatient rehabilitation of the alcoholic cost effective? Con position. Advances in Alcohol and Substance Abuse, 5:175, 1986.

Beeny S, Calderaro L, Miicke B, Schilling K. Nursing Care: Treatment Resistant Substance Abuse. Fair Oaks Nursing News, 14:3, 1986.

Brocar D. Patients in treatment for substance abuse: One nurse's viewpoint. Fair Oaks Nursing News, 14:1, 1986.

Curtis JL, Millman EJ, Joseph M. Prevalence rates for alcoholism, associated depression and dementia on the Harlem Hospital Medicine and Surgery Services. Advances in Alcohol and Substance Abuse, 61(1):45, 1986.

Fishman R (ed). Alcohol and Alcoholism. New York: Chelsea House Publishers, 1987.

Heather N, Robertson I, Davies P, (eds). The Misuse of Alcohol: Critical Issues in Dependence, Treatment and Prevention. New York: New York University Press, 1985.

Herrington RC, Jacobsen GR, Benzer DG (eds). Alcohol and Drug Abuse Handbook. St. Louis, MO: Warren H. Green, 1987.

Self-Study Exercises

Match the following:

1. ________ Stopping alcohol use results in specific signs and symptoms.
2. ________ Based on data that alcohol seems to run in families.
3. ________ Theory of alcoholism based on observation that different groups have different attitudes and rituals toward alcohol.
4. ________ A useful definition of alcoholism that associates addiction with resultant problem behaviors.
5. ________ The number of drinks that would cause a BAL of 0.1 mg% (legally intoxicated).
6. ________ BAL level that affects the entire motor area of the brain, causing staggering, ataxia, and emotional lability.

A. 5–6 drinks
B. 10–12 drinks
C. 0.3 mg%
D. 0.2 mg%
E. Psychological theory
F. Withdrawal
G. Dependence
H. WHO definition
I. DSM III-R criteria
J. Biological theory
K. Sociocultural theory

Identify two possible nursing diagnoses for a person with alcohol problems and formulate two short term goals (STG) (measurable and realistic) for each diagnosis.

7. Nursing Diagnosis 1: ________
   STG 1a: ________
   STG 1b: ________
8. Nursing Diagnosis 2:
   STG 2a: ________
   STG 2b: ________

Multiple Choice

9. When intervening with an intoxicated client it is useful to first:

   A. Let him or her sober up first.
   B. Decide on goals immediately, while the client is still in a good mood.
   C. Gain compliance by sharing your drinking habits with client.
   D. Ask what other drugs client might be taking.

10. Of the following difficult situations that Mr. Young might have to face, which might the nurse consider the *highest priority* for intervention?

    A. What his children will say to him.
    B. Being in situations or experiencing feelings which formerly led to drinking.
    C. What his mother will say to him.
    D. Embarrassment at having passed out while lying on his arm.

Short Answer

11. Name four principles of psychotherapeutic interventions with an alcoholic client.
    A. ______________________________
    B. ______________________________
    C. ______________________________
    D. ______________________________
12. Name two issues that a therapist needs to address when treating an alcoholic client.
    A. ______________________________
    B. ______________________________
13. Name and describe five therapeutic modalities used with alcoholic clients.
    A. ______________________________
    B. ______________________________
    C. ______________________________
    D. ______________________________
    E. ______________________________
14. Name four treatment outcomes that indicate effective recovery from alcoholism.
    A. ______________ B. ______________
    C. ______________ D. ______________

CHAPTER 24

People Who Depend Upon Substances Other Than Alcohol

Mary McAndrew

OUTLINE

KEY TERMS AND CONCEPTS ◆ ◆ ◆ ◆ ◆ ◆ ◆ ◆ ◆ ◆

The key terms and concepts listed here also appear in bold where they are defined or discussed in this chapter.

PSYCHOACTIVE SUBSTANCE USE DISORDERS
PSYCHOACTIVE SUBSTANCE ABUSE
PSYCHOACTIVE SUBSTANCE DEPENDENCE
TOLERANCE
WITHDRAWAL SYMPTOMS
POLYDRUG ABUSE
SYNERGISTIC EFFECT
ANTAGONISTIC EFFECT
NALOXONE (NARCAN)
TOXICOLOGICAL SCREENING
ANTIANXIETY AGENTS (MINOR TRANQUILIZERS, ANXIOLYTICS, SEDATIVE-HYPNOTICS)
PSYCHOMOTOR STIMULANTS (PSYCHOSTIMULANTS)
PSYCHOTOMIMETICS (HALLUCINOGENS)
SYNESTHESIA
NALTREXONE (TREXAN)
METHADONE (DOLOPHINE)
CLONIDINE
LAAM (L-ALPHA ACETYL METHADOL)
RESIDENTIAL THERAPEUTIC COMMUNITIES
EMPLOYEE ASSISTANCE PROGRAMS (EAPs)
PCP (PHENCYCLIDINE) INTOXICATION
FLASHBACK

Overview

The history of drugs in the United States begins with European explorers in the fifteenth and sixteenth centuries. Tobacco, cocaine, caffeine, opium, and LSD-like drugs were found in their travels to the New World and Asia and brought back home.

Columbus and other early explorers met Indians who carried rolls of dried leaves that they set on fire—and who then "drank the smoke" that emerged from the rolls. The Indians knew of the strange power of these leaves. Corti (1931) reported that the Indians, unable to give up their habit of smoking, always brought their supplies of tobacco with them. They found that nicotine produced a unique combination of effects—both stimulation and tranquilization. People then, as today, found that after they had smoked for a period of time they had to go on smoking or chewing tobacco or taking it as snuff (tobacco ground to a powder and inhaled), in order for their craving to be satisfied.

Many drugs used by North and South American Indians produced LSD-like effects. The effects of these drugs were considered a mystical and religious phenomenon, an experience that would bring humans closer to the gods and nature.

Thus we have evolved into a drug-oriented culture. We use a host of different drugs for a variety of purposes: to restore health, to reduce pain, to reduce anxiety, to increase energy, to create a feeling of euphoria, to induce sleep, and to enhance alertness. Many substances are available to alter mood or state of consciousness. People continue to take drugs today for other than medical reasons. Drugs may make them feel good. Drugs may relieve stress or tension or provide a temporary escape. Peer pressure is also a strong factor in the use of drugs by young people. In many parts of our society, the use of drugs has become a "rite of passage." Sometimes drug use is part of the thrill of taking a risk. From an early age we are "programmed" to accept drugs. The media tell us that drugs are part of the technology that can help make life a little better. They urge us to seek "better living through chemistry" (Resnick 1979).

DRUG ABUSE AND DRUG DEPENDENCE

There is a distinction between use and abuse of drugs. Almost everyone uses a psychoactive substance, even if it is a socially accepted substance such as coffee or tobacco, but not everyone misuses or abuses drugs. According to the Food, Drug, and Cosmetic Act, *a drug is defined as a substance intended for use in the diagnosis, cure, mitigation, treatment, or prevention of disease.*

However, the DSM III-R diagnostic category **psychoactive substance use disorders** refers to symptoms and maladaptive behavioral changes associated with those drugs that affect the central nervous system (APA 1987). Pathological use of a drug is classified as *substance abuse* and *substance dependence.* (Fig. 24–1).

Psychoactive substance abuse (drug abuse) includes (APA 1987) maladaptive and consistent use despite the following:

1. Social, occupational, psychological, or physical problems that are exacerbated by the drug; and/or
2. Recurrent use in situations that are physically hazardous (e.g., driving while intoxicated).

Psychoactive substance dependence (drug dependence) essentially includes the following (APA 1987):

1. Impaired control of drug use despite adverse consequences (as described above);
2. Development of **tolerance** to the drug (tolerance is a need for higher and higher doses to achieve intoxication or the desired effect);
3. **Withdrawal symptoms** occur as a result of continued use (withdrawal symptoms are the negative physiological and psychological reactions that occur when the drug is reduced or no longer taken).

Other associated characteristics of drug dependence include a compulsive need to spend more and more time in (1) getting the drug in any manner possible (e.g., theft), (2) taking the drug, and (3) recuperating from its effects. Important social, occupational, and recreational activities are given up in order to spend time with drug use. Figure 24–2 conceptualizes the process of drug abuse and dependence.

EFFECTS OF POLYDRUG ABUSE (POLYPHARMACY)

The taking of more than one drug at any given time is termed **polydrug abuse** or polypharmacy. This is seen in young, adult, and elderly clients. Polydrug abuse poses some real hazards to both the individual taking the drugs and the health care worker involved in treating a person who is intoxicated or in withdrawal. Polydrug use can have (1) synergistic effects and (2) antagonistic effects.

SYNERGISTIC EFFECT. Some drugs when taken together intensify or prolong the effect of either or both of the drugs. For example, the combination of alcohol plus a benzodiazepine, alcohol plus an opiate, or alcohol plus a barbiturate will all cause a synergistic effect. All these drugs are central nervous system (CNS) depressants. Two of these drugs taken together will result in far greater CNS depression than just the simple sum of the effects of each drug added together. Many unintentional deaths have resulted from lethal combinations of drugs.

ANTAGONISTIC EFFECT. Many people may take a combination of drugs to weaken or inhibit the effect of another drug. For example, cocaine is often mixed with heroin (speedball). The heroin (CNS depressant) is meant to soften the intense letdown of cocaine (CNS stimulant) withdrawal. **Naloxone (Narcan),** an opiate antagonist, is often given to people who have overdosed from an opiate (usually heroin), in order to reverse respiratory and CNS depression.

DRUG HISTORY. When a person is brought to the emergency room intoxicated or in severe withdrawal, it is vital to know what drug(s) the client has taken — and, if possible, the amount, route, and time of each drug. Each drug or category of drugs has unique properties requiring unique measures in case of an overdose or toxic reaction. For example, a person with a history of alcohol and heroin use may be brought into the emergency room stuporous or in a coma. Once the coma is

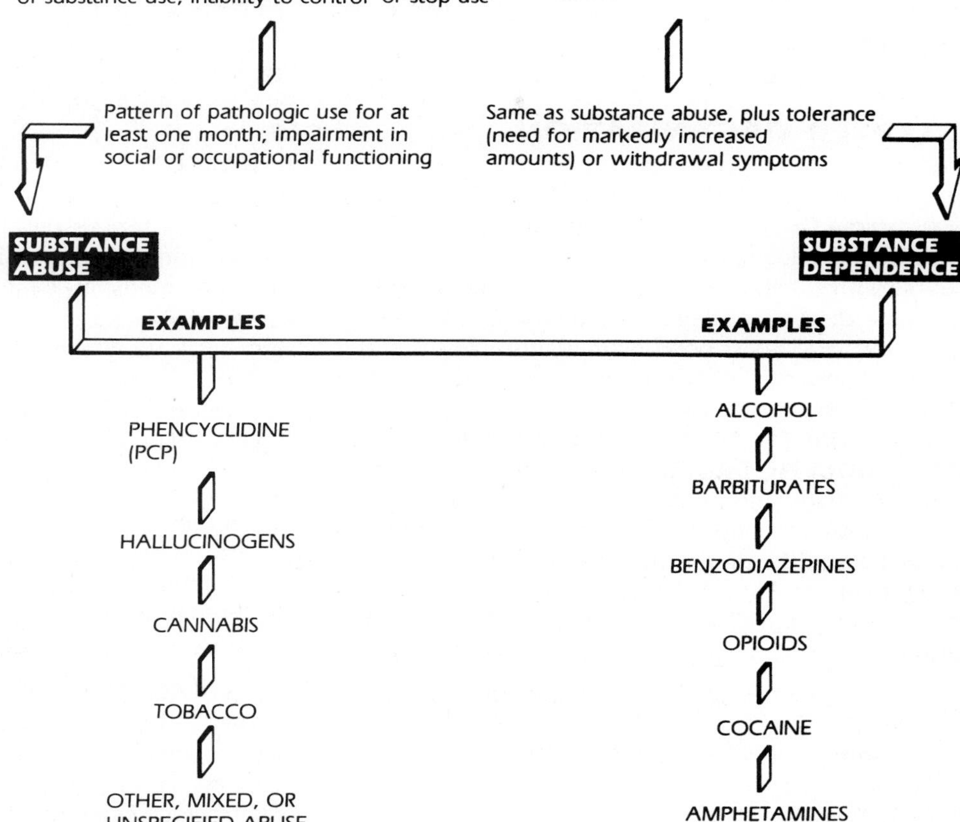

Figure 24–1. *Psychoactive substance use disorders*—DSM III. (*Adapted from* Janicak PG, Andriukaitis SN. DSM III: *Seeing the Forest Through the Trees. Psychiatric Annals,* 10(8):17, 1980, *and Diagnostic and Statistical Manual of Mental Disorders* [DSM III-R], *3d ed., revised. Washington DC: American Psychiatric Association,* 1987.)

reversed by naloxone, the client may go into alcohol withdrawal tremens 48 to 72 hours later. It is important for medical teams to know what other drugs the client has ingested. Friends and family members can supply this information.

DRUG SCREENING. Drug screening can indicate the presence of different drugs in a person's system. After consent for a **toxicological screening** is obtained, 100 ml of urine and 20 ml of blood are taken, and the specimens are collected in the presence of a witness (Bittle et al. 1986). Drug screening, however, is usually not available in time to help with an emergency drug overdose, but it is helpful in planning long term treatment.

NEUROLOGICAL EXAMINATION. It must be emphasized that whenever a person is brought into the emergency room in a coma, no matter what the drug history or presence of drugs on or in the body, ***a neurolog-***

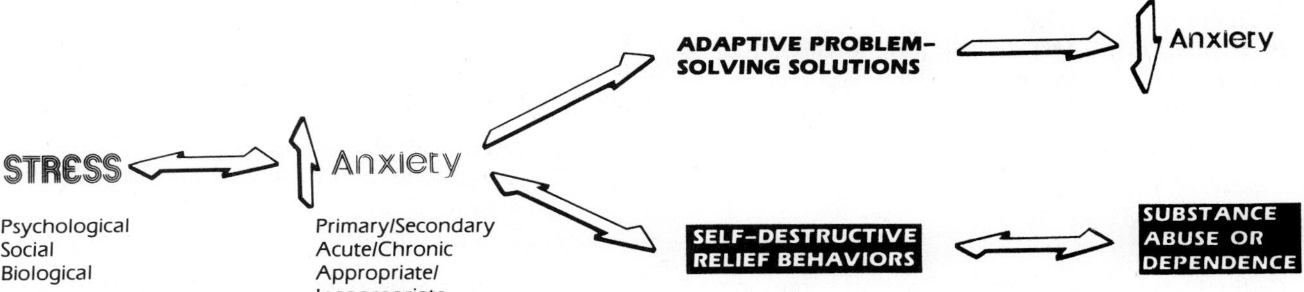

Figure 24–2. *Conceptualization of the process of substance abuse or dependence.*

ical examination should always be done. Some people, while intoxicated, get into fights or fall. This could result in a subdural hematoma or other neurological complications. If such complications are not diagnosed early, death may ensue.

CHAPTER ORGANIZATION

This chapter is divided into five sections. The first section, *General Guidelines*, provides general guidelines for assessment, diagnosis, planning, and treatment for people with substance abuse problems. The other four sections discuss antianxiety agents (sedative-hypnotics, or anxiolytics), psychostimulants, narcotics, and psychotomimetics. Brief descriptions of the four sections concerning drugs follow.

ANTIANXIETY AGENTS (SEDATIVE-HYPNOTIC OR ANXIOLYTIC DRUGS). A sedative is a drug that reduces activity and induces calmness. A hypnotic induces drowsiness and sleep. These drugs are known as **minor tranquilizers, antianxiety** agents, or **anxiolytics** (Kaplan and Sadock 1988).

These drugs are all prescription drugs. The **sedative-hypnotics,** or anxiolytics, include the following:

1. Benzodiazepines (e.g., Valium, Librium, Tranxene, Serax).
2. Barbiturates (e.g., Nembutal, Seconal).
3. Methaqualone (Quaaludes).
4. Chloral Hydrate.
5. Glutethimide (Doriden).
6. Meprobamate (e.g., Equanil, Miltown).

These drugs are medically prescribed to reduce pathological anxiety, tension, and agitation and, in some cases, to lower a person's convulsive threshold. They have a high potential for drug dependency. Anxiolytic substance abuse is high among teenage groups and young adults. They are also among the most common drugs of abuse used by health care professionals, along with narcotics and alcohol, all of which are CNS depressants. The benzodiazepines (e.g., Librium, Valium) are frequently used in the treatment of alcohol withdrawal (see Chapter 21).

PSYCHOSTIMULANTS. The psychostimulants, or **psychomotor stimulants,** that will be discussed in this chapter include:

1. Amphetamines.
2. Cocaine/crack.
3. Nicotine.
4. Caffeine.

Caffeine and nicotine are legal and in common use. Amphetamines, once prescribed loosely for weight reduction (diet pills) or energy (pep pills), are presently medically indicated only for narcolepsy and hyperactivity in children. Cocaine/crack is highly addictive, due to its rapid absorption and effect on the CNS. One main difference between the amphetamines and cocaine is that the amphetamines are long-acting and cocaine is short-acting. Both cocaine/crack and amphetamines are popular drugs of abuse, especially cocaine/crack.

NARCOTICS. Narcotic dependence is a world-wide concern. Every modern nation views narcotic dependency as a serious problem (Jaffe 1986).

Narcotics (opiates and opioids) are CNS depressants and used medically mainly for their analgesic effects. As drugs of abuse, they are used mainly for their euphoric effects, leaving the abuser indifferent to anticipated distress. Eventually a chronic user craves the drug more for warding off the effects of withdrawal than for the "high." Narcotics include:

1. Opium.
2. Heroin.
3. Morphine.
4. Codeine.
5. Methadone (Dolophine).
6. Meperidine (Demerol).

PSYCHOTOMIMETICS. Psychotomimetics, also known as **hallucinogens,** psychedelics, or psychodysleptics, produce abnormal mental phenomena in the cognitive and perceptual spheres. Such phenomena may include **synesthesia** (the hearing of colors or visualizing of sound), depersonalization, hallucinations, and paranoid or grandiose delusions. Lysergic acid (LSD), popular in the 1960's, was replaced by phencyclidine (PCP) in the 1970's. PCP is still used to a lesser extent. *Cannabis sativa* (marijuana, hashish), valued for its euphoric effect, shares many of the same qualities as LSD-type substances, although it lacks some of the consciousness-altering qualities of these drugs. The strength and dose of marijuana used in this country rarely produce hallucinations. Experimental use of the active ingredient in *Cannabis sativa*, tetrahydrocannabinol (THC), has proved effective in lowering intraocular pressure of glaucoma and in reducing nausea in cancer patients receiving radiation therapy or chemotherapy. Drugs falling in the category of psychotomimetics include the following:

1. PCP (phencyclidine).
2. LSD (lysergic acid) and LSD-like drugs (e.g., Mescaline and psilocybin).
3. *Cannabis sativa* (marijuana, hashish).

Alcohol, the most widely used legal drug of abuse, is discussed in Chapter 23.

General Guidelines

OBJECTIVES

After studying this section on general guidelines, the student will be able to:

1. Compare and contrast the terms substance abuse and substance dependence as defined by the *DSM III-R* (APA 1987).
2. Describe tolerance and withdrawal, and give a clinical definition of each.
3. Discuss the synergistic and antagonistic effects of drugs among polydrug abusers, and give an example of each.
4. Identify five theories that explain in part the phenomena of substance abuse.
5. Describe four components of the assessment process when working with a person who is chemically dependent.
6. Discuss health teaching on a primary and secondary level as it pertains to drug abuse.
7. Compare and contrast four methods for providing a therapeutic environment for a drug-dependent client, including the indications for each.
8. Identify three psychotherapeutic modalities found useful for substance abusers.
9. State four general goals that will potentiate the client's success at remaining drug-free.

Standard I: Theory

Hundreds of studies have focused on possible causes of substance abuse. Physical, social, developmental, psychological, cultural, and genetic studies have all failed to identify a single cause or group of causes (Bittle et al. 1986). No matter what the cause, once a person becomes dependent on a chemical agent, the person will continue to take the drug no matter what the physical, social, interpersonal, occupational, or legal consequences. A person will forsake family, friends, and lover and deny his or her own inner potential and talent in favor of the drug. The drug becomes the only thing that matters. The drug is taken initially to induce euphoria, increase feelings of self-esteem, and minimize problems and hurts. As time goes on, the drug is taken to relieve withdrawal symptoms. Therefore, continued use is reinforced by the positive presence of pleasure or to minimize the effects of withdrawal or both. As tolerance develops, more and more of the drug is needed to gain the desired effect. More of the person's time revolves around securing the drug, and many people do things they would not do ordinarily, to obtain the drug (e.g., prostitution, stealing, mugging, or even murder).

Some theories regarding a person's abuse of drugs follow (Donlon 1982; Cocaine Withdrawal Step By Step 1987; Frances and Franklin 1988).

GENETIC PREDISPOSITION. This theory has gained interest in studies of alcoholics and their children. It is thought by some researchers that alcoholism is caused by a genetically transmitted biochemical defect (see Chapter 23).

NEUROTRANSMITTER DEFECTS. Neurotransmitters are chemicals in the brain that transmit impulses from one cell to another. Certain drugs interfere with the work of neurotransmitters. Most research in this area at present is focused on the drug cocaine. Some researchers think that cocaine dependence is primarily associated with a deficiency in the neurotransmitters dopamine and norepinephrine. It is hoped that by correcting this deficiency an individual's craving for and withdrawal symptoms from cocaine can be reduced.

BIOCHEMICAL ASPECTS. The discovery of endogenous enkephalins and pituitary endorphins (the body's own opiate-like substances) have stimulated interest and information regarding biochemical mechanism underlying opiate actions and effects. The opiate receptors are found in the brain. Under normal conditions, a person's opiate receptors are exposed to certain levels of endorphins and enkephalins. When a person takes certain narcotics, these drugs block the body's opiate receptors and the body ceases to produce its own natural opiate-like substances, endorphins and enkephalins. When the opiate-like effects of the ingested substance wear off or cease, the body's own endorphin levels remain low, leaving the person dysphoric and in withdrawal.

SOCIOLOGICAL FACTORS. Cultural or peer pressure, especially during adolescence, appears to contribute to drug abuse. Some reasons adolescents give for taking drugs follow:

1. For acceptance.
2. To rebel.
3. From curiosity.
4. To relieve boredom.

SOCIOECONOMIC CLASS. Being a "drug addict" can give a person a place in a subculture where he or she can be accepted. This is most true in economically deprived and highly stressed and unstable environments, where drugs are taken to numb pervasive feelings of helplessness and to provide a person with a sense of belonging and identity.

SELF-MEDICATION. The myths that "happiness" should be an enduring state, and that anxiety, depression, and loneliness are unnatural and should be avoided at all costs, have contributed to the American "pill-popping" phenomenon. Over-the-counter medications are used by a large percentage of our population. Drug abuse, especially polydrug abuse, often is the result of an attempt to treat depression, solve problems, and escape intolerable situations.

Standard II: Data Collection

The nurse gathers data about substance abuse from assessing (1) *signs of intoxication/withdrawal*, (2) *level of physiological complications*, (3) *personal history and coping style*, and (4) *drug history*.

ASSESSING SIGNS OF INTOXICATION

Each drug has its own physiological signs and symptoms of intoxication and individual pattern of withdrawal symptoms. Therefore, specific, individual treatment is necessary when a person is in a coma, intoxicated, or in withdrawal. In the subsequent four sections of the chapter, specific symptoms of intoxications, overdose, and withdrawal are discussed.

ASSESSING THE LEVEL OF PHYSICAL COMPLICATIONS

Drugs of abuse can be lethal. The nurse needs to be aware of the physical side effects of specific drugs of abuse. Common physical complications related to drug abuse are listed in Table 24–1.

ASSESSING PERSONAL HISTORY AND COPING STYLE

The focus of the nursing history is to record the client's perceptions in the area of presenting problems and current lifestyle and to obtain a brief sketch of the client's current life, including family, friends, education, and employment history. The personal history includes having the client identify recent feelings of depression, anxiety, suspiciousness, or hopelessness.

Suicidal ideation is always assessed, especially in the case of toxicity or coma. The nurse needs to know if this was a suicide attempt or gesture. If the client appears to be suicidal, it should be determined whether there have been previous suicidal attempts or gestures. Information regarding suicide history of family members is also elicited. (Refer to Chapter 22 for assessment of suicidal potential.)

ASSESSING DRUG HISTORY

A history of substances abused includes all drugs taken, amount, length of use, route, and drug preference. It is important to determine how the drugs were used — that is, whether they were taken intravenously (IV) or intramuscularly (IM), intradermally ("skin-popped"), intranasally ("sniffed," "snorted"), smoked, or by mouth. Previous detoxifications and drug-free periods following detoxification also should be included, as well as factors that influenced the client's return to substance abuse.

Essentially, the nurse asks the following questions in a matter-of-fact, nonjudgmental fashion:

- *What drug(s) did you take before coming to the emergency room (hospital, clinic)?*
- *How did you take the drug(s)? (e.g.,* IV, IM, *orally, subcutaneously, smoking, intranasally)*
- *How much of the drug(s) did you take?*
- *When was (were) the last dose(s) taken?*
- *How long have you been using the drug(s)?*
- *How often and how much of the drug(s) do you usually take?*
- *Do you drink alcohol or smoke marijuana? (Often these are not considered drugs by some people.) How often? How much?*

Table 24–1 • POSSIBLE PHYSICAL COMPLICATIONS RELATED TO DRUG USE

DRUG	PHYSICAL COMPLICATIONS
Route: Intravenous*	
Narcotics (e.g., heroin) Phencyclidine piperidine (PCP) Cocaine/Crack	AIDS Hepatitis Bacterial endocarditis Renal failure Cardiac arrest Coma Seizures Respiratory arrest Dermatitis Pulmonary emboli Tetanus Abscesses—Osteomyelitis * **Note:** The preceding complications can result from any drug taken intravenously.
Route: Intravenous, Intranasal	
Cocaine	Perforation of nasal septum (when taken intranasally) Respiratory paralysis Cardiovascular collapse Hyperpyrexia
Route: Ingestion	
Caffeine	Acid indigestion Peptic ulcer Increased intraocular pressure in unregulated glaucoma Tachycardia Increased plasma glucose and lipid levels
Route: Smoking, Ingestion	
Marijuana	Impaired lung structure Chromosomal mutation—increased incidence of birth defects Micronucleic white blood cells—increased risk of disease due to decreased resistance to infection Possible long term effects on short term memory
Route: Smoking, Chewing	
Nicotine	*Heavy chronic use associated with* Emphysema Cancer of the larynx and esophagus Lung cancer Peripheral vascular diseases
Route: Intravenous	
Heroin	Constipation Dermatitis Malnutrition Hypoglycemia Dental caries Amenorrhea See *Route: Intravenous** for additional complications.
Route: Ingestion	
Phencyclidine piperidine (PCP)	Respiratory arrest See *Route: Intravenous** for additional complications.

If the person is not able to provide a drug history, look for indications of substance abuse such as dilated or constricted pupils, abnormal vital signs, needle marks, tremors, and history from family and friends (Brauerman and Shook 1987). Check clothing for drug paraphernalia.

The nurse should also gather data with regard to use or abuse of drugs among family members. Drug abuse by adolescents seems to be related to their parents' use and abuse of drugs, especially alcohol (Brooks 1983). Drug abuse by a family member may also be related to increase in anxiety or conflict within the family (e.g., threatened divorce or separation).

Standard III: Diagnosis

Nursing diagnosis for clients with psychoactive substance use disorders are many and varied, owing to the large range of physical and psychological effects of drug abuse or dependence upon the user and his or her family. Potential nursing diagnoses for people with psychoactive substance use disorders are as follows:

- Anxiety
- Ineffective individual coping
- Altered cardiac output
- Impaired communications
- Fear
- Hopelessness
- Potential for infection
- Altered parenting
- Ineffective breathing patterns
- Potential for self-harm
- Sexual dysfunction
- Sleep pattern disturbance
- Impaired social interaction
- Altered thought processes
- Potential for violence: self-directed or directed at others
- Altered family process
- Self-care deficit
- Disturbance in personal identity
- Diversional activity deficit
- Altered nutrition: less than body requirements
- Powerlessness
- Self-esteem disturbance
- Spiritual distress
- Impairment of skin integrity

Standard IV: Planning

CONTENT LEVEL—PLANNING GOALS

Nursing goals will vary widely depending on whether the client is in a coma or intoxicated, in withdrawal, suicidal, in need of learning more effective coping skills, or requiring specific referral information. Specific examples of long term and short term goals will be presented in each of the subsequent sections of this chapter.

PROCESS LEVEL—NURSES' REACTIONS AND FEELINGS

Although nurses may identify with and have sympathy for clients addicted to caffeine and/or tobacco, their responses to hard-core drug abusers may not be so sympathetic. Substance abusers, particularly repeat substance abusers, are subject to the disdain of many nurses. A client who has overdosed on heroin, LSD, or cocaine may be viewed by health care workers with disapproval, intolerance, moralistic condemnation and may be considered morally weak. Also, manipulative behaviors that are often seen in these clients lead nurses to feel angry and exploited (Zamora 1987b).

In some areas of the country, the recreational use of cocaine, cannabis, and speed is so common that the nurse may view this occurrence of intoxication or overdose as "rather normal" and may not have much emotional reaction. This attitude is as detrimental as strong emotional disapproval, because the nurse may underestimate the importance of supportive measures and client education and the need for follow-up psychotherapeutic intervention.

Perhaps the most detrimental attitude among nurses and other health care workers is that of *enabling* (supporting, or denying the seriousness of, the client's physical/psychological substance dependence). Bittle and coworkers (1986) describe several behaviors that signal enabling by the nurse. The nurse

1. Encourages denial by agreeing that the client only drinks/takes drugs "socially" or when a little nervous.
2. Ignores cues to possible dependency—steers away from drugs to topics more comfortable for the nurse (e.g., anxiety, depression).
3. Demonstrates sympathy for the client's "reasons" (work, family, financial problems) for abusing drugs rather than pointing out that these difficulties are

often the result of—not the cause of—substance abuse.

4. Preaches that the problem can be overcome by will power, thus minimizing the fact that the person is physically/psychologically chemically dependent and has lost control over the use of the drug.

Programs for Chemically Impaired Health Care Professionals

A nurse may deny drug abuse or dependence in others in order to reinforce denial of personal drug abuse or dependence. The problem of the chemically impaired health care professional is receiving more recognition and acknowledgement. Nurses and doctors appear to have higher rates of alcohol and prescription drug abuse than people in the general population (Jaffe 1985; Survey 1986). Programs for chemically dependent nurses have been developed in some states in response to a policy statement issued by the American Nurses' Association. The aim of these programs is to protect clients and to keep the nurse in active practice (perhaps with limitations) or to return the nurse to practice after suspension and professional help. Both the medical and nursing professions are formally recognizing this problem, and there is an increased commitment to the rehabilitation of chemically impaired health care professionals, in the form of self-help peer support groups, hotlines, crisis information, and treatment referral (Bittle 1986). See the section on antianxiety agents for further discussion of chemically impaired health care professionals.

Standard V: Intervention

V-A: PSYCHOTHERAPEUTIC INTERVENTIONS

Working with a person who is dependent on a psychoactive drug means working with behaviors that almost all substance abusers have in common. These behaviors include (1) dysfunctional anger, (2) manipulation, (3) impulsiveness, and (4) grandiosity (Zamora 1987b). These behaviors and suggested nursing interventions are discussed in Chapter 17. Working with clients who frequently display these behaviors can be challenging and, at times, frustrating. However, supervision, peer support, and team cooperation lessen anxiety and feelings of helplessness among staff and increase the client's opportunity to learn more adaptive coping styles.

Nurses with special training may teach interested clients relaxation techniques or self-hypnosis as an adjunct to other therapies. By offering an alternative coping behavior for anxiety reduction, the client may substitute a more adaptive action for lowering anxiety and, as a result, may gain a sense of control and self-esteem.

V-B: HEALTH TEACHING

People who abuse or are dependent on psychoactive drugs may develop a variety of physical illnesses (see Table 24–1). A client may need to be hospitalized when a complication is life-threatening (e.g., bacteria endocarditis, pulmonary embolus) or in need of long term care (e.g., hepatitis, severe abscesses).

Important health teaching with IV drug abusers includes (1) how to sterilize needles to minimize the risk of AIDS and hepatitis and (2) the use of condoms during sex to minimize the risk or spread of AIDS. (Some nurses find it difficult to accept these nursing care measures.) Essentially, health teaching for people who are abusing drugs and plan to continue use includes the following information:

1. How to administer the drug under antiseptic conditions if the IV route is being used.
2. Education as to the properties, side effects, and long term physical or emotional effects of the drug.
3. Referral information about community-based clinics, telephone numbers for hotlines, self-help groups, half-way houses, and so forth, for possible future use.
4. Nutritional information. Many people who use drugs suffer from malnutrition, either because of their lifestyle or because of the properties of the drugs themselves.

Primary Prevention

Primary prevention through health teaching can have an important impact on how youngsters and adolescents choose to solve problems and relate interpersonally. Resnick (1979) offers the following suggestions:

1. Involvement with programs that can strengthen interpersonal and social skills of individuals. An assertiveness training program is an example.
2. More drug education in schools and homes. Peer teaching is often most effective, especially among adolescents.

3. Availability of peer counselors for high school and college students. The normal issues adolescents deal with can be overwhelming for some—e.g., identity problems, setting occupational goals, heterosexual relationship issues, sexual issues, and drug concerns.
4. Increase in neighborhood recreational and occupational opportunities.
5. Support for families that aims to improve social conditions within the community.
6. Strong community interagency linkage, allowing sharing of resources.

Most communities have youth organizations such as scouting, 4-H clubs, and school clubs. It has been found that the young people who participate in these are at a lower risk for becoming substance abusers. Activities such as these help develop self-confidence and self-esteem in young people.

Part-time job placement can be an important alternative to substance abuse. Earning money on one's own can increase feelings of self-worth and confidence.

Health Teaching For Families

There has been a great deal of research on families with a chemically dependent member(s). Family intervention is often an important treatment modality in altering maladaptive drug use by one member. Family theorists view a crisis with one member as a signal of a family in distress.

It is believed that some forms of substance abuse may have their roots in the interpersonal context of family relationships (Klagsburn and Davis 1977). Certainly, once substance abuse is integrated into the family experience, the family responds. The response may favor both the abuse pattern and its consequences. In functional families, there is a coalition between the parents, and the children grow up knowing that the parents will stick together. The parental power is clear, and competing parent-child coalitions are absent (Beavers 1976). In sharp contrast, the marital partners in substance abusing families are typically not in coalition with one another. The power struggle of a spouse to control the substance abuse of the partner leaves its mark, with decreased caring and mutuality.

Conflict between the parents is postulated by Klagsburn and Davis (1977) as a cause of adolescent drug use. The child, by drawing attention to himself, may become a symbolic scapegoat for the unresolved feelings and tensions of the parents.

Clear ego boundaries for each family member are another characteristic of healthy families (Beavers 1976). In the substance abusing family there is a pattern of ego enmeshment. A child's fear of separation from the family may be an important dynamic in adolescent drug use, since substance abuse often serves to keep the child within or dependent on the family. To complicate matters, parents themselves often have not emancipated themselves from their families of origin (Weingarten 1980). Often there is no one member who consistently holds the power in a substance abusing family. In drug abusing families with adolescents, there is often inconsistent limit setting (Weingarten 1980). The married adult drug abuser often duplicates an earlier conflicted, ambivalent, and immature child-parent relationship with his or her spouse (Seldin 1972).

As substance abuse is integrated into the family, there may be a pattern of predictable roles for each of the members. Wegscheider (1981) describes six family roles:

1. The chemically dependent person.
2. The chief enabler.
3. The family hero.
4. The scapegoat.
5. The lost child.
6. The mascot.

The *chief enabler* is closest to the substance abuser and, in order to maintain the norms of family life, becomes increasingly responsible for fulfilling the duties left vacant by the abuser. The *family hero* feels responsible for the family difficulty and attempts to improve the situation. The *scapegoat* acts out of hurt in a defiant manner. The *lost child* withdraws into the self for comfort. The *mascot* uses wit to attract attention and survive in the family system.

Anger, ambivalence, fear, guilt, confusion, and mistrust are frequent feelings in substance abusing families. Conflict is a norm. Social isolation limits the energy derived from the larger community, and the family is entrapped with its own need to balance relationships. The adequate nourishment required for spontaneous, clear communication is lacking. Victimization caused by immature, impulsive members is frequent.

Counseling and support should be encouraged for all family members. Al-Anon and Al-a-Teen are self-help groups that offer support and guidance for adults and teenagers, respectively, in families with a chemically dependent member.

V-C: SOMATIC THERAPIES

There are times when medications are given in response to withdrawal from drugs. For example, the most well-known medical intervention is the methadone (Dolophine) maintenance programs developed in the 1960's. This form of treatment for heroin addiction is highly controversial.

Methadone (Dolophine) is a synthetic opiate that at certain doses (usually 40 mg) blocks the craving for and effects of heroin. However, it is itself highly addicting and when stopped produces withdrawal. **Naltrexone** (Trexan) is a nonaddicting narcotic antagonist that has allowed many addicts to live drug free. The use of **clonidine,** initially marketed for high blood pressure, has also proved to be an effective somatic treatment for some chemically dependent individuals when combined with naltrexone (Schloemer and Skidmore 1983; Frances and Franklin 1988). Clonidine is a nonopioid suppressor of opioid withdrawal symptoms; however, at this writing it has not been approved by the FDA for opioid detoxification. Clonidine is also nonaddicting. Other drugs used for clients intoxicated by or withdrawing from certain drugs can include diazepam (Valium) and antipsychotics such as haloperidol (Haldol). (Refer to each section for specific somatic therapies.)

Acupuncture has been an effective adjunct to treatment for withdrawal from nicotine, caffeine, alcohol, and narcotics for approximately 13 years (Zweig 1987). The success of acupuncture depends on supplemental lifestyle interventions and client commitment.

V-D: THERAPEUTIC ENVIRONMENT

DETOXIFICATION. The first step toward treatment is often detoxification. Each drug has unique properties, and each drug has individual interventions for safe withdrawal (see Tables 24–2 through 24–5). Many individuals do not go further in treatment than detoxification. For example, two out of three opiate dependent clients go back to using heroin within six months (Harvard Medical School 1987).

RESIDENTIAL THERAPEUTIC COMMUNITIES. Most residential therapeutic communities expect the addict to remain for 12 to 18 months. The goal of treatment is to effect a change in lifestyle, including abstinence from drugs. Other anticipated outcomes are the development of social skills and the elimination of antisocial behavior. Follow-up studies suggest that those clients who stay 90 days or longer exhibit a significant decrease in illicit drug use and recorded arrests and an increase in legitimate employment (Jaffe 1985). The residential therapeutic community is considered best suited for those individuals who have a long history of antisocial behavior (Klein and Miller 1986). Synanon, Phoenix House, and Odyssey House are three of the more familiar names among the more than 300 therapeutic communities in the United States.

OUTPATIENT DRUG-FREE PROGRAMS. These programs have the same goals as the therapeutic communities but aim to achieve these goals in an outpatient setting, thus allowing individuals to continue employment and family life. Outpatient drug-free programs are better geared to the polydrug abuser rather than the heavily addicted heroin client. These centers may offer vocational education and placement, counseling, and individual or group psychotherapy.

EMPLOYEE ASSISTANCE PROGRAMS. Employee Assistance Programs (EAPs) have been developed to provide the delivery of mental health services in occupational settings. Many hospitals and corporations have such programs for their professional staff. EAP programs deal with issues of alcohol and drug abuse and offer employee counseling, information, and referral services (Bittle et al. 1986; Brill et al. 1985).

V-E: PSYCHOTHERAPY

INDIVIDUAL. Individuals who have abused drugs for a period of time benefit more from analytical or supportive expressive psychotherapy than from standard drug counseling alone (Jaffe 1985). Other approaches that have proven effective for some are cognitive and behaviorally oriented therapies.

GROUP. Groups can help chemically dependent individuals break through denial and rationalization. Group members confront one another regarding drug and antisocial behaviors. Group cohesion fosters growth and commitment toward individual goals. Group interactions increase self-esteem and provide a sense of purpose and belonging. The group modality is especially effective with adolescents because peer relationships are often more acceptable than those of adult authority figures.

Other groups that are highly successful in supporting chemically impaired individuals are the self-help groups patterned after Alcoholics Anonymous (AA). Such groups include Pills Anonymous (PA), Narcotics Anonymous (NA), Cocaine Anonymous (CA), Valium Anonymous (VA), and many others.

FAMILY. Families who have a chemically impaired member need support, information, and guidance. The recovering addict usually has caused disruption, frustration, and confusion among other family members. These and other issues need to be addressed under the guidance of a trained therapist (e.g., nurse, social worker, psychologist). In fact some studies suggest that family therapy, in conjunction with regular urinalysis checks, is superior to standard day counseling in fostering a decrease in illicit drug use (Jaffe 1985).

Standard VI: Evaluation

Evaluation is a continuous process. Short term goals often include the substance abuser's physical safety when the individual's life is threatened, as may be the case in coma, intoxication, and withdrawal. Long term goals involve lifestyle changes, more effective coping methods, improvement in issues involving self-esteem and identity, and improvement in social and interpersonal relationships. Acee and Smith (1987) propose the following goals, which, when met, make possible alternate choices for a more satisfying and productive future.

The client will understand that

1. Chemical dependency is a progressively deteriorating disease if left unchecked.
2. Individuals are not responsible for their disease, but they are responsible for their recovery.
3. Clients cannot blame people, places, or things for their dependency. They must face their problems and their feelings.
4. Rehabilitation and recovery are life-long enterprises that begin with a commitment to a long term treatment effort.

Summary

Pathological use of drugs is divided into *substance abuse* and *substance dependence*. A person who abuses drugs is one whose social, occupational, psychological, or physical problems are exacerbated by the drug and/or whose continued use of the drug puts the person in physical danger. Drug dependence includes the preceding characteristics plus *tolerance* to or *withdrawal symptoms* when the body is deprived of the drug. The prevalence of polydrug abuse was discussed. The dangers of the *synergistic effect* were mentioned, as well as the *antagonistic effect* that drugs may have on each other. *Toxicological screening* is one way of indicating the presence of different drugs in the body.

Various theories of drug abuse were reviewed. No single theory has been found to explain the reasons for substance dependence and abuse.

Four areas of assessment are (1) signs of intoxication/withdrawal, (2) physical complications, (3) personal history and coping style, and (4) drug history. Since drug use can be precipitated by or be the cause of a wide range of psychological as well as physical problems, possible nursing diagnoses are numerous.

Goal planning reflects individual needs. Nurses' feelings need to be recognized and discussed with peers, since reactions to clients who are chemically dependent are often intense. Some common problematic responses are intolerance, moralistic condemnation, enabling, and denial.

A number of treatment modalities were covered, including detoxification, residential communities, outpatient drug-free programs, and employee assistance programs. Group, family, and individual interventions were addressed under psychotherapy. The greatest emphasis was placed on health teaching and primary prevention. Evaluating whether certain client-centered goals will be met depends in part on the client's being able to meet four basic goals compiled by Acee and Smith (1987).

The problem of drug abuse and dependence among health care professionals was addressed and will be discussed further in the next section.

Self-study exercises 1 through 15 at the end of the chapter will help you review the material presented in this section.

Antianxiety Agents (Sedative-Hypnotics, or Anxiolytics)

OBJECTIVES

After studying this section on antianxiety agents, the student will be able to:

1. Name four anxiolytics or antianxiety drugs often abused.
2. Discuss five physical and five psychological signs of sedative-hypnotic or anxiolytic intoxication.
3. Describe emergency medical and nursing treatments for a person who has overdosed, and identify five emergency situations that can occur in anxiolytic intoxication.
4. Discuss treatment for a person who is withdrawing from an anxiolytic CNS depressant.
5. Discuss some of the reactions a nurse might have when working with a chemically impaired nurse.
6. Identify six ways that you as a nurse can help a chemically impaired colleague.

Introduction

BARBITURATES

For centuries people have sought relief through drugs for anxiety and insomnia. During the nineteenth century, opiates had been prescribed to relieve these symptoms. Alcohol was also prescribed as the sedative or hypnotic of choice. Toward the end of the nineteenth century, two German scientists synthesized a new chemical called barbital, a derivative of barbituric acid. This drug was successfully used to facilitate sleep in clients and, given in smaller doses, it would decrease anxiety. In 1903 barbital was introduced into general medical practice under the trade name Veronal, and in 1912 phenobarbital was introduced under the trade name Luminal. Eventually, more than 50 barbiturates were synthesized and accepted for medical use. Long-acting barbiturates were developed for daytime sedation, and short-acting ones were used for prompt sedation and for inducing sleep without delay. These drugs are odorless and tasteless, and precise quantities can be dispensed in capsules or tablets.

During the 1930's and 1940's, it became apparent that these drugs were addicting. A person who became dependent on barbiturates suffers many of the same withdrawal symptoms as a person withdrawing from alcohol (see Chapter 21). Abrupt withdrawal of these drugs may prove fatal.

Eventually, states began outlawing nonprescription barbiturates. By the end of the 1940's, the United States, which had for decades used barbiturates sensibly for anxiety and insomnia, was persuaded that these drugs were "thrill pills." Unfortunately, for some people these warnings served as lures; illicit barbiturate use increased from year to year.

BENZODIAZEPINES

Diazepam (Valium) and chlordiazepoxide (Librium), both benzodiazepines, are known as anxiolytic, and antianxiety, medications. These drugs are also called minor tranquilizers. The effects of Valium, Librium, and other benzodiazepines are similar to those of the barbiturates. The major difference seems to be that a dose of a benzodiazepine (Valium or Librium) that is sufficient to calm anxiety seems to produce a little less sleepiness

Table 24–2 • SEDATIVE-HYPNOTIC OR ANXIOLYTIC AGENTS (ANTIANXIETY DRUGS)

DEFINITION: Known as minor tranquilizers, sedatives, hypnotics, and antianxiety agents. Reduce pathological anxiety, tension, and agitation without therapeutic effects on disturbed cognitive or perceptual processes. High potential for dependency; all act differently in the body but produce symptoms of intoxication and withdrawal similar to those of alcohol withdrawal.

		OVERDOSE		WITHDRAWAL	
DRUG	**INTOXICATION**	**Effects**	**Possible Treatments**	**Effects**	**Possible Treatments**
BARBITURATES Amobarbital (Amytal) Phenobarbital (Nembutal) Secobarbital (Seconal) **BENZODIAZEPINES** Diazepam (Valium) Chlordiazepoxide (Librium) Lorazepam (Ativan) Oxazepam (Serax) Alprazolam (Xanax) **CHLORAL HYDRATE** **METHAQUALONE** (Quaalude) **GLUTETHIMIDE** (Doriden) **MEPROBAMATE** (Equanil, Miltown)	PHYSICAL SIGNS: Slurred speech Incoordination Unsteady gait Drowsiness Decreased blood pressure PSYCHOLOGICAL/PERCEPTUAL: Disinhibition of sexual or aggressive drives Impaired judgment Impaired social/occupational function Impaired attention or memory Irritability	Cardiovascular or respiratory depression/arrest (mostly with barbiturates) Coma Shock Convulsions Death	IF AWAKE: Keep awake Induce vomiting Give activated charcoal to aid absorption of drug Every 15 minutes check vital signs (VS) COMA: Clear airway—endotrachial tube Intravenous (IV) fluids Gastric lavage with activated charcoal Frequent VS after client is stable for shock and cardiac arrest Seizure precautions Possible hemo- or peritoneal dialysis	CESSATION OF PROLONGED/HEAVY USE: Nausea/vomiting Tachycardia Diaphoresis Anxiety/irritability Tremors in hands, fingers, eyelids Marked insomnia Grand mal seizures AFTER 5 TO 15 YEARS' HEAVY USE: Delirium	Carefully titrated detoxification with similar drug, usually phenobarbital **NOTE: Abrupt withdrawal can lead to death**

Data from Grinspoon and Bakalar 1985; Smith 1984; Bittle et al. 1986; DSM III-R 1987.

than does a dose of barbiturates equally effective against anxiety. Benzodiazepines, like all anxiolytic drugs, are CNS depressants. Clients should be advised against the simultaneous ingestion of alcohol and other CNS depressant drugs (Table 24–2). Clients should also be cautioned against engaging in hazardous tasks requiring complete mental alertness, such as operating machinery or driving a motor vehicle. Withdrawal symptoms, similar to those for all sedative-hypnotic or anxiolytic drugs, occur following abrupt discontinuance. These include convulsions, tremors, abdominal and muscle cramps, vomiting, and sweating. Abrupt withdrawal from consistent long term use can prove dangerous, even fatal. Gradual withdrawal when coming off these drugs is safest.

METHAQUALONE

Methaqualone (Quaalude) is a nonbarbiturate sedative-hypnotic that was introduced into India in the 1950's as an antimalarial agent. It is a Schedule II drug, which means that it has dangerous potential for psychological and physical dependence. In humans the drug accumulates in fatty tissue and readily enters the brain, just as barbiturates do. High doses can cause psychological and physical dependence and dangerous withdrawal symptoms when the drug is stopped. Side effects include insomnia, abdominal cramps, headaches, anorexia, and nightmares. Severe grand mal convulsions may occur after sudden withdrawal from high doses (see Table 24–2).

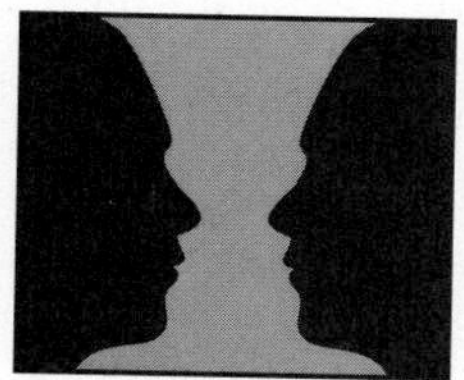

Case Study: Working With a Person Dependent on Valium

Elyse, a 34-year-old, recently divorced nurse was brought into the hospital emergency room by two friends who had gone to her apartment for a visit. They stated that they found Elyse lying on the couch; a half-empty bottle of vodka was open and near the couch. When her friends tried to talk to Elyse, she responded with slurred speech. When she attempted to walk, her gait was unsteady. The friends reported that when they questioned Elyse about her condition, she became extremely irritable.

Her friends stated that as they sat with Elyse they became increasingly alarmed, and phoned Elyse's physician, who encouraged them to take her to the hospital. On the way to the hospital, Elyse abruptly changed her mind and attempted to open the car door. Elyse's friends brought with them an empty bottle of Valium pills, which had recently been prescribed for Elyse.

Assessment

SIGNS OF INTOXICATION/WITHDRAWAL

Abuse of CNS depressants other than alcohol is determined by three major criteria; (1) a pattern of pathological abuse, (2) impairment in social or occupational functioning caused by the pathological use of the substance, and (3) duration of use, which requires that the disturbance last for at least one month. Use does not have to be continuous throughout a given month but must be frequent enough within a month's time to cause noticeable difficulties in social and occupational functioning.

Symptoms of intoxication include the following:

1. Mood lability
2. Disinhibition of sexual and aggressive impulses
3. Irritability
4. Loquacity
5. Slurred speech
6. Incoordination
7. Unsteady gait
8. Impairment of attention or memory
9. Impaired social judgment.

Continued misuse of any antianxiety drug has a cumulative toxic effect on the CNS that is life-threatening. In large doses, or in combination with other CNS depressants, antianxiety drugs may cause death.

During the assessment, the nurse determined that Elyse did display some symptoms of intoxication: namely, irritability, slurred speech, incoordination, unsteady gait, and impaired judgment. Because the continued misuse of CNS depressants has a cumulative effect on the CNS that is life-threatening, the staff had to determine immediately how much of the medication Elyse had consumed. Elyse was questioned and drowsily stated that she was not sure how many pills she had taken. The pharmacist was then called. During this time, vital signs were being taken, a gastric lavage was performed, and blood specimens were drawn.

PHYSICAL COMPLICATIONS

When a client has overdosed on or is quite intoxicated from CNS depressants, it is very important for the nurse to observe and record vital signs frequently. These include blood pressure, temperature, pulse, respirations, and neurological symptoms. It is also very important to assess respiratory functioning. An intoxicated client should be on seizure precautions; if the client does have a seizure, seizure activity should also be observed and recorded. If a seizure occurs, protect the client's head and limbs during the seizure, maintaining a patent airway. Always time a seizure and any periods of apnea. Urinary output is often monitored, and specimens saved for drug screening.

Another possible complication is pulmonary edema. The symptoms are anxiety and restlessness; gray complexion; cold, moist hands; cyanotic nail beds; incessant coughing; and noisy and moist breathing.

Elyse's blood pressure was 90/60; her pulse was 128; and her respirations were 8–10 per minute and shallow.

Continued on following page

Assessment *(Continued)*

PERSONAL HISTORY AND COPING STYLE

Because Elyse's verbal communication was impaired, the nurse gathered her data from Elyse's two friends and the pharmacist. When it was determined that Elyse's condition was not life-threatening, the nurse continued her assessment. She encouraged Elyse to describe her current problems and also gathered data from Elyse and her two friends about recent stresses in Elyse's life. The nurse learned that Elyse's brother had been killed recently in an automobile accident about a week before Elyse's divorce was finalized. Elyse's friends reported that Elyse had been quite depressed for the past few weeks, and that they had been quite concerned about her.

Elyse had been in charge of the intensive care unit at a nearby hospital. She was bright, ambitious, and respected by her peers. Her friends stated that they knew Elyse was sneaking Valium from the unit and were concerned, but they had no idea that her abuse of Valium was so serious. Elyse told her friends that the drug made her feel more relaxed and able to cope better with her problems and her job.

At this particular time, an accurate history of other substance abuse and length of use, as well as drug preference, could not be made because of Elyse's condition.

Because Elyse's situation could easily have been life-threatening, it was important to assess suicidal ideation and to determine if this was a suicide attempt or gesture. It appeared to the staff that this had been an actual suicidal attempt, since Elyse had taken a substantial amount of Valium pills with alcohol and had not been expecting visitors.

DRUG HISTORY

Elyse was unable to give any information at this time, and her friends were unaware of her use of any drugs other than Valium and alcohol.

Nursing Diagnosis

Some nursing diagnoses that pertain to Elyse follow:

1. *Impaired Verbal Communication* (slurred speech) related to CNS depressant effect of drug
2. *Potential for Self-Directed Violence* related to divorce, loss of brother, and drug dependence, as evidenced by drug overdose
3. *Self-Esteem Disturbance* related to divorce and loss of family members, as evidenced by substance abuse

Planning

CONTENT LEVEL—PLANNING GOALS

Goals relevant to each of the nursing diagnoses were established.

Nursing Diagnosis	Long Term Goal	Short Term Goals
1. *Impaired Verbal Communication* (slurred speech) related to Valium intoxication	The client will speak clearly by discharge.	1a. The client will talk with the nurse for 15 minutes each shift by (state the date). 1b. The client will name three personal strengths by (state the date).
2. *Potential for Self-Directed Violence* related to divorce, loss of brother, and drug dependence, as evidenced by drug overdose	The client will state that she wants to live by discharge.	2a. The client will make a no-suicide contract with nurse by (state the date). 2b. The client will agree to inform the staff of dysphoric feelings she is experiencing by (state the date). 2c. The client will discuss with the nurse what she can do to work out feelings.

Nursing Diagnosis	Long Term Goal	Short Term Goals
3. *Self-Esteem Disturbance* related to divorce, loss of family members, and drug dependence	Client will name two actions that she can take to improve her self-esteem and quality of life.	3a. Client will discuss with nurse effects of losses (husband and brother). 3b. Client will discuss with nurse extent of her substance abuse. 3c. Client will discuss with nurse and health team members long term treatment plans.

Some interventions planned to meet the set goals are listed here.

Short Term Goals	Interventions
1. Client will talk with nurse for 15 minutes each shift by (state the date).	1a. Approach client in a positive and open manner. 1b. Assist client to identify personal strengths. 1c. Give positive feedback.
2. Client will make a no-suicide contract with nurse by (state the date).	2a. Remove all possible or potential weapons, including glass bottles, belts, razors, and plastic bags. 2b. Assess immediate degree of suicidal risk and ask if client is thinking of harming herself. 2c. Keep client on one-to-one observation. 2d. Spend time with client for at least 15 minutes twice each day.
3. Client will discuss with nurse extent of her substance abuse by (state the date).	3a. During scheduled meetings, assist client in connecting beginning of Valium and alcohol abuse with feelings surrounding life events. 3b. Client will state when, how long she has been taking abused substance(s), as well as how much and what other drugs she has been taking.

PROCESS LEVEL—NURSES' REACTIONS AND FEELINGS

Word soon spread about a nurse having "overdosed." As accustomed as other nurses were to working with people who were intoxicated or in a coma related to substance abuse, this was different—nurses have strong feelings related to "one of their own." Many nurses had a highly moralistic, rigidly judgmental attitude: "She should have known better." "I hope they take her license away." "She's a disgrace." At the other extreme nurses were being enabling: "Poor thing, she had so many tough breaks . . . no wonder she needed something to get over her losses." Both these attitudes toward the chemically impaired nurses are defensive and not objective. Both attitudes can cause problems for the nurses that hold them, and certainly for the chemically impaired nurse-clients who might come under their care.

Chemical dependency is the number one health problem affecting nurses. Nurses have a 50% higher rate of chemical dependency than the general population.

An in-service education program was set up for the whole nursing staff, since this incident reflected concerns that hospital administrators had about their own staff. Attitudes, approaches, and resources were covered. It was stressed that a nurse who demonstrates behaviors consistent with drug abuse or dependence should be reported to a supervisor immediately. First,

Continued on following page

Planning *(Continued)*

this can prevent harm to clients under the nurse's care and, *second*, it may save a colleague's professional career and/or life.

The following guidelines were given to the nursing staff regarding dealing with a chemically impaired colleague (Jefferson and Ensur 1982):

Don'ts

There are some things that one should definitely NOT do, under any circumstances, when dealing with an alcohol- or drug-addicted nurse:

1. **Don't** lecture, moralize, scold, blame, threaten, or argue with the person about the problem. Document it and use it to counsel the person about job performance.
2. **Don't** lose your temper.
3. **Don't** "enable" the problem to continue by covering up the consequences, trying to protect the person, making excuses, or doing his or her job.
4. **Don't** give the person an easier work schedule.
5. **Don't** have a holier-than-thou attitude.
6. **Don't** be overly sympathetic. You are not a counselor or big sister/brother.
7. **Don't** accept what you know is a lie. When you know the person is lying, say so. Accepting lies only encourages more lying, and you will lose the person's respect at the same time.
8. **Don't** accept mere promises to "do better," and don't keep switching agreements. When you say that a job is in jeopardy (suspension or termination) if the person's performance does not improve, you must follow through.
9. **Don't** accept the responsibility of letting someone work on your unit or team if impaired by alcohol or drugs. Judgment is the first thing to go.
10. **Don't** put off facing the problem, hoping it will get better with time. It won't.

Helping the chemically impaired nurse is difficult but not impossible. The choices for actions are varied, and the only choice that is clearly wrong is to do nothing. Nurses who have worked with chemically impaired nurses state that the majority want to be helped and not protected.

Intervention

All sedative-hypnotics, including nonbarbiturate forms, can produce physical dependence and a barbiturate-like withdrawal syndrome, with convulsions, if the drug is taken in sufficient dosage over a long enough period. Symptoms of withdrawal include anxiety, tremors, nightmares, insomnia, anorexia, nausea and vomiting, seizures, delirium, and hyperactivity. The course depends on the particular drug (see Table 24–2).

Detoxification should be gradual, since abrupt withdrawal in a person who is physically dependent is dangerous. Supportive measures, including vitamins, restoration of electrolyte imbalance, and prevention of dehydration, are also used. Close observation of the client at this time is also essential (see Table 24–2).

Elyse was placed in the detoxification unit to treat the effects of her Valium and alcohol abuse. During the initial days of admission, she was on suicide precaution. She was rude and demanding, was contemptuous of the nursing staff, and demanded release from the unit. After several days passed, she became more withdrawn and depressed and started talking more with her primary nurse, Mrs. Brown. Mrs. Brown, who was 51 years old, had many years of nursing experience and had an intelligent and comfortable manner.

Dialogue	Therapeutic Tool/Comment
N: Elyse, I get the impression that life must have been getting very difficult for you lately.	Nurse validates and empathizes.
E: (*Silence*) . . . I don't think you would understand.	
N: I guess sometimes it feels like no one understands, but I would like to try.	Reflecting/empathy.
E: At times . . . I feel I can't go on any more . . . so many losses.	

Dialogue	Therapeutic Tool/Comment
N: Loss is difficult. Elyse, tell me about your losses.	Encouraging the client to share her painful feelings.
E: My brother's sudden death . . . We were so close . . . I depended on him so much.	
N: It must have been so difficult for you to lose him so suddenly.	Empathy.
E: (*Silence*) . . . No one knows . . . then Harry, he left . . . (*Elyse starts to cry*)	
N: Tell me what you are feeling right now.	Encouraging expression of feelings while feelings are close to the surface.
E: I don't know . . . angry maybe . . . Why does everyone leave me . . . I hate them . . . Oh, I wish I had a Valium now . . .	
N: And what does the Valium do to help you?	Begins to explore the drug dependence in a gently nonthreatening manner.

Elyse became less defensive as time went on and seemed to relate best to Mrs. Brown and the male social worker. He told Elyse about a Narcotics Anonymous (NA) group that was made up of chemically impaired people from the health care professions. He stated that substance abuse disorders among nurses and doctors is a widespread, recognized problem. Elyse still had a tendency to minimize her drug dependence, but she was willing to work on her feelings about her divorce and her brother's death.

By discharge, Elyse had attended two meetings of an NA group geared toward medical personnel and had started group and individual therapy, which she would continue on an outpatient basis.

Evaluation

On discharge, Elyse was no longer perceived as suicidal. She would continue group and individual therapy on an outpatient basis and agreed to attend NA on a regular basis.

Two weeks after discharge, Elyse wrote to the Director of Nurses to get her old job back. It was agreed that she would work as a staff nurse with the understanding that she would continue therapy and agree to periodic blood and urine testing. For a probationary period she was not to give medications or have access to the keys of the medication cabinet.

Three months later Elyse was doing well at work, was attending therapy regularly, and appeared less depressed and more hopeful regarding the future. She was able to admit that drugs had taken control of her life, and she was working hard to turn things around for herself.

Summary

Anxiolytic drugs have been used since 1903 to induce sleep and facilitate sleep in the form of barbiturates. Benzodiazepines (e.g., Valium, Xanax, Librium) have generally replaced the use of barbiturates because they have fewer sedative qualities and interfere less with motor activities. Methaqualone is another sedative-hypnotic in use. All these drugs are prescription drugs, are CNS depressants, produce tolerance and withdrawal symptoms, and have a synergistic effect when taken with alcohol. All drugs in this category, although different in action, produce similar withdrawal symptoms. They are all popular and dangerous drugs of abuse. Abrupt withdrawal in a chemically dependent individual can be dangerous, leading to grand mal seizures and death.

The case study highlighted the signs of intoxication and withdrawal of anxiolytic drugs and discussed some nursing responsibilities in the process of assessment, planning, and interventions. The issue of working with a chemically dependent colleague was briefly discussed, and some guidelines were outlined. Behaviors or performances suggesting chemical abuse or dependence need to be reported to a supervisor. Not only will the lives of clients be protected, but the lives and careers of colleagues can be preserved.

Psychostimulants

OBJECTIVES

After studying this section on psychostimulants, the student will be able to:

1. Identify four psychostimulants and state one unique quality of each.
2. Compare and contrast the signs of intoxication, overdose, and withdrawal symptoms from cocaine and amphetamine use.
3. Discuss three possible nursing interventions for a client addicted to cocaine.

Introduction

AMPHETAMINES

The drug known as amphetamine was first synthesized in 1887; however, medical uses were not known until 1927. Its effects in enlarging the nasal and bronchial passages and in stimulating the central nervous system were noted, and its effect on elevating blood pressure was discovered (Kramer 1969). This drug was marketed in 1932 under the trade name Benzedrine.

In 1937, researchers found that amphetamines had a paradoxical effect on some children whose functioning is impaired by hyperactivity and an inability to concentrate. It was found that amphetamines, instead of making them even more jittery, had a calming effect on many of these children and notably improved their concentration and performance (see Chapter 27).

By the end of 1971, there were at least 31 amphetamine preparations. These included amphetamine-sedative, amphetamine-tranquilizer, and amphetamine-analgesic combinations.

During World War II, the American, British, German, and Japanese armed forces were issuing amphetamines to their men to counteract fatigue, elevate mood, and heighten endurance. After World War II, many physicians prescribed amphetamines routinely for depression and weight loss and as energizers.

After World War II, with the expansion of the legal market for prescribed amphetamines, a modest black market in the drugs also started. Early black market patrons included truck drivers who were trying to maintain schedules that called for long over-the-road hauls without adequate rest periods. Soon truck stops along the main transcontinental routes were dispensing amphetamines as well as coffee and caffeine tablets to help drivers stay awake. Students were also using amphetamine "pep pills" when cramming for exams.

Stimulants have always been popular drugs of abuse with students, athletes, and entertainers. Now, because of their high potential for abuse and the quickness with which tolerance develops (8 to 12 weeks) legitimate use of amphetamines is limited to therapy for hyperkinesis in children and for narcolepsy (Kneisl and Ames 1986). Amphetamines can be dangerous. "Speed kills" is a common saying, and it has. Refer to Table 24–3 for the physical and psychological effects of intoxication from abuse of amphetamines and other psychostimulants, possible life-threatening results of overdose, and emergency measures for both overdose and withdrawal.

COCAINE AND CRACK

Cocaine is a naturally occurring stimulant extracted from the leaf of the cocoa bush. Once the drug of the rich and famous, cocaine use is now spreading to all socioeconomic groups. The drug acts on the CNS and changes the way a person thinks, feels, and behaves. Crack is a cheap, widely available alkalinized form of cocaine. Crack is smoked and takes effect in four to six seconds. Dependence on crack develops rapidly (Gold 1984). A popular rock star recovering from crack addiction stated, "If you are on crack, you have three choices: you can get off, you can go crazy, or you can die." The fleeting high obtained from crack (lasting five to seven minutes) is followed by a period of deep depression that reinforces addictive behavior patterns and guarantees continued use of the drug (New York State 1986). With the advent of crack, doctors are seeing a profound increase in the neurological and psychological complications associated with cocaine abuse.

Table 24–3 • PSYCHOSTIMULANTS

DEFINITION: Potent CNS stimulants with psychoactive and sympathomimetic effects—speeds up body processes.

		OVERDOSE		WITHDRAWAL	
DRUG	**INTOXICATION**	**Effects**	**Possible Treatments**	**Effects**	**Possible Treatments**
AMPHETAMINES (Long-acting) Dextroamphetamine (Dexedrine) Methamphetamine (Methadrine)	PHYSICAL SIGNS: Tachycardia Dilated pupils Elevated blood pressure Nausea and vomiting Twitching PSYCHOLOGICAL/ PERCEPTUAL: Assaultive Grandiose Impaired judgment Impaired social and occupational functioning Euphoria Increased energy SEVERE EFFECTS: Resembles paranoid schizophrenia Paranoia with delusions Psychosis Visual, auditory, and tactile hallucinations Severe/panic levels of anxiety Agitated potential for violence **NOTE:** **Paranoia and ideas of reference may persist for months afterward.**	Respiratory distress Ataxia Hyperpyrexia Convulsions Coma Death associated with hyperpyrexia, convulsions, cardiovascular shock	SUPPORTIVE MEASURES: Acidify urine (ammonium chloride) Phenothiazines to treat psychotic reactions MEDICAL AND NURSING MANAGEMENT FOR: Hyperpyrexia Convulsions Respiratory distress Cardiovascular shock	Depression Agitation Apathy Sleepiness Disorientation	Antidepressants for depression
COCAINE/CRACK (Short-acting) **NOTE:** *High obtained:* Snorted—3 minutes Injected—30 seconds Smoked—4–6 seconds (crack) *Average high lasts:* For cocaine—15–30 minutes For crack—5–7 minutes	PHYSICAL SIGNS: Tachycardia Dilated pupils Elevated blood pressure Insomnia Anorexia PSYCHOLOGICAL/ PERCEPTUAL: Elation Grandiosity Resistance to fatigue Impaired judgment SEVERE (*Chronic Use*): Paranoid thinking Disturbed concentration	Seizures Cardiac arrest Respiratory depression/arrest Convulsions Hyperpyrexia Death	MEDICAL AND NURSING LIFE-SAVING MEASURE FOR: Convulsions (prescribe Valium) Hyperpyrexia (use hyperthermia) Respiratory depression/cardiac arrest	Fatigue Depression Apathy Anxiety Chronic users often abuse or are dependent on a narcotic, alcohol, or an anxiolytic to lessen the withdrawal symptoms of cocaine/crack	DETOXIFICATION Experimental at present: 1. Amino acids 2. Dopamine agnostic 3. Antidepressants (Desipramine)

Table continued on following page

Table 24–3 • PSYCHOSTIMULANTS *Continued*

		OVERDOSE		WITHDRAWAL	
DRUG	**INTOXICATION**	**Effects**	**Possible Treatments**	**Effects**	**Possible Treatments**
	Psychosis Violent temper outbursts **Formication** (tactile hallucinations involving animals or bugs); "cocaine bugs" refer to the sensation some chronic users experience of bugs crawling under their skin CHRONIC USER COMPLAINTS: • Chronic insomnia • Chronic fatigue • Severe headaches • Nasal problems • Poor/decreased sexual performance • Potential toxic cardiovascular effects				
NICOTINE	None known; however, dependence caused by at least several weeks of smoking, 10 cigarettes (0.5 mg nicotine) per day			Cravings—"nicotine fits" Anxiety Restlessness Difficulty concentrating Disruption in sleep patterns Excessive eating Irritability Constipation Headaches Gastrointestinal disturbances	None known
CAFFEINE	PHYSICAL SIGNS: Restlessness Excitement Insomnia Flushed face Diuresis GI complaints Cardiac arrhythmias Psychomotor agitation Periods of inexhaustability Nervousness Rambling flow of thought			None known	

Data from Grinspoon and Bakalar 1985; Smith 1984; Bittle et al. 1986; DSM III-R 1987; Gold 1984; Cocaine 1987.

Psychological addiction to the drug is intense. Physical addiction is probable but at this time not proved conclusively. It is thought that the use of cocaine depletes the neurotransmitters dopamine and norepinephrine in the brain. Research is being conducted on correcting these biochemical alterations in an attempt to reduce the individual's craving for the drug and to alleviate some of the symptoms of withdrawal (Cocaine Withdrawal 1987). Refer to Table 24–3 for the physical, psychological, and withdrawal effects of cocaine/crack abuse.

NICOTINE AND CAFFEINE

Nicotine no longer has medicinal uses; when it is taken in tobacco, its effects are variable. It can act as a stimulant, depressant, or tranquilizer. Since nicotine is one of the most perniciously addicting drugs in common use, most tobacco users are "hooked" and, in effect, locked into the effects of tobacco.

Nicotine (cigarettes, snuff, chewing tobacco) and caffeine (coffee, tea) are common drugs used by people throughout the world. People who smoke over 10 cigarettes a day (containing at least 0.5 mg of nicotine) know how difficult it is to stop smoking once their bodies have become dependent upon the drug. It is well known that many medical conditions are associated with and most certainly caused by cigarettes (see Table 24–1). Despite this, many people continue to smoke and use other forms of tobacco because attempting to stop smoking involves enduring severe withdrawal symptoms (see Table 24–3).

Most Americans take caffeine by way of coffee or tea. People take coffee as a drug—"I've got to have two cups in the morning to function"; for social reasons—"Let's get together for coffee"; or as a reward—"After I finish this job, I'm going to take a coffee break." One cup of coffee contains 100 to 150 mg of caffeine. Intoxication is thought to result from ingestion of more than 250 mg of caffeine. Restlessness, excitement, cardiac arrhythmias, and nervousness are some of the signs of caffeine intoxication (see Table 24–3).

All stimulants accelerate the normal functioning of the body and affect the CNS. Common signs of stimulant abuse include dilation of the pupils, dryness of the oronasal cavity, and excessive motor activity.

When a person who has ingested a stimulant experiences chest pain, has an irregular pulse, or has a history of heart trouble, the person should be taken to an emergency room immediately. Otherwise, the person should be kept as calm and quiet as possible.

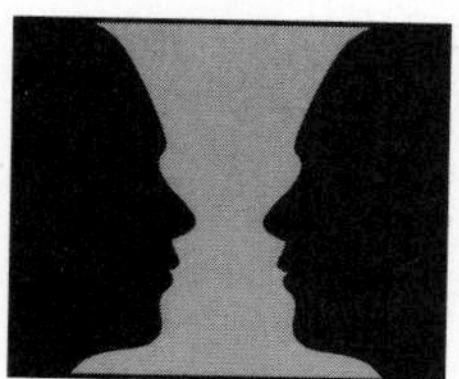

Case Study: Working With a Person Dependent on Cocaine

Fred, age 17, is an only child of parents who have been separated and divorced for over seven years. Prior to their divorce, the marriage had been described as very chaotic. The parents reportedly had frequent arguments in which they screamed at and occasionally hit each other.

Following the divorce, Fred's parents were awarded joint custody of Fred. Fred would spend two weeks each month with each parent. Fred's father, Mr. F., was an alcoholic whose own father had been distant and rigid. When drunk, Mr. F. would become belligerent and often fight with Fred. The arguments would be heated and occasionally physical.

Fred's mother was a passive-aggressive woman whose father was a belligerent alcoholic. Fred never appeared happy or at ease with either parent. Fred began using cocaine at the age of 15, when he had quite a bit of time on his hands because he had dropped out of school. During this period he usually spent his days "hanging out" at a nearby mall.

During the past seven months, Fred has been arrested three times for possession of cocaine. When questioned regarding his cocaine abuse, Fred states that at this point he believes that he has his addiction under control and is not in need of treatment. Mr. and Mrs. F. brought Fred to the hospital, stating that he is unmanageable. Fred was restless and talkative. He stated that he felt great and wanted to leave. His pupils were dilated and nonreactive to light, and his pulse and blood pressure were elevated. His clothes were soaked with sweat. His parents were very vocal, and his mother announced that the next time Fred was arrested, he would be charged as an adult and have a felony conviction.

Assessment

SIGNS OF INTOXICATION/WITHDRAWAL

In assessing Fred, the nurse observed the following signs of cocaine intoxication:

1. Psychomotor agitation
2. Elation

Continued on following page

Assessment *(Continued)*

3. Grandiosity
4. Loquacity
5. Hypervigilance
6. Tachycardia
7. Pupils dilated and nonreactive to light
8. Elevated blood pressure
9. Diaphoresis
10. Nausea and vomiting

PHYSICAL COMPLICATIONS

At present none were noted.

PERSONAL HISTORY AND COPING STYLE

From an interview, the nurse was able to assess Fred's perception of his cocaine use.

Dialogue	Therapeutic Tool/Comment
N: I understand you entered the treatment program yesterday afternoon after your court appearance.	Nurse places the event in time and sequence, validating the precipitating event.
F: Yeah—It was my Dad's idea.	
N: Well, what do you think of the idea?	Encouraging evaluation (actions first, thoughts, then feelings).
F: I don't like it. I don't need this place. I'm not a junkie—I just use cocaine, that's all. I can handle it.	
N: From what I've heard, your involvement with cocaine has gotten you into trouble.	Pointing out realities.
F: Yeah, well, I guess I can't deny that . . . but I still don't think I need this place.	
N: Are you saying that you don't think you need a treatment program?	Validating the client's perception.
F: Well, I don't know, I guess maybe I am messed up a bit.	
N: "Messed up."	Restating.
F: Yeah.	
N: What is one thing about you that's messed up?	Nurse encourages client to be specific rather than global.
F: *(Silence)* . . . I guess I feel like I don't belong anywhere.	
N: Talk more about that.	

DRUG HISTORY

Fred told the nurse that he started taking cocaine about two years ago at a party. Before that time he drank "with the guys" and "smoked a little pot." He said that now he took alcohol to soften the withdrawal from cocaine when he couldn't get Valiums or Quaaludes. He took the drug intranasally (snorted) and had been tempted to freebase (inhale specially prepared cocaine) but was frightened. He was presently taking the drug six or seven times a week intranasally. After talking to the nurse and weighing possible future legal complications, Fred agreed to enter the inpatient drug treatment program.

Nursing Diagnosis

Some nursing diagnoses pertaining to Fred follow:

1. *Dysfunctional Grieving* related to parental divorce
2. *Knowledge Deficit* related to detrimental effects of cocaine
3. *Diversional Activity Deficit* related to lack of motivation
4. *Ineffective Individual Coping* related to inadequate psychological resources

Planning

CONTEXT LEVEL — PLANNING GOALS

Fred and the nurse established goals relevant to each of the nursing diagnoses.

Nursing Diagnosis	Long Term Goal	Short Term Goal
1. *Dysfunctional Grieving* related to parental divorce	The client will gain an understanding of his underlying feelings regarding his parents' divorce by the time of discharge.	1. The client will meet with his parents in family counseling sessions and discuss his feelings by (state the date).
2. *Knowledge Deficit* related to detrimental effects of cocaine	The client will gain knowledge regarding substance abuse and its effects on the body and mind by the time of discharge.	2. The client will attend group educational sessions on substance abuse on four occasions (state the dates).
3. *Diversional Activity Deficit* related to lack of motivation	The client will have definite plans for his leisure time by the time of discharge.	3. The client will name three activities that interest him and that he would like to get involved in by (state the date).
4. *Ineffective Individual Coping* related to inadequate psychological resources	The client will state that he feels better able to cope with his feelings by the time of discharge.	4. The client will be able to cope with his painful feelings through participation in group therapy sessions by (state the date).

PROCESS LEVEL — NURSES' REACTIONS AND FEELINGS

The nurse had had to work out many of the personal feelings and reactions she used to have regarding a person dependent on an illicit drug. Her mother had had a serious alcohol problem and had abused valiums for many years. The nurse had found that going to Al-Anon and other support groups, as well as attending seminars geared toward understanding and working with people dependent upon a psychoactive substance, had helped her sort out many of her angry and confused feelings and had altered her initial reactions to people with substance abuse problems. She was aware that most nurses have strong, often negative, reactions to and feelings about people with drug dependence problems. When supervising her colleagues and peers, she encouraged discussion of personal feelings directed toward drug-dependent clients during staff meetings, in order to maximize the staff's therapeutic value.

Intervention

The inpatient unit combined a variety of appropriate educational programs, family involvement, group therapy with peers, and individual sessions with the primary nurse.

In relation to the short term goals listed, the nurse decided on a set of actions appropriate for reaching each goal. These nursing interventions should be seen as guidelines for all nursing staff working with the client to aid in maintaining continuity of care.

Short Term Goals	Interventions
1. The client will meet with his parents in family sessions and discuss his feelings by (state the date).	1a. Give the client positive support during one-to-one interactions. 1b. Discuss with the client his feelings toward his parents. 1c. Encourage client to participate actively in this phase of treatment.
2. The client will attend group educational sessions on substance abuse every other day, starting on (state the date).	2a. Discuss with the client the material from the educational sessions on an individual basis.

Continued on following page

Intervention *(Continued)*

	2b. Answer any questions the client may have. 2c. Reinforce the main points made during the educational sessions.
3. The client will name three activities that interest him and that he would like to get involved in by (state the date).	3a. Encourage the client to discuss activities that he has enjoyed in the past and that he is good at. 3b. Give client realistic feedback regarding his choices. 3c. Provide information regarding additional activities.
4. The client will cope with his painful feelings through participation in group and individual therapy sessions by (state the date).	4a. Approach the client in an open and positive manner. 4b. Encourage the client to name painful feelings in a supportive one-to-one session. 4c. Discuss with the client his support system.

Evaluation

Periodically, Fred and his nurse evaluate the goals.

Short Term Goal	Evaluation
1. The client will meet with his parents in family sessions and discuss his feelings and concerns by (state the date).	1. As of said date, the client and his parents met and have continued to meet in weekly sessions.
2. The client will attend group educational sessions on substance abuse every other day, starting on (state the date).	2. As of said date, goal was partially met. The client attended two of four sessions scheduled.
3. The client will name three activities that interest him and that he would like to get involved in by (state the date).	3. As of said date, goal was partially met. Fred decided on two activities and has started one—lifting weights in the gym.
4. The client will cope with his painful feelings through participation in group and individual therapy sessions by (state the date).	4. Goal was partially met. As of said date, client has been verbalizing his feelings in both group and individual sessions and is working on coping with these feelings.

The family met four times before Fred's dad dropped out. During a session that was evaluating family drug use, Fred's dad left, saying that Fred's problem had nothing to do with him. Fred's mother began to talk to the nurse about her own problems and decided to have individual therapy.

Fred decided to remain with his mother and visit his father periodically when his dad was not drinking. Fred and his mother began to talk a little more about themselves and their feelings and started to get to know each other for perhaps the first time. Fred continued his group sessions and was able to listen and share with peers who were experiencing many of the same feelings and were faced with similar problems. He began to feel less isolated and alone and had found one place where he got support and belonged.

Summary

Amphetamines have been around a long time as "diet pills" and "pep pills." They are often abused by students, athletes, and entertainers. Amphetamines are now medically indicated only for hyperkinesis in children and for narcolepsy. Intoxication includes euphoria, impairment in social and occupational functioning, increased energy, impaired judgment, and assaultiveness. Amphetamine psychosis results in symptoms similar to those seen in paranoid schizophrenia (e.g., paranoid delusions; visual, auditory, or tactile hallucinations; potential for violence; and panic reaction). Overdose of amphetamines and cocaine/crack can lead to hyperpyrexia, convulsions, respiratory depression, and cardiovascular shock. One difference between cocaine/crack and amphetamines is the rate of action. Amphetamines are long-acting and cocaine is short-acting, and dependence develops more rapidly with cocaine and crack.

Nicotine can act as a stimulant and is legal, and consistent use results in dependence on the drug. Despite the harmful effects of nicotine (see Table 24–1), people find it a difficult drug to give up.

The case study highlighted teenage addiction, assessment, planning, and interventions for a young man who was using cocaine.

Self-study exercises 27 through 39 at the end of this chapter cover the material on psychostimulants.

Narcotics

OBJECTIVES

After studying this section on narcotics, the student will be able to:

1. Compare and contrast the symptoms of narcotic intoxication with those of narcotic withdrawal.
2. Discuss the pros and cons of the following treatments for narcotic addictions, including which clients are most suited to each type of treatment:
   A. Methadone or LAAM (L-alpha acetyl methadol) maintenance
   B. Therapeutic communities
   C. Self-help abstinence-oriented model

Introduction

Opium is derived from the dried juice of the poppy, *Papaver somniferum*, and is an opiate. *Morphine*, *heroin*, and *codeine* are opiates and belong to the class called narcotics. *Methadone* and *meperidine* (Demerol) are narcotics referred to as opioids rather than opiates. Opium is a raw natural product, and morphine is the chief active ingredient in opium. Each grain of opium contains about one tenth of a grain of morphine. Heroin is produced by heating morphine in the presence of acetic acid (the acid found in vinegar). Heroin is converted back to morphine in the body.

Opium is usually taken orally or "smoked"—that is, it is heated, and its vapors inhaled. Morphine and heroin can also be sniffed, injected under the skin, into a muscle, or, for maximum effect, directly into a vein ("mainlined").

During the nineteenth century, opium was sold legally and was inexpensive. Opiates and countless pharmaceutical preparations containing them were freely accessible.

However, opiate use was frowned upon in some circles as immoral. Although deemed immoral, opiate use in the nineteenth century was not subject to the moral sanctions current today—for example, employees were not fired for addiction. Overall, addicts continued to participate fully in the life of the community. Thus, the nineteenth century escaped from one of the most disastrous effects of current narcotics laws and attitudes—the rise of a deviant addict subculture, cut off from respectable society.

During this time, opiates were prescribed for pain as well as for coughs, diarrhea, dysentery, and many other illnesses. It was not until 1906, when Congress passed the first Pure Food and Drug Act, that a major step forward was taken in control of opiate addiction. This act required that medicines containing opiates be so labeled. In 1914 Congress passed the Harrison Narcotics Act, which cut off altogether the supply of legal opiates to addicts, leading to the production and sale of

Table 24–4 • NARCOTICS (OPIATES AND OPIOIDS)

DEFINITION: An opiate derivative or synthetic that affects the CNS and the autonomic nervous system. Medically used primarily as analgesic (pain killer). Consistent use causes tolerance and distressing withdrawal symptoms.

		OVERDOSE		WITHDRAWAL	
DRUG	**INTOXICATION**	**Effects**	**Possible Treatments**	**Effects**	**Possible Treatments**
NARCOTICS Opium (paragenic) Heroine Meperidine (Demerol) Morphine Codeine Methadone (Dolophine) Hydromorphone (Dilaudid)	PHYSICAL SIGNS: Pupils constricted Decreased respiration Drowsiness Decrease in blood pressure Slurred speech Psychomotor retardation PSYCHOLOGICAL/ PERCEPTUAL: Euphoria Dysphoria Impairment of attention/memory Impaired judgment	*Pupils may be dilated due to anoxia* Respiratory depression/arrest Coma Shock Convulsions Death	Narcotic antagonist —e.g., naloxone (Narcan) quickly reverses CNS depression	Yawning Anorexia Insomnia Irritability Runny nose (rhinorrhea) Panic Diaphoresis Cramps Nausea "Bone pain" Chills Dilated pupils	Supportive measures if not life threatening short-acting Drugs—e.g., Heroine, Morphine Peak 48–72 hours Course 7–10 days Long-acting drugs—e.g., Methadone Peak 3–8 days Course several weeks

Data from Grinspoon and Bakalar 1985; Smith 1984; Bittle et al. 1986; DSM III-R 1987; Jaffe 1985.

adulterated, contaminated, and misbranded black-market narcotics.

Codeine is found in small quantities in opium; ordinarily it is taken orally. It is a narcotic and can be addictive if enough is taken. At one time many cough syrups contained codeine, such as turpin hydrate and codeine elixir, and addicts would buy large quantities. There are tighter controls on codeine cough syrups now, but there are still over 40 codeine mixtures on the market to treat coughs and colds or to provide pain relief.

Methadone (Dolophine) is a synthetic narcotic that generally resembles morphine and heroin in its effects but is not derived from opium. It was first synthesized in Germany in 1943, when opiate analgesics were not available because of the war. It was first called Dolophine. Methadone is an effective analgesic, and its physiological effects are the same as those of morphine and heroin. It is a narcotic and produces both psychological and physical dependence. Tolerance to methadone develops, then physical dependence as repeated doses are taken, and finally withdrawal symptoms when the drug is stopped or reduced. One of methadone's most useful properties is its cross-tolerance with other narcotics. When methadone reaches a sufficiently high level in the blood (40 mg), it can block the euphoric effects of heroin. Withdrawal symptoms of people physically dependent on heroin or morphine, including post-addiction craving, can be suppressed by oral administration of methadone. Doses range from 20 to 80 mg (sometimes up to 120 mg). Refer to Table 24–4 for signs of intoxication, overdose, and withdrawal and treatment.

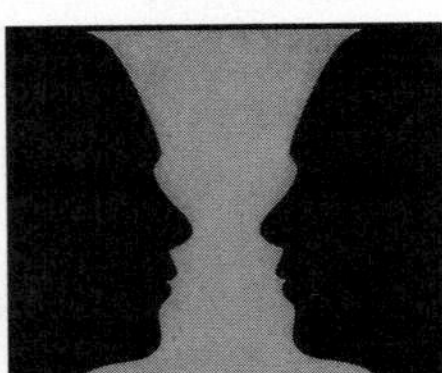

Case Study: Working With A Person Dependent on an Opiate

Bill K., a 20-year-old single man, was brought to the emergency room in a coma. He was accompanied by his mother, with whom Bill lives in a small apartment. Bill had been in his room at home. When his mother was not able to arouse him, she dialed 911 for an ambulance. A syringe and some white powder were found next to Bill.

Bill's breathing was labored, and his pupils were constricted. Vital signs were taken; his blood pressure was 60/40 and his pulse was 132. Bill's situation was determined to be life-threatening.

Bill's mother was extremely distressed, but she was able to report to the staff that Bill had a substance abuse problem and had been taking heroin for six months before entering a methadone maintenance program.

It was determined at this point to administer a narcotic antagonist, and naloxone was given intramuscularly. Following this, Bill's breathing improved and he began to respond to verbal stimuli, although his speech was slurred.

Bill's mother later told staff that Bill had been in the methadone maintenance program for the past year but had not attended the program or received his methadone for the past week.

Assessment

SIGNS OF INTOXICATION/WITHDRAWAL

In an emergency situation, when a patient has overdosed, a history taken from reliable family members, physical examination, and laboratory test (toxicological screening for drugs in blood and urine) as well as analysis of gastric contents provide data for the initial assessment. Bill's physical signs supported the diagnosis of heroin overdose:

1. Pupils constricted (in severe overdose, pupils will be dilated from anoxia)
2. Drowsiness
3. Slurred speech
4. Hypotension

Other signs and symptoms of intoxication include:

5. Euphoria
6. Dysphoria
7. Apathy
8. Psychomotor retardation
9. Impaired judgment

PHYSICAL COMPLICATIONS

Bill's mother stated that Bill had problems with constipation, but other than that he appeared healthy to her.

PERSONAL HISTORY AND COPING STYLE

The assessment of psychological status is a part of any nursing assessment, along with an assessment of the client's physical health.

In the case of Bill, due to the fact that his situation was life-threatening, an initial assessment had to be made very quickly. Initially an interview with Bill was not possible; therefore information had to be gathered from Bill's mother.

DRUG HISTORY

Bill had been attending a methadone maintenance program for the past year, after six months of heroin dependence. His mother stated that he also drank beer and whisky, but she did not know how much.

Nursing Diagnosis

Some nursing diagnoses that pertain to Bill, who has abused heroin, include the following:

1. *Ineffective Breathing Pattern* related to CNS depression due to heroin overdose
2. *Ineffective Individual Coping* related to substance abuse—heroin
3. *Methadone Noncompliance* related to lack of autonomy in health-seeking behaviors

Planning

CONTENT LEVEL—PLANNING GOALS

Some goals for the client who abuses narcotics follow:

Nursing Diagnosis	Long Term Goal	Short Term Goals
1. *Ineffective Breathing Pattern* related to CNS depression due to heroin overdose	Bill's breathing pattern will be stabilized within four hours.	1a. Bill's breathing pattern will be monitored every 15 minutes until stabilized.

Continued on following page

Planning
(Continued)

Nursing Diagnosis	Long Term Goal	Short Term Goals
		1b. Bill's vital signs will be within normal limits by (state the time).
2. *Ineffective Individual Coping* related to substance abuse —heroin	Bill will demonstrate two effective coping skills by discharge.	2. Bill will demonstrate one effective coping skill by (state the date).
3. *Methadone Noncompliance* related to lack of autonomy in health-seeking behaviors	Bill will realistically discuss short term goals and available treatment modalities with the nurse and health care team.	3a. Bill will discuss several treatment modalities with the nurse by (state the date). 3b. Bill will realistically discuss short term goals with the nurse in light of available treatment modalities.

Mr. Samuels, Bill's assigned nurse, identified nursing actions appropriate for reaching each goal. These nursing interventions should be seen as guidelines for all nursing staff working with the client, which maintain continuity of care. Some examples follow:

Short Term Goals	Interventions
1. Bill's breathing pattern will be stabilized within four hours.	1a. Observe the client closely. 1b. Take vital signs every 15 minutes and document findings. 1c. Maintain patent airway.
2. Bill's vital signs will be within normal limits within three hours.	2a. Support breathing. 2b. Continue to monitor vital signs. 2c. Observe for seizure activity.
3. Bill will demonstrate two effective coping skills by discharge.	3a. Approach the client in a positive and open manner. 3b. Provide information about local self-help groups for substance abusers. 3c. Discuss possible alternative behaviors when anxious or depressed.
4. Bill will discuss short term goals and available treatment modalities with the nurse by (state the date).	4a. Obtain a thorough history of substance abuse, including the particular drug(s) taken, length of use, route of administration, and drug preference. 4b. Present history to health care team and evaluate available treatment modalities and community resources. 4c. The health care team will meet with Bill regarding discharge planning.

PROCESS LEVEL—NURSES' REACTIONS AND FEELINGS

Mr. Samuels was a Vietnam veteran. During the war, he had seen many of his friends and colleagues become dependent on opiates. It was during this time that he became familiar with the physical and psychological effects of and long-term problems associated with opiate dependence. He had witnessed the disruption and negative changes in the lives of many of his friends. When he returned from the war, he decided to go into nursing. He believed that as a nurse he could be effective in helping people deal with the problems of drug dependence.

Intervention

Mr. Samuels knew that Bill's future ultimately rested with Bill. Mr. Samuels talked to Bill regarding his perceptions of his situation, where Bill wanted to go, and what Bill thought he needed to get there.

Dialogue	Therapeutic Tool/Comment
N: Bill, I was in the emergency room Friday afternoon when you were brought in by ambulance.	Nurse places the event in time and sequence, validating the precipitating event.
B: Were you? I guess a lot of people thought it was over for me.	
N: It certainly looked quite serious.	Emphasizing the reality—*prevents* minimizing situation.
B: Yeah. . . . I should have never left the program. . . . I was doing better, and I just didn't think I needed it anymore.	
N: You said you were doing well.	Reflecting.
B: Yeah. . . . I had a job, and I was beginning to save some money. Wow! I can't believe I blew this whole thing.	
N: I don't know that you really did. Your counselor for the program phoned Dr. L. this morning to find out how you were doing.	Pointing out reality.
B: Do you think they will take me back?	
N: Why don't we talk some more, and after we finish, I'll speak with the other staff about your situation. If you would like to get back into the program, you can call your counselor and we'll support your decision.	Gathering information.

Mr. Samuels met with the other members of the health care team and reviewed the following alternatives for opiate dependent individuals and discussed what might be suitable for Bill.

REVIEW OF ACCEPTED TREATMENTS FOR NARCOTIC ADDICTIONS

Essentially, there are three different models for the treatment of chemical dependency: (1) methadone maintenance, (2) therapeutic communities, and (3) self-help abstinence-oriented recovery (Klein and Miller 1986).

Methadone Maintenance

During 1980 there were an estimated 70,000 to 75,000 clients being treated with Methadone. **Methadone** is effective only for approximately 24 to 36 hours, so the client usually takes methadone every day.

In the mid-1970's, experimental clinical use began with a longer-acting drug called **L-alpha acetyl methadol,** or LAAM. **LAAM** is effective for up to three days (72 to 96 hours), so clients need only come in for their dose three times a week. This makes it easier for clients to hold down jobs and gives them more freedom than with methadone maintenance. LAAM is also an addictive narcotic: its therapeutic effects and side effects are the same as those of morphine, including withdrawal symptoms after tolerance has developed. (Ling and Blaine 1979).

Naltrexone (Trexan) is a relatively pure antagonist that blocks the euphoric effects of opioids. It has low toxicity with few side effects. A single dose provides an effective opiate blockade for up to 72 hours. Taking Naltrexone three times a week is sufficient to maintain a fairly high level of opiate blockade. For many, long term use results in gradual extinction of drug-seeking behaviors. Naltrexone does *not* produce dependence (Frances and Franklin 1988). In 1971, the United States Congress mandated a large-scale increase in research on narcotic antagonistic drugs. Naltrexone appears to be the best narcotic antagonist that has been developed to date.

Intervention
(Continued)

As mentioned, **clonidine,** widely used as an antihypertensive, has been found to be a nonopioid suppressor of opioid withdrawal symptoms (Frances and Franklin 1988). Several studies have demonstrated encouraging results using clonidine and naltrexone in treating opiate withdrawal (Charney et al. 1986; Frances and Franklin 1988); however, at this writing, clonidine has not been FDA approved for opioid detoxification.

Therapeutic Communities

Therapeutic communities, (TCs) or self-regulating communities, operate on the hypothesis that drug use is a symptom of an underlying character disorder or emotional immaturity. These programs have as a main goal a complete change in lifestyle: abstinence from drugs, elimination of criminal behavior, and development of employable skills, self-reliance, and personal honesty.

There are more than 300 residential TCs in the United States. The TC program includes encounter group therapy, various levels of educational programs, and assigned jobs within the community. TCs use self-government and group pressures, instead of relying on a professional therapeutic staff, to change immature behaviors. Residents of traditional TCs stay for at least 15 months.

Self-Help Abstinence-Oriented Model

Self-help groups patterned after Alcoholics Anonymous (AA)—for example, Narcotics Anonymous (NA), Chemical Dependency Anonymous (CDA), and Cocaine Anonymous (CA)—help teach individuals to face the seriousness of their problem and provide hope and support. Usually, the person first enters the detoxification unit, then may spend some time in the hospital, and finally is referred for outpatient therapy (usually group) and self-help groups.

Klein and Miller (1986) state that generally the *abstinence-oriented model* is best suited for individuals who are somewhat motivated and who are still in the early stage of drug dependence. The *therapeutic community* is best suited for individuals who have a long history of anti-social behavior, especially those ordered there by the court. The *methadone maintenance program* is appropriate for those who have failed at several attempts at abstinence and who are unable to stabilize their lives.

Evaluation

After reviewing Bill's history, the health care team decided that the self-help abstinence-oriented recovery treatment might be most helpful. Bill had not been on drugs a long time, he has a job, and he appears motivated. Naltrexone would be given in conjunction with outpatient psychotherapy and regular attendance at NA meetings.

Three months after discharge, Bill visited Mr. Samuels on the unit. He stated that his job was going well, he had made some friends in NA, and he was thinking of attending a local community college in the fall.

Summary

Opium, morphine, heroin, and codeine are opiates and belong to the class *narcotics*. Methadone (Dolophine) and Meperidine (Demerol) are nonopiate narcotics referred to as opioids. In 1914, the Harrison Narcotic Act banned the use of narcotics without a prescription.

Signs of intoxication include constricted pupils, drowsiness, decreased blood pressure, psychomotor retardation, and impairment in memory and social functioning. Overdose can lead to respiratory depression, shock, convulsions, and death. Treatment of overdose can be dramatically affected with a narcotic antagonist such as *Naloxone* (*Narcan*). Withdrawal symptoms include yawning, rhinorrhea, insomnia, diaphoresis, muscle cramps, "bone pain," chills, and dilated pupils. Treatment for withdrawal symptoms, which usually are not life-threatening, is mostly supportive.

Treatment modalities vary. Somatic treatment includes *methadone maintenance* (one dose effective for 24 to 36 hours) and LAAM (one dose effective for up to 3 days) as drugs of substitution. These drugs block the craving for and withdrawal symptoms from heroin and enable the addicted person to work and carry on a normal social life. One drawback is that these drugs also are addicting and can produce withdrawal symptoms. *Naltrexone* (*Trexan*), a narcotic antagonist, is an effective opiate blocker for up to 72 hours and has been a successful treatment modality for many.

Other modalities of treatment include therapeutic communities and self-help abstinence-oriented therapy. The indication for each form of treatment has been outlined in this section.

Self-study exercises 40 through 49 at the end of the chapter will help you review this section on narcotics.

Psychotomimetics

OBJECTIVES

After studying this section on psychotomimetics, the student will be able to:

1. Compare and contrast the signs and symptoms of low-dose, moderate-dose, and high-dose PCP (phencyclidine piperidine) intoxication.
2. Discuss what is meant by *synesthesia* and give two examples.
3. Define *flashback* and give an example.
4. Identify three possible long term results from heavy chronic marijuana use.

Introduction

Psychotomimetics, also known as hallucinogens or mind-altering drugs, were found all over the world by the early explorers. People have known and written about hallucinogens for centuries. Our discussion of the psychotomimetics includes PCP, LSD and LSD-like drugs, and *Cannabis sativa* (marijuana).

PCP

Phencyclidine piperidine (PCP) was first synthesized in 1926, and thirty years later experimental use on human beings began (Shulgin and MacLean 1976). Findings from research studies on humans led to the use of PCP for surgical anesthesia, and PCP was patented under the trade name *Sernyl* in 1960. After five years, it became evident that Sernyl produced many adverse side effects, including acute anxiety, agitation, hallucinations, delirium, muscle rigidity, and seizures (Burns et al. 1975). The acute anxiety experiences responded to brief therapeutic interventions, but acute psychosis caused by PCP resolves slowly (Table 24–5). The severity and frequency of these side effects soon led to the withdrawal of Sernyl from the market for human use.

Since 1967, PCP has been available legally only for use as an anesthetic in veterinary medicine. It was during this same year that its use as a street drug was first reported by Meyers, Rose, and Smith (1967–1968). In various regions of the country, PCP is known as the animal tranquilizer, angel dust, or the **p**ea**c**e **p**ill. It can be manufactured from a few readily available chemicals and is relatively simple to synthesize. The illegally produced PCP is manufactured in many forms: powders, pills, capsules, and liquids. It is smoked, sniffed, swallowed, injected, and even used as eye drops.

The route of administration plays a significant role in the severity of PCP intoxication. The onset of symptoms from oral ingestion occurs in about one hour. When taken intravenously, sniffed, or smoked, the onset of symptoms may develop within five minutes (APA 1987). The signs and symptoms of PCP intoxication may range from acute anxiety to acute psychosis. The cardinal signs of *both the* PCP *low-dose experience and the high-toxicity* experience include a "blank stare," ataxia, muscle rigidity, vertical and horizontal nystagmus, tendencies toward violence, and generalized anesthesia which lessens the sensations of touch and pain, making staff interventions difficult. H*igh doses* may lead to hyperther-

Table 24–5 • PSYCHOTOMIMETICS (HALLUCINOGENS)

DEFINITION: Produce *Abnormal Mental Phenomena* in the cognitive and perceptual spheres. For example, distortion in space and time, hallucinations, delusions (paranoid or grandiose), and synesthesia may occur.

		OVERDOSE		WITHDRAWAL	
DRUG	**INTOXICATION**	**Effects**	**Possible Treatments**	**Effects**	**Possible Treatments**
HALLUCINOGENS LSD (Lysergic acid diethylamide) Mescaline (Peyote) Psilocybin	PHYSICAL SIGNS: Pupils dilated Tachycardia Diaphoresis Palpitations Tremors Incoordination Temperature, pulse, respiration elevated PSYCHOLOGICAL/PERCEPTUAL: Fear of going crazy Paranoid ideas Marked anxiety/depression **Synesthesia**—e.g., colors are heard; sounds are seen Depersonalization Hallucinations although sensorium clear Grandiosity—e.g., thinking one can fly	Psychosis Brain damage Death	Keep client in room with low stimuli—minimal light, sound, activity Have one person stay with client—reassure client, "talk down" client **(NOT for PCP)** Speak slowly and clearly in low voice Valium or chloral hydrate for extreme anxiety tension **NOTE:** **PCP and LSD-like drugs have different treatment.**	None known	**NOTE:** **Tolerance develops quickly.**
PCP (PHENCYCLIDINE)	PHYSICAL SIGNS: Vertical or horizontal nystagmus Increased blood pressure, pulse, and temperature Ataxia Muscle rigidity Seizures Blank stare Chronic jerking Agitated, repetitive movements PSYCHOLOGICAL/PERCEPTUAL: Maladaptive behavior changes Belligerence, assaultiveness, impulsiveness, unpredictability Impaired judgment, social and occupational functioning SEVERE EFFECTS: Hallucinations, paranoia Bizarre behaviors—	Psychosis Possible hypertensive crisis/cardiovascular accident Respiratory arrest Hyperthermia Seizures	IF ALERT: Caution: If gastric lavage is used, can lead to laryngeal spasms or aspiration Acidify urine (cranberry juice, ascorbic acid); in acute stage, ammonium chloride—may continue for 10 to 14 days Room with minimal stimuli **Do NOT talk down!** Speak slowly, clearly, and in low voice *Diazepam* may be used for agitation *Haldol* may be used for severe behavioral disturbance **(*not* a phenothiazine)** MEDICAL INTERVENTION FOR: Hyperthermia	*Tolerance and withdrawal reactions have been reported:* Lethargy Craving Depression **NOTE:** **Takes from 24 to 48 hours to recover from a high** **Stays in urine for a week or more** **Long term effects of chronic PCP abuse may include** **• Dulled thinking** **• Lethargy** **• Loss of memory and impulse control** **• Depression**	

DRUG	INTOXICATION	OVERDOSE		WITHDRAWAL	
		Effects	Possible Treatments	Effects	Possible Treatments
	e.g., barking like a dog, grimacing, repetitive chanting speech Regressive behavior—e.g., public masturbation Violent bizarre behavior, including homicide and suicide Very labile behaviors		High blood pressure Respiratory distress Hypertension		
CANNABIS SATIVA (Marijuana, hashish)	PHYSICAL SIGNS: Tachycardia Conjunctional injection Increased appetite Impaired motor ability Talkative PSYCHOLOGICAL/ PERCEPTUAL: Euphoria Intensification of perceptions Apathy Excessive anxiety/ paranoia Impaired judgment Slowed perception of time Inappropriate hilarity Impaired memory Heightened sensitivity to external stimuli	Fatigue Paranoia Psychosis—rarely seen			Duration of effects: Smoking: 2–4 hours Ingestion: 5–12 hours **NOTE:** **Cannabis dependence is associated with such psychological symptoms as** • **Lethargy** • **Anhedonia (inability to enjoy life)** • **Difficulty concentrating** • **Memory problems**

Data from Grinspoon and Bakalar 1985; Smith 1984; Bittle 1986; DSM III-R 1987.

mia, agitated and repetitive movements, chronic jerking of the extremities, hypertension, and kidney failure. Persons with PCP intoxication may become stuporous with their eyes open, may be comatose, or may experience status epilepticus or respiratory arrest (Grinspoon and Bakalar 1985). (Refer to Table 24–5.)

The behavior of a client on PCP often presents difficult management problems for the nursing staff. Client safety is an important issue, since the client may fluctuate between immobility and aggressive outbursts. The amount of direct nursing care required varies with the amount of PCP ingested, route of administration, time lapse since last ingestion, and chronicity of use.

PCP Intoxication

LOW DOSE. Clients with PCP intoxication, even those requiring minimally restrictive care (those with low-dose toxicity, who have ingested 1–5 *mg of* PCP), sometimes place themselves in hazardous situations. This possible danger-to-self behavior requires that the client be placed in an environment with minimal, controlled stimuli (Peterson and Stillman 1979). Because of the possibility of paranoia in the client, the environment should be kept as unrestrictive as possible. Seclusion or restraints are indicated only when danger to self or others is present. Limited contact with one staff member should also be maintained with the client. When contact with the client is established, the nurse is careful not to violate the client's personal space.

Although only one person should interact with the client, no one person should be alone with the client. An adequate number of staff members should be present to manage the client if an assaultive situation develops.

The need for monitoring vital signs periodically should be assessed in terms of how agitated the person becomes. Often the physician will order Valium to reduce agitation and aid sleep. These clients may lose a significant amount of fluids through diaphoresis, and they should be encouraged to drink acidic fruit juices, such as cranberry juice, as replacement fluid. Substances such as cranberry juice, ascorbic acid, and ammonium chloride, which acidify the urine, encourage the excretion of PCP from the body (Burns et al. 1975).

MODERATE DOSE. Clients who have ingested 5 *to* 15 *mg* of PCP (moderate-dose toxicity) present more difficult management problems. Usually these clients are uncommunicative and very stimuli-sensitive. They also may exhibit sleep pattern disturbances, varying from continual drowsiness to wakefulness, and can quickly become agitated and combative. This assaultiveness often is accompanied by periods of amnesia, stupor, and other bizarre behavior (Cohen 1987). Ataxia, generalized twitching, and myoclonic rigidity are seen frequently during the waxing and waning psychotic episodes. Valium may be used for its tranquilizing effects and also to reduce severe convulsions. Haldol may be used to reduce the aggressive, combative behavior. *Phenothiazines should* NOT *be used, since they potentiate the anticholinergic actions of* PCP.

HIGH DOSE. When a client has ingested *over* 15 *mg of* PCP (high-dose toxicity), the situation is considered a severe psychiatric emergency, as this is the most-life threatening level of intoxication (Burns et al. 1975; Cohen 1987). This toxic drug state presents a very complex, confusing picture. The person's behavioral, mental, and physical status is unpredictable. Nurses, while maintaining a minimal amount of verbal and tactile stimulation, must resort to the most restrictive forms of physical restraint in order to prevent injury or harm to the client or others. Auditory hallucinations, mania, delusions, and severe agitation are typical symptoms (Luisada and Brown 1976). Mental states of disorientation, amnesia, and autistic thought processes also may be noted (Cohen 1987). These clients are also at physical risk because of the possibility of seizures, hyperpyrexia, respiratory distress, and coma. The client may need external respiratory assistance or external cooling to reduce dangerously high body temperatures. Blood pressure may have to be reduced to safe levels and convulsions controlled. After the coma lightens, the patient typically becomes delirious, paranoid, and violently assaultive.

Some chronic PCP users suffer from dulled thinking and reflexes, loss of memory and impulse control, depression, lethargy, and difficulty in concentrating (Grinspoon and Bakalar 1985). Refer to Table 24–5 for physical and psychological signs of PCP intoxication and withdrawal symptoms plus medical treatments. A saying on the street is: "PCP—not an upper or a downer but an insideouter."

LSD AND LSD-LIKE DRUGS

LSD (lysergic acid diethylamide), mescaline (peyote), and psilocybin are all hallucinogens. Mescaline and the mushroom *Psilocybe mexicana* (from which psilicybin is isolated) have been used for centuries in their religious rites by Indian peoples living in the southwestern United States and in northern Mexico. A term popular in the 1960's for the psychotomimetic drugs was "psychedelic," which in Greek means "for the soul to be manifest," emphasizing the subjective experience of expansion of consciousness reported by some users (Davison and Neale 1982). LSD was the drug of the '60's. The hallucinogenic experience was called a "trip." A good trip is characterized by a marked slowing of time, lightheadedness, images in intense colors, and visions in sound (*synesthesia*). People report experiences of spiritual ecstasy or of being united with humankind. During a bad trip, a person may experience severe anxiety, paranoia, and terror compounded by distortions in time and distance. The terrorized person may become violent, unpredictably suicidal, or dangerously grandiose (e.g., thinking he or she can fly). The trip ends when the effects of the drug wear off (8 to 12 hours for LSD). The best treatment for a person experiencing a bad trip is reassurance, companionship, and protection. Occasionally a tranquilizer (Valium, chloral hydrate) is indicated (Grinspoon and Bakalar 1985).

Flashbacks are a common effect of hallucinogenic drugs. Flashbacks are the transitory recurrence of psychotomimetic drug experiences when a person is drug-free. Such experiences as visual distortions, time expansion, loss of ego boundaries, and intense emotions are reported. Flashbacks are often mild and perhaps pleasant, but at other times individuals experience repeated recurrences of frightening images or thoughts (Davison and Neale 1982; Grinspoon and Bakalar 1985). Flashbacks are more likely to occur when a person is fatigued or after smoking marijuana. Prolonged adverse reactions have occurred, lasting 24 to 48 hours. Reactions have been described as an anxiety attack, depressive reaction, and psychosis.

MARIJUANA *(CANNABIS SATIVA)*

Cannabis sativa is an Indian hemp plant. Tetrahydrocannabinol (THC) is the active ingredient found in the resin secreted from the flowering tops and leaves of the *Cannabis* plant. THC has mixed depressant and hallucinogenic properties. Marijuana, the leaves from the *Cannabis* plant, is generally smoked ("joint," "reefer," "roach"), but it can be ingested. Some of the many and variable effects of marijuana are listed below. (Donlon and Rockwell 1982)

The desired effects:

1. Euphoria, detachment, and relaxation.
2. Sensations are intensified (e.g., sensory, auditory, visual).
3. Time is drawn out.

Concurrent effects:

1. Distance perceptions are distorted.
2. Tendency toward distractibility, sociability, and hilarity.
3. Increases appetite.

Undesirable effects:

1. Impairment in ability to drive a car.
2. Memory impairment.
3. With high doses, hallucinogenic phenomena begin to appear.

Possible effects of heavy chronic use:

1. Panic reactions.
2. Psychosis.
3. Flashbacks.

Individuals with schizophrenia, borderline, or affective disorders may have an exacerbation of symptoms after smoking marijuana. Marijuana users should be aware of the following facts about marijuana:

1. The effect in the lungs of smoking one marijuana cigarette is equivalent to the effect of smoking twenty tobacco cigarettes. Also, the tar produced by marijuana is considered more carcinogenic than the tar of tobacco (Bittle et al. 1986).
2. Studies suggest that marijuana may be harmful to the reproductive system, although the results as yet are not conclusive. People planning on bearing children might want to exercise caution in marijuana use (Frances and Franklin 1988).
3. People who have abnormal heart function could have difficulty, since marijuana increases the heart rate, sometimes dramatically.

Research is still needed, and often studies are conflicting. However, a pilot study found that marijuana dependent high school students had short term memory defects during the study and after six weeks of abstinence from the drug (McConnell 1988).

Marijuana is often used in conjunction with other drugs of abuse with which it may have a synergistic effect. For example, marijuana is often used with alcohol and cocaine. *Cannabis* is the most widely used illicit drug in the United States.

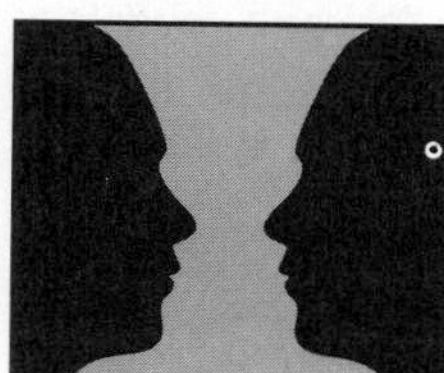

Case Study: Working With a Person in PCP Intoxication

Gina, a 14-year-old teenager, was brought to the emergency room after PCP ingestion. Gina presented with blunted affect. Her speech was incoherent at times, and she was disoriented to date and time. It also appeared that Gina was suffering from auditory and visual hallucinations, although Gina denied this.

This was Gina's first visit to the hospital, and she was accompanied by her parents, Mr. and Mrs. Tan.

Gina was described by her parents as having low self-esteem and thinking herself "ugly." They stated that she constantly strove to be accepted by her peers. Mr. and Mrs. Tan explained that recently Gina had been "hanging around" with a group of girls who appeared to them to be very involved in substance abuse. They believed that Gina had become involved with PCP through these girls, even though they had forbidden Gina to socialize with them.

Assessment

SIGNS OF INTOXICATION/WITHDRAWAL

The nurse noticed

1. Horizontal nystagmus
2. Ataxia

Continued on following page

Assessment *(Continued)*

3. Muscle rigidity
4. Some agitation
5. Gina's facial expression appeared blank

PHYSICAL COMPLICATIONS

None apparent at present.

PERSONAL HISTORY AND COPING STYLE

According to Gina's parents, this was Gina's first experience with drugs. Gina had been home for over an hour when the symptoms were first noticed. When the nurse asked Mr. and Mrs. Tan about Gina's other friends, Mrs. Tan said, "Well . . . not too many . . . you see we like her to stay home where we can keep an eye on her." The nurse asked both parents what Gina does when she gets upset. Again Mrs. Tan replied rather sharply, "Gina doesn't get upset—why should she?" When the nurse asked Mr. Tan if he could tell the staff anything about Gina's activities or friends, he evaded the nurse's eyes and stated, "I'm away a lot."

DRUG HISTORY

Gina's parents believed that this was Gina's first experience. Further data would be needed from Gina when the drug was out of her system.

Nursing Diagnosis

The nurse in the emergency room discussed her observations with the resident on duty. Both thought that Gina was experiencing low dose PCP intoxication. The physician suggested that Gina be monitored for an hour or so and then be discharged in the care of her parents. He agreed with the nurse that follow-up care for the family would be advisable and he would encourage family counseling. The nurse called the social worker and collaborated on plans regarding the following nursing diagnoses:

1. *Disturbance in Self-Esteem* related to giving into peer pressure in order "to belong."
2. *Altered Parental Role* related to anxiety over Gina's need to gain independence

Planning

CONTENT LEVEL—PLANNING GOALS

Goals relevant to the nursing diagnoses were formulated.

Nursing Diagnosis	Long Term Goal	Short Term Goal
1. *Disturbance in Self-Esteem* related to giving into peer pressure in order "to belong."	Gina will be involved with two school or community activities within six months.	1. Gina will meet with the school counselor within one week and work on developing activities and skills on an ongoing basis.
2. *Altered Parental Role* related to anxiety over Gina's need to gain independence	Both parents will state that they feel comfortable encouraging Gina in productive outside activities.	2. Family will meet with family therapist on a regular basis, starting this week, to address family fears, concerns, and frustrations.

PROCESS LEVEL—NURSES' REACTIONS AND FEELINGS

When the nurse first started to care for people with various drug dependent problems, she experienced annoyance and frustration at the behaviors and physical problems resulting from habitual drug abuse. It was through talking to other more experienced staff and through learning more about substance dependence that she began to feel less overwhelmed. She found that as her experience grew and her ability to interact more effectively increased, her frustration and old feelings of hopelessness regarding people with drug problems began to decrease. She felt especially hopeful for young people who were motivated and had access to community resources.

Intervention

Gina was given Valium to lower anxiety and agitation. The nurse placed her in a quiet, dimly lit room. Unlike a person who is intoxicated with LSD, mescaline, or other psychedelic drugs, reassurance and verbal support (talking down) is *rarely* useful with a person with PCP intoxication. In fact, increased environmental stimuli can trigger agitation and combativeness in some.

The nurse monitored Gina's vital signs every 15 minutes. Her blood pressure and pulse were moderately elevated (140/90 and 122, respectively) but stable. Because Gina was diaphoretic, the nurse offered her cranberry juice on several occasions.

During this time the nurse called the social worker and asked him to speak to Gina's parents regarding the observations of the health team and suggested interventions. Initially, Mrs. Tan seemed to bristle at the idea of family therapy but said she would go if it would help keep Gina away from drugs. Mr. Tan looked uncomfortable but also agreed to go. Their caring and concern for Gina appeared genuine.

After several hours, the physician re-examined Gina and said that she could go home in the care of her parents. The social worker would contact the school counselor the following day, and the family had an appointment for family counseling in two days.

Evaluation

Gina was fortunate. She had ingested only 1.5 to 2.0 mg of PCP, which is considered a low dose, and it had been her first. The nurse was alert to possible contributors to Gina's drug use, such as seeking belonging and experiencing rebellion through drug use. Other young people are not always so fortunate. People who smoke or ingest PCP more regularly may develop a tolerance to the drug and experience withdrawal symptoms consisting of lethargy, depression, and craving for the drug (Grinspoon and Bakalar 1985)

Three months after the PCP incident, Gina had joined a 4-H club and the school band, in which she was learning to play the drums. She seemed to involve herself easily in outside activities once she had parental encouragement and approval at home. She told the school counselor that her parents were more relaxed and learning to trust her. She had made friends in the 4-H club and was having a great time learning the drums in the school band, since the percussion section was made up of all boys, who turned out to be supportive and glad to have a girl in their section.

Summary

The psychotomimetics are drugs that produce abnormal mental phenomena in the cognitive and perceptual spheres. For example, there are distortions in space and time, depersonalization; with strong doses, hallucinations, delusions, and synesthesia (the "seeing of sounds" or "hearing of colors") may occur.

PCP intoxication, seen frequently in emergency rooms in the late 1970's, is still seen today. The route of administration plays a large role in the severity of PCP intoxication, as is the case with most drugs. The behaviors and nursing and medical interventions for low-dose, moderate-dose, and high-dose intoxication were discussed.

LSD, mescaline, and psilocybin were popular hallucinogenic drugs of the 1960's. Psychotomimetics have been used for centuries, often in religious rites. PCP, LSD, and LSD-like drugs can cause flashbacks for some users.

There are important differences in the treatment of people with PCP and LSD-like drug intoxication. In particular:

1. Persons with LSD-like drug intoxication respond to verbal support (talking down) if the person is panicky. One does *not* talk down a client with PCP intoxication. The person can become more agitated and assaultive.
2. Phenothiazines may be used at times with LSD-like drugs—but *never* with PCP—although Haldol may be used.

Other nursing measures for acute intoxication were covered.

Marijuana (*Cannabis sativa*) was discussed under psychotomimetics because they share many of the same properties. For the most part, hallucinations are not experienced with the type of marijuana smoked or ingested in this country. The various effects of marijuana were discussed, and some cautions for use were given. Marijuana is often used in conjunction with other drugs (e.g., alcohol, PCP, and cocaine). *Cannabis* is the most widely used illicit drug in the United States.

Self-study exercises 50 through 56 at the end of the chapter will help you review the material presented on psychotomimetics.

References

Acee AM, Smith D. Crack. American Journal of Nursing, 87(5):614, 1987.

American Psychiatric Association. Diagnostic and Statistical Manual of Mental Disorders, 3rd ed., revised. Washington DC: American Psychiatric Association, 1987.

Beavers WR. Athenetrial basis for family evaluation. *In* Lewis J, Beaucas WR, Gossit JT, Phillips US (eds). No Single Thread: Psychological Health in Family Systems. New York: Brunner/Mazel, 1976.

Bennett G, Vourahis C (eds). Substance Abuse. New York: John Wiley and Sons, 1983.

Bittle S, Feigenbaum JC, Kneisl CR. Substance abuse. *In* Kneisl CR, Ames SW (eds). Adult Health Nursing: A Biopsychosocial Approach. Menlo Park, CA: Addison-Wesley Publishing Company, 1986.

Brauerman BG, Shook J. Spotting the borderline personality. American Journal of Nursing, 87(2):200, 1987.

Brill P, Herzberg J, Speller JL. Employee assistance programs: An overview and suggested roles for psychiatrists. Hospital and Community Psychiatry, 36(7):727, 1985.

Brooks K, Adult children of alcoholics: psychosocial stages of development. Focus on Family and Chemical Dependency, 6(5):5, 1983.

Burns R, Lerner S, Gorrado R, Phencyclidine—State of acute intoxication and fatalities. Western Journal Of Medicine, 123:348, 1975.

Campbell C. Nursing Diagnosis and Intervention in Nursing Practice. New York: John Wiley and Sons, 1984.

Charney DS, Heninger GR, Kleber HD. The combined use of clonidine and naltrexone as a rapid, safe, and effective treatment of abrupt withdrawal from methadone. American Journal of Psychiatry, 143(7):831, 1986.

Cocaine withdrawal step by step. Editorial. Emergency Medicine, pp. 65–68, April 30, 1987.

Cohen AV. Alternatives to Drug Abuse: Steps Toward Prevention. Washington DC: National Institute on Drug Abuse, No. 14, Department of Health, Education, and Welfare, 1973.

Cohen S. PCP—New trends in treatment. Drug Abuse and Alcohol News, 7:7, 1987.

Count EC. A History of Smoking. London: George G. Harrap and Company, 1931.

Davison GC, Neale JM. Abnormal Psychology. New York: John Wiley and Sons, 1982.

Donlon PT, Rockwell DA. Psychiatric Disorders: Diagnosis and Treatment. Bowie, MD: Robert J. Brady Company, 1982.

Frances RJ, Franklin JF. Alcohol and other psychoactive substance use disorders. *In* Talbott JA, Hales RE, Yudofsky SC (eds). Textbook of Psychiatry. Washington DC: American Psychiatric Press, 1988.

Gold MS. 800-COCAINE. New York: Bantam Books, 1984.

Grinspoon L, Bakalar JB. Drug dependence: Nonnarcotic agents. *In* Kaplan HI, Sadock BJ (eds). Comprehensive Textbook of Psychiatry, 4th ed. Baltimore, MD: Williams & Wilkins, 1985.

Harvard Medical School. Opiate abuse—Part II. The Harvard Medical School Mental Health Letter, 3(8):1, 1987.

Hauschildt E. Addictions in nursing: Reality vs. image. The Journal, 15(12):12, 1986.

Hollister L. Phencyclidine use: Current problems. International Drug Therapy News, 14:5, 1979.

Jaffe JH. Opioid dependence. *In* Kaplan HI, Sadock BJ (eds). Comprehensive Textbook of Psychiatry, 4th ed. Baltimore, MD: Williams & Wilkins, 1985.

Jaffe JM. Drug addiction and drug abuse. *In* Goodman LS, Gilman A (eds). The Pharmacological Basis of Therapeutics, 5th ed. New York: MacMillan, 1975.

Jefferson LV, Ensur BE. Help for the helper: Confronting a chemically-impaired colleague. American Journal of Nursing, 82(4):574, 1982.

Kaplan HI, Sadock BJ (eds). Synopsis of psychiatry, 5th ed. Baltimore, MD: Williams & Wilkins, 1988.

Klagsburn M, Davis D. Substance abuse and family interaction. Family Process, 16:149, 1977.

Klein JM, Miller SI. Three approaches to the treatment of drug addiction. Hospital and Community Psychiatry, 37(11):1083, 1986.

Kneisl CR, Ames SW. Adult Health Nursing: A Biopsychosocial Approach. Menlo Park, CA: Addison-Wesley Publishing Company, 1986.

Kramer JC. Introduction to amphetamine abuse. Journal of Psychedelic Drugs, II:2, 1986.

Ling W, Blaine JD. The use of LAAM in treatment. *In* DuPont RC, Goldstein A, O'Donnell J (eds). Handbook on Drug Abuse. Washington DC: National Institute on Drug Abuse, Department of Health, Education, and Welfare, 1979.

Luisada P, Brown B. Clinical management of phencyclidine psychosis. Journal of Clinical Toxicology 9:539, 1976.

McConnell H. Marijuana update: Heavy use hits short term memory. The Journal, 17(7):9, 1988.

Meyers R, Rose A, Smith D. Incidents involving the Haight-Ashbury population and some uncommonly used drugs. Journal of Psychedelic Drugs, (Winter) 1:139, 1967–1968.

New York State Division of Substance Abuse Services. Report on crack. Albany: The NY State Division of Substance Abuse Services, 1986.

Peterson RC, Stillman RC. Emergency room treatment for phencyclidine (PCP) overdose. Resident Staff Physician, 25:116, 1979.

Resnick HS. It starts with people: Experiences in drug abuse prevention. Washington DC: National Institute on Drug Abuse, Department of Health, Education, and Welfare, (ADM). 1979.

Schloemer NF, Skidmore JW. Opiate withdrawal with clonidine. Journal of Psychosocial Nursing and Mental Health Services, 21(10):8, 1983.

Shulgin A, MacLean D. Illicit synthesis of phencyclidine (PCP) and several of its analogs. Journal of Clinical Toxicology, 9:553, 1976.

Smith MC. The client who is abusing toxic substances other than alcohol. *In* Lego S (ed). The American Handbook of Psychiatric Nursing. Philadelphia: J.B. Lippincott Company, 1984.

Survey uncovers widespread use of drugs among physicians. Editorial. Psychiatric News, 21(20):14, 1986.

Wegscheider S. From the family trap to family freedom. Alcoholism 1(3):36, 1981.

Weingarten N. Treating adolescent drug abuse as a symptom of dysfunction in the family. *In* Ellis BG (ed). Drug Abuse from the Family Perspective. DHHS Publication No. ADM 80-910, Washington DC: U.S. Government Printing Office, 1980.

Zamora LC. The client who generates anger. *In* Haber J, et al. (eds). Comprehensive Psychiatric Nursing. New York: McGraw-Hill Book Company, 1987a.

Zamora LC. Patterns of substance abuse. *In* Haber J, et al (eds). Comprehensive Psychiatric Nursing, New York: McGraw-Hill Book Company, 1987b.

Zweig C. Drug addicts, acupuncture and retraining. The Journal 16(3):12, 1987.

Self-Study Excercises

GENERAL GUIDELINES

Match the following:

1. ________ Includes the phenomena of tolerance and withdrawal. A. Psychotomimetics

2. ________ More of the drug is needed to get the desired effect.
3. ________ The combination of two drugs that enhance the effect of each other to a much greater degree than the sum of the effects of each drug when given alone.
4. ________ Naloxone (Narcan).
5. ________ Also known as minor tranquilizers or antianxiety agents.
6. ________ Causes abnormal perceptual and cognitive experiences.

B. Drug antagonist
C. Synergistic
D. Tolerance
E. Withdrawal
F. Substance abuse
G. Substance dependence
H. Synesthesia
I. Anxiolytic

Put P for primary or S for secondary health teaching.

7. ________ Increase in neighborhood recreational and occupational opportunities.
8. ________ Administration of drugs under antiseptic conditions.
9. ________ Increase in drug education at home, school—use of peer counselors.

Place T (true) or F (false) next to each statement.

10. ________ Therapeutic communities are well suited for individuals who have a long history of antisocial behavior and a poor record in methadone maintenance programs.
11. ________ Outpatient drug-free programs are well suited for persons who have a job and have intact family and/or who are polydrug abusers.

Complete the statements by filling in the appropriate information.

12. ________________ helps break down denial and rationalization and permits discussion of feelings in a supportive atmosphere.
13. ________________ in conjunction with urinalysis can be superior to drug counseling.
14. ________________ e.g., cognitive, analytic, supportive, psychoanalytic, are examples of this intervention strategy.

Short Answer

15. List four general goals a drug dependent (chemically impaired) person should meet in order to begin improving the quality of his or her life.
    A. ________________________________
    B. ________________________________
    C. ________________________________
    D. ________________________________

SEDATIVE-HYPNOTIC OR ANXIOLYTIC AGENTS

Match the following:

16. ________ Is less sedating than the barbiturates and causes less interference with motor activities.
17. ________ A nonbarbiturate sedative-hypnotic first introduced as an antimalarial agent.
18. ________ The first drug synthesized to facilitate sleep and reduce anxiety.

A. Barbiturates

B. Benzodiazepine (Valium, Librium)

C. Methaqualone (Quaaludes)

Indicate withdrawal (W), intoxication (I), or overdose (O).

19. ________ Unsteady gait, slurred speech, drowsiness.
20. ________ Tachycardia, marked insomnia, diaphoresis, irritability.
21. ________ Coma, shock, convulsions, respiratory or cardiovascular depression.
22. ________ Impaired social/occupational functioning, impaired judgment/memory.

Indicate treatment for overdose (O) or treatment for withdrawal (W).

23. ________ Maintain patent airway, take vital signs frequently, induce vomiting or gastric lavage if in coma.
24. ________ Administer gradually decreasing, titrated doses of the same or similar drug.

Short Answer

25. Write a paragraph regarding your possible reactions to a drug dependent client to whom you are assigned.

26. List six actions suggested in this section that you might take if working with a chemically dependent colleague (list in order of priority).
    A. ________________________________
    B. ________________________________
    C. ________________________________
    D. ________________________________
    E. ________________________________
    F. ________________________________

PSYCHOSTIMULANTS

Match the following:

27. ________ One of the first psychostimulants used and abused illegally. Medically indicated for hyperkinesis in children and for narcolepsy.
28. ________ A fast-acting drug of the 1980's; expensive, in wide use, and dangerous.
29. ________ An alkalinized form of cocaine acting in 4 to 6 seconds; intensely psychologically and perhaps physically addicting.
30. ________ A legal drug of addiction used nationwide since the time of Columbus.

A. Nicotine

B. Crack

C. Amphetamines

D. Cocaine

Indicate cocaine (C), amphetamine (A), or both (B).

31. ________ Overdose can result in respiratory depression/arrest, hyperpyrexia, seizures, cardiac shock/arrest, and death.
32. ________ Use of ammonium chloride to acidify urine.
33. ________ Short-acting; tolerance builds rapidly.
34. ________ Chronic users complain of runny nose due to erosion of nasal septum.
35. ________ Intoxication includes grandiosity, paranoia, impaired judgment, tactile or other hallucinations, and psychosis.
36. ________ Medicinal management and nursing care are vital in severe overdose.

Choose the answer that most accurately completes the statement.

37. Greta Turk, a highly successful editor, has been taking cocaine intranasally for four years and started freebasing two months ago. For the past week she has been locked in her apartment and has gone through $8000 worth of cocaine. She is unconscious when brought to the hospital. Nursing measures include all of the following EXCEPT:

    A. monitor vital signs every 15 minutes
    B. maintain a patent airway; give oxygen when indicated by physician
    C. observe for seizures and hyperpyrexia
    D. give ammonium chloride

38. After the drug is out of Greta's system, she will most likely experience

    A. hyperactivity and diaphoresis
    B. anxiety and depression
    C. marked insomnia and coarse, hard hands
    D. increased sexual impulses and euphoria

39. Greta was admitted to the inpatient treatment unit. As an adjunct to group and individual therapy, the nurse could work with Greta on all of the following EXCEPT:

    A. educating Greta about the psychological actions of the drug, its dangers, and latest research
    B. exploring strengths and activities that Greta enjoyed before becoming involved with the drug
    C. teaching Greta the indicators for and side effects and action of prescribed medications to ease withdrawal—e.g., antidepressants
    D. assuming an authoritarian leadership role, since Greta is now so dependent

NARCOTICS

Match the following:

40. ________ Different from most narcotics because it is synthetic and blocks craving for heroin.
41. ________ Found in many prescription cough syrups.
42. ________ Pupils constrict, blood pressure decreases, impaired concentration and judgment.
43. ________ Yawning, pupils dilated, "bone pain," rhinorrhea.

A. Signs of narcotic withdrawal

B. Signs of narcotic ingestion

C. Methadone or LAAM

D. Codeine

Place T (True) or F (False) next to each statement.

44. ________ Methadone maintenance at 40 mg or so can block craving for and withdrawal from heroin; effective for 24 to 36 hours.
45. ________ LAAM is effective for up to 3 days and is an addictive narcotic.
46. ________ Naltrexone (Trexan) is a narcotic antagonist effective for up to 72 hours.

Match the following:

47. ________ Best suited for motivated individuals in early stages of drug dependence progression.
48. ________ Best suited for those with long history of antisocial behavior.
49. ________ Best suited for those who have had several attempts at abstinence and are unable to stabilize their life.

A. Therapeutic community
B. Methadone maintenance
C. Self-help abstinence-oriented model

PSYCHOTOMIMETICS

Match the following regarding PCP.

50. ________ Ataxia, "blank stare," muscle rigidity, vertical and horizontal nystagmus, general anesthesia, and tendency toward violence.
51. ________ May be paranoid or assaultive; give cranberry juice and keep in area of low stimuli and least restrictive environment.
52. ________ Symptoms vary from drowsiness to agitative and combative; waxing and waning psychotic episodes marked by bizarre behaviors; amnesia and stupor. Valium or Haldol might be given.
53. ________ Psychiatric emergency—maximum restrictions needed to prevent injury to self and others; physical risks include seizures, hyperpyrexia, and respiratory distress; hallucinations and delusions flagrant.

A. Moderate dose (5–15 mg)
B. High dose (15 mg+)
C. Low dose (1–5 mg)
D. Cardinal signs at any dose

Place T (True) or F (False) next to each statement.

54. ________ A flashback is the transitory recurrence, when a person is drug-free, of an experience that a person had while taking a psychotomimetic (LSD-like drug, PCP, marijuana).
55. ________ Synesthesia is perceptual distortion, such as "seeing" sounds or "hearing" colors, triggered by some psychotomimetics.

Short Answer

56. If you were counseling a teenager who just started to use marijuana, as part of your health teaching what might be three possible long term physical effects that the teenager should be made aware of?
A. ________________________________
B. ________________________________
C. ________________________________

CHAPTER 25

People Who Defend Against Anxiety Through Eating Disorders

Michelle J. Conant

OUTLINE

KEY TERMS AND CONCEPTS

The key terms and concepts listed here also appear in bold where they are defined or discussed in this chapter.

FAMILY MODEL
Enmeshment
Overprotectiveness
Rigidity
Lack of Conflict Resolution

SYMPTOMS OF ANOREXIA NERVOSA

SYMPTOMS OF BULIMIA NERVOSA

INDICATIONS FOR INPATIENT TREATMENT FOR
Anorexia Nervosa
Bulimia Nervosa
Compulsive Overeating

BINGE-PURGE CYCLE

PSYCHOGENIC OBESITY
Developmental Obesity
Reactive Obesity

OBJECTIVES

After studying this chapter, the student will be able to:

1. Identify levels of anxiety by observing eating behaviors.
2. Discuss theories of etiology for eating disorders.
3. Describe five areas of assessment for persons with eating disorders, and briefly discuss three aspects of assessment for each area.
4. Compare and contrast the healthy need-satisfaction cycle and the disturbed need-satisfaction cycle.
5. Name at last three settings in which the nurse might encounter persons with eating disorders.
6. Recognize three indications for inpatient treatment for each of the following: anorexia nervosa, bulimia nervosa, and psychogenic obesity.
7. Identify major classifications of drugs used in the treatment of anorexia nervosa and bulimia nervosa.
8. Define anorexia nervosa and describe the "typical" anorexic.
9. Define bulimia nervosa and describe the "typical" bulimic.
10. Discuss obesity due to psychogenic compulsive eating.
11. Formulate nursing diagnoses for a client with anorexia nervosa, bulimia nervosa, and compulsive eating.
12. Construct nursing interventions for clients with each of the following: anorexia nervosa, bulimia nervosa, and compulsive overeating.
13. Identify three problems, apart from problems with eating, that might coexist in a person with an eating disorder.

The eating disorders to be discussed in this chapter are anorexia nervosa, bulimia nervosa, and obesity due to compulsive overeating. The disorders will be discussed as separate entities; however, it is believed that some common issues are at the core of all these disorders. Eating disorders cannot be placed on a wellness-illness continuum because it has not yet been determined that one is any more pathological than another. Hilde Bruch (1973) was the first to propose that deficits in learning to identify and express needs were present to some degree in all persons with eating disorders. Food and/or eating became a response of the person in dealing with anxiety (1973). The following conceptual model lists three eating disorders and the corresponding eating behavior that might be exhibited at each level of anxiety (Table 25–1). It is important to remember that eating behaviors are only one indication of the individual's anxiety level and that feelings of "loss of control" must be assessed.

Victims of anorexia and bulimia are usually white, middle class adolescent girls and women. However, increasing numbers of young women are seeking treatment for eating disorders from all economic and educational backgrounds (Dickstein 1985).

Table 25–1 • EATING DISORDERS ALONG THE ANXIETY CONTINUUM

LEVELS OF ANXIETY			
Mild	**Moderate**	**Severe**	**Panic**
Anorexia			
Rituals may be present.	—	—	Rituals used to control a total fast.
"Normal" but rigidly controlled meals are allowed.	Rigid diet—some calories taken.	Rigid fasting.	"Phobic" avoidance of food.
Bulimia			
Absent or only occasional binges of smaller amounts—some without purging; less physical discomfort felt after a binge.	Frequency of binges, amount of food, and subsequent purging.	—	Addictive nature of binge-purge cycle is extreme, i.e., more compulsive
Compulsive Eating			
Occasional and smaller binges with awareness of amounts eaten.	Frequency of bingeing with less awareness of amounts eaten.	—	"Mindless eating" with absence of control over eating.

The incidence of anorexia nervosa has greatly increased since the 1960's, and bulimia has shown a marked increase since the 1970's (Orbach 1985). A recent study has estimated one severe case of anorexia nervosa among every 200 adolescent women (Garner and Garfinkel 1985). In another study of normal college students, 13% reported binge eating, and 10% reported purge behaviors (Halmi 1981).

Because of the self-destructive and sometimes fatal outcome of these disorders, it is important for nurses to recognize, and have an understanding of, the dynamics of the eating disorders. Studies have shown a mortality rate for anorexia nervosa between 6.6% and 18% (Halmi 1988).

Some bulimics with vomiting behaviors have suffered fatal complications such as gastric dilation and gastric rupture (Mitchell et al. 1982). Severe electrolyte imbalances, especially hypokalemia, can lead to cardiac arrhythmias and cardiac arrest. Cardiac failure caused by cardiomyopathy as a result of ipecac (emetine) intoxication is being reported more frequently and often results in death (Halmi 1988).

At this time it is not possible to state the exact cause of eating disorders or to explain why persons exhibit one group of eating behaviors rather than another. For this reason, theories of etiology will be discussed as potentially underlying all three eating disorders, except for the biological theories, which are not within the scope of this chapter.

Since anorexia nervosa and bulimia affect mainly young women, individuals suffering from these syndromes will be referred to with the feminine pronouns. This chapter will address obesity only as it relates to compulsive eating, which is psychogenic in nature. Because the recent literature deals with this type of obesity from a female perspective, the feminine pronouns will be used.

Figure 25–1 conceptualizes the process of eating disorders as a self-destructive relief behavior.

Standard I: Theory

Although many biological etiologies have been suggested for the eating disorders, none has found uniform acceptance (Garfinkel and Garner, 1982). Theories such as genetic predisposition, hypothalamic dysfunctions, and psychomotor epilepsy have been proposed (Dickstein 1985). Research in this area is ongoing. None of the theories for a biological etiology for the eating disorders is widely accepted. This chapter discusses the following theories of etiology: (1) psychodynamic model, (2) family model, (3) sociocultural model, and (4) multidimensional model.

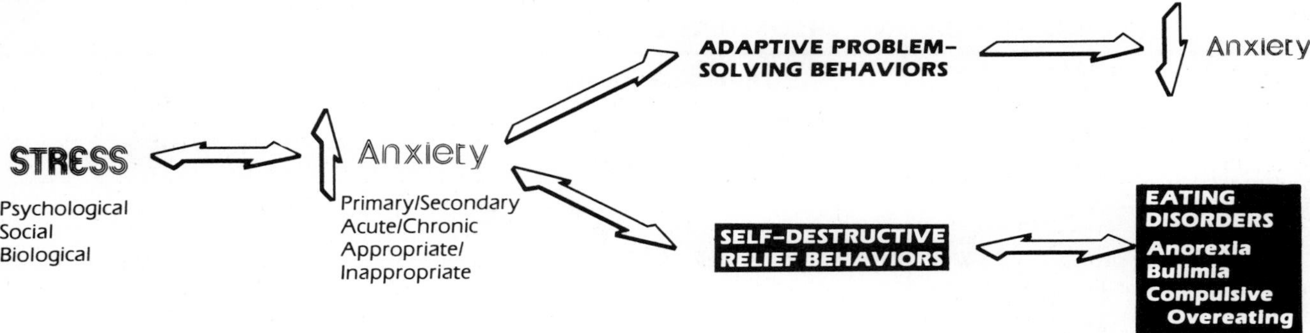

Figure 25-1. *Conceptualization of the process of an eating disorder.*

PSYCHODYNAMIC MODEL

The infant develops a healthy ego when the need-response cycle between infant and caregiver, usually the mother, is satisfying (Fig. 25-2). This child will move through the early months of life toward increasing differentiation from the mother, experiencing some separation anxiety and, later, some feelings of helplessness as this separation-individuation process is negotiated. This stage spans approximately six to 30 months of age. With support and encouragement from the mother, the child learns to handle the anxiety of separation. Disturbances in this stage of development occur if the child's need for separation-individuation is responded to with

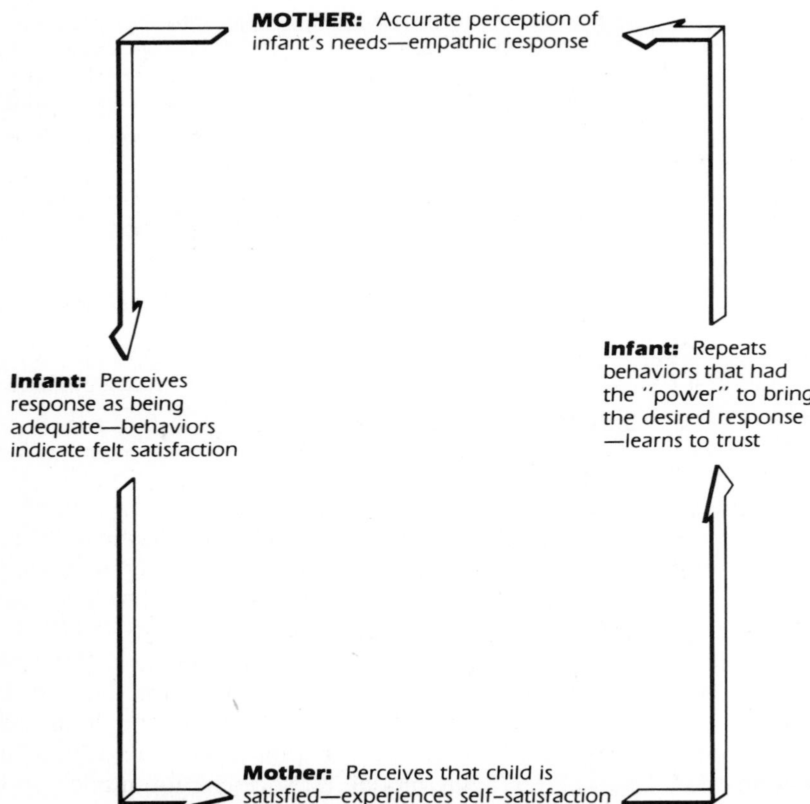

Figure 25-2. *Healthy need-response cycle.*

overprotectiveness and anxiety on the part of the mother (Fig. 25–3). It has been hypothesized that the mother, herself, may have experienced some difficulty in this stage of her development, making separation from the infant threatening. This results in the infant remaining undifferentiated from the mother, to some degree, and unable to view the self as separate with distinct bodily needs and feelings. This is extended even to emotional needs. The developing child does not learn to perceive and interpret her own emotional needs as separate from those of others. A distorted body image develops, along with a prevailing sense of ineffectiveness and helplessness in meeting individual needs. As the individual reaches later stages of development requiring increasing separation and independence, such as puberty or leaving the parental home, increased anxiety is experienced. Feelings of guilt and shame and fears of humiliation at the hands of others may be reawakened. These same feelings were often experienced in the past when moves toward separation from parents were attempted. Separation comes to be viewed as "bad."

A child develops the ability to use defense mechanisms and soothe herself to reduce anxieties and protect self-esteem. This is learned through "mirroring" or identifying with these behaviors in the parents (Geist 1982). For the individual who develops eating disorders, the development of healthy defense mechanisms is disturbed. The child becomes self-critical and is in constant conflict with inner drives and impulses. A sign of self-indulgence is met with self-deprecating thoughts and subsequent feelings of worthlessness. The body becomes the enemy, and it is denied any comfort. Control of the body and its biological needs, such as hunger, becomes a source of constant preoccupation. A break in the self-control arouses fears of a total loss of control, so that often the anorexic or bulimic is viewed as being phobic of food and fat. Because the bulimic and anorexic actually experience hunger—although it is suppressed more in the anorexic—they may also exhibit hunger-controlling behaviors, which can be in the form of obsessive thoughts and rituals around eating. This extreme need to control hunger is a response to poor impulse control, as seen in people with addictions.

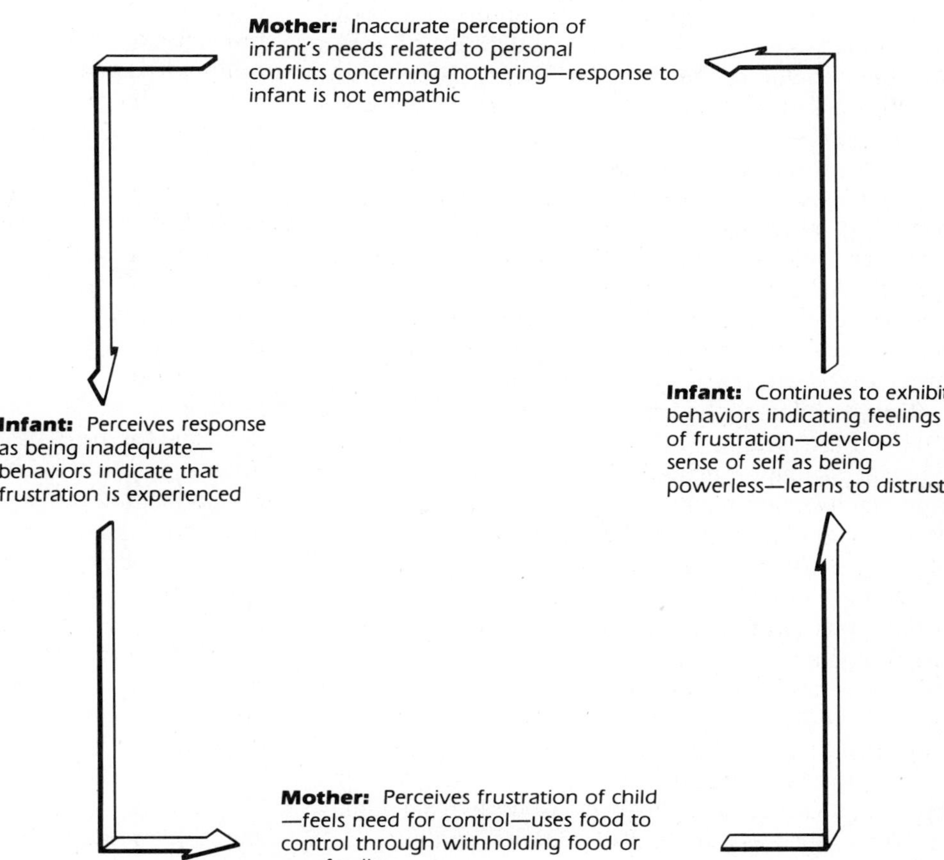

Figure 25–3. *Disturbed need-response cycle.*

FAMILY MODEL

When an individual exhibits destructive eating behaviors in the form of prolonged fasting, bingeing, or purging, these problem behaviors may become the primary concern of the family. The ways in which a family or its individual members deal with this problem may become the "reward" for the behavior and subsequently reinforce it. Therefore, the behavior results in secondary gains.

Five characteristics of the family with an anorexic member have been identified. These are *enmeshment, overprotectiveness, rigidity, lack of conflict resolution,* and *involvement of the sick child* in unresolved parental conflict (Minuchin 1978). Some or all of these characteristics may become exaggerated as the family attempts to deal with a person with anorexia nervosa or bulimia.

Enmeshment is characterized by difficulty of each family member to identify and meet his or her own needs apart from the others. There is an extreme awareness of how others feel and act, with subordination of personal priorities to those of "the family." The eating disorder, when exhibited, becomes "a family problem" rather than a problem for an individual family member. This can be seen in the example of parents wanting to "know exactly what is going on" in therapeutic sessions or in other family members changing their eating habits "for the benefit" of the identified client. Enmeshment signifies a lack of boundaries or separation between family members.

Overprotectiveness leads to a loss of autonomy and, subsequently, separation becomes difficult as the protected individual is left with feelings of incompetence and ineffectiveness when new tasks must be learned. An extreme example of this is panic when a personal checking account must be opened for the first time, or when a young woman is unable to shop for her own clothes without her mother's opinion.

Rigidity refers to the family's use of a narrow range of behaviors in dealing with all problems or situations. When an attempt is made to deal with a problem and it is ineffective, the family members may escalate their attempt rather than trying a new approach. An example of this would be attempting to limit a bulimic's food intake by limiting her spending money even after it becomes apparent that she will steal the food rather than stop bingeing.

Lack of conflict resolution can be seen in behavior such as "peacemaking" or abandoning the conflict prematurely. Often, in the case of the anorexic, the child is used as an ally against the other parent. The symptoms become the focus and may mask underlying family problems, such as a pre-existing marital conflict.

Mothers of women with eating disorders have been described as being preoccupied with weight and as having given up personal goals for dedication to fulfilling the needs of their families. This life of self-denial engenders anger exhibited through martyrdom, "nagging," or feelings of depression. This conflict is transmitted to the female infant through early feeding experiences that are often mismatched with the infant's needs. Overfeeding or underfeeding can occur as a response to the mother's feelings rather than the child's needs. Food then becomes the core of the conflict between mother and daughter and is seen as a means of control (Selvina-Palazzoli 1974).

It is not uncommon to hear of women with eating disorders spending inordinate amounts of time preparing food for others and gaining extreme satisfaction when it is eaten. In this way, food can become a means of controlling others, and their eating can vicariously satisfy her own hunger.

SOCIOCULTURAL MODEL

Ninety-five percent of those suffering from eating disorders are adolescent girls and women (DSM III-R 1987). The incidence of these disorders continues to increase (Mitchell 1985). The changing roles of women and the transmission of gender-appropriate role conflict from mother to daughter is believed by some theorists to be at the center of these phenomena. Mother is seen as a source of omnipotence and as the mediator of most of the infant's experiences. This is internalized by both male and female infants, but at this point the similarity ends. Girls go on to fear this internalized power and spend a lifetime attempting to control it so that they can "fit in" to society. The feminine ideal that society holds for women is that they be compliant and subordinate their needs to the needs of others. Open competition is allowed only in the arena of physical beauty. Since "slimness" is the current ideal, the groundwork has been laid for the development of eating disorders. Male infants, on the other hand, repress their feminine identity and fear it, projecting this fear onto all women and attempting to control women through their bodies. Therefore, many women today are faced with conflict. They want to compete and achieve in the world but are fearful of rejection by a society that approves and sanctions primarily the roles of wife and mother for women. Achievements outside the home are supported half-heartedly, and they are minimally supported as the primary role for women.

These conflicts can reveal themselves as an eating disorder. Obesity from compulsive eating, for example, can be viewed as a woman's unconscious attempt to rebel against societal pressure to be slim and powerless

(Orbach 1978). This rebellion through obesity exacts a price. Many obese women experience shame and self-hatred and are often punishing themselves for failing to maintain the feminine ideal. For these women, the rewards for independence and competence do not outweigh the pain of society's judgment (Millman 1980).

MULTIDIMENSIONAL MODEL

This model holds the position that the eating disorders are a product of a variety of influences at the biological, psychological, familial, and sociocultural levels of organization (Garfinkel and Garner 1982). Therefore, the clinical picture of various eating disorders could represent the end product of an interplay of a variety of influences, not just one etiological factor (Swift et al. 1986).

Standard II: Data Collection

When doing a psychiatric nursing assessment (Chapter 7) on a person with an eating disorder, areas such as (1) *weight*, (2) *eating*, (3) *activity*, (4) *family*, and (5) *physical signs and symptoms* need to be evaluated in depth. Physical signs and symptoms are an important part of the nursing assessment of eating disorders, because these disorders are potentially physically debilitating and even fatal. Since depression is often present in eating disorders, suicide potential may be an immediate concern.

ASSESSING WEIGHT

It is important to assess not only the present weight and how much the person has recently lost or gained but also the presence of distorted body image and the influence of mood (anxiety, guilt, depression) or events on weight status.

ASSESSING EATING

The nurse assesses not only the exact eating patterns but also the feelings and behaviors that surround the person's eating. Is there a **binge-purge cycle?** A binge-purge cycle is episodic, uncontrolled, rapid ingestion of large quantities of food over a short period of time often followed by "purging" (vomiting). Are there feelings of anxiety and shame? What is the degree of impulse control? Is the person aware of rigid or compulsive feelings around eating? Family patterns of eating, attitudes toward food, and eating in "secret" are areas in the nurse's assessment. The nurse also attempts to elicit the function of the bingeing, purging, and fasting behaviors. For the bulimic, the inability to control eating impulses may also suggest an inability to control other impulses as well. Lying, sexual promiscuity, compulsive drug use, and stealing are often present (Wilson 1982; DSM III-R 1987).

ASSESSING ACTIVITY

The presence of compulsive exercise is determined, and the function the exercise serves, both physically and emotionally, is evaluated.

ASSESSING FAMILY

Although there are similarities in family dynamics for the eating disorders, some researchers hypothesize differences in the styles of interaction between parents of bulimics and parents of anorexics. For example, some researchers state that families of bulimics tend to be more chaotic and disruptive than the families of anorexics. Parents of anorexics are often thought to be more rigid and controlling than those of bulimics. Therefore, the presence of overt marital conflict in the parents of the client is evaluated. The presence of poor impulse control (violence, drugs, alcohol) in family members is also assessed. How family members express anger, affection, sadness, and other emotions provides important data. Questions are asked to elicit the presence of competition for parental attention among siblings, the feelings and reactions of other family members to the client's eating behavior, parent's response to emotional needs of children, and so forth. Table 25–2 identifies some differences that may be found between an anorexic client and a bulimic client. There may be exceptions to these differences in individual cases.

ASSESSING PHYSICAL SIGNS AND SYMPTOMS

Since the eating disorders can be seriously debilitating and in some cases lead to death, careful physical assessment and awareness of specific signs and symptoms are crucial.

Some signs and **symptoms** often seen in a person who is severely **anorexic** are cachexia, hair loss, yellowish skin, cyanosis of the extremities, lanugo, cessation of menses, and peripheral edema.

Table 25–2 • CONTRASTING CHARACTERISTICS OF ANOREXICS AND BULIMICS

ANOREXIA	BULIMIA
Appearance	
Underweight; 25% below normal weight.	Normal or overweight.
Age	
13–22, average 18 years. Often younger than bulimics.	20's to 30's; often older than anorexics.
Signs	
Cachexia, hair loss, yellowish skin, lanugo, cyanosis of extremities, peripheral edema, amenorrhea.	Chipmunk facies (enlarged parotid glands), chronic hoarseness, dental caries, dehydration, electrolyte imbalance.
Family Environment	
Rigid and controlled; less overt evidence of marital discord.	More conflicts and overt fighting, chaotic, poor impulse control among family members, i.e., violence, drugs, alcohol.
Clinical Characteristics	
Introverted; more socially isolated than bulimics.	Extroverted, sexually active, high incidence of compulsive behaviors, i.e., promiscuity, drugs, stealing, suicide attempts.
Awareness of Disorder	
Denies hunger more often than bulimics. More denial of problem than in bulimics.	More aware of own eating disorder than anorexics. More distressed by symptoms than anorexics.

Data from Dickstein 1985; Johnson et al. 1984; Keltner 1984.

Some physical signs and **symptoms of bulimia** resulting from frequent vomiting are parotid gland enlargement (called chipmunk facies), chronic hoarseness/sore throat, dental caries from acid regurgitation, electrolyte imbalances (hypokalemia and alkalosis), and dehydration (Lucas 1982; Pyle et al. 1981).

The nurse also asks the client about the use of substances for purging (laxatives, diuretics) and evaluates for possible signs of anemia/malnutrition. Presence or absence of menses, as well as symptoms of premenstrual syndrome, is assessed.

Other forms of mental illness, such as depression, phobias, addictive diseases, and a range of obsessive-compulsive behaviors, are often present in someone with an eating disorder. These disorders are addressed in this chapter under DSM III-R *Classification* for each of the specific eating disorders.

A nursing assessment guide (Table 25–3) for a suspected eating disorder can be supplemental to a general psychosocial assessment (refer to Chapter 7). This assessment guide can be adapted for use with anorexia, bulimia, or compulsive eating. The sample questions are a guide, not necessarily appropriate or complete for all individuals in all settings.

Standard III: Diagnosis

Formulating nursing diagnoses for persons with eating disorders depends to a great extent upon the assessment. Some, but not all, nursing diagnoses appropriate for use with people with an eating disorder are discussed here.

One of the first concerns a nurse has when working with someone with an eating disorder is for his or her physical safety. For a severe anorexic, a priority of concern would be *altered nutrition: less than body weight* related to self-starvation. Physical safety for a client who is bulimic may be a priority when severe electrolyte imbalance threatens her life. Therefore, *cardiac output: decreased* related to excessive vomiting and dehydration is a relevant nursing diagnosis. Since depression is often present in people with eating disorders, and the suicide rate is high for this group, *potential for self-directed violence* related to identity crisis must be considered.

Young women with eating disorders usually have distorted self-concepts and low self-esteem. For example, for a person suffering from compulsive overeating, *dis-*

Table 25–3 • ASSESSMENT GUIDE FOR EATING DISORDERS

TO DETERMINE	SAMPLE QUESTIONS
Weight	
1. Presence of distortion/delusions about body image.	1a. What do you consider your ideal weight? 1b. Do you often "feel fat?"
2. Influence of moods or events on weight.	2a. How do you feel when you gain weight? 2b. What happens just before you decide to lose weight? 2c. (If purging) Would you be able to tolerate gaining ten pounds if you could stop purging?
3. Feelings about current weight.	3. What do you think about your present weight?
4. Fluctuations in weight over time.	4a. Have you recently lost weight? 4b. How much? In what period of time?
5. Past treatment history and response to past treatment.	5. Have you ever been treated for a weight disorder? Was it successful?
Eating	
1. Exact eating patterns, i.e., amounts and types of food eaten normally and during binges and mealtimes.	1a. What do you eat in a typical day? How much? When and where? 1b. What do you eat when you binge? How much? When and where? Why do you terminate binges? 1c. Do you ever induce vomiting after you have eaten? 1d. Do you ever fast? How long? How often?
2. Signs of "secret" eating or shame associated with bingeing.	2a. Do you prefer eating alone? 2b. How does your eating change when you are around people?
3. Perception of eating as a problem behavior.	3. Do you think your eating pattern is normal?
4. Degree of disabling affects on activities of daily living.	4a. How does eating (or not eating) interfere with your life? 4b. Do you find yourself thinking about food and calories often?
5. Anxieties precipitating bingeing and purging.	5a. Do you ever fear losing control over your eating? 5b. Do you feel you have any control over purging?
6. Function of the bingeing, purging, and fasting behaviors.	6a. How do you feel after your binge eat? How do you feel after you purge? 6b. How do you feel when you can fast?
Activity	
1. Presence of compulsive exercise as a form of purging.	1. Do you exercise? What type and how much each day?
2. Function exercise serves both physically and emotionally.	2a. How do you feel physically after exercising? Emotionally? 2b. How do you feel physically if you cannot/do not exercise? Emotionally?
Family (In the context of presenting problem)	
1. Presence of marital conflict in parents' marriage or with spouse if client is married.	1a. Do your parents appear to be happy? 1b. How would you describe your marriage?
2. Parental response to emotional needs of children, to separation/independence of children.	2a. How do members of your family express anger? 2b. Does your family show affection? How? Sadness? How? 2c. Describe a situation when you brought a problem to your mother/father. What did they do? How did you feel? 2d. How do you feel about expressing opinions that differ from those of your parents? 2e. How did your parents react when you finished high school? Left home for college?
3. Feelings and reactions of each family member, spouse, or significant person concerning client's eating behavior and weight.	3. What does your mother (father, sibling) do when you refuse meals? Eat too much? Purge?

Table continued on following page

Table 25-3 • ASSESSMENT GUIDE FOR EATING DISORDERS *Continued*

TO DETERMINE	SAMPLE QUESTIONS
Family (in the context of presenting problem)	
4. Presence of poor impulse control, i.e., drug/alcohol abuse or excessive tempers in family members.	4. Does anyone in your family abuse alcohol? Drugs?
5. Presence of overcontrol of appetites and feelings by family.	5. What do your mother, father, siblings do when they are upset, angry, happy, hungry, sad? How do you know when they are angry? Sad? Hungry? Happy?
6. Eating patterns of the family unit.	6a. Who plans the family meals? Who does the food shopping? Who pays for the food? 6b. Does your family eat meals together? 6c. Do you speak with each other at these times? 6d. How does it feel for you to eat meals with your family? 6e. How long does it take you to eat a meal?
Physical	
1. Signs and symptoms often associated with *anorexia nervosa*.	1. Is there presence of • cachexia/emaciation; • decreased body temperature; • peripheral edema; • cyanosis of the extremities; • constipation; • atrophic dry skin; • slow pulse; • yellowish skin; • amenorrhea; • hair loss; • lanugo on skin; • anemia/malnutrition.
2. Signs and symptoms often associated with *bulimia*.	2. Is there presence of • parotid gland enlargement (chipmunk facies); • dehydration; • chronic hoarseness/sore throat; • dental caries—loss of enamel on teeth; • rebound water retention (when purging stops); • anemia; • irregular menses/amenorrhea; • electrolyte imbalance, i.e., hypokalemia.
3. Presence of abuse of substances used for "purging."	3a. Do you use laxatives or diuretics to lose weight? How many? How often? 3b. Do you ever take amphetamines, caffeine/diet pills? How many? How often?

turbance in self-esteem or *chronic low self-esteem* as evidenced by obesity may be an appropriate nursing diagnosis.

Since the issues of control/lack of control are felt to be a central theme, *powerlessness* related to inability to stop the binge-purge cycle, or *ineffective individual coping* related to phobias and rituals surrounding eating could be used.

Often, a person with an eating disorder is consumed with guilt and shame and withdraws from others. Most people who are victims of these disorders are isolated and feel alienated. Building and rebuilding communications with others is an important long term goal. *Social isolation* related to obesity/low self-esteem/shame may be characteristic of some individuals with an eating disorder.

Standard IV: Planning

Planning interventions for people with eating disorders involves planning on the (1) content level and (2) process level. Planning on the *content level* is the actual setting up of client-centered goals and devising specific nursing interventions aimed at meeting those goals. The *process level* is a recognition of the kinds of reactions a client may stimulate in the nurse (countertransference) and awareness of how to deal effectively with these feelings and reactions. Skill and awareness on the part of the nurse to handle personal reactions and feelings help maintain mutual self-esteem and help facilitate the therapeutic process. Inability to recognize strong reactions to the client and deal with them professionally often leads to power struggles and deterioration of the therapeutic relationship.

CONTENT LEVEL—PLANNING GOALS

Interventions planned for clients with eating disorders directly relate to the specific goals set and outcomes desired. Some examples of possible short term goals are illustrated here. Specific goals and interventions are discussed under each specific disorder.

An extremely emaciated young girl with anorexia nervosa might have a nursing diagnosis of *altered nutrition: less than body weight* related to self-starvation. Some possible goals follow:

- Client will gain 1 kg per week.
- Client will demonstrate a minimum or absence of purging two weeks after treatment starts.

If suicidal thoughts are evident and *potential for self-directed violence* is used as a nursing diagnosis, some possible goals could be

- Client will remain safe with the aid of staff support and supervision.
- By (state the date) client will be able to name two people she can talk to when thinking of suicide.
- By (state the date) client will explore feelings of anger and hopelessness with the nurse.

People with eating disorders usually have distortions of body image and a poor self-concept. Negative self-evaluation often takes up much of the person's conscious thought. Therefore, assessing a person's self-concept is important in people with eating disorders. The nursing diagnosis of *disturbance in self-esteem* as evidenced by obesity may warrant some of the following short term and long term goals:

- Client will identify two personal strengths by (state the date).
- By (state the date) client will name three aspects of her personality that she admires.
- Client will name two personal accomplishments of which she is proud.
- Client will name one/two important goals she would like to attain in her life.

PROCESS LEVEL—NURSES' REACTIONS AND FEELINGS

Different behaviors often evoke specific reactions in people. Although the nurse may be aware of a variety of reactions and feelings aroused by a client with an eating disorder, some reactions may be expected. These specific countertransferential feelings will be dealt with separately under *Process Level* in the case studies dealing specifically with anorexia, bulimia, and compulsive eating. Health care professionals working with people who have eating disorders should always have supervision available to discuss transference-countertransference issues. Supervision also serves as a guide for validating perceptions and maximizing intervention strategies. Supervision may be informal, as in peer group supervision, or more formal, as with weekly reviews with other members of the health team. Without supervision, nurses may react to client's behavior emotionally rather than recognize the important underlying issues and intervene accordingly.

Standard V: Intervention

The nurse may work with a client with an eating disorder in a variety of settings and circumstances. In some settings, the eating disorders may be secondary to other medical disorders. For example, a client with diabetes admitted to a general medical unit for stabilization of insulin may also be obese because of a compulsive eating disorder. A young woman seen in an outpatient clinic because of irregular menses may also be bulimic. Severe cases of anorexia nervosa require hospitalization when malnutrition becomes life threatening. Eating disorders are treated in both inpatient and outpatient settings depending on the client's priorities of needs. The nurse may play a variety of roles when working with a person with an eating disorder.

V-D: SOMATIC THERAPIES

The use of medications for treating anorexia nervosa and bulimia is still being studied, although some medications have been used since the 1950's (Vandereycken 1984). Neuroleptics such as phenothiazines, and antidepressants in the tricyclic and MAO inhibitor groups are most often prescribed. For example, imipramine hydrochloride has been found to reduce the frequency and intensity of binges for some bulimic clients (Pope et al. 1983). The use of chlorpromazine (Thorazine) has been useful in the treatment of some severely obsessive-compulsive anorexic clients (Walsh et al. 1985).

Appetite regulators and anticonvulsant drugs have been used less frequently. In general, more controlled studies of any drugs used to treat these disorders are needed. Although there has been some improvement after beginning pharmacotherapy, it has not been determined conclusively that this is the result of the medication or the other treatment modalities used concurrently with the same clients. It is also unclear as to which symptom the medication is actually targeting. For example, it is known that phenothiazines decrease anxiety and that antidepressants relieve depression. Once these feelings underlying the maladaptive eating behaviors are relieved, the bingeing might subside.

Symptom relief is a great benefit to the client, but without a change in coping ability there is little reason to believe that once the medication is stopped, the eating behavior will not surface again. Any medication regimen must be monitored carefully, with special attention given to possible side effects or problems that are especially pertinent to this population. One problem is that purging will reduce the actual amount of medication assimilated by the client. For these clients, frequent monitoring of the drug level in the blood is necessary, if possible. Another problem is that hypothermia and hypotension, already found in anorexics, are increased by some medications.

V-E: THERAPEUTIC ENVIRONMENT

The decision to admit a person with an eating disorder to an inpatient unit, and the type of unit chosen — that is, psychiatric eating disorder unit or medical unit — depend on careful assessment and the client's immediate needs. Since physiological and safety needs must be addressed first, any acute physical distress needing immediate medical attention would warrant admission to a medical unit. Professionals staffing such a unit should have a sound base of knowledge of eating disorders. If the client's physical status is not life threatening, a psychiatric unit staffed by professionals specializing in treating eating disorders is recommended. There has been an increase in these types of units as the number of people suffering from eating disorders has increased. The types of therapeutic approaches used may differ, depending on the theory base used by the professionals in each unit. Indications for in-hospital admission and treatment approaches for (1) anorexia, (2) bulimia, and (3) obesity caused by compulsive eating are discussed subsequently.

Inpatient Treatment for Anorexia Nervosa

The main criteria for the admission of a person with **anorexia nervosa to an inpatient unit** are as follows:

1. Loss of over 15% of minimal normal weight, with signs of extreme resistance to take even a minimum of calories to maintain weight.
2. Medical emergencies, regardless of weight, such as serious arrhythmias.
3. Severe psychological distress, such as feelings of panic or suicidal ideation, which is persistent and is not relieved by outpatient treatment.

Inpatient treatment has a dual focus: nutritional rehabilitation and psychotherapy. A range of weight is set after consulting reliable height and weight charts and considering the person's body frame. This weight range can be set on the low normal end of the chart (Wooley and Wooley 1985). The client who is expected to achieve a low normal weight is not as likely to feel that she is being "fattened up."

An individualized diet that achieves a gain of two to three pounds per week will minimize the side effects of refeeding in anorexics (Fig. 25–4). Hyperalimentation and tube feeding are alternatives to be considered for individuals who do not successfully gain weight. Forcing clients to eat, using appetite stimulants, or using psychotherapy without addressing eating patterns are all inappropriate techniques that ignore the underlying dynamics of the disorder. Exercise for the purpose of maintaining full range of motion is encouraged, but compulsive exercise to "burn off" calories is discouraged.

Gaining weight is not the only goal. Establishing a normal pattern of eating is necessary so that weight can be maintained on an outpatient basis. Many clients agree to gain weight in order to be discharged but intend to lose the weight after discharge! For this reason, anxiety levels and attitudes during weight gain must be assessed and addressed during the psychotherapy sessions before discharge. One of the most effective methods of treatment for a severe anorexic is based on behavioral therapy. Behavioral therapists who treat clients with anorexia nervosa believe that behavior modification techniques are necessary while the person is suffering from physical starvation. The effects of starvation render the anorexic incapable of benefiting from insight-oriented types of therapy. Some of the effects of

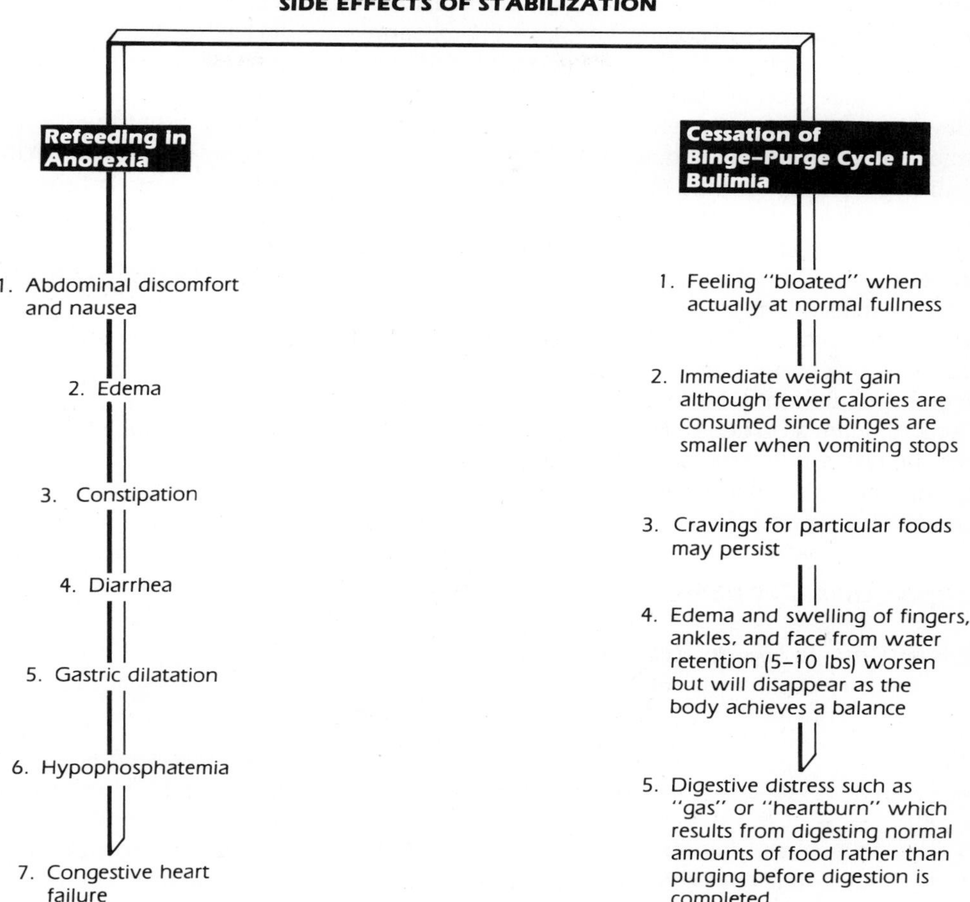

Figure 25–4. *Side effects associated with refeeding in anorexia and with cessation of the binge-purge cycle in bulimia.*

starvation are hyperactivity, irritability, and poor concentration and memory. Because of the repression of hunger and distorted body image, there is poor judgment, which makes meeting physical self-care needs difficult, if not impossible.

The following points are important for a behavior modification approach:

1. Weight gain, rather than eating behaviors, is reinforced.
2. A behavioral program must be individually suited to each client.
3. Only an enforceable program is effective, so a means of accurate monitoring must exist, such as regular "weigh-ins."
4. Psychotherapy can be integrated with a behavioral program, but the psychotherapist should not be the enforcer of the behavioral program. This helps avoid "power struggles" with the client.
5. Once weight gain commences and eating patterns appear normal, the client is allowed passes to eat in other situations, either alone or with family.

Inpatient Treatment for Bulimia Nervosa

Some **criteria for admission to an inpatient unit for a person with bulimia** follow:

1. Inability to interrupt a chronic and frequent binge-purge cycle in spite of outpatient treatment.
2. Medical emergencies, such as serious potassium depletion.
3. Psychiatric emergencies, such as persistent suicidal ideation.

The focus of inpatient treatment for normal weight bulimics will depend on the problems the individual presents, but generally, it will be re-establishment of a normal eating pattern, with avoidance of weight gain and a minimum of the physical side effects caused by the cessation of bingeing and purging (see Figure 25–4).

Because the bingeing and purging are actually signs of maladaptive coping with severe levels of anxiety and feelings of depression, it is common for these feelings to surface once the behaviors change. It is imperative that more adaptive ways of coping with anxiety are learned. Without the support and teaching by the nurse and other members of the treatment team, the bulimic may develop phobias, experience "anxiety attacks," or abuse drugs or alcohol to deal with anxiety. This work of learning healthier coping skills can begin during inpatient treatment, but long term follow-up consisting of ongoing psychotherapy is necessary to maintain any change.

Four areas of education for bulimics have been identified (Wooley and Wooley 1985). These are (1) physical effects of returning to a normal eating pattern, (2) weight regulation, (3) effects of starvation, and (4) effects of bulimia on health. This information is provided for the client in a structured and intensive program of group and individual sessions.

Inpatient Treatment for Obesity

Obesity due to compulsive eating that is psychogenic in nature is usually treated in an outpatient setting; however, there are some situations where **hospitalization** or residential treatment is recommended:

1. Need for interruption of chronic, uncontrollable eating.
2. Presence of potentially dangerous medical conditions that are aggravated by compulsive eating, e.g., diabetes, cardiac problems.
3. Need for rapid supervised weight loss to relieve conditions such as heart disease or to prepare for major surgery.
4. Treatment for obesity requiring surgery or drastic dieting.
5. Any psychiatric condition that requires inpatient treatment and exists concurrently with compulsive eating.

Regardless of whether the inpatient setting is medical or psychiatric, the nurse must maintain a holistic focus in his or her nursing practice. Addressing the "weight problem" and avoiding the client's emotional needs will reinforce for the client that her body is the "problem," and she will continue to deny her feelings. The client with compulsive eating behaviors must be viewed in the context of her need to cope with a poor self-image.

There has been a trend toward assessing each person's eating patterns and needs and formulating individualized plans that can be lifelong rather than focusing on quick weight loss diets. An exercise program may also be prescribed, but careful monitoring is necessary for those who have been leading sedentary lifestyles or who are extremely obese. Identifying the meaning food has in the person's emotional life and the function that compulsive eating serves is important in altering compulsive eating patterns. The advantage of a residential setting is that the client can begin working through all aspects of her problem in an intensive program and with the support of others who share her problem. This can be achieved through structured individual and group activities. A program such as this may last from one week to as long as a few months. As with other eating disorders, follow-up focuses on reinforcing and maintaining any progress made.

V-F: PSYCHOTHERAPY

There are several psychotherapeutic approaches that may be used, and the choice will determine the types of sessions — that is (1) individual, (2) group, or (3) family — the number of sessions, and the length of treatment. Two general issues are addressed, regardless of the specific approach used:

- Body image as it relates to self-image.
- Identification and effective expression of needs.

A nurse who is educated/certified in specific therapeutic modalities, usually at the master's level, may work with clients who have eating disorders in an outpatient unit, community mental health centers, or private practice. Three specific modalities are briefly discussed: (1) individual therapy, (2) group therapy, and (3) family therapy.

Individual Therapy

A number of theoretical models have been used effectively to treat individuals with eating disorders. Table 25-4 presents an overview of three theoretical models. The basic therapeutic approaches used in these models are also included.

Group Therapy

Group therapy for persons with eating disorders can be either time-limited, closed groups or long term, open groups. Closed groups do not admit new members once the groups begin meeting, and open groups do. The ideal size of therapy groups is from six to ten persons.

In the *short term groups* there is a didactic as well as a discussion component. Tasks, or "homework," are often prescribed, and each group session has a structured format and agenda. The group leader tends to

Table 25–4 • THEORETICAL MODELS FOR EATING DISORDERS

PREMISE	THERAPEUTIC APPROACH
Self-Psychology	
Person has a poorly developed sense of self and identity. When threatened, attempts to control anxiety, and "gaining control" takes the form of "controlling" food intake and weight. Anxiety is often stimulated when separation occurs, such as times of increased independence.	1. Explore situational crises (e.g., leaving home, divorce, success in career). 2. Explore meaning of the crisis. 3. Explore feelings when eating behaviors are used (fasting, bingeing, purging, compulsive exercise). 4. Assist connection between feelings and eating behaviors, e.g., **"YOU SEEM TO FEEL MUCH BETTER ABOUT YOURSELF WHEN YOU CAN AVOID A BINGE."**
Feminist Psychoanalytic Psychology	
The person is very ambivalent about her body. Messages transmitted by the mother that the body is to be feared and controlled and yet is the greatest source of approval from others. Messages hold that issues dealing with one's body (sexuality, power) are "taboo" or "wrong." The daughter learns to (1) withhold information about her problems and (2) deny her needs.	1. Establish a nonjudgmental alliance with client. Encourage the perception that the nurse is on the client's side. 2. Introduce consistency and reliability in scheduling sessions to establish trust. 3. Address the defensive behaviors of withholding or sullenness in a nonthreatening manner, e.g., **"IT MUST BE DIFFICULT TO TALK ABOUT PRIVATE MATTERS TO SOMEONE YOU JUST MET."** 4. Avoid power struggles. Do not become invested in whether or not the client gains weight. Refer client to physician to monitor client's weight and assess physical health.
Cognitive Theory	
The concept that people are motivated out of a belief system that is designed to increase feelings of self-esteem. People with eating disorders have faulty belief systems, e.g., food is all "good" or all "bad." This translates into all areas of the person's life, e.g., mistakes mean failure. FAULTY BELIEFS *Anorexics*—Being thin will solve problems. *Bulimics*—Food = comfort and removal of food control. *Compulsive eaters*—"fat" will protect one from intimacy and independence.	1. Establish a trusting relationship with client. 2. Explore client's belief system. 3. Introduce doubts about beliefs that lead to maladaptive behaviors, e.g., **"BEING THIN DOESN'T SEEM TO SOLVE YOUR PROBLEMS, SINCE YOU ARE THIN NOW AND STILL UNHAPPY."** 4. Explore functions the behavior serves, e.g., eating decreases anxiety. 5. Assist client in modifying false beliefs, e.g., **"BEING OBESE MAY POSE SOME PROBLEMS IN RELATIONSHIPS, BUT INTIMACY REQUIRES MORE THAN BEING THIN."**

Data from Garner and Bemis 1985; Geist 1982; Goodsitt 1985; Orbach 1985.

take a more directive role because of the time limits and structure of the group. There can also be encouragement of "networking" or a "buddy system" in which group members contact each other outside the group time for mutual support.

A second type of time-limited structured group is referred to as *repressive-inspirational therapy* (Lego 1982). Marathons and weekend retreats fall into this category and are offered to persons with eating disorders. These groups can focus either on control of the symptom, without focusing on the underlying dynamics, or on a specific dynamic such as "powerlessness." The problem with the former is that repressed feelings underlying the eating behavior will surface when the behavior is controlled prematurely. The disadvantage of the latter is that important issues and feelings are explored without enough time allowed for working through these issues and resolving feelings.

Analytic or intensive group therapy is long term and open. The dynamics underlying the eating behaviors are the main focus, and the group leader is, generally, a facilitator. Group members are encouraged to seek support and meet social needs outside the group membership by using skills learned in group sessions with friends and family. Group sessions are unstructured, with few "rules," and group members have primary responsibility for their use of group time and growth. For the person with eating disorders, this sense of personal responsibility and reaching out to others in mutual support are difficult to achieve, yet vital lessons to be learned.

Group experiences are invaluable for the client with an eating disorder, since social isolation is a common feature for many. Group therapy for women with eating disorders can facilitate communication about sex role socialization experience; choices and conflicts about school, work, and lifestyles; body image misperceptions; and eating patterns and defenses (Dickstein 1985). In the group setting, a person can learn that to be separate and autonomous, with personal needs and desires, is not only possible but encouraged.

Family Therapy

It can be assumed that food and eating have emotional meaning for families with a member who has an eating disorder. The overall goal of family therapy is to effect system changes. The focus is off the person with the eating disorder and on the family as a whole. The family is seen as a system whose parts are in constant interaction with each other. For these troubled families there has been an ineffectiveness in meeting needs—their own and each other's. This can be a result of faulty communication patterns, difficulties in boundaries and roles, and societal pressure when family norms are challenged. Family life is where separation and identity are learned and, in the case of families that include an anorexic or bulimic person, there seems to be little individuality. The person gets lost in the family system. This dysfunction in the family takes the form of an eating disorder. The functional family teaches its members to be unique and yet able to cooperate collectively with each other (Winstead-Fry 1982).

The family therapist functions as a participant-observer in the family process and treats the family in an understanding, empathetic, and nonjudgmental manner. It is important to enable the family members to become more differentiated. Using concepts of change theory as a guide, the family must be monitored by seeing differentiation as rewarding. Once differentiation has begun, there will be discomfort within the system until these changes become integrated. Positive feedback is important, along with compassion for any feelings of loss or separation anxiety experienced. Often, anger is expressed during this process, and this is an opportunity to assist the family in learning how to resolve conflict. The eating behavior will often change as this process unfolds. It is important to assist the family in making connections between changes in family patterns and the subsequent changes in the person's eating behaviors. This will reinforce that the disorder is a symptom of the dysfunctional family pattern. It is also important to point out that each individual is responsible for his or her own behavior. This will reduce the "guilt" experienced by parents and siblings and increase feelings of personal power in the person with the disorder by expecting her to "own" her own behavior.

Standard VI: Evaluation

The nurse evaluates the effectiveness of the interventions by determining whether the client-centered goals have been reached by the date set. Specific criteria for evaluating short term goals for clients will be discussed in each of the separate sections on anorexia, bulimia, and obesity due to compulsive eating.

Anorexia Nervosa

The medical term *anorexia* usually applies to a condition in which there is a loss of appetite. In the client with anorexia nervosa there may *not* be any loss of appetite or disinterest in food, and often the opposite is true. The anorexic is usually preoccupied with food and eating but will suppress her desire for food in order to control her eating. This preoccupation is seen in the anorexic's spending time in planning family menus; choosing restaurants where the family will eat; counting every calorie she ingests; and talking incessantly about food and weight-related issues. A preoccupation with exercise is often present, with the anorexic pushing herself beyond normal limits or needs in order to "work off" every calorie she might have ingested or to "allow" herself to eat a morsel of food.

Ninety-five percent of anorexics are women, and one in 250 teenagers becomes anorexic. Most develop the disorder between the ages of 13 and 22, with the most frequent age being 18. For most, weight was never an issue growing up, although some were slightly overweight. The typical anorexic comes from a white, middle- or upper middle–class family in which divorce or separation is rare. They are usually attractive and intelligent girls who are described as "never being any problem" as children. They tend to overachieve in studies and careers and spend a great deal of time in these pursuits. It is no wonder that the anorexic brings out feelings of confusion, anger, and helplessness in parents, friends, and professionals who must stand by and watch a gifted person, "for no reason," starve herself. In spite of pleas and even threats by concerned people, the anorexic maintains rigid control over her eating, and her only conscious goal is "not to eat." She avoids eating as though phobic of food and experiences anxiety approaching panic when her control is threatened. When she does relinquish control, even slightly, she subjects herself to harsh self-criticism for being "weak" and may experience feelings of hopelessness. In extreme cases, this can lead to suicide. Showing an anorexic the objective facts, such as her actual weight on a scale, her mirror image, or her calorie expenditure as compared with her calorie intake, only increases her need for control.

What would induce a young girl or woman with so many strengths to starve herself, sometimes to death, for the sake of a slim body? It is reported that 6.6 to 18% of anorexics die from self-starvation (Halmi 1988). The answer may lie in the possibility that the anorexic is controlling potentially disabling anxiety by controlling her eating. The exact source of this anxiety is different for each individual, but the conflicts most commonly encountered are ones of identity, separation, and autonomy.

DSM III-R CLASSIFICATION

The function of anorexia nervosa as a means of dealing with anxiety rooted in conflict is addressed in the DSM III-R (1987). This is seen in the following example in which the character disorder that underlies the eating disorder is placed on Axis II. The Axis II diagnosis indicates a personality or developmental disorder, whereas Axis I indicates a more acute problem.

Example: Axis I: Anorexia Nervosa
Axis II: Compulsive Personality Disorder

In the absence of a character disorder, a specific trait may be mentioned on Axis II.

Example: Axis I: Anorexia Nervosa
Axis II: Histrionic Personality Features

The criteria for a diagnosis of anorexia nervosa are specifically stated in the DSM III-R (1987) (Box 25-1).

Box 25-1. DIAGNOSTIC CRITERIA FOR ANOREXIA NERVOSA

A. Refusal to maintain body weight over a minimal normal weight for age and height, e.g., weight loss leading to maintenance of body weight 15% below that expected; or failure to make expected weight gain during period of growth, leading to body weight 15% below that expected

B. Intense fear of gaining weight or becoming fat, even though underweight

C. Disturbance in the way in which one's body weight, size, or shape is experienced, e.g., the person claims to "feel fat" even when emaciated, believes that one area of the body is "too fat" even when obviously underweight

D. In females, the absence of at least three consecutive menstrual cycles when otherwise expected to occur (primary or secondary amenorrhea). (A woman is considered to have amenorrhea if her periods occur only following hormone, e.g., estrogen, administration.)

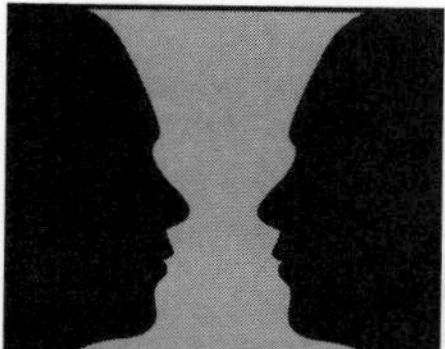

Case Study: Working With a Person Who Has Anorexia Nervosa

Jill is a 16-year-old high school student who has been admitted to an eating disorder unit of a local general hospital for anorexia nervosa. She is 5′7″ and weighs 90 pounds. Her parents report a usual weight of 125 pounds and say that she lost 35 pounds in the past five weeks. They report that she refuses to eat even her favorite foods. She was taken to the emergency room by her parents, who physically carried her from their home, against her protests. Jill was literally "kicking and screaming," protesting that she would "be forced to eat" and would "blow up like a blimp." During her initial assessment by her primary nurse, Ms. Heart, Jill was mute and avoided eye contact while maintaining a sullen look on her face. She fidgeted in her seat whenever a

Continued on following page

Case Study: Working With a Person Who Has Anorexia Nervosa *(Continued)*

question was asked but offered no verbal response. Ms. Heart noted that Jill's nail beds were blue and that she was shivering, although wearing clothing that was heavier than necessary for the well-heated room. Her hair was dull and limp, with some apparent bald patches, and her skin appeared dry with a yellowish tinge.

Assessment

Ms. Heart divides the data obtained during the initial interview with Jill into objective and subjective data.

OBJECTIVE DATA

1. Rapid weight loss
2. Emaciated appearance
3. Mute
4. Avoids eye contact
5. Sullen facial expression
6. Fidgety
7. Cyanosis of nail beds
8. Dry skin with yellow tinge
9. Shivering with heavy clothing
10. Dull, limp hair with bald patches
11. Physically carried to ER

SUBJECTIVE DATA (from parents, as client was mute)

1. "I'll blow up like a blimp."
2. "They'll force me to eat."
3. She was "kicking and screaming" (reported by parents).

Nursing Diagnosis

Ms. Heart reviews her data and formulates two nursing diagnoses in order of priority.

1. *Altered Nutrition: Less Than Body Requirements* related to self-starvation
   - Emaciated
   - Rapid weight loss
   - Cyanosis of nail beds
   - Dry skin, yellow tinge
   - Limp hair with bald spot
2. *Ineffective Individual Coping* related to anxiety over losing control and inability to trust
   - "They'll force me to eat"
   - Physically carried into ER
   - Mute
   - Avoids eye contact
   - Sullen facial expression

Planning

CONTENT LEVEL—PLANNING GOALS

Ideally, when planning care, short and long term goals are discussed and set with input from the client. Since Jill's physical starvation has altered her judgment and perception of her physical condition, Ms. Heart sets down the short term goals, with input from other members of the health team, and discusses them with Jill. Since Jill's self-starvation is life threatening, attention to gradual weight gain is given priority.

Nursing Diagnosis	Goals
1. *Altered Nutrition: Less Than Body Requirements* related to self-starvation	1a. Client will gain 0.5 to 1.5 kgm per week. 1b. Client will exhibit a minimum of adverse physical effects from refeeding and starvation during hospital stay (see Figure 25–3).
2. *Ineffective Individual Coping* related to inability to trust and anxiety over losing control	2a. Client will state she feels more in control within three weeks (state the date). 2b. Client will state she feels more comfortable with nurse and views nurse as a helping person by four weeks (state the date).

PROCESS LEVEL — NURSES' REACTIONS AND FEELINGS

Anorexic clients who exhibit behaviors such as being mute, withdrawn, and sullen may engender feelings of helplessness and subsequent anger in the nurse. The nurse can use insight into her feelings as a valuable tool in her nursing practice. A lack of self-awareness can interfere with the accepting and nonjudgmental attitude that is especially important in working with the anorexic client. This frightened young woman might be labeled "uncooperative" because of her defenses. Some behaviors, on the part of the nurse, that would indicate anger and need for supervision follow:

1. An avoidance of the client.
2. An increased attempt to control through primitive limit setting.
3. Any power struggles or argumentative interactions with the client.
4. Infantilizing the client or not providing appropriate limits to compensate for angry feelings.

Ms. Heart has been working with clients with eating disorders for two years and has become aware of the signs of covert anger on her part in relationship to the client's behaviors. She continues to be alert to her feelings and actions as clues to what is going on with her clients. Ms. Heart is in weekly supervision with the psychiatric nurse specialist assigned to her unit.

Intervention

Ms. Heart draws her nursing interventions from those outlined in Table 25–5. From these guidelines and input from the health team, Ms. Heart creates an individualized plan of care for Jill (Nursing Care Plan 25–1).

Evaluation

Ms. Heart continuously evaluates Jill's progress. She reviews the short term goals to determine whether they are realistic and to assure that the planned interventions are appropriate in meeting the goals. See Nursing Care Plan 25–1 for the frequent evaluation and outcome of Ms. Heart's nursing care.

Table 25–5 • NURSING INTERVENTIONS WITH ANOREXIA NERVOSA

NURSING INTERVENTION	RATIONALE
1. Monitoring temperature, respiration, and pulse (apical and radial) every day.	1. Increased risk of arrhythmias, bradycardia, and hypotension exists. Hypothermia is often present, therefore a slight elevation of body temperature above 98.6°F may be a high fever.
2. Observe for tetany or complaint of muscle cramping. Be aware of current electrolyte status.	2. Electrolyte imbalances are common. Subjective complaints of muscle cramping or observation of muscle stiffness in body movement is significant. Frequent electrolyte measures are necessary because of life-threatening complications of *hypokalemia*.
3. Observe caloric intake closely, i.e., (1) amount client eats voluntarily and (2) rituals that decrease amount eaten. 4. Observe closely after eating for signs of purging. 5. Observe activity level. 6. Measure urine and fecal output. 7. Weigh daily at the same time in light clothing.	3–7. Because of severe anxiety concerning eating and weight in controlled setting, some deception is to be expected. Therefore, objective as well as subjective data collection is essential.
8. Make contract for minimal safe weight range, which is a contingency for discharge. 9. Give assurance that quick weight gain is not desirable and slow controlled weight gain is the goal.	8–9. Participation in planning care increases feelings of control and compliance with treatment. A controlled diet can allay fears of too rapid weight gain.
10. Meet with client's nutritionist and physician on planning a diet to meet client's physical needs. Allow increasing control over types of food eaten after normal eating pattern is exhibited.	10. A team approach to planning diet ensures that physical and emotional needs are being addressed.

Table continued on following page

Table 25–5 • NURSING INTERVENTIONS WITH ANOREXIA NERVOSA *Continued*

NURSING INTERVENTION	RATIONALE
11. Respond to signs of distrust and anxiety by acknowledging these feelings in an empathetic manner—avoid interpretation or confrontation in initial stages of relationship.	11. Feelings of worthlessness and anxiety increase as weight increases. Client responds best to support and understanding of fears. To client, gaining weight may mean threat to survival.
12. Understand that behaviors of deception are expected. Avoid labels such as "bad client" or "liar."	12. View deceptive behaviors as a means of increasing self-esteem and "control." Avoid "power struggles" and negative judgments.

Nursing Care Plan 25–1 • A PERSON WITH ANOREXIA NERVOSA: Jill

NURSING DIAGNOSIS

Altered nutrition related to self-starvation

Supporting Data

- Emaciated.
- Rapid weight loss
- Cyanosis of nail beds.
- Dry skin with yellow tinge.
- Limp hair with bald spot.

Long Term Goal: Client's weight will be within safe limits by discharge.

Short Term Goal	*Intervention*	*Rationale*	*Evaluation*
1. Client will gain 0.5 to 1.5 kg per week.	1a. Observe caloric intake closely (amount eaten). 1b. Note rituals while eating. 1c. Observe after eating for signs of purging. 1d. Observe activity level. 1e. Measure urine and fecal output. 1f. Weigh daily at the same time in light clothing.	1a–f. Because of client's anxiety regarding eating and weight gain and being hospitalized against client's will, some deception is to be expected. For this reason, objective as well as subjective data collection is essential.	Goal Met. Week 1—0.5 kg. Week 2—0.7 kg. Week 3—0.9 kg. Week 4—1.1 kg. Week 6—1.2 kg, however two-pound ankle weight found in pants. Week 7—1.2 kg. Goal is being met, with a slow but steady weight gain.
	1g. Make contract with client for a minimal safe weight range, which is a contingency for discharge.	1g. Involvement in decision making increases sense of control and chances of compliance.	
2. Client will exhibit a minimum of adverse physical effects from refeeding and self-starvation during hospitalization.	2a. Daily monitoring of temperature, respiration, and pulse (apical and radial).	2a. Effects of starvation increase risk of arrythmias, bradycardia, and hypotension. Hypotension is often present.	Week 1—Within normal limits. Week 2—Nl limits. Week 3—Nl limits. Week 4—Nl limits. Week 5—Nl limits. Week 6—Nl limits. Week 7—Nl limits.
	2b. Observe for muscle twitching, facial twitching, wrist/ankle twitching, and cramping. Check current electrolyte status daily.	2b. Electrolyte imbalances can be life threatening.	Week 1—None. Week 2—complained of leg cramping, physician notified and potassium drawn. Week 3—None. Week 4—None. Week 5—None. Week 6—None. Week 7—None.

Short Term Goal	Intervention	Rationale	Evaluation
	2c. Observe for adverse side effects of refeeding: • abdominal discomfort • nausea • edema • constipation or diarrhea • gastric dilation • hypophosphatemia • congestive heart failure	2c. Adverse and possibly fatal effects can occur with overfeeding and too rapid weight gain.	Week 1—None. Week 2—complained of abdominal cramping × date. Week 3—complained of nausea, ankle edema × date. Week 4—None. Week 6—complained of constipation × date. Week 7—None.

Bulimia Nervosa

Bulimia nervosa is a clinical entity distinct from anorexia nervosa and compulsive eating. Bulimics can be divided into at least two different groups. The first are anorexics who have lost their rigid control over eating and who binge. Purging is an attempt to regain control. About 50% of anorexics engage in this behavior (Bruch 1985). The second group are persons who are normal weight or only slightly overweight who binge and then purge to maintain or lose weight. There has been an increase in this latter type in recent years, or at least an increase in the numbers seeking treatment. This group is the focus of this section.

The binge-purge cycle is compulsive in nature and may interfere with the individual's level of daily functioning to the extent that all of her waking time is spent or arranged around these behaviors. Jobs and relationships may be severely affected as the person becomes increasingly more preoccupied with bingeing and purging while simultaneously becoming more isolated. Binges may consist of thousands of calories consumed in a matter of minutes and end because of abdominal distress, sleep, or social interruption. In extreme cases, the person may eat until unconscious. Binge-purge behaviors may affect the lives of bulimics and their families in the same way that alcoholism or drug abuse affects other families. It is not uncommon for bulimic behaviors to surface in recovering alcoholics or for bulimia and substance abuse to exist simultaneously. Substance abuse and other forms of poor impulse control are frequently reported in family members of bulimics. This poor impulse control in the bulimic family is similar to the "uncontrollable" nature of the binge-purge cycle.

There is no clearly identified personality type among bulimics, but it has been proposed that there is an underlying depression in many (Halmi 1988). Signs and symptoms of depression, as well as reported suicide attempts and self-mutilation, are often present. The depression may be directly related to the loss of control the bulimic experiences over her eating or remain unchanged regardless of her improvement. A range of personality disorders has been identified in bulimics. Problems with interpersonal relationships, self-concept, and impulsive behaviors are common (Halmi 1988). Forms of poor impulse control include sexual promiscuity, kleptomania, compulsive spending, shoplifting, gambling, and compulsive lying. Other bulimics might guard against these impulses by exhibiting obsessive-compulsive behaviors such as "filling up every minute" to avoid temptation. Any slight deviation from their routine results in feelings of "emptiness" and anxiety.

Forms of purging may include self-induced vomiting, which can become spontaneous as the behavior persists. Food might simply be chewed and spit out without swallowing, and laxative abuse is common. A minority of bulimics may use diuretics for weight control.

It is thought that the bulimic has a "deficit in the sense of responsibility." The bulimic blames external events or other persons for her behavior. This belief may account for the "assumed helplessness" she ex-

Box 25–2. DIAGNOSTIC CRITERIA FOR BULIMIA NERVOSA

A. Recurrent episodes of binge eating (rapid consumption of a large amount of food in a discrete period of time)
B. A feeling of lack of control over eating behaviors during the eating binges
C. The person regularly engages in either self-induced vomiting, use of laxatives or diuretics, strict dieting or fasting, or vigorous exercise in order to prevent weight gain.
D. A minimum average of two binge eating episodes a week for at least three months
E. Persistent overconcern with body shape and weight

hibits. The power of others renders her powerless and unable to take charge of her own life (Bruch 1985).

DSM III-R CLASSIFICATION

The DSM III-R criteria for bulimia nervosa (Box 25–2) are very specific, but bulimics may vary greatly in their ability to adjust, so a diagnosis of bulimia nervosa, alone, may be misleading. There may be other, more serious, simultaneous diagnoses. The DSM III-R classification allows for this need to individualize the bulimic's treatment by using the following system:

Example: Axis I: Bulimia
Axis II: Borderline Personality Disorder with depressive features

A person with this diagnosis might present the binge-purge syndrome along with intense feelings of abandonment and depression that seem related to separation or loss. The treatment plan would need to address bulimia and depression and consider the dynamics of the borderline personality (see Chapter 17).

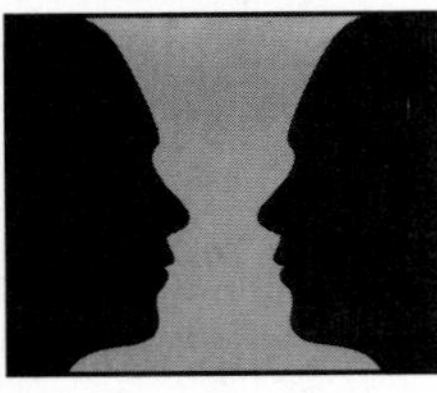

Case Study: Working With A Person Who Has Bulimia Nervosa

Nora is a well groomed 23-year-old woman who is a recent college graduate and living at home with her parents and 19-year-old sister. An older sister is married and lives nearby. Nora came to the Community Mental Health Center seeking counseling for "anxiety attacks." During the initial assessment by Mr. Hope, the psychiatric nurse clinical specialist, Nora reported "feeling panic before leaving home, even to go to work." She would manage to get to work only after "bingeing," but would purge once she arrived at her job. So far, she has been able to conceal this from her family and her employer but has received numerous warnings about her lateness. She has also experienced "sluggishness and irritability" after bingeing and purging. Nora works as a dietitian in a college cafeteria, which further complicates her situation, as she "sneak binges and purges" at least twice each workday. She reports "not being able to stop" this cycle and was tearful and speaking rapidly as she was interviewed.

Assessment

Mr. Hope observes that Nora is experiencing anxiety during the interview as she relates her distress over the emotionally and physically stressful binge-purge cycle. From the assessment, the nurse notes two important strengths: (1) Nora has achieved success in her education, and (2) she has remained employed in spite of a debilitating degree of anxiety. Nora's health status and employment status are being threatened, but she has some degree of good judgment in seeking assistance at this time.

OBJECTIVE DATA

1. Tearful with rapid speech
2. Employed at food-related job
3. Living at home with family of origin
4. Well-groomed
5. College graduate
6. Behaviors affect job
7. Behaviors kept secret from family and employer
8. Seems to be seeking help voluntarily

SUBJECTIVE DATA

1. "Panic" before leaving home
2. Reports binge-purge cycle that feels "uncontrollable"
3. "Sluggishness" and "irritability" after bingeing and purging

Nursing Diagnosis

From the data, Mr. Hope formulates the following nursing diagnosis:

Anxiety (*severe to panic*) related to separation issues
- "Panic" before leaving home
- "Uncontrollable" binge-purge cycle when under stress
- Tearful with rapid speech

Planning

CONTENT LEVEL—PLANNING GOALS

Mr. Hope spends time with Nora establishing long term and short term goals that are realistic, appropriate, and measurable.

Nursing Diagnosis	Long Term Goals	Short Term Goals
Anxiety (*severe to panic*) related to separation issues	Client will demonstrate use of two ways of coping with anxiety by (state the date).	1a. Within two weeks (state the date) client will identify specific events that increase her anxiety. 1b. Client will name two alternative coping skills for handling anxiety (other than bingeing and purging) within three weeks (state the date).

PROCESS LEVEL—NURSES' REACTIONS AND FEELINGS

The client with bulimia often has extreme anxiety because she feels she is out of control. Once the compulsive binge-purge cycle is in motion, there is a feeling of helplessness to control food. The helpless client may look to the nurse to solve her problems and may exhibit anger when this expectation is not met. Feelings aroused in the nurse from the client's helplessness and extreme dependency might set in motion the need to "take over" or "rescue" the client. These responses on the part of the nurse stem from a "need to be needed" or to "control" this person who feels she is unable to control her own life. Cues that signal the nurse is involved in a need to "rescue" the client are listed subsequently. These behaviors signal the need for supervision and can inhibit client progress.

1. Giving the client a diet to follow, believing that poor eating habits are "the problem."
2. Corroborating the client's belief that "food controls her" by telling her to avoid situations in which she might binge rather than focusing on the anxiety that is related to her behaviors.
3. Attempting to give the bulimic solutions or "pat answers" rather than using a problem-solving approach.

Intervention

Mr. Hope plans individual care for Nora, drawing from nursing interventions useful for a person with bulimia (Table 25–6).

Drawing from intervention guidelines and Nora's individual situation, Mr. Hope devised Nursing Care Plan 25–2.

Evaluation

Mr. Hope continuously evaluates the short term goals set for Nora. (1) He evaluates Nora's ability to identify situations that produce anxiety and make connections between perceptions, anxiety, and behaviors. (2) He evaluates alterations in her present coping skills and her use of alternative ways of handling stress. Refer to Nursing Care Plan 25–2 for specific observations in the evaluation of Nora on a weekly basis. During his interactions with Nora, he is watchful for any side effects resulting from the cessation of the binge-purge cycle (see Figure 25–4).

Table 25–6 • NURSING INTERVENTIONS WITH BULIMIA NERVOSA

NURSING INTERVENTION	RATIONALE
1. Communicate empathy; focus on feelings. Avoid comments that seem judgmental.	1. Establish a therapeutic alliance based on understanding in an atmosphere of openness and support.
2. Evaluate situation using a crisis intervention model, e.g., assess precipitating events, support system, and coping skills.	2. Ascertain strengths/weaknesses, coping skills, available resources, and potential crisis situations.

Table continued on following page

Table 25-6 • NURSING INTERVENTIONS WITH BULIMIA NERVOSA *Continued*

NURSING INTERVENTION	RATIONALE
3. Continuously assess • presence of an eating disorder, • family system.	3. Data collected in initial interview is not complete. Assessment is ongoing.
4. Assess for depression and potential suicidal risk.	4. Clinical depression common. Presence of anxiety and feelings of hopelessness indicate high-risk factors.
5. Assess for any immediate physical distress or potential health problems.	5. Immediate physical problem may warrant emergency treatment. Potential health problems warrant some immediate health teaching concerning effects of bingeing and purging.
6. Refer client to a physician of her choice for a complete physical examination.	6. An examination is warranted when bingeing and purging are frequent.
7. Refer to a psychiatrist for evaluation for possible pharmacotherapy.	7. Anxiety and possible depression may be relieved by medication, thus making outpatient treatment more manageable.

Nursing Care Plan 25-2 • A PERSON WITH BULIMIA NERVOSA: Nora

NURSING DIAGNOSIS

Anxiety (severe to panic) related to separation issues

Supporting Data

- Panic before leaving home.
- "Uncontrollable" binge-purge cycle when under stress.
- Tearful with rapid speech.

Long Term Goal: Client will demonstrate use of two ways of coping with anxiety by (state the date).

Short Term Goal	*Intervention*	*Rationale*	*Evaluation*
1. Within two weeks (state the date) client will identify precipitating events that increase her levels of anxiety.	1a. Assess for suicidal risk immediately.	1a. Underlying depression common. High anxiety and feelings of helplessness indicate possible suicidal ideation.	Goal met Week 1—(state the date) Not at risk at present.
	1b. Work with client on a one-to-one basis two times per week.	1b. Establish therapeutic relationship and evaluate for group participation with others who have eating disorders.	Week 2—(state the date) Client states she is beginning to see a connection between anxiety and family issues that involve separation, i.e., "growing up," "being different," "leaving home."
	1c. Communicate empathy; focus on feelings of anxiety. 1d. Avoid any comments that may seem judgmental.	1c–d. Establish therapeutic alliance based on understanding. Provide an atmosphere of openness and support. Help maintain self-esteem.	(State the date)—Since the client started group, validation from group and support have increased socialization. States she has two new friends with group encouragement.
2. Within four weeks (state the date) client will name two alternative coping skills when feeling increased anxiety.	2a. Evaluate client's situation using a crisis intervention model, e.g., assessing precipitating events, support system, and coping skills.	2a. To identify anxiety-provoking issues, adaptive and nonadaptive defenses, and possible resources for changes.	Plans to start back to school in fall for master's degree to fulfill dream of teaching dietitians. To date has three new supports:
	2b. Explore alternative coping skills—relation techniques, talking with friend, activities, problem solving.	2b. Help minimize need to utilize binge-purge cycle.	1. Group. 2. Increase in socialization (friends). 3. Plans for future.

Short Term Goal	Intervention	Rationale	Evaluation
	2c. Encourage participation and provide referred group therapy for eating disorders.	2c. Provide support and reduce feeling of isolation while learning new coping skills.	
	2d. Refer client to a physician for • complete exam, • possible pharmacotherapy.	2d. Treat or prevent physical damage from binge-purge behavior. Client's anxiety/depression may be relieved by medication, thus making outpatient treatment more manageable.	

Obesity Due to Compulsive Eating

Obesity is a physical condition that can have several possible etiologies. It can be the result of (1) a medical condition, (2) a lack of an adequate variety of foods, as seen in lower socioeconomic groups whose diets consist mainly of carbohydrates, (3) a side effect of pharmacotherapy such as steroid treatment, or (4) compulsive eating that is psychogenic in its origins. This latter type of obesity is discussed here and can be subdivided into two broad categories of either "developmental" or "reactive" obesity (Bruch 1985).

Developmental obesity is the type seen in persons who have been obese since childhood and is the result of overfeeding, beginning as early as infancy. **Reactive obesity** occurs later in life when compulsive eating becomes a maladaptive coping style at a time of stress. In either case, Hilde Bruch proposed that compulsive eating and obesity are defenses against feelings of depression or more unacceptable acting-out behaviors and that the premature removal of the eating behaviors and subsequent weight loss may allow these feared feelings and behaviors to surface.

If viewed in this way, compulsive eating and "being fat" may serve a similar function for the obese person that fasting and "being thin" serve for the anorexic. For example, a woman, who when in an obese state is withdrawn and isolated, blames her lack of close relationships on "being fat." If she were slim, she feels, she would be more physically attractive and would become outgoing. Although this change is desirable, it is also feared because obesity is, for her, a protection from the risks of intimacy. She feels that her "fat" is controlling her fate and, subsequently, denies responsibility for her own isolation. Like the anorexic, she believes that "if I were thin, all my problems would be solved." By holding onto this belief, she avoids the painful process of examining her own participation in her problems.

Like the anorexic and the bulimic, a person who uses food to maintain obesity may be experiencing conflicts about independence, autonomy, separation, and intimacy. Although there are many obese men, the current literature seems to focus on obese women, children, and adolescents. The reason for this is that these populations seek professional counseling for weight-related problems more often than adult males. Although there is a social stigma placed on "fat people" in general, obese women, children, and adolescents feel society's disapproval more acutely. Self-esteem is more dependent on body image among these populations. Feelings of shame and guilt, with subsequent depression, are frequent complaints. These feelings may be suppressed through an escalation of the compulsive eating and denial of the obesity. Obesity is denied when an obese person sees only her "better" parts in a mirror or avoids the mirror altogether.

DSM III-R CLASSIFICATION

Specific diagnostic criteria for obesity due to compulsive eating are not found in the DSM III-R. It is possible, however, to use one of two DSM III-R categories for diagnosis. (1) Atypical Eating Disorders or (2) Psychological Factor Affecting Physical Condition. An example of the former is:

Axis I: Atypical Eating Disorder
Axis II: Mixed Personality Disorder

and an example of the latter is:

Axis I: Psychological Factor Affecting Physical Condition
Axis II: Dependent Personality Disorder
Axis III: Obesity

Axis III is used, in this case, not only to identify obesity as a medical condition but also to emphasize that it is a result of a psychological condition.

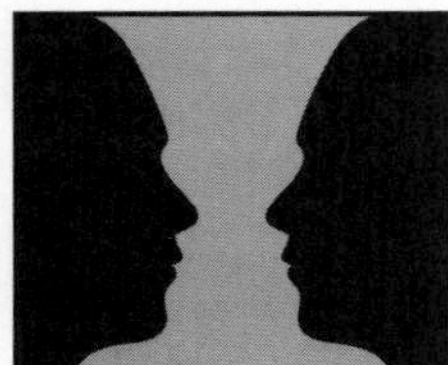

Case Study: Working With a Person Whose Obesity Is Caused by Compulsive Eating

Mary is a 45-year-old woman who was admitted to an inpatient mental health unit for depression. Her husband reported that she has not gone to her job for two weeks. Her reasons are vague, and physical complaints are general. She spends most of her days in bed but is awake most of the night. Her husband also reported an apparent increase in her eating, although she denies feeling hungry. The decision to hospitalize Mary was made after she verbalized passive suicidal ideation: "I really don't care what happens to me anymore."

Mrs. Worth, a staff nurse on the unit, saw Mary for the initial interview. Mary was despondent and became tearful when describing her feelings of "worthlessness." She stated, "I can't stand myself—I hate the way I look, but I can't do anything. I feel too ashamed to go to work and have people see me."

Mrs. Worth also noted that Mary appeared disheveled and wore tight-fitting clothing. Mary stated that she could no longer fit into her clothes. She had gained 45 pounds in the past two months and at 5′3″ weighed 175 pounds. She had no previous history of obesity but reported eating for comfort at times of stress. Mary began eating compulsively shortly after her father died following a long battle with cancer.

Assessment

Mrs. Worth divides her data into objective and subjective components.

OBJECTIVE DATA

1. Seclusive at home for two weeks
2. 45-pound weight gain in two months
3. Recent death of father
4. Appeared despondent and became tearful
5. Appeared disheveled
6. 5′3″ and 175 pounds.
7. Erratic sleep pattern
8. Increased eating without hunger

SUBJECTIVE DATA

1. "I really don't care what happens to me anymore."
2. Feelings of "worthlessness" and "self-loathing"
3. "Ashamed to have people see me."

Nursing Diagnosis

Based on her data, Mrs. Worth formulates the following nursing diagnoses:

1. *Dysfunctional Grieving* related to father's death, as evidenced by suicidal thoughts and feelings of worthlessness
   - 45-pound weight gain in two months (after father's death)
   - Seclusion and social isolation
   - Passive suicidal ideation
   - Feelings of worthlessness and self-loathing
2. *Disturbance in Self-Esteem* related to obesity, as evidenced by withdrawal and change in usual pattern of responsibility
   - Ashamed to be seen
   - Feeling worthless and expresses self-loathing
   - Disheveled appearance
   - Appears despondent and tearful
   - 5′3″ tall and 175 pounds

Planning

CONTENT LEVEL—PLANNING GOALS

After spending time with Mary, Mrs. Worth works out goals for her nursing diagnosis. Since Mary's physical safety is of utmost importance, priority of interventions is based on the data received from a thorough assessment of suicidal risk and intent (refer to Chapter 22).

Nursing Diagnosis	Long Term Goals	Short Term Goals
Dysfunctional Grieving related to father's death, as evidenced by suicidal thoughts and feelings of worthlessness	Within one year's time, client will state comfortably she remembers the good times and difficult times with her dad.	1a. Client will verbalize feelings about her father's death by the end of four days (state the date). 1b. Client will state she feels better about herself and name two specific strengths by (state the date).

PROCESS LEVEL — NURSES' REACTIONS AND FEELINGS

Clients who are obese and depressed are often suffering from low self-esteem and shame. When the nurse is confronted with a client who verbalizes self-loathing and self-deprecating statements, there is always a temptation to ease this pain or "take it away." This often indicates a need of the nurse to escape these feelings because they are almost as uncomfortable for the nurse as they are for the client. Some nursing behaviors that can interfere with the development of self-esteem in the client are listed subsequently. Evidence of these behaviors signals the nurse's need for supervision in order to maximize therapeutic intervention.

1. Telling the client that she is wrong about her evaluation of herself rather than exploring her strengths and weaknesses.
2. Giving the client compliments that are not genuine.
3. Telling the client "not to worry."
4. Focusing on her obesity as the main problem rather than on her feelings about herself. This reinforces her belief that her obese body is "shameful."

Intervention

There are a number of areas and levels of intervention that the nurse can use when working with a client who is obese. This chapter deals with obesity related to maladaptive coping responses. Therefore, the interventions focus on the underlying causes, such as depression, rather than on the physical manifestations, such as diets and exercise. Table 25–7 outlines nursing interventions useful for a client who is a compulsive eater.

Mrs. Worth plans individualized care for Mary (Nursing Care Plan 25–3) using some of the nursing guidelines but tailoring the plan to Mary's needs.

Evaluation

Mrs. Worth evaluates her goals during Mary's hospital stay. Evidence that appropriate grieving response has been activated would be seen in Mary's ability to talk more completely about the feelings experienced regarding her father's death. Mrs. Worth notes Mary's ability to share painful memories and feelings with her and significant others, and she evaluates appropriate affects regarding the grief reaction. A decrease in her thoughts about suicide and evidence of more spontaneous socialization are other indicators that the grieving process has been reactivated.

Signs of a more realistic self-concept and rise in self-esteem would be seen in statements to that effect from Mary and specific observations. Is Mary able to identify specific strengths? Does she speak less frequently about feeling worthless? Does she show an increase in control over eating behaviors? Have her hygiene and grooming improved? Evaluation of goals is noted on Mary's care plan (Nursing Care Plan 25–3).

Table 25–7 • NURSING INTERVENTIONS WITH COMPULSIVE EATING

NURSING INTERVENTION	RATIONALE
1. Assess suicidal risk.	1. Feelings of hopelessness and poor self-concept indicate high-risk factors.

Table continued on following page

Table 25-7 • NURSING INTERVENTIONS WITH COMPULSIVE EATING *Continued*

NURSING INTERVENTION	RATIONALE
2. Assess for depression.	2. Compulsive eating can be a way of handling depression and internalizing aggression.
3. Provide structured one-to-one sessions.	3. Frequent opportunities to verbalize feelings can diminish acting out through compulsive eating.
4. Provide structured activities.	4. Helps utilize empty time and control compulsive eating.
5. Provide group activities: formal (therapy) and informal (dance, art, etc.).	5. Provides feedback. Aids development of a more realistic self-image. Allows outlets to relieve tension and aggression.
6. Encourage physical evaluation by physician.	6. Evaluate any medical abnormalities resulting from obesity.
7. Encourage consultation by psychiatrist.	7. Evaluate need for psychopharmacology, i.e., antianxiety/antidepression medication.
8. Evaluate with client personal strengths and significant supports.	8. Assess present situation realistically. Emphasize strengths and evaluate need for support.

Nursing Care Plan 25-3 • A PERSON WITH PSYCHOGENIC OBESITY: Mary

NURSING DIAGNOSIS

Dysfunctional grieving related to father's death, as evidenced by suicidal thoughts and feelings of worthlessness

Supporting Data

- 45-Pound weight gain in two months (after father's death).
- Seclusion and social isolation.
- Passive suicidal ideation.
- Feelings of "worthlessness" and "self-loathing."

Long Term Goal: Client will start and continue to work through the grieving process.

Short Term Goal	*Intervention*	*Rationale*	*Evaluation*
1. Client will verbalize feelings about her father's death by the end of four days (state the date).	1a. Provide structure in client's day through one-to-one sessions with primary nurse. 1b. Provide structured activities throughout the day.	1a. Gives client opportunity to verbalize feelings of grief, loss, and separation. 1b. Helps to control compulsive eating.	Goal met Week 1—(state the date) Client's affect more appropriate; talking more freely of missing father. Week 2—(state the date) Continues to express feelings of sadness. Week 3—(state the date) Was able to express anger over father's leaving her—pounding fist on table. Grief process appears activated.

NURSING DIAGNOSIS

Disturbance in self-esteem related to obesity, as evidenced by withdrawal and change in usual patterns of responsibility

Supporting Data

- Ashamed to be seen.
- Disheveled appearance.
- Feels worthless and expresses self-loathing.
- 5′3″ and 175 pounds.
- Appears despondent and tearful.

Long Term Goal: Client will resume usual socialization and role-related responsibilities by (state the date).

Short Term Goal	*Intervention*	*Rationale*	*Evaluation*
1. Client will state she feels better about her situation and will name two strengths/supports in three weeks (state the date).	1a. Evaluate suicide potential and risk.	1a. Suicidal ideation and hopelessness result in high risk for self-destructive behavior.	Goal met Week 1—(state the date) Vague thoughts of "wanting to die"; suicide risk low.
	1b. Provide group activities: formal (therapy) and informal (dance, art, etc.).	1b. Group activities provide feedback. Aid development of more realistic self-image.	Week 2—(state the date) More spontaneous participation in group meetings. Hair clean and well groomed.
	1c. Evaluate with client number of personal strengths and supportive significant others.	1c. Potentially more realistic view of situation: • actual strengths, • actual supports available.	Week 3—(state the date) Appearance greatly improved—neatly dressed, nail care, and loss of 3 pounds. States feels better about self. States looks forward to going back to work and spending time with husband.

Summary

The eating disorders discussed in this chapter are (1) anorexia nervosa, (2) bulimia nervosa, and (3) obesity due to compulsive eating. There have been a number of theories proposed to explain the etiology of the eating disorders, e.g., psychodynamic, family, sociocultural, and multidimensional. A psychiatric nursing assessment on a person with an eating disorder includes the evaluation of specific areas. These are *weight, eating, activity, family*, and *physical signs and symptoms*.

Nursing diagnoses for a person with an eating disorder can cover a wide range of problem areas. General diagnoses often include *altered nutrition (less/more than body weight), disturbance in self-esteem, ineffective individual coping*, and *social isolation*. Planning effective nursing care involves planning on the *content level* (planning goals) and the *process level* (nurses' reactions and feelings).

Effective nursing intervention usually entails a variety of therapeutic modes. For example, medications may be used to treat an underlying depression. Inpatient treatment is often indicated when the physical status is life threatening. Examples include a person with anorexia nervosa whose low weight threatens her life and an obese person whose cardiac status is critical. Behavior modification has been found to be an effective approach for some people with eating disorders. Individual, group, and family therapy approaches are also important treatment modalities. Specific profiles of people with anorexia nervosa, bulimia nervosa, and psychogenic obesity were discussed. Specific interventions for each of these three eating disorders were outlined. The case studies demonstrated each eating disorder and nursing involvement within the framework of the nursing process.

References

American Nurses' Association. Standards of Psychiatric and Mental Health Nursing Practice. Kansas City, MO: American Nurses' Association, 1982.

Boskind-White M, White W Jr. Bulimarexia: The binge-purge cycle. Baltimore: John Hopkins University Press, 1985.

Bruch H. Eating Disorders: Obesity, Anorexia Nervosa and the Person Within. New York: Basic Books, 1973.

Bruch H. Four decades of eating disorders. *In* Garner DM, Garfinkel PE (eds). Handbook of Psychotherapy for Anorexia Nervosa and Bulimia. New York: Guilford Press, 1985.

Chernin K. The Hungry Self: Women Eating and Identity. New York: Times Books, 1985.

Dickstein LJ. Anorexia and bulimia: A review of clinical issues. Hospital and Community Psychiatry, 36:1086, 1985.

Fairburn C. Cognitive-behavioral treatment for bulimia. *In* Garner DM, Garfinkel PE (eds). Handbook of Psychotherapy for Anorexia Nervosa and Bulimia. New York: Guilford Press, 1985.

Garfinkel PE, Garner DM. Anorexia Nervosa: A Multidimensional Perspective. New York: Bruner/Mazel, 1982.

Garner DM, Bemis K. Cognitive therapy for anorexia nervosa. *In* Garner DM, Garfinkel PE (eds). Handbook of Psychotherapy for Anorexia Nervosa and Bulimia. New York: Guilford Press, 1985.

Garner DM, Garfinkel PE (eds). Handbook of Psychotherapy for Anorexia Nervosa and Bulimia. New York: Guilford Press, 1985.

Geist RA. Therapeutic dilemmas in the treatment of anorexia nervosa. (Available from Children's Hospital Medical Center), Boston, June, 1982.

Goodsitt A. Self-psychology and the treatment of anorexia nervosa. *In* Garner, DM, Garfinkel PE (eds). Handbook of Psychotherapy for Anorexia Nervosa and Bulimia. New York: Guilford Press, 1985.

Haber J, et al. (eds). Comprehensive Psychiatric Nursing, 2nd ed. New York: McGraw Hill Book Company, 1982.

Halmi KA. Eating disorders. *In* Talbott JA, Hales RE, Yudofsky SC (eds). Textbook of Psychiatry. Washington DC: American Psychiatric Press, 1988.

Halmi KA, et al. Binge eating and vomiting: A survey of college population. Psychosomatic Medicine, 11:697, 1981.

Johnson C, et al. The syndrome of bulimia: Review and synthesis. Psychiatric Clinics of North America, 7:247, 1984.

Keltner NJ. Bulimia: Controlling compulsive eating. Journal of Psychosocial Nursing and Mental Health Services, 22:24, 1984.

Lego S. Group-psychotherapy. *In* Haber J, et al. (eds). Comprehensive Psychiatric Nursing, 2nd ed. New York: McGraw Hill Book Company, 1982.

Lucas AR. Pigging out. Journal of the American Medical Association, 82:247, 1982.

Millman M. Such a Pretty Face: Being Fat in America. New York: Berkely Books, 1980.

Minuchin S. Psychosomatic Families—Anorexia Nervosa in Context. Cambridge, MA: Harvard University Press, 1978.

Mitchell J, et al. Gastric dilation as a complication of bulimia. Psychosomatics, 23:93, 1982.

Mitchell J, et al. Intensive outpatient group treatment for bulimia. *In* Garner, DM, Garfinkel PE (eds). Handbook of Psychotherapy for Anorexia Nervosa and Bulimia. New York: Guilford Press, 1985.

Orbach S. Accepting the symptom: Feminist psychoanalytic treatment of anorexia nervosa. *In* Garner DM, Garfinkel PE (eds). Handbook of Psychotherapy for Anorexia Nervosa and Bulimia. New York: Guilford Press, 1985.

Orbach S. Fat is a Feminist Issue. New York: Berkely Publishing Group, 1978.

Pope, et al. Bulimia treated with imipramine: a placebo-controlled, double-blind study. American Journal of Psychiatry, 140:554, 1983.

Pyle R, et al. Bulimia: a report of 34 cases. American Jounral of Clinical Psychiatry, 42:60, 1981.

Selvina-Palazzoli M. Self-starvation. London: Human Context Books, Chaucer Publishing Company, 1974.

Swift WJ, et al. The relationship between affective disorder and eating disorder: A review of the literature. American Journal of Psychiatry, 143:290, 1986.

Vandereycken W, Meerman R. Anorexia Nervosa: A Clinician's Guide to Treatment. New York: de Gruyter, 1984.

Walsh BT, et al. Bulima and depression. Psychosomatic Medicine, 47:123, 1985.

Webb LJ. DSM III Training Manual. New York: Brunner/Mazel, 1981.

Wilson CP, Mintz I. Abstaining and bulimic anorexics: Two sides of the same coin. Primary Care, 9:517, 1982.

Winstead-Fry P. Family therapy and application. *In* Haber J, et al. (eds). Comprehensive Psychiatric Nursing, 2nd ed. New York: McGraw Hill Book Company, 1982.

Wolman BB. Psychological Aspects of Obesity. New York: Van Nostrand Reinhold, 1982.

Wooley S, Wooley W. Intensive outpatient group treatment for bulimia. *In* Garner DM, Garfinkel PE (eds). Handbook of Psychotherapy for Anorexia Nervosa and Bulimia. New York: Guilford Press, 1985.

Self-Study Exercises

Choose the answer that most accurately completes the statement.

1. If the need-satisfaction cycle in early feeding experiences is healthy, the infant will develop

   A. feelings of frustration
   B. feelings of loss-of-control
   C. feelings of trust
   D. separation anxiety

2. Some factors in the development of eating disorders may be

   A. a disturbed family system
   B. inadequate socialization by the mother
   C. societal expectation
   D. a faulty belief system regarding weight and appearance
   E. all of the above

3. The most important goal for clients with eating disorders is

   A. achieving a normal weight
   B. the absence of maladaptive eating patterns
   C. the ability to identify and express their own feelings and needs
   D. the ability to have a sexual relationship

4. The typical anorexic or bulimic tends to deal with her imperfections

   A. by taking personal responsibility for her actions
   B. by harsh self-criticism and increasing efforts to be "perfect"
   C. by forgiving her shortcomings
   D. by objectively putting them in perspective

5. Family therapy for anorexics and bulimics would best focus on

   A. the problem of the eating disorder

B. the fact that the parents are to blame
C. separation-individuation of the family members
D. better nutrition for the family

Refer to the case study Working With a Person Who Has Anorexia Nervosa (*pp.* 693–696) *when answering questions* 6 *through* 10.

At mealtime, Ms. Heart observes Jill leaving her tray untouched for 30 minutes. Jill then begins cutting her food into tiny pieces and separating them into several piles on her plate. She then takes one piece at a time and chews it several times before swallowing. After a long pause, she drinks a glass of water and begins the process again.

6. Ms. Heart recognizes that Jill

   A. is using rituals to control her calorie intake
   B. is anxious about eating
   C. is trying to deny the hunger she feels
   D. is exerting control over the only area she feels she can control
   E. all of the above

7. Ms. Heart's most empathic intervention would be

   A. to spoon-feed Jill
   B. to set a time limit for meals
   C. to acknowledge that this is a difficult situation for Jill
   D. to consult with the physician about ordering tube feedings

8. Ms. Heart is aware that Jill may engage in the following behaviors after eating:

   A. rapidly pacing the halls
   B. vomiting
   C. sneaking a laxative
   D. weighing herself
   E. all of the above

9. The following physical signs are sometimes seen once eating is reestablished:

   A. edema
   B. hypothermia
   C. lanugo
   D. abdominal distention

10. Once Jill has begun gaining weight, Ms. Heart's priority regarding Jill's mental status is

    A. assessing for hallucinations
    B. assessing for hyperactivity
    C. assessing for purging
    D. assessing for signs of depression

Refer to the case study Working With a Person Who Has Bulimia Nervosa (*pp.* 698–701) *when answering questions* 11 *through* 15.

11. Before Nora will be able to give up her bingeing and purging behaviors without substituting other symptoms, she must

    A. be given a diet to follow
    B. learn and practice alternate ways of dealing with anxiety
    C. take antianxiety medication
    D. quit her job as a dietitian

12. Nora missed her first appointment after her initial interview. She tells Mr. Hope the following week that she was "too anxious to come in and binged and purged instead." The most helpful response, on Mr. Hope's part, would be:

    A. "You must keep your appointments to be responsible."
    B. "That must have been an uncomfortable feeling. Let's see if we can figure out what you were anxious about."
    C. "How much did you eat when you binged?"
    D. "There's no need to feel anxious about coming here."

13. During a session with Mr. Hope, Nora relates a situation in which she is "afraid to be around" a coworker she feels is "lazy" because she fears "losing control." The best response Mr. Hope could use would be:

    A. "It's okay—you won't lost control."
    B. "You can't do that or you'll lose your job."
    C. "Tell me more about how you feel when you're around him."
    D. "You can call me if you are afraid of losing control."

14. The following physical complaint, if offered by Nora, could warrant *immediate* medical intervention:

    A. swollen glands
    B. cramping and weakness of extremities with dizziness
    C. a "bloated feeling" after bingeing
    D. constipation

15. Mr. Hope realizes that he is feeling the temptation to placate Nora when she exhibits anxiety or anger during their session. This could indicate that

    A. he is a good role model
    B. he shares her fear that she is helpless
    C. he wants to help her
    D. he should medicate her

Refer to the case study Working With a Person Whose Obesity Is Caused by Compulsive Eating *(pp.* 702–705) *when answering questions* 16 *through* 18.

16. Considering Mary's signs of depression, Mrs. Worth's priority is to

    A. start Mary in group therapy
    B. start Mary on a 1500-calorie diet
    C. place Mary on close observation with suicidal precaution
    D. start Mary in a hygiene group

17. When Mary verbalizes that she feels "too ashamed" to be seen at work, Mrs. Worth's best response would be:

    A. "You have nothing to be ashamed of."
    B. "Work will help you keep your mind off your problems."
    C. "Tell me more about your feelings of shame."
    D. "You have a good husband and family to think about."

18. In a group therapy session, Mary verbalizes that she feels comfortable talking about her feelings to the group. Group therapy can provide all the following EXCEPT:

    A. opportunities to verbalize feelings
    B. aids in developing more realistic self-image
    C. providing feedback
    D. physiological safety

19. June is an obese woman of 30 whose family pattern indicates a history of overeating in response to stress. June is 5′2″ and has never weighed within a "normal" range for her size. Her obesity is probably

    A. reactive
    B. developmental
    C. organic
    D. all of the above

20. Compulsive eating may serve the function of

    A. reducing stress
    B. dealing with conflict
    C. punishment for guilt
    D. all of the above

PART THREE

MENTAL HEALTH ISSUES: SPECIAL POPULATIONS

POPULATIONS DEALING WITH UNIQUE ISSUES

UNIT VII

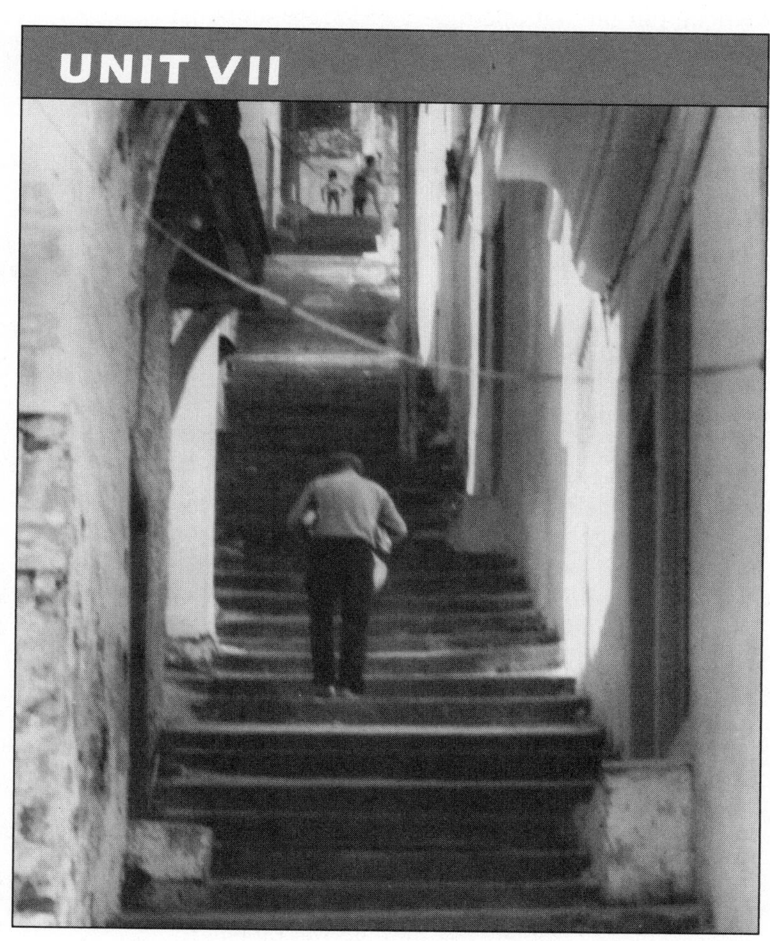

When you're halfway there, you stop disbelieving in there.

HUGH PRATHER

A Nurse Speaks

by Doris Hadley

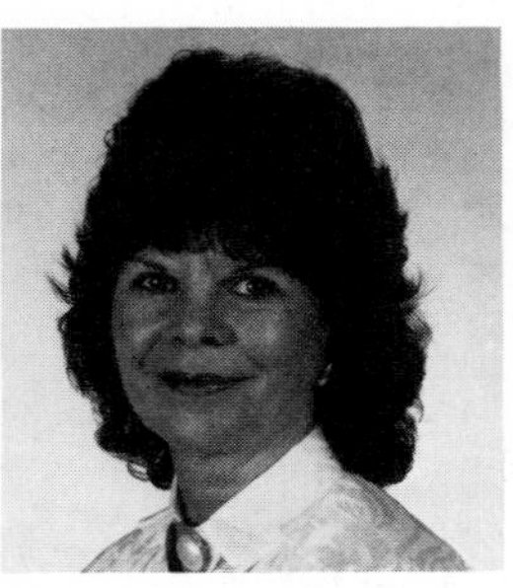

To David and Jeff and Kenny and Bill and Hillary and Gerry and Jackie—and on and on

I'm on the road again—flying from place to place. The flight has been delayed. It's Friday night and I won't get home until almost midnight. I started my day at 6:15 A.M. back in Florida; my week started with a 5:30 A.M. flight from San Francisco to Washington.

The weather is bad, and the flights bumpy. I've had bronchitis with a cough. I have not slept well in hotel and motel rooms with air conditioning. It's the hottest day of the year in Washington, D.C.—breaking 50-year-old records. No room service in Tampa and thunderstorms—I'll die without coffee. I'll refuse when they call me again. Why am I doing this?

I pick up my headphones and put on the tapes that David made for me. I'm so conditioned to relax when I put on that one tape by Alan Parsons that I immediately calm down. It has helped me through other bumpy flights. (I hate to fly! Why did I commit again?)

I do this because of David and all the others—all the other patients with AIDS who have given me focus for my life's work. I go to Topeka, Tampa, Marion, Tulare, Ft. Mead, Hot Springs, Gillette, and on because I'm an AIDS educator and believer—maybe even an activist.

I love teaching, and I'm good at it. I get high on it, especially if I get indications that what I say is received and possibly will be acted upon. "You were wonderful," a student says, "Thank you for coming." "I've got a better picture of what's happening." "I have a brother just diagnosed with AIDS. You've given me lots to help him." "I've got a son with AIDS. This course has helped me a lot—I now see why testing *without* consent is not good—what can I do to help?" "You've challenged me. Thank you. I went and shook the hand of the patient with AIDS on the panel—I couldn't have done that yesterday without running out to wash my hands." (Comments from nurses attending one workshop.)

And so, I'm on the road again, listening to the tapes David made for me and thinking about tomorrow and being good to myself because one of the songs is called "You Can't Take It With You." I've been living so much more since I started working with patients who are dying. They've taught me many, many things. They've taught me patience and acceptance and humor and honesty, and they have helped me decide what really counts in living and what is trivial.

"Going blind is awful," Tom said. "I never counted on this. I can't even see all of you anymore, but I recognize your voice and your touch."

"This dying is real hard, Doris," Ken said. "Man, it's hard." He died the next morning. Kenny could not speak at the end, but tears came to his eyes when I stood crying beside him and told him I would miss him—and I do.

David, back to you—I'll cry when you die. I'll never forget you. You've taught me about meditation and living with AIDS and how to survive bumpy plane rides. I'll travel over 50,000 miles this year, and I've said I won't do it again. (They've just announced more turbulence—here go the tapes again!)

I *wish* the epidemic would go away. I know it won't. I only hope the classes I teach and the many people I have contact with will reach out to their patients with compassion, to their communities with education, and to their families with facts. If that can continue to happen, I'll be on the road again for David and Jackie and Ken and Bill and Jeff and Jim and Tom and on and on, because it's the one weapon I have in this battle. It seems to be what I do well, and so here I go, bumping up and down through the night for my guys.

I've been in nursing for almost 30 years. This epidemic and caring for the patients with AIDS — living with it and dying with it — have changed my life. My interactions with the patients have been rewarding. These men have taught me about living day-to-day, about courage to try experiments, about their disease. I have become a patient advocate, hopefully changing people's attitudes about the disease, dispelling fears, and defending my own reasons for working in this stressful situation. Every week I see patients, their families, and friends who have come to grips with death, with discrimination, and with loss. I see most of them, despite their problems, being thoughtful of staff, maintaining a sense of humor, and enhancing our nursing care. Caring for them has bonded the staff together. We share their joys and their hopes, and we're sad when they have a relapse or die. These special bonds between nurses and their patients make up for the problems and frustrations we encounter.

CHAPTER 26

The Hospitalized Person

Jane B. Neese

OUTLINE

KEY TERMS AND CONCEPTS

The key terms and concepts listed here also appear in bold where they are defined or discussed in this chapter.

PSYCHIATRIC LIAISON NURSE

COPING

COPING STRATEGIES/MECHANISMS

PAIN

CHRONIC PAIN

STAGES OF RECOVERY FOR BURN CLIENTS
The Acute Stage
The Psychological Emergency
The Social Emergency
The Home Emergency

HIV (human immunodeficiency virus)
ARC (AIDS-related complex)
AIDS (acquired immunodeficiency syndrome)
ELISA
WESTERN BLOT

HIV-POSITIVE OR SERO-POSITIVE
AIDS-RELATED DEMENTIA/
HIV DEMENTIA COMPLEX/
HIV ENCEPHALOPATHY
CENTERS FOR DISEASE CONTROL (CDC)

STAGES IN THE PROCESS OF DYING
Denial and Isolation
Anger
Bargaining
Depression
Acceptance

OBJECTIVES

After studying this chapter, the student will be able to:

1. Discuss areas of stress encountered by a hospitalized person during the process of hospitalization.
2. Identify four positive coping strategies and four negative coping strategies that may be used by a hospitalized person.
3. Describe the role of the psychiatric liaison nurse.
4. Compare and contrast assessment of acute pain and assessment of chronic pain.
5. Explain five nursing interventions effective in reducing chronic pain.
6. Identify the four phases of recovery a severely burned person experiences.
7. Write four interventions for each of the above phases.
8. In a teaching plan, outline ways HIV *is* spread and ways it *cannot* be contracted.
9. Summarize staff needs and possible staff intervention needed when caring for people who are HIV infected.
10. Discuss at least four conflicts a hospitalized person with a cardiac dysfunction may experience. Discuss pertinent nursing interventions for both client and family.
11. Identify nursing interventions that may be useful to a dying person or his or her family during each of Kubler-Ross's five stages.

Physical and emotional crises occur every day in the medical setting. The stress of being physically ill greatly influences a person's psychological state and emotional reactions. An individual's particular personality structure as well as the nature of his or her illness plays a large part in the coping strategies a person employs to decrease stress. At times, a nurse working in the hospital environment may find that the client's anxiety or coping strategies negatively affect (1) an individual's health and (2) the nurse's ability to administer effective care. Understanding the stresses experienced and strategies used by the hospitalized person can greatly enhance the nurse's effectiveness.

This chapter looks at (1) possible sources of stress for the hospitalized person, (2) various coping strategies used by the hospitalized person, and (3) specific medical illnesses and possible emotional reactions to each. Six medical conditions that elicit unique emotional needs in a hospitalized person are presented here. The emotional needs of a person (1) in chronic pain, (2) with severe burns, (3) who has AIDS, (4) with cardiac dysfunction, (5) in an ICU, and (6) dying of terminal cancer are presented. The role of the psychiatric liaison nurse is discussed, because the liaison nurse is an important resource for staff when emotional difficulties arise with a medically ill client.

The Role of the Nurse

When the medically ill person experiences increased levels of anxiety, staff may need assistance in planning care. Most nurses possess sound psychosocial nursing communication skills. However, nurses working on medical or surgical units often become more task oriented and less comfortable with the socioemotional aspects of a client's needs. When this happens, a client's emotional needs may become ignored when the nurse plans care. The client's emotional reaction to his situation might, however, trigger frustration and confusion in the staff. Therefore, situations arise when a hospitalized client's behavior or emotional experience is beyond the skills of the nurse, and often of the medical team. In the general hospital there are several resources that nurses can contact to help in an emotional crisis. *First*, the psychiatrist diagnoses the psychiatric problem and recommends treatment; however, psychiatrists are only accessible by a physician's order. *Second*, the social worker is often aware of the family's history. The social worker is a useful resource regarding family dynamics and the family's financial situations. However, most social workers are unfamiliar with nursing interventions and lack knowledge of medical diseases. A *third* resource, who knows about medical illnesses, psychiatric illnesses, family dynamics, and the nursing process, is the psychiatric liaison nurse.

PSYCHIATRIC LIAISON NURSE

Psychiatric liaison nursing is a relatively new subspecialty of psychiatric nursing, initiated in the early 1960's (Johnson 1963; Lewis and Levy 1982; Robinson 1974). The **psychiatric liaison nurse** is usually a Master's prepared nurse with a background in psychiatric and medical-surgical nursing. A psychiatric liaison nurse functions as a nursing consultant in the management of psychosocial concerns, and as a clinician in helping the client deal more effectively with physical and emotional problems. Throughout the five steps of the nursing process (assessing, diagnosing, planning, intervening, and evaluating), a psychiatric liaison nurse assists the nursing and medical staff in caring for hospitalized, medically ill clients who are management problems or who have problems that impede client care (Fife 1983; Fife and Lemler 1983; Lewis and Levy 1982). Therefore, the psychiatric liaison nurse is a resource for the nursing staff who feel, for one reason or another, unable to intervene therapeutically with a client.

The psychiatric liaison nurse first meets with the nurse who initiated the consult. Then the liaison nurse reviews the medical records, talks with the physicians, and interviews the client. After interviewing the client, the liaison nurse discusses her or his assessment and suggestions with the referring nurse. If a psychiatric consultation is warranted, the psychiatric liaison nurse will generate the consultation by contacting the client's medical doctor. A case conference is sometimes needed to enhance communication and consistency in the care of a particular client.

Unique Assessment Strategies

Admission into the hospital often signifies that a medical condition is too complex to be treated in an outpatient setting. In emergencies, the client is immediately rushed to the hospital via ambulance. The client is generally unprepared for entrance into the hospital environment. There are a number of stressors that will increase anxiety in a person new to the hospital environment. Upon entering the hospital, the client begins to experience a loss of control and depersonalization. In the admitting office, the person is first asked his or her name and the name of his or her insurance company prior to any discussion regarding the presenting problem. The client is given a hospital number and an admitting diagnosis as methods of identification. Later, he may no longer be identified as "Mr. Smith," but as the man with cancer in Room 622.

After being admitted to a room, the client is given a hospital gown and requested to change. Indirectly, the client is beginning to understand that his or her role as provider, father, mother, or boss is changing to the "sick role." The sick role denotes giving up some independent functioning and assuming a more dependent position. A person rarely has time to comfortably adjust to the sick role. Usually within the first few days of hospitalization, the client has given up some identity and independent functioning.

ASSESSING STRESS AND ANXIETY RELATED TO HOSPITALIZATION

The reason for hospitalization generally is illness. The onset of an illness means loss of a previous health state. For some, hospitalization means the pre-existing illness is worsening. For others, hospitalization is their first encounter with a serious illness. Loss of health also affects how clients view themselves. If the illness entails surgery or any other mutilating procedure, the client's reaction may be a change in his or her body image and grief over his or her loss. An amputation severely affects a person's self-esteem and body image, especially if the amputation means loss of a job.

If the diagnosis has not been confirmed prior to admission, fear of the unknown can escalate anxiety to severe levels. In some cases, the diagnosis is made, yet the course of treatment is questionable, e.g., chemotherapy in oncology clients. The ultimate fear is the fear of death, especially if surgery is indicated.

Admission into the hospital means payment for medical services. Most clients are concerned about their insurance coverage. For prolonged hospitalizations, e.g., the burn client or cancer client, financial concerns become a primary focus and are a major source of stress for the family. The terminally ill client may worry about leaving his or her family with a financial burden after his or her death.

Hospitalization is a stressful period for the client and family and usually precipitates anxiety and confusion. The client's focus shifts from health to illness and from independence to dependence. One is separated from family and support systems. If the illness is terminal, grieving over loss of health, role, and life is stimulated. Fear of the unknown and financial worries may become the client's major concerns.

The nurse's assessment includes the stressors triggered by the process of hospitalization. When areas of client concern are identified, appropriate supports can be mobilized. Another important area to assess is the way the person copes with stress and anxiety.

ASSESSING COPING STRATEGIES

Coping differs from defense mechanisms in that *defense mechanisms are primarily an unconscious means to regulate internal emotional tension.* **Coping,** however, is a problem-solving behavior that is directed toward influencing, changing, or bringing about equilibrium to a threatening situation (Thornbury 1982; Weisman 1978). Generally, *coping is seen as a conscious means of altering a stressful event* in some manner by an individual. The ways people cope are a complicated mixture of how they initially perceive stress, how they behaviorally respond, and how they re-evaluate the stress and correct their response over a period of time (Weisman 1978). Lazarus (1982) defines coping as "not a single act but a constellation of many acts and thoughts engendered by a complex set of demands that may stretch over time" (Lazarus 1982, p. 178). Coping as a constellation is a helpful conceptual model, because individuals use various methods of coping in different situations at different times in their life and with different people. Basically, coping is the client's intervention with a stressor such as illness.

The action of *coping has several synonyms, e.g., coping skills, coping strategies, coping modes, coping patterns, and* **coping mechanisms.** For clarity, this chapter uses **coping strategies** to identify different techniques that physically ill clients use to deal with their illness. Clients are the best source in determining whether their coping has decreased their anxiety. Nurses can help by assessing the client's adaptive coping strategies and strengthening them by positive reinforcement. Open and honest communication helps facilitate positive coping abilities. Supportive, dependable relationships help clients to better adapt to their illness.

There are many factors that can influence one's ability to cope. For example, *interpersonal factors* include age, personality, intelligence, values, cultural beliefs, emotional state, and cognitive ability. *Disease-related factors* are type of illness, rate of onset, progression, functional impairment, and whether the disease or impairment is reversible. If a person's illness is a fast-growing malignancy with metastasis to the brain which renders him delirious, ability to cope would be seriously compromised. *Environmental factors* include the person's support system (family, friends, or community) and financial stability (Lipowski 1970). Each of these three determinants influences a person's choice of coping strategies.

Box 26–1. COMMON COPING STRATEGIES USED BY THE HOSPITALIZED PERSON

* 1. Seek information; get guidance.
* 2. Share concern; find consolation.
3. Laugh it off; change emotional tone.
4. Forget it happened; put it out of your mind.
* 5. Keep busy; distract yourself.
* 6. Confront the issue; act accordingly .
* 7. Redefine; take a more sanguine view.
8. Resign yourself; make the best of what can not be changed.
9. Do something, anything, perhaps exceeding good judgment.
10. Review alternatives; examine consequences.
† 11. Get away from it all; find an escape, somehow.
* 12. Conform, comply; do what is expected or advised.
† 13. Blame or shame someone, something.
14. Give vent; feel emotional release.
† 15. Deny as much as possible.

* Seen most in "effective copers"
† Seen most in "poor copers"

Data from Weisman A. The Coping Capacity: On the Nature of Being Mortal. New York: Human Sciences Press, 1984, pp. 36–37.

Weisman (1984) has described 15 commonly seen coping strategies (refer to Box 26–1).

Seeking information and obtaining guidance is the most commonly reported coping strategy. Nursing staff and physicians tend to reinforce this strategy and are more comfortable when the client does ask questions regarding his or her illness and treatment. The second coping strategy is even more adaptive, that of *sharing concern and finding consolation*. The third coping strategy, *changing emotional tone*, can be helpful or hurtful depending upon whether the client is laughing with someone or laughing at someone. Humor and laughter can defuse a tense situation or can escalate anxiety, depending upon how it is used. *Suppression* is the fourth coping strategy. Not only is suppression useful at times, it is necessary for clients if they are to continue to deal with their illness. This is especially true with cancer clients or terminally ill clients. *Keeping busy and distracting oneself* is also a common strategy. Usually this type of coping only postpones dealing with a different situation. Many times problems of self-worth are at the bottom of postponing dealing with the illness. The sixth coping strategy, *confrontation*, is the cornerstone of many coping strategies, since without confrontation, clients avoid the reality of their illness. Confrontation is not to be misconstrued as challenging in an angry manner. Confrontation in this case means to address the situation in a straightforward manner. *Redefinition* means to make virtue out of necessity or transform a deficit into a gain. A person redefines the situation to optimize the problem without compromising the truth. *Resignation* is the eighth coping strategy. Resignation entails acknowledging that the situation is beyond one's control. This is not the same as submitting to defeat, but means the ability to recognize one's limitations. Coping strategy number nine appears nonfunctional. Many people, however, take an *impulsive action*. An example of an impulsive action would be abuse of alcohol or attempted suicide. Number ten, *reviewing alternatives*, suggests that the client is taking the time to reflect on what has happened and re-evaluating the situation. "Now what are we going to do and where are we going?" are questions frequently asked. The eleventh coping strategy, *escape*, is probably contemplated by more clients than has been reported. No matter how well one copes, it is not surprising that the question "What if" is asked and left unanswered. Many clients have stated that they just want to get away from it all. However, few can escape their illness. *Conforming*

Table 26–1 • ASSESSMENT OF COPING SKILLS

QUESTIONS	RATIONALE
	Nurse obtains data on:
1. Have you ever been ill before? Has anyone in your family had this type of illness? What happened to them?	1. Past medical history and family history.
2. Before this illness, what has been the hardest thing for you to face in your life?	2. Perception of stressful events in person's life.
3. What was the situation like for you? What did you do? How did you feel? What helped you the most? What did not help you?	3. Coping strategies used in the past; which patient strengths can be maximized
4. How has this illness been a problem for you?. What has bothered you the most?	4. Person's perception of how illness affects his or her life.
5. What have you done about the problem? What are you going to do about the problem?	5. How realistic is patient's perception of illness. How effective are his or her problem-solving skills.
6. Whom do you rely on the most? How do they help you? (family, friends, religious affiliations).	6. Information on person's support system.
7. How do things generally turn out for you?	7. Patient's perception of optimism or pessimism regarding his or her life.
8. What do you know about your illness?	8. Level of patient knowledge and needs for patient teaching.
9. What has staff done to help you?/What has staff done that has not helped you?	9. Patient's perception of staff support and identification of individual needs still unmet.
10. What suggestions do you have for the staff, so that we can help you more?	10. This question encourages open communication and can give patient some sense of control over his or her situation.

Data from Weisman A. Coping with illness. *In* Hackett T, Cassem N (eds). Massachusetts General Hospital Handbook of General Psychiatry. St. Louis: C.V. Mosby Company, 1978.

and complying suggest a more passive stance. Most clients will comply just because compliance with the physician's suggestions is expected.

The thirteenth coping strategy, *blaming someone else*, is not necessarily adaptive, but is frequently seen. Crying or raving are examples of *giving vent or emotional release*. Even though the problem is not solved or altered using this coping strategy, the client may experience a reduction in tension. The last coping strategy is *denying as much as possible* and is the direct opposite of seeking information and sharing concern. Even though health professionals strongly oppose denial, denying as much as possible may have strategic temporary value. "Effective copers" tend to use coping strategies 1, 2, 5, 6, 7, and 12. They have a good relationship with the health care team and are optimistic and resourceful. On the other hand, "poor copers" use coping strategies 11, 13, and 15. In addition, poor copers have higher emotional distress and do not recognize their psychosocial problems (Weisman 1978).

Table 26–1 suggests questions that help the nurse assess a client's coping strategies. Through analyzing the data obtained from this assessment, the nurse can help maximize the client's strengths and identify the person's interpersonal supports.

Unique Intervention Strategies

Intervention strategies for hospitalized persons with specific medical conditions are presented later in this chapter under the six medical conditions discussed (i.e., chronic pain, burns, AIDS, cardiac dysfunction, intensive care, and terminal illness). Inherent in all of these situations are intense emotional reactions on the part of clients that often affect their behavior and even their progress.

However, there are many issues and concerns experienced by all hospitalized clients. The generalist is often an expert at identifying nursing diagnoses for the physically ill, yet it is vital that the nurse not limit the focus of care to the physical components of the client's condition. In doing so, crucial emotional needs may go unmet. This can result in prolonging recuperation or halting the process of recovery. The medical conditions discussed in this chapter are traumatic, extremely disruptive to the client and his or her family, and may involve a great deal of pain or fear of death. A competent assessment includes the client's acute concerns, coping strategies, and supportive system(s). Assessing the person's perception of his situation and the perception of his future is crucial in formulating nursing diagnoses concerning emotional needs and thereby identifying major areas for intervention. For example, a person who is dying may experience the anguish of *spiritual distress*. Grieving in this case may be imminent, and the process of dying may need to be facilitated and supported. A person who has had a myocardial infarction (MI) may have overriding concerns regarding *self-esteem* in relationship to self-concept, role performance, or personal identity. If these issues are not addressed, defensive maneuvers such as denial may have a direct impact on the person's medical compliance and could result in premature death. A person who is severely burned or in the ICU may experience extreme *social isolation* or *altered thought process* compounded by a lack of or distorted environmental stimuli among other things. *Potential for self-directed violence* should always be evaluated in a person who appears to feel hopeless. Suicide is not an uncommon phenomenon in a hospitalized person who feels overwhelmed, alone, fearful, and hopeless. *Powerlessness* is experienced to some degree by most all clients. If a sense of powerlessness is experienced by a person who has a high need to feel in control, nursing interventions need to be considered. All levels of *anxiety* will be seen in clients hospitalized for physical conditions. When levels of anxiety result in maladaptive or disorganizing behaviors, swift medical and nursing attention should be made available. Helping the client to lower anxiety to more comfortable levels allows for maximizing the person's ability to participate in his or her care, to problem solve, and to relate more productively to staff, family, and others. *Ineffective family coping* related to a hospitalized family member is also an area that may indicate specific nursing interventions.

Issues That Affect the Mental Health of Some Hospitalized Persons

A PERSON IN CHRONIC PAIN

Pain is an individual experience, which makes assessment and treatment complicated. Associated with the experience of pain are psychological, physiological, and cultural factors. Health professionals often attempt to define pain as purely physical or psychological (psychogenic) in nature. This view leads to confusion and frustration for both the staff and the client (Hackett 1978; Robinson 1974; Schmitt 1977). Zborowski's (1969) classic study described several cultural groups' responses to pain. Stoicism with little verbal and behavioral expression of pain was seen in the Old American and Irish population. People from Jewish and Italian backgrounds were most likely to be verbally expressive of their pain. A person's expression of pain often depends upon his or her cultural background.

Pain is an ancient warning system of the body, indicating that tissue damage has occurred. In some cases, tissue damage can occur without the person experiencing pain. Conversely, in some cases, even after tissues have healed, pain may continue to be experienced by the client (Robinson 1974; Schmitt 1977).

Pain can be classified into five categories: acute, subacute, recurrent acute, continuous, and chronic. In most cases, *acute pain* is the result of recent tissue damage and lasts up to a few days. *Subacute pain* lasts a few days to a few weeks. In *recurrent acute pain*, the client suffers from a disease which has exacerbations of pain followed by brief periods of remission, as seen in rheumatoid arthritis, migraines, and sickle cell disorders. An underlying malignant disease such as cancer is usually the cause of *continuous pain*. **Chronic pain** is classified as such when the client continues to be in pain for more than six months. Chronic pain can be the result of neck and back injuries, pancreatitis, or cancer (Escobar 1985). This section will focus on management of chronic pain.

For the nurse and the physician, assessment of chronic pain is difficult, since most pain models are based upon the concept of acute pain. *Acute pain differs from chronic pain in several ways*. In acute pain, the client exhibits more behavioral responses, including motor responses (writhing), vocal responses (crying), and social responses (withdrawal from others) (Robinson 1974). A person in acute pain gives the appearance of being in distress (Hackett 1978). Often nurses look for the behavioral responses to acute pain when assessing intensity of pain. Physiologically, a client in acute pain has an increase in pulse and blood pressure.

In contrast, a client in chronic pain does not manifest the same behavioral and physiological responses as the client with acute pain. Because of the chronic persistence of pain, a client may slowly adapt to the presence of pain without realizing it. Eventually, the client learns to accommodate to the pain and continues with his or her life while still experiencing pain. In addition, the body begins to adapt to chronic pain. Physiological responses are no longer inclusive data in determining intensity or presence of chronic pain. Often it is the person's adaptation to chronic pain that is the client's undoing. The staff may conclude that the client is not in pain if they are not able to adequately assess the symptoms for chronic pain (Hackett 1978). How does one measure chronic pain if a person does not behaviorally or physiologically manifest symptoms? It is the client who is the key. Chronic pain is an individual experience. Therefore the nurse needs to ask the client.

Myths Regarding Pain Control

Many nurses and other health professionals are hesitant to use narcotics for people with chronic pain. This hesitancy stems from fear of "addicting" the client to the narcotic. However, fewer than 1% of clients with chronic pain become physically dependent on medications. For classification of differences between drug abuse, drug dependence, drug tolerance, and physical dependence, see Table 26–2. These terms are misused

Table 26–2 • DEFINITION OF TERMS USED IN PAIN MANAGEMENT

DRUG ABUSE	Socially unacceptable voluntary use of drugs at dose levels and in circumstances and settings that are potentially harmful.
DRUG DEPENDENCE (Older Term: Drug Addiction)	Compulsive voluntary continuous or periodic use of a drug to experience its psychic effect or to avoid the discomfort of its absence.
DRUG TOLERANCE	Repeated use of a substance or drug, usually a narcotic, so that larger and larger dosages are needed to provide the analgesic effect obtained previously on smaller dosages.
PHYSICAL DEPENDENCE	Biochemical or physiological changes in the body that make continued use of the drug necessary to avoid a withdrawal syndrome.

Data from Vaillant GE. The alcohol-dependent and drug-dependent person. *In* Nicholi AM (ed). The New Harvard Guide to Psychiatry. Cambridge, MA: The Belknap Press of Harvard University Press, 1988.

commonly to describe the client's physiological response to narcotics.

Other **myths** regarding narcotic and analgesic usage follow (McGuire 1983; Rogers 1984):

1. The use of a potent narcotic can cause drug abuse or "addiction" dependence.
2. Withholding narcotics prevents drug abuse.
3. Drug tolerance and physical dependence are the same as drug abuse.
4. The client who "withdraws" is "addicted" or drug dependent.
5. PRN use of narcotics and analgesics is the best way to prevent drug abuse.
6. A client who asks regularly for medication is "addicted."
7. A client who needs more medication is becoming "addicted" drug dependent.
8. Demerol is the best injectable narcotic for pain relief.

There are also other misconceptions about pain control that influence nursing interventions—the misconception, for example, that pain caused by anxiety does not need to be treated. Keep in mind that the physically ill person's perception of pain is influenced by several factors. The *physiological* warning of tissue damage, *psychological* response, and *cultural* aspects all contribute to a person's perception of pain. Most people become anxious when they are in pain. Waiting for medication to relieve the pain, especially when the medication schedule is rigid, tends to increase anxiety and thereby increase pain. Anxiety and pain are closely entwined and both need to be treated. When the client in pain is anxious, the pain still needs to be alleviated through proper medical treatment. Another misconception is that a nurse is able to judge the "authenticity" of another person's pain. Some nurses have even stated that they can "tell" when a client is in "real" pain because they have worked with "so many" clients in pain. This erroneous belief may come from the nurse's fear of "addicting" a client, fear of being fooled, or personal need for control. This attitude only creates more distrust between nurses and the people under their care. Another misconception comes from giving a placebo in order to "test" whether the client is "faking" pain. Approximately one third of the hospitalized people with chronic pain will experience pain relief if given a placebo. Some possible reasons for this occurrence are that placebos work if the client trusts the staff. The client becomes less anxious after the placebo is taken. Also, placebos stimulate the body to produce endorphins, which are morphinelike brain chemicals. A placebo trial indicates only that the client can respond positively to a placebo; it *does not* separate psychogenic pain from organic pain. If clients discover that placebos are being used (and they generally do), clients feel tricked and begin to distrust staff. Placebo trials without the person's input can lead to destruction of the nurse-client relationship (Hackett 1978; McGuire 1983; Rogers 1984).

Assessment of Chronic Pain

Assessment of the pain is the first step in management of chronic pain. The nurse needs to find out the site, character, and duration of the pain. Is there anything that makes the pain worse or better? Does the client experience a change in mood because of the pain? Also, is the client newly diagnosed with a malignant disorder or is this a recurrent disease? Differentiate what type of pain the client is experiencing (i.e., acute, subacute, recurrent, continuous, or chronic). A thorough history of analgesic and narcotic usage needs to be taken. The history should include the drug, dosage, route, time interval, length of time on each drug, the effectiveness of each medication, and the side effects. Does one route work better than another route? Since these questions take a considerable amount of time, the nurse may ask the client to write a log documenting pain, type, medication, route, and such. The nurse can photocopy the log and return the original to the client. If the client does compile a log, the nurse can sit down, discuss the pain, and ask pertinent questions (Foley 1983; Hackett 1978; Rogers 1984).

In discussing the client's pain and previous interventions, the nurse must always accept the client's perception of pain, and never think of the pain as "imaginary." In order to alleviate the client's fear of abandonment, the nurse can assure the client that she or he will continue to assist in managing the pain even though there may not be any immediate results. It is also important to stress to the client that different methods of treating pain may not have "instant" results. In the treatment of chronic pain, the goal should be a decrease in the degree of pain. Some clients such as those with chronic pancreatitis will always have some degree of pain. Lessening the pain so that the client can continue functioning is the key to pain management.

Treatment of Chronic Pain

Biofeedback is useful in chronic back pain and headache by relaxing different muscle groups, thus releasing the tension that causes or aggravates the pain (Greenspan

1981; Hendler and Fernandez 1980; Schuman 1982). Even though biofeedback helps to reduce pain, the nurse does not have easy access to the machine and therapist. The nurse needs to be aware of the availability of biofeedback for the chronic pain client.

Teaching *relaxation techniques* is another intervention nurses can choose for their clients in chronic pain. Progressive muscle relaxation, rhythmic breathing, and guided imagery are three relaxation techniques that can induce the "relaxation response." Guided imagery is an effective means of deepening relaxation and desensitizing a person to a painful situation or experience. The client is taught to visualize a calm, beautiful place where he or she experiences peace and joy. When a deep sense of relaxation is reached, the client is taught to use images to reduce stress, promote healing, or reduce pain. Prior to teaching any relaxation technique, the nurse confers with the physician, then evaluates the client's readiness and past experiences with relaxation techniques. Refer to Chapters 9 and 15 for more detail on teaching relaxation techniques.

Hypnosis has also frequently helped to reduce pain. "Hypnosis depends almost entirely on the client. Only one in four subjects is able to achieve a state of concentration of sufficient magnitude for lasting pain control" (Hackett 1978). Even though hypnosis is more helpful in acute pain, some practitioners have taught autohypnosis (self-hypnosis) to clients who are suggestible. These clients are in a state of resting alertness and are able to block out painful sensations (Wain 1986).

Psychotherapy helps demoralized and desperate clients deal with the terror that pain comes to hold. Behavioral therapy and antianxiety and antidepressant drugs have proved useful. They do not eliminate the pain, but they make it easier to bear by relieving tension, fatigue, anxiety, and insomnia (Kleinman 1989).

When assisting the client with chronic pain, the nurse should accept the client's perception and experience of pain. Each client presents symptoms of pain differently. Promoting a trusting relationship with the client and openly discussing past attempts to control pain are helpful in determining a new approach to pain management. Medications are the most frequently used treatment intervention. Biofeedback and relaxation techniques such as guided imagery, rhythmic breathing, hypnosis, and progressive muscle relaxation (PMR) are other avenues that can help reduce the client's pain.

A 47-year-old single man, Jeff Tide, was admitted to the hospital for weight loss in addition to abdominal and back pain. Past history revealed that Mr. Tide had been shot in the abdomen by a student whom he had taught at a local technical college. As a result of the gunshot wound, Mr. Tide had a pancreatectomy, colostomy, and ileostomy. Several hospitalizations ensued to reverse the colostomy and ileostomy as well as to correct some abdominal adhesions. After the initial hospitalizations he attempted to return to work as a professor, but was unable to because of pain, nausea, vomiting, and weakness. Three years after the shooting, Mr. Tide was involved in a motor vehicle accident which injured his back. This present hospitalization focused on Mr. Tide's weight loss secondary to his inability to digest food without compatible pancreatic enzymes, and management of his chronic pain.

Initially Mr. Tide was placed on Percodan by mouth for pain, then changed to Tylenol #3 with codeine by mouth, and again to Demerol 50 mg by mouth, all to no avail. He continually asked for his pain medication every four hours and requested that the medication and schedule be changed. Soon Mr. Tide became frustrated and angry with the nursing staff. He constantly complained about his pain and the staff's poor quality of care. The nurses perceived Mr. Tide as demanding and manipulative. Several times the nursing staff entered his room to administer the pain medication and found him asleep. Exasperated, the nurses requested the psychiatric liaison nurse to assist them in dealing with this "demanding client."

During the interview the psychiatric liaison nurse assessed that Mr. Tide had chronic pain for more than five years *(assess the duration of pain)*. The client described that his pain was worse at night and after meals *(assess when the pain occurs)*. At home, he stated that he would take one to two Percodan tablets before meals and usually took two tablets before he went to bed *(assess previous medication schedule)*. He described that he was in pain most of the day (continuous), which periodically was intolerable. Normally, he rated his pain 4 on a 10-point scale *(assess the client's perception of the pain)*. If he missed taking his pain medication, his pain increased to the point where he would lie in bed the entire day. Mr. Tide stated that he was discouraged about controlling the pain and frustrated that no one was listening to his complaints.

After gathering all the data regarding the client's history, the psychiatric liaison nurse, the nursing staff, and the physician discussed the case and decided to implement the following. The client was to assess his pain on a 10-point scale every time he received pain medication (to continually assess pain and changes in pain). The pain medication was changed to his usual pain medication that he used at home incorporating his usual routine. Therefore, the client did not have to ask for pain medication (standing medication is more effective than PRN). He could refuse if needed. Mr. Tide would be encouraged to participate in physical therapy and to gradually increase his physical activity. The psychiatric liaison nurse would teach him progressive muscle relaxation (PMR), as well as guided imagery. Guided imagery was used to increase his sense of control and potentiate the effectiveness of the medications. The nursing staff were to check on the client every hour to see how he was doing in order to decrease staff avoidance and lessen Mr. Tide's sense of abandonment.

With the use of guided imagery, the client was able to decrease his use of Percodan to one tablet in the morning and two tablets at night. He also began talking more with the nursing staff. After compatible pancreatic enzymes were established, the client was able to eat without nausea, vomiting, and pain, which previously accompanied eating. He began ambulating more and was viewed by several nursing staff as an "enjoyable person." Possible discontinuation of his pain medication was discussed with the client, but was decided against at this time. The client was discharged with a 5-pound weight gain, an effective pain control plan, and a positive relationship with the staff. It was from Mr. Tide that this staff learned that a pain history and assessment are essential prior to the treatment of chronic pain.

A PERSON WHO HAS BEEN BURNED

The experience of almost being burned to death is one of the most frightening and devastating experiences a person can live through. Even a small burn strategically placed may cause significant emotional trauma (Goodstein 1985). Abruptly a person and his or her family are faced with an unexpected, painful, and life-threatening situation. For the family, the initial gratitude for their loved one surviving the trauma soon turns to thoughts of losing the loved one and fear of financial ruin. For the burn victim, feelings of helplessness, anger, fear, and guilt can become overwhelming (Mendelson 1983). Other issues that concern the burned client and the family are temporary or permanent loss of employment, pain, potential loss of limbs or other mutilating surgeries, loss of family role, separation from family, enforced dependency during a long treatment period, and the loss of the myth of invulnerability (Goodstein 1985).

The burn client needs to progress through four stages of recovery, which require different modalities of nursing interventions and medical treatment. Although one treatment or intervention may be very effective for one stage, the approaches and treatments are not exclusive for any one particular stage. The four stages are (1) *the acute stage*, (2) *the psychological emergency*, (3) *the social emergency*, and (4) *the home emergency*. As clients proceed through these four stages the nurse's compassion, empathy, guidance, interest, and support are crucial elements in the administration of effective health care (Mendelson 1983).

Stage One: The Acute Stage

The first 48 hours after a severe burn are characterized by shock. The client is usually fully oriented and deceptively calm and lucid, shows little or no anxiety, and appears emotionally dissociated from the situation (Goodstein 1985; Harper 1978). The client's calmness and lack of emotion can be upsetting not only to family but also to staff. Soon the physiological problems of severe burns are manifested, e.g., metabolic shock, electrolyte imbalance, edema, and infection, all of which may lead to disturbances in cerebral functioning (Jorgensen and Brophy 1975). Cerebral dysfunction is marked by emotional instability, exaggerated startle response, disorientation, clouding of consciousness, and daydreams and nightmares in which the injury is relived. In the more severely burned, delirium with disorientation and delusional thinking is rampant until the skin grafting reaches the 60% completion stage. Management of the delirious client includes avoidance of barbiturates, which impair cerebral functioning; frequent reorienting statements to the client; and symptomatic use of antipsychotic medications (such as Haldol) for agitation (Harper 1978). Refer to Chapter 21 for intervention with people who are delirious.

For the person who does not have a disturbance in sensorium, denial of the injury and its consequences may be the primary psychological defense. After two weeks, symptoms of anxiety resulting from nightmares about the cause of the burn (fire, hot fluid) may become manifest. Many people experience "flashbacks" of the trauma that are extremely stressful. Listening and allowing the person to discuss his or her nightmares help to decrease anxiety (Goodstein 1985; Harper 1978).

Shock is also a common reaction for the family during the acute phase. Unlike the client, the family begins to experience grief regarding potential losses. Even though the family rationalizes that the burns could have been fatal, ambivalence may exist about their loved one's survival versus possible disfigurement. The family may be torn as to whether to inform the burned victim of other deaths that occurred in the fire. Fear of disturbing the person or potentiating a "setback" may prevent the family from communicating with both the client and the staff. This lack of communication can lead to misinterpretation by the client.

Table 26–3 • THE BURN PATIENT: NURSING INTERVENTIONS DURING THE ACUTE STAGE

NURSING INTERVENTION	RATIONALE
1. Obtain past medical and psychiatric history from patient or family.	1. Past medical conditions can affect the person's present medical condition. Past psychiatric disorders such as schizophrenia, bipolar disorder, or anxiety disorder will affect the patient's present physical and emotional condition.
2. Orient patient frequently to place, person, time, and situation.	2. Frequently check the patient's orientation status (TxPxP). This orients the patient and decreases confusion. Gives the nurse opportunity to observe any changes in mental status (deterioration or improvement).
3. Allow frequent visits by family and close friends, especially when patient is confused.	3. Loved ones can help keep the person oriented and reduce confusion. A person responds more readily to familiar voices.
4. Explain procedures such as debridement to patient prior implementation.	4. Explanations to the patient of new experiences help better prepare him or her for a procedure, thus reducing fears and anxieties of the unknown.
5. Use an honest approach in speaking with the patient and family.	5. Establishing trust is paramount in patient care. Lack of honesty and genuine concern can hinder effective nursing care and positive response to treatments.
6. Inform family that confusion, hallucinations, and delirium are temporary. Explain the cause, e.g., electrolyte imbalance, etc.	6. Some families may believe that the patient has had a "nervous breakdown" if they witness the patient's hallucinations. An explanation of delirious symptoms helps allay fears.
7. Explain expected physical and psychological reactions patients have to burns.	7. Education of the family reduces their fears as well as helps them cope with this crisis. The family can assist in explaining what they have learned to the patient, thus reinforcing patient education previously done by the nurse
8. Use antipsychotic medications as ordered for agitation.	8. An agitated patient can be harmful to himself and others. Proper medication of agitated states is mandatory in securing the patient's safety.
9. Avoid the use of barbiturates.	9. Barbiturates alter cerebral functioning, causing oversedation, confusion, and a disturbed sensorium.

During the acute phase, the staff are involved with saving the client's life. After the client has stabilized, staff may begin to identify with the client. For example, if the client has lost other family members in the fire, the staff may become depressed and anxious about who will tell the client about the deaths. Usually surviving family members are responsible for informing the client of the tragedy (Goodstein 1985; Harper 1978). Refer to Table 26–3 for useful nursing interventions during the acute stage.

Stage Two: The Psychological Emergency

This second stage usually covers the next five to six weeks of hospitalization, after the client's condition has stabilized and the major grafting has begun. The success of the grafts or signs of infection influence the patient's mood, which can range anywhere from hope to despair. Depending upon the severity of the burn, *pain* associated with debridement and healing becomes the primary focus for the burned victim. Effective pain management is essential during this time. Pain is often associated with tanking and the necessary debridement to induce healing. Clients soon begin to dread the tanking procedure, where they are lowered into a tank of water and dead or infected skin tissue is removed to allow healthy tissue growth. Most clients become anxious and fearful in anticipation of this painful experience. Anxiety and fear may reach phobic proportions. Desensitization, behavior modification, and relaxation techniques can be helpful in lessening the client's pain or anxiety preceding the procedures (Goodstein 1985; Harper 1978).

While the tanking and grafting procedures continue, the burn client is continually being confronted with his or her appearance. Although he or she may still be periodically delirious, the client is now aware of the extent of the injuries, e.g., loss of limb(s), loss of genital functioning, inability to move. In addition to the physical losses, the client may be aware of the deaths of others in the accident. Grieving becomes the major psychological issue to address (Harper 1978).

Development of psychiatric complications, adjustment to his or her injuries, and commencement of the grief process have been associated with the person's (1) premorbid personality prior to the burn, (2) management problems, (3) the location of the burn, and (4) previous psychiatric history. Personality traits and characteristics do not change as a result of trauma; however, they can be intensified. If the client was demanding and controlling prior to the accident, the client may be even more controlling and demanding. Few severely burned clients acknowledge suicide attempts or previous self-destructive behavior; however, the possibility that the client unconsciously contributed to his or her injury needs to be explored (Harper 1978).

The length and frequency of delirium also influence the client's ability to adjust to injuries. Most clients experience some degree of delirium. If the delirium continues, the client will be cognitively unable to progress through the grief process.

Location of the burns also influences the length of emotional adjustment. With testicular loss, men can experience a syndrome associated with a decrease in testosterone that includes tearful episodes and feelings of helplessness. This syndrome is easily aided by testosterone replacement as well as psychotherapy. Since young men tend to represent the typical client in a burn unit primarily because of their occupational and recreational exposure, they find the immobility caused by the burn and the dependency particularly stressful. A person who previously dealt with stress through physical activity may regress and become uncooperative, disruptive, or dependent. Facial burns tend to prevent verbal communication, which can be extremely frustrating. A new method for communication needs to be developed between the client and the staff (Andreason 1974; Harper 1978).

Previous psychiatric disorders such as depression, schizophrenia, alcoholism, or a personality disorder will hinder a person's ability to cope during this stressful period. Andreason (1974) discovered that approximately 90% of the burn clients who had been diagnosed with a psychiatric disorder prior to the accident developed neuropsychiatric complications during hospitalization. The neuropsychiatric complications included severe depression, delirium, and severe regression.

During this period, the family also continues their grieving process. Their focus changes to the present day practicalities such as where to park, where to stay, travel arrangements, finances, insurance, and family relationships. During family visits focus is on the pain of the client, and how the staff is managing the pain. Since the family identify with the client, they may become frustrated and appear angry if they perceive that their loved one is not being adequately treated for pain. If the client is lethargic and uncommunicative, the family may also be frustrated and perceive the staff as overmedicating the client. In the family's attempts to help the client with his pain, they may inadvertently alienate the staff and end up feeling isolated and alone. The family's anxiety about survival diminishes after the grafts stabilize and the client is no longer delirious (Goodstein 1985).

The medical and nursing staff during this phase are constantly bombarded with questions by the family and the client—difficult questions that need to be answered in a warm, compassionate, and honest manner. Questions usually concern the client's appearance and future ability to function. Clients may ask, "How do I look?"; "Why can't I move my legs?"; "When will I be able to go back to work?" (Goodstein 1985).

Dealing with delirium, organic psychosis, depression, and dependency can be threatenting and difficult for staff to manage. The constant demand for staff's attention or pain medication is perceived by the staff as dependency and methods of "manipulating" the staff. When the client does attempt a premature move for independence, the staff may perceive the demand as a challenge for control. In this constant struggle between the client asserting independence on the one hand and demanding the fulfillment of his or her dependency needs on the other, the staff may begin to distance themselves, feeling disappointed and angry. Emotional tension can be further exacerbated if the overprotective family does not want the client informed of his or her losses, whether the losses are family members or potential losses of functioning (Goodstein 1985). Suggested nursing interventions during this stage are listed in Table 26–4.

Stage Three: The Social Emergency

During this stage, the client begins to concentrate on reintegration into family and work. Usually this phase begins approximately four weeks prior to discharge. By this time the client is medically stable and has more specific data from the staff regarding his or her condition. Sexuality may be tested first with staff. Clients request mirrors for a closer examination of their appearance and begin to recognize the "changed self" both

Table 26–4 • THE BURN PATIENT: NURSING INTERVENTIONS IN THE PSYCHOLOGICAL EMERGENCY

NURSING INTERVENTION	RATIONALE
1. Continue to assess the patient's pain. Rigorous pain management includes administering pain medications, relaxation exercises, and hypnosis.	1. The patient's pain will vary during different activities such as debridement and physical therapy. Medications are frequently administered prior to these procedures. However, relaxation exercises and hypnosis assist the patient in maintaining some control over his or her pain in addition to reducing the need for narcotics and analgesics.
2. Clarify the patient's misconceptions regarding tanking and debridement procedures.	2. Most patients initially do not understand the necessity of debridement. Since the goal of debridement is to enhance the circulation of the tissues so that new skin can continue to develop, all the old, burned skin must be removed.
3. Explain and describe patient's physical appearance when the person begins to ask questions about his or her appearance.	3. When patients begin to ask how they look or request a mirror, they are ready to begin adjusting to their new appearance. Describing their burned face or back helps prepare them and may reduce anxiety.
4. Encourage the patient to express his or her fears and concerns.	4. Verbally expressing personal fears can reduce the intensity of fear. Unjustified fears can be clarified by the nurse.
5. Allow patient to cry and express feelings of grief.	5. Expressing feelings or crying assist the grieving phase. Nurses must feel comfortable themselves when patients cry or the patients will quickly learn that they can not honestly express themselves. Grief is necessary if the person is to adjust to the burn.
6. Involve the patient in goal setting and decision making regarding his or her care.	6. Promotes independence and mutual communication between the nurse and patient. Aids in mutual evaluation of care.
7. Encourage adaptive coping strategies such as mobilization, hope, involvement with others, use of humor, participation in physical and occupational therapy, and in unit group activities.	7. Reinforces adaptive behavior and enhances adjustment to burn. Maintains healthier levels of self-esteem.
8. Initiate social work consultation with the family to answer their financial questions.	8. Family may proceed with needed assistance early in the patient's hospitalization.

visually and functionally. In coping with their disfigurement, clients may capitalize on their personality traits to rationalize their misfortune. In this phase the clients need to be active in making decisions regarding their care and long-term goals. The client renews contact with friends by allowing them to visit. Usually hope is maintained and humor has returned (Goodstein 1985).

Also by this time, the family have resolved their guilt and are hopeful. Family members are encouraged by the client's physical and emotional response to treatment. Cosmetics, physical functioning, and the client's psychological response to the injury are the family's primary focus. Even though staff are exclaiming that the grafts are "taking" and are "beautiful," the family still perceive the grafts as grotesque. It is hard to persuade the family that the red grafts will one day have the same normal flesh tones and texture as the client's skin. At this time, families will avoid emotional issues and tend to be very optimistic and reassuring (Goodstein 1985; Harper 1978).

In contrast, the staff may become very angry at the client's need for reassurance about personal appearance and sexual desirability. Mourning the client's impending departure can evoke anger and depression among staff members (Harper 1978). Refer to Table 26–5 for nursing interventions during this stage.

Stage Four: The Home Emergency

The true test of how clients redefine their identity and accept their injuries is determined upon discharge from

Table 26–5 • THE BURN PATIENT: NURSING INTERVENTIONS IN THE SOCIAL EMERGENCY

NURSING INTERVENTION	RATIONALE
1. Continue to encourage the expression of grief.	1. Assists the person to adjust to his or her injury.
2. Maintain close contact during this phase.	2. If the patient perceives the nurse as abandoning him or her during this phase, the patient may become more depressed or could begin exhibiting maladaptive behaviors.
3. Give positive reinforcement for selected behaviors (such as learning medication, participating in physical therapy, asking questions about his or her burns).	3. Continues to reinforce patient's adaptive behaviors to enhance adjustments to his or her injury. Positive reinforcement can be verbal praise or small rewards.
4. Confront the patient's inappropriate sexual advances in a firm but supportive manner. Ask the patient about his or her sexual concerns.	4. Initial supportive confrontation of the patient's sexual advances addresses the patient's problem and allows open discussion regarding the patient's feelings. If not confronted, the patient's sexual advances will increase in frequency and intensity, which usually enrage the nursing staff.
5. Assure patient that his or her concerns regarding attractiveness and desirability are a normal response and concern.	5. Helps reduce feelings of isolation and anxiety and encourages communication of concerns and feelings.
6. Encourage a visit from a well-adjusted burn patient.	6. Seeing and talking with a burn patient who is completely rehabilitated can be a great source of support and comfort. Helps decrease the patient's personal fears.

the hospital. Many clients will assume that discharge from the hospital denotes that their physical status is fine; however, reconstructive surgeries and continued physical therapy are scheduled after the initial discharge. Even though the skin grafts have healed, the wounds still appear red, raw, and painful to touch. Facially disfigured clients are high risks for "social death."

Several psychological problems can occur post discharge. Delayed grief is common when clients are constantly confronted with their losses upon returning home. The individual also mourns the loss of familiar and trusted relationships developed while hospitalized. Also, some clients do experience "flashbacks." In reliving the original trauma, insomnia, nightmares, loss of appetite, and phobias may result, adding more distress. Facing the outside world again with physical defects and disfigurement, redefining work and family roles, and discovering new financial resources are the major issues the burn client must resolve after discharge. Finding the courage to overcome these stressors will be determined by the client's coping abilities, in addition to strong family and social support.

Even though the family is relieved and excited about the client's homecoming, the emotional drain can soon become overwhelming. To most families discharge means that the client is well and will quickly resume his or her usual role. In some cases, clients are unable to fulfill their previous role in the family. The client's grieving and lack of energy may become a drain on the family. Often it is during this stage that the family need the most support at a time when they are away from the hospital staff who could provide support (Jorgensen and Brophy 1975). Refer to Table 26–6 for specific nursing interventions during the home emergency stage.

John, a 29-year-old married male, was admitted to the Burn Unit after sustaining 73% total surface area burns in a house fire. Initially, the client was classified as having 60% second-degree burns with the remaining third-degree burns involving his face, body, arms, and legs. The client suffered these burns while attempting to rescue family members remaining in the house. Initially the client was very lucid and calm, asking several questions about who survived the fire. At the time, he did not know that his four-year-old son died in the fire. Three days after the burn, the client became combative and disoriented; he screamed at the nursing staff and disconnected his various tubings. A psychiatric consultation was ordered to assist in managing John's combative behavior and assist him in adjusting to his burns. The psychiatric consultation revealed that John regularly abused alcohol, which had contributed to his combative behavior and electrolyte imbalance. To prevent alcohol withdrawal delirium (delirium tremons), the client was put on a medical detoxification schedule, which reduced the combativeness and hallucinations. However, John's confusion continued. Family members were encouraged

Table 26–6 • THE BURN PATIENT: NURSING INTERVENTIONS IN THE HOME EMERGENCY

NURSING INTERVENTION	RATIONALE
1. Continue to promote patient's positive personality traits and behaviors.	1. Reinforces the person's use of positive characteristics
2. Begin planning future goals, e.g., returning to work or retraining of new skills.	2. Mobilizes hope and assists reintegration into his or her previous family role.
3. Discuss possible reaction of others to the person's disfigurement.	3. Assists in preparing for inquiries and reactions from people in society.
4. Prepare the patient and family for more experiences of grief reactions (decreased energy, depression, decreased sleep, and loss of appetite).	4. Normal grief reactions may be relived when the patient returns home. Family may also experience grief upon the patient's return if the patient's role in the family has changed.
5. Discuss possible psychiatric complications, such as nightmares, severe anxiety, phobias of closed spaces and of noises and colors associated with the trauma, and insomnia, which would warrant a psychiatric evaluation.	5. Serves to educate the patient and family of possible symptoms that may warrant immediate evaluation, treatment, and counseling.
6. When necessary, vocational rehabilitation consultation.	6. Vocational rehabilitation consultation assists a person to examine other occupational opportunities and possible sources of funding.

to visit the client frequently and bring a calendar, clock, and pictures from home.

After the major grafts began to heal, John was consistently oriented and started asking questions about the fire and his appearance. Fearing that John would suffer a "setback," his wife refused to inform him of their son's death. Soon John became anxious, constantly asking questions about the fire, and demanding to see his three children. His anxiety reduced his appetite and ability to sleep. The psychiatrist and psychiatric liaison nurse worked closely with John's wife to assist her in discussing their son's death with John. In learning of his son's death, John became depressed for several weeks. He often expressed his feelings of guilt regarding his inability to save his son. His wife had taped the funeral service and a friend had taken pictures of the funeral and graveside service, which were shared with John in the hospital. The staff spent more time with the client listening to him retell the events of the fire.

During this period, John asked for a mirror to examine his face. Prior to viewing himself, John was told by his nurse about the discoloration of his skin and the areas that needed further grafting. John began asking questions about further surgery and how much return of function he would have in his legs. Physical therapy and occupational therapy consultations were made to discuss with John his future level of ability. An activity chart with progressive goals for walking and lifting weights was made with John's input. The chart was hung in his room to visually demonstrate his progress.

Once the depression associated with his son's death abated, John's major concern became going home. Since he previously was employed as a construction worker, he was worried about his ability to return to his job. During his hospitalization, he had lost weight and strength from his extensive wounds. The nursing staff pointed to his activity chart to reassure him that his strength was improving and that he was slowly accomplishing his goal.

John began flirting with the nursing staff and making sexual advances. At first, the nurses thought the flirting was a sign of recovery; however, the sexual advances became annoying. Nursing staff began to avoid John and spent little time interacting with him, which intensified his behavior. Finally, the head nurse asked John what was happening to cause him to behave in this manner. Blushing, John revealed that he was worried that his wife would not be attracted to him or find him sexually desirable. With the psychiatrist and nurses' help, John was able to begin discussing his fears with his wife.

After a seven-month hospitalization, John was discharged to continue his rehabilitation at home with outpatient physical and occupational therapy.

A PERSON WHO HAS ACQUIRED IMMUNODEFICIENCY SYNDROME (AIDS)

What AIDS is and How it is Detected

HIV (human immunodeficiency virus) is a slow retrovirus that is thought to be the causative agent in **AIDS**

(acquired immunodeficiency disease). Previously the virus was known as HTLV-III (human T-cell lymphotropic virus III) in the United States and as LAV (lymphadenopathy associated virus) in Europe.

The virus invades and eventually destroys helper T-lymphocytes, thus disrupting the body's immune response. Once the virus has invaded a helper T-lymphocyte, it may take from six weeks to 12 months or longer before the presence of HIV antibodies can be detected by testing.

HIV also directly attacks the central nervous system (CNS), resulting in a variety of neuropsychiatric symptoms. HIV *encephalopathy* or AIDS-*related dementia*, myelopathy, and neuropathy are possible sequelae. Personality changes include depression, psychosis, and inability to control aggressive impulses. The virus has been identified in blood, semen, tears, saliva, cerebrospinal fluid, and breast milk.

Presently, the **ELISA** (enzyme-linked immunosorbent assay) for the presence of HIV antibodies in the blood is the simplest, fastest, and least expensive detection method—more than 99% sensitive if antibodies are present. If positive, the ELISA should be repeated. If still positive, a standardized **Western blot** test can be administered to decrease any false-positive results.

It is important to note that the ELISA and Western Blot are not tests for AIDS, rather they detect the presence of antibodies to the AIDS virus (Perry and Markowitz 1988). A negative test result does not necessarily mean an individual is free of the AIDS virus. Antibody formation usually takes about four to 12 months to develop. However, a great many individuals develop antibodies by the sixth month, and in some cases, antibody formation can take up to a year to develop (Meisenhelder and LaCharite 1989). Therefore, individuals in high risk groups would need frequent testing (every three to six months) in order to ascertain the absence of antibody formation.

A positive test result *does indicate*, however, that (1) the *person is infected* with the virus and (2) the *person can infect others* with the virus through certain behaviors. Presently it is believed that not everyone who has a positive test result **(HIV-positive** or **sero-positive)** will necessarily develop AIDS. Rarely, a positive test result can turn out to be a false-positive. Perry and Markowitz (1988) suggest that the following statistics can be shared with people whose test results are positive (HIV-positive):

1. 1.5 million people in the U.S. are infected with HIV but less than 4% have developed AIDS.
2. Within the next 7½ years, of the people who are now HIV-positive
    - 35% will develop AIDS.
    - 40–45% will develop ARC (AIDS-related complex—immunodeficiency, fever, night sweats, fatigue, and lymphadenopathy).
    - about 20% will remain asymptomatic.

Box 26–2. SIGNS AND SYMPTOMS OF AIDS/ARC AND OPPORTUNISTIC DISEASES SEEN IN AIDS

Some Signs and Symptoms Seen in AIDS or ARC

Malaise
Persistent fevers
Persistent tiredness
Weight loss (more than ten pounds in short period of time)
Swollen glands (neck, armpits, groin)
Oral thrush
Persistent diarrhea
Coughing and/or shortness of breath
Skin rash, purple blotches or bumps on the skin
Bruising or bleeding
Neurological problems, difficulty concentrating, poor memory
Night sweats
Sore throat

AIDS diagnosis is made in the presence of sero-positive blood (HIV positive) and one or more life-threatening opportunistic diseases. Some possible opportunistic diseases are listed:

Herpes viruses
Cytomegalovirus (CMV)
Herpes simplex
Varicella zoster virus (VZV)—Herpes zoster (shingles) is caused by reactivation of VZV
Pneumocystis Carinii (PCP)
Toxoplasmosis
Mycobacterium tuberculosis
Kaposi's sarcoma
Lymphomas
Candida albicans (monilial infections)

Data from Gong V, Rudnick N. AIDS Facts and Issues. New Brunswick, NJ: Rutgers University Press, 1986, and Meisenhelder JB, LaCharite CL. Comfort in Caring: Nursing The Person With HIV Infection. Glenview, IL: Scott, Foresman and Company, 1989.

The incubation period (the time of HIV infection until the onset of symptoms) can be from six months to more than seven years. **ARC** (AIDS-related complex) suggests HIV-positive serum with or without generalized symptoms.

AIDS is diagnosed when a person who is sero-positive (HIV-positive) develops an opportunistic infection or neoplasm. The most common opportunistic diseases are *Pneumocystis carinii pneumonia* (PCP) and *Kaposi's sarcoma* (KS). *Pneumocystis carinii* pneumonia represents about 60% of the initial diagnoses among people with AIDS (Faulstich 1987). See Box 26–2 for signs and symptoms of AIDS/ARC and some life-threatening opportunistic diseases identified by the Centers for Disease Control (CDC).

However, once a person has been diagnosed with AIDS, the average lifespan is between six months and one year. Some people might live five years or longer, and some people who have ARC may never go on to develop the complete AIDS syndrome (Kaplan and Sadock 1988).

Who Should Be Tested

The **Centers for Disease Control** (CDC) suggests the high risk populations identified in Box 26–3 should be considered for HIV testing (Perry and Markowitz 1988). The chances of being sero-positive vary among these groups. A person's chances of testing HIV-positive vary with geographical areas (large East Coast and West Coast cities are presently the highest risk areas) although the incidence of AIDS is increasing all over the country. The sociodemographic groups of lower-income urban blacks and Hispanics are currently a high risk group (CDC 1986; Rogers and Williams 1987). However, estimated overall statistics for certain high risk groups have been compiled (CDC 1987). See Table 26–7.

The issue of testing or not testing is fraught with complex ethical and legal issues. Essentially, the issue of confidentiality versus the need to document and prevent the spread of AIDS to others is being intensely debated. The American Medical Association (AMA) and the American Psychiatric Association (APA) suggest that counselors may have an ethical duty to warn individuals who are known to be at risk of being infected by sero-positive clients. Notifying at-risk intimates may be indicated after all efforts have failed to induce clients to tell their at-risk partners. However, some argue that the public might be better served if HIV-infected individuals were assured of confidentiality. Perry (1989) believes that the lack of confidentiality could deter some HIV-infected individuals from seeking appropriate treatment. Education alone is often not enough to reduce high risk behaviors. Therefore, those who might change their high risk behaviors through psychotherapy may not seek treatment if they believed that confidentiality would not be maintained.

Box 26–3. AT-RISK GROUPS FOR AIDS

1. Men who at any time since 1978 have engaged in homosexual behavior.
2. Intravenous drug users, especially those who have shared needles or other equipment in "shooting galleries."
3. Recipients of blood and blood products between 1978 and March 1985.
4. Male and female sexual partners of those in the above risk groups.
5. Women who are considering pregnancy and who are at risk of having been infected by HIV or whose sexual partners may carry such a risk.
6. Subjects undergoing treatment for other sexually transmitted diseases.
7. Patients being evaluated for any medical, psychiatric, or neurological illness that may be due to an HIV infection as wells as patients who have even a remote chance of HIV exposure.
8. Heterosexual men and women who have had multiple sexual partners of unknown serological status, especially prostitutes.
9. Previously tested sero-negative individuals who continue to practice high risk behavior.
10. Emigrants from countries in which HIV prevalence is high.

Data from the Centers for Disease Control (CDC) as reported in Perry SW, Markowitz JC. Counseling for HIV testing. Hospital and Community Psychiatry, 39(7):733, 1988.

Table 26–7 • ESTIMATED OVERALL SERO-PREVALENCE AMONG SOME POPULATIONS

POPULATION	ESTIMATES OF AVERAGE OVERALL SERO-PREVALENCE*
1. Exclusively homosexual men	20–25%—May be as high as 68% in some locales
2. I.V. Drug abusers	Overall 50–65% *in* NYC *and* Puerto Rico. Can be as high as 72–80% in some samples
3. Persons with hemophilia in sero-prevalent areas *before* 1985	70% for hemophilia A 35% for hemophilia B
4. Bisexual men with infrequent homosexual encounters	5% sero-prevalence
5. Heterosexual partners of person with HIV infection or at risk of HIV infection	10–60% sero-prevalence
6. General population without identified risk	0.02% sero-prevalence

* Frequent sexual encounters, other socially transmitted diseases, open genital lesions, use of some drugs (e.g., alcohol, marijuana, steroids, and others) affect the risk of HIV infection.
Data from the Centers for Disease Control (CDC) as reported in Perry SW, Markowitz JC. Counseling for HIV testing. Hospital and Community Psychiatry, 39(7):733, 1988.

Many states stipulate that HIV testing cannot be used to discriminate against individuals who apply for housing, schooling, job placement, or job retention. However, in some states, the names and addresses of persons who tested sero-positive are reported to public health authorities (e.g., Colorado, Minnesota, and South Carolina) (Kaplan and Sadock 1988). At other times, the results of the ELISA and Western blot tests are recorded in a client's chart. Therefore, confidentiality is not always guaranteed. There are, however, anonymous testing sites, where testing is done using numbers and not names. In this way confidentiality is insured; however, the HIV-positive individual is left without test counseling and without referral information about support groups, therapy, and other kinds of available support.

What to Tell Clients About Transmission of the Disease

Most people know that HIV is transmitted from person to person via bodily fluids such as semen and blood and through intravenous (IV) use of contaminated syringes and needles. The two greatest at-risk groups are (1) homosexual and bisexual men and (2) IV drug abusers. Therefore, unprotected anal and vaginal intercourse is dangerous if either partner is HIV-positive. Also, sharing a needle with an HIV-positive individual is dangerous.

Many people also know that HIV is transmitted via the placenta at birth to babies having an HIV-positive mother. A newborn baby has a 30–70% chance of contracting an HIV infection from an HIV-positive mother (Perry and Markowitz 1988). Children who have contracted AIDS in the prenatal environment comprise about 77% of all children who have AIDS. Children with hemophilia or coagulation disorders comprise 6%, and 14% of children with AIDS are believed to have contracted the disorder through blood transfusions for other than hemophilia or coagulation disorders. The other 4% remain undetermined (L.K. 1988b).

However, *many people do not know* that HIV CANNOT be transmitted by

- fondling, hugging, dry-kissing, or mutual masturbation.
- contact with household items such as food, cookware, or toilet seats.
- mosquitoes.

And *no one knows* for sure whether the following activities can transmit HIV, since there is no hard evidence available at this time. Therefore, the following behaviors are questionable because they permit exchange of body fluids:

- Oral-genital contact (oral-vaginal/oral-penile/oral-anal).
- Kissing with saliva exchange (french kissing).

Status of Cure

Presently no effective treatment for the underlying immune deficiency or virus is in sight. Some drugs are being tested that inhibit an enzyme (reverse transcriptase) necessary for the replication of HIV. For example, one such drug, zidovudine (Retrovir, formerly known as AZT), is under study on sero-negative health care workers, who are given the drug soon after significant occupational exposure. Zidovudine does inhibit the growth of the human immunodeficiency virus (HIV). Zidovudine does not cure people with AIDS (PWA), but it may prolong life and decrease the number of infections that may occur with AIDS or ARC. It is hoped that administration of zidovudine early on can prevent HIV infection. The hypothesis is that Retrovir, if begun within a few days of HIV exposure and continued for a few weeks, may prevent HIV infection or at least alter the progression of the disease (L.K. 1988c). Currently, a number of drug trials are being conducted. Some of the experimental drugs are being given in combination with Retrovir (AZT). There is also research on developing an AIDS vaccine. Both research on drugs and on the development of a vaccine are in the very early stages.

Psychiatric and Neuropsychiatric Symptoms

Often nurses work with people with AIDS in a general hospital setting, although AIDS clients are frequently admitted into the psychiatric units as well. In either case, nurses want to know the kinds of behaviors they might see resulting, either directly or indirectly, from the disease AIDS.

People with HIV infection at any of its stages are faced with multiple concerns and existential dilemmas; loss of life, threat of pain, loss of function, social isolation, stigmatization, potential dementia, and economic ruin are at the fore.

Therefore, it is not surprising that feelings of hopelessness and fearful uncertainty can be expected. Compounding these feelings of hopelessness is the personal awareness by the HIV-infected individual of negative societal attitudes toward homosexual and bisexual practices, IV drug abusers, and the social stigma against AIDS itself. It is not surprising then that *suicide and suicide ideation* are clinical commonplaces.

Anxiety symptoms take the form of panic attacks, anorexia, tachycardia, insomnia, and agitation. *Intense anger* is frequently experienced and directed toward perceived public discrimination, dissatisfaction with governmental responses, and ineffective medical care (Faulstich 1987). Psychosis and paranoid behaviors may also be exhibited by some clients.

DSM III-R diagnoses include *depression* (reactive and major), which is the most common diagnosis. Other diagnoses include *adjustment disorder with depressed mood, dementia, panic disorder, paranoid reactions*, and *psychosis*.

Complicating the diagnosis of depression, is the possibility of AIDS-related dementia, also known as **HIV dementia complex** or **HIV-encephalopathy.** AIDS-related dementia seems to cluster into two broad categories (Perry and Markowitz 1986). One category mimics the signs and symptoms of depression. For example, forgetfulness, poor concentration, loss of libido, apathy, affective blunting, psychomotor retardation, anorexia, fatigue, and social withdrawal (AIDS Update 1988). The second category presents with subtle cognitive difficulties and acute psychotic presentation (e.g., delusions, hallucinations, psychomotor agitation, mania, and grandiosity). Around 60% of people with AIDS will develop some neurological symptoms, and in about 10% of cases it is the neurological symptoms that are the first indicators of HIV infection (AIDS Update 1988). Some neuropsychiatric symptoms of AIDS are listed in Box 26–4.

Box 26–4. NEUROPSYCHIATRIC SYMPTOMS IN PEOPLE WITH AIDS

Decrease in sleep
Decrease in appetite
Depressed mood
Withdrawal
Increased somatic complaints
Unkempt physical appearance
Disorientation
Difficulty with verbal expression
Feelings of hopelessness
Decreased feeling of self-worth
Feelings of helplessness
Decreased concentration
Suicidal thoughts
Decreased short term memory
Feelings of punishment
Slow verbal responses
Hallucinations
Delusions

Who Needs Intervention

The HIV-infected individual of course needs intervention. But often, care can be compromised if health care professionals, family, and friends are not properly educated and are without sufficient peer and outside support. Therefore, staff, the HIV client, and family and friends all need attention.

Staff. Although HIV risk for health care workers is stated as being low (4 out of 1,070 exposed) (L.K. 1988a), staff have significant concerns regarding their own safety. The present shortage of nursing staff, compounded with the increasing number of AIDS clients needing intensive physical as well as psychological care, raises many valid issues. Salisbury (1986) identifies many of these issues as contributing to staff burnout:

- fear of contagion/mortality
- young age of the afflicted
- repetitive deaths of clients
- deterioration of the client's physical condition and often of the psychological state
- need for extra precautions
- being the target of the client's anger

Many health care facilities are making an effort to deal with these staff issues, and offer support. One psychiatric unit that cared for AIDS/ARC clients found that staff significantly benefited from general meetings, small group meetings, individual supervision sessions, educational sessions, and opportunities to ventilate (Baer et al. 1987). Box 26–5 identifies some methods nurses can use to prevent burnout.

Education must include housekeeping and dietary staff, because often auxiliary staff refuse to enter the room of an HIV-infected individual for fear of contracting AIDS. Weekly staff discussion with the Department of Infection Control can decrease misperceptions among all staff.

Knowledge of and competence in implementing the hospital's infection control guidelines are crucial. Precautions usually include, among others, wearing gloves for contact with blood and body fluids, special precautions for reusable equipment and supplies, and disposing of used syringes in specially designated impermeable containers. **Each nurse should be very familiar with the disease control protocol practiced in his or her hospital.**

HIV-INFECTED CLIENT. A complicating factor is that often an HIV-infected individual's usual support system is affected or diminished. For example, a person whose support system consists of others in a high risk group may have witnessed many of his or her peers die of the disease already. Reactions of family and friends might be such that they are unable to support the individual because of their own fears and reactions. Therefore, for the same reason an individual has an increased need for abundant family support and love, little or none might be available.

Support groups for people with AIDS are designed to reduce isolation and personal rejection, and are able to provide educational, psychotherapeutic, and social interaction. Support groups can enhance self-esteem by allowing the person to manage his or her life by controlling personal attitudes and decisions in dealing with the disease (Menenberg 1987).

The gay community has been very responsive to the needs of AIDS victims; they have been active in fund raising, legislation, and research and development of community resources (Menenberg 1987).

Box 26–5. SUGGESTIONS FOR PREVENTING STAFF BURNOUT

1. Remember, rewarding and mutually beneficial relationships can be established with your AIDS patients.
2. Use AIDS network groups as a professional reference group to give *you* support.
3. Become familiar with the literature on death and dying and suicide.
4. Discuss and share and become aware of your own feelings about AIDS, people with AIDS (PWA), and death.
5. Expect to move through a process in which you feel deep despair before you gain a more balanced sense of reality.
6. Use a voluntary system of rotation with different types of patients.
7. Share feelings and maintain personal relationships with members of a specific nonprofessional community support and socialization group.

Data from Leukefeld C, Fimbres M. Introduction. *In* Leukefeld C, Fimbres M (eds). Responding to AIDS: Psychosocial Initiatives. Silver Spring, MD: National Association of Social Workers, 1987, as found in Leukefeld CG. Psychosocial initiatives in dealing with AIDS. Hospital and Community Psychiatry, 40(5):454, 1989.

Individual and group therapy are often useful in helping the HIV-infected client to work through depression and handle the many emotions that arise. Some issues concern guilt over sexual practices or drug abuse, possible social isolation, and associated fears or anger that arise over acknowledgment of the disease. Instructions in stress management and problem-solving techniques can be of benefit (Faulstich 1987). As mentioned, antidepressants may be given at times, and benzodiazepines are sometimes useful in reducing extreme anxiety and anxiety reactions. Psychiatric interventions for AIDS-related dementia are similar to the general management of the organic mental disorders. (See Chapter 21.)

Pastoral services can offer spiritual help and can provide a great deal of comfort. Social services provide discharge planning and any necessary referrals. Referrals include information on community resources, self-help groups, and finances.

Everyone needs to be continuously updated on the progression of AIDS and AIDS research — the general population, nurses, educators, and especially those who test HIV positive. Nurses should know about the *Morbidity and Mortality Weekly Report*, published by the Centers for Disease Control (CDC), in order to keep up to date on the rapid changes. Some guidelines for teaching clients and others follow:

1. *Mode* of HIV transmission *and* how HIV *is not* transmitted.
2. Behaviors that are *most effective in preventing* transmission or acquisition of HIV:
   - sexual abstinence
   - cessation of IV drug abuse
3. *Precautions that can reduce* HIV transmission or acquisition:
   - correct use of *latex* condoms with virucidal jelly
   - sterilization of needles and syringes: flushing out with chlorine bleach two times, then flushing out with clean water two times
   - do not share needles
   - avoid anal intercourse
   - avoid mucous membrane contact with blood, semen, vaginal secretions, saliva, urine, and feces
4. *Cautions* for people living with HIV-infected persons:
   - don't share toothbrushes
   - don't share razors
   - clean sero-positive blood from cuts with diluted chlorine bleach
   - dispose of sero-positive tampons in double plastic bags
   - avoid pregnancy if either partner is sero-positive

Frequent nursing diagnoses formulated for AIDS clients are identified in Table 26–8.

Table 26–8 • FREQUENT NURSING DIAGNOSES FORMULATED WITH AIDS CLIENTS

POSSIBLE NURSING DIAGNOSIS	RELATED FACTORS
Ineffective breathing pattern	*Pneumocystis carinii* pneumonia
Ineffective airway clearance	Respiratory and other opportunistic infections
	Anxiety
Altered nutrition: less than body requirements	Chronic diarrhea
Diarrhea	Lesions of the mouth and esophagus
Fluid volume deficit	Kaposi's sarcoma of the gastrointestinal tract
	Nausea and vomiting induced by medications
	Increased metabolic rate with fevers
Ineffective individual coping	Depression of chronic illness
Sensory-perceptual alterations	Social and physical isolation
Potential for self-directed violence	Psychological response to catastrophic illness
Spiritual distress	Infections or malignancies of the central nervous system
Social isolation	Imposed isolation requirements
Hopelessness/Powerlessness	Community/family/health care personnel's attitudes
Disturbance in self-esteem	Physical dependency
Anxiety/Fear	Poor prognosis
	Symptoms of acute infection
Impaired home maintenance management	Lack of community support services
Grieving	Inadequate home-care information
	Lack of people to assist with care
	Confusion or withdrawal of friends or family

Data from Gong V, Rudnick N (eds). AIDS Facts and Issues. New Brunswick, NJ: Rutgers University Press, 1986.

FAMILY AND FRIENDS. Families and friends also need to ventilate their concerns, get current medical information, and receive help with the exhausting work of caring for their loved ones at home (Baer et al. 1987).

Families and friends may also have to contend with unresolved issues concerning lifestyle or sexuality at the same time they are dealing with issues such as social stigma, contagion, and their own grief. Family members frequently need, and should receive, referrals for their own mental health treatment (Baer et al. 1987). Self-help groups for families and friends are available in many areas.

Epidemiologists predict that the AIDS epidemic is just beginning (Baer et al. 1987). Abundant resources are needed to mitigate this growing medical and psychological problem.

Richard was a 27-year-old male who was initially seen in the outpatient clinic for nausea, vomiting, and fever. Initially he was treated with antibiotics. For the next six months he would have periods of remission but the symptoms continued to recur. As the months passed, Richard began feeling depressed and fatigued, and lost interest in his job and usual activities with his friends. Finally, he was admitted to the hospital on a medical unit where he was found HIV positive and two days later was diagnosed with acquired immunodeficiency syndrome (AIDS).

When he learned of his diagnosis, Richard withdrew from the staff and was observed sitting for long periods of time in his room with the lights off and the curtains drawn. He was immediately placed in a single room on isolation precaution for blood and body secretions. The staff who had frequently visited Richard began avoiding his room. Many nursing staff and physicians were concerned and confused about proper gowning procedure when entering Richard's room. Several staff would put on gowns, gloves, masks, hairnets, and cover their shoes before entering; however, some staff just wore masks. Ancillary health professionals refused to enter his room to dispose of waste or to deliver his meals or mail. Soon Richard refused to see his family and would only answer questions in two-word phrases. A psychiatric liaison nurse consultation was initiated by the head nurse to assess and evaluate Richard for depression. The head nurse had asked Richard and he agreed to the consultation.

Initially, Richard was guarded and evasive when answering questions. After several visits, Richard told the psychiatric liaison nurse that he did not know what to tell his friends, family, and lover about the reason for hospitalization. Many of his friends and coworkers did not know that he was gay. He thought that his family was suspicious about his homosexuality, yet he had never confronted the issue with them. Since his father was a very conservative, traditional man, he was afraid of being rejected and "disowned" by his family. On the other hand, he believed his lover would accept his diagnosis, but felt extremely guilty for probably transmitting the disease to someone he loved. He stated he was angry at the staff for treating him like a "leper" and wondered why some of the staff used the full isolation technique and some wore masks. Those staff that used gowns, gloves, and masks prior to entering his room were perceived by Richard to be afraid of and disgusted by him. On the whole, he was angry at the staff for rejecting him and not coming into his room as often as they once did.

Richard was encouraged to contact his lover and discuss his fears with him. The psychiatric liaison nurse called the infection control nurse and scheduled a case conference for the staff. During the conference, the psychiatric liaison nurse presented the client's perception and feelings of rejection. The infection control nurse also reiterated and described hospital policy and procedure in working with people with AIDS.

After talking with his lover, Richard discovered that he was supported by him and felt encouraged to contact his family. His father was concerned about Richard's physical deterioration. Surprising to Richard, his family accepted his homosexuality and wanted to visit him in the hospital. The staff began visiting more often and began educating Richard about his disease and treatment. However, several staff members were still afraid of Richard's disease and did tend to avoid him. As Richard began feeling more supported by his family, lover, and the staff, he began talking more and his room was no longer dark and desolate. Continuing infection control inservice conferences were held to allay newcomers' fears and answer questions. The major nursing interventions were establishing rapport with Richard by returning to visit, listening to Richard's concerns, and accepting Richard's views nonjudgmentally.

A PERSON WHO HAS CARDIAC DYSFUNCTION

The heart has long been designated man's emotional core where feelings of love originate. In addition, the heart is where the life-blood is pumped to the rest of the body. When a person develops cardiac dysfunction, feelings of vulnerability and loss are intense.

Cardiac disease is one of the leading causes of nontraumatic deaths in the United States. An estimated 50% of all adult deaths are due to sudden cardiac death (Wells 1983). However, many people suffering from heart attacks do recover. Of those who recover from a myocardial infarction (MI), 25% will suffer persistent psychosocial difficulties (Croog 1984; Mayou 1984). For some people, an MI produces an emotional upheaval that results in personality disruption and maladaptive behaviors. The emotional upheaval and personality disruption are usually a result of underlying conflicts revolving around feelings of personal inadequacy (Visvanathan and Vizner 1984). Recovering from an MI can be a lengthy process that stresses both the client and his family. An understanding of the psychological components of cardiac dysfunction by the nurse can facilitate recovery.

A person's basic personality and usual coping strategies prior to an MI will greatly influence adjustment to his or her illness. Illness is a major source of stress. A person who has previously suffered a major depressive episode or anxiety disorder is most likely to have similar psychiatric problems during recovery and rehabilitation. A person who experienced sexual difficulties prior to the cardiac dysfunction is likely to continue to have sexual difficulties after the MI. More men than women have sexual problems such as performance anxiety or difficulties with arousal following an MI (Althof et al. 1984). In examining marital status, married persons tend to progress faster than single clients. Professional or nonmanual workers return to work sooner than manual workers (Croog 1984; Mayou 1984; Razin 1984). In addition, men return to work sooner than women (Althof et al, 1984). In summary, married professional men who have not had previous psychiatric disorders and have a balance of work and leisure activities tend to have a quick recovery and return to work.

Another factor that has been highly correlated with cardiac disease is Type A behavior pattern (refer to Chapter 15). These clients tend to have more difficulty adjusting to their perceived loss of control over their health and environment than other clients. Generally, the Type A person is internally driven to accomplish more tasks and tends to become inappropriately impatient with slowness. They are preoccupied with themselves, and evaluate their own worthiness by the number of their accomplishments. In their drive toward accomplishment, they are competitive even in areas that are noncompetitive. They wish to dominate every activity. Their speech is often explosive and pressured. Unfortunately for these individuals, they are often dissatisfied with their life and feel insecure regarding their status. In order to break their frenzied pace, some people tend to be self-destructive and may even be relieved when they have heart attacks so that they can stop (Blumenthal et al. 1984; Matthews 1982; Rosenman 1978). The Type A behavior pattern is often seen in clients who are business executives or professionals. When hospitalized, they may deny their symptoms and have difficulty assuming any characteristics of the "sick role."

In the event of an acute myocardial infarction, the person is usually rushed to the emergency room via ambulance. From there the client may be transferred to the coronary intensive care unit (CCU) for observation. Usual reactions to a heart attack are as follows. During the first two days, *anxiety* is the most frequent psychological response to the CCU environment. After the diagnosis is confirmed, the client usually becomes *depressed*. Fear of loss of health is confirmed by the diagnosis (Cassem and Hackett 1978; Hackett 1985). Even after the physicians have explained the diagnosis, some clients continue to deny their illness. Although initial denial can be adaptive, denial is not adaptive if the client leaves the hospital against medical advice (AMA). As illustrated in Box 26–6, several psychological factors have been linked to those clients who leave the cardiology service AMA. At times, minimal cardiac complications and low doses of medications may support the client's denial of the seriousness of his cardiac illness (Ochitill et al. 1985).

For the client who has *sudden cardiac death syndrome* or ventricular arrhythmias that are life threatening, the hospital course will vary. People who suffer from ventricular arrhythmias can be asymptomatic or symptomatic. Those who have symptoms such as syncope, palpitations, chest discomfort, or lightheadedness are forever wary of any indicator which heralds the onset of an arrhythmic episode. People who are asymptomatic may live in fear that at any moment they may lose con-

Box 26–6. PSYCHOLOGICAL FACTORS LINKED TO CARDIAC PATIENTS WHO LEAVE AGAINST MEDICAL ADVICE (AMA)

1. An increase in physical symptoms of chronic alcohol abuse.
2. A decrease in cardiac complications.
3. A decreased requirement of antihypertensive/diuretic medications while hospitalized.
4. An increase in somatic complaints prior to AMA.
5. An increase in apparent anxiety prior to AMA.
6. An increase in the use of psychotropic medication the day before AMA.

Data from Ochitill H, Havassy B, Byrd R, Peters R. Leaving a cardiology service against medical advice. Journal Of Chronic Disease, 38(1):78, 1985.

sciousness. Conventional and investigational medications are effective in 59–82% of this client population (Wells 1983). If conventional medications fail in controlling the ventricular arrhythmia, the investigational medications are tried one at a time and then dually. If the investigational medication fails, the client is "shocked" or cardioverted into a normal sinus rhythm. This procedure is done while the client is fully alert. This can be a terrifying experience.

If both conventional and investigational medications and cardioversion fail to control ventricular arrhythmias, surgery is the next consideration. For some clients a coronary bypass or a resection of a ventricular aneurysm is all that is necessary. However, the client who is a poor surgical risk may be a candidate for a pacemaker or an automatic implantable cardioverter defibrillator (AICD). For some clients who require investigational drug therapy or surgery, the hospital stay can be three months or longer.

If a person has been through many failed drug trials, the client and family become discouraged and depressed with lack of progress. It is important that the client and family are always informed of future treatment plans and an air of optimism is maintained. If hope does not prevail, depression may supersede the cardiac disease in severity. Treating the depressed *sudden cardiac death syndrome* client with antidepressant medication is difficult and tentative because of the presence of ventricular arrhythmias due to the medication's cardiovascular side effects. Supportive psychotherapy with emphasis on supporting adaptive coping strategies can be most helpful with this client population.

Nursing Interventions

Clarifying Myths. Nursing interventions for the heart attack client begin by clarifying general myths surrounding myocardial infarctions. Some commonly held myths are as follows:

Myths	Facts
1. People have to retire after an MI.	1. 80% of people with an MI return to work.
2. People have to give up sex or they will die.	2 Most people can resume normal sexual relations with spouse. Most deaths following orgasm involve sexual contact under unusual circumstances.

Since sex is a major concern for the cardiac client, education in this area is a necessity. The nurse is usually the person the client will begin to question about sex. Not only does the nurse need to educate the client in this area, but she or he also needs to inform the physician that the client is concerned about sexual activity. The physician will decide when the client can resume having sex. Usually, four to six weeks after an MI, a person can return to his or her previous sexual activity (Gondek 1983; Moore et al. 1984). Guidelines for counseling the post-MI client regarding sex are outlined in Box 26–7.

Myths	Facts
3. People die on the anniversary of a loved one's death or of their first heart attack.	3. This occurrence is extremely rare.

REDUCING ANXIETY. Other nursing interventions focus on reducing anxiety and preventing maladaptive coping following a heart attack. Initially, orienting the client to the coronary intensive care unit helps reduce anxiety. Since most clients are placed on cardiac monitors, the nurse can reassure the client that trained personnel are observing his or her cardiac rhythm and are nearby if needed. If the client lost consciousness during a cardiac arrest, the nurse needs to tell the client what has happened. The nurse asks if the client knows of anyone who has had a similar experience. If yes, the nurse can clarify misconceptions the person might have regarding his or her own situation. Once the nurse has determined that the client is ready to learn more about MI or cardiac disease, teaching can begin. Nothing helps the client more than an empathetic listener who is knowledgeable about cardiac disease. The client may ask the same question repeatedly when anxiety is moderate or severe. Answering questions in polite and reassuring tones will help lower anxiety (Tuggle 1982). If the client seems confused and disoriented, there may be delirium secondary to brain anoxia, psychotic reaction, or electrolyte imbalance. The nurse should alert the physician about the confusion and disorientation. Education should stop while the client is delirious.

INTERVENTION WITH FAMILY. Not only does the client experience anxiety following a myocardial infarction or sudden cardiac arrest, so also does the client's family. Keeping the family informed about treatments, procedures, and diagnoses and listening to their concerns help reduce their anxiety. As a result of anxiety, family members may not remember everything that the staff tells them; therefore, repeating information is often necessary. Whenever possible, provide a private room for the family to gather in and discuss their concerns. The nurse advises the family to limit the amount of visitors during the first three days of hospitalization.

Box 26–7. SEXUAL COUNSELING AFTER A MYOCARDIAL INFARCTION

The nurse:

1. Stresses it is normal for a person to feel weak, depressed, and anxious following a heart attack. These feelings do not mean the patient is rejecting his or her partner.
2. Explains the four stages of sexual response, (excitement, plateau, orgasm, and resolution). (Refer to Chapter 28).
3. Explains that the heart works the hardest during the orgasmic phase, which lasts only 10–15 seconds and is equivalent to walking up two flight of stairs.
4. Suggests cardiac rehabilitation programs that focus on increasing tolerance and assist the person in regaining strength.
5. Suggests ways to reduce stress during sexual intercourse. For example: Use familiar positions, use familiar surroundings, avoid extreme temperatures, avoid anal intercourse, avoid excessive alcohol intake or a heavy meal prior to intercourse (or wait three hours after a heavy meal), avoid unfamiliar partners, avoid strenuous activity after intercourse, foreplay will help prepare the heart gradually, and provide plenty of time.
6. Explains that nitroglycerin may be taken before intercourse to prevent chest pain. If chest pain occurs during intercourse, stop for awhile and take nitroglycerin before resuming.
7. Clarifies the symptoms of danger that need to be reported to the physician. These include: shortness of breath or increased heart rate for 15 minutes or more after intercourse, chest pain during or after intercourse, extreme fatigue the day following intercourse, sleeplessness following intercourse, and palpitations for longer than 15 minutes after intercourse. The patient should report any of these symptoms to his or her physician and ask the doctor specific questions.

Data from Gondek M. Post-MI sex: Those unspoken fears. RN, 46(5):61, 1983, and Moore K, Folk-Lighty M, Nolen M. The joy of sex after a heart attack: Counseling the cardiac patient. Nursing '84, April:104, 1984.

Even though visitors and family are genuinely worried, the client will be exhausted and need the rest.

Optimism also helps the family and client through this difficult time. False reassurance is very different from optimism. It is helpful to point out the positive aspects of the treatment, the diagnosis, and the staff's experience in treating people with cardiac disease. The sooner the person can be encouraged to become active, the sooner will be the return to productive patterns of living. Nurses can support the family to encourage the client to change or alter harmful patterns (e.g., smoking, excessive alcohol intake, and sedentary lifestyle), and alter high risk activities, which can help reduce the chance of recurrence of cardiac disease (Hackett 1985).

Mr. Topp, a 68-year-old retired Air Force general was hospitalized for a myocardial infarction (MI) that was complicated by malignant ventricular tachycardia. This was his first hospitalization and first major illness. He had retired from the military at age 65 to start his own international consulting firm. He found himself driven to an 18-hour workday. During the first month of hospitalization, he continued to carry on his business by two phones, which he demanded to have installed in his hospital room. Mr. Topp was constantly angry at the physicians for not having "cured the problem" during the first four weeks. He began complaining that the hospital was run so inefficiently, nothing was ever on time. His manner was abrupt, accusatory, extremely opinionated, and challenging. After several verbal battles with staff, a psychiatric liaison nursing consultation was ordered to help the staff deal more effectively with Mr. Topp. After several sessions the psychiatric liaison nurse discovered that Mr. Topp had intense fears of losing control of his body and of dying. Mr. Topp stated that he thought he would never recover, since the doctors had not found an antiarrhythmic medication that would prevent lethal ventricular tachycardia. Cardiac complications, lack of progress, loss of health, and loss of his business became major issues that eventually led Mr. Topp into a severe depression.

After asking Mr. Topp questions about his illness, the psychiatric liaison nurse assessed that the client had several misconceptions about his cardiac disease. The nurses devised a care plan around Mr. Topp's learning needs and began teaching him more about the heart and his particular problem. In addition, the rationales for different antiarrhythmic drug trials were explained. Soon, the client had progressed to the point where he could take his own medication and could tell the nursing staff the action and reason for taking the many medications that were prescribed. Mr. Topp and a staff nurse began leading a client medication group on the unit. Eventually, his anxiety lessened as he became more knowledgeable about his disease, and took more control over his medication regime. He was also included in making decisions about his daily schedule. Initially, Mr. Topp was extremely rigid in his outlook; however, as time progressed, he became more flexible.

Since Mr. Topp was a definite Type A personality, the psychiatric liaison nurse began some cognitive restructuring along with the staff, who began discussing methods of handling stress. Relaxation exercises were taught and reinforced. In addition, the nursing staff gave the client gentle but firm feedback regarding his aggressive behavior. When the client behaved assertively and directly, the nursing staff reinforced the behavior by talking with the client longer and by taking the client off the unit to the courtyard. (The client could not leave the unit unescorted by nursing personnel.)

Since none of the antiarrhythmic medications were able to control Mr. Topp's ventricular tachycardia, he became a candidate for the automatic implantable cardioverter defibrillator (AICD). Discharge plans were discussed with the client and his wife. Since Mr. Topp was unable to continue his job, which included a rigorous schedule, he decided to consult by phone to other agencies. Cardiopulmonary resuscitation (CPR) was taught to his wife and several close friends who lived nearby. Upon discharge, the client experienced some mild anxiety about leaving the safe environment in which he had become accustomed to living for three months. However, in general, his outlook was more optimistic and hopeful.

A PERSON IN AN INTENSIVE CARE UNIT (ICU)

Nothing quite prepares a person for admission into an intensive care unit (ICU). The environment of the ICU is filled with an air of urgency, danger, and heroism. The aim in the ICU is to maintain life and to resuscitate those clients whose tie to life is tenuous. Strange noises, odors, and bright, fluorescent lights fill the room and add to the confusion of a newly admitted client. Most ICUs are open, with client beds surrounding the core of activity, the nursing station. The client has little privacy and is able to observe life and death situations merely by glancing across the room. Even though a client is in plain view, he or she may be socially isolated. The medical jargon that is the predominant ICU language is totally alien. Isolation is the hallmark of the ICU setting (Cassem and Hackett 1978; Robinson 1974).

Many ICUs are centrally located to give easy access to the operating room, pharmacy, and laboratory. Therefore, they seldom have windows, which adds to disorientation for the client. Equipment that monitors fluid intake and heart rate are huddled around the client's bedside. The client is connected to these life support companions by a series of tubings. For the critically ill client, tubes seem to be connected to every appendage and orifice the client can supply. The ICU environment is terrifying and foreign for most clients. Those clients who have had little exposure to the hospital setting are particularly vulnerable (Cassem and Hackett 1978; Robinson 1974).

Being admitted to an ICU denotes a threat to life and evokes predictable psychological and emotional reactions in the clients. Not only is fear of death a common reaction, but also fear of being maimed by the various procedures needed to sustain life. With unfamiliar surroundings and unfamiliar people, the client may become panicked. "Nothing else distorts personality quite like panic" (Cassem and Hackett 1978). Staff are often amazed at the changes in personality when the client's panic subsides.

Intervention for Anxiety and Fear

Fear and anxiety are bound closely together in the ICU. Depression and delirium are additional psychological issues. During the initial two days, the client's anxiety is highest. Anxiety, illness, and admission to the ICU are closely linked. Fear of death is an imminent concern for the client and family. Fear and anxiety can be minimized by careful explanations and valid reassurance, as well as medications such as benzodiazepines (e.g., Valium). For example, when the nurse explains, "This medication will help your pain," the client's fears may be reduced. Panic levels of anxiety can produce a psychoticlike state. Depending on the situation, presence of a family member or antipsychotic medication can reduce psychotic symptoms.

Disorientation is common. The lack of adequate rest and the presence of sleep deprivation increase the probability of disorientation and misinterpretations of reality (illusions). Allowing the client to get uninterrupted intervals of sleep along with frequent orientation to person, place, time, and situation can help reduce disorientation.

Delirium is a frequent phenomenon in the surgical intensive care units. Delirious clients may exhibit psychotic behaviors such as severe agitation, hallucinations, and delusions. Levels of consciousness may also fluctuate. The client may be alert one moment, only to fall asleep the next. Delirium is usually organically caused from metabolic, vascular, hematologic, or endocrine abnormalities. In assisting a delirious client, the nurse should follow the interventions suggested with the disoriented client (Chapter 21). Clocks, calendars, adequate lighting, and family members can help the delirious client become better oriented. The extremely agitated and hallucinating client can be calmed by antipsychotic medication. The important initial medical intervention is determining the organic etiology of the delirium and correcting it as soon as possible.

The following highlights the fear and confusion a person may experience when admitted to an ICU.

A 55-year-old married male, Mr. Arnold, was admitted to the ICU after having a three-vessel coronary artery bypass. Mr. Arnold's surgery had taken longer than usual and necessitated his remaining on a cardiac pump for three hours. He arrived in the ICU without further complications. Upon awakening from the anesthesia, he heard the nurse exclaim, "I need to get a gas." Another nurse answered in a loud voice saying, "Can you take a large needle for the injection?" During this period of time, Mr. Arnold was experiencing the need to urinate and asked the nurse very calmly if he could go to the bathroom. Her reply was, "You don't need to go; you have a tube in." He again complained about his discomfort and assured the nurse if she would let him go the bathroom, he would be fine. The nurse informed Mr. Arnold that he could not urinate and that he had to keep the "mask" on so that she could get the "gas" and check his "blood levels." Upon hearing this, Mr. Arnold began to implore the nurse louder and stated that he saw the bathroom sign "over there." He assured the nurse that he would only take a minute. In reality "the sign" was an exit sign in the unit. To prove to him that a bathroom did not exist in the ICU and that the sign did not indicate a bathroom, the nurse took off the restraints and led Mr. Arnold to the sign. He abruptly broke away from the nurse's grasp and ran toward the entrance to the ICU. He discovered a door, which was the entrance to nurses' lounge, and barricaded himself in the room and pulled out his chest tube, Foley catheter, and IV lines. Needless to say, he found the bathroom that was connected to the lounge. Ten minutes later the nurses and security personnel broke through the barricade and escorted Mr. Arnold back to bed. When he became fully alert and oriented a day later, he told the nurses his perception of the previous events. Initially he thought he had been kidnapped and was being held against his will (the restraints were rather tight). When the nurse had yelled out about blood gas, he had thought she was going to kill him with noxious gas through his face mask (the reason he did not want to wear the face mask). All he could think about was escaping his tormentor and executioner. In this case, the nurse did *not* assess the alteration in Mr. Arnold's mental status and had allowed him to get out of bed. The medical jargon and loud voices had perpetuated his confusion and distortion of reality. The nurses could have told Mr. Arnold where he was, that the nursing staff were caring for him, and could have better explained the function of his Foley catheter. Furthermore, the staff could have brought in family members to help calm and orient Mr. Arnold.

A PERSON WHO IS DYING OF CANCER

Concerns of the Dying Person

Nothing in life adequately prepares a person for his or her own death. The experience of terminal illness intensifies painful feelings of loss: loss of personal existence and physical health, loss of loved ones and friends, and loss of financial resources are some of the losses a dying person confronts. One of the most profound losses for a victim of terminal cancer may be the loss of personal identity, secondary to physical changes. Prolonged radiation and chemotherapy may leave one confused, overwhelmed, and alienated from one's former sense of self and sense of purpose.

After being told the diagnosis, a person may experience intense emotional reactions, ranging from feelings of emptiness or disbelief to feelings of rage or loss of control. Suddenly a person is faced with fears unparalleled to any previous life experience. Fears of prolonged suffering, constant pain, imminent death, leaving financial burdens, and alienation and isolation are often mentioned by a dying person. The fear of abandonment may be a terrifying concern. Often the known family doctor transfers the person to an oncologist soon after the diagnosis of cancer has been made. If the person has had extensive hospitalization, friends and relatives who initially visited may no longer be available. Eventually a person may fear that everyone may leave him or her to die.

The fear of pain and of financial ruin may be well founded. With some of the more lethal carcinomas, the course of the disease is long, with only brief periods of remission. However, not all cancers are painful or result in death (Jerse et al. 1984). The nurse needs to be knowledgeable about the different types of cancer and the various prognoses. Armed with this knowledge and aware of the clients' understanding of their illness, the nurse is equipped to lend support and guidance for clients and their families.

Concerns of the Family

The family also experience painful and conflicting emotions as they begin to deal with the diagnosis. Not only must they concern themselves with their individual emotional reactions to the diagnosis, they must also deal with the client's response. They may react with disbelief with statements such as "Are you sure?" Fear of the future, anger, and guilt are all common responses. In addition, how to communicate the news to other family members and friends becomes an issue (Euster 1984).

Several helpful approaches have been identified for use when the medical staff discuss cancer with a client and family (Guttenberg 1983):

1. Discuss the prognosis with family and client in private and allow for plenty of time.
2. Encourage everyone to sit down.
3. Expect that the client and family will have strength. "Expecting success fosters success; expecting failure fosters failure."
4. Give the client and family reason to hope by being specific about the diagnosis and treatments, by describing staff role and efforts, by accentuating the positive, by displaying confidence, and by getting the client and family involved in daily activities and decision making.

These are only suggestions. It is very important to realize that the approach needs to be individualized to meet the client's needs and coping styles.

As the client's hospitalization continues, the family must constantly deal with disequilibrium. Generally, the family are unfamiliar with the hospital system. Consulting physicians who come and go may only increase confusion for the family. Even though the family may have met the oncologist, they are often unsure of what questions to ask. Even after learning some of the medical information, they are still unsure of its meaning. Eventually, the family are confronted with the physical realities of cancer, the weakness, the changes in skin coloring, the weight loss, and the physical mutilations. They are worried about their response to their loved one and how he or she will perceive their response. All these issues add to the family's frustration, fatigue, and feelings of helplessness as they attempt to deal with their own reactions to the cancer (Euster 1984).

Discharge of the client brings another set of problems for the client and family. "The continued stress of an ill family member creates feelings of anger in relatives" (Euster 1984, p. 432). Sometimes the illness necessitates role reversal, which may produce anger. Along with anger come feelings of guilt. Over time the family members who experience no relief become depleted of emotional support, physical assistance, and financial support. As time progresses their ability to cope may diminish along with social and financial support (Euster 1984).

Concerns Among Staff Members

Staff also has strong reactions when faced with a terminally ill cancer client. Some staff may withdraw from the client. Nursing staff may withdraw because they do not know what to say to the person or they may not be aware of what the person has been told. Ideally, the nursing staff should accompany the doctor when the diagnosis is being explained to the client and family. Physicians and nurses may also withdraw when they overidentify with the client. Members of the health care team often experience loss through personal identification with the client (Benoliel 1985).

Before planning interventions, staff must first examine their own reactions to a client who is terminally ill. The nurse's reactions are influenced by similar factors that influence the reactions of the dying person. Cultural, educational, and religious background affect the nurse's ability to deal with death. Past experiences with cancer clients, deaths of clients, and deaths of family members also play a role in how the nurses will interact with the dying client and family. Besides these factors, Adams (1984) suggested six other variables that play a major role in how nurses respond to dying clients, as seen in Table 26–9.

All these factors and variables are reflected in the nurses' delivery of client care. If nurses find that they are not able to cope with the dying client, or their response is negative, they should ask to be excused from the case.

Stages in the Process of Dying

Dying is a difficult and often emotionally painful topic to discuss. Until Kübler-Ross (1969) published her classic work on how people deal with their own death, little attention was paid to this often avoided subject. Even though Kübler-Ross named five distinct stages in the process of dying, her intent was not to "classify" the client into a stage, but merely to understand the emotions of a dying individual so that health care providers could be more empathetic. Needless to say, dying

Table 26–9 • FACTORS THAT INFLUENCE A NURSE'S REACTION TO A DYING PATIENT

FACTOR	REACTION
1. Length of hospitalization	The longer the hospitalization, the more time the nurse has to form a relationship with the client and family. Nurses may begin to experience their own sense of mortality and become uncomfortable and withdraw. Nurses who can accept personal feelings will develop more empathy and become more supportive.
2. Frequency of admissions	More frequent admissions to the hospital strengthen the relationship between the patient and staff. The closer the relationship, the more attached the nurse may become and the more grief will be experienced by the nurse when the patient dies. If the hospitalizations have been marked with prolonged pain and suffering, the nurse may experience a sense of relief when the client dies.
3. The role of the family	When the family is not available, the nurse may assume the role of the family. This tends to bond the nurse to the patient. If the family is present, the nurse may identify with the family, or avoid them if they react as his or her family would. If the family expresses their anguish openly, the nurse may feel like withdrawing, especially if the family is from a different culture.
4. The patient's condition	The nurse tends to withdraw or feel indifferent toward a person who is unconscious.
5. The patient's coping style	An angry or dependent coping style tends to promote withdrawal and avoidance in the nurse. Nurses accept better the person who utilizes intellectualization and rationalization as coping strategies.
6. The role of the subconscious	If the client's mannerisms stir a memory of someone else the nurse has known, then the nurse may react counter-transferentially to the client as if the client were that other person.

clients may skip stages or return to the first stage after completing the fourth stage. The most important aspect of these five stages is to understand the psychological dynamics that the dying person and family are experiencing so that the nurse can best facilitate adaptive coping and provide individualized client care.

STAGE ONE: DENIAL AND ISOLATION. The first stage usually begins after the person has just learned of his or her diagnosis. The initial reaction of *denial, shock, and disbelief* is experienced by almost all clients, not only during this first stage but also later on, from time to time. After being told about their terminal illness, people are in a temporary state of shock. Their affect may be blunted. The content of conversation is, "No, this can't be happening to me." Sometimes clients may even begin talking about death only to change the topic and contradict themselves later in the conversation. This denial leads to feelings of loneliness and isolation as they attempt to protect themselves against the onslaught of emotions. "Denial is usually a temporary defense and will soon be replaced by partial acceptance." (Kübler-Ross 1969, p. 40).

Mr. Dodds, a 50-year-old married man, was admitted to the hospital and diagnosed with adenocarcinoma of the pancreas. When told about his diagnosis, Mr. Dodds replied, "How can that be? I've never smoked. You must have the wrong client." His initial denial was replaced by anger after several unsuccessful operations to alleviate an obstructed pancreas.

STAGE TWO: ANGER. After the denial has dissipated, reality begins to take the form of *anger, rage, resentment, and even envy*. "Why me?" is the most frequently asked question and the most difficult one for family and staff to respond to. There is never an answer to this question. Anger may be internalized or displaced onto staff and loved ones. Projected anger can take the form of demanding or intimidating behavior toward staff and family. It is important that the nurse does not internalize the client's displaced anger but understands its source (Kübler-Ross 1969). Staff need to work on acceptance of the person during this stage, not to withdraw and leave the dying person feeling abandoned (Kübler-Ross 1969).

Mr. Dodds exhibited his anger by constantly complaining about his room, the nursing care, and his pain medication schedule. When the nurses entered his room with his pain medication, he would comment about their unprofessional appearance, or ask them to straighten the flowers in his vase. Finally, one of the nurses took the time to sit down and talk with him. Her response to his demands was, "It must be really frustrating for you now. How can I best help you?" Her response took Mr. Dodds by surprise since most people quickly left the room in anger after completing a task. Mr. Dodds began to discuss his fears and later asked the nurse to visit more often.

STAGE THREE: BARGAINING. Most of the *bargaining is made with God* in an effort to postpone the inevitable. Promises to be a better person may be associated with guilt, which may be the result of irrational fears. It is important that the nurse explore feelings of guilt and not brush these feelings aside. Usually this stage is marked by statements such as, "If I eat more, will you let me go?" and "If only I can live until my son graduates, I'll donate all my savings to the church" (Kübler-Ross 1969; Robinson 1974).

Sometimes bargaining helps the client muster the energy to accomplish a goal.

Mrs. Abrahams, a 65-year-old widow diagnosed with breast cancer with metastasis to the lung, had one wish. She had always talked about her only grandson graduating from high school. She wanted to be there in the auditorium when he walked up the steps to receive his diploma. Even though her lung involvement was extensive and restricted her, she did attend her grandson's graduation in a wheelchair. Twenty-four hours after returning to the hospital, she died.

STAGE FOUR: DEPRESSION. Soon the numbness of the denial and the rage of the anger are replaced by a great sense of loss. The dying client can no longer pretend there is nothing wrong or that surgery can cure the disease. *Depression becomes the emotional response* as the client begins to cope with the actual losses or impending losses. Depression is also "the preparatory grief that the terminally ill client has to undergo in order to prepare himself for his final separation from this world" (Kübler-Ross 1969, p. 86). During this phase, staff become more uncomfortable and may tend to avoid the client. Usually psychiatric consultations are generated when the staff begin to feel hopeless and helpless to "cure" the cancer.

Mrs. Jewel, a 52-year-old married mother of two, was diagnosed with adenocarcinoma of the pancreas with metastasis to the liver. She had been ill for almost two years without a definitive diagnosis. Upon learning of her diagnosis, the woman replied, "Well, I'm glad to finally know what's been making me sick for all these months. I had a feeling it was cancer." Her major concern was how to tell her husband and two daughters. She felt hopeless and helpless to change her prognosis. Eventually, she stopped interacting with the nursing staff. During the psychiatric liaison nursing consultation, the psychiatric liaison nurse learned of her concern about informing her family that she was dying. The nurse encouraged Mrs. Jewel to "role-play" communicating her diagnosis to her family. Mrs. Jewel also wanted to know if it was normal to be thinking of funeral arrangements. Mrs. Jewel discussed her wishes for her funeral and how to broach the subject with her husband. Two days after this interaction with the nurse, she shared her grief and last wishes with her family. Three weeks later, she died.

STAGE FIVE: ACCEPTANCE. This last stage signifies that the client has had enough time and assistance to work through the previous stages of denial, anger, and depression. The person has mourned his or her losses and is left tired and weak. This is a difficult time for both the client and family. By this time the person is void of feelings; the struggle is gone. The person withdraws and no longer desires to communicate. Many people like the quiet reassurance of someone sitting nearby just holding their hand (Kübler-Ross 1969). Those who see cancer as a challenge may fight this stage until, one day, they decide they are too weak and can no longer fight.

Mrs. Yolanda was a 68-year-old widow who was diagnosed with adenocarcinoma of the abdomen with extensive abdominal metastasis. She had been previously hospitalized several times in this particular unit and was well known to the staff. Prior to this admission, Mrs. Yolanda was known for her independent personality and her humorous jokes, which kept a constant stream of staff coming into her room. Her abdominal girth had extensively enlarged from her ascites, causing shortness of breath and dyspnea on exertion. She found it difficult to sleep lying down and could rest only by lying her head on the bedside table while sitting. Even though fluid was drawn from her abdomen numerous times, Mrs. Yolanda's girth continued to expand. She became increasingly uncomfortable and listless. Gone were her entertaining jokes and witty remarks to the staff. She confided *in the staff a week before she died that she "prayed to God to die. I'm no longer afraid . . . I'm ready to go; just let me go."*

Nursing Interventions

WHEN WORKING WITH A DYING PERSON. *During the first stage*, denial and isolation, the nurse needs to know what the physician told the client and family. Possible interventions include the following:

1. Stay with the client as the person expresses his or her anxieties.
2. Actively listen to the person and reflect emotions.
3. Give physical comfort if acceptable to the person, e.g., putting a hand on the client's arm.
4. Encourage the client to express thoughts and feelings and identify realistic problems.
5. Answer questions regarding the disease and treatments when asked.

Give essential information at this time and expect the client to ask the same question repeatedly (Ostchega and Jacob 1984; Robinson 1974; Wright 1985).

The client experiences anger and rage *during the second phase*. This phase may be difficult for staff. If the nurse internalizes the client's anger, the nurse may tend to withdraw or become angry with the client. Suggested nursing interventions include the following:

1. Recognize client's anger as being displaced.
2. Reflect and acknowledge his or her right to be angry.
3. Assist family members in dealing with client's anger.
4. If a client loses control, the nurse must take charge, talk with him or her in a quiet room, and give a sedative if necessary.
5. Involve the dying person in decision making, giving the person a sense of control over the situation.

During phase three, bargaining, the nurse continues to intervene by

1. Encouraging the client to discuss fears which may be related to feelings of guilt.
2. Suggesting clergy to assist in dispelling irrational religious beliefs.
3. Focusing on client's strengths and abilities to cope with situations in the past.
4. Giving the client some "time-out" from staff intervention.

During the depression stage, the nurse can be helpful to the client by evaluating when to intervene. "Sometimes dying persons need to feel the pain of their losses, and not have attempts made to relieve their suffering" (Benoliel 1985). Besides continued supportive listening and communication, useful nursing interventions are as follows:

1. Assist the client to discover ways of normalizing his or her life in the face of discontinuity and change (Benoliel 1985).
2. Keep the client informed of treatments, procedures, medications, and adverse side effects.
3. Develop small, obtainable, measurable goals with the client's input, (e.g., sitting up in the bed for ten minutes twice a day).
4. Be careful of withdrawing from or avoiding the client at this stage.
5. Request psychiatric consultation if the client becomes suicidal.
6. Refer the client to a support group such as Cancer Care.
7. Be available to explore philosophical questions the client has about life, religious beliefs, or life hereafter.
8. Continue to provide needed relief for pain control.

In the last stage of acceptance, the major goal for the nurse is to keep the client as comfortable as possible. Nursing interventions focus on maintaining dignity, especially if the client is mentally alert yet control of bodily functioning has been lost. Since most clients are exhausted and tired, shorter interactions are indicated in keeping the client informed of daily happenings and preserving strength. Table 26–10 summarizes nursing interventions during the five stages of dying for the client who is terminally ill.

When Working with the Family. (Refer to Chapter 18 for working with a grieving family.) Specifically, the nurse works with the family to deal with the physical realities of the diagnosis of terminal cancer. In order to assist the client, the nurse must also be aware of how the family is reacting to the crisis. Nursing interventions include the following:

1. Encourage the family to share their thoughts, fears, and feelings and help them identify problems.
2. Encourage the family to share their concerns with the dying member in order to facilitate open communication.
3. Orient the family to the hospital and unit, explaining visiting hours, parking, lodging, and other practical necessities.
4. Encourage the family to ask the doctor questions; writing down their questions on paper will help them to remember.
5. Give the family private time with the client to share feelings.
6. Involve the family along with the client in decision making regarding care, which helps foster a sense of control, and encourage the family members to give

Table 26-10 • WORKING WITH A PERSON WHO IS DYING

SUGGESTED NURSING INTERVENTIONS	RATIONALE
Stage One: Denial and Isolation	
1. Examine own feelings about death.	1. Personal defenses and fears can be projected onto dying person.
2. Encourage the patient's expression of feelings, concerns and fears: • Sit at bedside. • Actively listen, reflect client's feelings. • Hold hand, touch shoulder, etc., when appropriate.	2. If not identified and worked out. • Provides presence, decreases feelings of abandonment. • Lessens feelings of isolation—keeps channels of communication open. • For some, physical touch provides comfort and demonstrates concern.
3. Provide small amount of information at a time. Encourage questions when client is ready.	3. Having correct information can decrease anxiety and clarify information.
4. Encourage decisions regarding self-care.	4. Increases feelings of control and encourages functioning at optimum level.
Stage Two: Anger phase	
1. Acknowledge person's right to be angry.	1. Increases feelings of support and being understood.
2. Understand that anger directed at staff and family is not personal.	2. Feelings of helplessness and loss stimulate anger often projected onto staff and loved ones.
3. Work with client to rechannel anger into positive channels, e.g., making decisions, setting goals, fighting disease.	3. Can help rechannel energy in ways that help increase self-esteem, feelings of control, and sense of being supported by staff and others.
Stage Three: Bargaining	
1. Offer to contact clergy/rabbi.	1. May assist in dispelling irrational religious beliefs.
2. Encourage discussion of feelings, especially guilt and loss.	2. Decreases feelings of guilt and possible thoughts of being punished for past actions.
3. Encourage client's positive coping strategies used in past.	3. Positive reinforcement can strengthen positive behaviors.
4. Encourage periods of time to focus on more satisfying areas of life.	4. Periods of time away from discussion of disease and death helps person put life in broader focus.
Stage Four: Depression	
1. Focus on daily short term *obtainable* goals.	1. Emphasizes positive functioning and areas of independence.
2. Continue to spend time with client on regular basis.	2. Staff awareness of tendency to withdraw can help staff modify own behaviors.
3. Encourage client to participate in usual activities.	3. Can decrease time spent in brooding and offer broader focus of experience.
4. Encourage client to participate in support groups.	4. Discussion with others in similar circumstances can decrease feelings of isolation and increase feelings of being understood.
5. Maintain adequate pain control.	5. Physical comfort can increase ability to interact with others and may diminish tendency to withdraw.
Stage Five: Acceptance	
1. Sit with person—even when person doesn't want to talk.	1. Provides presence and support and decreases feelings of abandonment.
2. Allow appropriate privacy, e.g., during toileting, bathing.	2. Maintains sense of dignity.
3. Continue pain control.	3. Provides comfort during final stages of dying.

feedback to the staff about the client's likes and dislikes.

7. Encourage the family to prioritize problems and solve each problem one by one.
8. Discuss hospice care as a possible alternative in the terminal stages of the illness.
9. Encourage family members to attend a support group if available such as Cancer Care. This can help the family feel less isolated and alone during this time.
10. Include the children in the grieving process.

Working with a terminally ill client can be difficult. Communicating openly and honestly and offering a presence during a period when most people withdraw can be a profound experience for the nurse and the dying person. In assisting the client through the stages of dying, the nurse can gain a great deal from the client's experience and in the relationship with the dying person. An empathetic and caring relationship facilitates the person's progression through the dying process and can instill a sense of accomplishment and connectedness in the nurse. Although difficult and emotionally draining, working with a terminally ill client offers unique rewards.

Summary

Emotional reactions to physical illness are expected. Sometimes emotional reactions to physical illness can impede recovery and block effective nursing care. This can leave both the client and the staff in conflict or crisis. In many institutions it is the psychiatric liaison nurse who is available to help staff assess the client's situation and plan care more effectively with the client. The psychiatric liaison nurse has a knowledge of physical illness and the clinical skills to help people deal more effectively with emotional problems.

All nurses need to be aware of the stresses a person encounters when hospitalized for the first time. The nurse also needs to assess the particular coping strategies a client is using. By supporting and encouraging positive coping strategies while minimizing and undermining negative coping strategies, the nurse can greatly affect the way a person copes with his or her illness. Nurses need also to be aware of the specific emotional issues involved with common though complex medical illnesses and conditions. Such awareness can increase the nurse's ability to better evaluate for health teaching, empathize with the person's experience, formulate more meaningful nursing diagnoses, and plan effective nursing care.

The emotional experience a person may encounter during a specific medical illness and suggested nursing actions were discussed in this chapter. The specific medical illnesses include working with a person who is in chronic pain, who is severely burned, who suffers from AIDS, who has cardiac dysfunction, who is in an ICU, and, lastly, who is dying of cancer.

References

Adams F. 6 Very good reasons why we react differently to various dying patients. Nursing '84, 14:8, 1984.

AIDS Update. Know the early signs of HIV dementia complex. Nursing '88, 16(6): 18, 1988.

Althof S, Coffman C, Levine S. The effects of coronary bypass surgery on the female sexual, psychological and vocational adaptation. Journal of Sex and Marital Therapy, 10(3):176, 1984.

Andreasen N. Neuropsychiatric complications in burn patients. International Journal of Psychiatry in Medicine, 5(2):161, 1974.

Baer JW, Hall JM, Hulm K, Lewitter-Keohler S. Challenges in developing an inpatient psychiatric program for people with AIDS and ARC. Hospital and Community Psychiatry, 38(12):1299, 1987.

Benoliel J. Loss and terminal illness. Nursing Clinics of North America, 20(2):439, 1985.

Blumenthal J, O'Toole L, Haney T. Behavioral assessment of the type A behavior pattern. Psychosomatic Medicine 46(5):415, 1984.

Cassem N, Hackett T. The setting of intensive care. *In* Hackett T, Cassem N (eds). Massachusetts General Hospital Handbook of General Hospital Psychiatry. St. Louis: C.V. Mosby Company, 1978.

Centers for Disease Control. Current trends: Update on acquired immune deficiency syndrome (AIDS). United States Morbidity and Mortality Weekly Report, 31:507, 1986.

Centers for Disease Control. Acquired immunodeficiency syndrome (AIDS) among blacks and Hispanics. United States Morbidity and Mortality Weekly Report, 35:663, 1987.

Croog S. The heart patient after hospitalization: Social and psychological factors in life after a heart attack. Connecticut Medicine, 48 (10):633, 1984.

Escobar P. Management of chronic pain. Nurse-Practitioner, January: 24, 1985.

Euster S. Adjusting to an adult family member's cancer. *In* Roback H (ed). Helping Patients and Their Families Cope with Medical Problems. San Francisco: Jossey-Bass Publishers, 1984, pp. 428–452.

Faulstich ME. Psychiatric aspects of AIDS. American Journal of Psychiatry, 144(5):551, 1987.

Fife B, Lemler S. The psychiatric nurse specialist: A valuable asset in the general hospital. Journal of Nursing Administration, 13(4):14, 1983.

Fife B. The challenge of the medical setting for the clinical nurse specialist in psychiatric nursing. Journal of Psychiatric Nursing and Mental Health Services, 21(1):8, 1983.

Foley, K. The treatment of cancer pain. New England Journal of Medicine, 313(2):84, 1983.

Gondek M. Post-MI sex: Those unspoken fears. RN, 46(5):61, 1983.

Gong V, Rudnick M. AIDS Facts and Issues. New Brunswick, NJ: Rutgers University Press, 1986.

Goodstein R. Burns: An overview of clinical consequences affecting patient, staff and family. Comprehensive Psychiatry, 26(1):43, 1985.

Greenspan K. Biofeedback in the control of chronic pain. *In* Mark L (ed). Pain Control: Practical Aspects of Patient Care. New York: Masson Publishing, 1981, pp. 89–94.

Guttenberg R. Softening the blow: How to break bad news to a patient's family. Nursing Life, July/August: 17, 1983.

Hackett T. The pain patient: Evaluation and treatment. *In* Hackett T, Cassem N (eds). Massachusetts General Hospital Handbook of General Hospital Psychiatry. St. Louis: C.V. Mosby Company, 1978.

Hackett T. Depression following myocardial infarction. Psychosomatics (Supplement), 26(11):23, 1985.

Harper G. The burn unit. *In* Hackett T, Cassem N. (eds). Massachusetts

General Hospital Handbook of General Hospital Psychiatry. St. Louis: C.V. Mosby Company, 1978.
Hendler N, Fernandez P. Alternative treatments for patients with chronic pain. Psychiatric Annals, 10(12):25, 1980.
Jerse M, Whitman H, Gustafson J. Cancer in adults. *In* Roback H (ed). Helping Patients and Their Families Cope With Medical Problems. San Francisco: Jossey-Bass Publishers, 1984, pp. 251–284.
Johnson B. Psychiatric nurse consultant in the general hospital. Nursing Outlook, 2:728, 1963.
Jorgensen J, Brophy J. Psychiatric treatment modalities in burn patients. Current Psychiatric Therapies, 85 , 1975.
Kaplan HI, Sadock BJ. Synopsis of Psychiatry, Behavioral Sciences Clinical Psychiatry. Baltimore, Williams & Wilkins, 1988.
Kleinman A. Mental health and chronic pain. The Harvard Medical School Mental Health Letter, 8(2):4, 1989.
Kübler-Ross E. On Death and Dying. New York: Macmillan, 1969.
Lazarus R. Stress and coping as factors in health and illness. *In* Cohen J, Cullen J, Martin R (eds). Psychosocial Aspects of Cancer. New York: Raven Press, 1982, pp. 163–190.
Lewis A, Levy J. Psychiatric Liaison Nursing: The Theory and Clinical Practice. Reston, Virginia: Reston Publishing Company, 1982.
Lipowski Z. Physical illness, the individual, and the coping process. Psychiatry in Medicine, 1:91, 1970.
L.K. HIV risk (still) low for health care workers. American Journal of Nursing, 88(7):950, 1988a.
L.K. Incidence of AIDS among children. American Journal of Nursing, 88(7):951, 1988b.
L.K. Prophylactic retrovir study for health care workers. American Journal of Nursing, 88(7):950, 1988c.
Matthews K. Psychological perspectives on type A behavior pattern. Psychological Bulletin, 91(2):293, 1982.
Mayou R. Prediction of emotional and social outcome after a heart attack. Journal of Psychosomatic Research, 28(1):17, 1984.
McGuire L. Seven myths about pain relief. RN, December: 30, 1983.
Meisenhelder JB, LaCharite. Comfort in Caring: Nursing the Person with HIV Infection, Glenview, IL: Scott, Foresman and Company, 1989.
Mendelson I. Liaison psychiatry and the burn center. Psychosomatics, 24(3):235, 1983.
Menenberg SR. Somatopsychology and AIDS victims. Journal of Psychosocial Nursing, 25(5):18, 1987.
Moore K, Folk-Lighty M, Nolen M. The joy of sex after a heart attack: Counseling the cardiac patient. Nursing '84, April; 104, 1984.
Ochitill H, Havassy B, Byrd R, Peters R. Leaving a cardiology service against medical advice. Journal of Chronic Disease, 38(1):78, 1985.
Ostchega Y, Jacob J. Providing "safe conduct": Helping your patient cope with cancer. Nursing '84, April: 42, 1984.
Perry S. Debate: Warning third parties at risk of AIDS: APA Policy is a barrier to treatment. Hospital and Community Psychiatry, 40(2):158, 1989.
Perry SW, Markowitz JC. Psychiatric interventions for AIDS-spectrum disorders. Hospital and Community Psychiatry, 37(10):1001, 1986.
Perry SW, Markowitz JC. Counseling for HIV testing. Hospital and Community Psychiatry, 39(7):731, 1988.
Price W, Forejt J. Neuropsychiatric aspect of AIDS: A case report. General Hospital Psychiatry, 8:7, 1986.
Razin A. Coronary artery disease. *In* Roback H (ed). Helping Patients and Their Families Cope With Medical Problems. San Francisco: Jossey-Bass Publishers, 1984.
Robinson L. Liaison Nursing: Psychological Approach to Patient Care. Philadelphia: F.A. Davis Company, 1974.
Rogers A. 21 Problems in pain control—and ways to solve them. Your Patient & Cancer, September: 65, 1984.
Rogers MF, Williams WW. AIDS in blacks and Hispanics: implications for prevention. Issues in Science and Technology 3:89, 1987.
Rosenman R. The interview method of assessment of the coronary-prone behavior pattern. *In* Dembrowski T, Weiss S, Shields J, Haynes S, Feinleib (eds). Coronary-Prone Behavior. New York: Springer-Verlag, 1978.
Salisbury DM. AIDS psychosocial implications. Journal of Psychosocial Nursing, 24(12):13, 1986.
Schmitt M. The nature of pain with some personal notes. Nursing Clinics of North America, 12(4):621, 1977.
Schuman M. Biofeedback in the management of chronic pain. *In* Adrian C, Barker J (eds). Psychological Approaches to the Management of Pain. New York: Brunner/Mazel, 1982.
Thornbury K. Coping: Implications for health practitioners. Patient Counseling and Health Education, 4(1):3, 1982.
Tuggle D. Meeting the emotional needs of survivors of sudden cardiac death. Cardiovascular Nursing, 18(5):25, 1982.
Visvanathan R, Vizner T. The experience of myocardial infarction as a threat to one's personal adequacy. General Hospital Psychiatry, 6: 83, 1984.
Wain H. Pain control with hypnosis in consultation and liaison psychiatry. Psychiatric Annals, 16(2):106, 1986.
Weisman A. Coping with illness. *In* Hackett T, Cassem N (eds). Massachusetts General Hospital Handbook of General Hospital Psychiatry. St. Louis: C.V. Mosby Company, 1978, pp. 264–275.
Weisman A. The Coping Capacity: On the Nature of Being Mortal. New York: Human Sciences Press, 1984.
Wells G. Aggressive management of ventricular arrhythmia: With newer techniques to predict drug efficacy. Postgraduate Medicine, 74:145, 1983.
Wright L. Life threatening illness. Journal of Psychosocial Nursing, 23(9):7, 1985.
Zborowski M. People in Pain. San Francisco: Jossey-Bass, Inc., 1969.

Self-Study Exercises

Place a T (True) or F (False) next to each statement.

1. ________ Most people have plenty of time to adjust to "the sick role."
2. ________ A person is forced to give up parts of his or her identity and independent functioning during the first few days of hospitalization.
3. ________ Financial worries and distance from support systems can be major concerns for the hospitalized person.
4. ________ Fear of death is often the ultimate concern for a surgical patient.

Put a + (plus) for positive coping strategies or a 0 for negative coping strategies used by a hospitalized patient.

5. ________ Seek information, get guidance for decision making.
6. ________ Deny as much as possible.

7. ________ Share and discuss concerns, find consolation.
8. ________ Blame or shame someone or something for what is happening.

Choose the letter that best answers the following questions:

9. Chronic pain is different from acute pain. Which statement is false regarding chronic pain?

   A. A person slowly adapts to the pain.
   B. The patient is the key for assessing the level of intensity.
   C. A placebo does not work for a person in chronic pain.
   D. There may be no increase in pulse or blood pressure in chronic pain as there is in acute pain.

10. All of the following can be useful for the management of chronic pain. Which of the following would be the LEAST helpful in the management of chronic pain?

   A. Relaxation techniques, hypnosis, and guided imagery.
   B. Giving a placebo without the person's knowledge helps separate physical from psychological pain.
   C. Encouraging the person to take an active role in his or her own pain management.
   D. Always assess site, character, onset, and duration. Suggest that the patient keep a log.

Place the correct behavioral characteristics next to the stage of recovery in severe burns.

11. ________ Stage One
12. ________ Stage Two
13. ________ Stage Three
14. ________ Stage Four

A. Pain management is the physical focus and grieving the major psychological issue.

B. Delayed grief may appear. Redefining work and family role are major issues.

C. After initial calm, patient may become delirious and confused and "flashbacks" are common.

D. Patient may request mirrors to assess "changed self" and have concerns about sexual desirability.

Short Essay

15. For each of the four stages of recovery write down at least four interventions the nurse would consider when planning care for a client.

Place T (True) or F (False) next to each statement.

16. ________ A person with AIDS should be in isolation that requires staff to gown and glove.
17. ________ AIDS is restricted to those in the homosexual community and those who abuse IV drugs.
18. ________ Staff inservice conferences and frequent discussion of fears and myths regarding working with a person with AIDS reduce staff anxiety and can increase patient's emotional as well as physical comfort.
19. ________ Hugging, using the toilet, or eating off the dishes of an HIV-infected person can spread the disease.

Choose the letter that best answers the following questions:

20. Choose the answer that would trigger the LEAST amount of conflict or stress in a person with cardiac dysfunction.
    A. Sexual concerns regarding performance after myocardial infarction.
    B. Fear of loss of control or death may trigger denial of condition or medical noncompliance.
    C. Grieving may result in a clinical depression when hope is not sustained.
    D. Concern regarding hospital policy.
21. Which of the following is a common phenomenon in a surgical ICU?
    A. Dementia
    B. Delirium
    C. Phobia
    D. Somatization

Place the behaviors next to the corresponding stage in Kübler-Ross's five stages in the process of dying.

22. ________ Denial and Isolation
23. ________ Anger
24. ________ Bargaining
25. ________ Depression
26. ________ Acceptance

A. "If I take my medicine every day I will live."

B. "I feel so depressed. The staff seem to avoid coming into my room."

C. "I'm not afraid any longer, I'm ready to die now."

D. "I'm not dying . . . You have the wrong person."

E. "Why me? . . . How could God do this to me? It's not fair!"

27. For each of the above stages, name four nursing interventions and discuss the rationale for each.

CHAPTER 27

Children and Adolescents

Margaret H. Pipchick

OUTLINE

THE ROLE OF THE NURSE

Children

UNIQUE ASSESSMENT STRATEGIES
- Family
- Play
- Drawings
- Genogram
- General Observations
- Cultural and Religious Values

UNIQUE INTERVENTION STRATEGIES
- Psychotherapeutic Interventions
- Health Teaching
- Activities of Daily Living
- Somatic Therapies
- Psychotherapy

ISSUES THAT AFFECT THE MENTAL HEALTH OF SOME CHILDREN
- Mental Retardation
- Attention Deficit Disorder
- Conduct Disorder
- Separation Anxiety Disorder
- Pervasive Developmental Disorder—Autistic Disorder

Adolescents

UNIQUE ASSESSMENT STRATEGIES

UNIQUE INTERVENTION STRATEGIES
- Psychotherapeutic Interventions
- Health Teaching
- Activities of Daily Living
- Somatic Therapies
- Therapeutic Environment
- Psychotherapy

ISSUES THAT AFFECT THE MENTAL HEALTH OF SOME ADOLESCENTS
- Identity Disorder
- Adjustment Disorder
- Depression and Suicide
- Other Disorders

SUMMARY

KEY TERMS CONCEPTS

The key terms and concepts listed here also appear in bold where they are defined or discussed in this chapter.

ASSESSMENT OF THE CHILD
- Play Therapy
- Drawing
- Genogram

CHILD-ADOLESCENT PSYCHIATRIC NURSE SPECIALIST

PLAY THERAPY

MENTAL RETARDATION

ATTENTION DEFICIT DISORDER

CONDUCT DISORDER

SEPARATION ANXIETY

PERVASIVE DEVELOPMENTAL DISORDER—AUTISTIC DISORDER

ADOLESCENCE

MILIEU THERAPY

IDENTITY DISORDER

ADJUSTMENT DISORDER

ADOLESCENT DEPRESSION

The Role of the Nurse

Nurses draw from a broad range of theories in their work with children and adolescents. Theories include developmental (Erikson, Freud, Piaget), systems theory, psychoanalytic, interpersonal (Sullivan), and behavioral or cognitive (see Chapter 2).

John Bowlby (1988) stresses the influence on personality development and mental health of the child's and adolescent's sense of self and ability to relate and to handle adversity. Bowlby states that a child who grows up through adolescence with affectionate and responsible parents is provided with a secure base from which to explore the world and a place to return to in difficulty. This child is likely to grow up cheerful, socially cooperative, and an effective citizen, who will not break down in adversity. Unfortunately, the converse is often true. Children who are not provided the necessary support and encouragement are more likely to be less cheerful, to find life difficult, to have difficulty in intimate relationships, and to be vulnerable in conditions of adversity.

There is no theory that encompasses all aspects of human development. There are no answers for all children. Children differ in their rate of emotional and physical growth. They also tend to regress more quickly than adults, based on stress levels and degree of tiredness and pain. Loss of control and frustration easily lead to regressive behaviors in children. Therefore, symptoms in children do not have the same significance as in adults. Regressive symptoms in children may be the result of stresses that are inherent in development rather than true pathology. A fully established symptom may last for long periods of time and is not occasional in its occurrence.

Nurses observe children and adolescents and their families in a variety of settings. Nurses working with children in hospitals, well-child clinics, schools, camps, doctors' offices, and community health centers are in a position to identify potential developmental or emotional problems. Nurses can act as educators and provide needed resources and support for children, adolescents, and their families.

Nurses who work with children and adolescents in a psychiatric setting need to communicate with a variety of professionals regarding the types of problems they diagnose and treat. The level of independent assessment by nurses will depend upon their level of education. For example, nurses who are generalists may work with children in a variety of settings and should have a clear understanding of developmental theory. Nurses at the generalist level working in child psychiatric settings follow the same guidelines as they do for all other settings, as delineated in the *Standards of Psychiatric and Mental Health Nursing Practice* (1982). Essentially the nurse at the generalist level

1. Follows the steps in the nursing process, using sound scientific theory. Therefore, the nurse assesses, formulates nursing diagnoses, plans care and appropriate interventions, and evaluates client response to nursing action.
2. Uses specific interventions based on the following standards:
   - V-A *Psychotherapeutic interventions*
   - V-B *Health teaching* to families, groups, clients
   - V-C Fostering *activities of daily living*
   - V-D Administration of, recording of, and teaching involved with *somatic therapies*
   - V-E Assists in structuring a *therapeutic environment*

A specialist holds at least a Master's degree and is usually certified by the ANA in child and adolescent psychiatric nursing. Specialists may assume the generalist role as well as other specialists roles, samples of which follow (Grossman and Mayton 1988):

1. Participant in child, adolescent, family, or group psychotherapy
2. Clinical supervisor of client care, staff, and graduate nursing students
3. Educator of nurses and other child care personnel in a variety of academic and clinical settings
4. Consultant to professional and nonprofessional groups or individuals concerned with the general welfare, education, and care of children
5. Researcher who contributes to theory and practice of child and adolescent psychiatric nursing

Children

OBJECTIVES

After studying this section on children, the student will be able to:

1. Compare and contrast the functions of a nurse generalist with those of a nurse specialist when working with children with mental disorders.
2. Identify issues that can increase anxiety to crisis levels in families.
3. Discuss the following areas of assessment in child psychiatry:
   - A. Family
   - B. Play
   - C. Drawings
   - D. Genogram
   - E. General observations
   - F. Cultural and religious mores
4. Explain why play therapy, group work, and health teaching are especially useful interventions when working with children.
5. Describe the clinical characteristics in the following DSM III-R diagnostic categories and give a possible nursing diagnosis for each:
   - A. Mental Retardation
   - B. Attention Deficit Disorder
   - C. Conduct Disorder
   - D. Separation Anxiety Disorder
   - E. Pervasive Developmental Disorder—Autistic Disorder

The magnitude of children's mental health needs is overwhelming. It is estimated that at least 12% of children suffer from emotional or other problems that warrant mental health treatment (Pothier 1988). Mental health problems of children are often more difficult to identify than those of adults because of the need to distinguish between normal aspects of child development and mental health problems that could escalate if not treated (Pothier 1988).

Anxiety is a natural human phenomenon that has its early beginnings prior to birth and is inherent in the birth process. Throughout the stages of a child's development, anxiety is seen as a major and normal part of personality organization. Children experience a great deal of anxiety during the stages of normal development. Melanie Klein states that the principal task of the small child is to master the pressure of anxiety (1975).

Many children are at risk for mental illness due to societal and environmental issues, as well as cognitive or genetically inherited disorders (Pothier 1988). Some social and genetic issues responsible for alterations in a child's mental health are discussed briefly here.

SOCIAL ISSUES. There are many internal and external stresses that can increase anxiety within a family. When effective parenting skills, emotional or financial resources, or appropriate coping behaviors are not available, the mental health of a family is threatened. Some common external stresses follow.

Changes in Family Structure. A child is born into a family. Whatever structure that family may have, children need the family to facilitate their growth into loving, mature, flexible individuals who can adjust to an ever-changing future (Schuster 1986).

The tasks of the family are to provide security in emotional expression, sexual differentiation, and support for growth. The ability of the family to meet these tasks can foster or hinder the child's ability to master anxiety. Children are sensitive to the feelings of those around them.

The degree of anxiety that exists within parents or caretakers is often absorbed by the child. Changes in family structure can make meeting family tasks difficult. For example, some parents have increased financial or emotional burdens that may leave little energy free for helping children cope with normal developmental crises. The number of blended or stepfamilies is increasing in our society. Since this is a fairly new trend, role models for these parents are scarce, and the struggle to merge two families into one is tremendously taxing.

As more women return to work, younger children are in the hands of multiple caregivers, who, despite their qualifications and warmth, may frequently change. This increases the demands made on the child for handling additional stress and anxiety. Changes in family structure inevitably bring conflicts. Family members can experience tremendous growth when conflicts are worked through and each member is able to give and receive support through the changes. However, when insufficient support is available to an already anxious child, problems often occur and mental disorders may ensue.

Unemployment. The occurrence of sudden or chronic unemployment is a major stressor for families. This phenomenon is experienced at all levels of society. It can create a crisis because it leads to necessary changes in the family's financial status and frequently affects the self-esteem of all members.

Fear of Nuclear War. The threat of nuclear war affects the feelings of even young children regarding their belief in a future. Hopelessness and despair about the future create questions of whether life is or is not worthwhile. Adolescents particularly can become paralyzed by hopelessness during the time they should be looking toward and planning for a future.

Alcohol and Drugs. Dependency on alcohol and drugs is one of our country's largest health problems. Alcoholism and drug dependency are diseases that for many become ways of dealing with life's stresses. The family is affected when consequences of drugs or alcohol lead to ineffective parenting, inability to maintain relationships, and job loss. The child or adolescent is affected when use of substances interferes with the development of problem-solving skills, and the use of effective coping devices.

GENETIC FACTORS. Genetics can influence personality in relation to the development and functioning of the autonomic nervous system. A relationship has been demonstrated between genetic composition and a tendency toward introversion (more withdrawn) and extraversion (more outgoing). Genetic controls affect intelligence, motor skills, and personality (Pothier 1976). Irregularities in the genes can be the etiological factor in certain birth defects such as Down's syndrome, spina bifida, Tay-Sachs disease, and sickle cell anemia. Each of these effects of genetic components can lead to increased stress on the child and the family.

The specific disorders presented in this section on children are (1) mental retardation, (2) attention deficit disorder, (3) conduct disorder, (4) separation anxiety disorder, and (5) pervasive developmental disorder—autistic disorder.

Unique Assessment Strategies

When **assessing children,** the nurse needs to keep in mind (Fagin 1972):

1. Behaviors that are normal for a given age and developmental problems characteristic for that age. For example, it is normal for a two-year-old to cling to mother when faced with a stranger.
2. That there are individual deviations from the norm. One deviation or difference is not necessarily indicative of an emotional disturbance.
3. That repeated observations are necessary for an adequate evaluation.

A review of developmental age-related tasks is provided in Table 27–1 (Fagin 1972).

The assessment process occurs through clinical interviews of the child and family. Areas of assessment include (1) family, (2) play, (3) drawings, (4) genogram, (5) general observations, and (6) cultural and religious values.

FAMILY

During the family interview the nurse assesses (1) the presenting problem(s), (2) current family functioning, and (3) family attitude toward the child. Specific areas include

1. Commitment
   - What is the family's commitment to the child?
   - What is the family's commitment to understanding the symptom?
   - Is the family open to exploring some of the issues contributing to the problem?
2. Power
   - Who has the power in the family?
   - Is it the child with the symptom or the parents?
   - How do conflicts get resolved?
3. Closeness/Intimacy
   - How much sharing goes on in this family?
   - Are differences allowed?
   - What do the family members say about affection, talking, or closeness?
4. Ability to solve problems
   - What attempts have been made to resolve the current issue?

Table 27–1 • OUTLINE OF TOOLS AND TASKS BY ERAS OF DEVELOPMENT: CHILDHOOD

TASKS	TOOLS	IF TASKS NOT ACHIEVED
	Birth Through 1, 1½, 2 Years	
1. Learning to count on others to gratify needs, trust.	1. Crying and other prespeech vocalizations. 2. Mouth—used to express feelings (biting, spitting, pushing out) and satisfaction or dissatisfaction. 3. Empathetic observations, perceives feelings of other as his own. 4. Emergency reaction expressed by crying, increased motor activity, or apathy in the face of • fear • anxiety • rage 5. Experimentation, exploration, manipulation. 6. Autistic invention—allows for feelings of control, sees environment in highly personalized way.	If the child does not develop a strong sense of self, in later life problems of *mistrust, lack of self-confidence, dependency*, and *superficial relationships* may be experienced.
	1½ to 3 Years	
1. Learning to accept interference with one's wishes in relation to comfort. 2. Develops a sense of autonomy, sense of self.	1. Language—uses meaningful sounds to communicate. 2. Anus—tool used to give or withhold, control significant people in the environment to express feelings of power. 3. Experimentation, exploration, manipulation become more refined; behaviors seen: • exhibitionism • imitation • aggressive behavior • increased locomotion • masturbation	Autonomy does not develop. May express itself as excessive needs for control, order, overconforming behavior, and irrational rituals. Manifested in feelings of shame and doubt.
	3 to 6 Years	
1. Learning to separate from parents and socialize outside the family. • associates with age mates • imitates roles and responses • learns to stand alone • sexual identity 2. Develops a sense of initiative; learns to • select goals • persevere • recognize own worth • feel worthy and competent	1. Self—functions as it develops in terms of ego strengths and superego structure. 2. Emergency reaction; these are • shame • anger • guilt • doubt • anxiety	Child may lack initiative and belief in self-mastery. Problems can arise as to sexual or personal roles. Rigidity may be seen and the child may experience guilt. Reluctance to explore new skills, test abilities.
	6 to 9 Years	
1. Learns to form satisfactory relationship with peers. 2. Learns to win recognition by productivity. 3. Intellectually able to encompass the abstract, objective, or general event, e.g., — distinguishes fantasy and reality — rational connection between cause and effect	1. Competition—used to contest for affection and status. 2. Compromise—enables child to give and take in a reciprocal relationship to retain own position. 3. Cooperation—enables child to maintain own position by adjusting to wishes of others.	Child may have difficulty relating to peers. Feels inadequate and experiences a low self-esteem and inferiority which may persist into later life. Child may be unprepared for school. Reluctance to explore and form relationships and to explore the environment.

TASKS	TOOLS	IF TASKS NOT ACHIEVED
	6 to 9 Years	
4. Sees self in relation to others, e.g., — accepts reasonable restraints — begins to become self-reliant — begins to accept responsibility and take consequences for behavior — learns appropriate responses to situation	4. Experimenation, exploration, manipulation—further refined: • experiences learning as fun • cooperative play • recreational and sexual curiosity • becomes more aware of self and the world around him	

Adapted from Fagin C. Nursing in Child Psychiatry. St. Louis: C.V. Mosby Company, 1972, and Haber J. Developmental processes. *In* Haber J, Hoskins PP, Leach AM, and Sideleau BF (eds). Comprehensive Psychiatric Nursing, 3rd ed. New York: McGraw-Hill Book Company, 1987.

- How do family members communicate problems or concerns to each other?

5. Communication
   - How do members communicate with each other?
   - Are all members allowed to share?
   - Are feelings discussed?
   - Do family members listen to each other?

PLAY

Often children are unable to express themselves verbally. **Play** can be used by the nurse as a vehicle for communication as well as an arena for the child to act out internal conflicts.

Play sessions are held in an area where noise won't disturb others and normal accidents are acceptable (e.g., spilled paint). The room needs to be free from outside pressures. Some play materials that encourage freedom of expression are nursing bottles, dolls, doll houses, toy soldiers, cowboys or Indians, toy animals, puppets, crayons, paper, paints, clay, and cars. Games are useful for children who are too anxious to express themselves through play. The child's disturbing and often painful feelings are frequently revealed through projection onto play objects and through story telling.

DRAWINGS

Usually the child is asked to draw separate pictures of a house, a tree, and people. This provides data for assessing a child's interpsychic life. When a child draws a picture of a house, tree, and family interacting, family relationship problems can be revealed. Only individuals qualified to interpret drawings should do so. Nurses may ask the child to explain the drawings as a vehicle for communication but should not make assumptions about meanings unless specially trained.

GENOGRAM

A **genogram** is a systematic diagram of the three-generational relationships within a family system. It starts with the primary relationship in a nuclear family—*the parents. Children and brothers and sisters of the parents are added.* Squares are drawn to represent men, circles to represent women. Ages and dates of death are inserted in the respective squares or circles. Then the functioning of the family is reviewed. For example, which relationships are steady, which shift, which are functional? Attention is given to what was going on when the child was born and what was going on when the child's symptoms first appeared. Refer to Figure 27–1 for a sample of a genogram.

GENERAL OBSERVATIONS

The nurse also observes the child's verbal and nonverbal behaviors. Areas include affect and anxiety, mood, capacity to relate, cognitive level, and physical and neurological development. Refer to Table 27–2.

CULTURAL AND RELIGIOUS VALUES

Cultural and religious values should be considered part of the total assessment of the child. Questions the nurse might ask include the following (Pothier 1976):

- *What role does religion play?*
- *Does the family see their situation as hopeless?*
- *Is the family oriented to the present? Can they think about the future?*
- *Are they more action oriented?*
- *Is the good of the family more important than the individual?*
- *How similar is the functioning of this family to other families in their culture?*

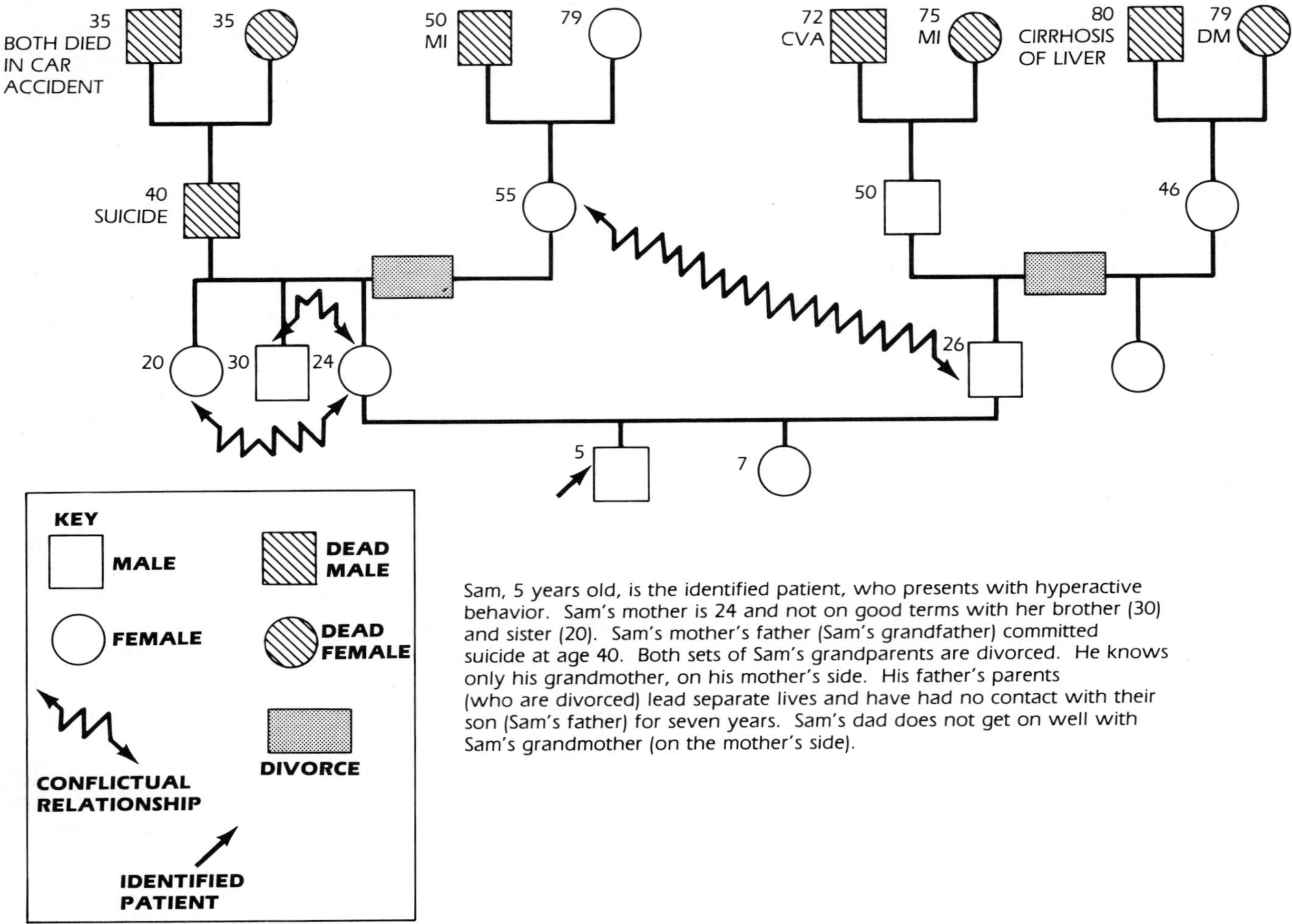

Figure 27–1. *Example of a genogram.*

The nurse needs to be aware of personal cultural values and be able to accept that clients may have different values.

Unique Intervention Strategies

During the clinical interview the nurse creates a warm, comfortable atmosphere. Genuinely attending to the child and family and preventing interruptions help facilitate communication. Uncomfortable feelings expressed by the members of the family as well as those experienced by the nurse need to be tolerated to understand what the family is experiencing on a day-to-day level. The nurse privately notes observations from the first moment of the first meeting. For example, who does the child stay close to? How does the child relate to other persons in the waiting area? Does the child come readily?

A major problem for nurses working with children is that of overinvolvement with the child. A nurse may easily become too subjective instead of maintaining therapeutic objectivity. Frequently when children's basic needs are not met, the nurse views the parents as villains. When this happens the nurse responds with attempts to rescue the child, rather than enlisting the parents as members of the same team.

Other reactions the nurse might have indicating overinvolvement include the following:

1. Telling children their feelings of anger are bad or not acceptable.
2. Wanting to hit the child.
3. Silently or verbally blaming the parents.

Table 27–2 • VERBAL AND NONVERBAL AREAS TO BE OBSERVED

AREA TO BE OBSERVED	SOME OBSERVATIONS TO BE NOTED
Affects and anxiety	How does the child use the environment? What emotions are observed? When do emotions change? Are affects appropriate during play? Are affects appropriate to child's age?
Mood	What is the overall emotional tone of the child? Is the child sad, happy, angry?
Capacity to relate	How does the child treat the nurse as a person? How much contact does the child initiate? Is the child affectionate, warm, aloof?
Cognitive level	Is the child able to move from an activity to talking about what is on his or her mind? How does a child tell a story? How far does the story progress?
Physical and neurological development	Child's posture Skin condition Height and weight Gait and balance Fine motor coordination Gross motor coordination Speech — lisps or stutters Quality and tone of voice Sensorimotor coordination Sensory intactness

When implementing nursing interventions, the nurse should guard against overinvolvement with the child.

PSYCHOTHERAPEUTIC INTERVENTIONS

The Child-Adolescent Psychiatric Nurse Specialist works with the family to identify dysfunctional behaviors, to modify or eliminate these behaviors, and to help the child develop more functional behaviors and to form satisfying relationships.

The child's symptoms are often a symptom of a dysfunctional family system. When this is the case, the ideal approach is to focus on the family. Children may need some individual sessions. The family will attempt to return to old ways of relating if interventions do not include the whole family.

Group therapy is a method of choice for children who share common problems. It is helpful for a child to know that other children experience the same feelings about such issues as divorce, chronic illness, or death of a parent. Isolation is diminished, common feelings are discussed, solutions are suggested, and sympathetic ties are formed during the group process.

Self-help groups can be extremely helpful for children and adolescents. Such groups as Alatot, Alateen, and many others exist nationwide. See the list of self-help clearing houses in the appendix.

HEALTH TEACHING

Primary prevention is one of the most important areas of nurses' work with children and families. Opportunities are always available in a health or hospital setting. Parents can be taught about their child's current developmental stage and be helped to prepare for the following stage.

Parents can also be taught to listen to their children's messages and be encouraged to talk about their own as well as their children's feelings:

- *How does your child express his feelings?*
- *What did you observe? How did he look?*
- *What did he or she say?*
- *What were your child's feelings? Did you check them out?*
- *What did you say to your child?*

When parents listen to their child and the child feels listened to, loneliness and anxiety are reduced and self-esteem increased. Destructive acting out behaviors become minimized as parents are better able to help channel their child's energy into more growth-producing ways.

Teaching parents and other adults who significantly influence the lives of our children needs to encompass the issues of sexual, aggressive, and race-related behavior. The following concepts set down by Francis (1972) provide an excellent basis for "orienting adults to their role in helping children." Adults need to know the following:

1. A child needs to be safeguarded from his immature judgments.
2. A child needs to depend on adults to fill in the gaps of his limited knowledge and experience.
3. A child needs to be recognized as a valuable and unique person.
4. A child does *not* need to be told that his spontaneous feelings and normal activities are bad.
5. A child does *not* need adult demands that he adjust to their world, for he must discover his own.
6. Persons who work with children need to know that curiosity about the human body, particularly the sexual organs, is normal and healthy.
7. They need to know that shaming, negative labeling, and physical punishment are psychologically destructive.
8. They need to know that anger is a normal, human emotion and that its verbal expression is psychologically healthy.
9. They need to know that altruism is not possible prior to adolescence and that children are normally self-centered.
10. They need to know that children are not born racist and that it is a crime against the child and against society to teach racist attitudes.

ACTIVITIES OF DAILY LIVING

Schools that concentrate on social and self-help skills exist for training moderately or severely mentally retarded children. Basic activities of daily living skills (ADL) are stressed.

SOMATIC THERAPIES

Children are occasionally placed on medication for the purpose of diagnosis or treatment. Pharmacological treatment needs to be used with caution. The lowest doses possible should be administered when medication is warranted.

Antipsychotics (phenothiazines) may help reduce disorganized thinking. Tricyclic antidepressants are sometimes used to treat childhood or adolescent depression. Ritalin (methylphenidate) and Dexedrine (dextroamphetamine) may be indicated in attention deficit disorders. The use of electroconvulsive therapy (ECT) with children is highly controversial.

PSYCHOTHERAPY

For the young child **play therapy** is often the medium in which a child can express hostility, fear, loneliness, or helplessness. Play therapy allows the child to experience and express intense or troubling emotions in a safe environment with a caring individual. For example, the therapist would set up a doll house with the same family configuration as the child's own. The child often portrays unconsciously the interpersonal conflicts which exist in his or her own home. The therapist might make comments such as "How does the little girl feel when the mother says she hates her?" or "How does the little boy feel when the daddy ignores him?" Family problems can be identified and alternative coping strategies can be acted out.

Issues That Affect the Mental Health of Some Children

MENTAL RETARDATION

Mental retardation has three essential features: (1) significant subaverage intellectual functioning (IQ of 70 or below), (2) deficits or impairments in adaptive functioning, and (3) onset before the age of 18. Children can be mentally retarded whether or not there is a coexisting mental or physical disorder.

CLINICAL FEATURES. Table 27-3 identifies the four levels of retardation from mild to profound. Clinical features associated with each level are also provided.

Rose is an eight-year-old retarded child with an IQ of 48. She is an only child and lives with her parents. When frustrated or angry Rose screams and throws objects as well as temper tantrums. Her mother dresses her and Rose is frequently incontinent. She can be friendly and likes to play with the neighbor's four-year-old boy. She is often hyperactive and requires a great deal of supervision when in a supermarket or department store. Rose attends a special school where the emphasis is on learning social and self-help skills.

Table 27-3 • DEGREES OF MENTAL RETARDATION

IQ LEVEL	CHARACTERISTICS
Mild Mental Retardation (Educable)	
50–70	1. Social and communication skills 2. Minimal impairment in sensorimotor areas 3. Academic skills to 6th grade level 4. Social and vocational skills, minimal self-support
Moderate Mental Retardation (Trainable)	
35–49	1. Poor awareness of social conventions 2. Can develop academic skills to about 2nd grade 3. May contribute to own support under close supervision
Severe Mental Retardation	
20–34	1. Poor motor development 2. Little speech 3. May learn to talk in school and learn hygiene 4. May be able to learn simple work tasks
Profound Mental Retardation	
Below 20	1. Minimal capacity for sensorimotor functioning 2. Some motor development and minimal self-care in school 3. Very limited self-care

Data from Diagnostic and Statistical Manual of Mental Disorders (DSM III-R), 3rd ed., revised. Washington DC: American Psychiatric Association, 1987.

SAMPLE NURSING DIAGNOSES AND GOALS. Possible nursing diagnoses for a mentally retarded child could include the following:

1. *Impaired verbal communication* related to mental retardation, as evidenced by problems finding the right words when speaking or inability to speak the dominant language.
2. *Altered growth and development* related to neurological impairment, as evidenced by inability/difficulty to perform age-related motor, social, or cognitive skills.

Depending on the child's potential and developmental level, possible goals may include the following:

Long Term Goals	Short Term Goals
1. Child will demonstrate two new tasks of ADL in three months.	1a. Child will put on shirt in three weeks. 1b. Child will put on pants in six weeks. 1c. Child will put on slip-on shoes in six weeks.
2. Child will go to the toilet by himself or herself in four months.	2a. Child will tell nurse/caregiver when he/she has to use the toilet (two months). 2b. Child will be able to pull down pants with the aid of nurse/caregiver (three months). 2c. Child will be able to pull down pants by self in four months.

ATTENTION DEFICIT DISORDER

Attention deficit disorder has been known in the past as hyperkinesis or minimal brain dysfunction. Attention deficit disorder is the most common condition receiving attention in the field of psychiatry today (Weiss 1985). Onset is before the age of seven.

This disorder is described in terms of behavior, but deeper problems cannot be overlooked and must be ruled out, e.g., depression, schizophrenia, or chaotic environment.

CLINICAL FEATURES. Behaviors observed more frequently in children with attention deficit disorder than in other children the same age follow (DSM III-R 1987):

1. Fails to finish things started.
2. Doesn't seem to listen.
3. Easily distracted.
4. Has difficulty concentrating on schoolwork or other tasks requiring sustained attention.
5. Often acts before thinking.
6. Shifts excessively from one activity to another.
7. May talk incessantly.
8. Has difficulty playing quietly.
9. Frequently calls out in class.
10. Has difficulty awaiting turn in games or group situations.
11. Runs about or climbs on things excessively.
12. Has difficulty sitting still or fidgets excessively.
13. Has difficulty staying seated.

Frankie is a six-year-old who daydreams in school. He listens while the teacher is present, but once she leaves he becomes bewildered. At lunchtime he runs around, bosses classmates, and calls to them from the other side of the room. At the end of the day his teacher asks him to stay and complete his work. He hands her all of the problems done with answers and numbers all over the page. At home he doesn't complete tasks started. He is a restless sleeper.

SAMPLE NURSING DIAGNOSES AND GOALS. Possible nursing diagnoses could include the following:

1. *Sensory perceptual alterations* related to neurological changes, as evidenced by restlessness and altered behaviors.
2. *Ineffective individual coping* related to sensory overload, as evidenced by alteration in social participation.

Possible goals might include the following:

Long Term Goals	Short Term Goals
1. Child will finish one short concrete task with a peer within three months with aid of medication and/or nurse/caregiver support.	1a. Child will be evaluated for appropriate medication if hyperactivity is severe. 1b. Child will complete one short concrete task with nurse/caregiver within two months. 1c. Child will be able to spend time with a peer for ten minutes without increased restlessness or outbursts. 1d. Within three months child and peer will be able to decide on one short concrete activity they both would enjoy.

CONDUCT DISORDER

The essential feature of a child with a **conduct disorder** is a repetitive and persistent pattern of conduct in which the basic rights of others or major age appropriate societal norms or rules are violated (DSM III-R 1987). Physical violence against persons or property and failure to establish a normal degree of affection, empathy, or bond with others are some manifestations of this disorder. Stealing, mugging, purse snatching, or armed robbery are frequently seen. Cruelty to others is usually noted. Poor frustration tolerance and temper outbursts are common. Lying, truancy, vandalism, frequent physical fights, and physical cruelty are some of the behaviors noted when making the diagnosis.

Conduct disorders are divided into *group type*, *solitary aggressive type*, and *undifferentiated type*. *Group type* is when conduct problems occur usually in the context of group activities with peers. *Solitary aggressive type* is predominately aggressive physical behavior toward peers and adults. *Undifferentiated type* is for children or adolescents who demonstrate mixed features of the conduct disorders.

Onset is before age 18. When seen in an adult the syndrome is called antisocial disorder. See Chapter 17.

CLINICAL FEATURES. Some clinical features seen in children with conduct disorders follow (DSM III-R 1987):

1. Physical violence against persons or property (vandalism, rape, breaking and entering, firesetting, mugging, assault).
2. Thefts outside the home involving confrontation with a victim (extortion, purse snatching, armed robbery).
3. Persistent serious lying in and out of home.
4. Repeated running away from home overnight.
5. Stealing not involving confrontation with a victim.
6. Often truant from school or work.
7. Physical cruelty to animals or people.
8. Often initiates physical fights.
9. Absence of guilt or remorse.

When Jeff was nine years old his mother was called into school when he beat up a seven-year-old girl. At ten he was constantly being lectured for "causing trouble" in class. During this time he took some toys from a friend's house. When he was asked about it he denied taking anything. However, his father found the missing toys in Jeff's closet. By the time he was 11 Jeff was caught with two older boys stealing a car. He no longer attended school regularly and took to "hanging out" with the gang.

Children and adolescents with conduct disorders pose a great challenge for nurses, parents and other people in the child's environment, e.g., teachers, clergy, peers, and neighbors. Working with the child or adolescent to develop appropriate and rewarding behaviors in place of inappropriate and destructive behaviors is important. A great deal of consistency, support, and patience is needed by the nurse/caretaker.

SAMPLE NURSING DIAGNOSES AND GOALS. For the nursing diagnosis of *potential for violence* related to antisocial character, as evidenced by history of overt aggressive acts, possible goals might include the following:

Long Term Goals	Short Term Goals
1. At the end of six months the child will use a positive coping strategy when he or she feels frustrated.	1a. At the end of one month the child will identify three situations that precipitate frustration or anger. 1b. At the end of two months the child will have identified three alternative coping strategies for anger or frustration (e.g., talking to specific person, punching bag, or going for "help"). 1c. At the end of three months the child will have role-played these strategies with nurse/caretaker using a variety of scenarios. 1d. At the end of four months the child will have replaced angry acting out with a positive coping strategy at least three times.

SEPARATION ANXIETY DISORDER

The essential feature of **separation anxiety disorder** is the child's excessive anxiety when separated from major attachment figures, home, or other familiar surroundings. The child may experience anxiety to the point of panic and his or her reaction is beyond that expected for the child's developmental level (DSM III-R 1987). Onset is before age 18, and persistence of anxiety concerning separation for at least two weeks is needed to make the diagnosis.

CLINICAL FEATURES. Some clinical features include the following:

1. Unable to visit friends, sleep at other's home, attend camp or school.
2. Unable to stay in room by self.
3. Physical complaints in anticipation of separation.
4. Morbid fear of being separated from caretaker or getting lost, kidnapped, or killed.
5. Sleep problems, nightmares involving separation.

Judy is eight years old; her older brother calls her a sissy because she is always clinging to her mother and has intense temper tantrums when her mother leaves the house even for short intervals to go shopping. Judy has been invited to a friend's sleepover birthday party. This is the first time she has been away from home by herself. She was able to stay at the party until bedtime, but then became anxious and frightened. Her parents had to come for her.

SAMPLE NURSING DIAGNOSES AND GOALS. For a child suffering from separation anxiety with a nursing diagnosis of *severe anxiety* related to separation from parent/caretaker, as evidenced by apprehension and temper tantrums, possible goals might include the following:

Long Term Goals	Short Term Goals
1. Child will be able to stay overnight at a peer's house experiencing minimal anxiety within two months.	1a. Child will stay at peer's house until 9 P.M. with parent by the end of two weeks. 1b. Child will stay at peer's house until 9 P.M. without parents by the end of one month. 1c. Child will stay at peer's house until 11 P.M. in pajamas by end of six weeks.

PERVASIVE DEVELOPMENTAL DISORDERS—AUTISTIC DISORDER

Pervasive developmental disorder is also called **autistic disorder.** Other terms used to describe this disorder in the past include childhood schizophrenia, childhood psychosis, and symbiotic psychosis. The disorder can range from mild to severe.

Autistic disorder is a disorder that is marked by failure

to develop interpersonal skills. The child is not responsive to others and does not develop verbal or nonverbal communication skills. The child treats people as objects and facial manifestations of recognition are not present. There is, however, often an attachment to objects such as a straw or rubber band. A fascination with mechanical objects is present, especially objects that spin, e.g., tops, fans, and records.

Motor behavior is affected; for example, a child displays stereotypical behavior such as flapping his arms, spinning around, or grimacing.

Language may be absent or take the form of echolalia, monologues, or unusual voice tones. Head-banging and self-rocking are common. These disorders usually appear in the first 30 months of life.

CLINICAL FEATURES. Some clinical features include the following:

1. Infant may not cuddle or respond when cuddled.
2. Language usually doesn't develop. If it does it is basic without much grammatical structure.
3. Involved with inanimate objects, never with people.
4. Compulsive need for following routines, e.g., dress routines, same route when going places, and keeping objects in organized places.
5. Head-banging and body-rocking are common.

Sam is six years old. He has been diagnosed as autistic since he was one year old. He doesn't speak but says "cookie, cookie, cookie" when angry or frustrated. He doesn't respond to the human voice and appears unaware of people around him. He spends hours turning a light switch on and off or watching a record go round and round. Once when Sam's mother got a new chair for the living room, Sam had a temper tantrum for hours until the old chair was replaced. Other than "cookie, cookie, cookie" Sam does not speak. He has been taught to use the toilet, feed, and wash himself.

Main nursing goals with the autistic child are to maintain an optimum level of functioning and prevent further regression. Goals are individually determined based on the present level of functioning and the severity of the disorder.

Refer to self-study questions 1 – 17 at the end of this chapter to review the material presented in this section on children.

Adolescents

OBJECTIVES

After studying this section on adolescents, the student will be able to:

1. Identify four areas of functioning a nurse assesses when working with adolescent clients.
2. Name two long term treatment objectives (goals) for work with adolescents.
3. Discuss four effective treatment modalities with adolescents.
4. Identify four personal qualities that will benefit a nurse working with adolescents.
5. Describe the clinical features of the following and give a nursing diagnosis for each category:
   A. Identity disorder
   B. Adjustment disorder
   C. Adolescent disorder

Anxiety continues to be a normal part of adolescent development, as the interplay between physical, psychological, intrafamilial, and social forces becomes more acute. However, adolescents tend to experience anxiety in unusually intense ways.

Normal adolescence, perhaps like no other phase in the life cycle, is marked by more acute self-consciousness, greater proneness to embarrassment, shyness and shame, and a deeper concern with questions about self-worth and self-esteem (Bleiberg 1988).

Not yet having an ego strong enough to recognize anxiety as a manifestation of internalized conflict, the adolescent uses many ways to defend against it, e.g., focusing on physical manifestations, projecting conflicts onto others, and displaying acting out behaviors. Rather than defending against anxiety, the goal for the adolescent is to experience minimal anxiety either by acting to alter an external situation directly or to produce a series of effective coping devices. A number of adolescents find it difficult to appropriately discharge their anxiety and act out their anxiety in maladaptive ways or become depressed.

Adolescents are extremely conscious of the physical manifestations of maturation, e.g., muscular tension, increased heart rate, widened pulse pressure, and feelings of overwhelming fatigue. They will often regard these as signs of physical illness rather than associate the feelings with a more sensitive awareness of bodily sensations.

Running away from home is a common way of handling conflicts and problems. Often, running away is a signal of existing family tension and turmoil. In some cases, running away can symbolize the conscious or unconscious wish of parents to relinquish family responsibilities and to "leave it all."

In many instances an adolescent who feels compelled to run away is seeking a release from intense dependency-independency conflict. Severe levels of anxiety lead to a desire to escape. On the one hand, the adolescent wants to prove his or her self-sufficiency. However, on the other hand, the adolescent secretly seeks to be taken care of. The runaway is both running from something (disappointment) and toward something (fantasized gratification).

Adolescents who feel rejected by parents may feel isolated, lonely, and empty. These adolescents are likely to plunge into premature loveless sexual relationships as an attempt to feel loved. The rate of teenage pregnancy continues to rise. Pregnancy often represents an attempt to feel whole and valuable and is not a desire for a baby (Miller 1974).

Experimentation with drugs often begins in adolescence or younger. Experimentation can progress to habitual use in order to escape frustrations and anxiety. Unfortunately, instead of providing an escape from problems, drug abuse becomes a problem in itself. Ego development is accomplished through confronting and learning to cope adaptively with reality. Habitual use of psychoactive drugs becomes a substitute for and avoidance of reality. Drug abuse impairs ego development and may conceal even poorer coping skills (Kaplan and Sadock 1988).

The personality strength the individual brings to adolescence is clearly the result of genetic endowment, interpersonal relationships within the nuclear family, and that family's relationships with its total environment.

The level of inner security and sense of family reliability that the latency age child brings into adolescence determine the adolescent's optimism regarding life and his or her capacity for emotional depth. A warm, loving family serves as a holding environment for the adolescent.

An adolescent's inner resources and the family's coping strategies determine the course of adolescence. The adult world is a source of conflict. Adolescents move toward peers for support in their demands for freedom and to validate their grievances toward their parents and the whole of the adult world. This group life helps adolescents cope with anxiety through camaraderie, humor, and continual action.

Unique Assessment Strategies

Assessment of the adolescent includes knowledge of adolescent development, adolescent functioning, normal family functioning and adolescent psychopathology, and the ability to relate to the adolescent and parent. Assessment is not a static process. Adolescents are evolving adults experiencing considerable fluctuation and shifts between the id, the ego, and the superego.

One of the essential yet most difficult questions to answer when assessing an adolescent is whether the problem is the result of a normal adolescent issue or the result of a developmental lag. During adolescence personality strengths and weaknesses are in constant flux. Normal adolescence involves a normal identity crisis that consists of turmoil and conflict to a limited degree. In normal adolescents, relationships with peers and parents are good. The adolescent has a sense of competence and self-esteem. There is a capacity for coping through the use of several adaptive mechanisms such as sublimation, a sense of humor, and anticipatory planning.

Assessment of the adolescent focuses on strengths and weaknesses of the personality (ego) and the family. Since the adolescent will have reached a higher level of ego functioning than the child, the nurse seeks the answers to the following questions:

- *What is the quality of interpersonal and peer relationships?*
- *What is the level of school interest, school involvement, and academic performance?*
- *Are there pathological indicators such as self-destructive, antisocial acting out or bizarre behavior?*

- *If psychotherapy is indicated, does the adolescent have the capacity and interest to observe self or the motivation to enter into a therapeutic alliance with the nurse/therapist?*

Table 27–4 outlines some tools and tasks for the preadolescent and adolescent.

It is beneficial to set up the initial interview with the adolescent rather than the parents in order to establish an alliance. The parents, however, do have a right to be involved in the process, even if the adolescent is antagonistic to their involvement. There are two focuses for the goals in adolescent counseling:

1. Remove obstacles to the normal growth and developmental process.
2. Improve relationships within the family in order to foster and support the process of growth.

The accomplishment of these goals usually involves a combination of individual and family sessions. Focus on communications, family conflicts, and the parental relationship is crucial.

Table 27–4 • OUTLINE OF TOOLS AND TASKS BY ERAS OF DEVELOPMENT: ADOLESCENCE

TASKS	TOOLS	IF TASKS NOT ACHIEVED
Preadolescence: 9–12 Years		
1. Moving to fully social state, e.g., • identifying self with peers of same sex • being more loyal to chum than to family members • relating closely to chum of same sex • expanding of interpersonal relationships	1. Capacity to love. 2. Consensual validation. 3. Collaboration. 4. Experimentation, exploration, manipulation.	Sense of self in relationship to others is not well developed, feelings of inferiority and isolation.
2. Seriously using learning to implement self for future life, e.g., • developing own value system • learning that recognition is won by directing activities toward constructive ends • becoming familiar with the rational and irrational ideas, values, and mores of his or her culture		Uncertainty about self, abilities, and where he or she fits into life.
Early Adolescence: 12–15 Years		
1. Working through developmental crisis of physiological and psychological changes and moving toward independence, e.g., • asserting self and challenging authority • evaluating own limitations and powers • examining and anticipating consequences of own decisions	1. Lust—awareness of sexual drive which stimulates the integration of situations affecting the genital zones. 2. Greater recognition of powers. 3. Experimentation, exploration, manipulation. 4. Anxiety.	Although a time of confusion and introspection for all at this age, the experience is especially pronounced and may persist into adulthood when the adolescent doesn't have the tools to negotiate this stage. The normal mood swings of adolescence may be intensified and prolonged.
2. Learning to establish satisfactory relations with members of the opposite sex, e.g., • accepting self as sexual object • finding suitable sexual objects • experimenting socially • learning healthy patterns for emotional release		Severe difficulty in heterosexual relationships is a result of identity confusion and low self-esteem.
Late Adolescence: 15 Years and Up		
1. Learning to become interdependent, e.g., • tolerating anxiety and using it constructively • establishing mature and reciprocal relationships with parents • accepting other people as individuals of worth	1. Genital organs. 2. Experimentation, exploration, manipulation. 3. Mature self-system.	Personal identity and role confusion result in — deficits in assuming responsibility — sense of inadequacy in controlling self — inability to compete successfully — dissatisfaction in personal relationships or isolation — difficulties in sharing and experiencing intimate relationships

TASKS	TOOLS	IF TASKS NOT ACHIEVED
Late Adolescence: 15 Years and Up		
2. Learning to integrate conscious values in harmony with practical, realistic, scientific world, e.g., • making decisions and choices of far-reaching importance for future • selecting mate and preparing for productive family life • learning to become economically, intellectually, and emotionally self-sufficient • achieving socially responsible behavior as a citizen of community, state, nation, and world.		
3. Forming durable sexual relationship with selected member of the opposite sex, e.g., wooing and winning mate with whom one develops the following: • willingness to share mutual trust • mutuality of sexual satisfaction • willingness to share procreation • willingness to regulate cycles of work and recreation • willingness to assume responsibility for others		

Adapted from Fagin C. Nursing in Child Psychiatry. St. Louis: C.V. Mosby Company, 1972, and Haber J. Developmental processes. *In* Haber J, Hoskins PP, Leach AM, Sideleau BF (eds). Comprehensive Psychiatric Nursing, 3rd ed. New York: McGraw-Hill Book Company, 1987.

Unique Intervention Strategies

PSYCHOTHERAPEUTIC INTERVENTIONS

In order to create a therapeutic system, the adolescent and the family must be able to recognize their communication styles. The nurse must recognize and experience the interactional patterns within the family and recognize the strengths of these patterns. The nurse addresses the adolescent's independent and autonomous components while at the same time recognizing the parents' executive position in the family (Minuchin 1974).

The whole process of assessment, diagnosis, and treatment should be explained to the family, and the family should take an active part in this process.

It is not easy to interview a troubled adolescent because of the high levels of anxiety, overt hostility, negativism, sullenness, withdrawal, silence, and surface compliance that an adolescent may bring to the interview. Long silences are not well tolerated by an adolescent. They only intensify anxiety.

The family and the nurse must come to an agreement on the nature of the problem and on goals needed for change. The contract may be initially limited, but it usually expands and changes over time.

HEALTH TEACHING

The health of future families depend on the health and vigor of adolescents today. Nurses are frequently the first health workers to have contact with adolescents using drugs because of their positions in schools, emergency rooms, hospitals, and home health agencies. Nurses working with youth have many opportunities through their observation skills, teaching skills, listening skills, and abilities to evaluate cues to identify problems, provide guidance, and make appropriate referrals. Nurses can work effectively with teenagers and families to help prevent alcohol and drug abuse, pregnancy, and sexually transmitted diseases. Involvement in community affairs and cooperation with parent-teacher organizations can be vehicles for the nurse to participate in prevention issues.

More specifically, nurses can help adolescents clarify values, teach communication skills, and provide information about sex and pregnancy. Learning alternate ways of handling stress is useful for adolescents.

ACTIVITIES OF DAILY LIVING

Structure is an important aspect of providing adolescents with a sense of security. The overwhelming conflicts adolescents may experience may make simple tasks like getting up in the morning complicated. Nurses can teach adolescents directly or work through their families to help them figure out simple tasks, such as how much time is appropriate for dressing, how frequent are their showers or baths, how much sleep do they need, and what foods are nutritious.

Recreational activities such as sports, drama, music, and crafts help develop self-confidence in individuals as well as provide opportunities to expand relationships.

SOMATIC THERAPIES

Adolescents frequently object to taking major tranquilizers because of drowsiness, fear of losing control, and the physical alteration of their bodies. As a result, the nurse needs to be aware that medications may be flushed down the toilet, thrown out, or accumulated for future use. Tricyclics in combination with psychotherapy can be helpful with adolescents who are depressed. Lithium may be used in some cases when a bipolar disorder is suspected. Anxiolytics (minor tranquilizers, e.g., benzodiazepines) are used with a great deal of caution with adolescents because of the drug abuse potential. Therefore, medication must be taken in front of the nurse. It is also essential for the nurse to explain the benefits and side effects to the adolescent. Collaboration with other health professionals is necessary in order to monitor the effectiveness of any medication.

THERAPEUTIC ENVIRONMENT

There are many theories about the best atmosphere in which to nurture adolescents and children while supporting independence and individuality through interpersonal relationships. One such environment is called **milieu therapy** (see Chapter 2). Many theorists have identified a need for and described such an environment. Each has subtle differences, but they all basically discuss the need for recognizing what aspects of the environment interfere with developmental growth and what changes are necessary to support the adolescent's needs and potential. Goals of milieu therapy include promotion of security, increase in self-esteem, and competence through learning skills. In milieu therapy activities such as meals, sleep, and play are conducted in a structured environment.

However, whether treatment is in an outpatient or inpatient setting, the home and family are the natural environment for the adolescent. All efforts must be directed toward treating the family as well as the adolescent.

OUTPATIENT SETTING. Adolescent problems that are precipitated by clear-cut external events such as the death of a family member, divorce of parents, or stress from a developmental crisis respond well to outpatient treatment. Family involvement and cooperation in ongoing treatment for any problem is also a good indication for outpatient treatment. An adolescent who recognizes an inner conflict and is motivated toward individual therapy should be considered for ongoing psychotherapy.

HOSPITAL TREATMENT. The decision to hospitalize an adolescent must be made with a great deal of caution since it can confirm the adolescent's worst fears about him- or herself. Positive results from hospitalization are difficult to achieve because the adolescent loses contact with and support of peers, and dependency conflicts are increased.

However, the structure of the hospital is essential for adolescents who need to live out their problems rather than discuss them. Brief hospitalization can help with suicidal or homicidal impulses, acute confusional states, evaluations, and drug therapy.

The adolescent's resistance to the process of introspection must be respected. The most conducive atmosphere for growth is through the creation of a therapeutic environment that is democratic rather than authoritarian, treatment oriented rather than custodial, humanitarian rather than oppressive, and flexible rather than rigid (Fagin 1974). Useful interventions include teaching concrete personal skills through which adolescents are expected (with help) to evaluate personal areas of poor functioning and to master a medication routine prior to discharge.

The term "milieu therapy" describes the exposure of an adolescent to a total environment that is designated for treatment. Ideally, every aspect of the environment is structured to provide treatment. Interactions are structured so that love and gratification are based on the adolescent's needs rather than what is "deserved."

Hospital treatment must include ongoing family therapy. The individual treatment of the adolescent must be a support for the treatment of the family.

RESIDENTIAL TREATMENT. Sometimes it is necessary to remove the adolescent from the home environment to a community residence. Community residences are small home-like residential centers for children, adolescents, and often adults who cannot cope with the stresses in their environment. Residences provide various degrees of protection, group therapy, and adjunct therapies. Behavior modification programs are often incorporated into the residential milieu, along with a variety of therapeutic modalities. Behavior modification is aimed at helping clients use more adaptive coping behaviors (Murray and Huelskoetter 1987). Therefore, residential treatment may be the treatment of choice for some adolescents. Two criteria for removal of an adolescent from the home are listed here.

1. The psychopathology of the adolescent (aggressive or severe acting out behavior) is self-destructive or dangerous to others.
2. The family situation is grossly inadequate (e.g., parents who have severe untreated alcoholism or addiction).

DAY HOSPITAL. Another environment for adolescent treatment is the day hospital. Most often this is used for adolescents whose emotional disturbance interferes with regular classroom activities. A day hospital provides specialized programs of study with a teacher-student ratio that is smaller than that in a regular school setting. The ultimate goal is to get the adolescent back into regular school. Therapeutic programs include behavior modification and group and individual counseling. Other courses are available to help develop skills in art, music, literature, and physical education. The whole program is geared toward growth and change.

PSYCHOTHERAPY

Theoretically, no single psychotherapy modality is the treatment of choice for all adolescent mental health problems. The three possible choices are family therapy, individual therapy, and group therapy. The choice may be a combination of the three to form an integrated approach. Any criteria for selecting or combining therapies will be based upon the assessment, nursing diagnosis, skills, and theoretical orientation of the nurse. For an overview of family, group, and individual therapy, refer to Chapter 2.

GROUP THERAPY. Group therapy works well and is often the modality of choice with adolescents because of the adolescent's natural turning toward peers. One form of group treatment of adolescents is *group psychotherapy*. Nurse therapists use the emotional interaction within the group to effect changes in personality dysfunction. A careful balancing of the group with attention to age, sex, intelligence, and personality style helps assure optimum group environment.

Nurse generalists (ADN or BS level) may run *human development* or *training groups* which have a more affective or cognitive focus and in which the goal of treatment is behavior change. These groups focus on particular issues, e.g., relationships of parental divorce. A third type of group is a *self-help group* such as Alcoholics Anonymous, Narcotics Anonymous, and Al-Anon. Self-help groups are usually composed of peers who are seeking assistance with specific handicaps or needs. A list of clearing houses for specific areas nationwide is found in the appendix.

A fourth group treatment for adolescents is the *peer pressure group*. In these groups hospitalized adolescents are encouraged to give constructive criticism and advice on the progress a particular group member is making toward fulfillment of treatment goals.

Working with adolescents can be very challenging for the nurse and the members of the health team. Adolescents have a way of hooking adults who are insecure within themselves into interactions that engage their vulnerabilities and ego deficits, rather than their competencies. When this happens, arguments ensue. A nurse working with adolescents should have the following characteristics:

1. A sense of contentment with his or her own life and the ability to acknowledge personal limitations and disappointments.
2. A capacity to confront adolescents. Encourage them to see that their ability to outsmart and manipulate others is better used to help themselves rather than belittle others.
3. A sense of humor.
4. A full outside life. The nurse needs to get emotional gratification from her or his outside life rather than looking to the adolescent for satisfaction.
5. Flexibility, along with an ability to relate to the social environment of the adolescent (e.g., questions about sports, TV programs, peers).
6. An ability to challenge adolescents to recognize the consequences of their behavior for themselves as well as the effect on others.

Issues That Affect the Mental Health of Some Adolescents

Some of the more prevalent disorders seen in adolescents today are presented here within the framework of the DSM III-R. Short vignettes are presented to illuminate the disorders, and possible nursing diagnoses are suggested.

IDENTITY DISORDER

CLINICAL FEATURES. The essential feature of an **identity disorder** is severe distress regarding the inability to integrate various aspects of the self into an acceptable sense of self. Uncertainty centers on a variety of issues, e.g., career choices, friendship patterns, sexual orientation, moral values, and long term goals. Evidence of an identity disorder usually appears in late adolescence (DSM III-R 1987).

The adolescent demonstrates impairment in social or occupational functioning (including academic) as a result of his or her symptoms. The disturbance must last at least three weeks before a diagnosis can be made (DSM III-R 1987).

Louie was a senior in high school when he began failing subjects that he had previously received A's in. He was unable to choose a college. He asked "Who am I?"; "I don't know what I want to do"; "Should I go to an all male or coed college?"; "What do I want to do with my life?" His grade point average was dropping and he began to withdraw from friends.

SAMPLE NURSING DIAGNOSES. Possible nursing diagnoses include the following:

1. *Ineffective individual coping* related to career choices/independence from family, as evidenced by inability to meet role expectations.
2. *Altered growth and development* related to loss of independence and autonomy, as evidenced by inability to make appropriate personal and career decisions.
3. *Powerlessness* related to inability to grow independent from family, as evidenced by dissatisfaction over inability to have control over personal and career decisions.

ADJUSTMENT DISORDER

An **adjustment disorder** is a maladaptive reaction to a specific psychosocial stressor. The disorder occurs within three months after the stressful event. There is impairment in social activities and relationships with others, and inability to function in school or work. Types of adjustment disorders include associated symptoms such as anxiety, physical complaints, depression, or conduct disturbances.

CLINICAL FEATURES. Depression, anxiety, or violation of the rights of others may be symptomatic of this disorder. Symptoms related to school work include inability to study or write. Whatever the symptoms they are in excess of normal reactions. The disorder does not last more than six months.

Suzy is 15 years old and her parents divorced two months ago. Suzy started to become jittery and obviously worried about anything and everything. She found she was unable to keep up with school assignments, write required reports, or study for examinations. She withdrew from friends and functioned poorly in her home chores. Suzy's parents are so upset they are unable to support Suzy at this time.

SAMPLE NURSING DIAGNOSES. Possible nursing diagnoses include the following:

1. *Severe anxiety* related to parents' divorce, as evidenced by inability to concentrate.
2. *Impaired social interactions* related to parents' divorce, as evidenced by inability to maintain peer relationships.
3. *Altered family processes* related to divorce, as evidenced by breakdown in family communications.

DEPRESSION AND SUICIDE

Since depression is so prevalent with our teenage population and suicide is the third leading cause of death among adolescents 15 to 24 years (homicide is number two), depression as it relates to children and adolescents is mentioned here even though Chapter 18 discusses depression at length. Depression in children and adolescents may be transient or situational, or may develop into a chronic long-standing state.

CLINICAL FEATURES. Symptoms such as difficulty in concentration, crying spells, insomnia, eating disorders, social isolation, and withdrawal are the same as for adult depression. However, acting out behaviors may mask depression in children and adolescents, e.g., school phobias, underachievement, truancy, temper outbursts, or use of drugs and alcohol. Nurses, parents, teachers, and others need to be alert for indications of suicidal intent in children and adolescents.

Children between three and twelve do think of suicide. Children of seven and eight have attempted to hang themselves. As mentioned, suicide is the number three cause of deaths among our teenage population, accidents being number one. Even then, it is thought that 50% of teenage motorcycle or automobile accidents are in fact suicide attempts or subintentional acts.

Adolescents who do commit suicide are more isolated, more hopeless, and less likely to communicate signals for help than those who do not commit suicide (Peck 1977). In a 1974 study of adolescents who killed themselves, 40–50% were abusing alcohol or drugs at the time of their death. Almost two thirds had stated they were not on good terms with their families, and 90% felt that their family did not understand them (Peck 1977). Studies have shown that among children and adolescents who exhibit suicidal behavior, family stress is the most important environmental factor (Peck 1977).

Box 27–1 outlines some behavioral manifestations and family characteristics which are statistically significant when assessing children and teenagers for risk of suicide.

Interventions with suicidal adolescents can involve many treatment modalities (family, group, individual). Various techniques can be used based upon the openness of the adolescent and recognition of the problem. The nurse can teach socialization skills, instill behavioral principles, and conduct peer pressure groups. The most important interventions focus on the adolescent's gaining self-confidence and the reduction of self-destructive wishes and behavior. The role is threefold: (1) convey a sense of hope that the situation can improve, (2) explore alternative ways of coping with stress, and (3) explore family patterns of communications and interactions.

Box 27–1. ADOLESCENTS AT RISK FOR SUICIDE

Characteristics of Adolescents

1. Family history of suicide
2. Previous suicide attempt
3. Chronic illness
4. Suffering bereavement
5. Alcoholism
6. Chronic use of drugs
7. Domestic difficulties
8. Depression in teenagers marked by acting out behaviors:
   - delinquent behaviors, i.e., stealing, vandalism, academic failure, promiscuity, fights at school, running away
   - escape behaviors, i.e., drugs, sex, withdrawal
9. Loss of girl/boyfriend

Characteristics of Family with Suicidal Teenager

1. Unproductive communications
2. Communications reveal much conflict between family members
3. Impaired problem-solving ability
4. Inconsistent positive reinforcements plus a greater number of negative reinforcements
5. Unstable home environment

Data from Hamlin WT. Adolescent suicide. Journal of National Medical Association, 74(1):25,1982, and Hart NA, Keidel GC. The suicidal adolescent. American Journal of Nursing, 79(1):80, 1979.

Corine is 17 years old and she recently moved from her family home in the city to start college on a rural campus. After being on campus one month she was found by her college roommate staggering and incoherent and near collapse. She was brought by ambulance to the nearest hospital. A note was found later in her room stating, "I feel so alone, no one cares for me anymore." After emergency treatment, Corine was able to say that she had taken about 8 analgesic pills with codeine and 25 aspirin tablets because she just "wanted some peace." After transfer from the intensive care unit to the adolescent unit, Corine stated that for about three weeks before the suicide attempt she had been exposed to a great deal of beer drinking, rudeness, and foul language, and an ongoing argument with her boyfriend from home. She told the nurse she had wanted to visit her family the weekend before, but the car broke down and no one could bring her home. Corine had chosen this college because of a tuition scholarship in music. She had a knee injury and had been on crutches for two weeks. She was feeling lonely, her boyfriend was not available, her parents were far away, and her roommate was busy with her own activities. She had no contacts at the college other than her roommate.

Corine was given the DSM III-R diagnosis of adjustment disorder with depressed mood.

SAMPLE NURSING DIAGNOSES. Possible nursing diagnoses would include the following:

1. *Potential for self-harm* related to separation from family and loss of significant support system, as evidenced by suicide attempt, and feelings of aloneness:
2. *Social isolation* related to moving to unfamiliar surroundings, as evidenced by no peer support and feelings of hopelessness.

OTHER DISORDERS

Conduct disorders were briefly addressed in the section on children. Obviously, as children reach adolescence, conduct disorders often persist and in adulthood are termed antisocial disorders (see Chapter 17). Borderline disorders are observed in adolescents, and this disorder is addressed in Chapter 17. Anorexia nervosa, a prevalent eating disorder among adolescents, is covered in

Chapter 25. Adolescent drinking and psychoactive substance abuse are factors affecting the mental health of our youth today. Alcohol use and psychoactive substance use are addressed in Chapters 23 and 24.

Refer to Self-Study Questions 18–30 at the end of this chapter to review the material related to adolescents.

Summary

Nurses observe children in a variety of settings and have ample opportunity to identify possible developmental or emotional problems. Therefore, the roles of the nurse generalist and nurse specialist were briefly outlined in the section on working with children and adolescents with mental problems. Most of the mental disorders seen in children are related to faulty life experiences or early relationship difficulties.

Anxiety is a normal part of negotiating the stages of growth and development. The task of the family is to provide security, support for growth, and sexual differentiation by helping a child deal with anxiety constructively. When the family is unable to provide emotional warmth and security, mental problems may ensue. A number of social and environmental stresses were discussed that can place a family in crisis.

An understanding of developmental, systems, psychoanalytic, interpersonal, and behavioral theories forms the background for nurses' work with children and adolescents. Assessment of a child involves such areas as the family, the child at play, the child's drawings, use of a genogram, and family cultural and religious beliefs. Various interventions specific for children were addressed.

Various DSM III-R disorders were discussed (mental retardation, attention deficit disorder, conduct disorders, separation anxiety, and infantile autism), and general characteristics and possible nursing diagnoses and goals were suggested. Vignettes were provided.

Adolescents experience anxiety in unusually intense ways. They cope with anxiety by focusing on physical manifestations, projecting conflicts onto others, and displaying acting out behaviors. If warmth, security, and stability are not present in an adolescent's family life, acting out behaviors may be maladaptive. For example, running away, loveless sexual relationships, experimentation with drugs, and depression/suicide are responses to adolescents' feeling unloved.

Assessment of the adolescent includes knowledge of adolescent development, adolescent functioning, normal family functioning, and adolescent psychopathology. Two long term treatment goals were mentioned. A variety of treatment modalities were discussed, e.g., hospital, outpatient, residential, day hospital, and various group modalities.

Three common disorders of adolescence were presented: identity disorder, adjustment disorder, and adolescent depression. Conduct disorders, also a problem seen in adolescents, may start in early childhood and was briefly covered in the first part of this chapter. Borderline disorder and the eating disorders are discussed in Chapters 17 and 25, respectively. Alcohol and psychoactive substance use disorders, also major problems among teenagers, are discussed in Chapters 23 and 24. Nursing diagnoses were suggested for each disorder.

References

Beitchman JH. Childhood schizophrenia: A review and comparison with adult-onset schizophrenia. Psychiatric Clinics of North America, 8(4), 1985.

Bleiberg E. Adolescence, sensed self and narcissistic vulnerability. Bulletin of Menninger Clinic, 52(3):5, 1988.

Bowlby J. Developmental psychiatry has come of age. American Journal of Psychiatry 145(1):1, 1988.

Bumbalo J, Siemon MK. Nursing assessment and diagnosis: Mental health problems of children. Topics In Clinical Nursing, 5(1):41, 1983.

Carpenito LJ. Handbook of Nursing Diagnosis, 2nd ed. Philadelphia: J.B. Lippincott, 1987.

Diagnostic and Statistical Manual of Mental Disorders (DSM III-R), 3rd ed., revised. Washington DC: American Psychiatric Association, 1987.

Fagin C. Nursing in Child Psychiatry. St. Louis: C.V. Mosby Company, 1972.

Fagin C. Readings in Child and Adolescent Psychiatric Nursing. St. Louis: C.V. Mosby Company, 1974.

Francis T. The crippling effects of racism. *In* Fagin C (ed). Nursing In Child Psychiatry. St. Louis: C.V. Mosby Company, 1972.

Greenspan S. The Clinical Interview of the Child. New York: McGraw-Hill Book Company, 1981.

Grossman J, Mayton K. Applying the nursing process with children. *In* Wilson HS, Kneisl CR (eds). Psychistric Nursing, 3rd ed. Reading, MA, Addison Wesley, 1988.

Haber J. Developmental processes. *In* Haber J, Hoskins PP, Leach AM, Sideleau BF (eds). Comprehensive Psychiatric Nursing, 3rd ed. New York: McGraw-Hill Book Company, 1987.

Kaplan HI, Sadock BJ. Synopsis of Psychiatry, 5th ed. Baltimore: Williams & Wilkins, 1988.

Keidel G. The suicidal adolescent. American Journal of Nursing, 79(1):80, 1979.

Kessler JW. Psychopathology of Childhood. Englewood Cliffs, NJ: Prentice-Hall, 1966.

Klein M. The Psychoanalysis of Children. London: Delacorte Press, 1975.

McBride AB. Coming of age: Child psychiatric nursing. Archive of Psychiatric Nursing, 2(2):57, 1988.

Miller D. Adolescence, Psychology, Psychopathology and Psychotherapy. New York: Jason Aronson, 1974.

Minuchin S. Families and Family Therapy. Cambridge, MA: Harvard University Press, 1974.

Murray RB, Huelskoetter MMW. Psychiatric/Mental Health Nursing, 2nd ed. Norwalk, Conn: Appleton & Lange, 1987.

Peck ML. Adolescent suicide. *In* Harron CL, et al (eds). Suicide: Assessment and Intervention. New York: Appleton-Century-Crofts, 1977.

Pothier PC. Child mental health problems and policy. Archives of Psychiatric Nursing, 2(3):165, 1988.
Pothier P. Mental Health Counselling With Children. Boston: Little Brown & Company, 1976.
Schneidman E. Preventing suicide. American Journal of Nursing, 1965.
Schuster CS, Ashburn SS. The Process of Human Development. Boston: Little, Brown & Company, 1986.
Standards of Psychiatric and Mental Health Nursing Practice. Kansas City, MO: American Nurses' Association, 1982.
Weiss G. Hyperactivity: Overview and new directions. Psychiatric Clinics of North America, 8(4):737, 1985.

Self-Study Exercises

CHILDREN

Place S (Specialist) or B (both specialist and generalist) next to each nursing role.

1. ________ Psychotherapeutic intervention.
2. ________ Psychotherapy (group, family, individual).
3. ________ Educator of nurses and other child care personnel in a variety of settings.
4. ________ Basic health teaching to families, groups, and clients.
5. ________ Researcher who contributes to theory and practice of child and adolescent psychiatric nursing.

Choose the letter that is the subject of each of the following definitions:

6. ________ Social issues that can increase anxiety in the family system.
7. ________ Helps identify what was happening when a child was born and the structure of generational relationships.
8. ________ Way to assess a child's interpsychic life and identify family relationship problems.

A. Drawings and play

B. Changes in family structure/unemployment

C. Capacity to relate and cognitive level

D. Genogram

Match the characteristics with the disorder

9. ________ Intellectual functioning subaverage and deficits in adaptive functioning.
10. ________ Easily distracted, runs about excessively, shifts from one activity to the other, acts before thinking.
11. ________ Violates the basic rights of others and social rules, physically violent against persons or property.
12. ________ Does not respond to people, only objects, rarely speaks, can be taught to perform some ADL.

A. Autism

B. Separation anxiety

C. Conduct disorder

D. Mental retardation

E. Attention deficit disorder

Place T (True) or F (False) next to each statement.

13. ________ It is important to focus on the child during therapy and pay a minimal amount of attention to other family members.
14. ________ Play therapy allows children to experience and express intense emotions in a safe environment.
15. ________ Primary prevention is one of the most important modalities of interventions with children and their families open to all nurses.
16. ________ Medication should be used with extreme caution in the treatment of children with mental disorders.

Short Answer

17. State one nursing diagnosis for each of the five disorders covered in the section on children.

ADOLESCENTS

Multiple Choice

18. Which of the following is NOT part of an adolescent assessment when assessing ego strengths?
    A. Quality of interpersonal relationships.
    B. Level of school interest, school involvement, and academic performance.
    C. Number of siblings the adolescent has.
    D. Evidence of destructive, antisocial, or bizarre behaviors.
    E. Motivation and ability to look at self (introspection).

Working with adolescents can be extremely challenging. Put T (True) or F (False) next to the following statements:

19. ________ Developmentally, adolescents are trying to separate from adults, and parental issues and inner conflicts can be projected onto the nurse.
20. ________ During this time the adolescents' peer group is most important and influential in their lives.
21. ________ Adolescents are generally confused and have poor problem-solving skills.
22. ________ Body and hormonal changes during this time can compound erratic behaviors.
23. ________ Nurses can and should plan on a major degree of personal gratification from their work with adolescents.
24. ________ A sense of humor is an important asset for a nurse to possess, especially when working with adolescents.

Match the clinical features with the disorder.

25. ________	Anxiety regarding inability to evaluate goals, sexual identity, choice of friendship patterns, etc.	A. Adjustment disorder

26. __________ Impairment in social, occupational, and relationship functioning related to an identifiable stressor.

27. __________ May be masked by antisocial or aggressive behaviors, truancy, phobias, taking drugs, and other behaviors.

B. Depression

C. Identity disorder

Short Answer

28. Make up one probable nursing diagnosis for each of the above-mentioned disorders.

29. Essentially, long term treatment goals are directed toward:

    A. ______________________________
    B. ______________________________

30. State one indication for the following type of treatment as it pertains to adolescents:

    A. Outpatient: ______________________________
    B. Hospital: ______________________________
    C. Residential Treatment: ______________________________
    D. Day Hospital: ______________________________

CHAPTER 28

Adult Relationships and Sexuality

Mary Jane Herron and William G. Herron

OUTLINE

KEY WORDS AND CONCEPTS

The key terms and concepts listed here also appear in bold where they are defined or discussed in this chapter.

INHIBITED DESIRE
PREMATURE EJACULATION
EJACULATORY INCOMPETENCE
EJACULATORY OR POSTEJACULATORY PAIN
ORGASMIC DYSFUNCTION
VAGINISMUS
PREMARITAL RELATIONSHIPS
OPEN MARRIAGE
BLENDED FAMILY
HOMOSEXUAL LIFESTYLE
TRANSSEXUAL
PARAPHILIAS
FETISHISM
PEDOPHILIA
EXHIBITIONISM
VOYEURISM
TRANSVESTISM
SADISM AND MASOCHISM

OBJECTIVES

After studying this chapter, the student will be able to:

1. Distinguish among levels of nursing education and appropriate assessment and intervention strategies.
2. Summarize the stages in the human sexual response.
3. Compare and contrast the major models of adult relationships discussed in this chapter.
4. Discuss the major sexual dysfunctions found among males and females.
5. Identify therapeutic interventions for the sexual dysfunctions.
6. Describe gender identity disorders and medical interventions for them.
7. Define the various nonstandard sexual behaviors.
8. Recognize the different sexually transmitted diseases by their symptoms.

The major mental disorders have been covered in the preceding chapters. However, there are several issues that can affect the mental health of some adults. Twentieth-century men and women face numerous social issues that cause conflict, anxiety, and stress in their daily lives and that may ultimately affect their mental health in a variety of ways. The number of stressors has increased as the world population has expanded and the personal and political boundaries between people have shrunk.

Social mores affecting the more personal aspects of people's lives have also changed dramatically in recent years. In earlier times, religious leaders were often responsible for setting standards of behavior and establishing expectations for personal life and loving. By the 1980's, however, religious affiliation among Americans had declined sharply and no new commonly accepted authority took the place religious leaders once held.

Standards for marriage, family life, and sexual practices have been particularly affected, with wide variations now being reported.

Americans, especially, have experienced numerous variations in standards, possibly due to the many different cultural and ethnic groups that make up our population. One of the early sexuality researchers, Havelock Ellis (1906), proposed that sexual customs are only relative to each individual society. Since we are a "melting pot" of cultures, our sexual practices are widely different. While these variations provide people with a wide range of possibilities, they also can create a sense of conflict about which choice to make.

Nurses are often the first to hear of concerns regarding sexuality that are affecting the mental health of clients. Changing family situations, worries about sexual development and desires, concerns about interpersonal relationships, sexual concerns about physical diseases, are all issues that many people have difficulty discussing, especially in a formal setting. Thus nurses can often encourage discussion by being aware of the importance of these concerns and by being receptive when clients make seemingly casual references to issues that are really of vital concern to them. Nurses can face the taboo which dictates that sexual issues are not the focus of "polite" conversation by encouraging questions and giving factual information when needed. This chapter focuses on interpersonal issues that may affect the mental health of some adults. The role of the nurse at different educational levels is defined. Guidelines for psychosexual assessment at the generalist level as well as appropriate interventions are presented.

The Role of the Nurse

Although foundations for nursing practice hold a holistic view, a client's sexuality is often not addressed in the treatment process. The nurse's background reflects education in the physical, social, and behavioral sciences, as well as theory and practice in counseling techniques. Because of this background training, the nurse is an ideal member of the health team to counsel clients in the sensitive and highly charged area of human sexuality (Zalar 1982).

Acute, chronic, or disabling conditions necessitate alterations in ways in which individuals express their sexuality. Adolescents and the aged have special issues and concerns regarding their sexuality. A nurse who is knowledgeable, nonjudgmental, and has good communication skills can play an important role in identifying potential problem areas and providing effective sex counseling or referral (Zalar 1982).

An example of need is identified in a study by Krueger et al. (1979) of premenopausal women who had hysterectomies for nonmalignant conditions. When asked for suggestions about how nurses could have assisted them with their sexual adjustment after surgery, 45 of 51 respondents indicated they would like nurses to provide more information about sexual adjustment after surgery (Zalar 1982). The crippling or disfigurement resulting from surgery, disease, or injury can negatively affect a person's sexual identity and sense of attractiveness. Since nurses spend more time with clients than perhaps any other member of the health team, they are in a prime position to assess, educate, and support clients in areas that threaten sexual identity or impair sexual function (Zalar 1982).

How does one define the nurse's role in helping selected clients meet their sexual needs? Masters and Johnson described nurses as intermediaries between physicians who are uncomfortable with the topic of sexuality and clients who lack the knowledge, or who have misconceptions about sexuality and sexual practices (Hogan 1980). The World Health Organization (WHO) describes the role of the nurse in terms of a supportive relationship with clients who have sexual problems and helping in such matters as feminine hygiene, family planning, helping parents deal with sexual behaviors and questions of their children, and assisting teachers with sex education (Hogan 1980). Many nurses have greatly expanded their roles and work with individuals who express unmet sexual needs and impaired functioning as sex therapists. Not all nurses will go on to become sex therapists, but all nurses should be knowledgeable about the bio-psycho-social aspects of sexuality throughout the life cycle, about the effects of various illnesses on sexual functioning, and about the effects of psychological and sociocultural deprivations on human sexual functioning (Hogan 1980).

Four levels of sexual counseling have been described (Annon 1978; Zalar 1982):

1. *Permission*: Reassurance that the client's sexual practices are normal, and professional "permission" to continue his or her usual practice. Permission can prevent the escalation of a major problem.
2. *Limited information*: Providing information directly related to the client's concerns is within the nurse's domain. Limited information directly relating to the client's problem can effect significant changes in attitudes and behaviors.
3. *Specific suggestions*: Direct attempts to assist the client to change behavior in order to reach stated goals is the third level. At this level the nurse offers specific suggestions related to the client's particular problem.
4. *Intensive therapy*: The fourth level includes intensive therapy when brief therapy has not been effective. At this level the client is often referred to a professional with specific knowledge, experience, skills, and time to devote to specialized treatment.

Nurses working in acute or chronic care settings, schools, or nursing homes, on the generalist level, "should be able to competently assist clients with needs involving (1) permission and (2) limited information. These aspects of sexual health care are usually preventive in nature" (Mims 1977). Interventions on these levels include limited sex education and limited information about sexual feelings, behaviors, and myths (Zalar 1982). The other two levels, (3) specific suggestions and (4) intensive therapy, can be carried out by nurses with more specific training and advanced knowledge in the area of human sexuality, for example, a nurse educated at the practitioner level or at the master's level prepared in the area of human sexuality and therapy. The important prerequisites for a nurse in counseling a client about human sexuality on any level are knowledge, skill, and ease in discussing sex as an activity of daily living (Schuster et al. 1982).

Many nursing leaders encourage more sex education for nursing students in the nursing curricula, and believe that without training in sexuality, students might not have the necessary skills needed for sensitive and effective counseling. For example, students might not have the cognitive knowledge needed, the ability to recognize personal feelings, or the sensitivity to respond in an effective manner to reduce anxiety and enhance positive change. It is also believed that when sexuality has been altered, affected, or denied during the acute or chronic phases of illness, nurses should become aware of special problems their clients might be experiencing (Magenity 1975; Jacobson 1974; Zalar 1982).

Unique Assessment Strategies

There may be times when a physical condition or the result of surgery will alter or impair a person's sexual desire, ability to function, or sexual self-concept.

During the process of people's lives, there are many situations that can increase sexual tension and alter sexual drive; for example (Felstein 1986):

- Move to a new house/apartment
- Move to a new town/country
- Increase in traveling in one's occupation
- Starting a new career
- Regular or heavy gambling
- Drug and alcohol intake

For a person struggling with a physical or emotional problem, entering adolescence or advanced age, difficulties and concerns with sexual functioning are valid and vital concerns.

A variety of physical conditions as well as medical interventions can alter sexual functioning, and require counseling and information in order for the client to find alternative and satisfying means to attain his or her goals. The following are only a sample of common recurring health problems that can alter sexual function and greatly affect a person's sense of attractiveness and identification as a sexual being.

For example, clients who have experienced a myocardial infarction (MI) will have concerns with sexual function (refer to Chapter 15 case study, as an example). The most common cause of sexual dysfunction is lack of knowledge resulting in fear. A client often believes that sexual intercourse will cause another heart attack. Fatigue, pain, and shortness of breath related to cardiovascular disease may also cause sexual dysfunction (Stier 1986).

Clients who have had a leg amputated may be able to function sexually, but may see themselves as less attractive and worry about their partner's reactions.

Clients with disorders of the musculoskeletal system may also experience sexual dysfunction and disturbance in self-concept related to prolonged hospitalization, traction, casts, deformity, and pain. Sexual dysfunction can also be related to depression and anxiety as a result of the musculoskeletal disorder. Often, problems occur when the partner's perception of the client as a sexual being is altered, affecting their usual sexual relationship (McCausland 1986).

Clients with nervous system dysfunction may complain of sexual dysfunction as a result of insult to parasympathetic fibers from spinal cord segments S-2, S-3, and S-4; sympathetic fibers from the lumbar spine; or peripheral nerves from these segments (Markarian 1986).

Surgical procedures such as ostomies, mastectomies, hysterectomies, and prostatectomies can profoundly affect a person's self-concept, and require definite sexual counseling and encouragement of expression.

Often, other side effects of a variety of medications can cause sexual dysfunctions. For example, drugs that may cause *impotence* or *delayed ejaculation* in men and *decreased responsiveness* in women are:

- *Phenothiazines* (e.g., Mellaril, Thorazine, Prolixin).
- *Sedatives-Hypnotics-Opiates* (e.g., morphine, barbiturates, diazepam, lithium carbonate).
- *Tricyclic Antidepressants* (e.g., imipramine, desipramine).

Drugs that may induce *depression*:

- Antihypertensive drugs (e.g., reserpine, methyldopa, propranolol).
- Ethyl alcohol.

The following suggestions have been outlined by Cole and colleagues (1979) to help the nurse obtain information regarding sexual concerns or dysfunctions the client may be experiencing:

1. Do not force the person to talk about sex.
2. Place sexuality in the context of other problems.
3. Do not place your own moral standards on the client.
4. Conduct discussions in a clear and frank manner.
5. Do not assume that once the topic has been talked over it is resolved.

Hogan (1980) suggests that the nurse have an introductory statement prepared. For example, "As a nurse I am concerned about all aspects of your health. However, we often neglect helping clients in what may be a very important part of their lives—their sexual needs. I'm going to ask you some questions in this area."

Woods (1984) has suggested using a three-question form called "A Brief Sexual History" to obtain information about a person's sexual functioning and concerns. The first question asks about sexual *roles*, the second question identifies the person's *sexual image*, and the third, *sexual functioning*.

1. Has anything (illness, pregnancy, health problems) interfered with your being a (wife, husband, mother, father)?
2. Has anything (heart attack, mastectomy) changed the way you feel about yourself as a (man, woman)?
3. Has anything (surgery, disease) changed your ability to function sexually?

Table 28–1 suggests some statements the nurse can use to facilitate communication for identifying more specific areas and opening up channels for future teaching and clarifying.

It is important for the nurse to use correct terminology, even though the client may use slang words for parts of the body or sexual acts. Slang or street terms often have emotionalized connotations for the person using them. For the nurse to use such terms can cast doubts on the nurse's professionalism or competence. Always "check out" words the client may use to make sure both the nurse and the client are talking about the same thing (Hogan 1980).

Table 28–1 • STATEMENTS TO FACILITATE COMMUNICATION

SITUATION BEING EXPLORED	FACILITATING STATEMENT
Giving rationale for question	As a nurse, I'm concerned about all aspects of your health. Many individuals have concerns about sexual matters, especially when they are sick or when they are having other health problems.
Giving statements of "generality" or "normality"	Most people are hesitant to discuss . . . Many people worry about feelings . . . Many people have concerns about . . .
Identifying sexual dysfunction	Most people have difficulties some time during their sexual relationships. What have yours been?
Obtaining information from an unmarried individual	The degree to which unmarried persons have sexual outlets varies considerably. Some have sexual partners, others have none, some relieve sexual tension through masturbation, others need no outlet at all. What has been your pattern?
Identifying sexual myths	While growing up, most of us have heard some sexual myths or half-truths that continue to puzzle us. Are there any that come to mind?
Identifying feelings about masturbation	Many of us grown-ups have heard a variety of stories about masturbation and what problems it supposedly causes. This can cause worry even into adulthood. What have you heard?
Determining if homosexuality is a source of conflict	Some say homosexuality is a mental disorder, others an emotional block, others a crime or sin. What is your attitude toward your homosexual orientation?
Identifying older individuals' concern about sexual functioning	Many people, as they get older, believe or worry that this signals the end of their sex life. Much misinformation continues this myth. What is your understanding about sexuality during the later years? How has the passage of time affected your sexuality (sex life)?
Obtaining and giving information (miscellaneous areas)	Frequently people have questions about . . . What questions do you have about . . . What would you like to know about . . . ?
Closing the history	Is there anything further in the area of sexuality that you would like to bring up now? I hope that if questions or concerns do come to mind in the future we'll be able to discuss them.

Adapted from Green R. Human Sexuality: A Health Practitioner's Text. Baltimore: Williams & Wilkins, 1975.

Unique Intervention Strategies

From the sample of possible situations a nurse may encounter in the hospital setting, a number of nursing diagnoses become apparent. First, the obvious *altered sexuality patterns* or *sexual dysfunctions* related to a variety of pathophysiological conditions, treatment modalities, or situations is often present. Some problems may be due to a *knowledge deficit*. Problems identifying sexual identity should be assessed for and may take the form of *disturbance in self-esteem*. Not only may the individual experience *ineffective coping*, but a disruption of usual sexual patterns and methods of sexual expression in one partner may lead to *altered family processes*. When a person is left with a deformity or altered body image (mastectomy, ostomy), *grieving* is a natural reaction, one which can also alter a person's sexual desire or ability to function.

Nurses intervene in areas of sexuality on a variety of levels. Watts (1979) has identified various levels of assessment and levels of interventions appropriate for certain levels of training (Table 28–2). At the generalist level the nurse screens for sexual functions and dysfunctions. Nurse generalists will intervene at level one, which entails education, limited information about sexual feelings, behaviors, and myths. Nursing knowledge includes a sound understanding of sexual development, reproduction, sexual expression, sexual dysfunction, and disease.

Hogan (1980) stresses awareness of beliefs, attitudes, and values, since these directly influence how a person interacts with others. Values clarification on such topics as masturbation, dating, petting leading to orgasm, abortion, and homosexuality are important areas for self-evaluation. As nurses, we are entitled to our own feelings, attitudes, beliefs, and standards regarding sexuality; however, clients under our care are equally entitled to theirs, without censure or criticism.

Specific sex education and counseling, sex therapy, and individual and marital therapy are appropriate for nurses with postgraduate training in sex education and above. Therefore, nurse generalists need to recognize when referrals are indicated and know whom to contact.

Hogan (1980) goes on to stress that skill and sensitivity in understanding the client's concerns and relating

Table 28-2 • LEVELS OF ASSESSMENT AND INTERVENTION

PROFESSIONAL COMPETENCE REQUIRED	LEVELS OF ASSESSMENT	LEVELS OF THERAPEUTIC INTERVENTION
	Level 1	
Nurse generalist	Health history • Screen for sexual function and dysfunction	Limited education • Limited information about sexual feelings, behaviors, and myths • Refer to levels 2 or 3 if necessary
	Level 2	
Professional nurse with postgraduate training in sex education and counseling	Sexual history	Sex education and counseling • Specific information about sex and sexuality • Concise suggestions about sexual fears and adaptations to illness and anticipatory guidance • Refer to level 3 if necessary
	Level 3	
Professional nurse, physician, psychologist, social worker, all qualified as trained sex therapists	Sexual problem history	Sex therapy • Individual or group therapy • Couple therapy • Refer to level 4 if necessary
	Level 4	
Psychiatric nurse clinician with an MSN, physician, psychologist, social worker, all with subordinate specialty in sex therapy	Psychiatric and psychosexual history	Eclectic approach • Intensive individual psychotherapy, sex therapy, and marital therapy

There is linear relationship between the depth of a patient's sexual problems and the kind of professional competence that is needed to assess and treat them.

Watts DJ, Dimensions of sexual health. Copyright 1979 American Journal of Nursing Company. Reprinted from American Journal of Nursing, September, 1979, Volume 79, No. 9. Used with permission. All rights reserved.

empathically to them are as important as specific knowledge to answer client's concerns. Nurses are needed to promote sexual health in the home, schools, clinics, hospitals, nursing homes, and extended care facilities. Nurses at all levels are in prime positions to educate parents, community groups, school groups, and teachers on sexually transmitted diseases (STDs), especially AIDS (refer to Chapter 26).

In the discussion to follow, dealing with psychosexual disorders, specific interventions are the province of the professional staff with specific training in sexuality and therapy — nurses, social workers, psychologists, or psychiatrists.

Issues That Affect the Mental Health of Some Adults

RELATIONSHIPS PEOPLE CHOOSE

People today are more unlikely than in the past to accept a static, unsatisfying marriage. Changing economic needs and societal norms are such that we are more open to a variety of patterns. Concerns about the development of intimacy (close personal relationships) are widely discussed phenomena which affect the lifestyle choices of many adults (Herron and Rouslin 1984). Some of the choices we make will be discussed with an emphasis on how they affect our general mental health.

Premarital Relationships

Once believed to be the legal and moral right of only the married, sexual activity is now considered by some to be completely acceptable for any consenting adults. According to a report published by the National Center for Health Statistics (1985) more than 75% of American women are beginning sexual activity prior to marriage with almost all males doing so. This is a sharp increase from a previous survey in the early 1960's which showed 48% of women delaying intercourse until marriage. Indeed, the practice has become so commonplace that the Roman Catholic Council of Cardinals, meeting in 1985, felt it necessary to reiterate that premarital intercourse was not permitted according to that church's law.

For the young people involved, a new emotional difficulty has sometimes replaced the old one of "should we or shouldn't we?" It consists of a feeling reported especially by young women that they *must* have intercourse after a few dates. If one does not engage in sex, his or her maturity is suspect. The pressures of fear of pregnancy are largely dismissed (unrealistically, as one in every five babies born in the United States is out of wedlock and usually unplanned). The fear of the spread of disease does not appear to be sufficiently high to alter most heterosexual behavior, although the advent of AIDS has changed sexual practices for many. Most young people do marry and thus the premarital sex issue is put to rest for them. There is, however, an increasingly large group of adults who have never married.

The Never-Married Adult

The ranks of the never-married adult are steadily increasing in the industrialized nations. This relatively new phenomenon has not been evident long enough to afford us much statistical information, but the impact of the group seems to be increasingly powerful. By 1980, nearly 18 million Americans were living alone, although some of these had been previously married (Wolfe 1982). Typically, upon completion of as much schooling as was thought desirable, young people would begin to actively look for marriage partners. While this is still true in many cases, it has become much more acceptable for men and women to reach age 25 or older without having married. Economic independence and opportunity have dramatically changed the lifestyles of many in this group, affording them the opportunity to live independent of their family of origin. Sexual activity is frequent and the stereotypical "old maid" image has all but disappeared. Varieties of problems do exist for this group as they begin to age and find fewer societal supports for themselves than do other groups. Potential partners often leave the group for marriage, making it increasingly hard to find suitable choices. As members of the family of origin die or move, single adults may find themselves lonely and lacking for companionship. Worries about who will care for them in their old age become significant, and financial support in times of trouble is more tenuous than for those with a more comprehensive family network. Nonetheless, more and more adults are making the choice to never marry and many report satisfaction with their independent and self-sufficient life.

Traditional Marriage

Traditional marriage was, at one time, the goal of most of the American population. During most of this century it was considered inappropriate and even unlawful to have sex outside of marriage. Career choices outside of motherhood were very limited for women and unmarried men beyond a certain age were often regarded with suspicion. Cross-racial and cross-religious unions were unusual and divorce was considered quite scandalous and reserved for only the most serious of reasons.

A typical traditional marriage today contains many of these features, although there have been some significant changes. According to the National Center for Health Statistics (1985), the large numbers of people born after World War II (the "baby-boomers") have postponed marriage in order to further their education and careers. The marriage age for both men and women has been moving upward with men having a first marriage at age 24 and women at 21. Once married, the age of women having their first baby has also risen, and the total number of children born to a married couple has declined. Wives are much more likely to work outside of their home in today's marriage with over 50% of married women so employed. Thus a typical modern marriage might be like that of Ellen and Joe.

Ellen is a 24-year-old dental assistant. She has an AA degree from a community college and is taking a night course working toward another degree. She works for a local dentist four days a week. She and Joe have been married for two years. They live in a condominium on which they have a large mortgage. Joe is a technician for a public utility. He has had two years of college. As a union member his job is secure although his hours are long and he must work overtime during emergencies. Joe and Ellen met during high school. He was raised a Catholic and she a Protestant. They attend services at her parents' church on Easter and Christmas. They plan to have children in a few years when they can better afford a maternity leave for her.

Joe and Ellen had been seriously involved with other people during college. Although neither was a virgin at the time of their marriage they expect that they will be sexually exclusive with one another. One area of conflict for them has been Joe's desire to continue to "hang out" with his buddies from work after hours. He often will stop for a beer or to watch a game with them. Ellen feels this interferes with their relationship as a couple and reminds him that both their sets of parents had their spouses as their best friend.

Otherwise, they agree on most issues. Ellen does most of the housekeeping chores although Joe does help her. Although their parents are pressuring them for grandchildren, they are very satisfied with their decision to wait a few more years. They have sex three or four times a week and have no fear of pregnancy since Ellen is on the Pill.

Open Marriage

Open marriage is the name given to a relatively new concept that accepts free sexual interaction with those other than one's spouse. First popularized in the sixties (O'Neill and O'Neill 1972), it does not mean marital "cheating" in which one partner engages in extramarital sex without the knowledge or consent of the other. Instead, a couple agrees that together or separately, they will be involved in sexual activity with others. Although the phenomenon of open marriage has received a great deal of publicity, it does not appear to be prevalent in reality. In several surveys only between 2% and 4% of married couples reported having engaged in this activity (Hunt 1974; Taruis and Sadd 1977). Typical comments from couples who have attempted open sexual activities include such things as, "We hardly have time for sex with each other let alone outsiders," and "It has taken so long to build an intimate and warm relationship with one partner. I wouldn't want to take the chance of destroying it," and the practical and true, "The risk of picking up a disease just isn't worth it." Those few who do participate in open marriages over a period of time, however, seem very enthusiastic. Members of The Lifestyle Organization (TLO) based in Anaheim, California, actively promote open marriage and alternative lifestyles in human sexuality. They report enhancement of their marriages, relief from boredom, and openness and spontaneity, which they feel did not exist for them previously. They say, it is far better for a marriage to proceed on a foundation of honesty about sexual desire for others than to fall prey to the "cheating" type of extramarital behavior that prevails in so many traditional marriages. Both Kinsey and Hunt found that around 45% of men and 20% of women had at least one secret incident of extramarital sex. This kind of clandestine affair is much more devastating if discovered than an open sexual arrangement. Thus far, the social and legal codes of conduct of most cultures do not permit "open marriages" nor does this seem likely to change in the immediate future.

Divorce

Not many years ago divorce was considered so unacceptable that it was grounds for expulsion from "polite society." Politicians who divorced were considered unelectable and many legal statutes made it next to impossible to dissolve a marriage without grave cause. Yet divorce has become almost commonplace today with approximately 45% (almost half) of all American marriages ending in divorce (Glick 1980). Government studies show that 20% of first marriages end in divorce within five years (up from under 10%, ten years ago) indicating that there is less interest than in earlier years in "sticking it out."

Societal attitudes toward divorce have changed as the numbers of divorced people have increased. There is little if any taboo or social censure if children are not involved. Divorced persons almost always begin dating and resume sexual activity within a year of divorce, with 100% of the men and over 80% of the women reporting active sex lives.

Many divorced people express dissatisfaction with their lives, however. Society does not have a role for them and many feel a sense of personal failure at not having made their marriage work. Financial pressures are often an additional burden in the form of alimony and child support issues. Loneliness can become a problem and many divorced people begin to look for new partners as soon as possible. In fact those divorced people who do remarry tend to do so within five years of their breakup. Today about a third of all marriages involve at least one partner who has been married before (Glick 1980).

LIFESTYLE CHOICES

Remarried Family— Blended Family

As the divorce rate has risen, so has that of the family in which one or both partners may have children from a former marriage. Given many names such as "stepfamilies," "blended families," "remarried families," most of the participants seem to prefer to be thought of just as a "family." Since about three-quarters divorced parents do remarry (Calderone and Johnson 1981), as do most widows and widowers with young children, many children become someone's stepchild for at least a portion of their lives.

The task of these new family units becomes complicated as a variety of new roles are created. There may be stepsiblings present in the home. New babies become a challenge as a half-sibling and as a bond between the adult partners which the older children may resent or fear. Some children end up with many sets of relatives, "old" and "new" grandparents, cousins, friends, and even homes.

Donna and Rory are examples of parents who have created a blended family. Donna was divorced three years ago from John. She receives child support payments from John who has the children visit every other weekend and for one month in the summer. John has remarried a young woman who is expecting a baby in several months. Rory is divorced from Cathy. He has joint custody of his son who spends Monday through Thursday with his mother and Thursday through Sunday with Rory. Cathy has remarried Jim who has a 16-year-old daughter who lives in a distant state and who spends two weeks at Christmas and the entire summer with her father.

Donna and Rory would like to have a child together but fear the complication. At present their combined three children have several sets of parents and siblings to deal with. It is virtually impossible to arrange family vacations, as Donna's children are with their father when Rory's son is with him and the involvement of the new spouse's children make it impossible to change plans.

The children in this "remarried" family must deal with a variety of adults in different ways. Family rules and customs often vary from house to house. Religious convictions and financial status may differ, sometimes making the children feel as if they must fend for themselves in constantly changing situations. The parents involved have the problem of divided loyalty between new spouse, original child, new spouse's children by a previous marriage, and possibly new children produced in the new marriage. When former partners are hostile or still involved in disputes concerning finances or child custody the situation may become almost unworkable.

In intact families it can be expected that family members will help one another in times of stress and difficulty. Each person's problem creates a network of responses that usually lead to emotional balance. The family becomes the mediator between its members and the world. This kind of response is altered in the blended family, but it does not mean that it must disappear. Some extended family groups are able to continue to function in supportive ways even though traditional patterns have changed. Despite some times of confusion, the larger numbers of people involved can supply a variety of resources and emotional experiences for those involved.

Single Parent Family

Quite the opposite of the many adults usually found in a blended family is the ever growing number of families led by one parent. Once almost exclusively the result of death or divorce, single parenthood has become an option of choice for more and more people.

As mentioned earlier, many adults are now choosing to never marry but this may not mean a choice not to raise children. It is becoming more commonplace for women to have children although unmarried, and pregnancies are sometimes arranged via artificial insemination or unknowing partner with no thought that more than one parent will raise the child. Adoption by single people has become a possibility, especially in the case of the "hard-to-place" child. Despite media attention to the single father or deliberately pregnant single actress, the overwhelming majority of single parents are women and most have reached that status accidentally, that is via an unplanned pregnancy or divorce. About 45% of children today spend some or all their early years with only one parent (Calderone and Johnson 1981).

Often the situation is one of stress and discomfort for both parent and child. Unless finances are no problem, a child may be left unattended or in an inadequate day care or babysitting arrangement while the parent works. Without a partner to confide in or share burdens with, a single parent can become overly confiding in the child and may give the child too many responsibilities too soon. In many two-parent families at least one parent is available, either part or full time during the day and so is able to participate in school functions and activities. This is rarely the case for the single parent and can create added conflict.

The single parent who lives in close contact with an extended family or network of friends seems to have the best situation. If others are available to help with childrearing and finances, the job is made easier.

Homosexuality

Although sexual activity between those of the same sex has been evident throughout history and in almost every culture (Ford and Beach 1951), it has usually been considered immoral, illegal, or both. Even today, many states legislate against "unnatural sexual activity," and social acceptance of openly gay people is still far from complete, especially away from major urban areas.

In recent years, the spread of diseases such as AIDS has given rise to a new surge of antihomosexual feeling with comments such as "it's what they deserve," and "lock them all up" not uncommon. The fact that homosexual women (lesbians) are in the lowest AIDS risk group is ignored. Indeed the fact that female homosexuals exist is often ignored both in law and in social recognition.

The number of people involved in homosexual activity is difficult to estimate. Sometimes the activity is only situational and exists because there are no other partners available, as might be the case with a person in prison. On the other hand, there might be a person who is firmly convinced that he or she is homosexual and whose sexual fantasies only involve partners of the same sex. Due to religious or social pressure the person may choose never to act on these fantasies, and yet could probably be called homosexual. We do know that about 37% of all men and 13% of all women have had at least one sexual same-sex experience (Kinsey 1948, 1953). Among these, approximately 60% of both sexes have lived in a coupled relationship or a single one with numbers of partners, which they considered satisfactory (Bell and Weinberg 1978). In fact, over 50% of the men in Bell and Weinberg's lengthy study (1978) reported that they had had more than 500 sexual partners each.

The origin of homosexuality as a sexual choice is an area of great debate. Theories range from the concept that such a sexual preference is somehow genetically determined, hormonally influenced, the result of abnormal development as a child, or perhaps a matter of conditioning. For most people involved in homosexual behavior, the origins don't really matter. Of more importance is the finding of a partner and the need to develop a satisfactory lifestyle in a society with few guidelines or supports for them. One lifestyle of a homosexual male can be seen in the case of Jack.

Homosexual males

Jack was born the third child and only son of middle-class Catholic parents. From early childhood he had a strong interest in the games of his sisters and in his earliest sexual fantasies he almost exclusively chose other males as his partners. When Jack went away to college, he was approached by an older boy who initiated his first sexual experience. Six years later, Jack is living about 50 miles from his home town in a large city. He has had numerous partners, most of them met in gay bars. Recently, fearing disease, he has limited his activity to mutual masturbation. He would like to live in a permanent relationship with another man but hasn't found the right one yet. Jack has told his sisters about his homosexuality but fears telling his parents who are quite religious. Because his parents don't know about Jack's sexual orientation, Jack rarely visits home in an attempt to avoid questions about whom he is dating, and what he does in his free time. He once went to a gay men's rap group but felt uncomfortable with the politically active nature of the group. He has not "come out" at work for fear of ridicule. Although one of his sisters encouraged him to enter psychotherapy and "cure" his homosexuality, he has no desire to do so.

Jack's experience is typical of the way most gay men lived until quite recently. Fear of legal and social repercussions kept them "in the homosexual closet," and the desire to protect family from unpleasantness made them afraid to be open with parents and relatives.

For many gay men, Jack's kind of situation still exists, but in increasing numbers gay men are coming out and living their lives in a more open manner. Since the late 1960's the gay liberation movement has had an ever growing effect on the personal and political mores of the United States. Laws regarding consensual adult activity are increasingly being liberalized, and discrimination of any kind based on sexual orientation is less tolerated and is illegal in some states. Personal liberation has occurred for many people who are able to accept their homosexuality as natural, and who live their lives openly and happily. One such couple can be seen in the story of Jamie and Rhoda.

Homosexual Females

Jamie was 20, married, and attending a local college when she met Rhoda. They quickly became friends and greatly enjoyed the political discussions begun in their history class. Jamie had been married to Ron at 18 at her parents' urging. They believed a traditional role was best for women and were long-time friends of Ron's well-to-do parents. Jamie did not have much sexual experience when she was married and assumed that her lack of interest in sex with Ron was "just the way it is" for most women. Otherwise, her marriage was happy enough and she and Ron were good friends.

Rhoda had been involved with both men and women before she met Jamie. She was politically active in the campus women's movement and was becoming convinced of her own lesbianism. She was attracted to Jamie from the start and began to encourage her to join her friends in their activities. After a few months, Jamie and Rhoda became lovers. Jamie found sex with a woman an entirely different and better experience than with Ron. About one year after the women met, Ron and Jamie had their marriage annulled. Jamie immediately moved in with Rhoda and has been with her for 11 years. The women have been quite active in the lesbian liberation movement and Rhoda, who became a teacher, successfully sued the city board of education for the right to be a classroom teacher even though openly gay. Jamie occasionally sees Ron, who has remarried, and neither bears any resentment.

Because of the somewhat dramatic nature of the marriage breakup, Jamie never had to worry about when to "come out" to her parents. They knew from the start. At *first they were very upset and unaccepting, but as the years went by and their daughter seemed happy and in a stable relationship their attitude softened. Rhoda and Jamie are quite content in their life together and have a large circle of friends both straight and gay.*

The possibility of living in an open and accepted living relationship makes the quality of life for Rhoda and Jamie much better than for Jack. As more people gain knowledge about homosexuality and some of the homophobic bias of the past diminishes, it should be possible for more gay people to create a happy life for themselves.

SEXUALITY

Becoming a Sexual Being

We have come a long way since the late 1800's when Freud first made the apparently shocking point that sexual feelings and response did not just burst upon the scene in adolescence. Sex, it turned out, was present from birth, and in a much more complex and encompassing way than had ever been previously imagined. *First*, human sexuality is an evolving concept that includes cognitive, affective, social, and instinctual-psychological responses. Second, this development takes place in stages that build upon and can affect each other, both positively and negatively. Review Chapter 2 for psychosexual stages of development.

Sexuality is a part of human behavior throughout the life cycle. Now we know that infants, toddlers, and elementary school children are just as much sexual beings as adolescents and adults. We also know that the way parents and other adults respond to children affects subsequent psychosexual development. Yet, many people remain reluctant to accept the facts of sexual development. Denial is too frequent and ignorance about sexual behavior is found on all socioeconomic and educational levels. Nurses can help resolve a number of these problems with a straightforward presentation of facts that will help clients understand their children's needs. As Freud (1905) noted, children have sexual instincts that motivate a great deal of their lifelong behavior.

What Freud saw as a preadolescent latency period in regard to sex actually contains considerable private sexual activity. We are also learning a great deal about female sexuality, an area in which the early psychoanalysts had their confusions. In this regard, Masters and Johnson (1966) have shown the validity, and value, of the clitoral orgasm as opposed to the previously suggested superiority of the vaginal orgasm. Freud's greatest contribution was opening up the discussion of sexuality and sexual development. Previously, little was known or discussed and as a result parents had no idea how to view the sexual development of their children. We are now aware of the importance of our reactions as a child passes through the various stages. These early experiences in emotional relating have important consequences in later years. A positive and accepting attitude by parents provides a background for the child to have satisfactory adult relationships. An informed nurse is aware of developmental patterns, and uses his or her knowledge to help parents adjust to the child in different ways at different times. For example, if a mother of a two-year-old expresses dismay at the child's unexpected resurgence of clinging behavior, it can be explained that this is a part of necessary reassurance and is to be expected, not feared. When working with adult clients it is useful to relate their current state to earlier patterns. If the adult did not satisfactorily pass through each stage he may become stuck or fixated at a given level. This may occur because of parental errors, misfortunes, or pathologies and can range from severe to mild. Refer to Chapters 2 and 27 for problems that can develop when there are difficulties negotiating various stages of growth and development.

The Human Sexual Response

The importance of events in the early years of life on an adult's sexual patterns is indeed striking. For years, psychoanalytic theory has struggled with these issues in an attempt to assist adults in making fuller lives for themselves. Only recently, however, have we had adequate physiological knowledge of what occurs during a normal sexual response cycle.

In 1966, William Masters and Virginia Johnson published the results of their 12-year research project with almost 700 subjects (Masters and Johnson 1966). Using such devices as an electrocardiograph to measure changes in heart rate, a pH meter to measure acidity of the vagina, an electromyograph to measure muscular contractions, and an artificial penis complete with a recording apparatus inside, they began to collect the first verifiable data on the sexual response cycle during intercourse and masturbation. Over 10,000 sexual cycles were observed in men and women under conditions including fatigue, drug use, pregnancy, and old age. The resulting information is of profound importance to the field of sexology and has provided a factual basis for the relatively new techniques of sex therapy. Basically, Masters and Johnson discovered that there is one sexual response pattern for males and three basic patterns for females (Figs. 28–1 and 28–2).

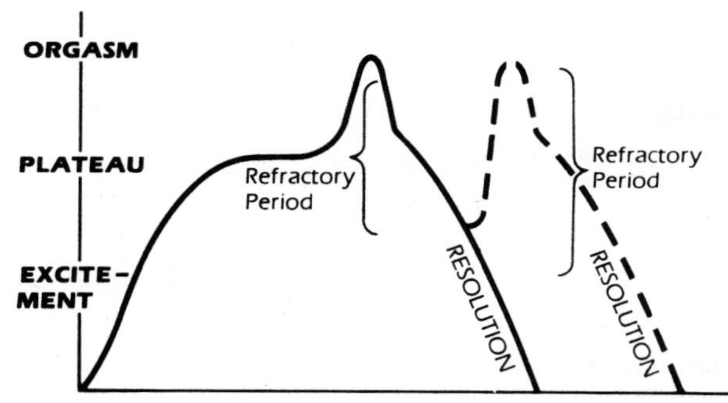

Figure 28–1. *Male sexual response cycle.* (Redrawn from Masters WH, Johnson VE. *Human Sexual Response.* Boston: Little, Brown & Company, 1966.)

In both males and females, the sexual response cycle begins with *stage one, the excitement phase.* During the onset of erotic feeling, males will experience erection of the penis and females will begin vaginal lubrication and often have swelling of the breasts and labia and "tenting" of the cervix and uterus. Blood pressure and pulse increase and some people experience a reddening of the skin called "sex flush." This leads to *stage two,* called *plateau,* if effective stimulation is continued. Here sexual tensions are intensified and will lead to the relatively brief *third stage* of *orgasm.* A sense of orgasmic inevitability is produced in which the person cannot stop the orgasm. During these 10 seconds or so males will usually expel semen and females will often experience uterine contraction.

After orgasm, both men and women will proceed to *stage four,* that of *resolution.* In males this is usually rapid, with the penis returning to its unstimulated size. The female clitoris will also return to normal position, and the orgasmic platform and uterus begin to shrink. This phase generally takes 15 to 30 minutes in women, longer if they have been stimulated but have not had an orgasm.

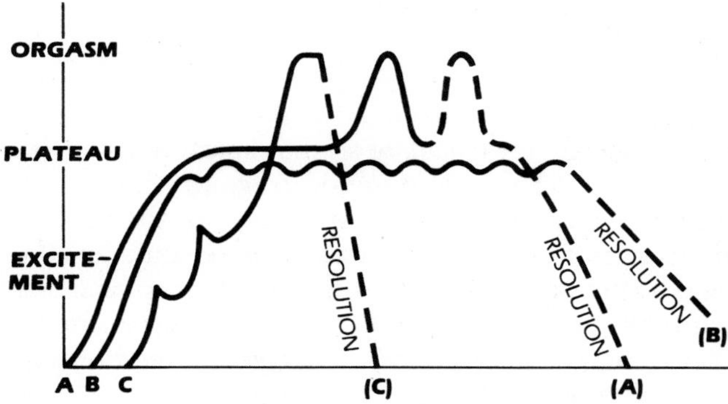

Figure 28–2. *Female sexual response cycle.* (Redrawn from Masters WH, Johnson VE. *Human Sexual Response.* Boston: Little, Brown & Company, 1966.)

During the resolution stage, males will enter the refractory period during which they cannot be aroused again. Age, culture, and expectation seem to determine the length of this period, which varies from minutes to days and from male to male.

The information the sexology community obtained from this research has both educational and therapeutic value. Indeed, one of the primary motives for conducting these studies originally was in order to aid those experiencing some kind of sexual dysfunction. Masters and Johnson have estimated that over 30% of American couples suffer a dysfunction (Masters and Johnson 1970), and they and other sexologists have developed a number of very specific techniques to deal with a variety of male and female sexual dysfunctions.

Sexual Dysfunctions

Refer to Figure 28–3 for an overview of the DSM III-R classification of psychosexual disorders.

In both male and female charts, a disorder called **inhibited desire** is listed. Kaplan (1979) contends that this disorder is the most common among couples requesting sex therapy. The DSM III-R refers to this disorder as *hypoactive sexual desire disorder.* Lack of desire is typified by deficient or absent sexual desire or fantasies, and a decline in sexual activity with no particular wish for this to improve. In cases where both partners, man and woman, suffer from this problem, there is usually no conflict. Only if there is a desire for a child, or if one of the partners becomes dissatisfied with the minimal or nonexistent sexuality is a sex therapist consulted. This dysfunction is sometimes situational, for example, occurring during times of unusual stress at work or upon the birth of a child. Sometimes it can be accounted for when one of the partners becomes involved sexually elsewhere. Thus, a man having a secret love affair may not be suffering from the sexual disorder of inhibited desire but rather from the marital problem of no longer being interested in his wife. For married couples sexual intercourse two to three times a week is considered average. Substantially less sex than this or failure of the male to have or maintain an erection 25% of the time or failure of the woman to lubricate much of the time are all symptoms of inhibited desire (Kaplan 1974).

SEXUAL DYSFUNCTION—MALES. *Sexual aversion disorder* is a disorder characterized by persistent or recurrent extreme aversion to, and avoidance of, all, or almost all, genital sexual contact with a sexual partner.

Erective incapacity is a disorder of the excitement phase of the sexual response cycle, which is included in inhibited desire but which can be separate from it. Formally

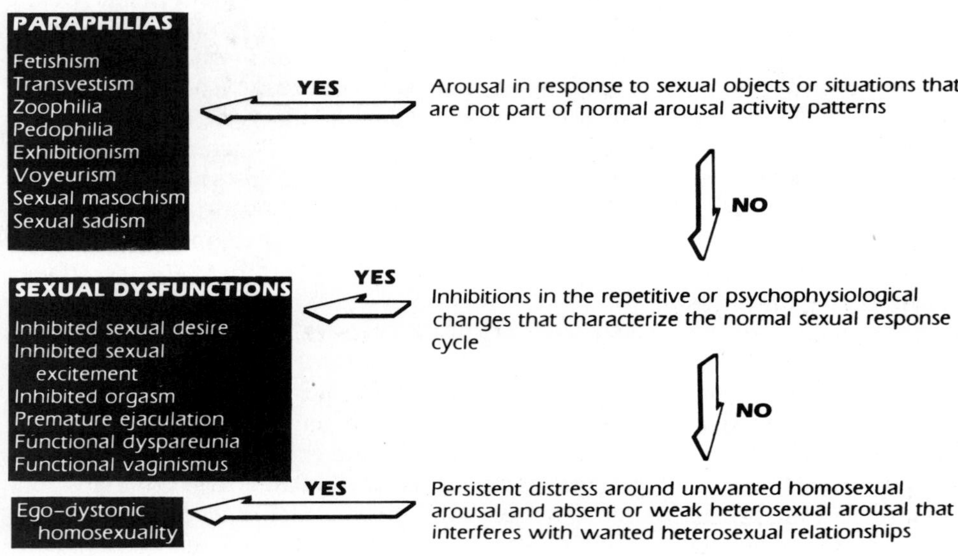

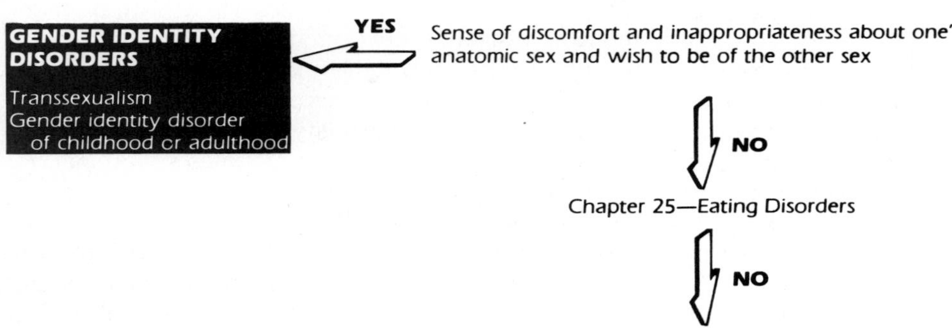

Figure 28–3. *Psychosexual disorders. (Adapted from* Janicak PG, Andriukaitis SN. DSM III: *Seeing the Forest Through the Trees. Psychiatric Annals,* 10(8):17, 1980, *and Diagnostic and Statistical Manual of Mental Disorders* [DSM III-R], *3rd ed., revised. Washington* DC: *American Psychiatric Association,* 1987.)

referred to as impotence, it is estimated that over half of the male population has had this experience some of the time.

Premature ejaculation used to be the most commonly presented sexual difficulty of males, but the effective therapeutic techniques used with this difficulty have reduced it to second place, behind inhibited desire. There are many ways to define what is premature. Some have suggested that any ejaculation occurring before the partner is satisfied is premature. Others suggest that ejaculation occurring before the man wishes it to more than 50% of the time is premature. However, this could include those who wish to engage in sex for hours before they ejaculate so that hardly seems a fair description. The usual duration of coitus is between four and seven minutes, so anything less than a two-minute erection more than half the time could be considered premature. It is not uncommon for some males who suffer from this difficulty to come to orgasm immediately on entering the vagina or even before they can proceed from foreplay to intercourse.

Ejaculatory incompetence, or retarded ejaculation, is a relatively rare phenomenon in which the male becomes repeatedly erect and wishes to ejaculate but cannot. This occurs in 1 in 700 men and is called in the DSM III-R *inhibited male orgasm*. Pain in the testicles will often occur after a length of time of erection with no ejaculatory release.

Ejaculatory or **postejaculatory pain** can also lead to sexual dysfunction as the experience of intercourse becomes more and more unpleasant. While not very common, those afflicted can suffer for minutes or even hours. See Table 28–3 for overview of male sexual dysfunctions.

SEXUAL DYSFUNCTION—FEMALES. In females, *inhibited desire* or *hypoactive sexual desire* is typified by lack of vaginal lubrication and a lack of interest in sex. Often referred to as "*frigidity*," this disorder seems to affect many women at times of stress or physical illness, but only a small number of women all the time.

Orgasmic dysfunction, or inhibited female orgasm, is the most commonly presented female problem. Some of those women involved are not interested in any case, but many are very interested in being able to fully enjoy sex. These women are taking an increasingly active role in assuring themselves this experience.

Sexual Pain Disorders. Vaginismus is the disorder in which the vaginal muscles involuntarily go into spasms during intercourse. This can cause great pain and lead to inhibited desire as well.

Dyspareunia is persistent genital pain in either a male or female before, during, or after sex. Table 28–4 gives an overview of female sexual dysfunctions.

CAUSES. The difficulties people have in creating a satisfactory sexual life can often be treated through a variety of behavioral and psychodynamic techniques by a professional with special training in this area. Many nurses have joined other health professionals in taking the additional training needed to become a certified sex educator/therapist through the American Association of Sex Educators, Counselors and Therapists (AASECT), based in Washington, D.C.

It is believed that *biological causes* of sexual dysfunction occur in only 20% or less of presenting cases. Biological causes include general illness, e.g., the flu, colds, or fatigue, and certain diseases, in addition to those mentioned earlier, such as diabetes, hepatitis, and multiple sclerosis. Hormonal disorders in which medications cause a drop in androgen such as hypopituitary problems and the feminizing of testicular tumors also may cause sexual dysfunction. Alcohol and hard drug use (cocaine and heroin) decrease sexual drive. As mentioned, hypertensive drugs and the phenothiazines can affect sexual performance in some clients. Other physical conditions that can cause pain are arthritis, back pain, obesity, vaginal infection, or late stages of pregnancy. Age can be a factor in sexual dysfunction in several ways. Postmenopausal women may need more lubrication and older men may find they do not ejaculate as frequently as they did when they were younger. Also, if a partner is lost through death or divorce and the one remaining has no sexual activity for a period of years, he or she may find it hard to regain sexual function. Age in itself does not cause dysfunction, however, and many couples report active and satisfactory sex lives well into their eighties.

Psychological causes of sexual dysfunction can be attributed to the following:

1. Ignorance as to what actions are stimulating for oneself or partner.
2. Anxiety due to fear of failure.
3. Demand for performance or an excessive need to please the partner.
4. Perceptual and intellectual defenses that get in the way of eroticism, such as "not feeling."
5. Turning off with judgmental thoughts and becoming engrossed in self-observation instead of participation.
6. Poor relationship choices that can result in partner rejection, lack of trust, power struggles, and other sexual sabotage that virtually guarantee that sex will not be rewarding.

Various schools of psychology take different approaches to the causes of sexual problems. Adherents of psychoanalytic theory explore unconscious conflicts connected to critical childhood experiences, such as guilt regarding sexuality, incestuous wishes, and the inability to trust and love another person. Adherents of systems theory emphasize the pathological transac-

Table 28–3 • SEXUAL DYSFUNCTIONS OF THE MALE

PROBLEM	PHASE	MAJOR SYMPTOM
Inhibited desire	Arousal-excitement	No erection, no sexual interest
Erective incapacity	Arousal-excitement	No or partial erection 50% of the time
Premature ejaculation	Orgasmic	Ejaculation before he wishes 50% of the time
Ejaculatory incompetence	Orgasmic	No or rare ejaculation
Ejaculatory pain	Orgasmic	Pain upon or just after ejaculation much of the time

Table 28–4 • SEXUAL DYSFUNCTIONS OF THE FEMALE

PROBLEM	PHASE	MAJOR SYMPTOM
Inhibited desire	Arousal	No lubrication, little interest
Orgasmic dysfunction	Orgasmic	Inability to have orgasm most of the time
Vaginismus	Orgasmic	Involuntary, painful spasms during intercourse

tions between partners that can create a sexually destructive environment, and behavior theorists see specific conditioned reactions impairing sexual response as a result of adversive contingencies that have followed sexual behavior.

TREATMENT. Treatment of the various dysfunctions is based on much of the pioneering efforts of sexologists like Masters and Johnson and Helen Singer Kaplan. Specially trained nurses and other sex therapists seem to blend behavioral and psychodynamic techniques.

When a couple decides on sexual counseling, a sexual history will become part of the general history taken in the first session or two. Particular emphasis is on trying to ascertain specific details as to what the couple actually does sexually. The therapist will want to rule out organic causes or require a medical consultation if in any doubt. She or he will want to determine what stage of the response cycle is impaired and if the problem is primary and one or both partners have never performed satisfactorily or if it is secondary and not always in force. The couple's interaction, as in their communication patterns and expectations, will give the therapist clues as to the psychodynamic relationships. Sometimes what is presented as a sexual difficulty may also be a greater problem in that the entire relationship is distressed. Also it is important to be alert for unconscious deceptions on the part of the couple. For example, many self-reported cases of female lack of orgasm can be more properly diagnosed as premature ejaculation. Also, often unconsciously, one or both partners may suffer from cultural attitudes which prohibit enjoyable sex. "Sex is for procreation not recreation" is an idea that still inhibits many people.

The therapeutic intervention required in all the possible cases of dysfunction will usually include anxiety reduction and a certain amount of "permission giving." The attitude that it is all right to enjoy sex is vital for successful treatment. Couples are urged to openly discuss their sexual needs and desires and to take turns, from time to time, in concentrating on giving pleasure to one or the other partner. The problem is treated as "theirs" not just his or hers. Information and education is considered crucial as is the need for open communication in order to change destructive patterns.

Sex therapy cannot be very successful if the relationship is not a good one. Indeed, this is one of the reasons for discontinuing the use of surrogates, a procedure which was once thought more appropriate. The sexual area is but one in the complexity of a total relationship and, while important, is not exclusively the issue.

Gender Identity Disorders

Gender, the physical fact of maleness or femaleness, is usually the first significant item to be known about a person. Social groups immediately begin prescribing different role models for males and females. Boys and girls are treated differently from birth (Rubin et al. 1974), from areas such as choice of toys and clothing to the amount of handling and cuddling each receives.

The child becomes aware early on of the psychological as well as physiological differences between the sexes and most are firmly committed to the societal expectations for their gender as early as 18 months of age. In rare cases where gender was misassigned at birth due to physical abnormality or where accidental damage has been suffered, it is considered almost impossible to reassign a child to the opposite sex after age one and a half. By then the sense of gender identity, of being male or female, is too firmly rooted to change (Money and Ehrhardt 1972).

For most people, the private sense they have of themselves as being male or female matches their physical makeup. As children grow into adolescence and become aware of sexual interactions they are clearly aware that they are a man or a woman, and, regardless of heterosexual or homosexual preferences, they will be satisfied in their gender identity.

TRANSSEXUALISM. There are, however, other people who do not have this match between biological gender and psychological gender identity. These people, called **transsexuals,** have an early and persistent feeling that they are trapped in a body with the wrong genitals. In reality, they believe, they are and were always meant to be of the opposite sex. Experts at the Erickson Educational Foundation, which studies transsexualism, have estimated that there are approximately

10,000 such people in the United States. About 2000 of these have undergone sex reassignment surgery to correct what they believe to be their physically flawed bodies (Slavitz 1976). Although both males and females are found in the greater group of transsexuals, men seem to outnumber women by about seven to one (Levine and Lothstein 1981).

Little is known of the origins of transsexualism, but childhood patterns seem to be fairly consistent. Typically, the child who becomes transsexual relates better to the other sex. Boys will prefer female friends and activities and will cross-dress whenever possible. Girls will develop masculine type behavior and refuse to be involved in those activities usually assigned to females. Of course, not all children with such childhood behavior become transsexuals. At puberty, the true transsexual will be quite horrified at the physical changes taking place. This is not true for most homosexuals or transvestites. The opposite sex behavioral style continues on into adulthood with transsexuals and often leads them to a desire for sexual reassignment as they find partners with whom they wish to live or marry.Transsexuals never consider themselves to be homosexual. The biological female who falls in love with a woman believes herself to really be a man who loves that woman. Thus a desire for congruity in gender identity and physiology becomes important for many.

Until 1964, Americans wishing such surgery were forced to go to other countries. In the last twenty years, however, such reassignment has been permitted at selected hospitals and clinics within the United States.

Treatment generally begins with psychotherapy for about two years. If the client is considered a potential candidate for surgery, he or she is urged to live in the cross-gender role for two years, e.g., dressing in the clothing of the opposite sex, or using make-up. After a period of time (two years), if the client is still considered a good candidate for surgery, then hormone therapy is begun. Hormone therapy (males taking estrogen and females androgen) helps develop the bodily characteristics desired, for example, hips and breasts in the biological male, and body hair and lack of menstruation in the biological female. The client continues cross-dressing and otherwise living as the "new" sex and continues psychotherapy. Legal and social arrangements are made, such as name change on various documents, and new employment if it is necessary to leave a former job owing to discrimination. Relationship issues are discussed in therapy such as what to tell parents, children, and former spouses. Only after it appears that a successful outcome is likely is surgery performed. Then the male will undergo castration for removal of the penis and a vagina and cosmetic clitoris will be made. The female will have a mastectomy and hysterectomy. Phalloplasty, the construction of an artificial penis, has been attempted but with little success. The organ produced has no sensation and is able to become erect only with an artificial device. The clitoris is retained as it is the only source of orgasm for the "new" man. At this time there is no possibility of transplanting the reproductive organs so the "new" men and women are always sterile.

Professionals debate the value of this type of sex surgery, with conflicting studies making the issue rather unclear. Some transsexuals seem to live happy and productive lives without undergoing this expensive and painful surgery, while others seem unable to function without it. The number of people involved is so limited that each case must be treated individually, and until more information becomes available few conclusive statements can be made about the desirability of sexual reassignment surgery.

Two different adaptations to transsexualism can be seen in the following vignettes:

Male To Female Transsexual

Susan, age 43, is a nurse who lives alone. In her earlier life she was Steve, a biological male, who always disliked his body and wished he were a girl. As a little child he used to tell his mother that he wanted his penis to fall off. He refused to stand while urinating, preferring to sit as his mother did. He stayed close to home, often helping his mother around the house and "dressed up" in her clothing and make-up whenever she would allow it. At first his parents permitted these activities thinking it was "cute," but when he began school they made some attempts to limit his feminine behavior. Steve adapted by hiding women's clothing in his room and used it whenever he could. He continued to play with the girls and in adolescence developed a crush on the captain of the football team. Steve's masculine body was very distressful to him, and consciously he did all he could to feminize it and yet still appear in such a way as to be accepted at school and home. By age 17, Steve was very anxious for sexual contacts and began to frequent gay bars. Although this provided him with some male partners he was not satisfied with his appearance or their statements regarding "gay pride." Steve did not feel gay but rather that he was a woman looking for a husband. During nursing school Steve learned of sexual reassignment surgery and immediately felt it would be right for him. He applied to Johns Hopkins University's Gender Clinic and was accepted. Steve followed the usual program for sex change and was surprised at the hostile reactions he received. When informed of his plans, his parents legally disowned him and have refused to see him since. He went ahead with the surgical procedure and changed his first name to Susan. Subsequently, he suffered from loss of promotion at work, where many staff members refused to associate with him, and he is presently planning to relocate to another state where he will attempt to keep his former identity a secret. Thus far, Susan has not found a husband but reports, "I would do it all again. My body looks as it should and I am content for the first time in my life."

Female To Male Transsexual

Laura, a female transsexual, has made a somewhat different adaptation. Like Steve, she felt cursed with the wrong body from early childhood. She was a "tomboy" from an early age and managed to wear dresses only when forced to. She was embarrassed by her developing breasts and hips at puberty and has always affected a mannish hairstyle and walk. Laura became involved with Patty, a slightly older woman, in college. Patty was quite feminine but disliked men. She had an earlier lesbian relationship which she had enjoyed and was happy to become involved with Laura. The couple have now lived together for nine years. Laura has not chosen sexual reassignment surgery since she can appear fairly masculine without it. She and Patty have fallen into rather traditional husband and wife roles. Laura is somewhat disturbed that others might consider her a lesbian, but since Patty is satisfied she accepts that label. Her inner belief is that she was meant to be Patty's husband and plans to continue their "family" as long as Patty will have her.

Sexual Disorders

For some adults the preferred expression of sexuality will include unusual behavior often found unpleasant or bizarre to the majority of people. Even when engaged in by consenting adults, these activities are usually criticized or even made illegal by the greater society.

The bias against these nonstandard behaviors is such that there is an assumption by both the public and professional communities that the participants are disturbed and unable to relate well to others. These **paraphilias,** as they are often called, are described officially as those activities which are unconventional and which diminish the capacity of the person to have a close relationship with another (American Psychiatric Association 1987).

Some people, of course, do find that having a strong desire or need to engage in unconventional sexual behavior is a problem. They may suffer from guilt, fear of ridicule, and may have difficulty finding partners. Others, however, do not experience these problems and are resentful of the mental health community's wish to "cure" them. The situation for many is similar to that of homosexuals not so many years ago. As long as a certain sexual activity is scorned and considered both illegal and disturbed, its adherents may suffer. As the general public becomes more educated and aware of their bias, more and more participants are free to be open and honest about the nature of their lives. As with all other groups, some people with a paraphilia may be unable to relate to others and are nongiving, whereas others may have few if any life difficulties.

Many people have no real wish to actually perform nonstandard behaviors but are sexually aroused by the fantasy. It is important to remember that this group of people also suffer and may be encumbered by guilt and shame.

The majority of people involved in the various paraphilias are male. There is no certainty as to why this is although explanations include genetic, hormonal, and social influences. Perhaps as women become better educated sexually and more free to determine their own desires in terms of behavior, they will become involved in greater numbers.

Certainly, culture and experience play a role in what is considered a paraphilia. For someone who has never seen a male dressed in other than trousers or jeans, a flowing silk gown might be considered abnormal wear. Yet, in many countries and eras such a gown would be appropriate for a man. In some cultures, a casual kiss between acquaintances on the street is the norm. Elsewhere, such behavior could be considered lewd, immoral, and reason for arrest. We often see a conflict between the stated norms such as, "sex should be reserved for marriage," and the actuality where the majority of adults have been involved in sexual experiences outside of marriage. Standards regarding what is the norm and what is not are always changing, so it is difficult to predict what will be acceptable and what will not in future years. Currently the following are considered unusual enough to be called paraphilias: fetishism, pedophilia, exhibitionism, voyeurism, transvestism, sadism and masochism, and zoophilia.

FETISHISM. A person with a sexual fetish will find it necessary to have some external object present, either in fantasy or reality, in order to be sexually satisfied. The fetish may be mild and quite socially acceptable such as black lace undergarments being worn by a woman as a necessary part of sex life with her husband. For many couples this would not present a problem but for some it might. If the fetish becomes more unusual and the partner needed his wife to wear a tightly fitting rubber corset, for example, she might well refuse. Some fetishists also develop problems when they do not have cooperative partners. They may assault women in public because they are wearing the fetish object or may commit robbery in an attempt to get a particular object.

Most fetishes develop during adolescence with the object often associated with the mother or other significant females. In some cases the fetish takes the form of objectification of a part of the body, such as the foot. This variation is known as partialism and often is undetected, especially if the object of excitement is also viewed as sexual by others (such as breasts and buttocks).

PEDOPHILIA. Pedophilia involves the desire or fantasy of an adult (16 years or older) to have sex with a prepubescent child generally 13 years old or younger. The DMS III-R states there has to be at least five years, age difference. Almost universally prohibited, it is nonetheless an activity that has occurred both cross-culturally and over the centuries. In recent years, a great deal of attention has been paid to this sexual abuse of children, and it is now thought that approximately 80% of the victims know the adult as a family member, friend, or neighbor (Sanford 1980). The sexual activity often includes fondling and masturbation, with intercourse occurring more rarely. Because those involved often know one another, it is believed that large numbers of cases of pedophilia are unreported. Some of those involved maintain that the activity is not necessarily harmful to the child and that a responsible adult participant will become sexual only with a consenting young partner. The age at which a child can truly give consent is, of course, open to question. Most people would agree that a seven-year-old cannot, but the ability of a 15-year-old to understand and desire sex is more debatable. Both are legally children, however, and thus are not able to engage in sexual activity with an adult according to the law.

Due to the secrecy about pedophilia, we do not have accurate information regarding its incidence or well-defined profiles of the pedophile. It is known, however, that the partners usually know one another and that the adult is often a married, somewhat conservative man. In cases of pedophilia among family members, which is called *incest*, the vast majority of cases include father or stepfather and daughter. Cases between mother and child are extremely unusual, with brother-sister incest believed to be more common.

EXHIBITIONISM. The intentional exhibition of one's genitals in a public place is deemed more harmless than many of the other paraphilia. Although exhibitionism is illegal, the exhibitionist is usually not interested in sexual assault or rape and prefers to startle his victims and then move on. This compulsive need to display the penis seems to often be triggered by stress in otherwise sedate, middle-class males. Females have been thought not to be involved as exhibitionists although one might argue that the intent behind some strippers and porno models could be the same as the street flasher.

VOYEURISM. "Peeping" at others while they make love or watching a woman undress is considered a paraphilia only when this activity becomes compulsive and preferable to other sexual activity. The voyeur is thought to be almost always a heterosexual, middle-class male who wishes no contact with those upon whom he is spying. Often the man is described as shy, socially unskilled, without close friends. A man who enters a building where these activities are going on, however, can be dangerous and he may commit crimes such as rape or robbery (Gebhard et al. 1965).

TRANSVESTIC FETISHISM. Transvestism involves obtaining sexual satisfaction via dressing in the clothing of the opposite sex. Thought to be an almost exclusively male activity, the desire to use woman's clothing is related to fetishism but often goes beyond the use of one particular object. Those involved usually develop their interest in female clothing early, and, unlike transsexuals, they have no doubt as to their masculinity or a wish to be female. Usually heterosexual, many transvestites only cross-dress in specific sexual situations and are often surprised to receive the cooperation and support of their female partners in obtaining clothes and other feminine articles.

SEXUAL SADISM AND MASOCHISM. Sexual sadism and masochism are two related paraphilias which include the giving **(sadism)** and receiving **(masochism)** of psychological or physical pain or domination. While statistics show that actual involvement in sadomasochistic activity (S/M) is not too prevalent, the fantasy of such behavior is quite frequent among both homosexuals and heterosexuals (Masters and Johnson 1979). For some, roles are never switched, with the desire always the same — to be the dominant or to be the submissive. More often, however, there is some mixing of roles with pain not necessarily a feature. Activities may range from mild restraint or biting to much more severe activity including inflicting bodily harm (Herron and Herron 1982). Both homosexual and heterosexual people are involved in sadomasochistic lovemaking, and many do not follow the sex-role stereotypes which might be expected. So, males who are thought to be more aggressive and dominant, in a psychological and social sense, are often interested in masochistic behavior. The same is true for females who wish to be sexually dominant (Herron et al. 1983).

Criminal acts of rape, assault, and other sexual violence are often described as sadistic or masochistic. While this may be the intent in some cases, one should no more link these crimes to S/M activity than one would link rape to intercourse. The vast majority of people involved in S/M are interested in having consenting, adult partners. In fact, in many S/M support groups, such as the Eulenspiegel Society of New York and the Society of Janus in San Francisco, the preparation of elaborate scripts outlining what kind of behavior is acceptable from person to person is commonplace.

OTHER PARAPHILIAS. There are numerous other nonstandard sexual behaviors that some people engage in as either a part of or their major source of pleasure. As with the other paraphilias discussed they may or may not cause a problem for the participant, depending on the availability of consenting partners and the societal norms at the time.

Some of these behaviors are zoophilia, or sexual contact with animals; coprophilia, klismophilia, and urologia are all associated with elimination of feces, enemas, or urine; necrophilia, in which a corpse or immobile partner is desired; scatophilia, where obscene language is used; and frotteurism, where sexual gratification occurs in rubbing up against a stranger.

INTERVENTIONS. Many of the people involved in nonstandard sexual practices find no need for therapy. If their sexual activities are carried out with a consenting, adult partner and do not involve any illegality, or are not physically or emotionally harmful to either partner, they are in no more need of counseling than any other person might be.

If, however, the person is experiencing relationship difficulties, wishes to change sexual orientation, or does become involved in illegal activity, or is physically or emotionally harming others or is being harmed, then therapy is indicated.

The most usual treatment design used specifically with paraphilias is behavior therapy. An attempt will be made to help the person learn a new sexual response pattern that will eliminate the need for the activity that is causing the problem. Techniques range from positive reinforcement for appropriate object choices to aversion techniques where mild electric shocks may be used at inappropriate choices. The most successful treatments seem to be those that include psychodynamic techniques designed to help the patient understand the origin of the paraphilia. Substitution can be helpful, as in the case where a pedophile's wife agreed to play the role of a child in dress and manner during some sexual encounters. In this way, the man was able to achieve sexual satisfaction in a legal way and his wife came to enjoy her role in helping him be involved with her instead of molesting children.

For many, however, therapy does not appear to alter criminal behavior. A relatively poor success rate has been shown for many sex offenders who have undergone treatment programs in prison.

Sexually Transmitted Diseases (STDs)

Any disease that can be contracted by sexual contact can be classified a sexually transmitted disease (STD). STDs are also called venereal disease, and there are a variety of types, which range from merely annoying to life threatening.

AIDS. Recently an enormous amount of attention has been paid to the usually sexually transmitted disease of AIDS or acquired immunodeficiency syndrome. Because the HIV (human immunodeficiency virus) can incubate anywhere between six months to ten or more years, there is grave concern among many people that they were exposed to AIDS years ago and now they live with the dread of developing AIDS years after the fact.

AIDS involves a disruption of the body's immune system. The virus attacks certain white blood cells called T-4 lymphocytes, leaving the person open to many serious diseases. Weight loss, diarrhea, lesions that do not heal, cancers, infections, and severe motor dysfunction are all possibilities on the road to almost certain death. (Refer to Chapter 26 for further discussion of AIDS.)

The United States leads the world in reported cases of AIDS. In 1988 it was estimated that a million and a half persons in the United States were infected and that 100 new cases of AIDS per day were being reported (Jones 1988). The Center for Disease Control states that approximately 73% of AIDS victims are homosexual or bisexual males, 17% intravenous drug users, 1% hemophiliacs, 1% heterosexuals, 1% blood transfusion recipients, and 7% others. During sexual intercourse infected semen enters the partner's bloodstream through abrasions in the mucous membranes. Intravenous drug users can be contaminated when the blood from one infected user is passed via a shared needle to another. Caretakers and relatives of AIDS victims are rarely at risk. The virus, which must enter a person's bloodstream to cause infection, is carried in the highest concentration in blood and semen and in low concentration in saliva and sweat. A caretaker is rarely in contact with the former and is thus not likely to contract the disease.

There is enormous public outcry and fear regarding the disease. Hospitals have refused to accept AIDS victims as clients, and school systems throughout the country have rejected AIDS students in response to boycotts led by fearful and angry parents. Some nations have considered requiring screening blood tests for any foreigners wishing to visit.

Although safe sex practices can be taught, and early studies showed the gay community significantly changing its sexual habits (National Center for Health Education 1985), there is disturbing evidence that education is not eradicating the problem to the extent formerly hoped for. Although dramatic behavior changes have occurred, especially in the gay community, infection of intravenous drug users and a smaller number of homosexuals continue. In spite of massive health education programs aimed at high risk groups, there are those who pay no more attention to these programs than many do to other health issues, such as cessation of smoking (Stall 1988). Meanwhile, research efforts are continuing in an effort to find a way to combat this dreaded disease. (Refer to Chapter 26).

HERPES. Another sexually transmitted disease that has received widespread attention in recent years is herpes simplex virus (HSV, or *Herpesvirus hominis*). The United States Public Health Service (1982) reports that there is at least a tenfold increase in cases in the last ten years and that there is no cure for the viral infection as yet. At present, herpes genitalis is not a reportable disease. It is most often found in the 15–30 age group.

Herpes genitalis is an infection resulting in rupture of vesicles causing painful ulcers. Systemic symptoms include fever, malaise, and inguinal node enlargement. Symptoms occur approximately two to seven days after incubation.

The ulcers are usually present on the medial aspects of the labia minora, clitoris, vagina, urethra, and cervix. They can last from four to six weeks (Wardell 1986). The first attack tends to be the most severe and about two-thirds of herpes victims do not have any more outbreaks although the virus does remain in the system. One-third of the victims do have recurring infections, which are contagious as long as the symptoms are present. Although there is no known cure, Acyclovir (Zovirax), can reduce pain and itching and may reduce the duration of the first attack.

Other side effects of herpes can include keratitis where the virus is transferred to the eyes. An association with cervical cancer and the infection of infants born vaginally to mothers with an outbreak of the disease is suspected. Psychological effects can also be quite profound with some people losing all sexual desire because of fear of contracting or spreading the disease. Among some single adults the question; "Are you clean?" has become part of dating procedure, with the herpes client consequently left feeling most undesirable.

Health care professionals can do a great deal to educate the public about the prevention of herpes. Those with an outbreak can be taught to avoid sexual activity. Mothers can be encouraged to deliver their babies by cesarean section if an outbreak occurs. Washing of hands and towels and sheets can help prevent the spread of the virus.

GONORRHEA. Gonorrhea is one of the most common STDs. Gonorrhea is a bacterial infection (*Neisseria gonorrhoeae*) which enters the body through warm, moist areas such as the genitals or mouth. Approximately one million cases are reported each year and three million are suspected. Males tend to experience pain when urinating and discharge; about 50–75% of females have less obvious early indications and may be asymptomatic, while others may experience painful urination and discharge. Sterility can be caused by untreated gonorrhea in both men and women.

Since the early stages are not obvious in women, it is likely that the disease will not be treated and secondary infections such as inflammation of the pelvis (PID) can occur. A baby born to an infected mother will become blind if the bacteria enters his or her eyes. Therefore all newborns' eyes are now treated with tetracycline or silver nitrate to prevent possible blindness.

Early diagnosis of gonorrhea is painless and important. Uncomplicated cases are treated with a single dose of aqueous penicillin G procaine (4.8 mil units intramuscularly) divided and given in two sites, and probenecid (Benemid) (1.0 g by mouth) (Campbell and Frisse 1983). Streptomycin hydrochloride may be used if the client is allergic to penicillin or the organism is penicillin resistant. A repeat culture should be taken two weeks after pharmacological treatment. Treatment is relatively simple with effective antibiotics. Gonorrhea is twice as prevalent as it was 15 years ago.

Use of condoms, washing of the genitals, and visual inspection of a partner's genitals can help prevent the spread of this and other sexually transmitted diseases.

SYPHILIS. Syphilis is caused by the spirochete *Treponema pallidum*, and remains a serious sexually transmitted disease, with over 25,000 cases reported each year between 1980 and 1986 (CDC 1986). Penicillin or other antibiotics are able to cure the disease at any stage, although damage that has already been caused by the disease cannot be reversed.

Syphilis appears to have existed for many centuries in all parts of the world. It is a chronic infection, which can be transmitted via the mouth, genitals, anus, or even a small lesion. It travels through the blood stream to all parts of the body and can take many years to develop completely into a serious and life-threatening illness.

In its *primary stage*, syphilis can be detected by dark-field examination after the incubation period of 10 to 90 days. The only symptom is a painless sore called a chancre, which usually appears near the mouth, anus, or genitals within a week to several months after infection. The chancre grows for one to eight weeks and generally is open at the top with a band of hard tissue around the base. Because it is quite painless or in females may be growing internally, this sore is often ignored or not seen. If it is not treated at this stage the ulcers will heal in three to nine weeks and the disease goes on to the second stage.

The *second stage* lasts between two and ten weeks while the disease spreads with sores or lesions appearing on the vulva, mouth and pharynx, axilla, and under the breasts. During this stage systemic symptoms may occur such as fever, sore throat, and headache. All these symptoms disappear even without treatment, and the disease can still be unknown to its victim.

The *third or latent stage* of syphilis can last for decades. No longer contagious, except to a child born of a carrier parent, the disease nonetheless may attack various parts of the body including the circulatory and nervous system.

Only in the *fourth, late stage* of syphilis does its presence become obvious. Serious illness, blindness, and mental and cardiovascular problems can all be present.

The treatment of syphilis in the primary and secondary stages is with penicillin G benzathine (2.4 mil units in a single dose) (Campbell and Frisse 1983). Probenecid (Benemid) is given 30 minutes before injection to help maintain plasma concentration of the penicillin. Clients allergic to penicillin may be given tetracycline hydrochloride (500 mg by mouth 4 times a day for 15 days) (Campbell and Frisse 1983).

Fear of syphilis has waned some with the advent of more effective treatment procedures. Still there are hundreds of thousands of cases reported in the United States each year and possibly many more which go undetected until it is too late to cure them.

Summary

Nurses at the generalist level can take a health history and screen for sexual function and dysfunction. Nurses at this level are in key positions to teach others (parents, community, adolescents) about sexually transmitted diseases, bio-psycho-social aspects of sexuality throughout the life cycle, and the effects of certain illnesses on sexual functioning.

Many adults in our society experience stress surrounding changing social mores, relationship issues, and sexual behavior. In order to recognize these issues and to help clients come to terms with them, the nurse should become aware of the various kinds of difficulties and the developmental basis for them.

Personality patterns and sexual awareness and reactions begin to develop in the very early years. A typical pattern will include a relatively smooth transition from one stage to the next with the child first experiencing the world and the relationship via the primary caretaker, and might include many years as a single adult due to divorce, death, or never-married status, and often includes single parenting. If remarriage occurs, the issues of blending the two former families into one can be difficult.

For some adults, sexual orientation can cause life stress problems or relationship difficulties. Homosexuals are just beginning to gain legal and social acceptance, and those who engage in other nonstandard behaviors are often shunned and live in fear of legal action.

Prevalent sexual dysfunctions among men and women have been discussed. Specific sexual disorders (paraphilias) were mentioned. An overview of prevalent sexually transmitted diseases was presented.

Issues such as those discussed in this chapter are of great importance to individuals in their quest to obtain a satisfactory adult life. Knowledge and empathy regarding these formerly little discussed areas are needed in order for nurses to assist clients in improving the quality of their lives.

References

American Psychiatric Association. Diagnostic and Statistical Manual of Mental Disorders, 3d ed., revised. Washington DC: American Psychiatric Association, 1987.

Annon JS. The PLISSIT model: A proposed conceptual scheme for the behavioral treatment of sexual problems. Journal of Sex Education and Therapy, 2:1, 1978.

Bell AP, Weinberg MS. Homosexualities. New York: Simon & Schuster, 1978.

Bohannan P. Divorce and After. Garden City, NY: Doubleday, 1968.

Calderone MS, Johnson EW. The Family Book About Sexuality. New York: Harper & Row, 1981.

Campbell JW, Frisse M (eds). Manual of Medical Therapeutics. Boston: Little Brown and Company, 1983, pp. 897–899.

Centers for Disease Control. Statistical data re syphilis. Morbidity and Mortality Weekly Report, pp 356–362, 1986.

Cole CM, Levin EM, Whitley JO, et al. Brief sexual counseling during cardiac rehabilitation. Heart Lung, 8:124, 1979.

Ellis H. Studies in the Psychology of Sex. New York: Basic Books, 1938.

Fairbairn WP. An Object-Relations Theory of the Personality. New York: Basic Books, 1952.

Felstein I. Understanding Sexual Medicine. Lancaster, England: MTP Press Limited, 1986.

Ford C, Beach F. Patterns of Sexual Behavior. New York: Ace, 1951.

Freud S. Three essays on the theory of sexuality. The Standard Edition Of The Complete Psychological Works of Sigmund Freud, 7. London: Hogarth Press, 1905, 125–145.

Gebhard P, Gagnon JH, Pomeroy WB, Christenson CV. Sex Offenders: An Analysis of Types. New York: Harper & Row, 1965.

Glick PC. Remarriage: Some recent changes and variations. Journal of Family Issues, 1:455, 1980.

Hamilton R. The Herpes Book. Los Angeles, CA: JP Tarcher, 1980.

Herron MJ, Herron WG. Meanings of sadism and masochism. Psychological Reports, 50:199, 1982.

Herron MJ, Herron WG, Schultz CL. Sexual dominance/submission, gender and sex-role identification. Perceptual and Motor Skills, 56:931, 1983.

Herron WG, Rouslin S. Issues in Psychotherapy, Vol 1. Washington DC: Oryn, 1984.

Hogan R. Human Sexuality, A Nursing Perspective. New York: Appleton-Century-Crofts, 1980.

Hunt M. Sexual Behavior in the 1970's. Chicago: Playboy Press, 1974.

Jacobson L. Illness and sexuality. Nursing Outlook, 22:50, Jan. 1974.

Jones JM. Section Introduction. Psychology and AIDS. American Psychologist, 43(11):899, 1988.

Kaplan HS. The New Sex Therapy. New York: Brunner/Mazel, 1974.

Kaplan HS. Disorders of Sexual Desire. New York: Simon & Schuster, 1979.

Kinsey A, Pomeroy W, Martin C. Sexual Behavior in the Human Male. Philadelphia: W.B. Saunders Company, 1948.

Kinsey A, Pomeroy W, Martin C, Gebhard P. Sexual Behavior in the Human Female. Philadelphia: W.B. Saunders Company, 1953.

Kolodry RC, Masters WH, Johnson VE. Textbook of Human Sexuality for Nurses. Boston: Little, Brown & Company, 1979.

Krueger JC, Hassell J, Goggin DB, et al. Relationship between nurse counseling and sexual adjustment after hysterectomy. Nursing Research, 28:145, 1979.

Ladas AK, Whipple B, Perry JD. The G Spot. New York: Dell, 1981.

Levine S, Lothstein LM. Transsexualism or the gender dysphoria syndromes. Journal of Sex and Marital Therapy, 7:85, 1981.

Magenity J. A plea for sex education in the nursing curriculum. American Journal of Nursing, 75:1171, 1975.

Markrian MF. The nursing process for clients with nervous system disorders. *In* Kneisl CR, Ames SW (eds). Adult Health Nursing. Reading, MA: Addison-Wesley Publishing Company, 1986.

Masters WH, Johnson VE. Human Sexual Response. Boston: Little, Brown & Company, 1966.

Masters WH, Johnson VE. Human Sexual Inadequacy. Boston: Little, Brown & Company, 1970.

Masters WH, Johnson VE. Homosexuality in Perspective. Boston: Little, Brown & Company, 1979.

McCausland LH. Surgical approach to musculoskeletal system dysfunction. *In* Kneisl Cr, Ames SW (eds). Adult Health Nursing. Reading, MA: Addison-Wesley Publishing Company, 1986.

Mims FH. Sexuality in the nursing curriculum. Nursing Education, 11:23, 1977.

Money J, Ehrhardt A. Man and Woman, Boy and Girl. Baltimore: Johns Hopkins Press, 1972.

National Center for Health Education. The emerging pandemic of AIDS. Center, 3:3, 1985.

National Center for Health Statistics. National survey of family growth. Washington DC: National Center for Health Statistics, 1985.

O'Neill GO, O'Neill N. Open Marriage. New York: M. Evans, 1974.

Rubin J, Provanzano F, Luria Z. The eye of the beholder: Parent's view on sex of newborns. American Journal of Orthopsychiatry, 44:512, 1974.

Sanford LT. The Silent Children. Garden City, NY: Dell, 1980.

Schuster EA, Unsain IG, Goodwin MH. Nursing practice in human sexuality. Nursing Clinics of North America, 17(3):345, 1982.

Sexton RE, Sexton VS. Intimacy: A historical perspective. *In* Fischer M, Stricker G (eds). Intimacy. New York: Plenum Press, 1982.

Slavitz H. Transsexualism: A radical crisis in gender identity. *In* Gordon S, Libby R. (eds). Sexuality Today and Tomorrow. North Scituate, MA: Doxbury Press, 1976.

Stall R, Coates T, Hoff C. Behavioral risk reduction for HIV infection among gay and bisexual men. American Psychologist, 43(11):878, 1988.

Stier FL. The nursing process for clients with major blood vessel dysfunction. *In* Kneisl CR, Ames SW (eds). Adult Health Nursing. Reading, MA: Addison-Wesley Publishing Company, 1986.

Taruis C, Sadd S. The Redbook Report on Female Sexuality. New York: Delacorte Press, 1977.

U.S. Public Health Service. Sexually transmitted diseases: Treatment guidelines. Morbidity and Mortality Weekly Report, 17:356, 1982.

Wardell DW. Specific disorders of the female reproductive system. *In* Kneisl CR, Ames SW (eds). Adult Health Nursing. Reading, MA: Addison-Wesley Publishing Company, 1986.

Watts RJ. Dimensions of sexual health. American Journal of Nursing, 79(9):1570, 1979.

Weinberg JS. Sexuality, human needs and nursing practice. Philadelphia: W.B. Saunders Company, 1982.

Wolfe L. The good news. New York Magazine, 15(7):33, 1982.

Woods NF. Human Sexuality in Health and Illness, 3rd ed. St. Louis: C.V. Mosby Company, 1984.

Zalar MK. Role preparation for nurses in human sexual functioning. Nursing Clinics of North America, 17(3):351, 1982.

Self-Study Exercises

Using Watts Levels, identify the following levels with either the assessment or the intervention level:

1. ________ Takes a psychiatric and psychosocial history.
2. ________ Is a professional nurse with postgraduate training in sex education and counseling.
3. ________ Sex therapy—individual or group.
4. ________ Imparts limited information about sexual feelings and behaviors.
5. ________ Screens for sexual function and dysfunction.

A. Level 1
B. Level 2
C. Level 3
D. Level 4

Match the stages in the human sexual response.

6. ________ The sex organs return to normal.
7. ________ Orgasm occurs.
8. ________ Build up of sexual tension.
9. ________ Onset of erotic feelings.

A. Stage 1—Excitement

B. Stage 2—Plateau

C. Stage 3—Orgasm

D. Stage 4—Resolution

Match the following paraphilias with their definition:

10. ________ Need for a specific object.
11. ________ Public display of genitals.
12. ________ Sexual arousal when cross-dressing.
13. ________ Pain or humiliation and sex.
14. ________ Sex with a child.

A. Sadomasochism

B. Pedophilia

C. Fetishism

D. Exhibitionism

E. Transvestic fetishism

Complete the statements by filling in the appropriate information.

15. Masters and Johnson discovered that males but not females have a ________ period in a typical sexual response cycle.
16. Approximately ________ % of American women begin sexual intercourse prior to marriage.
17. Approximately ________ % of all American marriages end in divorce.
18. The gender identity disorder resulting in a person believing he or she is really the other sex is called ________.
19. ________ is considered the most common sexual dysfunction.
20. Helen Singer Kaplan advocates a blending of ________ and ________ techniques in treating sexual dysfunction.

Brief Essay

21. Write a paragraph comparing and contrasting a person who has a homosexual lifestyle with a person who is a transsexual living a cross-gender role.

CHAPTER 29

The Elderly

Sally Kennedy Holzapfel

OUTLINE

KEY TERMS AND CONCEPTS

The key terms and concepts listed here also appear in bold where they are defined or discussed in this chapter.

AGEISM

ZUNG SELF-RATING DEPRESSION SCALE

SOCIAL DYSFUNCTION RATING SCALE (SDS)

REMOTIVATION THERAPY

REMINISCING THERAPY

GROUP PSYCHOTHERAPY

DAY CARE PROGRAMS

DIAGNOSTIC RELATED GROUPS (DRGs)

MEDICARE

MEDICAID

LIVING WILLS

HOSPICE PHILOSOPHY

HIGH RISK SUICIDE FACTORS IN THE ELDERLY

OBJECTIVES

After studying this chapter, the student will be able to:

1. Discuss five myths on aging.
2. Compare the purpose, format, and desired outcomes among the following group treatments: remotivation, reminiscing, and psychotherapy.
3. Explain two advantages and two disadvantages of the DRGs.
4. Compare and contrast the differences between Medicare and Medicaid.
5. Recognize guidelines a nurse can employ in approaching issues of life and death with a client.
6. Discuss ways in which the nurse may assist families of a dying client.
7. List three goals of Living Wills.
8. Summarize the concept of the Hospice Program.
9. Identify the elder group at highest risk for suicide.
10. Describe the characteristics of two types of elderly alcohol abusers.

The growing number and proportion of elderly in the United States have a significant impact on our economic, social, and health institutions, and mental health services. For example, at the turn of the century, 4% of the total population was over 65 (Schneider and Emr 1985). In 1983, 11.7% of the total population was over 65, and by the year 2000, 13.2% of the population will be over 65. By the year 2040, estimates indicate 20.5% of the population will be over the age of 65 (Price and Feldman 1983).

The trend in the health of the elderly has shown that chronic illness and disability are the major threats to the older person's health as opposed to acute illnesses. At least 80% of individuals over 65 report at least one chronic condition; many elderly have multiple chronic conditions (Price and Feldman 1983). The likelihood of developing one or more chronic illnesses increases significantly with age: individuals 75 years of age and older are the most prone to chronic illnesses and functional disabilities. Chronic illness is responsible for more than 70% of all deaths (Kayser-Jones 1986).

The life expectancy for males increased from 46 years at the turn of the century to 74 in 1983; females' life expectancy climbed from 48 to 78 years in the same period. In 1983, there were 149 women for every 100 men in the over 65 category. The female-male sex ratio increases with age. Women's greater longevity has significant ramifications for society and for the health care professions in particular. More older women with more severe functional limitations are the people the health professions will be working with, both in the community and in nursing homes (Caserta 1983).

It is meaningful to separate the needs of persons in the older age groups, particularly the group 85 and older, from those of other aged persons; there are noticeable differences between individuals in their sixties (old) and people in their eighties (old-old). The younger group is relatively healthy; the older group is much more profoundly affected by the chronic diseases and disorders of aging. In fact, the fastest expanding age group is the group 85 years or older. Presently 1% of the population is over 85 years of age; it may increase as much as eightfold in the next 40 to 50 years (Schneider and Emr 1985).

The following list identifies specific facts about mental health and the aged (Cohen 1980; Burnside 1988):

1. Mental illness is more prevalent among the elderly than among younger persons (18–25% of the elderly have mental problems).
2. Psychosis increases significantly after age 65.
3. Suicide occurs more frequently among the elderly than in any other age group.
4. Senile dementia is the fourth leading cause of death among the elderly.
5. Fifteen percent of the elderly have chronic physical problems that can result in negative psychological responses.

Dementia and depression are two major mental health concerns among the elderly.

Alzheimer's disease, an organic mental disorder, is the most common form of dementia in the elderly. Individuals in their sixties and early seventies have a 4% chance of developing Alzheimer's disease; there is a 10–15% risk of developing Alzheimer's when people reach their late seventies and early eighties; in the 85 and older age group, the risk is between 20 and 30%. Schneider and Emr (1985) predict Alzheimer's disease to be the leading cause of death in the next century. See Chapter 21 for a discussion of Alzheimer's disease.

The population of elderly persons has been increasing so steadily that questions of elder care are highly apparent whenever issues about health care delivery are raised. Unfortunately the elderly receive little attention in the positive areas of health education aimed at prevention and rehabilitation; they receive a great deal of notice in tertiary care, high technology care, and, finally, institutional care (German 1981).

The increasing number and population of elderly persons are having a significant impact on the utilization and cost of health care services, and this has important implications for nursing (Kayser-Jones 1986), especially in hospitals and nursing homes.

The Role of the Nurse

Nurses have much to contribute to the care and promotion of health in the elderly. However, questions arise as to whether student nurses are given accurate information and sufficient exposure to the elderly. If not, sufficient theory and principles needed to provide safe and excellent care to elders are deficient (Burnside 1988). Lack of specific information necessary for a student nurse to make sound decisions in regard to elderly clients is in part a result of the following:

- Negative faculty attitudes toward the old.
- Lack of exposure and lack of clinical emphasis with older persons.
- Negative student attitudes toward the elderly due to information based on myths and stereotypes.
- Unfamiliarity with gerontological information and resources.

One of the factors that contribute to the negative view that nurses (generalists, educators, students) as well as the general population have toward the elderly are the myths that surround being old. These myths and stereotypes of the aged underlie the phenomenon of ageism.

AGEISM AND THE ELDERLY

Ageism has been defined as a bias against older people based solely on their age (Gambert 1983); it is a system of destructive, erroneous beliefs. In essence, ageism reflects a dislike by the young of the old (Preston 1986), depicting the disparaging effect of society's attitudes toward the elderly (Austin 1985).

Ageism differs from other forms of discrimination in that it cuts across gender, race, religion, and national origin (Neussel 1982). Old age does not award a desirable status or membership in a sought-after club; rather, it is a social category with negative connotations (Matthews 1979). Butler (1975) has written:

> Ageism is manifested in a wide range of phenomena, both on individual and institutional levels—stereotypes and myths, outright disdain and dislike, or simply subtle avoidance of contact; discriminatory practices in housing, employment, and services of all kinds; epithets, cartoons, and jokes.

Effects of ageism can be observed throughout different levels of society; even health care providers are not immune to its effects. Their attitudes reveal in many instances society's values as a whole, which are characterized by negativism and stereotyping (Benson 1982). Participating in the therapeutic milieu, they cannot easily dissociate themselves from the predetermined disapproval of society's attitudes toward the elderly (Heller and Walsh 1976). Negative values can surface in a myriad of ways in the health care system. Financial and political support for programs for the elderly are difficult to obtain; the needs of the elderly come second to those of smaller but younger population groups.

Studies have shown that almost all health professionals prefer to work with children or young adults, and that few choose to specialize in geriatrics (Green 1981). Student nurses and nurses prefer to work with clients of age groups other than the old (Gomez et al. 1985).

Medical care of aged clients has been characterized by pessimism, defeatism, and professional aversion (Spence et al. 1968). Such negative attitudes and stereotyped thinking have been found both among professionals and ancillary personnel in nursing homes and other institutional settings (Adelson et al. 1982).

Bower (1981) found that there is a relationship between nurses' attitudes, the characteristics of their elderly clients, the setting in which the nursing care takes place, and the educational background of the nursing personnel. It also appears that the longer nurses worked with older clients, the more likely they are to hold stereotypical views of them. Gerontological nursing education and sensitization to the needs of the elderly can help change these attitudes and bring about a more positive approach.

According to Elliot and Hybertson (1982), the social conduct of older clients and their level of functional independence have a bearing on the feelings of, and approach taken by, nursing personnel. Nursing assistants expressed negative feelings about caring for extremely dependent elderly clients. Independence in self-care and pleasing client conduct elicited more positive feelings; socially unacceptable behaviors provoked unfavorable attitudes.

There is a need to foster more positive attitudes among nurses who provide direct service to their elderly clients (Benson 1982). Two interrelated reasons support this objective. First, the increase in the number of geriatric clients requiring nursing services has been accompanied by a decline in the number of nurses interested in working with elderly clients. Negative attitudes toward the elderly may be a contributing factor to this shortage (Penner et al. 1984). Second, it has been suggested that nurses who work with elderly clients and harbor such negative attitudes will engage in actions harmful to the best interests of their clients (Bower 1981).

Two types of inservice programs are recommended to improve negative attitudes: (1) *provide factual information about the aging process*; (2) *address and isolate the attitudes related to client care* (Elliot and Hybertson 1982). Educational programs need to discuss misconceptions about the elderly; this may increase the number of new nurses who are willing to work with elderly clients. These educational and training programs must address the dynamics of the nurse/staff-client interactions. Nursing personnel need to be made cognizant that their own actions may augment the very behaviors that they dislike in the elderly. Furthermore, consideration must be given to the effects that organizational policies and practices may have on the staff and their interaction with elderly clients (Penner et al. 1984).

Even though advanced levels of education appear to be associated with decreased stereotyping of the aged, it does not seem to increase preference for working with the aged. Positive attitudes toward the elderly and to caring for them need to be instilled during basic nursing education; this should be included in the curriculum (Gomez et al. 1985).

A better understanding of the aging process and the ability to differentiate between normal and abnormal, e.g., dementia versus normal aging, is necessary for a productive and positive interaction between nursing-care givers and their aging clients.

In defining one of the objectives of nursing care of the elderly, Preston (1986) comments:

> We must resist the ease of paternalism, which weakens our relationship with the elderly. We must endeavor to study them and their particular problems as vigorously as we study diseases. And we should love them, for that is the only way we can love ourselves when we take their places.

Refer to the Quiz: *Facts and Myths of Aging* in Table 29–1. Answers are on page 820.

GENERALIST NURSING PRACTICE VERSUS GERONTOLOGICAL NURSING

McConnell (1988) states that elements of nursing practice remain the same between generalist nursing prac-

Table 29–1 • QUIZ: FACTS AND MYTHS OF AGING

T	**F**	1. The majority of older adults past the age of 65 are demented.	**T**	**F**	11. The aged are well off and no longer impoverished.
T	**F**	2. The senses of vision, hearing, touch, taste, and smell all decline with age.	**T**	**F**	12. Many individuals experience difficulty when they retire.
T	**F**	3. Muscular strength decreases with age.	**T**	**F**	13. The elderly are prone to fall victim to crime.
T	**F**	4. Sexual interest declines with aging.	**T**	**F**	14. Most elderly are infirm and require help with daily activities.
T	**F**	5. For the older adult, regular sexual expressions are important to maintain sexual capacity and effective sexual performance.	**T**	**F**	15. Older individuals are more dependable and have fewer accidents than younger persons.
T	**F**	6. At least 50% of restorative sleep is lost as a result of the aging process.	**T**	**F**	16. The majority of older adults are socially isolated and lonely.
T	**F**	7. As a group, the elderly are major consumers of prescription drugs.	**T**	**F**	17. Medicaid is a federally assisted program providing health care benefits to anyone over the age of 65.
T	**F**	8. Older adults are not able to learn new tasks.	**T**	**F**	18. The term "ageism" reflects society's positive views toward the elderly.
T	**F**	9. The elderly have a high incidence of depression.	**T**	**F**	19. Widowers are more likely to remarry than widows.
T	**F**	10. As individuals age, they become more rigid in their thinking and set in their ways.	**T**	**F**	20. Older widows appear to adjust better than younger ones.

Answers found on page 820.

Table 29–2 • NURSES PREPARED TO CARE FOR THE ELDERLY

FUNCTION	EDUCATION
Nurse Practitioner (NP)	
Performs "medical acts" • Prescribes medications • Diagnoses disease • Manages chronic disease	1. Certificate programs open to any RN regardless of level of preparation 2. Master's level programs 3. RNs certificated jointly by state boards of nursing and medicine
Clinical Specialist	
Advanced practitioner of nursing/clinical teacher	Master's degree (MSN, MN), also RNs
Nurse Scientist	
Nurse researcher or nurse educator	Doctor of Nursing Science (DNS) or Doctor of Philosophy (PhD) Nursing or PhD in psychology, sociology, physiology, anthropology

Adapted from McConnell ES. A conceptual framework for gerontological nursing practice. *In* Matteson MA, McConnell ES. Gerontological Nursing: Concepts and Practice. Philadelphia: W. B. Saunders Company, 1988, p. 35.

tice and gerontological nursing practice. For example:

1. Goals of nursing
2. Generic nursing process and methods
3. Professional practice roles:
   - Follow standard of practice
   - Code of Ethics
   - Accountability to clients

Nurses in the levels of nursing practice shown in Table 29–2 have specific knowledge of aging and the interaction of health, aging, and illness as well as knowl-

Box 29–1. SKILLS FOR GERONTOLOGICAL NURSING

Gerontological nurses should be skillful in applying generic nursing methods to care of the aged and be able to do the following:

- Utilize research findings from gerontology as well as nursing and the biomedical and behavioral sciences to inform nursing practice
- Interact with individuals who have sensory loss
- Perform multidimensional assessment of the elderly person using existing standardized tools and individualized approaches
- Implement rehabilitative nursing techniques
- Help clients integrate past life with present
- Include the older person and family members in developing goals for nursing care, even if the individual has significant communication or cognitive impairments
- Modify the environment to maximize the older person's ability to function independently
- Provide excellent palliative, supportive, and spiritual care for those who are dying
- Give counsel to the grieving
- Consider ethical dilemmas encountered by old people, their kin, and their health care providers
- Help families and communities overcome hostilities toward the elderly
- Participate in professional activities designed to improve health care for the elderly
- Supervise the efforts of paraprofessional and lay caregivers in providing nursing care to the aged
- Teach paraprofessional and lay caregivers and old people about the impact of the aging process and the disease process on self-care abilities and requisites of older persons
- Teach paraprofessional and lay caregivers and old people about techniques to achieve self-care objectives
- Establish developmentally appropriate criteria for evaluation and nursing care

Data from Matteson MA, McConnell ES. Gerontological Nursing: Concepts and Practice. Philadelphia: W. B. Saunders Company, 1988, pp. 37–38.

Table 29–3 • THE NURSING PROCESS AND THE CARE OF THE ELDERLY CLIENT

	ASSESSMENT	IDENTIFYING PROBLEMS	ESTABLISHING GOALS	INTERVENTION	EVALUATION
1. Physiological Needs Food/Fluid Shelter/Warmth Air Rest/Sleep Avoidance of pain Sex	Usual and present nutritional, eliminational, sleep, and sexuality patterns Physical activity exercise pattern Emotional pain and discomfort Suicide potential Physical health Medications	**Altered patterns of urinary elimination** **Altered nutrition** Dehydration **Constipation** **Sleep pattern disturbance** **Sexual dysfunction** **Knowledge deficits** Medications or physical illnesses that may cause depression **Potential for self-violence**	Establishing and maintaining adequate biological functioning in areas of sleep, nutrition, and elimination Relief from emotional pain and discomfort Elimination of drug- or disease-induced depression	Assist with ADLs Support of self-care abilities Encouragement to start a physical activity regime Teach side effects of antidepressants Treat medical problems under poor control Change medications that may cause depression	Feelings of physical satiation Homeostasis Optimal physical health
2. Safety and Security Needs Feel free from danger Need for a predictable, lawful, orderly world Need to feel in control	Home environment assessment Mental status exam Assessment of visual acuity and hearing Knowledge of disease process Physical mobility	**Ineffective individual coping** **Powerlessness** **Fear** **Sensory/perceptual alterations** **Impaired physical mobility** **Self-care deficit**	Establish predictability and structure in environment Maintenance of a safe environment Realistic understanding of disease course and expected outcome Reversal of treatable confusion	ECT, hospitalization, antidepressive medications for the severely depressed Avoid relocations when possible Correct environmental hazards Encourage a structured daily routine Instruct about disease course and prognosis	Feeling in control of one's disease and optimistic about the future Confidence in the future Feelings of safety, peace, security, protection, lack of danger and threat
3. Need for Love, Belonging, and Affection Need for contact and intimacy Need for friends Need for feeling of having a place, "belonging" Need for interactions with others	Family relationships and members Friends that are supportive Recent losses Present and past social interactions	Disruption in significant relationships **Social isolation** Lack of contact with, or absence of, significant others **Impaired social interactions**	Maintenance of significant relationships with family and friends Establish community support system Resumption of previous level of social activity	Encourage social interactions that have been enjoyed in the past Encourage interactions with family members, friends, and health caregivers Provide reassuring, supportive atmosphere	Feelings of loving and being loved, of being one of a group, of acceptance
4. Need for Esteem and Self-Respect Need for achievement, mastery, and competence Need for reputation or prestige, appreciation, and dignity Need for love of self	Amount of pleasurable pursuits Emotional or mood assessment Role patterns Coping—stress tolerance pattern Attitude about self, the world, the future	**Disturbance in self-esteem** Loss of significant roles Unrealistic self-expectations **Anxiety** Lifestyle change Dependency on others	Acceptance of realistic limitations Establish appropriate roles Achieve self-acceptance Accept ownership of consequences of one's own behavior	Teach problem-solving skills Cognitive therapy Promote self-care Counseling Behavior therapy Relaxation techniques	Feelings of self-confidence, worth, strength, capability and adequacy, of being useful and necessary in the world
5. Need for Self-Actualization Need for beauty Need for self-expression Need for new situations and stimulation	Occupation, job history Value-belief patterns	Loss of zest for life **Spiritual distress** **Grieving**	Expression of self through meaningful recreational activities Exploring new interests	Encourage a nonrestrictive environment Provide beauty in environment Read to the sick or hard of hearing Music	Autonomy Freshness of appreciation Creativeness Spontaneity Feelings of self-fulfillment

From Ronsman K. Therapy for depression. Journal of Gerontological Nursing, 13(12):21, 1987.

edge and skill to modify and implement nursing methods. See Box 29–1 for gerontological nursing skills.

Psychiatric nurse specialists who work with the elderly experiencing mental health problems also need to know about normal aging and interactions between aging and illness. Ronsman (1987) provides an overview of the nursing process in the care of elderly client (Table 29–3).

Unique Assessment Strategies

Nurses who work with the elderly benefit from specific knowledge about normal aging, drug interactions, and chronic diseases. Those who work with the elderly population who have mental health problems also need to have special skills, e.g., interviewing, assessment, and knowledge of effective treatment modalities. Lekan-Rutledge (1988) outlines approaches to the elderly person during the initial assessment. Since examination and interviews can produce anxiety in the elderly, and since the initial interview is often in unfamiliar surroundings, the guidelines in Table 29–4 are useful no matter what the setting or purpose of the interview.

Because effective coping, problem solving, and adaptive behaviors are necessary for healthy social functioning, the degree of social dysfunction needs to be assessed. The **Social Dysfunction Rating Scale** (Table 29–5) is widely used for this purpose.

Depression and substance abuse among the elderly are both major health problems. Since they both affect each other, a special scale for detecting the presence of depression among the elderly has been devised. **Zung's Self-Rating Depression Scale** is one of the most widely used (Table 29–6). The client rates himself, unless he is illiterate or has vision problems. The score is derived by dividing the sum of the 20 items by 80 (the maximum score) (Lekan-Rutledge 1988). Scores above .38 or a raw score of 50 and over signify depression requiring hospital treatment (Zung 1965).

Unique Intervention Strategies

Pfeiffer (1978) emphasizes that the majority of older persons are well. Those that do present with mental problems are treatable and responsive. He does stress

Table 29–4 • GUIDELINES FOR THE FIRST INTERVIEW

APPROACH	PROCESS COMMENTS
1. Approach the client: note appearance, posture, spontaneous activity, grooming, hygiene, comfort, presence of others, facial expression, attentiveness, interest.	1. Cues gathered about musculoskeletal, neurological, genitourinary (GU), gastrointestinal (GI), cardiovascular, and pulmonary systems, cognitive and emotional function, senses, social support.
2. Address the client by name. Introduce self: "My name is . . . I prefer to be called . . . What do you like to be called?"	2. Hearing. Ability to respond to social situation, cues about cognitive and affective function.
3. Offer to shake hands or grasp client by the hand.	3. Neuromuscular function, strength, skin temperature, texture.
4. Establish eye contact, ask about visual ability and use of glasses. Position self in full view of client. Adjust lighting for brightness, but avoid glare.	4. Assess vision.
5. Ask client about any hearing difficulties and if client can hear you clearly. Ask about the use of hearing aid, lip reading, better hearing in one ear than the other.	5. Cues about hearing and cognitive function.
"How are you feeling today?" If a clinic visit, "What brings you here today?" or "Is anything troubling you lately?" Probe specifically with open-ended questions, e.g., "Oh, you're hurting, tell me more about that."	Self-assessment of health, symptoms assessment, cognitive and verbal function, communication skills, optimism, emotional response.
"What would you like help with today?" Note the issues identified and the order of concerns.	Cues about client's priorities, expectations, response to health, or social problems or concerns.
6. Summarize the interaction so far. "Mrs. J., we have approximately 45 minutes together to address your concerns. I think that will give us time to deal with the concerns you have voiced. I would like to proceed now by asking you a few more questions and then do the following exam procedures for these reasons."	6. Establish trust, contract for and set mutual expectations for the encounter, prioritize concerns, validate inferences with the client.

From: Matteson MA, McConnell ES. Gerontological Nursing: Concepts and Practice. Philadelphia: W. B. Saunders Company, 1988, p. 80.

Table 29–5 • SOCIAL DYSFUNCTION RATING SCALE

Directions: Score each of the items as follows:
1. Not present 2. Very Mild 3. Mild 4. Moderate 5. Severe 6. Very Severe

Self-esteem

1. ______ Low self-concept (feelings of inadequacy, not measuring up to self-ideal).
2. ______ Goallessness (lack of inner motivation and sense of future orientation).
3. ______ Lack of a satisfying philosophy or meaning of life (a conceptual framework for integrating past and present experiences).
4. ______ Self health concern (preoccupation with physical health, somatic concerns).

Interpersonal System

5. ______ Emotional withdrawal (degree of deficiency in relating to others).
6. ______ Hostility (degree of aggression towards others).
7. ______ Manipulation (exploiting of environment, controlling at other's expense).
8. ______ Overdependency (degree of parasitic attachment to others).
9. ______ Anxiety (degree of feeling of uneasiness, impending doom).
10. ______ Suspiciousness (degree of distrust or paranoid ideation).

Performance System

11. ______ Lack of satisfying relationships with significant persons (spouse, children, kin, significant persons serving in a family role).
12. ______ Lack of friends, social contacts.
13. ______ Expressed need for more friends, social contacts.
14. ______ Lack of work (remunerative or nonremunerative, productive work activities that normally give a sense of usefulness, status, confidence).
15. ______ Lack of satisfaction from work.
16. ______ Lack of leisure time activities.
17. ______ Expressed need for more leisure, self-enhancing, and satisfying activities.
18. ______ Lack of participation in community activities.
19. ______ Lack of interest in community affairs and activities that influence others.
20. ______ Financial insecurity.
21. ______ Adaptive rigidity (lack of complex coping patterns to stress).

PATIENT: ______________ RATER: ______________ DATE: ______________

From Linn MW, et al. A social dysfunction rating scale. Journal of Psychiatric Research, 6:299, 1969.

Table 29–6 • ZUNG SELF-RATING DEPRESSION SCALE*

	NONE OR LITTLE OF THE TIME	SOME OF THE TIME	A GOOD PART OF THE TIME	MOST OR ALL OF THE TIME
1. I feel down-hearted, blue and sad	1	2	3	4
2. Morning is when I feel the best	4	3	2	1
3. I have crying spells or feel like it	1	2	3	4
4. I have trouble sleeping through the night	1	2	3	4
5. I eat as much as I used to	4	3	2	1
6. I enjoy looking at, talking to and being with attractive women/men	4	3	2	1
7. I notice that I am losing weight	1	2	3	4
8. I have trouble with constipation	1	2	3	4
9. My heart beats faster than usual	1	2	3	4
10. I get tired for no reason	1	2	3	4
11. My mind is as clear as it used to be	4	3	2	1
12. I find it easy to do the things I used to do	4	3	2	1
13. I am restless and can't keep still	1	2	3	4
14. I feel hopeful about the future	4	3	2	1
15. I am more irritable than usual	1	2	3	4
16. I find it easy to make decisions	4	3	2	1
17. I feel that I am useful and needed	4	3	2	1
18. My life is pretty full	4	3	2	1
19. I feel that others would be better off if I were dead	1	2	3	4
20. I still enjoy the things I used to do	4	3	2	1

*A raw score of 50 or above is associated with depression requiring hospital treatment.
From Zung WK. Zung self-rating depression scale. Archives of General Psychiatry, 12:63, 1965.

that psychotherapeutic approaches need to be simplified and modified for older clients. Certain psychotherapeutic techniques are useful for the elderly client:

1. Crisis intervention techniques (Chapter 10).
2. Empathetic understanding.
3. Encouraging ventilation of feelings.
4. Re-establishing emotional equilibrium if the anxiety is out of hand.
5. Explaining alternate solutions.

Burnside (1988) offers specific guidelines for caring for an elderly client. She urges nurses to pace themselves, *not* to move quickly, rush, or joggle the client. She also urges nurses to "truly listen" and make the quality of their time important, not the quantity. Specific guidelines in the one-to-one relationships and interviews are listed subsequently (Burnside 1988):

1. Select a setting that provides privacy for the interview.
2. Make certain that the client is physically comfortable.
3. Ask the client what name he or she prefers to be called and then use it often.
4. Touch can be effective in getting the client's attention.
5. Assess the client's mental status, e.g., observe for any deficits in recent or remote memory and determine if any mental confusion exists. Be aware of **all** medications that the client is taking and their effects, any side effects, and possible drug interactions. A patient taking many medications can be confused.
6. Ascertain the status of the client's sight and hearing faculties. If the client has a hearing aid or glasses or both, make certain that they are being worn.
7. Lighting in the interview setting is important, as the older adult needs three times more light to see than the teenager. Do not allow sunlight or bright lights to shine directly into the client's face, as the older adult's eyes are very sensitive to glare.
8. Sit close to and speak directly to any clients who have hearing deficits. Maintain direct eye contact with the client when sitting or standing not more than five feet away. When speaking, do *not* exaggerate lip movements; as this action distorts the mouth and what is being said. Talk in a moderate voice with a slower than normal rate of speech. Do *not* shout. This action accentuates the vowel sounds and obscures the consonants, which are already hard for the elderly person to hear.
9. Observe the client for any signs of fatigue. Gauge his or her attention span, and keep the interview short if necessary.
10. Pace the interview, slowing it, if necessary, to match the client's needs. At the same time, allow the client enough time to think and respond to any questions, instruction, or discussions.
11. Try to include the client in all decisions.
12. Explain clearly to the client all the possible options from which to choose when making a decision. (Remember that choices may be more limited for the aged.)
13. When possible, use reminiscing strategies to keep obtaining information. Stimulate memory chains by attempting to recall patterns of association that will improve the client's recollection.
14. If the client verbalizes low self-esteem or negative views of aging, pick up on his or her strengths and point them out.
15. *Give instructions to the client slowly and clearly; print them in letters large enough to be read later, when the client's anxiety level may be lower.* If you are using handouts, make sure that the type is large enough for the client to read.
16. Make an appointment for the next meeting. The client should understand what is expected both of the interviewer and of the client before the next meeting.
20. If possible, include family members in part of the interview for added input, clarification, support, and reinforcement.
21. Be an advocate for the elderly.

INPATIENT SETTINGS

When clients are institutionalized, group therapy is an economical way to provide therapeutic intervention. **Remotivation therapy, reminiscing therapy,** and **group psychotherapy** are three group modalities often led by nurses who have special training or education. Table 29–7 outlines the purpose, format, and desired outcomes for each type of group. Table 29–8 gives an example of a remotivation therapy session.

COMMUNITY-BASED PROGRAMS

The hazards of institutionalization are numerous and include increased mortality, decreased social opportunity, and "learned helplessness." The purpose of many community-based long term care services is to promote the elder's independent functioning and reduce stress on the family system (Henderson and McConnell 1988). One such program for the elderly is the **day care program.**

As a result of rising institutional costs and ever-longer waiting lists for in-home care, interest in alternatives to long term care is increasing. Much too often

Table 29–7 • USEFUL GROUP MODALITIES FOR ELDERLY CLIENTS

REMOTIVATION THERAPY	REMINISCING THERAPY (LIFE REVIEW)	PSYCHOTHERAPY
Purpose of Group		
• Resocialize *regressed* and *apathetic* clients.	• Share memories of the past. • Increase self-esteem. • Increase socialization. • Increase awareness of the uniqueness of each participant.	• Alleviation of psychiatric symptoms. • Increase ability to interact with others in a group. • Increase self-esteem. • Increase ability to make decisions and function more independently.
Format		
• Groups are made up of 10–15 clients. • Meetings held once or twice a week. • Meetings are highly structured in a classroomlike setting. • Use of props. • Each session discusses a particular topic. • See Table 29–8 for the five basic steps used in each session.	• Groups are made up of 6–8 people. • Meetings once or twice weekly for one hour. • Topics include holidays, major life events, birthdays, travel, food, and more.	• Group size 6–12 members. • Group members should share similar a. problems b. mental status c. needs d. sexual integration. • Group meets at regularly scheduled times (number of times a week, duration of session) and place.
Desired Outcomes		
• Increases participant's sense of reality. • Offers practice of health roles. • Realizes more objective self-image.	• Alleviates depression in institutionalized elderly. • Through the process of reorganization and reintegration provides avenue by which elderly can a. achieve a new sense of identity b. achieve a positive self-concept.	• Decreases sense of isolation. • Facilitates development of new roles and re-establishes former roles. • Provides information for other group members. • Provides group support for effecting changes and increasing self-esteem.

Data from: Matteson MA, McConnell ES. Gerontological Nursing: Concepts and Practice. Philadelphia: W. B. Saunders Company, 1988.

individuals and their families can no longer afford the expense of a nursing home, and frequently institutionalization is not the best answer. Therefore, help from federal, state, and local governments is required. The idea of establishing day care facilities should be seriously considered (Butrin 1985).

The concept of day care is not new. It started in England in the early 1940's and came to the United States about a decade later. Essentially there are two types of day care programs: (1) supervised daytime recreation and social activities and (2) inclusive health care and rehabilitative programs (Koenen 1980). The boundaries of these programs do blend and overlap (O'Brien 1981).

The first program affords the participants the opportunity for recreation and social interaction; they usually do not receive rehabilitative care. This is the more common type and less expensive to operate (Koenen 1980). The second program goes beyond meeting recreational and social needs; it provides restorative and posthospital care, health promotion, health maintenance and services for the high risk elderly, and psychosocial services to the frail aged (O'Brien 1981). Nursing personnel, pharmacists, physicians, physiotherapists, occupational therapists, social workers, lay persons, and volunteers are available, forming a broad base of support necessary for such care. This program aims to prevent or slow down any mental, physical, or social deterioration, in order to thus maximize the older adult's full potential regardless of disease or condition (Koenen 1980).

Day care centers of one sort or another exist in nearly every state. Nationwide there are more than 1200 such centers, which is a great increase from the dozen that were present in 1970. With a combined annual budget of about $150 million, these centers care for an estimated 28,000 elderly. Approximately 75% are nonprofit institutions run by either hospitals, centers for the elderly, or churches (Ansberry 1986).

Although the number of adult programs is growing, most limit themselves to recreation and social orientation. Even though many states are interested in developing health rather than social models, they look to the federal level for direction and participation in funding; this has slowed down the process. Funding, or lack of it, continues to be a primary issue in the development of day care facilities (O'Brien 1981).

Charges for day care usually range from $10 to $70 a day, often not enough to cover fully the actual costs of services; subsequently, many centers require outside

Table 29–8 • EXAMPLE OF A REMOTIVATION SESSION (BODIES OF WATER)

STEP 1: Climate of Acceptance
The leaders personally welcomed each participant as he or she arrived at the group session. After the leaders introduced themselves, each group member made a self-introduction. The leader used a calendar to orient the members to the date and time of the current remotivation session. The theme for session 4 was introduced by the leader as "bodies of water—rivers, lakes, and oceans." All group members had some familiarity with bodies of water because of their residence in Seattle.

STEP 2: Creating a Bridge to Reality
The world globe was used as a visual aid to stimulate discussion on bodies of water. The leader asked questions, for example, "How are bodies of water formed from glaciers?" Pictures of glaciers, rivers, and lakes were shown.

The leader read poems about tide pools, sea shells, and fishing written by anonymous grade school children. Discussion was stimulated by the leader asking, "What can we do at the ocean?" Visual aids and props were provided for direct sensory stimulation. Some examples of these aids and props included (1) different types of sea shells, (2) fishing tackle and bait, (3) suntan lotion, (4) sun hat, and (5) sunglasses.

A poem by an anonymous author about fishing was read to the group. This was followed by recorded music with lyrics about fishing experiences.

STEP 3: Sharing the World We Live In
Group discussion focused on jobs related to bodies of water. Topics the participants discussed in regard to self or others included crabbing, clamming, shrimping, and fishing. Visual aids were provided to stimulate further discussions on past related experiences involving bodies of water. Pictures of river-rafting, canoeing, scuba diving, and sailing were shared.

STEP 4: An Appreciation of the Work of the World
This time was used for the members to think about work in relation to others. More experiences in past related work roles were discussed as well as hobbies and pastimes. The group then participated in singing a familiar, old song, "Love Letters in the Sand," written in 1931 by J. Fred Coots and revived in 1957 when sung by Pat Boone.

STEP 5: Climate of Appreciation
The group members were thanked individually by the leaders for coming to the group and sharing their experiences. The following remotivation session theme and meeting date were announced prior to terminating the session.

Group Response to Session 4
Most members of the group appeared to enjoy discussing their experiences in relation to bodies of water. Many members recalled fishing and boating experiences. Other members expressed interest in this topic by their nonverbal participation in touching and smelling some physical props, and observation of visual aids. All but two participants touched the seashells and smelled the fish eggs. One lady in the group stood up and modeled the sun hat and glasses, while a man demonstrated how to reel in the line on a fishing pole. Several participants remarked on how beautiful the pictures of the glaciers were. All but a couple of group members sang to the recorded lyrics on fishing. One member stood up and danced to the music, while many others clapped to her movements.

From Janssen JA, Giberson DL. Remotivation therapy. Journal of Gerontological Nursing, 14(6):31, 1988.

funding (Ansberry 1986). Most socially oriented centers derive their funding from clients, donations, and fund raising by the center (O'Brien 1981). Many of the medical models are funded through private insurance, Medicaid, or other sources. Because of these funding sources, they are highly regulated; admission requirements are strictly followed.

Part of the problem of reimbursement may lie with the haphazard regulation and licensing of many of the socially oriented centers. Only 15 states require licensing; 13 others have certification requirements. In the other states, day care centers do not have to meet any requirements. If public funds are used for subsidizing centers, then, of course, more stringent standards must be met (Ansberry 1986). This is often the case with the medical model.

Adult day care does provide a vital function for older adults and their families, thereby permitting them to continue their present living arrangements and to maintain their social ties to the community; this relieves families of the burden of 24-hour daily care for their elderly dependents. If institutionalization becomes necessary, day care staff can work with their clients and their families to assess the present situation and make recommendations for placement (O'Brien 1981).

Financial Issues That Affect Quality of Care

Quality and availability of care for the elderly are also affected by changes in the health care system. One significant factor in the quality of care an elderly person will receive as well as the availability of specific resources is the person's finances. The Diagnostic Related Groups, or DRGs, is a system by which Medicare payments are made to the hospitals and appears to be having an enormous impact on the extent of medical care to the elderly. Method of payment, Medicare/Medicaid, can also greatly affect the quality of care an elder client may receive. Therefore DRGs and Medicare/Medicaid will be briefly discussed in this section.

DRGs AND THE ELDERLY

Health care expenses in the United States have significantly increased since the introduction of Medicare in 1965, with costs rising much faster than the overall rate of inflation. Hospital charges, in particular, have zoomed upward, exceeding any other health care cost (Knowing Your Rights 1985). The rate of hospital admissions for the elderly also increased, as did the average length of hospitalization (Lueckenotte 1987).

In the past, by using a retrospective based payment or per-diem method, hospitals were paid for whatever services they provided during the client's stay, which was viewed as one of the main factors causing the exorbitant rise in hospital care costs. Although subject to internal review boards, the per-diem method did not provide hospitals with a real incentive to eliminate unnecessary tests, treatments, and extended hospital stays (Warren 1984; Knowing Your Rights 1985).

Concerned with spiraling medical costs, Congress introduced, in 1983, a new hospital payment system for Medicare clients, replacing the per-diem method. Based on a prospective (in advance) method of reimbursement (PPS), clients are charged in accordance with the so-called **Diagnostic Related Group (DRG).** This change means that the reimbursement rate to the hospital is determined in advance at the time of a person's hospital admission. Instead of paying the actual costs, a person is charged at a predetermined rate based on his or her diagnosis. Thus, reimbursement for hospitalization is no longer based on the length of stay nor on actual costs incurred by the hospitals (Staley and Luciano 1984). The fee schedule is established by using one of the 467 categories of DRGs. In the event that a client's diagnosis is changed during hospitalization, the appropriate new DRG category would be applied (Harron and Schaeffer 1986).

Cost curtailment is the key advantage of the DRGs, forcing hospitals to operate on a more cost-efficient basis. As a result, clients undergo fewer, and frequently unnecessary, tests and procedures. This cost-cutting may lead to shorter hospital stays, which in turn makes it less likely that clients will suffer from iatrogenic diseases (Champlain 1985). When it comes to costs, DRGs ensure equity among clients; the same fees are charged for comparable services. Competition within the hospital industry is encouraged (Warren 1984).

There are, however, also disadvantages. Tight cost control may influence the decision-making process. Rapid, aggressive medical care and speedy discharge may be the least suitable care for the elderly. The older adult requires additional consideration: the institution and health care providers should take into account the physical and psychosocial changes of the aging, the presence of chronic disease, and the impact of acute illness. This combination produces significant clinical difficulties: How to provide high-quality, cost-effective care for the elderly in an acute care setting (Lueckenotte 1987).

Other concerns have emerged. Because the DRGs encourage efficiency, there is a strong incentive for undertreatment by the hospitals, since money received under a given DRG and not spent in the treatment of a client can be retained as profit. Furthermore, the system may induce hospitals to deny admission to clients who have complicated medical problems and whose treatment costs will far surpass the DRG reimbursement (Fleck 1987). As a rule, hospitals are adjusting their services to the DRG's reimbursements (PPS Shortchanging 1985). The elderly who are at an advanced age are particularly at risk for not receiving quality care. They often have serious multiple medical problems and are thus considered unwanted income losers. Therefore, hospital management might be tempted to select a short stay client over a high cost elderly client (Floyd and Buckle 1987).

According to the U.S. General Accounting Office, under the DRGs hospitals are discharging Medicare clients sooner and often in poorer condition than was the case under the former per-diem retroactive system (Champlain 1985). This has resulted in a reduction of quality care for some clients (PPS Shortchanging 1985).

Since hospitals tend to limit, whenever feasible, the duration of hospitalization to what is reimbursable under the DRGs code, clients have been told that they must leave because their allocated number of days have run out (Kelly and Bankhead 1985). This is a misleading statement. It is, rather, the hospital that allows a certain number of days for the client, since any excess would result in unreimbursable expenses (Carlson and Oriol 1986).

The DRG system does not concern itself with the psychosocial consequences of hospitalization, since hospitals are reimbursed only for treating the client's physical ailments. Social, rehabilitative, or psychological care is not necessarily provided. However, without such therapeutic services, many hospitalized elderly may eventually become institutionalized (Champlain 1985).

Because of the financial pressures on hospitals, medical teams cannot afford time-consuming diagnoses but must make a rapid assessment of the client and his or her condition on admission. Such a quick process can leave the older client in a state of confusion. This, in turn, can influence the treatment team's decision as to whether a client may go home or should be discharged to a nursing home (Champlain 1985).

The discharge of a Medicare client to a nursing home can create a difficult situation. Nursing homes are reluctant to accept Medicare clients for whom they receive a more limited reimbursement than for private clients. A *Catch*-22 situation may arise: the frail older adult is discharged early by the hospital and therefore needs nursing-home care, but the nursing home is reluctant to take the client. Medicare pays only for the first 20 days of nursing home care and only if the client was hospitalized for at least three days prior. Many nursing homes are not geared to receive clients who require more intensive treatment. Many nursing homes lack the sophisticated equipment and staff needed to provide the intensive care required (PPS Shortchanging 1985).

Although DRGs have induced hospitals to perform on a more cost-efficient basis, which, in turn, has helped to curtail runaway hospital costs, the older adult may be caught in the middle. "It is a program for the masses, but it involves individuals—clients, doctors, hospitals. The diagnoses are clear, all 467 of them. But their impact on the individual represents the great unknown prognosis." (Kelly and Bankhead 1985).

MEDICARE/MEDICAID AND THE ELDERLY

Illness, considered one of the greatest perils of old age, is the paramount financial concern of the aged. Comprising only 11% of the population, the elderly contribute more than 30% of the total personal health care expenditures (Ebersole and Hess 1981).

In 1965, Medicare (Title 18) and Medicaid (Title 19) were introduced into the Social Security Act. Under **Medicare,** medical care is provided for the elderly (65 and older) without regard to their financial condition (Ebersole and Hess 1981), assisting them to meet the high cost of health care. Medicare payments do not go to the client directly but to the private sector providing the care (Gibson et al. 1984). Most Medicare funds are used for acute hospital care, physician services, and some short term, home health services, and only minimally for long term care (Caserta 1983; Fleck 1987).

Three factors contributed to Medicare's introduction. *First*, many elderly were denied access to the health care system because they could not afford it. *Second*, prior to the 1960's, resources and medical advances were not readily available for treatment of specific problems affecting the elderly, e.g., stroke, cancer, chronic obstructive pulmonary disease, and heart disease. Medical advances have allowed improved management and treatment of chronic health care problems. *Third*, many elderly in need of medical attention were without insurance as retirees (Fleck 1987).

Medicaid, on the other hand, was designed to provide coverage for the impoverished who could not afford either the expense of Medicare contributions or who had used up their Medicare benefits. Unlike Medicare, Medicaid is not administered on the federal level but is left to the discretion of the states. Medicaid is the largest single provider of institutional long term care funding, but is provided only in the case of the poor elderly (Caserta 1983; Fleck 1987). Refer to Table 29–9 for similarities and differences between Medicare and Medicaid.

Because the state regulatory agencies set the Medicaid reimbursement rates, they perform an important role in determining the quantity and quality of care rendered in nursing homes to Medicaid supported clients. Their rulings also influence wages, and the number and mix of employed registered nurses, licensed practical nurses, and nurses' aides. These decisions have crucial ramifications for the clients in long term care (Grimaldi and Sullivan 1981).

Because Medicaid coverage varies from state to state, services may be inconsistent in quality and extent (Ebersole and Hess 1981); thus, Medicaid reimbursement continues to be a concern. Many health agencies and physicians either do not accept Medicaid clients or they limit the number of clients, since Medicaid does not repay for all the services rendered (Tesfa 1982).

The Down Side of Medicare/ Medicaid

In both Medicare and Medicaid, exploitation and inequalities exist, with providers profiting at the elders' expense. For example, under Medicare, the providers are not required to follow established rates; almost 50% of them do not accept the assignment. When the providers charge what they deem appropriate, the elderly clients must seek partial payment from Medicare and then make up the difference themselves, often a serious hardship (Ebersole and Hess 1981).

When Medicare was introduced over 25 years ago, no one could have predicted the dramatic rise in its costs, since medical advances were not predictable. The unlimited flow of money into Medicare provided the financial means to encourage and back medical research. New medical breakthroughs were utilized, thereby increasing the charges and driving medical costs even higher. Society became the scapegoat of its conscientious intentions and good works (Fleck 1987).

Medicare expenditures exceeded $75 billion in 1986.

Table 29–9 • COMPARISON BETWEEN MEDICARE AND MEDICAID

	MEDICAID—TITLE 19	MEDICARE—TITLE 18
To Secure Data	Contact the Welfare Office.	Contact the Social Security Office
Objective	A public assistance program to pay medical bills.	An insurance program to pay medical bills.
Eligibility	For specific groups of indigent and low income individuals: ● The adult, over age 65. Some older adults may receive both Medicare and Medicaid benefits. ● The blind, the disabled. ● Members of families with dependent children.	Individuals over 65 years of age, regardless of income.
Services Provided	All inpatient services paid. ● Total coverage.	Hospital insurance or inpatient care. Medicare pays roughly ⅓ of inpatient costs. $300 deductible. Ninety days for each benefit interval. Skilled Nursing Home: Client must be hospitalized before admission. Restrictions regarding number of days, amount of reimbursement, and type of illness. Home Health Care: Hospital insurance can reimburse the permitted costs of visits. Individual must be confined to home and meet certain criteria. Services include: skilled nursing care, physical and speech therapy, and some other services.
Areas Not Covered	● None known.	● Full-time professional nursing care. ● Homemaker service. ● Medications. ● Routine physical examinations.
Financing	Financed by 20% county, 20% state, and 60% federal funds.	Financially supported by the Social Security Trust Fund. Employee and employer both make contributions. Insured individual must also pay monthly premium. Additional funds come from federal tax general funds.
Supervision	State governments administer the program with their own criteria and federal guidelines. The Federal Health Care Administration is accountable for federal aspects of Medicaid.	Federal government administers program under the Health Care Financing Administration of the U. S. Department of Health and Human Services.
Eligibility Test or Test Given	Yes.	No.

Adapted from Baines E. Medicare vs. Medicaid. Journal of Gerontological Nursing, 10(2):36, 1984.

Even though predictions are that the system will go bankrupt between 1993 and 1995, many believe that reducing expenditures is morally wrong and economically a hardship to the elderly (Fleck 1987). America is graying and its elderly population is expected to increase by close to 125% by the year 2030. Today there are about four workers for every individual receiving Medicare. In 2030 this will have to change to two workers per Medicare recipient, in effect doubling the worker's tax burden (Crozier 1985).

The Catastrophic Coverage Act, passed by Congress in 1988, was envisioned as a way to protect the older adult against the cost of devastating illness. In return for an additional premium of under $5.00 per month (to increase to $13.50 by the year 1993), Medicare will cover an unlimited number of days of hospitalized care, with the recipient paying a limited amount per year (Newswatch 1989; Pear 1987). Seniors, in addition, now must pay a surtax of $22.50 for each $150.00 of taxes owed. Many elderly are angry about the surcharge and respond that they are not receiving any additional financial assistance with this bill. In spite of paying for their own additional insurance coverage, they also must now pay these increased costs (Newswatch 1989).

Besides the burden on society in general, the institutionalized elderly, and their families in particular, have to cope with the high costs, often facing financial ruin. Of the $35 billion spent on nursing home care in 1985, more than half came from the elderly and their families. A major portion was also borne by Medicaid. Medicare paid for less than 2%; contributions from private insurers were negligible.

Nursing home bills typically cost about $22,000 a year. A lengthy nursing home stay can be immensely costly and can leave little for the noninstitutionalized spouse. According to one study, *two out of three elderly who live alone will run out of money after only 13 weeks in a nursing home* (McGrath 1987).

Alternatives for the Future

The Catastrophic Coverage Act (1988) provides a few benefits in long term care, particularly in guarding against spousal impoverishment (Newswatch 1989). The noninstitutionalized spouse is allowed to keep some income in assets, but the bill's overall long term benefits are sparse (Newswatch 1989).

Another approach would be a relatively new program of nursing home or long term care insurance. It would be an important option for the elderly, differing from Medicare and Medigap (private insurance designed to pay the deductible and coinsurance portions of Medicare). Depending on the policy and the state in which it is provided, long term care insurance regularly reimburses set amounts for services of skilled, intermediate, or custodial care at nursing homes. In some situations, it also pays for home health care (Sloane 1987). Until long term care insurance becomes more widespread, individuals admitted to nursing homes must pay for their own care unless they become eligible for the Medicaid program. Since they must divest themselves of most of their assets to receive Medicaid benefits, they and their families become destitute. It is a heartbreaking situation for all.

Issues That Affect the Mental Health of Some Elderly

The issues chosen here for discussion are three of the most prevalent problems for many elders: (1) *Death and dying* of the elderly poses complex legal and ethical issues for the elder client, the family, doctors, and nurses; (2) *suicide* is a growing phenomenon among the elderly; and (3) *alcoholism* is a "neglected disease" affecting both the physical and the mental health of some elderly. Elder abuse, another serious problem for many elders, is covered in Chapter 14.

DEATH AND DYING AND THE ELDERLY

Life is bounded by two milestones: birth and death. To some, death is the completion of a life process; to others it is a passage to another life. For all though, the thoughts and fears of death and its irreversibility have a particular significance.

As recently as 50 years ago, the elderly approaching death found themselves not in the hospital or nursing home but at home, with death usually taking place in the familiar surroundings of home. The individual could thus progress through the dying process in the intimate environment of home (Olson 1981), with death to some extent being part of living.

More recently, lower mortality rates and increased life expectancy have made death "less visible, less meaningful and less controllable than it was in the past" (Ross 1981). For many persons death has been "transposed, insulated, technologicalized, decontextualized" (Ross 1981). There is a growing concern that death in America is too often controlled by machines rather than by nature (Wallis 1986). Our technical knowledge and our utilization of artificial support of circulation, respiration, and other systems have made it possible to prolong the lives of those who otherwise would have died sooner (Olson 1981). This technical expertise is often applied regardless of mental capacity. Today, approximately 80% of all people die in hospitals or nursing homes, often surrounded by life-extending apparatuses (Wallis 1986).

As a youth oriented society, Americans view death as not being of immediate concern but rather as a remote prospect. By turning their sick over to the medical experts, they expect the advanced technologies to answer all problems, including death. Thus they insulate themselves from death (Ross 1981). Polls have been conducted on themes of death and prolonging life. When members in a retirement community were asked to assess the extent of intervention they would like should they be dying, the majority desired only comfort care; they were not interested in the life-extending processes. Many wanted to insure that their wishes were followed by having a written document of such wishes accessible to their physicians (Snow and Atwood 1985). A Louis Harris poll of over 1000 adults found that 86% thought terminally ill clients ought to be able to tell their physicians to let them die; almost an equal percentage favored withdrawal of feeding tubes, if this was the client's desire (Wallis, 1986).

Another group was asked what they would desire if they had severe memory loss, were unable to care for themselves, or had no chance of recovery. A much greater percentage of older persons as compared with younger individuals said they would refuse ICU care or tube feeding (Patients ponder 1985).

Living Wills

"A **Living Will** is an expression by a person, while competent, which states the individual's preference that life-sustaining treatment be withheld or withdrawn if he or she becomes terminally ill and no longer able to make health care decisions" (Weiler and Buckwalter 1988).

A Living Will is one guide in deciding the course of treatment and can serve to ease the conscience of families. A Living Will can, in some states, help shield those providing care and making medical decisions as well as the hospital itself from legal liability. The Living Will concept originated (1968) as a tool to develop individual guidelines pertaining to medical intervention at times when the technology or treatment that keeps a person alive cannot advance a reasonable quality of life or chance of recovery. Living Wills have meaningful legal value; during times of crisis, they sway the course of therapy. Although a majority of states have Living Will laws, some are still without them. In these states the physician is not bound to follow a Living Will (Understanding the Living Will 1986). However, its existence reflects a person's desire and thus should be used as a guideline.

Physicians are having a difficult time making decisions affecting the care of their dying clients. The American College of Physicians' Ad Hoc Committee on Medical Ethics stated that a physician has a responsibility to make certain that his or her hopelessly ill client dies with dignity and with as little suffering as possible (Jenike 1984). The committee thus affirmed that a person's wishes, as best can be determined, should be respected and his or her dignity maintained. Even food and water were on the list of treatments that could be withheld under these circumstances (Wallis 1986).

The committee also commented that cardiopulmonary resuscitation should be used for the prevention of sudden unexpected death. If, however, such efforts would only prolong the dying process, a decision to write a "do-not-resuscitate" order would be deemed ethically proper. The committee emphasized that age alone does *not* justify coding a client "do-not-resuscitate." Clients who are mentally competent adults have the legal right to accept or refuse any form of treatment, and their wishes must be recognized and honored by their physicians. Only the clients can decide whether or not they wish to be resuscitated if faced with a terminal event (Jenike 1984).

These recommendations are not always easy to follow. Physicians feel compelled to apply treatment regardless of the client's prognosis—unless the client specifically objects or has written a Living Will (Kleiman 1985). This is what nurses and physicians have been trained to do, and what is dictated by law. The physician's and nurse's education and training all emphasize positive actions to sustain and prolong life (Wanzer 1984). In addition, withholding treatment from hopelessly ill clients may open the physician to malpractice charges. A Living Will, if recognized in the state, can give the physician guidance in situations in which the clients can no longer speak or act for themselves (Kleiman 1985).

Our society has never before faced the problem of so many people living for so long with such severe impairment. No specific cure exists for many of the chronic diseases afflicting the elderly, e.g., senile dementia, stroke, osteoporosis, rheumatic disease, advanced cancer, and arteriosclerosis (Nelson 1982).

Because of advances in medicine, the ability to extend life may carry "overwhelming emotional hardships, agonizing pain, and devastating financial costs" (Kaufman 1985). A point may be reached in which the balance of what is to be "saved," when weighed against emotional and financial ruin, favors the latter. The question should be asked: "Should the quality of life become a weightier consideration than mere survival?" (Nelson 1982).

Society has increasingly turned to the legal system for direction. In the Karen Ann Quinlan decision (1976), the New Jersey Supreme Court permitted the removal of life-sustaining treatment from a terminally comatose woman if her family and attending physician agreed. In addition, a hospital ethics committee had to agree that there was no reasonable possibility that she would emerge from her "comatose condition to a cognitive, sapient state" (Kaufman 1985). She lived for 10 years more without a respirator. If the client is in a completely unresponsive state, e.g., coma, and has given no specific directions previously, the physician and family are faced with a difficult dilemma.

In 1985, the New Jersey Supreme Court ruled that all life-sustaining medical treatments, including feeding tubes and respirators, could be withheld or withdrawn not only from terminally ill clients who are incompetent but also from those who are competent. And, furthermore, consent of the client's guardian, family members, and physicians, as well as state administrative agencies, was required before life-saving treatment could be withdrawn (Kaufman 1985).

Next to the client, who has the right to accept or refuse treatment, the physician has a major role in the decision-making process. Medical ethics have only recently started to look into questions surrounding the intent of decreased medical intervention. Physicians are strongly influenced by their personal values and unconscious motivations and a fear of legal liability, which often can interfere with the ability to make the best choice for the elders under their care (Wanzer et al. 1984).

The concept that a person may be better served by doing less, not more, is not easily accepted. A decision to pull back is much more difficult to make than one to go ahead with aggressive support. The advanced and complex medical technology leads physicians into making use of all resources available, which is a temptation that needs to be understood and recognized when deciding how much or how little to do for a client (Wanzer et al. 1984).

Monetary cost to society and the use of scarce treatment resources in the care of the hopelessly ill must be taken into account. In the past, expense rarely was an important factor in decision making. Today, however, as society tries to contain the skyrocketing cost of health care, the physician is subject to insistent demands for constraint that cannot be ignored. The financial disaster of the client's family, as well as the strain on resources for others who are not hopelessly ill, needs to be weighed in this decision-making process. The client's well-being does obviously remain foremost (Wanzer et al. 1984).

Hospice Care

One alternative to dying in hospitals or nursing homes is the hospice approach. The **hospice philosophy** is characterized by the acceptance of death as a natural conclusion to life; the clients have the right to live and die in a way decided by them, rather than one set by the care providers (MacElveen-Hoehn and McIntosh 1981). One goal of hospice care is to establish a special bond between the individual who is dying and the family (Burggraf and Stanley 1989). Terminally ill clients thus receive supportive care in their homes or in a homelike setting. The focus is on keeping dying people comfortable, free of pain, as active as possible, and close to their families. They need not fear being subjected to prolonged medical care against their wishes. The hospice approach may constitute for many an acceptable equilibrium between the clients' needs and wishes and the emotional financial strain on their relatives.

Nurse's Role In The Decision-Making Process

Nurses may be in the best position to know whether or not "the remaining life is worth the suffering of the client." Not only do they spend more time with the client than the physician and often even family members, but they also have a broader understanding of the client because of their communication skills and concerns with the sociological and psychological basis of illness and health. The nurse is often involved in decisions whether to treat the client aggressively or to allow the client to die without the use of life-support equipment (Olson 1981). Box 29–2 offers guidelines relating to issues of life and death.

In working with the client's family, the nurse should orient family members and significant others about the ethico-legal policies of the institution and assist them to live with, and understand the concepts of, dying and death (Alford 1986). The nurse should explain that the family need not feel morally obligated to provide for all possible medical care extending only the suffering of the client. This is especially true when such extraordinary measures do not represent the client's values and beliefs (Sherlock and Dingus 1984).

Maintaining an open and continuing dialogue among the client, family, nurse, and physician is of principal importance. The nurse should serve as an advocate for the competent clients in their decision making, and be supportive of the client's surrogate when determinations need to be made (Alford 1986).

Any indication the clients might have given in the past about their views toward death and dying should have a bearing on their medical care. Existence of a Living Will is also an indication of their wishes. *Old age alone ought not to be a factor*. Age becomes significant only as expressed by the client, e.g., "I'm tired; I'm too old; I want to go" (Gadow 1979).

Each institution should have a written policy on "coding" to serve as a guideline for physicians and

Box 29–2. GUIDELINES FOR RELATING TO ISSUES OF LIFE AND DEATH

1. Understand that it is the client's will, not health, that is all-important.
2. Assess the client for ethico-legal factors, e.g., Living Wills, guardianship, competency.
3. Know the state's nursing practice act and understand the state laws and the institution's policies concerning death and the termination of life support systems.
4. Follow the ANA Code of Ethics and the ANA Standards of Gerontological Nursing.

Data from Alford D. Managing ethical and legal dilemmas in the care of the elderly. Presentation at Current Directions in Gerontological Nursing, Bethesda, MD, September 26, 27, 1986.

nurses. Affected clients should have orders in effect for implementation. **The nurse should never accept verbal "no-code" orders from physicians** (Alford 1986).

Should a situation arise in which the physician, on one hand, and the nurse, on the other, develop a fundamental difference as to what is in the best interest of the client, the nurse should talk to the Director of Nursing and might even turn to the institution's ethics committee. It is advisable to keep written documentation of any such discussions.

If the institution does not have an ethics committee, it should be encouraged to form such a body, preferably to consist of a nurse, a physician, a lawyer, a community member, and a religious advisor. It is important that any guidelines and policies be continually updated to reflect new legal decisions.

SUICIDE AND THE ELDERLY

In spite of recent publicity attesting to the growing number of suicides among the young, suicide rates of the elderly in the United States are 50% higher and continue to be the highest of any age group (McIntosh 1985; Osgood 1988). Comprising about 13% of the population, the elderly account for 25% of the total number of annual suicides (Eliopoulos 1987; McIntosh 1985). Refer to Chapter 22 on suicide.

A study of this phenomenon identifies despair as the major motive for suicide (Burnside 1988). Other significant factors are feelings of hopelessness and uselessness. For the older adult, suicide may be seen as a final gesture of control at a stage when independence is at risk or activities are limited. For this reason, a suicide attempt is more likely to succeed. Unlike with younger persons, there may be no history of previous suicidal gestures or attempt (Ebersole and Hess 1981).

Money can be a contributing factor to the high suicide rate. Federal cuts in programs like Medicare, Medicaid, and food stamps, along with state ordered medical-aid cuts, cause many elderly Americans to worry about their future. An inverse relationship between economic conditions and suicide rate has been identified (Marshall 1978).

Statistically, among the elderly the white male consistently has the highest suicide rate, particularly if he is over 75 years of age (Burnside 1988; Eliopoulos 1987; Forbes and Fitzsimons 1981; Whall 1985). This rate seems to reflect the significant role that position and achievement play in the lives of the older white male. In old age, they may suffer more fundamental losses than women do. For example, a man may lose status, contact with fellow workers, wage and station, while many older women retain many of the roles that they had during their earlier years (Ebersole and Hess 1981). Since men have been more likely to achieve and associate with social standing more than women, a loss in status at retirement or otherwise can be more traumatic for them, although this is changing with the change in women's roles.

The characteristics of the older white male at risk for suicide point to a white, Protestant male between the ages of 65 and 70, father of two children. He would be likely to have had a domineering parent, would not have finished high school, and would be retired from a low income job. As a loner, not socially active, without hobbies, he would be living with a friend or relative at the time of suicide. His situation would be aggravated by a strong dependence on drugs, chronic insomnia, or depression. He would kill himself with a gun and leave behind a note and a will (Miller 1978). These features should be borne in mind when caring for the older adult.

Assessing Suicide Risk in the Elderly

Other **high risk** situations that may intensify the potential for *suicide among the elderly* are (1) *widowhood*, (2) *illnesses and intractable pain*, (3) *status change*, and (4) *losses*. With respect to the latter, losses may be personal in nature (death of a family member or close friend), economic (loss of earnings or job), or social (loss of prestige or position) (McIntosh 1985; Boxwell 1988). The potential for suicide is intensified by these changes and losses.

Old age has been described as a "season of losses." Frequently, multiple losses accompany the aging process (Osgood 1988). These losses increase stress at a time when the older adult may be the most vulnerable and least resistant to stress, precipitating a depressive state. Nevertheless, the majority of older adults are able to function despite their losses. Those who give in may do so because of hopelessness (Boxwell 1988).

In assessing suicide risk, the health care provider must examine prior suicidal behavior and understand that the elderly make fewer suicidal gestures than the population at large. An inquiry into the client's idea of the future should also be examined (Boxwell 1988).

Depression puts the client at an increased risk for suicide (Friedman 1976). It is the most frequent functional psychiatric disorder of later life, causing two-thirds of the suicides among the elderly (Gurland and Cross 1983). It has also been the most underdiagnosed and undertreated disorder (St. Pierre et al. 1986).

Depression versus Dementia

Depression is often confused with dementia. This is an important fact for nurses to keep in mind. Unlike dementia, depression is treatable with medication and other interventions. Depression is not always recognized as such. Assessment may be difficult because the depressed elderly may appear demented. They may show profound memory and other intellectual impairments, become very unsociable, or agitated, and appear to be demented. A careful systematic assessment, therefore, is necessary to properly identify the illness (St. Pierre et al. 1986). Some distinguishing characteristics of dementia and depression are listed in Table 29–10.

In making assessment, the health care provider needs to be familiar with the symptoms of later life depression, which may include one or more of the following (Osgood 1988):

- Changes in sleep patterns and symptoms of insomnia.
- Changes in eating patterns—particularly loss of appetite.
- Weight loss.
- Excessive fatigue.
- Increased concern with bodily functions.
- Alterations in mood.
- Expression of apprehension and anxiety without any reason.
- Low self-esteem, feelings of insignificance, pessimism.

A careful evaluation of the etiology of any presenting depression is also necessary. Depression can be caused by drugs such as reserpine, rauwolfia derivatives, steroids, and phenothiazines as well as by metabolic and endocrine diseases like hepatitis, and adrenal and thyroid insufficiency. Generally, chronic health problems may also augment the suicide potential (Osgood 1988).

Antidepressants and the Elderly

In choosing a drug to treat depression in the elderly, primary emphasis should be placed on avoiding possible side effects rather than on efficacy. When starting therapy, low antidepressant dosages are generally recommended; they then can be slowly and gradually increased. Orthostatic hypotension is of particular concern to the elderly. *Nortriptyline* and *doxepin* are two drugs reported to have low orthostatic effects. The elderly male may have a pre-existing condition of prostatic hypertrophy. Desipramine and trazodone have the fewest anticholinergic effects on urinary retention. Drugs with a high degree of sedation such as doxepin or trazodone may be less desirable than desipramine or nortriptyline in the treatment of the elderly with coexisting symptoms of psychomotor retardation or hypersomnolence (Neshkes and Jarvik 1986).

Social networks to reduce suicide potential have not been as successful among older adults as they have for younger persons (Ebersole and Hess 1981). The elderly with suicidal tendencies infrequently seek help; they have difficulty admitting that they have a weakness (Gottashalk 1986). They may be reluctant to turn to others because of the ethical and moral stigma of suicide and suicide ideation or the social embarrassment of psychiatric illness. Instead of looking for assistance from the mental health professional, the suicidal geriatric client would rather go to his or her primary care provider and complain of depressive or somatic manifestations. Primary care providers, therefore, must have sensitive assessment skills for suicidal risk and be

Table 29–10 • DEMENTIA VERSUS DEPRESSION

DEMENTIA	DEPRESSION
Insidious onset	Onset often quick
Symptoms present for lengthy period of time	Symptoms often present for short period of time
Low suicide risk	High suicide risk
Attempt to hide deficits	Highlights deficits and disabilities
Mental status questions answered incorrectly; attempt to conceal errors	Lack of interest in responding to such questions; frequently answers "I don't know" or "I don't care"
Symptoms more conspicuous at night	Symptoms not typically worse at night
History of psychiatric disturbances uncommon	Frequent history of psychiatric disturbances
Cognitive impairment comparably stable, with a steady worsening over the years	Cognitive impairments may vary greatly
Vacillation in mood and behavior	Constant depressed mood; agitation may be superimposed

Adapted from St. Pierre J, et al. Late life depression: A guide for assessment. Journal of Gerontological Nursing 12(7):5, 1986.

knowledgeable about methods of intervention (Boxwell 1988).

Right to Suicide

One concern of nursing is the question of whether an elderly individual has the right to commit suicide. Intensifying the ethical and moral dilemma of suicide is the distinction that must be made between suicide and voluntary active euthanasia (Boxwell 1988). Although society frowns on suicide in general, there seems to be a growing recognition that elderly persons with terminal illnesses should be able to take their own lives. If an elderly alert client is confronted with an intractable, lingering, and painful illness, with no hope of relief except for suicide, is the intervention of the health care provider to prevent suicide justifiable? If the determination is made to intervene, e.g., by hospitalization and physical restraint, it could be suggested that the health care provider has placed a higher value on the client's life than the client has (Boxwell 1988).

Although suicide is discussed in Chapter 22, there are specific factors which concern the elderly, such as retirement related difficulties, physical illness, economic problems, loneliness, social isolation, and ageism. Innovative methods to deal with these factors need to be developed for the elderly. Education of the public in general and health care providers in particular is necessary to raise the level of awareness of this geriatric problem (McIntosh 1985).

ALCOHOLISM AND THE ELDERLY

Alcoholism, the country's most neglected disease, is a particular concern for the older adult (Lasker 1986). There are *two major types of alcohol abusers*: (1) the "*aging alcoholic*" and (2) the "*geriatric problem drinker*." The *aging alcoholic* has had alcoholic problems intermittently throughout most of his early life with regular alcohol abusive pattern starting to evolve in late middle or older age. The *geriatric problem drinker*, on the other hand, has no history of alcohol-related problems but develops an alcohol abusive pattern in response to the stresses of aging (Dupree et al. 1984).

The stressful, or "reactive factors," that precipitate late-onset alcohol abuse are often caused by environmental conditions that may include retirement, widowhood, and loneliness. The geriatric problem drinker's inability to cope with these situations may cause him to turn to alcohol as an escape from realities. Widowers comprise the largest proportion of late-onset elderly alcoholics (Price and Andrews, 1982).

Alcohol and Aging

Excessive consumption of alcohol can create particular problems for the elderly. The older adult has an increased biological sensitivity to, or conversely, a decreased tolerance for, the effects of alcohol. This diminished resistance, combined with age-related changes such as weakened manual dexterity, balance, and postural flexibility, can increase the likelihood of falls, burns, or other accidents (Valanis et al. 1987).

Some drinkers, as they get older, note changes in their response to alcohol, e.g., headaches, reduced mental abilities with memory losses or lapses, and a malaise rather than a feeling of well-being. These problems start to occur at lower levels of consumption than used to be the case in earlier years. Older persons are likely to drink more frequently but in lesser quantities than younger individuals, who tend to drink larger amounts less often (Gomberg 1980). Thus, the possibility of alcohol abuse in cases of only moderate ingestion by the elderly is not frequently recognized by the alcoholic's friends or family (Alcohol and the elderly 1984).

With aging, the body becomes less resilient; healing from injury or infection is slower, and stress is more likely to cause a loss of physiological equilibrium. As the proportion of fatty tissues to lean body mass increases with age, the individual's metabolic rate usually slows down, increasing the amount of time it takes the body to eliminate drugs (Schuckit 1982).

Alcohol and Medication

The interaction of drugs and alcohol in the elderly can have serious consequences. There is a decreased functioning of the liver enzymes that break down the alcohol, which on a short term basis has the effect of prolonging the action of many medications potentiating their effect. On the other hand, chronic ingestion of alcohol enhances the metabolism of many drugs by causing faster turnover of medication.

Older individuals can expect higher blood alcohol levels than younger persons for an equivalent intake of alcohol (Schuckit 1982). Alcohol's effects on the brain may be one reason that alcohol abuse sometimes mimics or exacerbates normal changes of aging, since even a moderate intake of alcohol can impair the cognition and coordination skills that are already decreased with age.

The effects of alcohol can be particularly harmful if an older person is taking antidepressants or tranquilizers (Hartford and Samorajski 1982). Extreme care is required in treating the older alcoholic with any medications. For example, the therapeutic use of disulfiram

(Antabuse) to cause disagreeable psychological and physiological reactions when alcohol is drunk is not recommended because of possible cardiovascular side effects (Gulino and Kadin 1986).

Alcohol consumption produces a change in a person's sleep pattern, particularly affecting the older adult. Unlike younger persons, the elderly take longer to fall asleep and do not sleep as restfully. While alcohol may decrease the time it takes to fall asleep, this benefit is offset by causing frequent awakenings during the night (Hartford and Samorajski 1982).

Symptoms of Aging Versus Symptoms Seen in Alcohol Dependence

Health practitioners working with the elderly need to be concerned with, and sensitive to, possible alcohol abuse among their older clients. Careful assessment of the conditions is necessary to differentiate the normal physiological changes of the aging from those due to excessive drinking. Some of the symptoms of alcohol abuse are poor coordination, visual disturbances, slurred speech, gastrointenstinal complaints; they may often mimic the normal aging process (Guilino and Kadin 1986). Confusion and disorientation in an older client is not always caused by dementia or Alzheimer's disease but may be due to alcohol abuse (Hartford and Samorajski 1982).

Treatment for the Elder Alcoholic

Because many elderly do not live in big families or have work-related contacts, they are less likely to be referred for treatment compared to younger drinkers (Gulino and Kadin 1986). Too often, by the time the elderly alcoholic comes to the notice of any treatment agencies, the client's support systems and resources are severely decreased or depleted. Declining social, physical, and psychological performances are frequently found in the elderly alcoholic, thus exacerbating the difficulties of loneliness, depression, monotony, accidents, social conflict, loss, and physiological changes of aging (Burns 1988).

Treatment plans for the elderly problem drinker should emphasize social therapies. Elderly alcoholics tend to be more passive than younger alcoholics and may benefit from interpersonal involvement with professional health care personnel (Burns 1988). The old respond easily to emotional and social support (Gulino and Kadin 1986). Family therapy should be encouraged. Group therapy made up of middle-aged and older alcoholics can be effective (Gomberg 1980).

The older alcoholic who does seek help may be confronted with serious gaps and inadequacies in the health care delivery system (Gulino and Kadin 1986). Substance abuse counselors, therefore, must be in contact with other agencies providing services to the elderly so that their help can be coordinated. They should be cognizant of the financial and transportation abilities of their elderly client (Gomberg 1980).

The aging alcoholic is difficult to treat. On the other hand, prognosis for the geriatric problem drinker—a person who had led his life up to this point without recourse to alcohol and whose drinking is caused by losses and stress—is excellent. It is important that health care providers recognize this recovery potential. Proper education and awareness of a positive outcome for the geriatric problem drinker could increase the availability of resources: if the prognosis is good, providers and agencies should be more willing to spend resources on treatment. This knowledge is valuable to share with the older client, since restorative outcome is so frequently a self-fulfilling prediction (Gomberg 1980).

Of the health care providers, nurses are in an excellent position to assess the elderly client with alcoholic problems. They can educate the problem drinkers, families, physicians, and emergency room and other health personnel (Gomberg 1980). A great educational effort is needed to alter the pervasive negative attitudes toward the elderly drinking person (Gulino and Kadin 1986). Nursing should share its realization of the presence of an alcohol problem with older clients in a nonjudgmental manner.

Considering the magnitude of the problems and the likelihood that numbers of older abusers will continue to increase, efforts need to be intensified to identify the causes and to develop appropriate interventions to treat alcohol dependence among the elderly. If not, such dependence can overwhelm those charged with meeting the health and social-service needs of the older adults (Brown 1982).

Summary

There are a number of issues that older adults face as they age and many myths existing that foster negative attitudes. Ageism is found in all levels of society and even among health care providers, thereby affecting the way they render care to their elderly clients.

Nurses who care for the elderly in a variety of settings may function at various levels, e.g., generalist, nurse

Table 29–1 • ANSWERS TO QUIZ: FACTS AND MYTHS OF AGING

1. **False.** Ninety percent of older adults possess a healthy mental ability; 5% exhibit symptoms of chronic mental dysfunction; and another 5% display signs of acute mental impairment (Courtenay and Suharat 1980).

2. **True.** All the senses decrease with aging. Many of the changes begin slowly when the individual is in his or her mid-forties and increase with aging. (1) Vision: Particularly affected are peripheral vision, visual acuity, adaptation to dark, and accommodation (presbyopia). (2) Hearing: Decreased ability to hear high frequency sounds with later changes possibly involving middle and low frequency sounds (presbycusis); males tend to show hearing loss earlier than women. (3) Taste: The number of functioning taste buds is reduced, which particularly affects the ability to taste sweet and salty flavors. (4) Touch: Simultaneously occurring with age are the loss of receptors and an increased threshold for stimulation; pain and pressure are thus not as easily sensed. (5) Smell: A decline in the number of fibers in the olfactory nerve has been reported, leading to speculation that smell also undergoes age-related changes (Eliopoulos 1987; Saxon and Etten 1978).

3. **True.** As one ages, muscle fibers atrophy and decrease in number with fibrous tissue slowly displacing muscle tissue. Overall muscle mass, muscle strength, and muscle movements decrease. The arm and leg muscles, which become particularly flabby and weak, show these changes as well. Exercise is important to minimize the loss of muscle tone and strength (Eliopolous 1987).

4. **False.** Sexual interest and activity continue to play a pivòtal role in providing life satisfaction (Pfeiffer 1978).

5. **True.** Masters and Johnson in their work on human sexuality found that regular sexual expressions for the older adult are important for maintained sexual capacity and effective sexual performance (McCarthy 1979).

6. **True.** Changes in sleep patterns occur along the entire life span. Restorative sleep declines rapidly with aging and by age 50 is reduced by 50%. It not only takes the elderly more time to achieve restorative sleep than the younger adult, but with aging, sleep is less effective (Lerner 1982).

7. **True.** Comprising 11% of the population, the elderly accounted for 25% of all prescription drugs sold. This is not a surprising finding, since the incidence of chronic diseases among the elderly is high and prescription drugs are often used with chronic disease (Raffoul et al. 1981; Burggraf and Stanley 1989).

8. **False.** All age groups can learn. Limited, of course, by any physical limitations, older adults can usually master anything others can do if allowed a little more time. Jobs involving manipulation of objects or symbols or requiring discrete and clear responses are particularly well performed by older people (Atchley 1977; Burggraf and Stanley 1989).

9. **True.** Clinical depressive disorders increase in both prevalence and intensity with age. It may be called the "common cold" of the elderly and is expected to further increase in the years ahead (Steffl 1984; Bettis 1979).

10. **False.** The ability to change and adapt has little to do with one's age but more with one's character (Judson 1985).

11. **False.** Although a small number of aged are very well off, and many are moderately comfortable, a large segment remains poor. According to government statistics, 14% of older adults live in poverty (Binstock 1983).

12. **True.** One out of three retirees encounters difficulty adjusting to retirement. Adapting to a diminished income and no longer being in a job-related environment were two of the most frequently listed causes of difficulty (Atchley 1977).

13. **True.** In May 1982, the House Select Committee on Aging conducted a study on crimes and fraud. Senior citizens make up 11% of the population but constitute about 30% of the victims of crime. Business and investment frauds rank high on the list of white-collar crimes perpetrated against the elderly (Business and investment frauds 1982).

14. **False.** Eighty percent of older adults are healthy enough to carry on their normal lifestyles; 15% have chronic health conditions interfering with their lives; about 5% are institutionalized (Ebersole and Hess 1981).

15. **True.** Older persons are more reliable workers; their accuracy, performance, and stability are better and the number of accidents is lower except in situations requiring rapid reaction time (Palmore 1979).

16. **False.** Most elderly have relatives, friends, and organizations that are significant to them. About two-thirds do not consider loneliness a problem (Ebersole and Hess 1981; Wershow 1981).

17. **False.** Medicaid is a federally assisted state administered program that provides health care benefits to low income persons. Medicare, on the other hand, provides health insurance basically to individuals 65 and over (Baines 1984).

18. **False.** The term "ageism" reflects the negative prejudicial views of older people that pervade our youth oriented society (Adelson et al 1982).

19. **True.** Nearly twice as many widowers wed annually as compared with widows in spite of the fact that older widows outnumber older widowers by four times. In addition, half of those widowers who do remarry choose wives under 65 years of age (Atchley 1977).

20. **True.** Sociologists have found that for the older widow, widowhood is viewed as ordinary with supports available from family, friends, and the community. The younger widow, however, is viewed differently: widowhood is not a normal occurrence. The younger the widow, the more problems she encounters (Atchley 1977).

practitioner, and a clinical specialist in gerontological nursing. Nurses working with the mentally ill elder client should know about aging and about psychotherapeutic approaches to the elderly. Nurses with special training and education may lead remotivation, reminiscing, or psychotherapy groups geared toward the special needs of this population.

The health care system has undergone great changes in the last 20 years; the introduction of Medicare and Medicaid has led to long overdue health insurance and public assistance for the elderly. The positive aspects of the DRGs have been undermined by their negative impact on the elderly and their hospitalization.

Older adults face increasing problems of alcohol and suicide. When it comes to dying and death, the elderly's wishes (and those of their families) are frequently ignored. Living Wills and opting for hospice care can afford some clients death in dignity.

References

Adelson R, Nasti A, et al. Behavioral ratings of health professionals' interactions with the geriatric patient. The Gerontologist 22(3):227, 1982.

Alcohol and the elderly. Geriatrics 39(12):28, 1984.

Alford D. Managing ethical and legal dilemmas in the care of the elderly. Presentation at Current Directions in Gerontological Nursing, Bethesda, MD, September 26, 27, 1986.

Ansberry C. Day care centers for the elderly spring up as alternatives to costly nursing homes. Wall Street Journal, Dec. 8, 1986, p. 29.

Atchley R. The Social Forces in Later Life. Belmont, CA: Wadsworth Publishing Company, 1977.

Austin D. Attitudes towards old age: A hierarchical study. The Gerontologist, 25(4):431, 1985.

Baines E. Medicare vs. Medicaid. Journal of Gerontological Nursing, 10(20):36, 1984.

Baker R. Attitudes of health care providers toward elderly patients with normal aging and disease-related symptoms. The Gerontologist, 24(5):543, 1984.

Benson E. Attitudes toward the elderly: A survey of recent nursing literature. Journal of Gerontological Nursing, 8(5):279, 1982.

Bettis S. Depression: The "common cold" of the elderly. Generations, 3:15, Spring, 1979.

Binstock R. The aged as scapegoat. The Gerontologist 23(2):136, 1983.

Bower HT. Social organization and nurses' attitudes toward older persons. Journal of Gerontological Nursing, 7(5):293, 1981.

Boxwell A. Geriatric suicide: The preventable death. The Nurse Practitioner, 13(6):10, 1988.

Brown B. Professionals' perceptions and alcohol abuse among the elderly. The Gerontologist, 22(6):519, 1982.

Burggraf V, Stanley M. Nursing the Elderly: A Care Plan Approach. Philadelphia: J. B. Lippincott Company, 1989.

Burns B. Treating recovering alcoholics. Journal of Gerontological Nursing, 14(4):18, 1988.

Burnside I. Nursing and the aged. A Self-Care Approach. New York: McGraw-Hill, 1988.

Business and investment frauds perpetrated against the elderly: A growing scandal. A Report by the Chairman of the Select Committee on Aging. Comm. Pub. No. 97-347. Washington DC: U.S. Government Printing Office, 1982.

Butler R. Why Survive? Being Old in America. New York: Harper & Row, 1975.

Butler R, Lewis M. Aging and Mental Health. St. Louis: C.V. Mosby Company, 1977.

Butrin J. Day care. A new idea? Not really. Journal of Gerontological Nursing, 11(4):19, 1985.

Carlson E, Oriol W. DRGs surviving Medicare's new obstacle course. Modern Maturity, 27:87, 1986.

Caserta J. Public policy for long term care. Geriatric Nursing, 4(4):244, 1983.

Champlain L. DRGs: Putting the squeeze on your older patients. Geriatrics, 40(7):77, 1985.

Cohen G. Prospects for mental health and aging. *In* Biren J, Sloane R (eds). Handbook of Mental Health and Aging. Englewood Cliffs, NJ: Prentice Hall, 1980.

Courtenay B, Suharat M. Myths and realities of aging. Athens, GA: University of Georgia, Georgia Center for Continuing Education, 1980.

Crozier D. Data watch. Health Affairs, 4:115, 1985.

Dupree L, Broskowski H, et al. The gerontology alcohol project: A behavioral treatment program for elderly alcohol abusers. The Gerontologist, 24(5):51, 1984.

Ebersole P, Hess P. Toward Healthy Aging. St. Louis: C. V. Mosby Company, 1981.

Eliopoulos C. Gerontological Nursing. Philadelphia: J. B. Lippincott Company, 1987.

Elliot B, Hybertson D. What is it about the elderly that elicits a negative response? Journal of Gerontological Nursing, 8(10):568. 1982.

Fleck L. Decisions of justice and health care. Journal of Gerontological Nursing, 13(3):12, 1987.

Floyd J, Buckle J. Nursing care of the elderly. The DRG influence. Journal of Gerontological Nursing, 13(2):20, 1987.

Forbes E. Fitzsimons V. The older adult: A process for wellness. St. Louis: C. V. Mosby Company, 1981.

Friedman J. Cry for help: Suicide in the aged. Journal of Gerontological Nursing, 2(3):28, 1976.

Gadow S. Advocacy nursing and new meanings of aging. Nursing Clinics of North America, 14:81, 1979.

Gambert S. (ed). The geriatric patient: Effective management of behavioral and mental disorders. Spring House, PA: McNeil Pharmaceutical, 1983.

German P. Delivery of care to older people: Issues and outlooks. Topics in Clinical Nursing 3(1):1, 1981.

Gibson M, Levit K, et al. National health expenditures, 1983. Health Care Financing Review 6(20):1, 1984.

Gillis M. Attitudes of nursing personnel toward the aged. Nursing Research, 22(60):517, 1973.

Gomberg E. Drinking and problem drinking among the elderly. Publ. #1 Alcohol, Drugs and Aging: Usage and Problems. University of Michigan: Institute of Gerontology, 1980.

Gomez G, Otto D, et al. Beginning nursing students can change attitudes about the aged. Journal of Gerontological Nursing, 11(1):6, 1985.

Gottashalk E. Ending it all. Wall Street Journal, July 20, 1986.

Green C. Fostering positive attitudes toward the elderly: A teaching strategy for attitude change. Journal of Gerontological Nursing, 7(3):169, 1981.

Grimaldi P, Sullivan T. Medicaid reimbursement of long term nursing care. Geriatric Nursing, 2(2):133, 1981.

Gulino C, Kadin M. Aging and reactive alcoholism. Geriatric Nursing, 7(3), 148, 1986.

Gurland B, Cross P. Suicide among the elderly. *In* Aronson MK, et al (eds). The Acting Out Elderly. New York: Haworth Press, 1983, pp. 456–465.

Harron J, Schaeffer J. Drugs and the intensity of skilled nursing. Geriatric Nursing, 7(1):31, 1986.

Hartford J, Samorajski T. Alcoholism in geriatric population. Journal of American Geriatric Society, 30:18, 1982.

Heller B, Walsh E. Changing nursing students' attitudes toward the aged: An experimental study. Journal of Nursing Education, 15(5):9, 1976.

Henderson ML, McConnell ES. Gerontological care in community settings. *In* Matteson MA, McConnell ES (eds). Gerontological Nursing. Philadelphia: W. B. Saunders Company, 1988.

Janssen JA, Giberson DL. Remotivation therapy. Journal of Gerontological Nursing, 14(6):31, 1988.

Jenike M (ed). Ethical considerations in the care of the hopelessly ill patient. Topics in Geriatrics, 3(4):13, 1984.

Judson D. Attitudes toward aging. Current Consumer and Lifestudies, September: 14, 1985.

Kaufman I. Life and death decisions. New York Times, Oct. 6, 1985, p. 21.

Kayser-Jones J. Doctoral preparation for gerontological nurses. Journal of Gerontological Nursing, 12(3):19, 1986.

Kelly J, Bankhead C. DRGs: How are they stacking up? Medical World News, March 11, 1985, p. 80.

Kleiman D. Uncertainty clouds care of dying. New York Times, Jan. 18, 1985, p. B1–2.

Knowing Your Rights: Medicare's Prospective Payment System. Washington DC: AARP Health Advocacy Services Program Department, 1985.

Koenen R. Adult day care: A northwest perspective. Journal of Gerontological Nursing, 6(4):218, 1980.
Lasker M. Aging alcoholics need nursing help. Journal of Gerontological Nursing, 12(1):16, 1986.
Lekan-Rutledge D. Functional assessment. *In* Matteson MA, McConnell ES. Gerontological Nursing. Philadelphia: W. B. Saunders Company, 1988.
Lerner R. Sleep loss in the aged: Implications for nursing practice. Journal of Gerontological Nursing, 8(6):323, 1982.
Linn MW, et al. A social dysfunction rating scale. Journal of Psychiatric Research, 6:299, 1969.
Lueckenotte A. Sharpen skills in hospital settings. Journal of Gerontological Nursing, 13(3):12, 1987.
MacElveen-Hoehn P, McIntosh E. The hospice movement: Growing pains and promises. Topics in Clinical Nursing, 3(3):29, 1981.
Marshall J. Changes in aged white male suicide: 1948–1972. Gerontologist, 33:763, 1978.
Matteson MA, McConnell ES. Gerontological nursing in acute care settings. *In* Matteson MA, McConnell ES. Gerontological Nursing, Concepts and Practice. Philadelphia: W. B. Saunders Company, 1988.
Matthews S. The social world of old women: Management of self-identity. Sage Library of Social Research 78. Beverly Hills, CA: Sage Publications, 1979.
McCarthy P. Geriatric sexuality: Capacity, interest and opportunity. Journal of Gerontological Nursing, 5(1):20, 1979.
McConnell ES. A conceptual framework for gerontological nursing practice. *In* Matteson MA, McConnell ES. Gerontological Nursing. Philadelphia: W. B. Saunders Company, 1988.
McGrath A. The financial agony of long term illness. U. S. News & World Report, Feb. 9, 1987, pp. 53–57.
McIntosh J. Suicide among the elderly: Levels and trends. American Journal of Orthopsychiatry, 55(2):287, 1985.
McMahon M, Miller P. Behavioral cues in the dying process and nursing implications. Journal of Gerontological Nursing, 6(1):16, 1980.
Miller M. Toward a profile of the older white male suicide. Gerontologist, 18(1):80, 1978.
Moore I. Ending it all. Suicide in old age. Nursing Times, Feb. 12, 1986, pp. 48–49.
Murray R, Wilson M, et al. The nursing process in later maturity. Englewood Cliffs, NJ: Prentice Hall, 1980.
Nelson L. Questions of age. Doctors debate right to stop "heroic" effort to keep elderly alive. Wall Street Journal, Sept. 7, 1982, p. 20.
Neshkes R, Jarvik L. Depression in the elderly: Current management concepts. Geriatrics, 41(9):51, 1986.
Neussel F. The language of ageism. The Gerontologist, 22(3):273, 1982.
Newswatch: Is the Catastrophic Care Bill a catastrophe? Geriatric Nursing, 10(2):58–59, 1989.
O'Brien C. Adult day care and the bottom line. Geriatric Nursing, 2(4): 283, 1981.
Ogg E. The right to die with dignity. Public Affairs Pamphlet, 587. New York: Public Affairs Committee, 1980.
Olson J. To treat or allow to die: An ethical dilemma in gerontological nursing. Journal of Gerontological Nursing, 7(3):141, 1981.
Osgood N. Suicide in the elderly: Clues and prevention. Carrier Foundation Letter #133, April 1988.
Palmore E. Advantages of aging. Gerontologist, 17:220, 1979.
Patee J. Uncovering the elderly 'hidden' alcoholic. Geriatrics, 32(2):145, 1982.
Patients ponder the right to die. Medical World News, March 11, 1985, p. 124.
Pear R. Reagan, apostle of less, assures expended health care for elderly. New York Times, Feb. 15, 1987, sect. 4, p. 1.
Penner L, Ludenia K, et al. Staff attitudes: Image or reality. Journal of Gerontological Nursing, 10(3):110, 1984.
Pfeiffer E. Sexuality in the aging individual. *In* Solnick R (ed). Sexuality and Aging. CA: University of Southern California Press, 1978.
PPS shortchanging Medicare patients? Medical World News, March 25, 1985, p. 17.
Preston T. Ageism undermines relations with elderly. Medical World News, Dec. 8, 1986, p. 26.
Price D, Feldman J. Living longer in the United States: Demographic changes and health needs of the elderly. Milbank Memorial Fund Quarterly—Health and Society, 61:362, 1983.
Price J, Andrews P. Alcohol abuse in the elderly. Journal of Gerontological Nursing, 8(1):16, 1982.
Raffoul P, Cooper J, et al. Drug misuse in older people. The Gerontologist, 21(2):146, 1981.
Ronsman K. Therapy for depression. Journal of Gerontological Nursing, 13(12):18, 1987.
Ross H. Society/cultural views regarding death and dying. Topics in Clinical Nursing 3(3):3, 1981.
St. Pierre J, et al. Late life depression: A guide for assessment. Journal of Gerontological Nursing, 12(7):5, 1986.
Saxon S, Etten J. Physical change and aging. A guide for the helping professions. New York: The Tiresias Press, 1978.
Schneider E, Emr M. Alzheimer's disease. Geriatric Nursing, 6(3):136, 1985.
Schuckit M. A clinical review of alcohol, alcoholism, and the elderly patient. Journal of Clinical Psychiatry, 43(10):396, 1982.
Sherlock R, Dingus M. Families and the gravely ill: Roles, rules and rights. Journal of the American Geriatrics Society, 33:121, 1984.
Sloane L. Nursing home insurance. New York Times, August 1, 1987, 40.
Snow R, Atwood K. Probably death: Perspectives of the elderly. Southern Medical Journal, 78:851, 1985.
Spence D, Feigenbaum E, et al. Medical students' attitudes toward the geriatric patient. Journal of the American Geriatrics Society, 16:976, 1968.
Staley M, Luciano K. Eight steps to costing nursing services. Nursing Manager, 15:35, Oct. 1984.
Steffl D. Handbook of Gerontological Nursing. New York: Van Nostrand Reinhold Company, 1984.
Sullivan R. Right to die rule widened in terminal cases. New York Times, Jan. 18, 1985, p. A1, B2.
Tesfa A. What does it take to let them go home. Journal of Gerontological Nursing, 8(12):692, 1982.
Understanding the living will. Senior Medical Review. AARP, 1(3):4, 1986.
Valanis D, Yeaworth R, et al. Alcohol use among the bereaved and nonbereaved older persons. Journal of Gerontological Nursing, 13(5):26, 1987.
Wallis C. To feed or not to feed? Time, Mar. 31, 1986, p. 60.
Wanzer S, Aldelstein S, et al. The physician's responsibility toward hopelessly ill patients. New England Journal of Medicine, 310(15):955, 1984.
Warren J. An uncertain future for the state's innovative hospital free system. New York Times, Dec. 9, 1984, NJ Sect. p. 42.
Weiler KA, Buckwalter KC. Care of the demented client. Journal of Gerontological Nursing, 14(7):26, 1988.
Wershow H. Controversial issues in gerontology. New York: Springer Publishing Company, 1981.
Whall A. Suicide in older adults. Journal of Gerontological Nursing, 11(8):40, 1985.
Whall A. Alcoholism in older adults. Journal of Gerontological Nursing, 12(1):36, 1986.
Zung WK. A self-rating scale. Archives of General Psychiatry, 12:63, 1965.

Self-Study Exercises

Place T (True) or F (False) next to each statement.

1. ________ The elderly are prone to be crime victims.
2. ________ "Ageism" reflects society's positive view of the elderly.
3. ________ Older adults are able to learn new tasks.
4. ________ Most elderly are infirm and require help with daily activities.

Match the type of group—R (Remotivational), REM (Reminiscing), and P (Psychotherapy)—with the following descriptions:

5. ________ Shares memories of past events, helps increase esteem and socialization.
6. ________ Can help resocialize regressed and apathetic clients. Structured setting with set agenda.
7. ________ Problems are discussed among people with similar problems; aim is to relieve psychiatric symptoms and solidify functioning.

Short Answer

8. List two types of inservice programs to improve negative attitudes toward the elderly.

   A. ________________________________

   B. ________________________________

9. List two advantages of the DRGs.

   A. ________________________________

   B. ________________________________

10. List three disadvantages of the DRGs.

    A. ________________________________

    B. ________________________________

    C. ________________________________

11. Define a Living Will.

    ____

    ____

12. In issues of death and dying, the nurse should be aware of guidelines. Name at least four sources for them.

    ____

    ____

    ____

    ____

Place T (True) or F (False) next to each statement. Correct the false statements.

13. ________ Medicare is an insurance program to pay medical bills for individuals between the ages of 60 and 65.
14. ________ Medicare pays the complete costs of any hospitalization.

15. __________ Medicaid assists the elderly poor with their health care.
16. __________ Medicare is administered on a state-wide level. Therefore, the criteria for eligibility differ among states.
17. __________ Nursing home insurance is a newly developing program to provide financial assistance with institutionalization.
18. __________ Fatty tissues decrease with age, thereby slowing down the elimination of alcohol.
19. __________ Alcohol provides a beneficial night's sleep.
20. __________ Alcohol can mimic the normal changes of aging.
21. __________ Alcohol exacerbates all chronic conditions.

Circle the characteristics of an elderly person who is most likely to commit suicide (Miller 1978).

A. Catholic
B. Black
C. Married
D. No children
E. Used drugs to kill himself
F. Active socially in church
G. Male
H. Age 63
I. Did not finish high school
J. Left a note

CHAPTER 30

The Mentally Ill Who Are Chronically Homeless

Jeffrey S. Grunberg

OUTLINE

KEY TERMS AND CONCEPTS

The key terms and concepts listed here also appear in bold where they are defined or discussed in this chapter.

CHRONIC DISAFFILIATION
CHRONIC HOMELESSNESS
SHELTERS

OBJECTIVES

After studying this chapter, the student will be able to:

1. Explain what is meant by chronic homelessness.
2. Explain what is meant by the process of homelessness.
3. Describe the nurse's role in the interdisciplinary treatment team process as explained in the section on the day care center for the mentally ill.
4. Discuss the various types of mental illness common among the homeless.
5. Explain the importance of team assessment when working with the chronically homeless.
6. Describe how chronically homeless people may perpetuate their condition.

Homelessness — The Broad Picture

Homeless people come from every race, are of every age, and are both male and female. This chapter will consider those people who chronically reside in public shelters where to be homeless is to suffer more than just the absence of a home. It is to suffer from a lifestyle completely ravaged by **chronic disaffiliation,** that is, cut off and estranged from family, community, and peer support and involvement. In fact, to the extent that a shelter resident is disaffiliated, to that extent, for the purposes of this chapter, he or she is homeless. Homelessness then, for many, is a lifestyle problem. Homelessness is a process that exists on a continuum, one that leads to long term residency in a mental hospital or public shelter. Many of the people who currently suffer from this lifestyle problem once had residences of their own or shared dwellings with family members or with friends. In fact, it is not uncommon when working with homeless clients to see them return again and again after their discharge. Each discharge, no matter how carefully worked out, has failed. What can be stated then, here at the very beginning, is that this population is not a simple one to understand. Those people who today are considered the *chronically homeless*, are a complex people. And so are their problems. To best illustrate this, it will be necessary to briefly discuss some of the various subgroups that comprise these sheltered homeless.

The description of these subgroups will reflect the primary diagnoses of the persons involved. The reader should keep in mind that the problems of the people discussed here are not limited to their primary diagnoses.

There are three main categories of chronically homeless people from which many subcategories can be identified: (1) *the general population*, (2) *the mentally disabled*, and (3) *the handicapped*, all of which can be subdivided by age. Among the *general population* are those who may have problems with veteran or welfare benefits, substance abuse, housing, or employment, as well as legal difficulties.

Among the *mentally disabled*, there are those who share the same problems with the general population, as well as those with a primary diagnosis of mental illness. Usual DSM III-R diagnoses found among the homeless population include psychotic disorders (schizophrenia, bipolar and depression disorders), personality disorders (borderline, dependent, or antisocial), organic mental dysfunctions, and others.

Among the *handicapped*, there are those who share the same problems with the general population or the mentally disabled, as well as having a physical disability. Chronic or dormant and untreated problems may include active tuberculosis, hepatitis, diabetes, and AIDS.

Frequent problems among all groups are often compounded by previous or current dependence on alcohol or other substances, which in itself can lead to nutritional and other medical problems. All of these conditions are further exacerbated by various degrees of disaffiliation or estrangement from families, society in general, and peers. Often, the chronically homeless have limited education, have been imprisoned at some time or another, and suffer from differing degrees of institutionalization.

Before the 1970's, the stereotype of a middle-aged, chronically alcoholic man as the image of a homeless person was perhaps accurate. However, the homeless today average 34 years of age (Bassuk 1987) and comprise both men and women, families, the very young, and the very old. The National Coalition for the Homeless estimates that the homeless population in this country has swelled to two or three million (J.O.C. 1988).

MENTALLY ILL HOMELESS ADULTS. Psychosis among the mentally ill is estimated to affect from 25–50%. One-third to one-half of homeless persons are dependent upon alcohol or other substances. The adult population of homeless people include many who are referred to as "the young adult chronic patient" population. This young adult chronic population consists of men and women in their twenties who may have a primary diagnosis of schizophrenia, bipolar disorder, or borderline or antisocial personality disorder among other mental health problems. Characteristics common to the young adult chronic population include a fragile ego development, vulnerability to stress, and impairments in thinking, perception, attention span, and concentration. Pathological defenses against anxiety are evidenced by frequent incidents of suicide, violence, substance dependence, retreat to psychosis, or complete denial of needing help. These young adults also demonstrate tremendous deficits in their ability to form satisfactory interpersonal relationships, their social skills, and their competence in performing activities of daily living (Brunger 1986).

HOMELESS FAMILIES. Families now constitute about 20% of the homeless population, whereas before 1980 it was unusual to see a family on the streets (Bassuk 1987). One study found that the majority of homeless families comprised a young, single woman with two or three children who were receiving Aid for Dependent Children (AFDC). One-third of these homeless mothers have been physically abused, about one-fourth had been reported to the Department of Social Services for probable child abuse and neglect. Many of these mothers had a total work history of less than one month, and most felt profoundly isolated and disconnected from the community. Not surprisingly, the children had a wide range of psychological, social, and cognitive problems. Severe anxiety, depression, and learning difficulties were common (Bassuk 1987).

HOMELESS/RUNAWAY YOUTHS. Robertson (1988) refers to the phenomenon of homeless adolescents as a hidden crisis whereby a million or more adolescents are living on the streets annually. More than 900,000 of these youths are involved in prostitution. In fact, the most common survival strategies are prostitution, pornography, and dealing drugs. One study found that more than half of these youths had left home by age 13, and since that time had averaged nine moves a year (Bassuk 1987). Most studies support that these youths come from chaotic families, with the majority having a parent with a criminal history or substance abuse problem, and one-half being physically abused (Bassuk 1987).

Homelessness is not, therefore, the result of not having a home or shelter. For many people, homelessness is the most recent stage in a lifelong or long term series of problems (Brent and Dattalo 1988). Homelessness is a process that does, however, respond to intervention. The treatment may be lengthy and require a great deal of patience, but it can be successful.

THE PROCESS OF HOMELESSNESS

Usually, the term **chronic** refers to a situation that has existed for a significant length of time. Disaffiliation, arrested social development, dealings with clinics and social workers, conflict with employers, being on welfare, psychosexual difficulty, limited insight, and self-mutilation are life experiences that thousands of homeless men and women share across the country. A *Scientific American* study (Bassuk 1984) found that 74% of shelter residents had no family relations and 73% had no friends. The figure jumps to 90% for those homeless who also had psychiatric histories. The study concluded that **chronic homelessness** is often the final stage in a lifelong series of crises and missed opportunities, the culmination of a gradual disengagement from supportive relationships and institutions.

Many chronically homeless people experience many social workers and social work settings. Many chronically homeless are treated by a number of hospitals and clinics, and over a period of time a homeless person may be given a number of psychiatric diagnoses. For example:

- Dysthymic disorder
- Atypical psychosis
- Schizophrenic disorder, paranoid type
- Paranoid personality disorder
- Dependent personality disorder
- Borderline personality disorder
- Histrionic personality disorder

This does not point to psychiatric confusion nor to a lack of communication among treatment facilities, as much as it makes a case for the complexity of the chronically homeless person. A look at the hospital records indicates that while a person presented the appropriate array of symptoms to warrant a specific diagnosis, the person does not usually stay in any one place long enough to allow for any sort of diagnostic fine-tuning to take place. Before anything more accurate can be developed, great and prolonged care in the development of a therapeutic alliance must be established. Since the persons who suffer from homelessness as a lifestyle problem are severely and actively disaffiliated and estranged from themselves, others, and their environment, one or two hours, or even one or two sessions are not enough to develop the necessary therapeutic alliance. It may take several months or up to a year or more before substantial treatment or even diagnoses can be established. This fact should warn the practitioner against false or premature confidence, or rigidity when approaching the treatment of the homeless person.

Complicating this already complex picture is the unfortunate occurrence of caseload transfers or the introduction of new or replacement treatment staff. While a homeless person may be involved in effective treatment, if a new staff person takes over all or part of his or her treatment, a brand new therapeutic alliance must be established. This will prolong treatment.

FUTURE DIRECTIONS

Everybody seems to be getting involved in helping the many thousands of homeless men and women throughout the United States. Politicians and advocates are joined by the Pentagon, by architects, welfare workers, psychiatrists, the religious, the casinos, organizers, and others. The more that they participate, the more city, state, and federal funding will follow. More and more chronic mentally ill homeless will crowd more and more shelters. As more programs will open up there will be a growing job market for those who wish to work with this population. There will be a need for experienced professionals to "change gears" and accept specialized training with this "new" population. Colleges are already beginning to teach subjects both directly and indirectly related to the problem, and some offer specialty degrees in the field of homelessness. Politicians are very careful to publish policy statements regarding the homeless, and significant portions of public debates are devoted to the subject.

If the problem is seen as a new one, there may be a solution. That is, if deinstitutionalization is considered the primary cause, reinstitutionalization will be seen as the solution. If the lack of low-cost housing is considered the main cause, a housing solution will be sought. Unfortunately, such a complex problem will not be corrected by any one single solution. If, however, one looks at this problem and defines it as an encompassing lifestyle problem that results in severe and chronic disaffiliation, then possible solutions become clearer.

Carol Johnson, director of the homeless services for the Massachusetts Department of Mental Health, stated that "mental health issues are an integral part of the experience of homelessness . . . you can't separate homelessness, mental illness, and bureaucratic structures . . . the opposite of homelessness is community, not shelter" (J.O.C. 1988, 29).

Some of the homeless should be reinstitutionalized, many should be offered low-cost housing, many need forced residency drug or alcohol rehabilitation, others need to be returned to prison; prisons and their release policies and after-care programs need to be made more effective. The welfare system needs to be revamped, as does our education system. The family needs to be strengthened. Problematic as it is, because most of the homeless have multiple problems, there just will not be any single solution for any one person. Chronic homelessness is a lifestyle problem. Programs will need to be set up in nearly every one of the above-mentioned centers of treatment, each with the understanding of this lifestyle problem.

The Role of the Nurse

Nurses function within an evolving society challenged by complex medico-psycho-social phenomena. The American environment is greatly affected by the ravaging effects of family abuse, substance abuse, the AIDS epidemic, and the phenomenon of homelessness. Each one of these factors is vastly complex, raising difficult questions and demanding innovative, creative, and most likely complex interventions in the search for solutions. Each problem mentioned draws heavily upon the human services and touches not only the mental health of those directly involved but affects families, friends, communities, and the health care staff of those who come in contact with affected individuals.

The mentally ill homeless come in contact with the health care system in a number of settings: the emergency room, hospital surgical and medical units, prison settings, and community health care settings. Although the phenomenon of homelessness is seen mostly in large urban areas at present, the possibility exists that smaller communas the homeless population continues to grow. There are, unfortunately, no "interventions" or "fixed solutions" that can possibly be useful or even effective in the care of all of these clients. Their problems are numerous, overwhelming, and include often overlapping medical, financial, social, and emotional issues.

Nurses are trained in both medical and psychosocial aspects of care and are carving out a variety of new and creative roles to deal with complex mental health problems. The role of the nurse who works with the mentally ill, chronically homeless population is presently evolving. For example, nurses are increasingly assuming the role of case managers in the area of community health (Brunger 1986; Davidson et al. 1988). The nurse's role of caring is more suited to providing nurturance to long term chronic mentally ill clients than is the curing role of the medical model (Brunger 1986).

Some cities have allocated psychiatric beds solely for the purpose of caring for the mentally ill homeless. In New York City a mobile psychiatric team (Project HELP) goes out into the street to function as an "emergency room (ER) in the street for high-risk patients" who are referred by the police. The team conducts a psychomedical assessment. The program is intended for that segment of the homeless population who are mentally and physically ill, and who are found to be a danger to themselves or others. This particular approach has raised questions from the American Civil Liberties Union regarding infringement of a person's civil liberties. However, at the very least, concern is being generated by public officials to provide funding and support for new and nontraditional approaches in the search for solutions.

Some nurses are opting to care solely for the homeless mentally ill client, either on an inpatient basis or as part of a mobile unit assessing psychomedical emergencies. Many nurses work in community shelters in a variety of functions. Some work within the framework of the traditional medical model, assessing clients' health needs, administering medications, making appointments in outpatient clinics for follow-up, and running hygiene and health seminars. Other nurses may function more as socializing agents conducting activity or orientation groups, teaching basic social skills, and working with clients informally on a one-to-one basis or in small groups with the hope of establishing trust ties, decreasing alienation, and increasing socialization and self-esteem.

Not all nurses will be working directly with the mentally ill homeless. However, it is useful for all nurses to better understand the phenomenon of the chronically homeless mentally ill.

Specific interventions and "how to" is beyond the scope of this chapter, if indeed specific interventions exist. It is hoped that the reader will be able to better understand some of the dynamics and experiences of the chronically homeless, and through a vignette of one individual, view the plight of the chronically homeless with more insight and understanding. As to what is involved in effective treatment, insight is the first step, in any event, to intervention with this population. Lamb (1988) states that there can be gratification working with the chronically mentally ill, without perhaps achieving high levels of functioning for the client. Mental health workers can help change chaotic, dysphoric lifestyles into lives that are characterized by some degree of stability, contentment, and satisfaction.

Homelessness—A Closer Look

SHELTERS FOR THE HOMELESS

A shelter is not a desirable place to live. As an alternative, it is usually safer than being on the street and might save a person's life. A shelter is a place where positive human contact may take place either with a peer or with a staff member, or with an entire program of both staff members and peers. To treat the problems of alienation in any sort of isolated situation would be ineffective. It is only within an environment of peers that treatment is possible. Shelters do not provide a person with adequate privacy, and often they do not even provide adequate accommodations. However, for many, some hope does lie within the shelter's walls.

A life can go either way in a public shelter system. A person can become more chronically entrenched, or one can take on a different momentum, one of improvement and reconfiguration. Often, the longer one stays in a shelter setting the less likely one is to emerge from it. However, treatment can be effected even after several years of residency have elapsed.

Essentially, **shelters** are institutions. The very structure that appeases the anxiety of the new resident only serves to exacerbate his or her chronicity. The longer individuals abide by the rules, the less they will think for themselves and the less they will see themselves as effective problem solvers who share the burden of responsibility for their very condition.

Shelters do, however, provide a forum for human interaction, for affiliation. Therein lies their efficacy.

A TREATMENT CENTER WITHIN ONE SHELTER SYSTEM

Regulated as to funding by the State Office of Mental Health and monitored as to functioning by the City Department of Mental Health, the program under discussion here is a Community Support Services (CSS) treatment program in New York City. It is designed to treat an enrolled psychiatric population of homeless men. All of these men reside in this particular shelter and all are 18 years of age or older. *Psychiatric impairment* resulting in an inability to function independently is the eligibility requirement. That is to say, the primary diagnosis of each enrolled patient must be a psychiatric one.

The CSS team is staffed by a program director, a clinical coordinator (MSW), two case managers, a recreational therapist, a rehabilitation counselor, a nurse (RN), a half-time psychiatrist, three rehabilitation aides, an administrative assistant, and a file clerk. It is an interdisciplinary team and all of the clients are treated by all staff.

The physical environment consists of offices and treatment rooms as well as a dayroom with a television, stereo, pool table, ping-pong table, and card tables. Every day begins in this room with a one-hour community meeting attended by all staff and clients. It is during these meetings that clients may be observed and assessed for any acute changes in status requiring medical or crisis intervention. It is also an opportunity for the residents to focus in on their peers, as well as the community outside of the shelter. For example, staff may introduce lively discussions of current events, bring up incidents occurring in the shelter, make staff announcements, deal with client complaints or inquiries, or any other general matter. Discussion of specific personal problems is frowned upon, as it would be in any community meeting, unless it can be related to the whole.

During the course of the day, shelter residents may remain in the dayroom and take part in a number of activities, or they may need to see some of the other staff. In any case, the dayroom serves as a living room.

Shelter residents may also go to the nurse's office where, in addition to obtaining medication, clients may weigh themselves, have their blood pressure taken, inquire as to personal health concerns, or attend classes where slides are shown and lessons are given by the nurse on the effects of alcohol, marijuana, or other drugs. There is a recreation office where special crafts projects are undertaken and where a library is housed. A model apartment with a built-in kitchen and a sofa-bed is where the rehabilitation counselor teaches activities-of-daily-living-skills such as budgeting, shopping, cooking, and housekeeping. Lastly, there is a therapy room where the clinical coordinator holds various smaller group sessions.

Figure 30–1 demonstrates the treatment philosophy of both the shelter and the day treatment program. In circle "A" the client is shown in an uncertain world with many issues to face. Circle "C" shows how people cope with an uncertain world; they create an inner circle of greater certainty, one consisting of family and friends, one that enhances a person's self-respect, personal resources, developing skills, new outlooks, confidence, and honesty. It has already been discussed how this inner circle of greater certainty for the chronically homeless person is either extensively damaged or nonexistent. Circle "B" demonstrates some of the functions of the shelter. A temporarily stabilizing inner circle is created. Certainty is offered by the various rules and regulations of the shelter itself. It is the function of all staff to attempt the development of a more permanent inner circle of certainty as in circle "C" and then to help the person's transition into it. How and in what form these attempts are made are topics addressed in the next section, Strategies for Working With A Person Who Is Homeless.

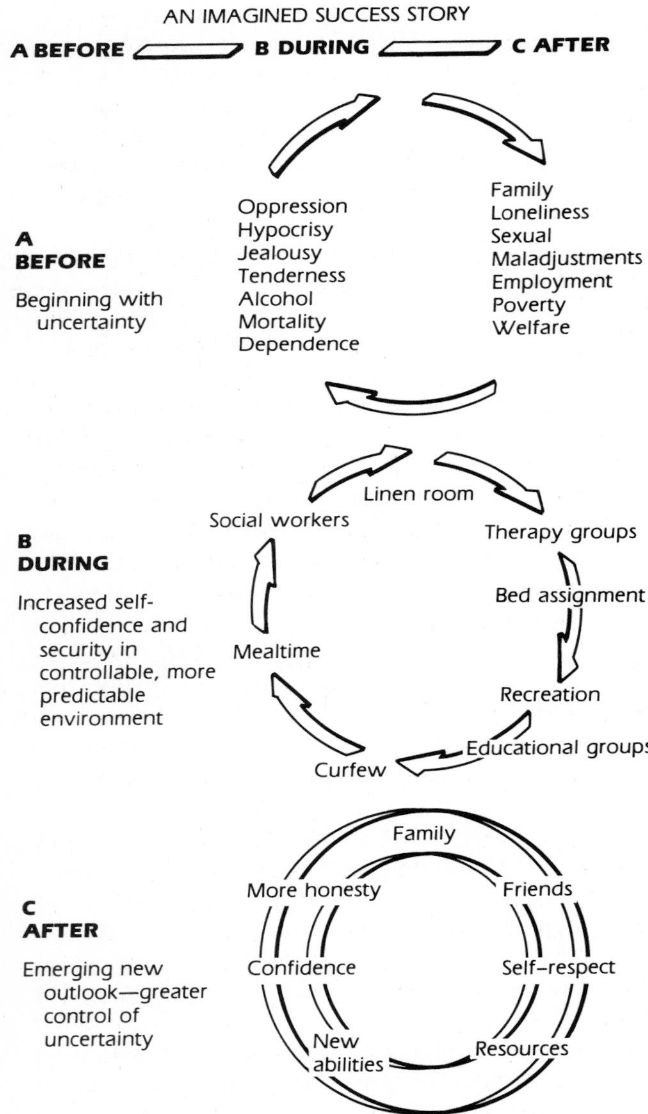

Figure 30–1. *Treatment philosophy of a day treatment program.*

STRATEGIES FOR WORKING WITH A PERSON WHO IS HOMELESS

Most nurses will be caring for homeless men and women in acute care facilities. There are times when such clients' compliance, personal attitudes, and behaviors will trigger anxiety and frustration in the nurse. An understanding of the process of chronic homelessness may help reduce both anxiety and frustration. Attitudes and approaches toward the homeless hospitalized person will be explored in this section.

A biographical sketch of one man will be presented. His life and progress in a day-treatment program will be followed. It is true that not all homeless men and women have the same story. However, many parallels can be drawn between the homeless man presented here and the issues of all mentally handicapped chronic homeless. Issues include severe isolation, lack of independence, abrasive public behavior, difficulties with authority, and limited insight. Physical problems include poor hygiene, medical problems, substance abuse, and poor nutrition. Social problems encompass financial deficits, job difficulties, domicile problems, and lack of family or community affiliations.

Biographical Sketch

George Chapman, the youngest of five, was born in 1955. His parents, Jewish-Russian immigrants, came to the United States a year before George was born. Soon after moving to the United States, George's father developed "emotional problems" and "back problems." Because of these two disabilities he was unable to work. George attended high school and received his high school diploma in 1972. He speaks of those years as ones during which he was basically a loner who was always picked on for not being a fighter:

> My family always had to protect me. In fact, all the teachers and all the kids in school called me a loner. But

they also called me one of the nicest kids around. They used to say to me "George, do you enjoy being alone?" and I would say, "Yes." Then they would say "Why is that?" and I would answer, "Because people don't really give a shit about you. People try to use you and take advantage of you. It's a self world." And I meant it. I had absolutely no friends to trust.

The summer after completing high school he got a job in a department store as a stock clerk. During these three months of employment, he remembers getting sick often. In fact, he says, all during his school years and especially during that summer, he always had stomach problems. He left that job after the summer and later that fall, at the age of 17, he began working in May's department store. He worked there for a period of four months until he was fired for "not listening to the assistant manager." Soon after that, he took a job at Seaman's bank, where he worked as clerk for three months until he was fired because he "couldn't get along with the public." At 18, he joined the Air Force. About six weeks later he was discharged for not being able to adjust to military life:

I had been having problems getting along with the Drill Instructor.

George than returned home and lived with his parents. He collected unemployment benefits, and when the time ran out he turned to welfare roles:

I was referred to the Office of Vocational Rehabilitation. There they sent me to a psychiatrist to see why so many people complained about me, why I got all those bad references. You see, everybody said that I was demanding, overpowering, and overbearing. I like to feel in control. Also, I have to go to the bathroom a lot. That's also why I was fired so much. Also, I was depressed because I had no friends and no one liked me.

In 1975, George's father suffered a stroke and died. George's mother moved into a nursing home shortly thereafter. In 1978, at the age of 23, George was hired as a subway token clerk for the New York City Transit Authority. During the next 22 months, he was hired and fired three times by the Transit Authority, the first two times for arguing with his supervisors and coworkers, and the last for stealing subway tokens and selling them for personal profit. He returned to welfare roles.

In October of 1981, his mother passed away. A little later that year he started pulling out his hair in fistfuls while shaving other parts of his body. An employment counselor referred him to a psychiatrist who offered him antidepressant medication. In his words:

I went home and immediately took 100 mg of the drug. I tried to kill myself but I should have taken more because it only caused me to sleep fourteen straight hours. I called my sister. She told me to come over. When I got there I took my clothes off to show her how I had shaved every single hair off my body. She called her boyfriend and they took me to the hospital. Officially, I was hospitalized because I shaved all the hair off my body and was throwing away clothes and other things because I noticed that there were imperfections in them. I was distraught and depressed and unhappy. I remember going over to see my sister on the subway. Everybody was afraid of me because of how I looked. But look, you'd be depressed too if you were by yourself all the time.

He was hospitalized for 13 days in November. Upon release, he began shaving himself again and was rehospitalized for 7 days. Then he was transferred to another hospital where he remained for four and one-half months. Here, his hospitalization came to a halt because:

The doctor threw me out in the street. He said I was a pain in the ass and anyway he was having trouble getting me into a community residence because of the problems he had getting paid from Medicaid. So, he threw me onto the street and I stayed at a welfare hotel in midtown Manhattan for a couple of weeks. Then, I was told I could move into the community residence in Brooklyn. I lived there for four months before being transferred to a midtown Manhattan location.

After six months at his new location, he was found to be disagreeing too often with the management's rules and regulations. He was soon placed in another residence. This time:

It was an old folks' home. I hated it and just left. I went to New York and got into one of those shelters on Park Avenue. Two shelters later, I ended up at this shelter. That was in '83.

While in this new shelter, through his social worker's efforts, he applied for reinstatement of his Social Security disability benefits and eventually was granted $473 per month. Next, he was helped to find a hotel room and, after three months in the shelter, was on his own again. Three weeks later, he was thrown out because he couldn't get along with the management. He then started moving around to different rooming houses and shelters and ended up at the same shelter where he had originally applied for his benefits.

Seven years after officially entering the New York City shelter system, he is still in it. And this despite having, at his estimate, "over 800 different social workers."

At present, George is 35 and living in an 800-bed shelter for homeless men. He is enrolled in a day treatment program that serves up to 100 different mentally ill residents of the shelter.

In the next section, we will examine what type of efforts do and do not work in the treatment of George's homeless lifestyle and mental illness. We will see that these are not unrelated concerns. We will also see that progress is slow, unpredictable, and elusive, although it is incrementally present.

Assessment

When a client is first referred to the program by the shelter's social service department, the client is asked to spend some time in the dayroom. There, the new member mingles with the other residents and is observed by the staff. During his first few days in the program area, he will be drawn into conversation with various staff members and be more formally interviewed by the program director, the clinical coordinator, the nurse, and the psychiatrist. It is in this way that suitability to the program is determined. The clinical coordinator, during the intake interview, draws extensively on the client's history of treatment, notes which other treatment facilities' records should be sent for, and, after conferring with other staff members, drafts a treatment plan (see Table 30–1). This is reviewed by the program's director. Staff assignments that facilitate the development of rapport with the new resident are made.

ASSESSING HABITS, BEHAVIORS, AND NEEDS. A typical day begins for George at approximately 7:00 A.M. Lying in his bed in a room shared with nine others, he opens his eyes to the sounds of his fellow residents coughing or opening their lockers, or of the shelter's staff making their maintenance rounds, or security checks. Usually still in his clothes from the day before, he quickly uses the bathroom but does not wash up. He makes his way to the cafeteria where, after waiting in line and speaking to no one, he sits at an empty table with his tray. Still not having talked to anyone, he eats, returns his tray and goes to the building where the day treatment program has its basement wing. There, he joins others who are sitting around, smoking cigarettes, engaging in conversation, watching an early morning television talk show, or playing pool. George, still not having showered or washed, might approach a staff member and make a few comments regarding which staff are or are not coming in that day, or he might go into the bathroom down the hall and using the mirror there, pull out any facial hairs that have appeared since the day before. If there are too many he might go back upstairs and shave them off. He is especially careful to keep his eyebrows shaved.

By 8:45 A.M. the community meeting starts. It is here, in the program's dayroom, that staff and clients sit along the perimeter of the room and discuss recent announcements, problems, and treatment issues. George is often the loudest and most vocal. He usually complains of staff not paying enough attention to him or showing him enough respect, and of how his fellow clients make fun of him. In turn, his fellow clients make more fun of him. He seems to enjoy it, laughing often, snapping his fingers together to make pronouncements, and generally having a good time. After the meeting ends an hour later, he goes out into the hallway and signs up on every waiting list so that he can be one of the first seen by each staff member. While waiting for his name to be called, he pops in and out of the secretarial office making comments about how beautiful he finds the secretaries. In addition to this, he frequently opens the door to the program director's office demanding to be seen because he has some very important things to discuss about how unhappy he is with the staff. He will also go in and out of the dayroom to play pool, watch little bits of different television programs, and complain that he feels he is being made to wait too long for whatever it is he wants.

When it is his turn to see the nurse, he usually goes into her office and demands that it be cleared so he can get proper attention. Then, while taking his vitamins with a glass of juice, he complains of stomach problems and asks for some pills for constipation. He might prod the nurse into making a comment regarding his missing patches of hair or his bleeding eyebrows and then admit to her that this is all part of his "perfection thing." While continuing to talk with her he hears his name called out to see the case manager. He rushes over there and spends the next hour complaining that he should not have to pay back an overpayment received from the Social Security Administration. He draws into the conversation anyone who may enter the room in an effort to rally support for his rigid and very angry stance regarding his problem with his benefits. Should the staff's clinical coordinator or the program director enter the room, he might leap up and ignore the case manager, beginning instead to alternately joke and argue with the others, snapping his fingers to help make his points. During all his interactions with staff and clients he often punctuates his comments with various forms of physical contact ranging from slaps on the back and quick neck rubs to two-handed hugs or short arm punches. After his series of meetings he returns to the dayroom area, though he will continue to open any closed doors and demand to be seen by whoever is busy. After a one-hour lunch break, he returns to the program area for a virtual repeat of his morning's activities. He is usually one of the last clients around at closing time, still full of energy. After the program's staff leaves for the day, he goes to the cafeteria and waits for dinner to be served; he then goes up to the sleep area looking for conversation. There are usually one or two people to talk to about the day, including gossip about the staff and what he plans to accomplish the next program day. If several clients gather around, he becomes embroiled in arguments or sometimes friendly and sometimes not too friendly roastings. By bedtime, still not having washed and still not having changed his clothes, he lies down hours before he is tired so he can be alone. He falls asleep by midnight and does not wake up until around 7:00 the next morning.

ASSESSING RELATABILITY. The program is set up in a way that gives George a reason to relate to each staff member. The availability George has to staff, however, poses an obstacle: he immediately comes face to face with the poor quality of his social interaction skills. While the staff wish to address this problem, they do not want him to experience too much failure too soon, for he might turn away and leave the program. It must be kept in mind that he is not involuntarily hospitalized. To the contrary, he may leave the shelter at any time, without needing anyone's consent. The staff also know that since it is common for people to experience some anxiety when confronted with a new social situation, it is likely that George will act the way he always has when feeling tense. They expect to quickly experience his personality quirks. With this in mind, fully aware of the delicate nature of their *initial* interactions with him, the staff will spend the first several days engaging in relatively safe conversations.

STAFF AWARENESS DURING THE ASSESSMENT PERIOD. The most important aspect of working with the chronically homeless population is the development of a relationship. The relationship often begins, as any other, with small talk. Attention must be focused on an effort to reflect the importance placed on the new client as an individual. Humor is a safe and affectionate way to make this point, so long as the humor is relevant and respectful. After several short conversations, each of which draws upon the previous one, staff provide feedback and evidence that he has been listened to. This also provides staff the opportunity to model appropriate conversational and interpersonal skills. Gradually the range of conversation may be broadened, all the while reinforcing the client's positive aspects. Although the context of the conversation may be focused on solving problems, it is the relationship staff hope to foster, and one it is hoped the client desires to continue. The relationship must be based upon mutual respect. The understanding that staff wish to convey is not one of an authority figure but of a person who simply wishes to know another. The client already knows that staff's job is to work with him, but despite this, if interest is genuine, he will wish to develop an affiliation. As basic trust develops and the client knows that staff believe in him, and he senses he is cared for, staff can more clearly define mutual goals regarding treatment and begin to establish clear roles. In George's case, it will be necessary to remind him of the staff's role in his life. George is quick to "forget" who staff are and what they have set out to accomplish with him. Actually, consistent repetition of staff's role in his life serves to assuage his ever-renewed interpersonal anxiety. Reiterations provide interpersonal structure. As time passes, George will need less and less repetition of that sort, but whenever crisis develops, and it is *his perception of crisis that is essential here*, his need for staff to justify their role will intensify. Relationships with George should provide him with consistency, and they need to be largely supportive in nature. These relationships will have at their roots the fact that he can trust certain staff and feels that they find him likable. When he finds the affiliation satisfactory, he will seek its maintenance even under stress. Then, and only then, can the relationship(s) serve as a treatment leverage. The very fact that he will not want the satisfactory affiliation to be disturbed will serve as both a motivator and measuring stick in regard to his responsiveness to treatment.

Box 30–1 depicts an actual conversation between George and the program director only hours after he entered the dayroom his first day in the program.

In this short exchange, a relationship with some established parameters has begun with the program director. Many things emerge as relevant regarding George, issues that the treatment staff must keep in mind during their time with him. He has a temper easily triggered. He is aware that he is demanding, and is willing to be somewhat confronted but only when first sided with. Also he must be allowed to be somewhat confrontational himself. He has been in hospitals and has received medication and is proud that he is not on any at present. He has Social Security problems that he considers extremely important. Employment is a concern and there is some issue regarding women. What could not be seen from the transcript of this conversation was George's physical condition. The program director entered in his casenote the fact that George was unevenly shaven and had many small facial wounds still freshly scabbed. His left eye twitched frequently and he maintained intense eye contact throughout the conversation. He wore no socks and his shirt was badly stained with smudge marks. His body odor was strong and his breath stale.

These facts, drawn from just one exchange, will be the partial focus of staff's concern during the days to follow. During daily meetings, each staff member will be formulating the groundwork for on-going relationships and will attempt to touch upon key issues appropriate to their professional discipline.

Because of the nature of George's personality, and his level of disaffiliation as a chronically homeless man, there is ample opportunity for staff to actively engage him. Every time he makes demands he is, after all, inter-

Box 30–1. INITIAL CONTACT

DIRECTOR: Excuse me, you're new in this program, aren't you?
GEORGE: Damn right I'm new here but I don't need anymore of this bullshit. All I want is to get the hell out of this place.
DIRECTOR: Well it's about time.
GEORGE: What do you mean it's about time? I don't belong here.
DIRECTOR: Well it's about time that I finally met someone who knows he shouldn't be living in a place like this.
GEORGE: Damn right I know that, I'm not like these other guys, these bums.
DIRECTOR: Do you think you'll ever get out of here? I mean a lot of people come into this program, act like they're crazy, and then decide they like it. By the way, are you crazy?
GEORGE: No, I am not crazy and I've never been crazy. I never should have been sent into the hospital and I never should be here. I don't take any medication and, in fact, every single doctor who has ever treated me has admitted that I've never been crazy. I'm only here because sometimes I do get a little demanding. Oh yeah, and overpowering. Oh, but the only reason that I am really here is because I have a Social Security problem. I want you to get my checks started up again. They claim it's my fault that they overpaid me but it's their fault. They screwed up my whole life.
DIRECTOR: What did you say your name was?
GEORGE: George Chapman.
DIRECTOR: George let me tell you something. I am the Director of this program, but I do not know about your Social Security problem. I could have my staff look into things and figure a way to help you. I will make sure my staff takes the time to get to know you and then, with you guiding them, they can put together the best strategy for you to successfully attack your Social Security problem. In fact, we have to make sure we take the time to get to know you because, you know, people are complex and it's my theory that no man ends up in a place like this just because of one problem. Am I right? I mean, you do have more than one problem don't you? You are complex, right?
GEORGE: Damn right I am. I got a lot more than just one problem. I've got personality difficulties I think they're called, and I need a girlfriend and I need a damn job.
DIRECTOR: You see what I mean? I am going to make sure that the staff does not rush into anything. I am going to make sure they ask you everything they should so that they can really help you. Staff has to get to know a man before they can help him the right way.
GEORGE: Damn right.
DIRECTOR: I'll probably sit down with you myself before this week is out and we'll talk some more. Listen, good luck.

acting. His many approaches, as abrasive as they may initially be, will be transformed by the staff into positive interactions. After a series of positive interactions, a sound assessment can be made, then each staff member can begin the intervention included in the treatment plan.

Formulating a Treatment Plan

An initial treatment plan was drawn up for George Chapman four days after he first entered the dayroom (Table 30–1). The plan will be reviewed by the clinical coordinator approximately one month after its initiation. At that time the staff will begin meetings to discuss a more structured, comprehensive treatment plan.

The comprehensive treatment plan is formally reviewed every six months during the client's first year of treatment, and once a year thereafter. Staff are expected to make monthly casenotes reflecting their interactions with the client's progress toward goal attainment. A daily record documenting the amount of time spent with each client is recorded on statistical forms. The casenotes, treatment plans, intake data, psychiatric exams, and medical records make up the client's chart. Chart audits are conducted yearly by the City Depart-

Table 30–1 • TREATMENT PLAN

1. *Ineffective individual coping*	Related to helplessness, as evidenced by frequent angry complaints about SSA benefits.
Long term goal:	Client will gain self-reliance for benefit-related problems.
Short term goal:	Client will discuss SSA problems only in the office of the social worker.
Modality:	Delay gratification for complaints by enforcing use of social worker sessions and point out negative behavior in group settings using peer feedback.
2. *Constipation*	Related to emotional disturbances, as evidenced by chronic constipation.
Long term goal:	Client will demonstrate self-reliance regarding treatment of constipation as well as understanding some causative factors and preventive techniques.
Short term goal:	Client will provide medical history and keep physical examination appointments upon each complaint.
Modality:	Individual sessions and self-care groups with nurse.
3. *Ineffective individual coping*	Related to inadequate psychological resources, as evidenced by becoming overbearing in interpersonal situations.
Long term goal:	Client will ask questions of peers and reflect on answers.
Short term goal:	Client will refrain from interrupting others without first asking permission and displaying some patience.
Modality:	Group sessions—negative behavior pointed out and discussed vis-a-vis peer comments regarding it.

ment of Mental Health to ensure quality care and suitability of treatment.

The problems identified by staff are expressed in concrete, specific terms. As can be seen in this sample treatment plan (Table 30–1), problem number 2 is to be attended to by the nurse. The problem is chronic constipation. This has been present for many years in George's life. It has caused him to lose one job and was the catalyst in his being discharged from the military. It has also allowed him a safe area of expression of need: it is a legitimate problem and usually leads to attentiveness from the staff. It is a recurrent problem and it appears to be stress-related. It is also a physiological expression of his emotional problems, that is, he has difficulty expressing feelings, which get pent up until they are explosively released. This leads to his experiencing great levels of tension relief and greater amounts of attention from the staff. When deciding on treatment for his chronic complaint of constipation it is essential that it is seen as an aspect or expression of homelessness as a lifestyle. For example, when George complains of constipation, demanding that staff stop whatever they are doing in order that they may resolve his discomfort, the nurse can make it clear to George that in order to deal properly with his problem, George must first provide a thorough medical history, agree to sign whatever release of information forms are necessary, and keep whatever appointments are set up for him. The nurse will also explain the connection between stress and his problem. If George refuses, the nurse can question the authenticity of George's complaints, or if they were real, he would want to comply. The nurse validates the seriousness of his discomfort and need for a resolution. It is important for the nurse to understand the history of the problem and previous attempts at treatment. This process of assessment and establishing rapport may span several sessions and as many days. During this time the nurse may give George some over-the-counter medication.

Throughout the relationship great care is taken to acknowledge George's successes, regardless of how small they may be. The nurse's speaking tone will reflect several things:

- Concern for the client's lifestyle difficulties and physical pain.
- The attitude that ultimately he is responsible for his own treatment.
- The belief that he is a complex person who will take some time to get to know.

After George was assessed by the psychiatrist, he was given the diagnosis of *borderline personality disorder*. (Refer to Chapter 17). This confirmed the staff observations and reaffirmed the need to set clear limits in a neutral nonthreatening manner.

Regardless of how well the care plan is designed, it will be ineffective if the staff cannot establish an interpersonal affiliation with George. It is crucial to develop a positive working relationship with the client before introducing new strategies necessary for change. In order to do this, the nurse and other staff must *avoid* being drawn into a defensive position. Staff attendance at treatment planning sessions is ongoing in order to coordinate joint efforts. This is vital to avoid any severe differences among staff with regard to treatment approach.

Intervention

The chronically homeless person represented here by George Chapman often shares some of the same qualities of cognition that a paranoid person possesses. For example, a paranoid person has a lack of trust along with a general sense of suspiciousness. These two qualities can perpetuate the paranoia and heighten levels of disaffiliation and estrangement, thus blocking the development of healthier ways of evaluating reality and interacting with others. For the chronically homeless, a lack of trust and a general sense of suspiciousness are necessary qualities if they are to survive in the streets. The fact that there is nobody to turn to will heighten an individual's sense of isolation, thereby deepening one's disaffiliation. The inability to trust and general sense of suspiciousness are both a cause and a natural outcome of his condition, the homeless lifestyle problem.

Because affiliation or emotional bonding between staff and client is the goal, extraordinary care must be taken not to exacerbate the client's sense of disaffiliation and isolation. Staff must be very direct with homeless clients. Eye contact should be unobtrusive, and the tone of voice, regardless of what is being said, should be sincere. Staff must be able to articulate the rationale behind their decisions and avoid being vague. Clients must be regarded as ultimately responsible for their treatment in so far as they need to actively participate in it. This will actually give the staff greater credibility in the clients' eyes and will, in time, empower the clients to gradually effect positive change.

Disaffiliated persons do not want to be bothered by anyone who is ingenuine. That is to say, their suspiciousness will be intensified if they sense any false demonstrations of genuine interest. If one lacks an ability to be direct with a homeless client, is condescending in any way, or is not appropriately assertive, then treatment may be ineffectual. At all times, the staff attempts to model appropriate problem-solving behaviors, even when the client is exasperating and provocative. If the staff can respond in a pleasant but out of the ordinary way, perhaps with humor, then there is a possibility of breaking through the negative defenses which perpetuate the chronic homeless lifestyle. For example, staff can focus on ignoring the negative aspects of what is said, and then rephrase the more positive commentary.

Although the client's approach may be perceived as negative, demanding, crude, or vulgar, the client is often just looking for the staff member to demonstrate belief in him or understanding and attention. The following interaction between George and his social worker took place just after George burst into the office and very loudly began making demands. Box 30–2 shows how the staff member used the context of George's stated problems to refocus on the process.

In this example the staff worker has successfully shifted the focus to the "here and now." Instead of focusing on why it was that George defined his world around him as "garbage," and instead of falling into a defensive posture, and instead of immediately disciplining him for his behavior, the staff member used positive affiliation as a treatment tool. He got right to the heart of the matter by engaging George, but he did not do it on George's terms. Instead, he responded in a manner that surprised George and made him listen and respond to the present. At the same time, the staff member was able to explain to George some of the ramifications of his behavior, but not until their alliance was established.

As regards the care plan, an effort was made to help George establish a capacity for self-observation. Dozens, perhaps hundreds, of similar exchanges over many months of treatment might actually effect an improvement in George's ability to modify his behavior. At the very least, it is a less stressful way for staff to assert themselves and, at the same time, demonstrate through modeling an understanding of the disaffiliative core of homelessness as a lifestyle. The client on some level will feel understood.

The most effective intervention tool possible when some degree of affiliation or relatedness occurs is the interactions with peers. During community meetings, or more casually during the day, it is George's peers that the staff will turn to for support of their observations. When George confronts a staff member in the hallway in a demanding way, staff can turn to other clients who are nearby for help in dealing with George. They can throw their hands up and ask for some help as to how they should respond to him or, after George accuses a staff person of not paying enough attention to him, the staff person can turn to the other clients and ask them if they feel that George does not get enough attention. Their responses will invariably put George "in his place." Other clients will have been developing their own notions of George, not too different from those that some of George's previous employers or relatives or therapists have held. This can be useful in a long term setting after a solid relationship has been developed between a staff member and a client. It is done in such a way that it is clear to the client the purpose is for realistic feedback, not to put him down or as a license for others to ridicule him.

Often it's the other clients who will confront George in ways that the staff can then mediate. The disaffiliate cares a great deal about what his peers think of him. In time, surprisingly, George finds himself experiencing

Box 30-2. REFOCUS ON THE PROCESS

GEORGE: I want to be seen by you and I want to be seen now. I'm tired of all this garbage. Why should I wait for everything. Damn it, I am so tired of all this garbage. Garbage! That's all I ever get. Damn it I'm tired of it.

STAFF: I think that's why they went on strike.

GEORGE: What the hell are you talking about?

STAFF: The sanitation workers. They said it in the news the other day. They were sick of all that garbage. You know, maybe we can get you a job as a sanitation man. Think of all the people that will agree with you then.

GEORGE: Don't make jokes of a serious thing. I'm serious and you're making jokes. Now how am I supposed to get help?

STAFF: You think I'm joking? I'm serious. You and the sanitation men think alike. They could probably use you to head up their union. Then they would get justice.

GEORGE: Damn right and I'd be a damn good union head. I'd be a better worker than you. You're always making jokes.

STAFF: And if I didn't, how would you know I care? Hey, you can only make jokes with the people who you like to see laugh. Maybe I just like having you around sometimes.

GEORGE: (*Smiles*) I'm the best, right?

STAFF: Listen George. When you come in the room demanding all sorts of things and yelling at me I don't know what else to do. So, I make a joke or two. Then we become two people enjoying a laugh. Then you calm down and we can get down to serious business. You know, if you came into my office calm, then we could get down to serious business sooner. So, next time, we can still have a laugh or two, but let's do it without the screaming. In fact, next time you come in and yell at me, I wouldn't be surprised if I just refused to talk to you because, I mean, I know you don't want to give me headaches. I know you really want me concentrating on how to help you and not where I can find some aspirin.

GEORGE: I know, I know. I always do that. I scream, then I get calm. But you got to admit it. I am the best. (*Snaps his fingers several times and hits his knees while smiling broadly.*)

moderate success at a series of relationships both with staff and some of the other patients. He feels some hope, however slight, and begins to experience a mild re-evaluation of his personal abilities. Though these feelings are somewhat artificial in nature, since the relationships he has formed have been created as if in a "laboratory," they do provide the basis for highly visible practice at social interactions. Staff, right along with the client, get to experience first hand some of the themes that have contributed to George's homeless lifestyle. He does experience pleasure at his new found social successes. Once this pleasure is acknowledged in a variety of ways, the interpersonal stressors can then be strategically offered and a less contrived struggle can begin. The overall goal is to strengthen his emerging social skills to a less protected, more realistic environment. The staff enforce this treatment strategy to encompass every major area of his life. For example, the nurse will implement this basic strategy around the areas of self-care, medication, and health care issues.

While the first part of this strategy may take only two or three weeks to establish, the second phase may need to continue for many months or until George shows himself resilient enough to be referred to another, more risky residential setting such as a co-ed group home in the community. It is there that this treatment will continue.

Evaluation

Frequent evaluation of the care plan by the homeless client, staff, and supervisor is crucial. Invariably new staff may plan goals which may seem to be short term, but are actually long term in view of the client's capacity. Realistic goals require a multidisciplinary approach. Client input when setting goals is vital, although at times tricky. Often the client is unable to assess his abilities or tolerate societal constraints. For example, a young adult client may say that all he wants is to get a job—but refuse to alter his poor grooming habits and sloppy dress. Therefore a creative and client-centered approach needs to be taken by the staff in order to establish more realistic and mutually acceptable initial goals. Evaluation is ongoing and constant. Often one finds that a variety of intervention strategies need to be tried. Often the initial "short term goal" and intervention strategies undergo radical change before progress starts. Constant evaluations are crucial for both client and staff. For the client, if the goal is not within his abilities, discouragement and hopelessness are reawakened. For the staff, frustration, hopelessness, and burnout ensue. Frequent informal as well as formal staff conferences are mandatory for the success of any program. Staff conferences provide the opportunity for shared observations and the planning of creative collective goals and treatment approaches. When this is undertaken within a setting of mutual support and respect, staff burnout is minimized and client progress can be maximized.

Summary

Homeless people come from every race, are of every age, and are both male and female. The history of many mentally ill chronically homeless people reflects a long process of which homelessness is the final stage. A mentally ill, chronically homeless person is disaffiliated (estranged from) society and personal supports.

Nurses play various roles in their work with the homeless population. Many settings allow for less traditional, more creative roles. Roles for the nurse working with the homeless population are continuing to evolve.

Shelters for the homeless were discussed and an example of a day treatment program for the mentally ill sheltered homeless was explored. Treatment philosophy, assessment strategies, and intervention modalities were presented through a clinical example of a chronic young adult homeless man. The many problems he encounters and needs he presents mirror the problems and needs of the homeless population in general, although personality, behaviors, and individual strengths and deficits may require different individualized plans of care.

When working with a mentally ill homeless person, it is even more crucial than usual to establish a very concrete interpersonal connection. If there is no relationship other than the severely limited and traditional one of staff to client, then there will be no treatment. Much as when working with the person suffering from a borderline personality disorder, the psychiatrist must often abandon analytic distance and become more "caring" in the client's eyes, so must the nurse or the social worker abandon the constraints of their traditional roles when treating the homeless client. It is important when attempting treatment of someone like George to develop a functional understanding of this unique personality matrix, homelessness-as-lifestyle. It is necessary to understand the various indices of homelessness as a lifestyle mainly in terms of its disaffiliating qualities. It stands to reason, then, that the makeup of the treatment program, and the methods of the people employed in it, will be affected by this understanding.

References

Bassuk EL. The homeless problem. Scientific American, 251(1):40, 1984.

Bassuk EL. Homelessness. The Harvard Medical School Mental Health Letter, 3(7):4, 1987.

Brent BB, Dattalo P. Homelessness: Consequences of a crisis or long term process. Hospital and Community Psychiatry, 39(8):884, 1988.

Brunger JB. The young chronic client in mental health today. Nursing Clinics of North America, 21(3):451, 1986.

Davidson RE, Factor R, Grundlach E, Adler K. Psychiatric nursing role in a community mental health center. Community Mental Health Journal, 24(1):83, 1988.

J.O.C. Building a sense of community cooperation among agencies key to helping the homeless. Psychiatric News, 23(8):29, 48, 1988.

Lamb HR. Community psychiatry and prevention. *In* Talbott JA, Hales RE, Yadofsky SC (eds). Textbook of Psychiatry. Washington, DC: American Psychiatric Press, 1988.

New York launches effort to remove mentally ill from streets. Psychiatric News, 23(2):8, 32, 1988.

Robertson JM. Homeless adolescents: A hidden crisis. Hospital and Community Psychiatry, 39(5):475, 1988.

Self-Study Exercises

Choose the answer that most accurately completes the statement.

1. People who are chronically homeless are best helped by

   A. a clean and safe shelter
   B. a suitable job

C. companionship and "buddies"
D. multiple interventions to complex problems

Place T (True) or F (False) next to each statement.

2. __________ Long term stays in shelters can potentiate a barrier to a more independent future.
3. __________ People who are chronically homeless just need proper shelter.
4. __________ People who are chronically homeless often perpetuate their problems despite sound interventions and planning.
5. __________ It is possible to help initiate positive directions in the lifestyles of many chronically homeless.
6. __________ The process of chronic homelessness and disaffiliation can be traced to early childhood development.
7. __________ The personality characteristics that keep a person relatively safe on the street are the same characteristics that can hinder positive relationships.
8. __________ More politicians, educators, and aspects of society are becoming more involved with finding avenues to help the growing number of homeless.
9. __________ The more attention is focused on the homeless population, the more state, federal, and city support may be available.
10. __________ The best approach with the chronically homeless is the conservative and analytic approach.

Write short answers to the questions that follow:

11. Name four important aspects a nurse should keep in mind when INITIATING a relationship with a chronically homeless person.

    A. ____________________ B. ____________________
    C. ____________________ D. ____________________

12. Name four benefits the nurse and client gain from close work with an interdisciplinary team.

    A. ____
    B. ____
    C. ____
    D. ____

13. Name four common mental disorders found among the chronically homeless population.

    A. ____
    B. ____
    C. ____
    D. ____

APPENDIX I

Self-Help Clearinghouses

(for help in finding or forming a mutual aid self-help group)

CALIFORNIA SELF-HELP CENTER 1-800-222-LINK or (213) 825-1799, U.C.L.A., 405 Hilgard Avenue, Los Angeles, CA 90024. Gerald Goodman & Marion Jacobs, Co-Directors. Provides information on local clearinghouses in the state, a few of which are:

> **NORTHERN REGION SELF-HELP CENTER** (916) 456-2070, Mental Health Assn of Sacramento, 5370 Elvos Ave., Suite B, Sacramento, CA 95819.
>
> **BAY AREA REGION SELF-HELP CENTER** (415) 921-4401, Mental Health Association, 2398 Pine Street, San Francisco, CA 94115.
>
> **CENTRAL VALLEY REGION SELF-HELP CENTER** (209) 723-8861, Mental Health Association of Merced County, P.O. Box 343, Merced, CA 95341.
>
> **SOUTHERN REGION SELF-HELP CENTER** (619) 297-2861, Mental Health Association of San Diego, 3958 Third Ave., San Diego, CA 92103-3003

CONNECTICUT SELF-HELP/MUTUAL SUPPORT NETWORK (203) 789-7645, Consultation Center, 19 Howe Street, New Haven, CT 06511. Vicki Spiro Smith, Director.

ILLINOIS SELF-HELP CENTER 1-800-322-M.A.S.H. (in Illinois only) or (312) 328-0470, 1600 Dodge Avenue, Suite S-122, Evanston, IL 60201. Daryl Isenberg, Director.

KANSAS SELF-HELP NETWORK (316) 689-3170 Campus Box 34, Wichita State University, Wichita, Kansas 67208-1595. David Gleason, Director.

MASSACHUSETTS CLEARINGHOUSE OF MUTUAL HELP GROUPS (413) 545-2313, Massachusetts Cooperative Extension, 113 Skinner Hall, University of Massachusetts, Amherst, MA 01003. Warren Schumacher, Director.

MICHIGAN SELF-HELP CLEARINGHOUSE (517) 484-7373, 1-800-752-5858 (in MI only), Michigan Protection & Advocacy Service, 109 West Michigan Ave., Suite 900, Lansing, MI 48933. Ms. Toni Young, Coordinator.

> **CENTER FOR SELF-HELP** (616) 925-0594, Riverwood Center, 1485 Highway M-139, Benton Harbor, Michigan 49022.

MINNESOTA MUTUAL HELP RESOURCE CENTER (612) 642-4060, Wilder Foundation Community Care Unit, 919 Lafond Ave., St. Paul, MN 55104.

MISSOURI KANSAS CITY SUPPORT GROUP CLEARINGHOUSE (816) 361-5007, Kansas City Association for Mental Health, 1020 East 63rd St., Kansas City, MO 64110.

NEBRASKA SELF-HELP INFORMATION SERVICES (402) 476-9668, 1601 Euclid Ave., Lincoln, NE 68502. Barbara Fox, Director.

NEW JERSEY SELF-HELP CLEARINGHOUSE 1-800-367-6274 (in NJ only), (201) 625-9565, TDD (201) 625-9053, St. Clares-Riverside Medical Center, Pocono Rd., Denville, NJ 07834. Edward J. Mandara, Director.

NEW YORK STATE SELF-HELP CLEARINGHOUSE (518) 474-6293, N.Y. Council on Children & Families, Empire State Plaza, Tower Building, Albany, NY 12223. Mary Huber, Coordinator. Provides information on additional local self-help clearinghouses in N.Y. (upstate) other than those listed below:

NEW YORK CITY SELF-HELP CLEARINGHOUSE, INC. (718) 596-6000, P.O. Box 022812, Brooklyn, NY 11202. Dianne Metzger, Director.

WESTCHESTER SELF-HELP CLEARINGHOUSE (914) 347-3620, Westchester Community College, 75 Grasslands Rd, Valhalla, NY 10595. Leslie Borck, Director.

LONG ISLAND SELF-HELP CLEARINGHOUSE (516) 348-3030, N.Y. Institute of Technology, Central Islip Campus, Central Islip, NY 11722. Pat Verdino, Director.

OREGON NORTHWEST REGIONAL SELF-HELP CLEARINGHOUSE (503) 222-5555, 718 W. Burnside Ave., Portland, OR 97209. Doreen Akkerman, Coordinator.

PENNSYLVANIA SELF-HELP GROUP NETWORK OF THE PITTSBURGH AREA (412) 247-5400, 710 1/2 South Avenue, Wilkinsburg, PA 15221. Betty Hepner,Coordinator.

PENNSYLVANIA SELF-HELP INFORMATION & NETWORKING EXCHANGE (717) 961-1234, S.H.I.N.E., Voluntary Action Center of Northeast Pennsylvania, 225 N. Washington Ave., Park Plaza, Lower Level, Scranton, PA 18503. Eric Fetterolf, Director.

SOUTH CAROLINA MIDLAND AREA SUPPORT NETWORK (803) 791-9227, Lexington Medical Center, 2720 Sunset Blvd., West Columbia, SC 29169. Becky Stone, Coordinator.

TEXAS For an update on the development and availability of a statewide self-help clearinghouse in Texas, contact the Mental Health Association in Texas, 1111 W. 24 St., Austin, Texas 78705, telephone (512) 476-0611, Christine Devall, contact person. An already existing regional clearinghouse is:

DALLAS SELF-HELP CLEARINGHOUSE (214) 871-2420, Mental Health Association of Dallas County, 2500 Maple Avenue, Dallas, TX 75201-1998. Carol Madison, Director.

VERMONT SELF-HELP CLEARINGHOUSE 1-800-442-5356 in VT only, or (802) 241-2249, c/o Parents Assistance Line, 103 South Main Street, Waterbury, VT 05676. Donna Carpenter, Coordinator.

WASHINGTON, D.C. SELF-HELP CLEARINGHOUSE OF GREATER WASHINGTON (703) 536-4100, Mental Health Assn. of N. Virginia, 100 N. Washington St., Falls Church, VA 22046.

NATIONAL INFORMATION—U.S.

SELF-HELP CLEARINGHOUSE (201) 625-7101; TDD (201) 625-9053, St. Clares-Riverside Medical Center, Denville, NJ 07834. Publishes the Self-Help Sourcebook directory of national groups.

NATIONAL SELF-HELP CLEARINGHOUSE (212) 840-1259, City University of New York Graduate Center, 33 West 42nd St., New York, NY 10036. Frank Riessman, Director.

SELF-HELP CENTER (312) 328-0470, 1600 Dodge Avenue, Suite S-122, Evanston, Illinois 60201. Daryl Isenberg, Director.

CANADA

CANADIAN COUNCIL ON SOCIAL DEVELOPMENT (613) 728-1865, P.O. Box 3505—Station C, Ottawa, Ontario, Canada K1Y 4G1. Publishes national newsletter, *Initiatives*. Hector Balthazar.

CALGARY FAMILY LIFE EDUCATION COUNCIL (403) 262-1117, 233 12th Avenue S.W., Calgary, Alberta, Canada T2R OG9. Sonia Eisler, Executive Director.

MONTREAL CAMAC, CENTRE D'AIDE MUTUELLE (514) 484-7406, C.P. 535, Succ. Desjardins, Montreal, Quebec, Canada H5B 1B6. M. Jean-Claude Boisvert, President.

NOVA SCOTIA THE SELF-HELP CONNECTION (902) 422-5831, 5739 Inglis Street, Halifax, Nova Scotia B3H 1K5. Margot Clarke, Coordinator.

SASKATCHEWAN SELF-HELP DEVELOPMENT UNIT (306) 652-7817, 410 Cumberland Avenue North, Saskatoon, Saskatchewan, Canada S7M 1M6. Richard Wollert, Director.

SELF-HELP CLEARINGHOUSE OF METRO. TORONTO (416) 487-4355, 40 Orchard View Blvd, Suite 215, Toronto, Ontario, Canada M4R 1B9. Lori Kociol, Director

WINNIPEG SELF-HELP RESOURCE CLEARINGHOUSE (204) 589-5500 or 633-5955, NorWest Coop & Health Center, 103-61 Tyndall Avenue, Winnipeg, Manitoba, Canada R2X 2T4.

OVERSEAS

Each of the following can provide information on additional self-help clearinghouses and networks in that country or region of the world:

AUSTRALIA WESTERN INSTITUTE OF SELF-HELP phone (09) 383-3188. Address: 80 Railway Street, Cottesloe, 6011, Western Australia. Cheryl A. Dimmack, Contact Person.

EUROPE INTERNATIONAL INFORMATION CENTRE ON SELF-HELP AND HEALTH E. Van Evenstraat 2C, B-3000 Leuven, Belgium. Provides information on clearinghouses and projects throughout Europe. Jan Branckaerts, Director.

ENGLAND NATIONAL SELF-HELP SUPPORT CENTRE NCVO, 26 Bedford Square, London WC1B 3HU. Mai Wann, Director.

GERMANY Nationale Kontakt- und Informationsstelle zur Amregung und Unterstutzung von Selbsthilfegruppen Albrecht-Achilles-Strasse 65, D-1000 Berlin (West) 31. Klaus Balke, Director.

ISRAEL SELF-HELP CLEARINGHOUSE phone 661231, American Jewish Joint Distribution Committee, Inc., J.D.C. Hill, Jerusalem, Israel 91034. Martha Ramon, Director.

JAPAN SOCIETY FOR STUDY OF SELF-HELP GROUPS Dept. of Soc. Welfare, Faculty of Humanities, Sophia University, 7-1 Kioicho, Chiyoda-ku, Tokyo 102, Japan. Tomofumi Oka, Director.

From Mandara EJ. How to ideas. *In* Mandara EJ, Meesc A (eds). The Self-Help Sourcebook: Finding and Forming Mutual Aid, 2nd ed. Denville, NJ: Self-Help Clearinghouse, 1988.

APPENDIX II

Table 7–4 • NURSING DIAGNOSTIC CATEGORIES

Pattern 1: Exchanging

Altered Nutrition: More than body requirements
Altered Nutrition: Less than body requirements
Altered Nutrition: Potential for more than body requirements
Potential for Infection
Potential Altered Body Temperature
Hypothermia
Hyperthermia
Ineffective Thermoregulation
Dysreflexia
Constipation
Perceived Constipation
Colonic Constipation
Diarrhea
Bowel Incontinence
Altered Patterns of Urinary Elimination
Stress Incontinence
Reflex Incontinence
Urge Incontinence
Functional Incontinence
Total Incontinence
Urinary Retention
Altered (Specify Type) Tissue Perfusion (Renal, cerebral, cardiopulmonary, gastrointestinal, peripheral)
Fluid Volume Excess
Fluid Volume Deficit (1)
Fluid Volume Deficit (2)
Potential Fluid Volume Deficit
Decreased Cardiac Output
Impaired Gas Exchange
Ineffective Airway Clearance
Ineffective Breathing Pattern
Potential for Injury
Potential for Suffocation
Potential for Poisoning
Potential for Trauma
Potential for Aspiration
Potential for Disuse Syndrome
Impaired Tissue Integrity
Altered Oral Mucous Membrane
Impaired Skin Integrity
Potential Impaired Skin Integrity

Pattern 2: Communicating

Impaired Verbal Communication

Pattern 3: Relating

Impaired Social Interaction
Social Isolation
Altered Role Performance
Altered Parenting
Potential Altered Parenting
Sexual Dysfunction
Altered Family Processes
Parental Role Conflict
Altered Sexuality Patterns

Pattern 4: Valuing

Spiritual Distress (distress of the human spirit)

Pattern 5: Choosing

Ineffective Individual Coping
Impaired Adjustment
Defensive Coping
Ineffective Denial
Ineffective Family Coping: Disabling
Ineffective Family Coping: Compromised
Family Coping: Potential for Growth
Noncompliance (Specify)
Decisional Conflict (Specify)
Health-Seeking Behaviors (Specify)

Pattern 6: Moving

Impaired Physical Mobility
Activity Intolerance
Fatigue
Potential Activity Intolerance
Sleep Pattern Disturbance
Diversional Activity Deficit
Impaired Home Maintenance Management
Altered Health Maintenance
Feeding Self-Care Deficit
Impaired Swallowing
Ineffective Breastfeeding
Bathing/Hygiene Self-Care Deficit
Dressing/Grooming Self-Care Deficit
Toileting Self-Care Deficit
Altered Growth and Development

Table continued on following page

Table 7–4 • NURSING DIAGNOSTIC CATEGORIES *Continued*

Pattern 7: Perceiving	
Body Image Disturbance Self-Esteem Disturbance Chronic Low Self-Esteem Situational Low Self-Esteem Personal Identity Disturbance	Sensory/Perceptual Alterations (Specify) (Visual, auditory, kinesthetic, gustatory, tactile, olfactory) Unilateral Neglect Hopelessness Powerlessness
Pattern 8: Knowing	
Knowledge Deficit (Specify)	Altered Thought Processes
Pattern 9: Feeling	
Pain Chronic Pain Dysfunctional Grieving Anticipatory Grieving Potential for Violence: Self-directed or directed at others	Post Trauma Response Rape-Trauma Syndrome Rape-Trauma Syndrome: Compound Reaction Rape-Trauma Syndrome: Silent Reaction Anxiety Fear

From North American Nursing Diagnosis Association. Classifications of nursing diagnosis: Proceedings of the Eighth Conference.

APPENDIX III

Drug Information

ANTIPSYCHOTIC/NEUROLEPTIC

PHENOTHIAZINE

CHLORPROMAZINE

(Thorazine, Chlorazine)

USES:

1. Management of acute psychotic disorders (schizophrenia, manic phase of a bipolar disorder) and to maintain remission of these psychotic disorders.
2. Management of severe behavioral disturbances in (a) children or (b) clients with organic mental disorders.
3. Other: Intractable hiccups, acute intermittent porphyria, tetanus, preoperatively, or to control nausea and vomiting.

ACTION: Blocks postsynaptic dopamine receptors in the cerebral cortex basal ganglia, hypothalamus, limbic system, brain stem, and medulla. Therefore, there is inhibition or alteration of dopamine release, which is thought to be related to the suppression of the clinical manifestations of schizophrenia.

DOSAGES & ROUTES

	PO	IM	RECTAL SUPPOSITORY
Adult	10 to 50 mg twice daily to every 4 hours	25 to 50 mg 1–4 times daily	50–100 mg 3–4 times daily
Child	0.55 mg/kg every 4–6 hours	None	1.1 mg/kg every 6–8 hours
Elderly	(Debilitated) 25 mg 3 times daily		

CONTRAINDICATIONS: Comatose states, alcohol or barbiturate withdrawal states, bone marrow depression, pregnancy, lactation.

CAUTIONS: Seizure disorders, diabetes, hepatic disease, cardiac disease, glaucoma, prostatic hypertrophy, asthma.

REMARKS: A "low potency" neuroleptic (low neurological symptoms [EPS]), but high sedation and autonomic side effects (e.g., hypotension, cardiac, allergic). Food or antacids decrease absorption. Liquid preparation more rapidly absorbed.

SIDE EFFECTS

AUTONOMIC: Dry mouth, nasal congestion, constipation or diarrhea, urinary retention or urinary frequency, inhibition of ejaculation and impotence in men.

CNS: *Extrapyramidal Symptoms* Pseudoparkinsonism, akathisia, dystonia. Possible vertigo or insomnia.

CV: Orthostatic hypotension, hypertension, vertigo, EEG changes.

ENDOCRINE: Changes in libido, galactorrhea in women, gynecomastia in men.

OCULAR: Photophobia, blurred vision, aggravation of glaucoma.

OTHER: Weight gain, allergic reactions such as eczema and skin rashes.

ADVERSE REACTIONS **CNS:** *Acute dystonias* (painful neck spasms, torticollis, oculogyric crisis, convulsions, and so forth). *Tardive dyskinesia* (choreiform movements of the tongue, face, mouth, jaw, and possibly extremities). Elderly and those on drug for extended periods more susceptible; often the condition is irreversible.

HEMATOLOGIC: Agranulocytosis—drug immediately stopped.

HEPATIC: Jaundice; clinical picture resembles hepatitis.

NEUROLEPTIC MALIGNANT SYNDROME (NMS): Rare life-threatening syndrome. Includes severe rigidity, fever, increased white count, unstable BP, renal failure, tachycardia, tachypnea. Hold all drugs. Immediate administration of dantrolene sodium and bromocriptine most successful somatic prescription.

NURSING MEASURES:

1. Take BP lying and standing (withhold if systolic 90 or below) and notify MD.
2. Hold dose if EPS or jaundice.
3. Check frequently for urinary retention.
4. Check for constipation (avoid impaction).
5. Observe for fever, sore throat, and malaise and monitor CBC, indicating a blood dyscrasia.

INFORM CLIENT:

1. Rise slowly to sitting position and dangle legs five minutes before standing to minimize orthostatic hypotension.
2. Avoid sun. Use sunscreen when in direct light to avoid skin blotching.
3. Avoid sun. Client may experience severe photosensitivity. Advise wearing sunglasses to minimize photophobia.
4. Avoid use of alcoholic beverages, as they enhance CNS depression.
5. Do not operate machinery if drowsiness occurs.

HALOPERIDOL

(Haldol, Haldol Decanoate-Peridol)

ANTIPSYCHOTIC/NEUROLEPTIC

BUTYROPHENONE

USES:

1. Management of psychotic disorders.
2. Helps control remissions in schizophrenia.
3. Controversial use for children with combative, explosive hyperexcitability.
4. Control of tic and vocal utterances of Gilles de la Tourette's disorder.
5. Useful in acute mania and acute and chronic organic psychosis.
6. Management of drug-induced psychosis (LSD).

ACTION: Blocks the binding of dopamine to the postsynaptic dopamine receptors in the brain.

DOSAGES & ROUTES

	PO	IM
Adult	0.5–2.0 mg 2–3 times daily	(SEVERE) 3–5 mg every 1–8 hours to control symptoms, then give PO
Child	Not for children under 3 years. For children 3–12 years, 0.05–0.15 mg/kg/day in 2–3 divided doses.	
Elderly	Elderly or debilitated clients may require smaller doses than adults.	

CONTRAINDICATIONS: Hypersensitivity, Parkinson's, depression, seizures, coma, alcoholism, and during lithium therapy.

CAUTIONS: The elderly, clients on anticoagulant therapy, clients with glaucoma, prostatic hypertrophy, urinary retention, or asthma.

REMARKS: A "high potency" neuroleptic; higher incidence of EPS but lower incidence of sedation and orthostatic hypotension. Haldol Decanoate given IM can have lasting effects from one to three weeks.

SIDE EFFECTS

AUTONOMIC: Dry mouth, nasal congestion, constipation or diarrhea, urinary retention or urinary frequency, inhibition of ejaculation and impotence in men.

CNS: *Extrapyramidal Symptoms*: pseudoparkinsonism, akathisia, dystonia, vertigo, insomnia, headache.

CV: Orthostatic hypotension, hypertension, dizziness, EEG changes.

ENDOCRINE: Changes in libido, galactorrhea in women, gynecomastia in men.

OCULAR: Photophobia, blurred vision, aggravation of glaucoma.

OTHER: Weight gain, allergic reactions such as eczema and skin rashes.

ADVERSE REACTIONS

CNS: *Acute dystonias* (painful neck spasms, torticollis, oculogyric crisis, convulsions, and so forth. *Tardive dyskinesia* (choreiform movements of the tongue, face, mouth, jaw, and possibly extremities). Elderly and those on drug for extended periods more susceptible; often irreversible.

HEMATOLOGIC: Agranulocytosis — drug immediately stopped.

HEPATIC: Jaundice; clinical picture resembles hepatitis.

NEUROLEPTIC MALIGNANT SYNDROME (NMS): Occurs within 24–72 hours. Fever, rigidity, renal failure, arrythmias, and more. Give dantrolene sodium or bromocriptine immediately.

NURSING MEASURES:

1. Check for signs of tardive dyskinesia (protrusion of tongue, puffing of cheeks, chewing or puckering of the mouth) and report them to MD immediately.
2. Observe for other signs of EPS and jaundice.
3. Check for orthostatic hypotension (take BP lying and standing). Withhold if systolic 80 or below.
4. Check frequently for urinary retention.
5. Check for constipation (avoid impaction).
6. Observe for fever, sore throat, and malaise, and monitor CBC, indicating a blood dyscrasia.
7. Monitor renal function during long-term therapy.
8. Monitor blood levels every week.

INFORM CLIENT:

1. Rise slowly to sitting position and dangle legs five minutes before standing to minimize orthostatic hypotension.
2. Use sunscreen when in direct light to avoid skin blotching.
3. Avoid use of alcoholic beverages, as they enhance CNS depression.
4. Refrain from operating machinery if drowsiness occurs.

BENZTROPINE MESYLATE

(Cogentin)

ANTIPARKINSON

USES:

1. Treating Parkinson's disease.
2. Treatment of extrapyramidal symptoms (except tardive dyskinesia) due to use of neuroleptic/antipsychotic medications.

ACTION: Cogentin is an anticholinergic agent. This drug increases and prolongs the action of dopamine activity in the CNS, thereby correcting neurotransmitter imbalances and minimizing involuntary movements.

DOSAGES & ROUTES

	PO	IM
Adult	0.5–2 mg every day initially. Gradually increase to 4–6 mg/day. For drug-induced extrapyramidal symptoms, 1–4 mg once or twice a day IM or PO.	For acute dystonic reactions 0.5–2 mg IM or IV.
Elderly	Use lower doses.	

CONTRAINDICATIONS: Narrow-angle glaucoma, pyloric or duodenal obstruction, peptic ulcers, prostatic hypertrophy, obstructions of bladder neck, myasthenia gravis, and children under three (3) years. Rarely indicated for children.

CAUTIONS: The elderly and clients with cardiac, liver, or kidney disease or hypertension. Also used with caution in clients taking barbiturates or alcohol.

REMARKS: The effects of benztropine are cumulative and may not be evident for two or three days. After four to six months of long term maintenance antipsychotic therapy, antiparkinsonian drugs can be used on a prn basis or withdrawn. Some clients respond best to the medication given every day. Others do better with divided doses. Long term use of benztropine with a neuroleptic can predispose a patient to tardive dyskinesia.

SIDE EFFECTS

AUTONOMIC: Dry mouth, blurred vision, nausea, restlessness.

CNS: Sedation, vertigo, paresthesias.

CV: Palpitations, tachycardia.

GI: Nausea, vomiting, constipation, paralytic ileus.

GU: Dysuria, urinary retention.

OCULAR: Blurred vision, mydriasis, photophobia.

OTHER: Anhidrosis (abnormal deficiency of sweat).

ADVERSE REACTIONS

CNS: CNS depression, mild agitation, hallucinations, delirium, toxic psychosis, muscle weakness, ataxia, and numbness of the fingers.

NURSING MEASURES:

1. Monitor intake and output. Observe for urinary retention.
2. Give medication after patient voids to reduce possibility of urinary retention.

3. Monitor for constipation; abdominal pain or distention may indicate potential for paralytic ileus.
4. Indications of CNS toxicity (depression or excitement, hallucinations, psychosis, or other) warrant withholding the drug and informing the physician immediately).

INFORM CLIENT:

1. Avoid driving or operating hazardous equipment if drowsiness or dizziness occurs.
2. Tolerance to heat may be reduced owing to diminished ability to sweat. Plan periods of rest in cool places during the day.
3. Stop taking the medication if CNS toxic effects, or difficulty swallowing or speaking, or vomiting occurs. Inform MD immediately.
4. Monitor urinary output and watch for signs of constipation.
5. Consult with MD prior to using any medication, prescribed or over the counter, once started on Cogentin.

DIAZEPAM

(Valium)

ANXIOLYTIC (ANTIANXIETY) AGENTS

BENZODIAZEPINE

USES:

1. Management of anxiety disorders, for short term relief of anxiety symptoms.
2. Presurgical sedation to allay anxiety and tension.
3. Alcohol withdrawal.
4. Seizure disorders.
5. Anticonvulsant.
6. Relief of skeletal muscle spasticity.

ACTION: One action of the benzodiazepines is to increase the action of gamma-aminobutyric acid (GABA). The benzodiazepines help GABA open a chloride channel in the postsynaptic membrane of many neurons, thereby reducing the neuron's excitability.

DOSAGES & ROUTES

	PO	IM/IV
Adult	Anxiety—2–10 mg 2–4 times daily	2–10 mg 2–4 times daily
	Muscle relaxant—2–10 mg 2–4 times daily	5–10 mg every 3–4 hours
	Convulsions—2–10 mg 2–4 times daily	5–10 mg at 10-minute intervals
	ETOH withdrawal—10 mg 3–4 times daily	10 mg initially, followed by 5–10 mg every 3–4 hours
Elderly	2.5 mg twice daily	For convulsions, 2–5 mg (increase gradually as needed)

CONTRAINDICATIONS: Acute narrow-angle glaucoma, untreated open-angle glaucoma, during or within 14 days of MAO inhibitor therapy, depressed or psychotic patients in the absence of anxiety, first trimester pregnancy, breast-feeding, shock, coma, acute alcohol intoxication.

CAUTIONS: Epilepsy, myasthenia gravis, impaired hepatic or renal function, drug abuse, addiction-prone individuals. Injectable diazepam used with extreme caution in the elderly, the very ill, and people with COPD. May elicit rage reactions in some clients.

REMARKS: The benzodiazepines can produce psychological and physical habituation, dependence, and withdrawal. Therefore the benzodiazepines are recommended for short term therapy (two to four weeks). These drugs need to be used with caution in individuals who have histories of addiction. Withdrawal from these drugs should be gradual in order to minimize withdrawal symptoms.

SIDE EFFECTS **CNS:** Sedation, vertigo, weakness, ataxia, decreased motor performance, confusion.

OCULAR: Double or blurred vision.

SKIN: Urticaria, rash, photosensitivity.

GI: Change in weight, dry mouth, constipation.

ADVERSE EFFECTS **CNS:** Benzodiazepines are CNS depressants. They are fairly safe when used on their own, but when used in combination with other CNS depressants, they can cause death.

CV: Tachycardia to cardiovascular collapse.

METABOLIC: Changes in liver or renal function tests.

INJECTION SITES: Can cause venous thrombosis or phlebitis at injection sites.

NURSING MEASURES:

1. Obtain drug history of prescribed and over-the-counter (OTC) medications.
2. Periodically monitor blood cell count and liver function test during prolonged therapy.
3. Assess for unexplained bleeding, petechiae, fever, and so forth.
4. IM therapy: Aspirate back, administer deeply into large muscle mass; inject slowly; rotate injection sites.

INFORM CLIENT:

1. Avoid alcohol or any other central nervous system depressants (anticonvulsants, antidepressants) while taking a benzodiazepine—can lead to respiratory depression. Check with MD before taking.
2. Avoid driving or operating hazardous machinery if drowsiness or confusion occurs.
3. Avoid abrupt withdrawal of benzodiazepine.

IMIPRAMINE HYDROCHLORIDE

(Tofranil)

ANTIDEPRESSANT

TRICYCLIC

USES:

1. The principal indication for tricyclic antidepressants (TCAs) is the treatment of depression (major, bipolar, or dysthymia).
2. Imipramine is effective in some organic affective disorders and obsessive-compulsive disorders.
3. Imipramine is used as adjunctive treatment in childhood enuresis and in bulimia.
4. Found useful in the treatment of agoraphobia with panic attacks and generalized anxiety disorder.

ACTION: TCAs block the reuptake of norepinephrine and serotonin into their presynaptic neurons.

DOSAGES & ROUTES

	PO	IM
Adult	50 mg/day to start, given in 1–4 divided doses up to 200 mg daily for outpatients	Do not exceed 100 mg/day in divided doses
Child	For childhood enuresis, 25 mg before bedtime; for depression in children *over* 12 years, 30–40 mg daily initially	
Elderly	Used with caution—usually start at lower dose	Geriatric clients start on 30–40 mg daily initially

CONTRAINDICATIONS: Recent myocardial infarction or cardiac disease, severe renal or hepatic impairment. Death may occur if used with an MAO inhibitor. However, the two may be cautiously used together in cases of refractory depression. Tricyclics may also cause fatal cardiac arrhythmias in clients with hyperthyroidism. Use with caution in children and adolescents. Special cautions for the elderly, especially those with cardiac, respiratory, cardiovascular, hepatic, or GI diseases.

CAUTIONS: Other cautions include people with renal or hepatic disease and those with narrow-angle glaucoma. The potential for suicide must be assessed. Tricyclics lower the seizure threshold: any client with a seizure disorder needs careful monitoring.

REMARKS:

1. Before receiving the TCAs, clients need a thorough physical and cardiac workup.
2. Patients need to know that mood elevation may not occur for two to four weeks.

SIDE EFFECTS

ANTICHOLINERGIC: Dry mouth and nasal passages, constipation, urinary hesitancy, esophageal reflux, blurred vision.

CV: Orthostatic hypotension, hypertension, palpitations.

CNS: Tachycardia, vertigo, tinnitus, numbness and tingling of extremities, stimulation.

ENDOCRINE: Galactorrhea, increased or decreased libido, ejaculator and erectile disturbances, and delayed orgasm.

OTHER: Weight gain and impotence, cholestatic jaundice, fatigue.

ADVERSE REACTIONS

AUTONOMIC: Intracardiac conduction slowing.

CV: Myocardial infarction, congestive heart failure, arrhythmias, heart block, cardiotoxicity, cerebrovascular accident, shock.

CNS: Ataxia, neuropathy, EPS, lowered seizure threshold, delirium.

HEMATOLOGIC: Bone marrow depression, agranulocytosis.

PSYCHIATRIC: Hallucinations, shift to hypomania, mania, exacerbation of psychosis.

NURSING MEASURES:

1. Monitor BP (both lying and standing) every two to six hours when initiating therapy.
2. Observe suicidal clients closely during initial therapy.
3. Supervise drug ingestion to prevent hoarding of drug.
4. Assess for urinary retention.
5. Monitor liver function tests and complete blood count (assess for signs of cholestatic jaundice and agranulocytosis).
6. Small amount of drugs should be dispensed if client is to be discharged.
7. Diabetic clients should be closely monitored, especially during early therapy, since hypo- or hyperglycemia may occur in some clients.
8. All clients on the tricyclics need to be observed for the occurrence of hypomania or manic episodes, urinary retention, orthostatic hypotension, and seizure activity.

INFORM CLIENT:

1. Rise slowly to prevent hypotensive effects.
2. Do not drive or use hazardous machinery if drowsiness or vertigo occurs.
3. Do not use over-the-counter (OTC) drugs in conjunction with a TCA without a physician's approval.
4. The effects of alcohol and imipramine are potentiated when used together, and alcohol use should be discussed with MD before taking drug.
5. One to four weeks may pass before you experience therapeutic effects.

ANTIDEPRESSANT

MONOAMINE OXIDASE INHIBITOR (MAOI)

PHENELZINE SULFATE

(Nardil)

USES:

1. MAOIs are used primarily for depression that is refractory to tricyclic (TCA) therapy.
2. MAOIs are particularly effective in atypical depression, agoraphobia, or hypochondriasis.
3. Panic disorders.

ACTION: Antidepressant effect thought to be due to irreversible inhibition of MAO, thereby increasing the concentration of epinephrine, norepinephrine, serotonin, and dopamine within the presynaptic neurons and at the receptor site.

DOSAGES & ROUTES

	PO
Adult	15 mg 3 times daily. Increase rapidly to 60 mg daily until therapeutic level is noted.
Elderly	Are prone to side effects. Not used with children.

CONTRAINDICATIONS: MAOIs can cause untoward interactions with certain foodstuffs or cold remedies, which may produce hypertensive crises, CVA, or hyperpyrexia states that can lead to coma or death. Therefore, a confused or noncompliant client is at risk with an MAOI.

Other contraindications include people with congestive heart failure, cardiovascular or cerebrovascular disease, impaired renal function, glaucoma, history of severe headaches, liver disease, elderly or debilitated patients, and people who are pregnant or who have paranoid schizophrenia.

CAUTIONS: Depression accompanying alcoholism or drug addiction, manic-depressive states, suicidal tendencies, agitated clients, and people with chronic brain syndromes or history of angina pectoris.

REMARKS: Because of the severe interactions of some foodstuffs and medication, clients need comprehensive teaching, teaching aids, and supervision.

High-tyramine foods include beer, red wine, aged cheese, dry sausage, fava beans (Italian green beans), brewer's yeast, smoked fish, any kind of liver, avocados, and bologna. Chocolate and coffee should be used in moderation.

Drugs causing severe medication interactions include Demerol, epinephrine, local anesthetics, decongestants, cough medications, diet pills, and most over-the-counter medications.

SIDE EFFECTS

GENERAL: Constipation, dry mouth, vertigo, orthostatic hypotension, drowsiness or insomnia, weakness, fatigue, weight gain, hypomania, mania, blurred vision, skin rash. Muscle twitching common.

ADVERSE REACTIONS

HYPERTENSIVE CRISIS: Intense occipital headache, palpitation, stiff neck, fever, chest pain, brady/tachycardia, intracranial bleeding.

HEPATIC: Jaundice, malaise, right upper quadrant pain, change in color or consistency of stools.

NURSING MEASURES:

1. Monitor BP for orthostatic hypotension every two to four hours during initial therapy.
2. Assess for other potential signs of hypertensive crises.
3. Observe for marked changes in mood, e.g., hypomania, mania.
4. Monitor intake and output and frequency of stools.
5. Have client dangle legs five minutes before standing.
6. Depressed persons are at risk for suicide; continue to monitor and observe for potential suicidal behaviors.

INFORM CLIENT:

1. Inform client and family clearly and carefully as to foodstuffs and medications to avoid. REVIEW IN DETAIL.
2. Instruct clients taking MAO inhibitors to wear a medical identification tag or bracelet.
3. Caution client to avoid all over-the-counter (OTC) drugs unless approval of MD has been obtained.
4. Caution client to avoid all alcohol.
5. Encourage client and family to go to ER immediately if signs and symptoms of hypertensive crises are suspected. Phentolamine (Regitine) can be given for hypertensive crises.

FLUOXETINE HYDROCHLORIDE

(Prozac)

ANTIDEPRESSANT

USES:

1. Prozac is a relatively new antidepressant medication that is chemically unrelated to tricyclics or MAOIs.
2. Has been found effective in clients with bulimia.

ACTION: Is a potent serotonin reuptake blocker, whose use results in an increase in the amount of active serotonin within the synaptic cleft and at the serotonin receptor site. Increased serotonin in these areas appears to modify affective and behavioral disorders.

DOSAGES & ROUTES

Adults	20 mg per day. May reach 40–60 mg in divided doses. Do not exceed 80 mg daily.
Elderly	Same as for adults. No dosage for children as yet established.

CONTRAINDICATIONS: None known.

CAUTIONS: Use with clients with concomitant systemic illness has not been studied extensively. Caution should be used with pregnant women or women who are breast-feeding, children, and the elderly. Caution should also be used with clients with liver disease or renal impairment or in a client with a recent MI.

REMARKS: Prozac, like the tricyclics and MAOIs, takes from two to five weeks to produce an elevation of mood. Advantages of this drug are that there are fewer anticholinergic side effects and that there is a low incidence of cardiovascular effects. However, Prozac may impair judgment, thinking, and motor skills.

SIDE EFFECTS **GENERAL:** The most common side effects reported with fluoxetine hydrochloride are nausea, nervousness and anxiety, insomnia, and vertigo. When these side effects are severe, the drug is discontinued. If a rash or urticaria or both develop, the drug should be discontinued. Anorexia may appear in some people.

ADVERSE REACTIONS See side effects.

NURSING MEASURES:

1. Fluoxetine hydrochloride is given in early A.M. without consideration to meals.
2. Clients who are potentially suicidal are assessed for suicidal thoughts or actions. Carefully observe taking of medication.
3. If client is underweight and experiences anorexia, MD should be alerted to re-evaluate continuation of medication.

INFORM CLIENT:

1. If rash or urticaria appears, notify MD immediately.
2. Do not drive or operate machinery if drowsiness occurs.
3. Avoid alcoholic beverages.

ANTIMANIC

LITHIUM

LITHIUM CARBONATE/CITRATE

(Carbolith, Eskalith, Lithane, Lithizine, Lithonate, Lithobid)

USES:

1. Primarily used to control, prevent, or diminish manic episodes in people with bipolar depression (manic-depressive psychosis).
2. Used *experimentally* in alcoholism, premenstrual syndrome, drug abuse, phobias, and eating disorders.

ACTION: Lithium is an alkali metal salt that behaves in the body much like a sodium ion. Lithium acts to lower concentrations of norepinephrine and serotonin by inhibiting their release and enhancing their reuptake by neurons. The therapeutic effects, as well as the side effects and toxic effects, of lithium are thought to be related to the partial replacement of sodium by lithium in membrane action.

DOSAGES & ROUTES

	PO
Adult	Acute mania, 600 mg 3 times daily; maintenance dose 300 mg 3 times daily or 4 times daily.
Child	Not labeled for pediatric use.
Elderly	Reduce to 600–900 mg daily to produce low serum concentration of about 0.5 mEq/l.

CONTRAINDICATIONS: Pregnancy, nursing mothers, significant cardiovascular or renal disease, schizophrenia, severe debilitation, dehydration, or sodium depletion.

CAUTIONS: The elderly, thyroid disease, epilepsy, concomitant use with haloperidol or other antipsychotics, parkinsonism, severe infections, urinary retention, diabetes.

REMARKS: Serum lithium levels must be monitored during drug therapy. The therapeutic range is very narrow, and potential for toxic effects is high if blood levels are not monitored. During acute stage, blood levels are raised to 1.00–1.4 mEq/l. Maintenance therapy blood levels run from 0.8–1.2 mEq/l. Side effects and toxic effects are common at higher doses (1.5 mEq/l or more). Before starting a patient on lithium, a BUN, T4, T3, TSH, and ECG should be taken.

SIDE EFFECTS: The major long-term risks of lithium therapy are hypothyroidism and impairment of the kidney's ability to concentrate urine.

Below 1.5 mEq/l. Polyuria, polydipsia, lethargy, fatigue, muscle weakness, headache, mild nausea, fine hand tremor, and inability to concentrate. May experience ankle edema. Symptoms disappear during continued therapy.

ADVERSE AND TOXIC EFFECTS

1.5–2.0 mEq/l. Vomiting, diarrhea, muscle weakness, ataxia, dizziness, slurred speech, confusion.

2.0–2.5 mEq/l. Blurred vision, muscle twitching, severe hypotension, persistent nausea and vomiting. Thyroid toxicity is common.

2.5–3.0 mEq/l or more. Urinary and fecal incontinence, seizures, cardiac arrhythmias, peripheral vascular collapse, death.

NURSING MEASURES:

1. If serum lithium levels are above 1.5 mEq/l or if client has persistent diarrhea, vomiting, excessive sweating in hot weather, infection, or fever, check with MD before giving dose.
2. Check urine specific gravity periodically and teach patient to do so at home (normal: 1.005–1.025).
3. Administer with meals.
4. Assure that client is well hydrated.

INFORM CLIENT:

1. Drink plenty of liquids (2–3 liters/day) during initial therapy and 1–1.5 liters/day during remainder of therapy.
2. Know the side effects and toxic effects of lithium therapy and seek out MD immediately if problems arise.
3. Have blood lithium levels taken at regular intervals as directed in order to regulate dosage and prevent toxicity.
4. Maintain a regular diet, thus maintaining average salt intake (6–8 g) required to keep serum lithium in the therapeutic range.
5. Avoid alcohol.
6. Be aware that antibiotics (Flagyl and tetracycline) and nonsteroidal anti-inflammatory agents (Indocin) can increase lithium levels.
7. Know that caffeine can lower lithium levels.

Key to Self-Study Exercises

Chapter 1

1. C
2. A
3. E
4. H
5. B
6. F
7. D
8. G
9. True (Table 1–2)
10. True (p. 8)
11. True (p. 8)
12. True (p. 8)
13. False (p. 10)

Chapter 2

1. D (pp. 16–21)
2. A (p. 16)
3. C (p. 17)
4. C (pp. 16–17)
5. D (p. 18)
6. A (p. 18)
7. C (p. 20)
8. C (p. 21 and Table 2–3)
9. E (p. 21 and Table 2–3)
10. G (p. 21 and Table 2–3)
11. H (p. 21 and Table 2–3)
12. B (p. 21 and Table 2–3)
13. F (p. 21 and Table 2–3)
14. A (p. 21 and Table 2–3)
15. D (p. 21 and Table 2–3)
16. D (p. 23 and Table 2–4)
17. A (p. 23)
18. C (p. 22)
19. B
20. D
21. C
22. A
23. D
24. B
25. Behavior modification (p. 27)
26. Gestalt (p. 28)
27. Classical psychoanalysis (p. 27)
28. Transactional analysis (p. 27)
29. Short term dynamic psychotherapy (p. 27)
30. Psychoanalytic psychotherapy (p. 27)
31. See pp. 28–29
32. See pp. 29–30

Chapter 3

1. D (p. 45)
2. C (p. 45)
3. A (p. 46)
4. H (p. 58)
5. G (p. 58)
6. True (p. 40)
7. True (p. 40)
8. Review pp. 41 and 56
9. Review pp. 41–45
10. Review inside front cover

Chapter 4

1. Refer to pp. 66–67
2. Refer to pp. 67–68
3. Refer to p. 68
4. Refer to pp. 69–70, note Fig. 4–1, pp. 71–72
5. Refer to pp. 70–75
6. Refer to pp. 75–78

Chapter 5

1. The two world wars revealed record numbers of persons with mental illness. The public began to recognize the link between stress and mental illness: anyone could have a "breaking point."
2. Pennsylvania Hospital, Philadelphia, 1752. Psychiatric care was a component of total hospital care.
3. (1) Nursing was a family function, expected of all women. (2) A religious duty to perform "good works." (3) An occupation, characterized by apprenticeship training and employment for wages.
4. Feudal manorial relationships provided the model for hierarchical relationships within hospitals. Living on the premises; institution run as a self-sufficient entity; patients carrying out domestic duties.
5. Characteristics of public hospitals as closed systems: Some had their own police, fire department, post offices, etc. Staff often lived on premises. Some hospitals had farms or dairies. Patients provided labor to run institution.
6. Teaching self-control to patients by persuasion; work programs, leisure-time activities.
7. 1841. The public responded by building hospitals for the mentally ill.
8. To hide the mentally ill; fear of the mentally ill; belief that fresh air, rest, and quiet were healing; land for hospitals was cheaper.
9. Linda Richards started the first nurses' training school in a hospital for the mentally ill.
10. In 1909 recommendations were made that all nursing training programs include psychiatric experience. In 1953 the NLN adopted curriculum guidelines that implemented the recommendations.
11. Harriet Bailey. The emphasis on disease.
12. Carry out medical prescriptions. Assist in medical treatments. Provide activities; serve as companions. Provide "habit training."
13. Bolton Act; three programs; 1943.
14. Shortage of qualified faculty; unclear definitions of "advanced nursing," few textbooks.
15. 1953; seven decades.
16. Whether psychiatric nurses should provide psychotherapy. Only nurses with advanced education and supervised training provide psychotherapy.
17. Integration grants supported a psychiatric nurse faculty member to integrate psychosocial sensitivity into all nursing education.
18. 1963: Journal of Psychosocial Nursing; Perspectives in Psychiatric Care.
19. Before 1950's nurses kept busy at tasks and physical care; after 1950's nurses talked to patients.
20. pp. 103–104
21. Table 5–2
22. (1) Anything that goes on may be talked about; talking may increase understanding; understanding may change behavior. (2) Language influences thought, thought influences actions; feelings arise in relation to thoughts and actions.
23. Scholarship; research
24. Descriptive theories; intrapersonal theories, interpersonal theories; systems theories; social science theories.
25. p. 106
26. p. 106
27. Self analysis
28. p. 108
29. Board of Nursing is part of state government; boards associated with state organizations are voluntary and have no force of law.

30. Figure 5–1 and Standards of Psychiatric and Mental Health Nursing.

Chapter 6

1. False (p. 114)
2. True (p. 114)
3. True (p. 114)
4. False (p. 114)
5. Nonverbal (pp. 115–116)
6. Verbal (pp. 115–116)
7. Nonverbal (pp. 115–116)
8. Verbal (pp. 115–116)
9. Review Tables 6–2 and 6–3
10. Review Tables 6–2 and 6–3
11. Review Tables 6–2 and 6–3
12. Review Tables 6–2 and 6–3
13. Review Tables 6–2 and 6–3
14. Social (pp. 124–125)
15. Intimate (pp. 124–125)
16. Intimate (pp. 124–125)
17. Therapeutic (pp. 124–125)
18. Social (pp. 124–125)
19. Therapeutic (pp. 124–125)
20. Intimate (pp. 124–125)
21. Termination (p. 126)
22. Orientation (p. 126)
23. Working (p. 126)
24. True (p. 126)
25. True (pp. 126–127)
26. True (p. 127)
27. Review Table 6–5
28. Review Table 6–5

Chapter 7

1A. Gathering data (p. 141)
1B. Verifying data (p. 141)
2A. Problem (p. 152)
2B. Probable cause (related to) (p. 152)
2C. Identifying data (as evidenced by) (p. 152)
3A. Determining desired outcomes (LTGs and STGs) (p. 154)
3B. Identifying appropriate nursing care (p. 154)
4A. Validating the care plan (p. 156)
4B. Giving nursing care (p. 156)
4C. Continued data collection (p. 156)
5A. Evaluating goals (p. 163)
5B. Reassessment of care (p. 163)
6. Process (pp. 141–149)
7. Content: history (pp. 141–149)
8. Content: mental/emotional (pp. 141–149)
9. Process (pp. 141–149)
10. Content: mental/emotional (pp. 141–149)
11. Content: history (pp. 141–149)
12. Content: history (pp. 141–149)
13. Content: mental/emotional (pp. 141–149)
14A. Refer to pp. 150–154
14B. Refer to pp. 150–154
14C. Refer to pp. 150–154
15A. Refer to pp. 154–156
15B. Refer to pp. 154–156
15C. Refer to pp. 154–156
16. Refer to pp. 164–165 and Box 7–2
17A. Stated in measurable terms (p. 155)
17B. Short, specific, and realistic (p. 155)
17C. Have specific time set (p. 155)
17D. Stated in positive terms (p. 155)
18A. Partially met; still hears voices but they no longer tell her to kill herself or threaten her
18B. Partially met; can name two resources: (1) continue with nurse therapist, (2) weekly visits to brothers
18C. Met; client now completes self-care

Chapter 8

1. True (p. 174)
2. False (p. 175)
3. False (p. 174)
4. A
5. H
6. C
7. G
8. D
9. B (p. 180)
10. E (p. 180)
11. A (p. 180)
12. C (p. 180)
13. D (p. 180)
14. D (pp. 177–180)
15. E (pp. 177–180)
16. B (pp. 177–180)
17. A (pp. 177–180)
18. C (pp. 177–180)
19. Refer to Table 8–2
20. Severe
21. Moderate
22. Panic
23. Mild
24. Moderate (review Table 8–3)
25. Severe (review Table 8–4)

Chapter 10

1. B
2. C
3. A
4. B
5. C
6. A
7. False (pp. 201–210)
8. False (pp. 201–210)
9. True (pp. 201–210)
10. False (pp. 201–210)
11. True (pp. 201–210)
12. False (pp. 201–210)
13. True (pp. 201–210)
14. False (pp. 201–210)
15. Refer to pp. 210–211
16A. Ability to care (p. 214)
16B. Ability to listen (p. 214)
16C. Ability to be creative and flexible (p. 214)
17A. Identify personal feelings during interaction (p. 214)
17B. Hearing what the client says and leaves out (p. 214)
17C. Monitoring what goes on in the interaction (p. 214)
18. Review Table 10-2, p. 213
19. A (p. 215)
20. C (p. 215)
21. B (p. 215)
22. A (p. 215)
23. See p. 221
24. Maturational; situational; adventitious

Chapter 11

1. D
2. C (see Box 11–1, p. 229)
3. E (p. 229)
4. G (pp. 229–230)
5. A (pp. 229–230)
6. F (pp. 229–230)
7. C (pp. 229–230)
8. D (pp. 229–230)
9. B (pp. 229–230)
10. G (pp. 229–230)
11. E (pp. 229–230)
12. A (Tables 11–3, 11–4, 11–5, 11–6)
13. B (Tables 11–3, 11–4, 11–5, 11–6)
14. A (Tables 11–3, 11–4, 11–5, 11–6)
15. C (Tables 11–3, 11–4, 11–5, 11–6)
16. B (Tables 11–3, 11–4, 11–5, 11–6)
17. C (Tables 11–3, 11–4, 11–5, 11–6)
18. A (Tables 11–3, 11–4, 11–5, 11–6)
19. A, D (Tables 11–3, 11–4, 11–5, 11–6)
20. A (p. 232)
21. B
22. A
23. True
24. True
25. True
26. False
27. False

Chapter 12

1. True (pp. 251–252)
2. False (pp. 251–252)
3. False (pp. 251–252)
4. False (pp. 251–252)
5. False (pp. 251–252)
6. True (pp. 251–252)
7. True (pp. 251–252)
8. False (pp. 251–252)
9. True (pp. 251–252)
10. True (pp. 251–252)
11. D (Table 12–2)
12. D
13. D
14. Refer to pp. 258–259
15. Review Table 12–3
16. Refer to p. 262
17. Crisis
18. Crisis
19. Crisis
20. Internal change
21. Internal change
22. Crisis
23. Internal change

Chapter 13

1. True (pp. 270–271 and Table 13–2)
2. True (pp. 270–271 and Table 13–2)
3. False (pp. 270–271 and Table 13–2)
4. False (pp. 270–271 and Table 13–2)
5. False (pp. 270–271 and Table 13–2)
6. False (pp. 270–271 and Table 13–2)
7. False (pp. 270–271 and Table 13–2)
8. False (pp. 270–271 and Table 13–2)
9. Acute (p. 272)
10. Long Term (p. 272)
11. Acute (p. 272)
12. Long Term (p. 272)
13. Acute (p. 272)
14. Long Term (p. 272)
15. Acute (p. 272)
16. D (pp. 276–278)
17. B (pp. 276–278)
18. D (pp. 276–278)
19. D (pp. 276–278)
20. D (pp. 276–278)
21. D (pp. 276–278)
22. Review p. 275
23. Review p. 274

Chapter 14

1. D (pp. 288–289)
2. X (p. 290)
3. O (p. 290)
4. O (p. 290)
5. X (p. 290)
6. O (p. 290)
7. O (p. 290)
8. A, B, C, E, F, H, J
9. See p. 292
10. See p. 292
11. See p. 290
12. See p. 293
13. See pp. 294–295
14. See p. 291
15. See p. 294
16. True
17. False
18. True
19. False
20. False
21. False
22. True
23. False
24. True
25. True
26. True
27. False

Chapter 15

1. E
2. D
3. B
4. C
5. F
6. True
7. True
8. False
9. True
10. False
11. True
12. True
13. False
14. Secondary (p. 322)

15A. p. 323
15B. p. 324

16. p. 325
17. p. 326
18. p. 329
19. p. 329

Chapter 16

1. K
2. C
3. F
4. N
5. J
6. D
7. E
8. G
9. H
10. M
11. L
12. B
13. C
14. D
15. A
16. A
17. B
18. C
19. E
20. F

Chapter 17

1. True
2. False
3. True
4. False
5. p. 394
6. Box 17–2, p. 392
7. p. 398
8. D
9. E
10. C
11. C
12. D
13. True
14. False
15. True
16. False
17. True
18. False
19. True
20. True
21. False
22. True
23. Kernberg
24. Constitution
25. Masterson
26. D
27. p. 413
28. p. 410
29. Table 17–8, p. 410
30. A, B, D, F

Chapter 18

1. Developing awareness (p. 426)
2. Restitution (p. 426)
3. Shock (p. 426)
4. False
5. True
6. False
7. D
8. C
9. A
10. E
11. B
12. F
13. Unsuccessful
14. Successful
15. Unsuccessful
16. Successful
17. C
18. C
19. Table 18–2, p. 430
20. Table 18–2, p. 430
21. Table 18–2, p. 430
22. Major depression (p. 433)
23. Dysthymic (p. 433)
24. Major depression (p. 433)
25. Dysthymic (p. 433)
26. Biological (pp. 435–437)
27. Cognitive (pp. 435–437)
28. Psychoanalytical (pp. 435–437)
29. Learning theory (pp. 435–437)
30. See pp. 438–440
31. See pp. 438–440
32. See pp. 438–440
33. See pp. 438–440
34. See pp. 438–440
35. See pp. 438–440
36. Refer to pp. 442–443
37. Refer to pp. 442–443
38. Refer to pp. 442–443
39. Non-productive
40. Productive
41. Productive
42. Not helpful (Table 18–5, p. 446)
43. Not helpful (Table 18–5, p. 446)
44. Not helpful (Table 18–5, p. 446)
45. Helpful (Table 18–5, p. 446)
46. Not helpful (Table 18–5, p. 446)
47. Not helpful (Table 18–5, p. 446)
48. See Table 18–6, p. 447
49. See Table 18–6, p. 447
50. See Table 18–6, p. 447
51. See Table 18–6, p. 447
52. C
53. See Table 18–8, p. 449
54. C
55. D
56. B

Chapter 19

1. D
2. C
3. See p. 472
4. See p. 472
5. See p. 472
6. Refer to p. 474
7. Refer to p. 474
8. Refer to p. 474

9. See p. 474
10. See p. 474
11. See p. 474
12. See p. 474
13. Refer to Table 19–3, p. 477
14. Refer to Table 19–3, p. 477
15. Refer to Table 19–3, p. 477
16. Refer to Table 19–3, p. 477
17. See p. 478
18. See p. 478
19. See p. 478
20. Refer to p. 479
21. Refer to p. 479
22. Refer to p. 479
23. Helpful (Table 19–2, p. 476)
24. Helpful (Table 19–2, p. 476)
25. Not helpful (Table 19–2, p. 476)
26. Not helpful (Table 19–2, p. 476)
27. Not helpful (Table 19–2, p. 476)
28. Helpful (Table 19–2, p. 476)

Chapter 20

1. D (pp. 493–495)
2. C (pp. 493–495)
3. E (pp. 493–495)
4. B (pp. 493–495)
5. E (pp. 493–495)
6. C (pp. 493–495)
7. A (pp. 493–495)
8. False
9. True
10. False
11. True
12. Refer to p. 497
13. Feeling (p. 501)
14. Refer to p. 502
15. Refer to p. 504
16. A, B, D
17. A, B, C, D, E
18. A, B, D
19. Hallucinations (pp. 506–507)
20. Hallucinations (pp. 506–507)
21. Hallucinations and delusions (pp. 506–507)
22. Hallucinations (pp. 506–507)
23. Delusions (pp. 506–507)
24. Hallucinations and delusions (pp. 506–507)
25. Hallucinations (pp. 506–507)
26. Hallucinations and delusions (pp. 506–507)
27. Hallucinations and delusions (pp. 506–507)
28. False (pp. 508–513)
29. True (pp. 508–513)
30. False (pp. 508–513)
31. True (pp. 508–513)
32. True (pp. 508–513)
33. False (pp. 508–513)
34. True (pp. 508–513)
35. True
36. True
37. True
38. True (pp. 515–516)
39. True (pp. 515–516)
40. False (pp. 515–516)
41. True (pp. 515–516)
42. C
43. C
44. C
45. C
46. D
47. B
48. Refer to p. 504
49. Refer to Table 20–10, p. 526

Chapter 21

1. Syndrome (p. 535)
2. Syndrome (p. 535)
3. Disorder (p. 535)
4. Syndrome (p. 535)
5. Disorder (p. 535)
6. Delirium (Table 21–4, p. 549)
7. Dementia (Table 21–4, p. 549)
8. Dementia (Table 21–4, p. 549)
9. Delirium (Table 21–4, p. 549)
10. Dementia (Table 21–4, p. 549)
11. Delirium (Table 21–4, p. 549)
12. Dementia (Table 21–4, p. 549)
13. Delirium (Table 21–4, p. 549)
14. E (Table 21–3, p. 547)
15. B (Table 21–3, p. 547)
16. A (Table 21–3, p. 547)
17. F (Table 21–3, p. 547)
18. F (pp. 551–552)
19. G (pp. 551–552)
20. D (pp. 551–552)
21. C (pp. 551–552)
22. B (pp. 551–552)
23. Refer to pp. 541–542
24. Refer to pp. 552–553
25. Refer to p. 554
26. See Tables 21–6, 21–7, 21–8
27. See Tables 21–6, 21–7, 21–8
28. Refer to p. 560

Chapter 22

1. True (p. 579)
2. False (p. 579)
3. False (p. 579)
4. False (p. 579)
5. False (p. 579)
6. True (p. 579)
7. True (p. 579)
8. D
9. C
10. D
11. D
12. C
13. C
14. Tertiary
15. Secondary
16. Secondary
17. Tertiary
18. Primary
19. Secondary
20. Refer to pp. 585–586
21. Refer to pp. 585–586
22. Refer to pp. 586–587

Chapter 23

1. F
2. J
3. K
4. H
5. A
6. D
7. See pp. 613–616
8. See pp. 613–616
9. A
10. B
11. See p. 618
12. See p. 622
13. See p. 623
14. See p. 624

Chapter 24

1. G
2. D
3. C
4. B
5. I
6. A
7. Primary (p. 641)
8. Secondary (p. 641)
9. Primary (p. 641)
10. True (p. 643)
11. True (p. 643)
12. Self-help groups
13. Family therapy
14. Psychotherapy
15. Refer to p. 644
16. B (pp. 645–646)
17. C (pp. 645–646)
18. A (pp. 645–646)
19. Intoxication (Table 24–2, p. 646)
20. Withdrawal (Table 24–2, p. 646)
21. Overdose (Table 24–2, p. 646)
22. Intoxication (Table 24–2, p. 646)
23. Overdose (Table 24–2, p. 646)
24. Withdrawal (Table 24–2, p. 646)
26. Refer to p. 650
27. C
28. D
29. B
30. A
31. B (Table 24–3)
32. A (Table 24–3)
33. C (Table 24–3)
34. C (Table 24–3)
35. B (Table 24–3)
36. B (Table 24–3)
37. D
38. B
39. D
40. C
41. D
42. B
43. A
44. True (p. 663)
45. True (p. 663)
46. True (p. 663)
47. C
48. A
49. B
50. D
51. C
52. A
53. B
54. True
55. True
56. Refer to p. 669

Chapter 25

1. C
2. E
3. C
4. B
5. C
6. E
7. C
8. E
9. A (Fig. 25–4, p. 689)
10. D
11. B
12. B
13. C
14. B
15. B
16. C
17. C
18. D
19. B
20. D

Chapter 26

1. False
2. True
3. True
4. True
5. Plus (Box 26–1, p. 718)
6. Negative (Box 26–1, p. 718)
7. Plus (Box 26–1, p. 718)
8. Negative (Box 26–1, p. 718)
9. C
10. B
11. C (pp. 724–729)
12. A (pp. 724–729)
13. D (pp. 724–729)
14. B (pp. 724–729)
15. Refer to pp. 724–729
16. False
17. False
18. True
19. False
20. D
21. B
22. D
23. E
24. A
25. B
26. C

Chapter 27

1. Both specialist and generalist (p. 753)
2. Specialist (p. 753)
3. Specialist (p. 753)
4. Both specialist and generalist (p. 753)
5. Specialist (p. 753)
6. B
7. D
8. A
9. D
10. E
11. C
12. A
13. False
14. True
15. True
16. True
17. See text
18. C
19. True
20. True
21. False
22. True
23. False
24. True
25. C
26. A
27. B
28. See text
29. Refer to p. 766
30. Refer to pp. 768–769

Chapter 28

1. D (Table 28–2, p. 781)
2. B (Table 28–2, p. 781)
3. C (Table 28–2, p. 781)
4. A (Table 28–2, p. 781)
5. A (Table 28–2, p. 781)
6. D
7. C
8. B
9. A
10. C
11. D
12. E
13. A
14. B
15. Refractory (p. 787)
16. 75% (p. 781)
17. 45% (p. 783)
18. Transsexualism (p. 790)
19. Inhibited desire (p. 787)
20. Behavioral; psychodynamic
21. Refer to pp. 784–786 and pp. 790–792

Chapter 29

1. True (p. 820)
2. False (p. 801)
3. False (p. 820)
4. False (p. 820)
5. Reminiscing (p. 808)
6. Remotivational (p. 808)
7. Psychotherapy (p. 808)
8. Refer to p. 802
9. Refer to pp. 810–811
10. Refer to pp. 810–811
11. Refer to pp. 813–814
12. Refer to Box 29–2, p. 815
13. False (p. 811)
14. False (p. 811–812)
15. True (p. 811)
16. False (p. 812)
17. True (p. 813)
18. False (p. 818)
19. False
20. True
21. True
22. G, I, J (p. 816)

Chapter 30

1. D
2. True
3. False
4. True
5. True
6. True
7. True
8. True
9. True
10. False
11. Refer to p. 833
12. Refer to pp. 834–835
13. Refer to p. 826

INDEX

Note: Page numbers in *italics* refer to illustrations; page numbers followed by *t* refer to tables.